Third Edition

Physician Assistant

A Guide to Clinical Practice

Third Edition

Physician Assistant

A Guide to Clinical Practice

Ruth Ballweg, MPA, PA-C

Associate Professor;
Director, MEDEX Northwest,
Physician Assistant Program,
University of Washington School of Medicine,
Seattle, Washington

Sherry Stolberg, MGPGP, PA-C

Consultant;
Adjunct Associate Professor,
Drexel University Physician Assistant Program,
Lincoln, Massachusetts

Edward M. Sullivan, MS, PA-C

Physician Assistant,
J. Kirkland Grant Obstetrics and Gynecology Practice,
Mesquite, Texas

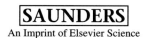

An Imprint of Elsevier Science

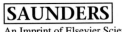

An Imprint of Elsevier Science

The Curtis Center
Independence Square West
Philadelphia, Pennsylvania 19106

PHYSICIAN ASSISTANT:
A GUIDE TO CLINICAL PRACTICE,
Third Edition

ISBN 0-7216-0017-4

NOTICE

Physician Assistant is an ever-changing field. Standard safety precautions must be followed, but as new research and clinical experience broaden our knowledge, changes in treatment and drug therapy may become necessary or appropriate. Readers are advised to check the most current product information provided by the manufacturer of each drug to be administered to verify the recommended dose, the method and duration of administration, and contraindications. It is the responsibility of the licensed prescriber, relying on experience and knowledge of the patient, to determine dosages and the best treatment for each individual patient. Neither the publisher nor the author assumes any liability for any injury and/or damage to persons or property arising from this publication.
Previous editions copyrighted 1999, 1994

Managing Editor: Thomas Moore
Acquisitions Editor: Shirley Kuhn
Developmental Editor: Peg Waltner
Publishing Services Manager: Pat Joiner
Senior Project Manager: Karen M. Rehwinkel
Senior Designer: Mark A. Oberkrom

Printed in the United States of America

Last digit is the print number: 9 8 7 6 5 4 3 2 1

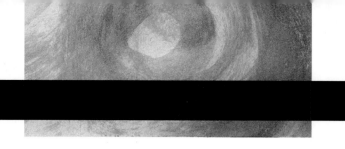

Contributors

David P. Asprey, PhD, PA-C
Associate Professor and Program Director,
Physician Assistant Program,
University of Iowa,
Iowa City, Iowa

Patrick C. Auth, MS, PA-C
Director,
Physician Assistant Program,
MCP Hahnemann University,
Philadelphia, Pennsylvania

Ruth Ballweg, MPA, PA-C
Associate Professor;
Director, MEDEX Northwest,
Physician Assistant Program,
University of Washington School of Medicine,
Seattle, Washington

Susan Blackwell, PA-C
Senior Physician Assistant,
Thoracic Oncology Program,
Duke University Medical Center,
Durham, North Carolina

Dennis M. Bruneau
Physician Assistant,
Gilliam County Medical Center,
Condon, Oregon

Geraldine A. Buck, MHS, PA-C
Director,
Advanced Physician Assistant Studies Program,
MCP Hahnemann University,
Physician Assistant Program,
Philadelphia, Pennsylvania

Tom Byers
Former Deputy Mayor,
Seattle, Washington

R. Scott Chavez, PhD (c), MPA, PA-C, CCHP-A
Vice President,
National Commission on Correctional
   Health Care,
Chicago, Illinois

John L. Chitwood, LtCol, USAF, MS, MPAS, MA, PA-C
Assistant Professor,
Interservice Physician Assistant Program;
Assistant Professor,
Saint Francis University,
Loretto, Pennsylvania

Linda M. Dale, MSOD, PA-C
Site Coordinator,
MEDEX Northwest,
Yakima, Washington

Lee A. Daly, PA-C, MHS
Senior Physician Assistant,
Multidisciplinary Breast Program,
Division of Hematology and Oncology,
Duke University Medical Center,
Durham, North Carolina

Ann Davis, MS, PA-C
Director of State Government Affairs,
American Academy of Physician Assistants,
Alexandria, Virginia

William R. Duryea, PhD, PA-C
Director,
Master of Medical Science Program,
Saint Francis University,
Loretto, Pennsylvania

Timothy C. Evans, MD, PhD
Medical Director and Assistant Professor of
    Medicine,
MEDEX Northwest,
University of Washington School of Medicine,
Seattle, Washington

Nicole Gara, MA
Vice President,
Government and Professional Affairs,
American Academy of Physician Assistants,
Alexandria, Virginia

Ronald D. Garcia, PhD
Assistant Dean for Minority Affairs,
Associate Director, Primary Care
    Associate Program,
Stanford University School of Medicine,
Stanford, California

F. J. Gino Gianola, PA-C
Clinical Coordinator,
MEDEX Northwest,
Physician Assistant Program,
University of Washington School of Medicine,
Seattle, Washington

Anita Duhl Glicken, MSW
Associate Professor of Pediatrics;
Child Health Associate,
Physician Assistant Program,
University of Colorado Health Sciences Center,
Denver, Colorado

J. Kirkland Grant, MD
Chairman,
Department of Obstetrics and Gynecology,
Mesquite Community Hospital,
Mesquite, Texas

Jim Hammond MA, PA-C
Professor and Director,
Physician Assistant Program,
James Madison University,
Harrisonburg, Virginia

Kenneth R. Harbert, PhD, CHES, PA-C
Chair,
Department of Physician Assistant Studies;
Associate Professor,
University of Sciences in Philadelphia,
Philadelphia College of Osteopathic Medicine,
Philadelphia, Pennsylvania

Nelson Herlihy, MHS, PA-C
Volunteer Faculty,
Primary Care Associate Program,
Stanford University School of Medicine,
Palo Alto, California;
Private Practice,
Anderson Rowe MD,
San Ramon, California

Roderick S. Hooker, PhD, MBA, PA-C
Chief,
Division of Health Services Research;
Associate Professor,
Department of Physician Assistant Studies,
University of Texas, Southwestern Medical Center at
    Dallas,
Dallas, Texas

Jeffrey Hummel, MD, MPH
Clinical Assistant Professor,
University of Washington Department of Internal
    Medicine;
Director for Research and Clinical Improvement,
University of Washington Physicians Network,
Seattle, Washington

Robert W. Jarski, PA-C, PhD
Director, Complementary Medicine and Wellness
    Program;
Associate Professor,
Oakland University School of Health Sciences,
Rochester, Michigan

Steven Johnson, PA-C
Physician Assistant,
Palo Alto Medical Foundation,
Palo Alto, California

David Jones, BA, PA-C
Physician Assistant,
Gilliam County Medical Center,
Condon, Oregon

P. Eugene Jones, PhD, PA-C
Chairman and Professor,
Department of Physician Assistant Studies,
The University of Texas Southwestern Medical
    Center at Dallas,
Dallas, Texas

Timothy J. King, PA-C
Faculty, Southwest Georgia Area Health Education
    Center,
Albany Area Primary Health Care, Inc.,
Albany, Georgia

David H. Kuhns, PA-C, MPH
Consultant in refugee and international health,
Cumberland Center, Maine

Paul Lombardo, MPS, RPAC
Program Chair,
Department of Physician Assistant Education,
University of Stony Brook,
Stony Brook, New York

H. James Lurie, MD
Associate Professor,
MEDEX Northwest,
Physician Assistant Program,
University of Washington School of Medicine,
Seattle, Washington

Ann M. Meehan, RHIA
Project Manager,
Health Information Management Services,
HCA,
Nashville, Tennessee

Dawn Morton-Rias, PD, PA-C
Assistant Professor and Chairperson,
Physician Assistant Program;
Interim Dean,
College of Health Related Professions,
Downstate Medical Center,
Brooklyn, New York

Venetia L. Orcutt, MBA, PA-C
Vice Chair and Associate Professor,
Department of Physician Assistant Studies,
University of Texas Southwestern Medical Center at
    Dallas,
Dallas, Texas

Donald M. Pederson, PhD, PA-C
Director,
Physician Assistant Program,
University of Utah School of Medicine,
Salt Lake City, Utah

Vyjeyanthi S. Periyakoil, MD
Director, VA Geriatrics Clinic;
Associate Medical Director, VA Hospice
    Care Center,
Palo Alto VA Health Care System,
Palo Alto, California

Paula Phelps, MHS, PA-C
Assistant Professor and Physician Assistant,
Physician Assistant Program,
Idaho State University,
Pocatello, Idaho

David J. Pillow, Jr., MD, FACEP
Medical Director Emergency Department,
Saint Paul University Hospital,
Dallas, Texas

Michael Powe
Director,
Health Systems and Reimbursement Policy,
American Academy of Physician Assistants,
Alexandria, Virginia

Michael Rackover, PA-C, MS
Associate Professor and Academic Coordinator,
Physician Assistant Program,
Philadelphia University,
Philadelphia, Pennsylvania

Richard R. Rahr, EdD, PA-C
Professor and Chair,
Physician Assistant Program,
University of Texas Medical Branch,
Galveston, Texas

Maryann Ramos, MPH, PA-C
DiLorenzo Tricare Health Clinic,
The Pentagon,
Washington, DC

Nanci Cortright Rice, PhD, MF, BF
Vice Chairperson and Graduate Program Director,
Masters of Science and Healthcare Policy
    Management Program,
SUNY at Stony Brook,
Stony Brook, New York

John M. Schroeder, PA-C, JD
Director,
Physician Assistant Program,
Idaho State University,
Pocatello, Idaho

Albert Simon, MEd, PA-C
Chair,
Department of Physician Assistant Sciences,
Saint Francis University,
Loretto, Pennsylvania

Martin L. Smith, STD
Chief, Clinical Ethics Service;
Associate Professor, Critical Care Medicine,
Clinical Ethics Service,
The University of Texas M D Anderson Cancer
Center,
Houston, Texas

Sherry Stolberg, MGPGP, PA-C
Consultant;
Adjunct Associate Professor,
Drexel University Physician Assistant Program,
Lincoln, Massachusetts

Henry Stoll, PA-C
Senior Lecturer,
MEDEX Northwest,
Physician Assistant Program,
University of Washington School of Medicine,
Seattle, Washington

Ernest L. Stump, ACSW, LCSW
Assistant Director and Behavioral Scientist,
Altoona Family Physicians,
Altoona Hospital,
Altoona, Pennsylvania;
Instructor,
Saint Francis University,
Loretto, Pennsylvania

Kimberly Suggs, MS, RHIA, CCS
Director, Strategic Initiatives,
HCA Health Information Management Services,
Spring, Texas

Edward M. Sullivan, MS, PA-C
Physician Assistant,
J. Kirkland Grant Obstetrics and Gynecology Practice,
Mesquite, Texas

Peggy A. Valentine, EDD, RN, PA-C
Associate Dean,
Howard University,
Washington, DC

Mary Em Wallace, FNP, PhD
Primary Care Associate Program,
Stanford University School of Medicine,
Palo Alto, California

Durward A. Watson, PA-C
Clinical Physician Assistant,
Southwest Infectious Disease Associates,
Dallas, Texas

John R. White, Jr., PharmD, PA-C
Associate Professor,
Washington State University College of Pharmacy,
Pullman, Washington

Lynda White, MHS, PA-C
Associate Director,
University of California, Davis;
Family Nurse Practitioner,
Physician Assistant Program,
Sacramento, California

Emily WhiteHorse PA-C, MA
Assistant Professor and Academic Coordinator,
Physician Assistant Program,
Philadelphia University,
Philadelphia, Pennsylvania

Keren H. Wick, PhD
Research Coordinator and Editor,
MEDEX Northwest,
Physician Assistant Program,
University of Washington School of Medicine,
Seattle, Washington

Chantelle Wolpert, MBA, PA-C, CGC
Physician Assistant and Genetic Counselor,
Center for Human Genetics,
Duke University Medical Center,
Durham, North Carolina

Gwen Yeo, PhD
Co-Director, Stanford Geriatric Education Center,
Stanford University School of Medicine,
Palo Alto, California

Sarah F. Zarbock, PA-C
Medical writer/editor,
Lakeville, Connecticut

We dedicate this text to PA students: past, present, and future.
You inspire us with your curiosity, motivation, and commitment to patient care.
We hope that this project will contribute to your education,
and that you will use it to contribute
to the lives and well-being of your patients.

Foreword

Thirty-one years ago doctors were in short supply. Nurses were even scarcer. The old model of the doctor, a receptionist, and a laboratory technician was inadequate to meet the needs of our increasingly complex society. Learning time had disappeared from the schedule of the busy doctor. The only solution that the overworked doctor could envisage was more doctors. Only a doctor could do doctors' work. The lengthy educational pathway (college, medical school, internship, residency, and fellowship) must mean that only persons with a doctor's education could carry out a doctor's functions.

I examined in some detail the actual practice of medicine. After sampling the rich diet of medicine, most doctors settled for a small area. If the office was set up to see patients every 10 to 15 minutes and to charge a certain fee, the practice conformed. If the outcome was poor, or if the doctors recognized that the problem was too complex for this pattern of practice, the patient was referred.

Doctors seeing patients at half-hour or 1-hour intervals also developed practice patterns and set fee schedules to conform. The specialists tended to treat diseases and leave the care of patients to others. Again, they cycled in a narrow path.

The average doctors developed very efficient patterns of practice. They operated 95% of the time in a habit mode and rarely applied a thinking cap. Because they did everything that involved contact with the patients, time for family, recreation, reading, and furthering their own education disappeared.

Why this intense personalization of medical practice? All doctors starting practices ran scared. They wanted to make their services essential to the well-being of their patients. They wanted the patient to depend on them alone. After a few years in this mode, they brainwashed themselves and actually believed that only they could obtain information from the patient and perform services that involved physical contact with the patient.

During this time I was building a house with my own hands. I could use a wide variety of materials and techniques in my building. I reflected on how inadequate my house would be if I was restricted to only four materials. The doctor restricted to a very slim support system could never build a practice adequate to meet the need of modern medicine. He or she needed more components in the system. The physician assistant was born!

Nurses, laboratory technicians, and other health professionals were educated in their own schools, mostly hospital related. The new practitioner (the PA) was to be selected, educated, and employed by the doctor. The PA—not being geographically bound to the management system of the hospital, the clinic, or the doctor's office—could oscillate between the office, the hospital, the operating room, and the home.

A 2-year curriculum was organized at Duke Medical School with the able assistance of Dr. Harvey Estes, who eventually took the program under the wing of his department of Family and Community medicine. The object of the 2-year course was to expose the student to the biology of humans and to learn how doctors rendered services. On graduation, PAs had learned to perform many tasks previously done only by licensed doctors and could serve a useful role in many types of practices. They performed those tasks that they could do as well as their doctor mentors. If the mentor was wise, the PA mastered new areas each year and increased his or her usefulness to the practice.

Setting no ceilings and allowing the PA to grow have made this profession useful and satisfying. Restricting PAs to medical supervision has given them great freedom. Ideally, they do any part of their mentors' practice that they can do as well as their mentors.

The PA profession has certainly established itself and is recognized as a part of the medical system. PAs will be assuming a larger role in the care of hospital patients as physician residency programs decrease in size. As hospital house staff, PAs can improve the quality of care for patients by providing continuity of care.

Because of the close association with the doctor and patient and the varied duties of the PAs, they have an intimate knowledge of the way of the medical world. They know patients, they are aware of the triumphs and failures of medicine; they know how doctors think and what they do with information collected about patients. For these reasons, they are in demand by all businesses that touch the medical profession. One of the first five Duke students recently earned a doctoral degree in medical ethics and is working in education. The world is open, and PAs are grasping their share.

We all owe a debt of gratitude to the first five students who were willing to risk 2 years of their lives to enter a new profession when there was little support from doctors, nurses, or government. From the beginning, patients responded favorably, and each PA gained confidence and satisfaction from these interactions. Patients made and saved the profession. We hope that every new PA will acknowledge this debt and continue the excellent work of the original five.

EUGENE A. STEAD, Jr, MD
Florence McAlister Professor Emeritus of Medicine
Duke University Medical Center
Durham, North Carolina

Preface

The physician assistant profession was established to bring quality primary health care to patients, particularly those in underserved urban and rural communities. PAs have been successful in meeting this goal and, as the profession has expanded, in moving into medical and surgical specialties and many other professions related to medicine. This text provides a comprehensive description of the PA profession and how PAs practice.

The first edition was published at a time of expansion in PA programs and in the number of PA graduates. It served as the only comprehensive text about the profession that included detailed chapters on the core competencies and skills required for clinical practice. Intended primarily for PA students, the text was also used by administrators, employers, PA graduates, and PA applicants. Its publication signaled a new level of maturation in the PA profession, and its success encouraged the development of a variety of other texts for PAs. The second edition was expanded and updated to reflect the growth of the PA profession.

The third edition has been improved by the addition of eight new chapters. Each chapter includes *Case Studies* that illustrate the narrative in "real-life" terms. *Clinical Applications* at the end of each chapter consist of questions to stimulate thought, discussion, and further investigation. The *Resources* section of each chapter provides an annotated list of books, articles, organizations, and/or websites for follow-up research.

Many PA programs find the text useful for professional issues courses and as a supplement to other core courses, such as physical diagnosis and clinical skills courses. PA students have found the chapters on specific specialties helpful in preparing for clinical rotations. PA graduates thinking about changing jobs or encountering new challenges in credentialing will find a number of relevant chapters. Health care administrators and employers can benefit from an overview of the profession, as well as information specific to PA roles and job descriptions. Policy analysts and health care researchers will find a wealth of information about PAs at the micro and macro levels. Finally, potential PAs can be informed and inspired by the accomplishments of the profession.

The text is organized in five sections:

- *Overview* of the physician assistant profession includes the profession's history, a description of PA education, and a chapter about credentialing and licensing.
- *Core Competencies* in the physician assistant profession consists of 18 chapters on the knowledge and skills that form the foundation of PA clinical practice. Ranging from medical ethics to history and physical examination skills to dealing with stress, this section serves PA students and graduates for first-time learning or for review. The addition of chapters on Medical Legal Issues and Practicing Evidence-Based Medicine acknowledges the importance of these core competencies.
- *The Health Care System* provides seven chapters about the organization of health care in the United States and analysis of how PAs practice in various components of health care. Students will find this section a useful overview of health care, both at the macro and micro levels. This section should be of particular interest to health care administrators and policy analysts for its information about the PA profession, as well as to PAs interested in

moving from one sector of health care to another. The Managed Care chapter has been substantially revised and renamed to reflect shifts in the health care insurance industry and resulting issues of patients' access to services.

- *Roles and Settings* includes 15 chapters on PA practice in a variety of specialty areas, ranging from internal medicine to surgery. Chapters include a sample of core knowledge and "pearls" from each specialty, as well as a description of PA practice, including sources of challenge and satisfaction. This section provides helpful tips for students preparing for clinical rotations and for PAs interested in changing employment. Potential employers and supervising physicians can learn how a PA could enhance their practice settings. Four chapters have been added as a result of the evolution of the PA profession and emerging PA roles: Orthopedics, Dermatology, Oncology, and Infectious Disease Medicine.

- *Current Issues* consists of eight chapters that focus on current issues in the PA profession and emerging key issues in health care. Ranging from PAs in international health care to dying and death, this section provides a brief sample of topics of interest to PA students, graduates, and others. This section is enhanced by three new chapters, which reflect developments in the art and science of medicine and the importance of the PA role in prevention: Genetics in Primary Care, Complementary and Alternative Medicine, and Violence Prevention.

The editors are delighted to include the foreword by Dr. Eugene Stead, one of the founders of our profession. Dr. Stead continues to be a revolutionary thinker and advocate for change in the health care system. As Gandhi said, *"We must be the change we wish to see in the world."* Encouraged by Dr. Stead and by countless colleagues, students, and patients, we hope this text can continue to serve as a resource and inspiration for the PA profession.

Acknowledgments

The support of our colleagues, students, friends, and loved ones has helped to make this text a reality. The patience and good humor of our spouses/partners, Arnold Rosner, Ben Wells, and Cindy Sullivan, and the enthusiasm of our children, Dayan Ballweg and Pirkko Terao, Jesse Lyons, and Chris Sullivan, kept us going during many long days and nights.

The authors who contributed their time and expertise have made this text a success. These are busy people who care about the PA profession, and their commitment has been an inspiration during each stage of the project.

Contributors to the first and/or second editions of this text deserve our appreciation for their participation: Beth Anderson, Phyllis Barks, Stephen Bartholomew, Pat Connor, Steven Curley, Bill Finerfrock, Diana Garcia, David Gwinn, Paul Jacques, Jimmie Keller, Debbie Jalbert, Martha Kelly, Gerald Marciano, Anthony Miller, Venetia Orcutt, Jay Slotkin, Karen Sadler Sparkes, Walter Stein, and John Yerxa. A special acknowledgment goes to David Buck, our deceased colleague and friend, who loved the PA profession and enriched us all with his commitment to excellence.

Thanks to the faculty and staff of the MEDEX Northwest PA Program at the University of Washington, particularly to Keren Wick and Sally Mantz, and to the PA Program at Drexel University. Their advice, support, and tolerance helped us through this project.

The pioneers who founded this profession deserve our recognition and gratitude. The PA profession has been fortunate to have many friends in medicine, government, and other health professions who have helped to advance the profession while reminding us of our roots. PA educators in every program around the country continue this commitment every day through their creative and humanistic involvement in the professional growth of their students.

We gratefully acknowledge our editors, Shirley Kuhn and Peg Waltner, for their belief in this project. Peg's creativity, attention to detail, and continuous encouragement resulted in substantial improvements in this edition.

Finally, we need to recognize the contributions of the patients who have been part of the learning process of all the authors. We are all students of medicine and life, and we continue to learn and grow with the cooperation of the people we care for. We entered the PA profession to help patients, and we hope that this text can further that goal.

Contents

Section V   Current Issues

Appendices

Third Edition

Physician Assistant

A Guide to Clinical Practice

CHAPTER 1

History of the Profession

Ruth Ballweg

INTRODUCTION

What was to become the physician assistant (PA) profession has many origins. Although it is often thought of as an "American" concept—using former military corpsmen to respond to the access needs in our health care system—the PA has historical antecedents in other countries. Feldshers in Russia and barefoot doctors in China served as models for the creation of the PA profession.

Feldshers in Russia

The *feldsher* concept originated in the European military in the 17th and 18th centuries and was introduced into the Russian military system by Peter the Great. Armies of other countries were ultimately able to secure adequate physician personnel; however, because of a physician shortage, the large numbers of Russian troops relied on feldshers for major portions of their medical care. Feldshers retiring from the military settled in small rural communities, where they continued their contribution to health care access. Feldshers assigned to Russian communities provided much of the health care in remote areas of Alaska during the 1800s.[1] In the late 19th century, formal schools were created for feldsher training, and by 1913, approximately 30,000 feldshers had been trained to provide medical care.[2]

As the major U.S. researchers reviewing the feldsher concept, Victor Sidel[2] and P.B. Storey[3] described a system in the Soviet Union in which the annual number of new feldshers equaled the annual number of physician graduates. Of those included in the feldsher category, 90% were women, including feldsher midwives.[3] Feldsher training programs, which were located in the same institutions as nursing schools, required 2½ years to complete. Outstanding feldsher students were encouraged to take medical school entrance examinations. Roemer[4] found in 1976 that 25% of Soviet physicians were former feldshers.

The use of Soviet feldshers varied from rural to urban settings. Often used as physician substitutes in rural settings, experienced feldshers had full authority to diagnose, prescribe, and institute emergency treatment. A concern that "independent" feldshers might provide "second-class" health care appears to have led to greater supervision of feldshers in rural settings. Storey[3] describes urban feldshers, whose roles were "complementary" rather than "substitutional," as limited to primary care in ambulances and triage settings and not involving polyclinic or hospital tasks. Perry and Breitner[5] contrast the urban feldsher role with that of U.S. physician assistants:

> Working alongside the physician in his daily activities to improve the physician's efficiency and effectiveness (and to relieve him of routine, time-consuming tasks) is not the Russian feldsher's role.

China's Barefoot Doctors

In China, the *barefoot doctor* originated in the 1965 Cultural Revolution as a physician substitute. In what became known as the "June 26th Directive," Chairman Mao called for a reorganization of the health care system. In response to Mao's directive, China trained 1.3 million barefoot doctors over the subsequent 10 years.[6]

The barefoot doctors were chosen from rural production brigades and received their initial 2- to 3-month training course in regional hospitals and health centers. Sidel[2] comments that the barefoot doctor is considered by his community, and apparently thinks of himself, as a peasant who performs some medical duties rather than as a health care worker who performs some agricultural duties.

Although they were designed to function independently, barefoot doctors were closely linked to local hospitals for training and medical supervision.

Upward mobility was encouraged, in that barefoot doctors were given priority for admission to medical school. In 1978, Dimond[7] found that one third of Chinese medical students were former barefoot doctors.

The use of feldshers and barefoot doctors was significantly greater than that of physician assistants in the United States. Writing in 1982, Perry and Breitner[5] noted:

> *"Although physician assistants have received a great deal of publicity and attention in the United States, they currently perform a very minor role in the provision of health services. In contrast, the Russian feldsher and the Chinese barefoot doctor perform a major role in the provision of basic medical services, particularly in rural areas. The 'discovery' in the United States that appropriately trained nonphysicians are perfectly capable of diagnosing and treating common medical problems had been previously recognized in both Russia and China."*

Developments in the United States

In the United States beginning in the 1930s, former military corpsmen received on-the-job training from the Federal Prison System to extend the services of prison physicians. In a 4-month program during World War II, the U.S. Coast Guard trained 800 purser mates to provide health care on merchant ships. The program was later discontinued, and by 1965, fewer than 100 purser mates continued to provide medical services. Both of these programs served as predecessors of federal physician assistant training programs at the Medical Center for Federal Prisoners, Springfield, Missouri, and Staten Island University Hospital, New York.

In 1961, Charles Hudson, MD, proposed the concept at a medical education conference of the American Medical Association (AMA). He recommended that "assistants to doctors" should work as dependent practitioners and should perform such technical tasks as lumbar puncture, suturing, and intubation.

By 1965, Henry Silver, MD, and Loretta Ford, RN, had created a practitioner training program for baccalaureate nurses working with impoverished pediatric populations. Although the Colorado program became the foundation both of the nurse practitioner movement and of the Child Health Association PA Program, it was not transferable to other institutions. According to Gifford, this program depended . . . "on a pattern of close cooperation between doctors and nurses not then often found at other schools."[8] In 1965, therefore, practical definition of the physician assistant concept awaited establishment of a training program in local circumstances that could be applied to other institutions.

Developments at Duke University

In the late 1950s and early 1960s, Eugene Stead, MD, developed a program to extend the capabilities of nurses at Duke University Hospital.[9] This program, which *could* have initiated the nurse practitioner movement, was opposed by the National League of Nursing. The League expressed the concern that such a program would move these new providers from the ranks of nursing and into the "medical model." Simultaneously, Duke University had also had experience with training several firemen, ex-corpsmen, and other non–college graduates to solve personnel shortages in the clinical services at Duke University Hospital.[9]

The Duke program and other new PA programs arose at a time of national awareness of a health care crisis. Carter and Gifford[10] described the conditions that fostered the PA concept as follows:

1. An increased social consciousness among many Americans that called for the elimination of all types of deprivation in society, especially among the poor, members of minority groups, and women.
2. An increasingly positive value attached to health and health care, which produced greater demand for health services, criticism of the health care delivery system, and constant complaints about rising health care costs.
3. Heightened concern about the supply of physicians, their geographical and specialty maldistribution, and the workloads they carried.
4. Awareness of a variety of physician extender models, including the community nurse-midwife in America, the "assistant medical officer" in Africa, and the feldsher in the Soviet Union.

5. The availability of nurses and ex-corpsmen as potential sources of manpower.
6. Local circumstances in numerous hospitals and office-based practice settings that required additional clinical support professionals.

The first four students—all ex–Navy corpsmen—entered the fledgling Duke program in October 1965. The 2-year training program's philosophy was to provide students with an education and orientation similar to those given the physicians with whom they would work. Although original plans called for the training of two categories of PAs—one for general practice and one for specialized inpatient care—the ultimate decision was made to focus on skills required in assisting family practitioners or internists. The program also emphasized the development of lifelong learning skills to facilitate the ongoing professional growth of these new providers.

Concepts of Education and Practice

The introduction of the PA presented philosophical challenges to established concepts of medical education. E. Harvey Estes, MD,[11] of Duke, described the hierarchical approach of medical education as being "based on the assumption that it was necessary to first learn 'basic sciences,' then normal structure and function, and finally pathophysiology. . . ." The physician assistant clearly defied these previous conventions. Some of the early PAs had no formal collegiate education. They had worked as corpsmen and had learned skills, often under battlefield conditions. Clearly, their skills had been developed, often to a remarkable degree, before the acquisition of any basic science knowledge, or any knowledge of pathologic physiology.

The developing physician assistant profession was also the first to officially share the knowledge base that was formerly the exclusive "property" of physicians:

> Prior to the PA profession, the physician was the sole possessor of information, and neither patient nor other groups could penetrate this wall. The patient generally trusted the medical profession to use the knowledge to his benefit, and other groups were forced to employ another physician to interpret medical data or medical reasoning.

The PA profession was the first to share this knowledge base, but others were to follow—such as the nurse practitioner.[11]

Thirty years later, it is common to see medical textbooks written for PAs, nurse practitioners, and other nonphysician providers. Such publications are relatively new approaches for gaining access to medical knowledge.

The legal relationship of the PA to the physician was also unique in the health care system. Tied to the license of a precepting physician, the PA concept received the strong support of establishment medicine and ultimately achieved significant "independence" through that "dependence." In contrast, nurse practitioners (NPs), who emphasized their capability for "independent practice," incurred the wrath of many physician groups, who believed that NPs needed supervisory relationships with physicians to validate their role.

Finally, the "primary care" or "generalist" nature of physician assistant training, which stressed the acquisition of strong skills in data collection and problem solving, as well as lifelong learning, made the PA extraordinarily adaptable to almost any patient care setting. The dependent status of PA practice provided PAs with ongoing supervision and almost unlimited opportunities to expand skills as needed in specific practice settings. In fact, the adaptability of physician assistants has had both positive and negative impacts on the PA profession. Although PAs were initially trained to provide health care to the medically underserved, the potential for the use of PAs in specialty medicine has been "the good news and the bad news." Sadler and colleagues[12] recognized this concern early on, when they wrote (in 1972) that

> The physician's assistant is in considerable danger of being swallowed whole by the whale that is our present entrepreneurial, subspecialty medical practice system. The likely co-option of the newly minted physician's assistant by subspecialty medicine is one of the most serious issues confronting the PA.

A shortage of physician assistants in the early 1990s appeared to aggravate this situation and confirmed predictions by Sadler and colleagues[12] that

> Until great numbers of physician's assistants are produced, the first to emerge will be in such demand that relatively few are likely to end up in primary care or rural settings where the need is the greatest. The same is true for inner city or poverty areas.

Although most PAs initially chose primary care, increases in specialty positions raised concern about the future direction of the PA profession. The Federal Bureau of Health Professions was so concerned about this trend that training grants now encourage training programs to require that all students complete clinical training assignments in medically underserved areas.

Military Corpsmen

The choice to train experienced military corpsmen as the first physician assistants was a key factor in the success of the concept. Sadler and colleagues[12] pointed out, "The political appeal of providing a useful civilian health occupation for the returning Vietnam medical corpsman is enormous."

The press and the American public were attracted to the PA concept because it seemed to be one of the few positive "products" of the Vietnam War. Highly skilled, independent duty corpsmen from all branches of the uniformed services were disenfranchised as they attempted to find their place in the U.S. health care system. These corpsmen, whose competence had truly been tested "under fire," provided a willing, motivated, and proven applicant pool of pioneers for the PA profession. Robert Howard, MD,[14] of Duke University, in an AMA publication describing issues of training physician assistants, noted not only that there were large numbers of corpsmen available, but also that using former military personnel prevented transfer of workers from other health care careers that also were experiencing shortages:

> "... the existing nursing and allied health professions have manpower shortages parallel to physician shortages and are not the ideal sources from which to select individuals to augment the physician manpower supply. In the face of obvious need, there does exist a relatively large untapped manpower pool, the military corpsmen. Some 32,000 corpsmen are discharged annually who have received valuable training and experience while in the service. If an economically sound, stable, rewarding career were

available in the health industry, many of these people would continue to pursue such a course. From this manpower source, it is possible to select mature, career-oriented, experienced people for physician's assistant programs."

The decision to expand these corpsmen's skills as physician assistants also capitalized on the prior investment of the U.S. military in providing extensive medical training to these men.

Richard Smith, MD, founder of the University of Washington's MEDEX program, described this training:

> The U.S. Department of Defense has developed ways of rapidly training medical personnel to meet its specific needs which are similar to those of the civilian population.... Some of these people, such as Special Forces and Navy "B" Corpsmen, receive 1,400 hours of formal medical training, which may include nine weeks of a supervised "clerkship." Army corpsmen of the 91C series may have received up to 1,900 hours of this formal training.
>
> Most of these men have had 3 to 20 years of experience, including independent duty on the battlefield, aboard ship, or in other isolated stations. Many have some college background; Special Forces "medics" average ½ year of college. After at least 2, and up to 20, years in uniform, these men have certain skills and knowledge in the provision of primary care. Once discharged, however, the investment of public funds in medical capabilities and potential care is lost, as they work as detail men, insurance agents, burglar alarm salesmen, or truck drivers. The majority of this vast manpower pool is unavailable to the present medical care delivery system because, up to this point, we have not devised a civilian framework in which their skills can be put to use.[15]

Other Models

Describing the period 1965 to 1971 as "Stage One—The Initiation" of Physician Assistant Programs, Carter and Gifford[10] have identified 16 programs that pioneered the formal education of physician assistants and nurse practitioners. Programs based in university medical centers similar to Duke emerged at Bowman Gray, Oklahoma, Yale, Alabama, George Washington, Emory, and Johns Hopkins and used the Duke training model.[8]

As was previously mentioned, a dramatically different training model developed at the University of Washington, pioneered by Richard Smith, MD. Assigned to the Pacific Northwest by Surgeon General William Stewart, Smith was directed to develop a physician assistant training program to respond uniquely to the health manpower shortages of the rural Northwest. Garnering the support of the Washington State Medical Association, Smith developed the MEDEX model, which took a strong position on the "deployment" of students and graduates to medically underserved areas.[15] This was accomplished by placing clinical phase students in preceptorships with primary care physicians who agreed to employ them after graduation. The program also emphasized the creation of a "receptive framework" for the new profession and established relationships with legislators, regulators, and third party payers in order to facilitate the acceptance and utilization of the new profession. Although the program originally exclusively recruited military corpsmen as trainees, the term *MEDEX* was coined by Smith not as a reference to their former military roles but rather as a contraction of "*Med*icine *Ex*tension."[16] In his view, MEDEX, as a term of address, avoided any negative connotations of the word *assistant* and any potential conflict with medicine over the appropriate use of the term *associate*. MEDEX programs were also developed at University of North Dakota School of Medicine, University of Utah College of Medicine, Dartmouth Medical School, Howard University College of Medicine, Charles Drew Postgraduate Medical School, Pennsylvania State University College of Medicine, and Medical University of South Carolina.[17]

In Colorado, Henry Silver, MD, began the Child Health Associate Program in 1969, providing an opportunity for individuals without previous medical experience but with at least 2 years of college to enter the physician assistant profession. Students received a baccalaureate degree at the end of the second year of the 3-year program and were ultimately awarded a master's degree at the end of training. Thus, it became the first physician assistant program to offer a postgraduate degree as an outcome of PA training.

Compared with the pediatric nurse practitioner educated at the same institution, the child health associate, both by greater depth of education and by law, could provide more extensive and independent services to pediatric patients.[10]

Also offering nonmilitary candidates access to the physician assistant profession was the Alderson-Broaddus program in Phillipi, West Virginia. As the result of discussions that had begun as early as 1963, Hu Myers, MD, developed the program, incorporating a campus hospital to provide clinical training for students with no previous medical experience. In the first program designed to give students both a liberal arts education and professional training as physician assistants, Alderson-Broaddus became the first 4-year college to offer a baccalaureate degree to its students. Subsequently, other PA programs were developed at colleges that were independent of university medical centers. Early programs of this type included those at Northeastern University in Boston and at Mercy College in Detroit.[18]

Specialty training for physician assistants was first developed at the University of Alabama. Designed to facilitate access to care for underserved populations, the 2-year program focused its entire clinical training component on surgery and the surgical subspecialties. Even more specialized training in urology, orthopedics, and pathology was briefly provided in programs throughout the United States, although it was soon recognized that entry-level PA training needed to offer a broader base of generalist training.

Controversy About a Name

Amid the discussion about the types of training for the new health care professionals was a controversy about the appropriate name for these new providers. Silver of the University of Colorado suggested *syniatrist* (from the Greek *syn,* signifying "along with" or "association," and *iatric,* meaning "relating to medicine or a physician") for those health care personnel performing "physician-like" tasks. He recommended that the term could be used with a prefix designating a medical specialty and a suffix indicating the level of training (aide, assistant, or associate).[19] Because of his background in international health, Smith believed that *assistant* or even *associate* should be avoided as

potentially demeaning. His term *MEDEX* for "physician extension" was designed to be used as a term of address as well as a credential. He even suggested a series of other companion titles, including "Osler" and "Flexner."[15]

In 1970, the AMA-sponsored Congress on Health Manpower attempted to end the controversy and endorse appropriate terminology for the emerging profession. The Congress chose *associate* rather than *assistant* because of its belief that *associate* indicated a more collegial relationship between the PA and supervising physicians. *Associate* also eliminated the potential for confusion between PAs and medical assistants. Despite the position of the Congress, the AMA's House of Delegates rejected the term *associate,* holding that it should be applied only to physicians working in collaboration with other physicians. Nevertheless, PA programs such as those at Yale and Duke called their graduates *physician associates,* and the debate about the appropriate title continued. A more subtle concern has been the use of an apostrophe in the PA title. At various times, in various states, PAs have been identified as *physician's assistants,* implying ownership by one physician, and *physicians' assistants,* implying ownership by more than one physician; they are now identified with the current, more appropriate title *physician assistant.* The June 1992 edition of the *Journal of the American Academy of Physician Assistants* contains an article by Eugene Stead, MD, reviewing the debate and calling for a reconsideration of the consistent use of the term *physician associate.*[20]

The issue concerning the name resurfaces regularly, particularly among students who are less aware of the historical and political context of the title. Although most PAs would agree that the title *assistant* is less than optimum, the greater concern now is that the process to change it would be cumbersome, time consuming, and potentially threatening to the PA profession. Every attempt to "open up" a state PA law, with the intent of changing the title, would bring with it the risk that outside forces (e.g., other health professions) could modify the practice law. Similarly, the bureaucratic processes that would be required to change the title in every rule and regulation in each state and in every federal agency would be incredibly labor intensive. State and national PA organizations would be seen by policymakers as both self-serving and self-centered if such a change were attempted. Thus, until such time as there is a restructuring of all titles for all professionals, it is unlikely that this title will change.

PROGRAM EXPANSION

From 1971 to 1973, 31 new PA programs were established. These startups were directly related to available federal funding. In 1972, Health Manpower Educational Initiatives (U.S. Public Health Service) provided more than $6 million in funding to 40 programs. By 1975, 10 years after the first students entered the Duke program, there were 1282 graduates of physician assistant programs.

From 1974 to 1985, nine additional programs were established. Federal funding was highest in 1978, when $8,686,000 assisted 42 programs. By 1985, the American Academy of Physician Assistants (AAPA) estimated that 16,000 physician assistants were practicing in the United States.[21] A total of 76 programs were accredited between 1965 and 1985, but 25 of those programs later closed (Appendix Table 1-1). Reasons for closure range from withdrawal of accreditation to competition for funding within the sponsoring institution and adverse pressure on the sponsoring institution from other health care groups.[22]

PA programs entered an expansion phase beginning in the early 1990s when issues of efficiency in medical education, the necessity of team practice, and the search for cost-effective solutions to health care delivery emerged. The American Academy of Physician Assistants urged the Association of Physician Assistant Programs (APAP) to actively encourage the development of new programs, particularly in states where programs were not available. Beginning in 1990, APAP began a process for new program support, including new program workshops, and ultimately a program consultation service (PATH, Program Assistance and Technical Help) to promote quality in new and established programs.

There has been a burgeoning in new programs to the point where there is now a lively debate concerning new program development. (Currently, more than 130 programs are accredited, compared with just more than 50 programs in the 1980s.) A concern is the issue of potential "oversupply." The difficulty lies in the impossibility of making accurate predictions about the future health workforce, a problem that applies to all health professions. Expanded roles of PAs in academic medical centers (as resident replacements), in managed care delivery systems, and in enlarging community health center networks have created unpredicted demand for physician assistants in both primary and specialty roles. The major variable, aside from the consideration of the ideal "mix" of health care providers in future systems, has to do with the *numbers* of people who will receive health care and the *amount* of health care that will be provided to each person. If only a few people will get health care and they will receive only limited health care, then we probably already have enough providers. On the other hand, if everyone will get health care and will receive even a moderate amount of health care, then we clearly need more of all types of providers.

Other features of the debate include concerns about the locations of new programs (heavily concentrated in the Northeast), the nature of sponsoring institutions (liberal arts colleges unattached to academic health centers), and the access to academic degrees (community colleges). Current policy studies from a variety of sources (APAP Blue Ribbon Report, the Pew Report on PAS in Managed Care) recommend careful monitoring of the supply of PAs, along with other health care providers. Although neither the AAPA, the APAP, nor the Accreditation Review Committee on Physician Assistants (ARC-PA) can stop the development of new PA programs, the trend is to recommend caution in preventing the overdevelopment of new programs based on careful analysis of employment trends.

FUNDING FOR PROGRAMS

The success of the Duke program as well as of all developing PA programs was closely tied to external funding. At Duke, Stead was successful in convincing the federal government's National Heart Institute that the new program fell within its granting guidelines. Subsequently, Duke received foundation support from The Josiah Macy, Jr. Foundation, the

Carnegie and Rockefeller foundations, and the Commonwealth Fund.[10]

In 1969, federal interest in the developing profession brought with it demonstration funding from the National Center for Health Services Research and Development. With increasing acceptance of the physician assistant concept and the demonstration that PAs could be trained relatively rapidly and deployed to medically underserved areas, the federal investment increased. In 1972, the Comprehensive Health Manpower Act, under Section 774 of the Public Health Act, authorized support for PA training. The major objectives were education of PAs for the delivery of primary care medical services in ambulatory care settings; deployment of PA graduates to medically underserved areas; and recruitment of larger numbers of residents from medically underserved areas, minority groups, and women to the health professions.[23]

PA funding under the Health Manpower Education Initiatives Awards, and Public Health Services Contracts from 1972 to 1976 totaled $32,669,565 for 43 programs. From 1977 to 1991, PA training was funded through Sections 701, 783, and 788 of the Public Health Service Act. Grants during this period totaled $87,927,728. According to Cawley in 1992,[23] "this legislation has supported the education of at least 17,500, or over 70% of the nation's actively practicing PAs."

During the period of program expansion, the focus of federal funding support has become much more specific. Tied to the primary care access goals of the Health Resources and Services Administration (HRSA), PA program grants commonly support less program infrastructure and more specific primary care initiatives and educational innovations. Examples of activities that may be eligible for federal support include clinical site expansion in urban and rural underserved settings, recruitment and retention activities, and curriculum development on topics such as managed care or geriatrics.

An important trend has been the diversification of funding sources for PA programs. In addition to federal PA training grants, many programs now benefit from clinical site support provided by other federal programs such as Area Health Education Centers (AHECs) or the National Health Service Corps (NHSC). Also, many programs have benefited from expanded state funding, based on state workforce projections of an expanded need for primary care providers.

ACCREDITATION

Accreditation of formal PA programs became imperative because the term *physician assistant* was being used to label a wide variety of formally and informally trained health personnel. Other leaders of the Duke program—E. Harvey Estes, MD, and Robert Howard, MD—asked the American Medical Association to determine educational guidelines for physician assistants. This request was consistent with the AMA's position of leadership in the development of new health careers and its publication of "Guidelines for Development of New Health Occupations."

The National Academy of Science's Board of Medicine had also become involved in the effort to develop uniform terminology for physician assistants. It suggested three categories of physician assistants. Type A was defined as a "generalist" capable of data collection and presentation and having the potential for independent judgment; type B was trained in one clinical specialty; type C was determined to be capable of performing tasks similar to those performed by type A, but not capable of independent judgment.

Although these categories have not remained as descriptors of the PA profession, they helped the medical establishment move toward the support of PA program accreditation. Also helpful were surveys conducted by the American Academy of Pediatrics and the American Society of Internal Medicine determining the acceptability of the PA concept to their respective members. With positive responses, these organizations, along with the American Academy of Family Physicians and the American College of Physicians, joined the AMA's Council on Medical Education in the creation of the "educational essentials" for the accreditation of physician assistant training programs. The AMA's House of Delegates approved these essentials in 1971.

Three PAs—William Stanhope, Steven Turnipseed, and Gail Spears—were involved in the creation of these essentials as representatives of the Duke, MEDEX, and Colorado programs, respectively. The AMA appointed L.M. Detmer administrator of the accreditation process. In 1972, accreditation applications were processed and 20 sites were visited in alphabetical order, 17 of which received accreditation. Ultimately, the accreditation activities were carried out by the Joint Review Committee, which was a part of the AMA's Committee on Allied Health Education and Accreditation (CAHEA). Later, the Joint Committee was renamed the Accreditation Review Committee (ARC). In 2000, the ARC became an independent entity, apart from the CAHEA, and changed its name to the Accreditation Review Commission. Current members of the ARC include the Association of Physician Assistant Programs, American Academy of Physician Assistants, American Academy of Family Physicians, American Academy of Pediatrics, American College of Physicians, American College of Surgeons, and American Medical Association. In 2001, more than 130 PA programs held accreditation.

CERTIFICATION

Just as an accreditation process served to assess the quality of PA training programs, a certification process was needed to ensure the quality of individual program graduates. In 1970, the American Registry of Physician's Associates was created by programs from Duke University, Bowman Gray School of Medicine, and the University of Texas, Galveston, to construct the first certification process. The first certification examination, for graduates from eight programs, was administered in 1972. It was recognized, however, that the examination would have greater credibility if it was administered by the National Board of Medical Examiners. During this same period, the AMA's House of Delegates requested the Council of Health Manpower to become involved in the development of a national certification program for PAs. Specifically, the House of Delegates was concerned that the new professional role should be developed in an orderly fashion, under medical guidance, and should be measured by high standards. The cooperation of the AMA and the National Board of Medical Examiners ultimately resulted in the creation of the National Commission on Certification of Physician Assistants (NCCPA), which brought together representatives of 14 organizations as an independent commission. Federal grants contributed $715,000 toward the construction and validation of the examination.[10]

In 1973, the first NCCPA national board examination was administered at 38 sites to 880 candidates. In 1974, 1303 took the examination; in 1975, there were 1414 candidates. In 1992, 2121 candidates were examined. In 1997, the examination was administered to 3728 candidates.

Now administered only to graduates of AMA-accredited PA programs, the NCCPA board examination was originally open to three categories of individuals seeking certification:

➤ "Formally trained PAs . . . eligible by virtue of their graduation from a program approved by the Joint Review Committee on Educational Programs for Physician's Assistants.

➤ Nurse practitioners are eligible provided they have graduated from a family or pediatric nurse practitioner/clinician program of at least 4 months' duration, affiliated with an accredited medical or nursing school.

➤ Informally trained PAs may sit for the examination provided they have functioned for 4 of the past 5 years as PAs in a primary care setting. Candidate applications and detailed employment verification by current and former employers provide data for determination of eligibility.[24]

Since 1986, only graduates of CAHEA-accredited PA programs have been eligible for the NCCPA examination.

The NCCPA's assignments include not only the annual examination but also technical assistance to state medical boards on issues of certification. The NCCPA publishes an annual directory of certified PAs, which is available to licensing boards.

The NCCPA also administers a re-certification process, which includes requirements to complete and register 100 hours of continuing medical education (CME) every 2 years and to sit for re-certification examinations every 6 years. The first re-certification examination was given in 1981. The move toward re-certification was seen as placing PAs in a leadership position among health professionals; both CME and examination were included as a quality assurance mechanism.

Re-certification quickly became a focus of controversy among PAs, many of whom were concerned that a primary care examination potentially discriminated against specialty PAs. The supporters of the re-certification examination stressed the primary care role of PAs, even in specialty practice. After years of internal controversy within the PA profession, an alternative pathway for re-certification that does not require a proctored examination was approved in 1991. Despite this new option, the issue of re-certification remains a major controversy.

ORGANIZATIONS
AAPA

What was to become the American Academy of Physician Assistants was initiated by students from Duke's second and third classes as the American Association of Physician Assistants, incorporated in North Carolina in 1968. With E. Harvey Estes, Jr., MD, as its first advisor and William Stanhope serving two terms as the first President (1968-69 and 1969-70), the organization's original purposes were to educate the public about PAs, to provide education for PAs, and to encourage service to patients and the medical community. With initial annual dues of $20, the Academy created a newsletter as the official publication of the AAPA and contacted fellow students at the MEDEX program and at Alderson-Broaddus.

By the end of the second year, national media coverage of emerging PA programs throughout the United States was increasing (Fig. 1-1), and the AAPA began to plan for state societies and student chapters. Tax exempt status was obtained, the office of President-Elect was established, and staggered terms of office for board members were approved.

Controversy over types of PA training models offered the first major challenge to the AAPA. Believing that students trained in 2-year programs based on the biomedical model (type A) were the only legitimate PAs, the AAPA initially restricted membership to these graduates. The Council of MEDEX Programs strongly opposed this point of view. Ultimately, discussions between Duke University's Robert Howard, MD, and MEDEX Program's Richard Smith, MD, resulted in an inclusion of graduates of all accredited programs in the definition of *physician assistant,* and thus in the AAPA.

At least three other organizations also positioned themselves to speak for the new profession. These were a proprietary credentialing association, the American Association of Physician Assistants (a group representing U.S. Public Health Service PAs at Staten Island); the National Association of Physician Assistants; and the American College of Physician Assistants, from the Cincinnati Technical College PA Program. AAPA President Paul Moson provided the leadership that "would result in the emergence of the American Academy of Physician Assistants as the single voice of professional PAs" (W.D. Stanhope, C.E. Fasser, unpublished manuscript, 1992).

This unification was critical to the involvement of PAs in the development of educational standards and the accreditation of PA programs. During Carl Fasser's term as AAPA President, the American Medical Association formally recognized the AAPA, and three Academy representatives were formally appointed to the Joint Review Committee.

During the AAPA presidency of Tom Godkins and the APAP presidency of Thomas Piemme, MD, the two organizations sought funding from foundations for the creation of a shared national office. Funding was received from the Robert Wood Johnson Foundation, the van Ameringen Foundation, and the Ittleson Foundation. Because of its 501(3)c tax exempt status, APAP received the funds for the cooperative use of both organizations.[25] "Discussions held at that time between Piemme and Godkins and other organizational representatives agreed that in the future, because of the limited size of APAP, . . . funds would later flow back from the AAPA to APAP" (W.D. Stanhope, C.E. Fasser, unpublished manuscript, 1992). Donald Fisher, MD, was hired as executive director of both organizations, and a national office was opened in Washington, D.C. According to Stanhope and Fasser, "a considerable debt is owed to the many PA programs and their staff who supported the early years of AAPA."

AAPA constituent chapters were created during President Roger Whittaker's term in 1976. Modeled after the organizational structure of the American

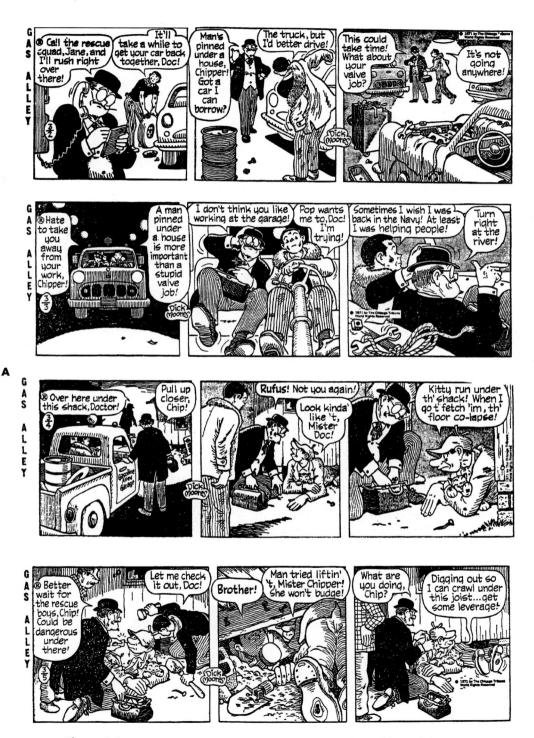

Figure 1-1 © *Tribune Media Services. All rights reserved. Reprinted with permission.*

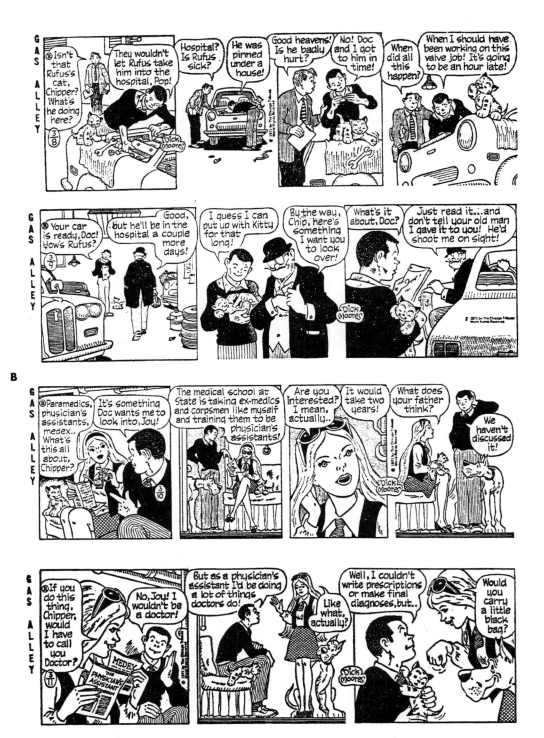

Figure 1-1, cont'd For legend see p. 11.

Academy of Family Physicians, the AAPA's constituent chapter structure and the apportionment of seats in the House of Delegates were the culmination of initial discussions held in the formative days of the AAPA. The American Academy of Family Physicians hosted the AAPA's first Constituent Chapters Workshop in Kansas City, and the first AAPA House of Delegates was convened in 1977.

Throughout its development, the American Academy of Physician Assistants has been active in the publication of journals for the profession. As the first official journal of the AAPA, *Physician's Associate* was originally designed to encourage research and to report on the developing PA movement. With the consolidation of graduates of all programs into the AAPA, the official academy publication became *The PA Journal, A Journal for New Health Practitioners*. In 1977, *Health Practitioner* became the official magazine of the AAPA, followed by *Physician Assistant* in 1983 and *The Journal of the American Academy of Physician Assistants* in 1988. *Clinician Reviews* and *Physician Assistant,* published by external publishers, also offer medical articles and coverage of professional issues for PAs.

According to its current Bylaws,[26] the American Academy of Physician Assistants is committed to

1. Encouraging its membership to render quality services to the health professions and to the public.
2. Developing, sponsoring, and evaluating continuing medical or medically related education programs for the physician assistant.
3. Assisting in the development of role definition for the physician assistant.
4. Assisting with the coordination and standardization of curricula for the physician assistant.
5. Participating in the accreditation of physician assistant training programs.
6. Participating in the development of criteria leading to certification of the physician assistant.
7. Developing, coordinating, and participating in studies having an impact either directly or indirectly on the physician assistant profession.
8. Serving as a public information center with respect to its members, health professions, and the public.

Governed by a 13-member Board of Directors, including officers of the House of Delegates and a student representative, the Academy includes ten standing committees and three councils. Specialty groups and formal caucuses bring together academy members with a common concern or interest.

The AAPA's Student Academy is composed of chartered student societies from each PA training program. Each society has one seat in the Assembly of Representatives, which meets at the annual conference and elects officers to direct Student Academy activities.

The annual conference serves as the major political and continuing medical education activity for PAs, with an average annual attendance of 5000 to 6000 participants. A list of past and present AAPA presidents is provided in Appendix Table 1-2. A history of conference locations is given in Appendix Table 1-3. Appendix Table 1-4 lists presidents of the Student Academy (SAAPA) from the AAPA.

Legislative and leadership development activities for the Academy take place at an annual Constituent Chapter Officers Workshop (CCOW) in September of each year. CCOW also provides an opportunity for lobbying of state congressional delegations in Washington, D.C. AAPA regional meetings also provide annual opportunities for leadership development and skill building. Key to the success of the American Academy of Physician Assistants is a dedicated staff at the national office in Alexandria, Virginia. Under an Executive Vice President who is responsible to the AAPA Board of Directors, six vice presidents manage Academy activities related to governmental affairs, education, communications, member services, accounting, and administration.

APAP

Composed of member programs rather than individuals, the Association of Physician Assistant Programs evolved from the original American Registry of Physician's Associates, which was formed in collaboration by training programs at Duke University, Bowman Gray School of Medicine, and the University of Texas, Galveston. The Registry was originally created "to determine the competence of Physician's Associates" through the development of a national certifying examination. After these functions were subsequently assumed by the National Board of Medical Examiners, and ultimately the National Commission on Certification of Physician Assistants (NCCPA) in 1972, the Registry became the Association of Physician Assistant Programs.

Led by Alfred M. Adler, Jr., MD, its first President, the Association of Physician Assistant Programs evolved as a network within which member programs could work on "curriculum development, program evaluation, [and] the establishment of continuing education programs"; the APAP also was developed to "serve as a clearing house for information and define the role of the physician assistant."[5]

Like the Association of American Medical Colleges, the Association of Physician Assistant Programs represents educational programs, whereas the American Medical Association and the American Academy of Physician Assistants represent individual practitioners.

APAP offices are located in the AAPA building in Alexandria, Virginia, and provide a contracted service with the Academy. The APAP, governed by a six-member Board of Directors, holds its major annual meeting in October, as well as meetings in conjunction with the AAPA Annual May Meeting. The APAP is also organized by regional consortia, which meet on an individual schedule to consider regional training and professional issues. Activities are carried out by both standing and ad hoc committees. APAP Presidents are listed in Appendix Table 1-5.

The APAP offers an on-line directory of PA programs as a resource for program applicants. In 2001, APAP began a nationwide centralized electronic application process (CASPA) to streamline PA program application. So far, not all programs have participated in CASPA; however, the hope is that this service will serve the same function as the American Medical College's Application Service (AMCAS) process used extensively by U.S. medical schools, both for the medical school admissions process and for data collection regarding the applicant pool.

A major function of the APAP is support of PA program faculty. An on-line newsletter, *APAP Update,* provides information on APAP activities and educational opportunities. APAP's formal publication, *Perspectives of PA Education,* offers articles on a range of PA educational issues. APAP also promotes scholarly activity through the Faculty Development Research Institutes.

TRENDS

Although the first PA programs were developed with the primary purpose of training male military corpsmen, the demography of the profession soon changed, largely because the PA profession developed in historical context with both the women's and the civil rights movements.

Early articles and promotional materials for PAs described the new provider almost universally as "he." In 1966, Eugene Stead, MD, explained, "Our intent is to produce career oriented graduates. Since the long-range goals of most females remove them from continued and full time employment in the health field, we anticipate that the bulk of the student body will be males. This is not meant to exclude females, for those who can present credentials which would assure the Admissions Committee of proper intent should be considered in the same light as male applicants."[27]

In fact, there were many "career oriented" women seeking exactly this type of training. By the mid-1970s, the PA profession was quickly evolving—fueled not only by the need for changes in the health care system but also by the attraction to the profession of strong, motivated women seeking a new and open-ended health career. PA program brochures included photographs of both male and female students, and marketing for the PA profession began to focus on the diversity of individuals entering the profession. In 1972, 19.9% of PA students were women; in 1976, 32.8% were women; and by 1981-82, the distribution of graduates was nearly equal.[28, 29] The percentages of women entering U.S. medical schools for the same years were 16.8%, 23.8%, and 30.8%, respectively.[30] By the late 1990s, there was some concern that the PA profession might become a female-dominated profession because women filled more than 60% of the training slots. The move to master's degrees seems to have accelerated the increase in the number of women in PA programs. Researchers have yet to fully explore this phenomenon and its potential impact on the PA profession.

PA programs also immediately focused on recruiting minority candidates for physician assistant training. PA programs to train Native Americans and Alaska Natives were established at Indian Health Service hospitals in Phoenix, Arizona, and Gallup, New Mexico. Programs were also established at Drew University, Howard University, and Harlem Hospital with initiatives to train African-Americans for inner city practice. In addition, federal funding guidelines encouraged other PA programs to emphasize the recruitment and training of minority physician assistants. Since 1987, 20% of all PA students have been minorities. Nevertheless, the recruitment of minorities into the PA profession is an ongoing issue. In 1977, Ruth Webb of the Drew Program challenged "each and every PA to accept the responsibility for seeking out five minority applicants during the coming year. Your minimum goal would be to have at least one of them accepted into your parent program."[31] This challenge is equally appropriate as an ongoing issue.

NATIONAL HEALTH POLICY REPORTS

Two national reports, one by the Institute of Medicine in 1978 and the other by the Graduate Medical Education National Advisory Committee (GMENAC) in 1981, had a major impact on both physician assistants and nurse practitioners.

In 1978, the National Academy of Sciences Institute of Medicine (IOM) issued its "Manpower Policy for Primary Health Care." Strongly supporting PAs and NPs, the IOM statements included the following recommendations[32]:

➤ For the present time, the numbers of PAs and NPs being trained should remain at the current level.

➤ Training programs for family physicians, PAs, and NPs should continue to receive direct federal, state, and private support.

➤ Amendments to state licensing laws should authorize, through regulations, PAs and NPs to provide medical services, including prescribing drugs when appropriate and making medical diagnoses. PAs and NPs should be required to perform the range of services they provide as skillfully as physicians, but they should not provide medical services without physician supervision.

Emphasizing the value of primary care, the IOM report stressed that even with the projected increase in the supply of physicians, physician assistants and nurse practitioners have an important role to play in the delivery of primary care.[32]

Charged by the U.S. Secretary of Health, Education and Welfare, a national advisory committee began in 1976 to examine the physician supply issue. The report by GMENAC, published in 1981 and seen as a major turning point in the history of American health care,[33] projected an oversupply of physicians by 1990. Strategies for correcting this oversupply included reducing medical school enrollments, limiting the utilization of foreign-trained physicians, and reviewing the need to train nonphysician providers. According to Cawley,[23] "many people who supported PAs during the times of physician shortage viewed an excess of physicians as signaling the discontinuation of federal funding for PA programs and the exit of PAs from the medical scene." Although federal funding was not completely eliminated, it was significantly reduced, from $8,262,968 in 1980 to $4,752,000 in 1982. The reduced funds could assist only 34 programs, rather than the previous 43, and the amounts per program were significantly cut.

In retrospect, there were significant flaws in the assumptions of the GMENAC process. Among the issues that could not be predicted were the impact of the human immunodeficiency virus (HIV), the greater utilization of physician services, the shortening of physician workweeks, and the changing lifestyles of physicians. As a result, questions remain about the existence of a physician shortage, and the general understanding is that the United States has a physician maldistribution. As Cawley states, "any perceived negative impact of the rising physician numbers on the vitality of the PA profession has failed to occur."[23] According to Schafft and Cawley, "the most significant outcome of the study was a gradual awareness that the profession would have to reevaluate its mission and redirect its efforts to validate its existence."[33]

FUTURE EVENTS

Two physician assistant symposia in the mid-1980s looked toward the future of health care and the position of PAs in that future. The American Academy of Physician Assistants sponsored an October 1984 symposium, entitled "The Future of Health Care: Challenges and Choices." In the foreword to the Symposium's Executive Summary,[35] 1984 AAPA President Judith Willis described the event and its outcomes:

➤ In bringing together the symposium panelists, health care practitioners, and policymakers, the American Academy of Physician Assistants hoped to explore concrete problems facing the health care sector in the coming decades—manpower, services, financing technology—as well as provide a forum to focus on the challenge for the future of health care in the United States.

➤ If there were a consensus from the symposium presentations and workshops, it would be that the future of health care is dependent not so much on biomedical techniques, but rather on how care is delivered and who controls the practice of medicine.

In 1986, the Association of Physician Assistant Programs formed an Ad Hoc Futures Committee, devoted its mid-year meeting to the study of the Physician Assistant of the Future, and created a vision document recommending directions for PA education. Portions of the vision document read as follows[34]:

➤ *Professional and Practice Characteristics:* The physician assistant career will include expansion into many different roles: clinical, nonclinical, and combinations of the two. There will be more horizontal and vertical career mobility than at present. Physician assistants will continue to be dependent practitioners in the sense of being supervised by physicians, but will have increased performance autonomy. Physician assistants will be part of a multidisciplinary approach to community medical practice. PAs will become more active in anticipating and meeting the health care needs of society.

➤ *Public Policy Issues:* Physician assistants will respond by mastering the political skills necessary to become more involved in policy decisions affecting health care delivery. Such skills and involvement will be directed toward establishing great uniformity of laws and regulations governing PA practice and facilitating practice reciprocity among states.

➤ *Entering the Profession:* Applicants and entering PA students will have strong prior academic preparation. . . . More students will enter with bachelor's degrees than now, and some will enter seeking graduate level education.

➤ *Education:* Primary care will remain the focus of entry-level education for the PA profession. Baccalaureate degrees will remain the most common credential awarded for entry-level education, but other kinds of credentials will be preserved for some students. Programs will employ as faculty physician assistants who are trained as teachers, and physicians will continue to be integrally involved in PA education. The number of postgraduate residency programs in clinical specialties will increase. Some postgraduate training will follow a fellowship model and some will offer a master's degree upon completion.

From the vantage point of the 1990s, the predictions of both the AAPA and the APAP future projects provided accurate guidance for the further development and evolution of the PA profession.

CURRENT ISSUES AND CONTROVERSIES

The development of any new career brings with it controversies and concerns. The late 1960s heralded the creation of the physician assistant and the successful implementation of the pilot projects that would serve as the foundation for subsequent PA training. In the 1970s, enthusiastic new PAs pioneered the role in a variety of settings, practice acts were put in place in most states, and professional organizations were established at national and state levels. The 1980s saw both the continued training of PAs and questions about where PAs fit in the health care system. Although the GMENAC report resulted in a backlash against PAs and nurse practitioners through fewer federal dollars for training, the late 1980s found PAs being used in a wider range of practice settings than had ever been dreamed of by the founders.

During the 1990s, our attention focused on training and utilization; however, there was new appreciation for the political context of health care in a rapidly changing society. Federal health workforce policy documents were paralleled by similar state documents that acknowledged the state-specific issues. Most frequently, these documents called for a maintenance or expansion of the primary care workforce and acknowledgment of the valuable roles that PAs have to play in any health care system, based on their generic primary care training, their adaptability, and their willingness to rapidly respond to the needs of specific health care "niches."

Demand

In a health care system with either a shortage or at least a maldistribution of physicians, determination of the appropriate number of physician assistants and nurse practitioners involves a controversial calculation. PAs and NPs speak with a louder political voice than in the past, but their relatively small numbers compared with more powerful physician organizations sometimes leave their message muffled by comparison.

Development of managed health care systems and greater attention to accessible, cost-effective, and high-quality care make physician assistants desirable in many clinical settings. PA training programs find that many new graduates have signed employment contracts prior to graduation. Other graduates have a difficult time making choices between a variety of job opportunities.

We had all hoped that one outcome of the health reform process would be some "reality-based" workforce projections. Unfortunately, the groups that worked on this issue were limited by the impossibility of such a prediction (see the previous discussion of this issue in this chapter). The Council on Graduate Medical Education, an arm of the Division of Medicine of the Health Resources and Services Administration, convened the Advisory Group on Physician Assistants and the Workforce in 1994.[36] The result is a report, in *Physician Assistants in the Health Workforce,* that projects future needs for PAs but falls silent (as do other workforce reports of the time) on the actual numbers of providers needed in the "new" health system. The recommendations of the report included the following:

1. Expand the output of PA educational programs.
2. Increase the level of federal grant support for PA educational programs.
3. Provide increased funding to expand the supply of PA graduates.
4. Retain primary care as the dominant theme of PA education.
5. Provide incentives in Title VII–authorized PA grant programs that encourage sponsoring academic institutions to integrate clinical educational experiences among various health professions.
6. Include incentives in federal grants supporting PA educational programs to reward, maintain, and improve efforts in the recruitment of students and faculty from minority, disadvantaged, and ethnic groups.
7. Provide incentives in federal PA and other grant programs to encourage the recruitment of PA students from rural areas and the use of rural preceptorships that facilitate the return of these graduates to rural practice.
8. Recommend that the Secretary of Health and Human Services develop a plan encouraging PA educational programs to recruit and retrain honorably discharged military personnel, particularly those from underrepresented minority and ethnic groups.
9. Promote health services research that examines clinical effectiveness, patient outcomes, and resident-substitution ratios when PAs are used in graduate medical education staffing positions.

Although some of these recommendations may have served as the basis for some of the "debates" described earlier, the primary intent of the report was to provide greater clarification about the important role of PAs in meeting the nation's health care needs. A secondary intent was to create a policy document that would prevent some of the backlash against PAs and NPs that had occurred as a result of the GMENAC report.

Primary Care Versus Specialization

Physician assistants were created to respond to the primary care access problem in this country. Although changing job patterns reflect in part the high demand for a relatively small number of available physician assistants, many leaders are concerned that the move away from primary care will lead to decreased federal support for PA training and utilization. Other PA leaders actively encourage the move toward specialization as a strategy to enhance what they see to be the visibility and status of the profession.

In the midst of this controversy are many unanswered questions. There is little research about the actual tasks of PAs within specialty practices. Many specialty PAs contend that they are hired by specialists to provide "primary care" to the specialist's patients. If this is the case, a myriad of secondary questions need to be answered about the reimbursement levels for these services, as well as the specialist's ability to supervise services that he or she may not have been trained to provide. Similarly, what role does the "primary care" function of the PA in a specialty practice play in retaining patients in the specialty practice, and is that role appropriate?

Federal and state policymakers continue to be concerned about training physician assistants for the purpose of providing primary care, especially to underserved populations. Federal training initiatives not only place increasing importance on training in medically underserved clinics (urban and rural) but also promise to put more pressure on programs to encourage students to seek employment in these settings. These trends have a significant impact on recruitment, selection, and training patterns of PA programs. They also have the effect of putting PA educators in direct conflict with those PA leaders who believe that the future of PAs lies exclusively in the specialties and subspecialties.

A broader view of the "primary care versus specialization" issue is to see both trends as a positive demonstration of the flexibility of PAs to respond to a rapidly changing health care system. The generalist nature of PA training, required by accreditation, allows PAs maximum mobility within the health care system. Compared with physicians, whose relatively early specialization leaves little opportunity for re-direction, PAs may move back and forth from primary care to the specialties throughout their careers. Research tracing PA career patterns may

help us to better understand the implications of these transitions.

Who Speaks for Us

The growth of the PA profession has also brought with it the expansion of professional organizations, both nationally and at the state level. PA training programs are often seen as the source of information about state or regional issues. State medical boards and the NCCPA also provide information about PA roles and utilization.

There is always an ongoing tension—which is probably not limited to PAs—about who speaks for our profession and the consistency of the messages that are delivered. Lobbying efforts by the AAPA in Washington, D.C., benefit from input from both constituent chapters and individual PAs. Professional staff members cannot be expected to be the exclusive voices of the PA profession. PA programs and state chapters must work together to provide consistent messages. This reality requires the willingness of PAs to be visible and involved not just in health care but in the political process as well.

Degree Issues

In the closing moments of the AAPA Cincinnati Conference in 1987, the House of Delegates passed a resolution supporting a baccalaureate degree as the entry-level credential for physician assistants. Immediately following that action, the membership of the APAP passed an opposing resolution stating that the AAPA stance was "premature." The significance of degrees continues to be a subject of ongoing and heated controversy.

The proponents of bachelor's degrees for PAs hold that the lack of a degree requirement decreases the credibility of the PA profession and has been a barrier to the expansion of PA practice in some states. Opponents of the degree requirement believe that it limits entry to PA training, especially for rural "second career" applicants, who have little access to formal academic prerequisites.

Proponents of degrees further maintain that the requirement of degrees gives PAs upward mobility, particularly within federal and academic systems. Opponents, citing trends away from primary care in other professions associated with advanced degrees, assert that the focus on degrees is a move away from the primary care mission of the PA profession.

In fact, the relationship of the PA to other professionals is a key aspect of this controversy. Nurse practitioner program accreditation is now mandating that all current graduates be "master's prepared" as part of their independent practice model. Proponents of the degree requirement for PAs fear unfavorable comparison with nursing and nurse practitioners if it is not adopted. Opponents of the degree requirement feel strongly that the degree trends in nursing have led to maldistribution and internal dissension within the profession; they predict similar conflict within the PA community if the degree requirement is adopted.

Central to this issue is the definition of the "gold standard" for PA training and certification. Passing the NCCPA entry-level examination, coupled with graduation from a CAHEA-accredited program, is currently the recognized credential for practice in most states. Proponents of degrees believe that degrees give PAs credibility in addition to that provided by NCCPA certification. Opponents of the degree requirement point out that many other professions, including physicians, are credentialed by competency-based training and examination rather than by degree.

The 1992 AAPA House of Delegates again considered the degree requirement as part of the required "Sunset Review" of policies. After heated discussion, they tabled the position paper on degrees prepared by the Education Council. In 2000, the AAPA House of Delegates adopted resolutions stating that PA education should be conducted at the graduate level and supporting credentials awarded to students that are reflective of the graduate level of education.[37] A policy paper prepared by the Association of Physician Assistant Programs in the same year acknowledged the increasing numbers of master's degree programs and supported the movement of programs to this degree level, but also recognized that individual programs must maintain their unique missions of service and access. It was acknowledged that advanced degrees could be a barrier to this mission.

At this writing (2002), 58% of PAs responding to the AAPA's annual census hold a bachelor's degree and 31% have received master's degrees.[38] Many new PA programs have chosen the master's degree as their level of education. In many cases, this decision has been made internally within the institution without the input of the PA educational community. As a result, particularly in some regions of the country, there is a "trend" toward the master's degree. Those in support of this "trend" argue that the master's degree increases the credibility of PAs. Those who do not support this trend make the case that the graduate education process (wherein research and administrative courses may have a higher priority than full-time clinical training) has the potential to decrease clinical training hours and detract from the strong primary care experience of PAs. There is also the concern that graduate programs decrease access to PA programs for many candidates, particularly those from diverse backgrounds and rural communities. Regardless of one's opinion on this issue, PA program graduates from programs at all levels must be monitored so that any trends, positive or negative, can be discerned for graduates with differing academic credentials.

Interactions With NPs

PAs have been involved with physician organizations both formally and informally since their beginning; however, more recently, interactions of PAs with nurse practitioners have been considered. Relationships between PAs and NPs, at least at the academic or professional organization level, have been fraught with tension; however, at the clinical level, PAs and NPs have often recognized and emphasized their similarities rather than their differences. The changing health care system, as well as common concerns for access and primary care services, encourages alliances between PA and NP organizations. These alliances are facilitated by what is now a clearer definition of similarities and differences between them. Although NPs regard "independent practice" as an essential feature of the professional identity of nursing, PAs continue to believe that "independence through dependence" and strong relationships with physician preceptors are essential features of their profession. NPs have chosen to define themselves as "master's prepared" as a critical issue, especially as an aspect of their independent practice. PAs recognize the NCCPA examination as the "gold standard" of their profession. NPs now limit admission to their profession to those with baccalaureate degrees in nursing, but PAs have broader entry criteria encompassing both first career and second career individuals. Both groups believe that competent nonphysician providers can increase access to care, especially primary care services. Both groups believe that nonphysician providers are part of the cost-effective solution to our health care crisis. Each group can benefit from a better understanding of the other's education/training and practice issues. Frequent liaisons between PAs and NPs, particularly in recognition of their similarities and differences, will benefit us all.

Relationships With Physicians

It is also important that PAs be clear about their relationships with physicians. Because of concern that physician assistants might be lumped into the excessively generic term, *nonphysician providers,* AAPA President William H. Marquart clarified the AAPA's position on independent practice in a letter to John L. Clowe, MD, President of the American Medical Association, dated May 11, 1993; he wrote, in part:

➤ Physician assistants do not seek independent practice, direct reimbursement from third party payers, or federal preemption of state practice acts. . . .

➤ All actions affirm positions held by the profession since its inception 25 years ago: that PAs practice with physician supervision and that third party coverage of PA services should be paid to the PA's employer.

➤ PAs and advance practice nurses are frequently referred to as nonphysician or mid-level providers, and, regrettably, people sometimes fail to draw a distinction between the two professions. We felt it would be appropriate at this time to let you know that PAs maintain a strong belief in the need to work closely with physicians.

M. Roy Schwarz, MD, the AMA's Senior Vice President for Medical Education, responded on May 25, 1993, to the letter as follows:

"I am very pleased to have an official confirmation of your posture concerning independent practice. . . . Having been involved in the original development of the MEDEX Program at the University of Washington, and having watched the physician assistant movement develop, I could not be more pleased with its evolution and the performance of its people.

You have undoubtedly seen me quoted in newspapers concerning the nursing agenda and their quest for the independent practice of primary care. I never intended [to include], nor have I included physician assistants in those comments. . . . I have clearly indicated in every interview that physician assistants do not have this as their goal, that they are completely satisfied with their present role, and that their relationship with medicine is an excellent one. Your letter reaffirms that conviction, and I appreciate having it.

My best to you and your colleagues as you go about serving America's needs."

CASE STUDY 1-1

The history of the PA profession in Washington State illustrates how critical, and positive, interaction with a state medical association has facilitated the development of PA practice.

1968: The Washington State Medical Association (WSMA) was a partner with the University of Washington School of Medicine in the creation of the MEDEX Northwest physician assistant program. This support was based on the need for health care in rural communities and the premise that the additional support and care provided by MEDEX graduates would result in the retention of rural physicians within the communities.

1971: The Washington State Medical Association sponsored an amendment to the medical practice act allowing physician assistants to practice under the supervision of a practicing physician. This pioneering legislation was sponsored by a physician/legislator, James McDermott, MD, who now serves in the U.S. Congress.

1977: With the endorsement of the WSMA, the Board of Medical Examiners amended its Rules and Regulations to allow physician assistants to write prescriptions.

1982: Physician assistants were invited to join the Washington State Medical Association. The Washington Academy of Physician Assistants (WAPA) was allowed a voting seat in the WSMA House of Delegates, and WAPA became a participant in the Interspecialty Council.

1986: The Washington State Medical Association House of Delegates passed a resolution to place a physician assistant on the Board of Medical Examiners.

1987: The Washington State Legislature passed legislation to place a PA on the Board of Medical Examiners who would vote on PA matters.

1990: Washington PA status is changed from "registered" to "licensed" by legislative action, with the support of the WSMA. The PA on the Board of Medical Examiners is given full voting privileges.

1991: Again by legislative action, with the support of the WSMA, a PA is added to the Medical Disciplinary Board and is given full voting privileges.

1993: Washington passes "Single Licensure Law" for PAs, thus increasing the flexibility of PA utilization.

CONCLUSION

The social change theory, which holds that "it takes society 30 years, more or less, to absorb a new technology into everyday life,"[39] can be applied to physician assistants. Created during a time of chaos within the health care system, PAs are now, more than ever, a solution to access, efficiency, and economic problems in health care. Consumers are not yet 100% informed about physician assistants, but more and more have been the recipients of PA care. Current transitions to managed care or managed competition require that physician assistants be part of the provider formula. The range of opportunities for PA employment is limitless in both primary care and the specialties. Maintaining a responsive and flexible stance in this rapidly evolving health care system is the most important strategy for the profession as PAs look to the future.

CLINICAL APPLICATIONS

1. Research the history of the PA profession in your state. What, if any, was the involvement of the state medical association in the creation of the practice "environment"? Who were the key PAs in the formation of the state academy? If one does not exist, prepare a chronological list of state academy presidents and conference locations.

2. Keep a longitudinal diary of the issues that are your personal, local, state, regional, and national concerns regarding the PA profession. These might include specific licensure or reimbursement issues, or even your personal reflections on the changes occurring across time. Use this diary as a personal history of your PA career. You might want to include your successful application to PA school as the first item in this diary.

REFERENCES

1. Fortuine R. Chills and Fevers: Health and Disease in the Early History of Alaska. Fairbanks: University of Alaska Press, 1992.
2. Sidel VW. Feldshers and feldsherism: the role and training of the feldsher in the USSR. N Engl J Med 1968;278:935.
3. Storey PB. The Soviet feldsher as a physician's assistant. Washington, DC: Geographic Health Studies Program, 1972. US Dept of Health, Education, and Welfare Publication No. (NIH) 72–58.
4. Roemer MI. Health Care Systems in World Perspective. Ann Arbor, MI: Health Administration Press, 1975.
5. Perry HB, Breitner B. Physician Assistants: Their Contribution to Health Care. New York: Human Sciences Press, 1982.
6. Basch PF. International Health. New York: Oxford University Press, 1978.
7. Dimond EG. Village health care in China. In: McNeur RW (ed). Changing Roles and Education of Health Care Personnel Worldwide in View of the Increase in Basic Health Services. Philadelphia: Society for Health and Human Values, 1978.
8. Gifford JF. The development of the physician assistant concept. In: Alternatives in Health Care Delivery: Emerging Roles for Physician Assistants. St Louis: Warren H. Green, 1984.
9. Fisher DW, Horowitz SM. The physician assistant: profile of a new health profession. In: Bliss AA, Cohen ED (eds). The New Health Professionals: Nurse Practitioners and Physician's Assistants. Germantown, MD: Aspen Systems Corp, 1977.
10. Carter RD, Gifford JF. The emergence of the physician assistant profession. In: Perry HB, Breitner B (eds). Physician Assistants: Their Contribution to Health Care. New York: Human Sciences Press, 1982.
11. Estes EH. Historical perspectives—how we got here: lessons from the past, applied to the future. In: Physician Assistants: Present and Future Models of Utilization. New York: Praeger, 1986.
12. Sadler AM, Sadler BL, Bliss AA. The Physician's Assistant Today and Tomorrow. New Haven, CT: Yale University, 1972.
13. PA Training Grant Kit. Rockville, MD: Bureau of Health Professions, Health Resources and Services Administration, 1991.

14. Howard R. Physician Support Personnel in the 70s: New Concepts. (Burzek J [ed].) Chicago: American Medical Association, 1971.

15. Smith RA, Vath RE. A strategy for health manpower: reflections on an experience called MEDEX. JAMA 1971;217:1365.

16. Smith RA. MEDEX. JAMA 1970;211:1843.

17. Lawrence D, Wilson W, Castle N. Employment of MEDEX graduates and trainees. JAMA 1975;234:174.

18. Myers H. The Physician's Assistant. Parson, WV: McClain Printing Company, 1978.

19. Silver HK. The syniatrist. JAMA 1971;217:1368.

20. Stead EA. Debate over PA profession's name rages on. J Am Acad Physician Assist 1992;6:459.

21. First Annual Report on Physician Assistant Education Programs in the United States, 1984-85. Arlington, VA: Association of Physician Assistant Programs, 1985.

22. Third Annual Report on Physician Assistant Education Programs in the United States, 1986-87. Arlington, VA: Association of Physician Assistant Programs, 1987.

23. Cawley JF. Federal health policy and PAs: two decades of government support have contributed to professional growth. J Am Acad Physician Assist 1992;5:682.

24. Glazer DL. National Commission on Certification of Physician's Assistants: a precedent in collaboration. In: Bliss AA, Cohen ED (eds). The New Health Professionals: Nurse Practitioners and Physician's Assistants. Germantown, MD: Aspen Systems Corp, 1977.

25. Stanhope WD. The roots of the AAPA: the AAPA's first president remembers the milestones and accomplishments of the Academy's first decade. J Am Acad Physician Assist 1993; 5:675.

26. American Academy of Physician Assistants: Constitution and Bylaws. In: Membership Directory 1997-1998. Alexandria, VA: American Academy of Physician Assistants, 1997.

27. Stead EA. Conserving costly talents providing physicians' new assistants. JAMA 1966;19:182.

28. Light JA, Crain MJ, Fisher DW. Physician assistant: a profile of the profession, 1976. PAJ 1977;7:111.

29. Selected Findings from the Secondary Analysis: 1981 National Survey of Physician Assistants. Rosslyn, VA: American Academy of Physician Assistants, 1981.

30. American Medical Association. Annual report on medical education in the United States, 1987-88. JAMA 1988;260:8.

31. Webb R. Minorities and the PA movement. Physician Assist 1977;2:14.

32. Stalker TA. IOM report: the recommendations and what they mean. Health Pract Physician Assist 1978;2:25.

33. Schafft GE, Cawley JF. The Physician Assistant in a Changing Health Care Environment. Rockville, MD: Aspen Publishers, 1987.

34. Physician Assistants for the Future: An In-depth Study of PA Education and Practice in the Year 2000. Alexandria, VA: Association of Physician Assistant Programs, 1989.

35. A Symposium: The Future of Health Care: Challenges and Choices, Executive Summary. Alexandria, VA: American Academy of Physician Assistants, 1984.

36. Physician Assistants in the Health Workforce, 1994. Rockville, MD: Bureau of Health Professions, Health Resources and Services Administration, 1994.

37. AAPA House of Delegates. AAPA Policy Manual, H-P-200.2.1 and H-P-200.2.2. Adopted 2000.

38. AAPA Physician Assistant Census Report, page 2. Alexandria, VA: AAPA, 2001.

39. Cringely RX. Accidental Empires. New York: Harper Collins, 1993.

RESOURCES

Hooker RS, Cawley JF. Physician Assistants in American Medicine. New York: Churchill Livingstone, 1997. *This detailed account of the development of the PA profession provides valuable and accessible resource material on PA history. The material contained in this publication is equally valuable to students, practicing PAs, and employers.*

Physician Assistants in the Health Workforce, 1994. The Advisory Group on Physician Assistants and the Workforce. Rockville, MD: Council on Graduate Medical Education (COGME), Bureau of Health Professions, Health Resources and Services Administration, 1994. *This federal document summarizes many of the discussions that took place at the federal level during the health reform period and recommends policies for the expansion of PA programs and the continuation of federal support for PA education.*

Annual Report of Physician Assistant Educational Programs in the United States. Alexandria, VA: Association of Physician Assistant Programs (APAP), updated and published annually. *APAP's annual publication contains extensive data on PA programs, including information on faculty, students, and program resources. Each yearly publication also examines current trends in PA education and practice.*

Advisory Committee on Training in Primary Care Medicine and Dentistry: A report to the Secretary of U.S. Department of Health and Human Services and Congress. Health Resources and Services Administration, November 2001. *Report on the past and present of Bureau of Health Professions training grant activities includes accomplishments of primary care programs, including PA programs, in a state-by-state format. The advocacy document was prepared to support re-authorization and expanded funding for Title VII, Section 7 of the Public Health Service Act.*

CHAPTER 2

Education

Jim Hammond

INTRODUCTION

This chapter presents some of the contributions and characteristics of physician assistant (PA) education and PA educators during the past three decades. The views presented are based on the author's experience as a PA participating in PA education from the 1970s to the present. The chapter portrays PA education as a vibrant, creative, and responsive component of professional health care education.

PA education is a powerful force affecting the future of the profession. The influence of education lies in the determination of what knowledge, skills, and attitudes will be presented to PAs during the formative, student stage of their careers. The first responsibility of PA education is to be responsive to the needs of society.

PA education was founded and resides within universities, which dedicate themselves to respond to the needs of society, not to the needs of a particular profession. For the PA profession to succeed, it must respond to society. This response is most effective when all members of the profession are working toward the same goals.

Four time periods are considered in this chapter discussion—the mid-1960s through the 1970s, the 1980s, the 1990s, and the 2000s. Within each period, four factors are examined:
➤ Social forces influencing the period.
➤ Key features of PA education.
➤ Characteristics of PA educators.
➤ Attributes of PA students.

THE MID-1960s THROUGH THE 1970s—PIONEER PERIOD

Social Forces

Before the PA profession existed, and thus before PA education was born, society needed improved access to quality medical care. Across the country, a few visionaries responded to this need and dreamed of creating a new type of medical provider who could extend the service of physicians. Working with physicians, these new providers would perform the most fundamental yet complex tasks in medicine—the diagnosis, treatment, and prevention of a wide array of diseases and disorders—tasks not commonly done by nursing or allied health professionals. They would improve access to medical care and make care available to rural and underserved populations. They would counsel and educate patients and their families. They would provide the same quality of services performed by physicians. The new providers would begin work after about 2 years of medical education. They might or might not have any previous health care education or experience. It was quite a set of dreams.

To understand how these dreams originated, a historical perspective is needed. The forces for change in society during the 1960s were as great as at any time since the Great Depression. Hundreds of thousands of people openly demonstrated for equal rights, equal economic opportunities, personal recognition, and a better place in society. Tens of millions more quietly hoped for these changes. Other millions resisted change. Fears that the fabric of American society was being rent were pronounced daily by news commentators and civic leaders. A mix of fear and hope was visible on faces across the strata of society. Among the many responses of the state and federal government was the declaration of war—a war on poverty and inequality.

Within this context of broad social change came a dramatic expansion of health care delivery. Medicare and Medicaid were born. These two programs provided the means by which millions could obtain health care, which previously had been out of reach. Millions of new patients entered this health care nonsystem. An already stretched medical profession could not meet the demand. Many of the newly enfranchised people resided in rural and inner city areas, the very areas with the fewest physicians.

The dreamers were compassionate, creative individuals who sought answers to society's needs. For every PA program, there was at least one visionary founder. By 1971, the U.S. Department of Health, Education, and Welfare reported that 80 institutions were pursuing the development of PA programs.[1] Some institutions did not open programs; others opened and closed them after only a few years of operation. By the end of the 1970s, the number of programs had stabilized at about 50.

It was one thing to dream the dreams. It was another to bring them to reality. For this, the dreams were entrusted to educators.

Education

The designers of PA educational programs required answers to a number of key questions:

➤ What segments of the population would this new type of provider serve?
➤ What would be the mission, values, and identity of the new providers?
➤ What would be the role of these new providers?
➤ What would be their relationship with physicians?
➤ How does an educational program teach a physician/PA relationship for which no role models exist?
➤ What should be the depth, breadth, and priorities of the curriculum?
➤ What should be the length and intensity of the curriculum?
➤ What backgrounds and characteristics of applicants would be associated with successful students?
➤ What methods of teaching would be most successful?
➤ How do educational programs create markets to employ graduates?
➤ What factors would lead students to choose positions in specialties and geographic areas that would meet the needs of the targeted portions of society?
➤ How do educational programs create acceptance for the new role among patients, physicians, and other health care professionals?

Although the answers to many of the questions seem apparent now, there was no clarity at the time. The manner in which the educational features were combined and implemented resulted in new approaches to medical education. These approaches were based on a philosophy of educating people to meet a specific societal need—increased availability of quality health care. The values that the early program leaders projected upon PA education and subsequently upon the profession were strongly service oriented.

Although programs shared a fairly consistent set of goals, they chose a variety of methods to achieve them. Thus there were different models for PA programs. Even programs sharing the same basic model created variations to meet local needs or to use different resources. This created significant individuality between programs tempered by an equally strong camaraderie.

Given the breadth of their responsibilities, early educators needed vast amounts of energy and a broad set of skills. In addition to persuading universities and medical communities to start a program and participate in this experiment, they had to find the people and funding to make it happen. They designed and implemented curricula that had never been attempted. Before PAs existed, they were frequently called upon to describe the PA role to legislators and health policymakers. As meager numbers were educated, it fell to the educators to convince physicians and other employers to hire the newly graduated PAs. Before sufficient PAs became available to lead the profession, the early educators were responsible for establishing methods to ensure the quality of PA education. They did this by forming a national network of PA educational programs that eventually developed into the Association of Physician Assistant Programs (APAP), and by participating in the development of a national accrediting body for PA educational programs—the Committee on Allied Health Education and Accreditation (CAHEA) of the American Medical Association.

As with many new educational endeavors, PA programs went through an initial period of development that was largely experimental. As with most experiments, not all elements proved successful. However, several early features remain prominent within PA education today.

Compact Curriculum A commonly heard description of PA education is that it is 75% of medical school in 50% of the time. This intensity is necessary to keep educational costs down. Many students also were coming out of the workforce to return to school and sought to reenter the workforce as soon as possible. Several factors made compactness possible:

➤ All elements of the curriculum had to contribute to meeting the mission of the program. Mission statements identified the role of graduates and the populations the program intended to serve.

➤ PAs were educated to make professional judgments involving the health and well-being of others. The breadth and depth of the curriculum ensured a foundation in the arts and sciences sufficient to support understanding of the scientific and behavioral components of the medical information.

➤ Every course was examined to eliminate superfluous content, reduce redundancy, and maintain practicality. Topics were integrated between courses that were offered simultaneously and those sequenced throughout the curriculum.

➤ The outcome-based philosophy of the program mission was applied to clinical rotations and didactic courses. Courses were designed and students were evaluated against competency-based outcomes delineated in the learning objectives for every course, often for every lecture and clinical experience.

➤ Practicality was achieved by coursework that required the same processes and skills that would be needed upon graduation. Lecture topics were frequently presented in a case-based format.

➤ Community participation in PA education increased practicality. Community-based clinicians presented a large portion of the medical lectures. Many programs required clinical rotations away from teaching hospitals and in community settings where students were assigned to precepting physicians whose only teaching responsibility at the time was one PA student. This one-on-one approach increased the intensity of learning and the weight of decision making for the student. It also allowed the student to perform in all the settings he or she might experience as a graduate, such as an office, a hospital, or a public health clinic.

➤ Programs used standardized patients to help instruct students in interviewing techniques, history taking, physical examination, and clinical problem solving. By the late 1970s, videotaping of students to critique their interviewing skills was widespread.

➤ The utilization of instructors from a wide variety of disciplines exposed students to the multidisciplinary nature of clinical practice.

Diversity of Education   One danger of a compact, intense curriculum was that programs would all adopt identical curricula. Such "sameness" was contrary to the philosophy of PA education. Several factors guarded against this possibility:

➤ With its first set of accreditation standards published in 1971, the accrediting agency firmly established a competency-based approach for PA education.[2] Promotion of diverse educational approaches among programs with insistence on basic standards became a hallmark of PA education. This has continued to breathe vitality and experimentation into PA programs.

➤ The practice of programs being sponsored by different types of institutions—general universities, hospitals, colleges, and medical schools—helped to ensure a diversity of educational approaches that fostered creativity and expansion of the profession in a multitude of directions.

Psychosocial Emphasis   Many of the early leaders of programs were not physicians. They viewed medical care from a consumer's perspective. They were critical of what they judged to be a lack of interpersonal skills on the part of many physicians. They ensured that PA education would not suffer from this deficit by including strong psychosocial components in the curriculum:

➤ Curricula were evaluated and lecturers were chosen to ensure a patient-centered focus.

➤ Interviewing and counseling skills were given strong emphasis.

➤ Programs selected students who already had well-developed interpersonal skills.

➤ This people-centered philosophy was reinforced by example as programs developed extensive support systems to help students cope with the pressures inflicted upon them by the compact, intense educational system.

Devotion to Underserved Populations   This value was part of the foundational philosophy of many programs. It manifested itself in several ways:

➤ It was widespread in program mission statements.

➤ Several programs were specifically designed to educate PAs who would work with inner city, rural poor, or Native American populations.

➤ Many programs made strong efforts to recruit and select students from underserved populations in the hope that they would return there to practice.

➤ A number of programs concentrated the clinical education of students in clinics, hospitals, and public health services devoted to serving the underserved.

Educators

Initially, the PA profession lay in the hands of educators, none of whom were PAs and many of whom were not clinicians. There was, however, some commonness to their sense of mission—determination to make a difference in health care delivery. They did not set out to establish a new profession, but to respond to the needs of society and to actualize the vision of the founders of each program.

These early PA educators came from a variety of backgrounds, including medicine, social work, nursing, biology, and chemistry. Some had been primarily educators, whereas others were clinicians. Although their educational and professional backgrounds varied considerably, some personal characteristics were important to their success. They had a pioneering spirit—strong on conceptualization, doggedly determined to succeed, willing to take personal risks, anxious to experiment, and boundless in energy. They were creative people, as well as skilled team builders, with substantial powers of persuasion.

Students

The diversity of both the mission and the educational approach among PA programs resulted in the admission of groups of students with a wide variety of academic and experiential backgrounds. Nonetheless, some generalizations seem relevant.

Because PA was a new profession, it opened new avenues for people already working in health care but looking for a role with greater decision making or more direct work with patients. Although many early students had been military corpsmen, PA programs also attracted large numbers of nurses, medical technologists, radiology technologists, respiratory therapists, and others with substantial prior experience who were looking for added knowledge and responsibility.[3] Students with no prior clinical experience were also admitted. Case Study 2-1 provides examples.

CASE STUDY 2-1

Miriam was 32 years old when she heard about the PA program in her city. She knew it was the right career for her. After 4 years at a liberal arts college, Miriam had joined the Peace Corps and worked in family planning in the South Pacific for 2 years. She returned to the United States and became active as a health educator in the women's community for several years. Miriam wanted to do more in health care but did not want to be a physician or a nurse. With the goal of working in obstetrics and gynecology, Miriam applied to the PA program and was accepted.

John came to the PA program at age 30 with 6 years of experience as a Navy corpsman, including one tour of duty in Vietnam. John was 19 years old when he was drafted, and he gained considerable medical experience in the service, which was not transferable into civilian jobs. After 5 years of occasional college courses and a variety of short-term jobs, John realized that he missed patient care, and he found out about the PA profession from a physician friend. He applied, but was told that his college grades were too erratic. He spent a year bringing up his grade point average and was accepted the following year with the goal of working in a rural family practice setting.

Maria was 20 years old and had 1 year of college when she applied to the PA program. Maria had been the primary caregiver for her mother for 5 years until her death a year before. Caring for her

mother and getting involved in advocacy for patients with multiple sclerosis had convinced Maria that she wanted a medical career with a focus on patient education. Although she was by far the youngest student in her class, with the least formal medical experience, Maria was very successful in the PA program.

Fred was a 45-year-old medical technologist who had risen through the ranks to become the director of laboratory services at the local hospital. Fred had dreamed of becoming a physician but never had the financial resources. When the first PA was hired in the hospital, Fred discovered the PA profession. After several long conversations, Fred realized that he might have a chance to work in medicine as a PA with direct patient contact and make his dream come true. He took a few science courses to brush up on his study skills and began the PA program with the goal of returning to his community hospital as the second PA in the department of medicine.

Well into the 1970s, most states did not have laws governing the practice of PAs. Students attracted in the early years were risk takers. As they entered PA programs, they knew there was no guarantee they would be allowed to practice upon graduation.

Students in this era often relished the opportunity to serve as pioneers. Following graduation, many established state and national PA organizations, addressed professional issues such as quality assurance, worked for passage of legislation enabling practice, and fought for reimbursement. Some became the first generation of PAs to educate other PAs.

THE 1980s—MATURATION PERIOD
Social Forces

The 1980s witnessed a strong resurgence of business values in society. It was widely proclaimed that everything from churches and government to universities, medical practice, and health care delivery could be vastly improved if they operated on the profit-based principles of modern business. The early 1980s saw the enrollment of large numbers of students in graduate programs at business schools across the land. By the mid-1980s, many business graduates had found their way into health care. It was the time of health maintenance organizations (HMOs), preferred provider organizations (PPOs), and diagnosis-related groups (DRGs). Health care was to be "managed" for the welfare of society by those trained in business, that is, the stockholders.

The PA profession was well positioned to benefit from some aspects of this environment. PA was establishing itself as a profession of cost-effective, high-quality medical care providers. PAs were steeped in the concepts of team practice. As those in charge of health care corporations sought to expand their businesses, keep costs under control, and raise earnings, they discovered PAs. The demand for PAs grew throughout the decade.

As the health care industry developed new systems, it created positions with new foci such as expanded geriatric care, a return to medical care home visits, broader patient education, case management, and more comprehensive occupational medicine. While searching for people with broad-based, primary care education and flexible attitudes to fill the new positions, it discovered PAs.

Within these developing health care systems, employers were looking for multi-skilled individuals who combined a medical background with a background in areas involving business, law, education, management, and finance. They discovered PAs. Because PA education is brief compared with physician education, it attracts people with extensive backgrounds and conversely allows practicing PAs to pursue further education in complementary fields.

Physician specialists also discovered PAs. During the decade, virtually every medical specialty came to include PAs.

Hospitals were faced with several problems. Some teaching hospitals faced reductions in the number of physician residents available to them. Others experienced monthly fluctuations in the quality of care as residents rotated to new services. Still others needed to provide additional support to attending physicians to prevent them from straying to competing hospitals. In looking for solutions, hospitals discovered PAs.

By the 1980s, the profession had grown sufficiently to become a visible part of the health care system.

Education

PA education came of age during the 1980s. Growth in the number of practicing PAs and in the diversity of employment situations for PAs resulted in changes in education. Because of variations within the institutions sponsoring PA programs, changes were not uniform across all programs or regions. However, several trends seem apparent.

Acceptance of Programs   The number of operational PA programs stabilized at around 50. Educational institutions began to view PA programs less as educational experiments and more as permanent units. Universities began finding homes for programs within the administrative structure. For some institutions, this meant elevation of programs to departmental status. For others, it involved deciding whether the PA program should be a component of medical or allied health education. The creation of regular, tenure track positions for PA faculty members began a trend toward graduate degree requirements for faculty positions. The commitment to attain graduate degrees led many PA faculty members to decide on education as the primary component and clinical practice as the secondary component of their career.

Curriculum Development   Through the use of incentives in training grant programs, the federal government prompted changes in the education of primary care providers. PA programs were induced to incorporate additional health promotion and disease prevention topics in their curricula and to improve student knowledge and skill in serving specific patient populations, such as the aging, racial and ethnic minorities, and those affected by the human immunodeficiency virus (HIV).

Postgraduate Programs   The rise in the percentage of PAs working in medical specialties led to a number of efforts. With the exception of three entry-level programs that prepared students to work in general surgery, entry-level PA programs became limited to a primary care focus. Entry-level programs in orthopedics, urology, radiology, and other specialties closed. Postgraduate programs appeared in a variety of specialties, including occupational medicine, emergency medicine, general surgery, neonatology, and geriatric medicine. Most were 1 year in length and were modeled on residencies in medical education. Most offered a certificate of completion as the credential. A few offered academic master's degrees as the graduation credential.

Issues of Standardization

Debate over a minimum academic degree for entry into the PA profession occurred sporadically throughout the 1980s. Generally, the debate took place among practicing PAs and within the American Academy of Physician Assistants (AAPA). It was focused on whether or not the baccalaureate level should be adopted as the minimum degree. However, while that question went unresolved, events within some of the programs took a different turn.

A small but increasing number of programs began offering master's degrees as the entry-level credential. They did so in response to several factors. As some universities began requiring PAs to hold at least a master's degree to accept a faculty position, it was readily apparent that few PAs held master's degrees. Second, as institutions reviewed the curricula of their PA programs, some determined that the length of college education and the level of learning inherent in PA education were more compatible with the master's degree than with the baccalaureate degree. Finally, factors in the job market began to demonstrate that the responsibility level of PAs was akin to that of other health care professions that awarded master's degrees.

There were also reasons not to offer the master's degree. Extending the length and cost of PA education would limit the people who could attend PA programs and would reduce the cost effectiveness of the profession. It would reduce the pool of people from rural and inner city backgrounds who could qualify for admission, and thus would negatively influence the distribution of PAs to these areas of need. The competency-based rather than degree-based philosophy of the accrediting body also weighed against adoption of a uniform entry-level degree. Although there was no final resolution of the issue, the percentage of programs offering a master's degree as entry into the profession would gradually increase.

Educators

The shift toward business values in medical care, specialization for PAs, and competition for PAs with other health care professions were widely discussed in PA education circles. As is often the case, educational institutions moved more slowly than the general society. PA programs continued to adhere to the service values upon which they were founded, resisting the move to new values. Likewise, they were slow to respond to the expansion of the job market late in the decade. This slow response created a backlog of pressure that would result in the rapid expansion of programs in the 1990s.

Perhaps the most consequential developments in PA education in the 1980s were linked to gradual changes in the makeup of the faculty. During the 1960s and 1970s, most directors of PA programs were not PAs. Likewise, the array of instructors and preceptors included few PAs. As more PAs became available in the 1980s, the percentage of PAs in education rose dramatically. Eventually, the majority of directorships were held by PAs, and virtually all programs had a core of full-time PAs serving as faculty. Physicians and other clinicians continued to be heavily involved as guest lecturers and clinical preceptors.

The new educators had been students in PA programs during the pioneer period of the 1970s. Often, they had created the first clinical positions they held. Many were the first to work in a particular town, county, hospital, or clinic. They were creative, determined people with an overwhelming sense of ownership of the PA profession. They brought these values and energies to PA education. This shift of personnel at the center of PA education had a number of consequences:

➤ The PAs came with solid clinical credentials. They also had professional connections with many physicians in the medical community. The medical director was no longer the only person at the program qualified to judge the quality and appropriateness of the medical component of the curriculum. Medical director roles generally became more collaborative or diminished in scope and prominence.

➤ The teaching styles of PAs were less traditionally academic and more clinical. They converted patient-centered clinical practice to student-centered faculty practice. They developed personal commitments to each student and felt obligated to provide intervention strategies for every educational problem that occurred. This led to an educational approach that was heavily student centered.

➤ These educators had been socialized into the service values of the profession when they were trained as PAs. When they found themselves on the admission committees of programs, they exercised their influence and continued to search for candidates with an altruistic or service orientation. PA educators were trying to create new PAs in their own image.

➤ The heavily student-centered approach taken by faculty provided a great deal of support for students who were often struggling to meet the demands of the most intense education they had ever experienced.

➤ As programs were granted departmental status, PA teaching positions often were converted to formal faculty positions. PAs were now faced with meeting the standard requirements of university faculty to teach, perform service, do research, and hold a terminal degree, preferably a doctorate. Because PA instructional positions often did not fit the usual university faculty mold, a period of adjustment was required for programs and faculty. Teaching and performing service were not generally a problem. However, most faculty did not hold doctorates and had not been trained to do research. Through the 1980s and to the present, some programs still struggle to design and maintain faculty positions that meet the needs of PAs, the programs, and the universities.

➤ The fact that universities encouraged and often supported faculty to perform professional service proved to be a boon to many state and national PA organizations. Faculty often had the skills, the connections, and the time to devote to these activities.

Students

As was true for most helping professions, the 1980s were marked by fluctuations in the number of people applying to PA programs. The decade began with a sufficient pool, but there was a dip in the size of the pool by the mid-1980s. Finally, the late 1980s saw a rise in numbers that became dramatic in the 1990s.

A shift also occurred in the characteristics and motivations of the applicants. The initial wave of applicants in the 1960s and 1970s consisted predominantly of people with substantial prior clinical experience and a pioneering or altruistic career focus. This ratio continued into the early 1980s. With the climate in the country moving away from altruism toward job security and personal income, the characteristics of applicants changed. The number of applicants seeking PA as a first career rose, although this group still did not predominate. A shift of motivation placed greater value on career income, status, and security. In keeping with these values, more graduates gravitated toward higher paying specialties in middle and upper middle class practices. Fewer went to rural and underserved areas.

THE 1990s—BOOM OR BUST TIME
Social Forces

At work for decades, the social energy for health care reform realized its greatest impact in the 1990s. Years of steadily rising health care insurance costs provided a strong incentive for large corporate employers to find a more affordable solution. Health care experienced steady movement toward larger delivery systems. Mergers and buyouts continued to be the mode of operation. Many small rural hospitals closed, forcing patients to travel to distant centers for care. Likewise, many physician practices were owned or managed by hospitals or large provider organizations. This diminished the presence of service-oriented values at the table of corporate decision making. The focus shifted toward serving the stockholder and away from the consumer and the provider.

Despite substantial reform, health care in the United States could not be characterized as a system. Rather, it consisted of a patchwork quilt of many local, regional, and national systems. Although there were benefits to this situation, it also created problems of access and availability for people with special or expensive problems, the poor, the working poor, and those living in physically or culturally remote corners of society. The rapid growth of large managed care systems and the rising influence of insurance providers dominated the 1990s.

Simultaneously, growth also occurred in another segment of society. The medically underserved portion of the population expanded.

Another focus of change was the building of primary care services. Efforts were made to reverse the ratio of primary care to specialty physicians and to create a majority of primary care providers. With government funding supporting this change, primary care became the watchword of many health care professions. Competition between professions for the primary care niche increased.

By the 1990s, the PA profession enjoyed high demand, and salaries rose. Early in the decade, the number of positions available for PAs significantly outdistanced the supply. The variety of positions also continued to increase as health care delivery underwent dramatic developments. National publications pointed to PA as a hot career that would not cool down for years to come.[4]

Although early in the decade the number of clinical positions available for PAs was reportedly high nationwide, by the mid- and late 1990s, the situation seemed less clear. Rapid changes in health care delivery seemed to be simultaneously creating surpluses and shortages of positions on a regional or local basis.

Education

Expansion, proliferation, and growth were the hallmarks of PA education in the 1990s. Never had change been so dramatic for PA education. Although slow to respond to the increasing demand for PA jobs in the late 1980s, universities expanded programs in the 1990s. The decade began with 51 accredited PA programs[5]; by 1999, there were 120.[6] Established programs also increased capacity. The average number of applicants per program was fairly stable at 85 to 100 from 1984 through 1989. The number rose dramatically between 1990 and 1995, peaking at about 420, then fell steadily to a low of about 240 by the end of the decade. During this period, the average number of students enrolled per annual class per program rose from 24 (1984) to a high of 43 (1995 & 1998), then dropped off to 39 by 1999.[6] Between 1983 and 1999, the percentage of minority students increased from 13.8% to 22%. In 1995, there were 9.8 applicants on average for each student enrolled.[7] By 1999, the ratio was reduced to 5.6:1.[6]

This rapid growth in educational programs was not restricted to PAs. Nurse practitioner programs also expanded. Simultaneously, community-based medical education, pioneered for more than 20 years by PA educators, was recognized as an effective method of increasing the distribution of graduates to rural and underserved areas. Success is not always a plus. Government funding incentives requiring that students of health professions perform some of their clinical education in underserved areas created competition among programs and between professions for community-based clinical education sites.

Growth created significant problems for PA education in the 1990s, but problems of success. Not the least was the challenge of maintaining the quality of education in the face of significant shortages of program faculty and leadership. Competition between programs, new roles for PAs, and proportionately diminishing government support also occurred. These seemingly negative forces were more than offset by new energy and initiatives to meet the challenges and by an influx of new educators bringing fresh ideas, new skills, and an enthusiastic spirit. Individually and collectively, programs responded with a number of initiatives, including the following examples:

➤ Faculty recruitment was addressed jointly by the APAP and the AAPA through presentations at the national spring meetings. These informational and skill-building sessions were aimed at getting practicing PAs involved on a part-time or full-time basis with local PA programs.

➤ Faculty/staff development projects enhanced the skills of clinical PAs coming into programs as clinical coordinators and classroom teachers. Other projects focused on assisting faculty members to develop the research skills needed in their positions. These efforts included sessions at national meetings, independent workshops of several days' duration sponsored by APAP with support from the federal government, and other projects mounted by groups of educators.

➤ With support from the federal government, APAP conducted studies on the recruitment and retention of minority faculty.

➤ Leadership development also included annual independent workshops, as well as sessions at national meetings.

➤ Excellence in education was addressed through a set of services called PATH (Program Assistance and Technical Help) offered by APAP. Services included confidential consultation, annual national workshops, and publication of written materials.

➤ Networking, perhaps the most valuable tool for educators, was fostered by APAP and aided by new communication technologies.

➤ Educators created an annual, comprehensive, self-assessment examination (PACKRAT) to provide both students and programs with indicators of the educational preparation of students.

➤ The Accreditation and Review Committee on Education for the Physician Assistant revised the standards for PA educational programs.[8] The committee also spearheaded a process for reviewing developing programs prior to admission of students. This provided a level of quality assurance to the initial students.

➤ The National Commission on Certification of Physician Assistants modified the certification examination for those entering the profession.

➤ AAPA with the support of APAP initiated a major project to explore the changing roles of PAs by comparing what students were taught with what PAs did in practice. The project was intended to lead to refinements in both entry-level and continuing education for PAs.

➤ The number of new programs offering a master's degree, coupled with the addition of older programs converting to a master's degree, continued to drive the discussion about establishing an entry-level degree.

It is clear from this brief list that PA education responded vigorously to the challenges presented in the dynamic decade of the 1990s.

Educators

The growth of PA education saw the incorporation of many new people. Doubling the number of programs stressed the pool of available talent for faculty positions. This stimulated institutions to broaden the faculty by including non-PAs with more diverse backgrounds. The increase in diversity strengthened the education offered. Programs also used a greater number of clinically based PAs as guest lecturers, mentors, and preceptors, thus reducing the need for full-time PA faculty.

Students

Larger applicant pools in the beginning of the decade caused increased competition for admission. Although presumably this led to students who were better qualified, it is too early to determine whether it resulted in PAs who practice better. Case Study 2-2 provides examples of PA students in the 1990s.

CASE STUDY 2-2

Lisa first heard about the PA profession in high school, when her older brother, Curtis, became a PA. He lived at home while attending school, so Lisa met his classmates and heard stories about his rotations. When Curtis got a job in a local hospital emergency department, he encouraged Lisa to start volunteering. Lisa continued to volunteer and completed an emergency medical technician (EMT) course while in college. She started college as a pre-med major with the goal of becoming a physician but became discouraged by the competitive attitude of the other pre-med students. She enjoyed her time with the local ambulance squad and dropped out of college after her sophomore year to work full time in prehospital care. After 2 years, Lisa decided to become a PA to work in emergency medicine, but with a broader scope of practice. She applied to several programs and was accepted on the waiting list of one program. She continued working and took additional college courses while applying again. Upon applying for a second time, Lisa was accepted to the PA program that Curtis had completed.

Luis had been a police officer for 15 years before being disabled by a knee injury. While in the police department, he had completed 2 years of college toward a degree in political science. Throughout his police career, Luis had been an active volunteer in a variety of health-related community groups; he had cared for homebound elders and people with the acquired immune deficiency syndrome (AIDS). After completing his rehabilitation, Luis decided to pursue his lifelong interest in medicine. He worked as a security guard at night to support his family while taking science and other prerequisite courses. After 2 years of taking courses and continuing his community service, Luis was accepted into a PA program. His goal upon graduating was to work in primary care in the urban community where he grew up.

Janice was a high school teacher for 4 years and started a peer counseling program at her high school for students with alcohol and drug problems. Through this project, Janice became interested in health care and started volunteering at a residential community center for homeless and runaway teens. She met a PA student who was doing a community service project at the teen home and started to learn about the PA profession. After 2 years of volunteering and taking additional science courses, Janice was accepted at a PA program with the goal of working in adolescent medicine.

David was an emergency department nurse for 5 years. While working alongside PAs and physicians in the emergency department, David realized that he was interested in diagnosing and treating patients and found himself drawn to the PA profession. He admired the competence and compassion of the PAs and decided to apply to PA programs. David's grades in nursing school had been mediocre, although his performance evaluations and recommendations were outstanding. After being rejected once, David took courses on a part-time basis for 2 years to improve his academic credentials and was accepted. Although he had always enjoyed emergency medicine, David's goal was to find a family practice position in which he could follow patients and their families over time and provide continuity of care.

THE 2000s—MOVING FORWARD
Social Forces

As this is written in 2002, the new decade is still young. Most current social forces are continuations of those of the 1990s. New forces such as the September 2001 advent of major terrorist actions on American soil and the national response of a global war on terrorism have not matured to the point of impacting health care and the education of PAs.

Education

There have been, however, three developments in PA education that merit discussion. All have begun to change PA education. One has the potential to change the profession to a greater degree than it has altered education.

First, in May of 2000, the AAPA adopted two resolutions concerning the level of academic degree it thought should characterize PA education.

Standard Professional Degree, 2000-B-16a
The American Academy of Physician Assistants believes that a graduate degree, professional or academic, [should] be awarded by all accredited PA programs to students who successfully complete the program.
Standard Professional Degree, 2000-B-16b
The Speaker communicates to the AAPA and the Accreditation Review Commission for PA Education (ARC-PA) representatives the Academy's desire to make a graduate degree, professional or academic, a requirement represented in the *Standard* (AAPA House of Delegates, May 2000).

In October 2000 at its annual meeting, APAP adopted the following policies:

The Association of Physician Assistant Programs (APAP) recognizes that PA education in accredited programs is conducted at the graduate level and recommends that PA programs grant students a credential reflective of this level of curriculum.
The credential granted should reflect the institutional mission and needs of the local and regional communities served by the program, and maintain the academic integrity of the curriculum and the competency of students. The Association shall . . . assist programs with conversion to granting a graduate credential (*Minutes, APAP Business Meeting, October 26 & 29, 2000, Washington, D.C.*).

Though these actions establish no requirement for PA programs to offer graduate degrees and set no date by which such a requirement would take place, they captured the existing mood of many programs that had or were converting to master's degrees and accelerated the process for many other programs.

In 1987, there were 48 PA educational programs in the United States. Only 4.2% awarded a master's degree. By 1990, the number of programs had risen to 55, and the percentage of programs awarding a master's degree had nearly doubled to 9.1%. By 1995, the number of programs was 80, and the percentage awarding a master's degree had doubled again to 18.75%. By 1999, the percentage had nearly doubled again to 35.83% of the then-120 PA programs. As of 2001, there were 126 PA educational programs in the United States, and 42.86% offered a master's degree.[9,10]

The move to graduate level degrees for entry into the PA profession has many consequences. It affects the qualifications for entrance into programs and the cost of education. This in turn alters the accessibility of PA education to segments of the population. It places the impression of the depth and breadth of PA education on a plane with other professions making similar changes—nurse practitioners, physical therapists, and occupational therapists. It may increase the cost of health care to the consumer as it raises the cost of education.

The second development occurred in 2001, when the APAP introduced a centralized application service for candidates applying for admission to PA programs. Called CASPA, this service, which was used by little more than half the programs in its inaugural year, should make the application process more efficient for applicants. It facilitates application to multiple participating programs. In time, it should provide the first extensive data on the national applicant pool. Analysis of this information should assist individual programs and PA education in general to make wiser decisions about recruitment. These efforts in turn should lead to a more diverse and more talented student body that is better suited to meet future challenges that will face the profession.

The third factor under way in the early part of the decade is a rise in the number of programs and students participating in international placements for clinical rotations as part of the educational process. Though this option has been exercised by a handful of programs and students for many years, recent years have seen increased interest and implementation. Aside from the benefits to the individual students, the visibility this creates for the profession in other countries may rekindle and enhance the episodic efforts of a few PA educators over the years to introduce the concepts of PA education to other countries, especially medically underserved countries. PA programs in other countries would undoubtedly look much different than programs in the United States because they would have to be designed and implemented by natives of those countries to ensure sensitivity to health care culture and needs in those countries. Nevertheless, the basic concepts of intense, high-quality education leading to widespread distribution of primary care–educated clinicians working as team members with physicians and other providers could greatly expand the availability and accessibility of health care in areas with great need.

Educators

The growth of PA education in the 1990s created the need for a significant increase in the number of PA educators. The response to this need brought many PAs from clinical practice into PA education. The challenge of the 2000s will be to retain them in PA education and equip them with the credentials and skills to have rewarding careers as programs move to the graduate level.

THE FUTURE

What will PA education of the 2000s and beyond look like?

Social Forces

The first aspect to investigate is what society will look like. We hear much about the age of technology, rapid communication, the plethora of information available to consumers, medical advancements in prevention and treatment, the maturing of managed care, and more.

Some not-so-startling changes to look forward to include the following:

➤ The Internet will continue to keep patients better informed, and it will allow them to consult with clinicians around the world, independent of their personal providers.
➤ The Internet will create more opportunities for clinicians to educate their patients and the public at large.

➤ Patients will have access to an increasing array of kits for home laboratory tests.

➤ The clinician/patient relationship will change as patients are better informed and have access to better communication with a larger number of clinicians from coast to coast.

➤ Some office visits, especially follow-up visits, will take place via technology, decreasing the need for patients to reside near their clinicians.

➤ Managed care will mature and become more competitive, better balancing quality care and profit.

➤ Population shifts that increase the numbers of people with minority backgrounds, advanced years, and languages other than English will create the need for new skills among clinicians.

➤ Managed care will change the PA profession by narrowing its scope of practice and weakening its unique bond with the physician.

➤ As clinicians from many professions vie for larger shares of the primary care arena, PAs may experience a relative shift toward specialty care as was seen in the 1980s and was reversed in the 1990s. This is a reflection of the breadth and depth of PA education.

➤ PAs working in primary care will continue to serve rural and underserved populations to a greater extent than other professions.

➤ Alternative modalities of medical care will increase in appeal to the public, competing for the primary care arena.

➤ The move to graduate degrees for entry-level PAs will move PA away from its traditional niche of cost-effective care. As PA vacates that claim, other professions will be started or expanded to fill the niche.

All of this and more will probably come to pass for those with the money, societal class, and education to participate. However, if present trends continue, there will also be greater separation within society, that is, a widening gap between the "haves" and the "have nots." Apparently, the number of citizens without access to health care in our country has been increasing during the 1990s and into the 2000s. This will continue unless other forces intervene. If this continues, it will provide challenges and opportunities for

PA, a profession that takes pride in its ability to adapt to new opportunities.

Education

The future for PA education may include the following:

➤ PA education will be exported to other countries, where its methods for intense medical education will be adapted to meet the needs of other cultures.

➤ Programs in the United States will lengthen, as they find it impossible to include more complex technological skills with the already compact medical curricula.

➤ The trend toward requiring a baccalaureate degree for admission to a PA program will decrease the numbers of rural and minority students in programs as the applicant pool falls.

➤ The lengthening of programs and the trend toward awarding master's degrees may lead to the fulfillment of at least one early PA visionary. Namely, medical education may become stepped, so that people with bachelor's, master's, and doctoral degrees may be able to practice at different levels and proceed to the next educational level without going back to step one.

➤ The number of PA programs will peak in the early 2000s and will fall back slightly before restabilizing.

➤ Large health care delivery systems will continue to view the cost of educating physicians, PAs, nurses, and other providers as detrimental to profits. This will pressure the government to reimburse these systems for providing clinical sites for the education of health professionals.

➤ Unfortunately, this may also set up a struggle between universities and health care systems for control of the direction of education of health professionals.

In 1996, APAP hosted a meeting on the future of PA education. Some of the previously mentioned items were drawn from the report of that project.[11] Whether some, all, or none of these opinions come to pass, it is clear that the future will be filled with challenges for the next generation of PA educators. If the past is an indication, it is also apparent that they will face the challenges with creativity, energy, and vision.

Educators and Students

Who will be the educators of PAs in the future? What characteristics will describe them? They will not come from the vision of PA educators of today. Rather, they will be shaped by those currently considering a career in PA education.

CONCLUSION

In the 1960s, it began with a simple concept—people with or without medical experience could be educated to perform many of the tasks previously reserved for physicians; this education could be offered in a format briefer than medical school, and the new graduates would assist overworked physicians and extend services to underserved patients. More than 40 years later, these ideas have led to a nationwide network of about 130 PA programs graduating more than 3000 new clinicians each year. PA education and the PA profession have grown and prospered because they have been responsive to society's need for available, cost-effective, quality medical care. These remain strong needs in society. To continue to prosper, PA must position itself as a leader in solving these problems.

From its infancy to the present, this educational network of programs has continued to provide broad-based medical education that graduates could apply to a wide spectrum of medical areas. PAs provide medical services to all segments of the population while serving primary care and rural and underserved areas in higher percentages than other medical disciplines.

Programs have offered this foundation through innovative curricular designs that rely on collaboration with educators from other disciplines and with community-based clinicians. This collaboration accounts for much of the energy, flexibility, and continuous renewal common to PA education. PA education is presently growing in many ways—more programs, larger programs, more students, new waves of clinicians becoming faculty members, and new curricular elements. There are new challenges from society requiring new responses—an increasing number of medically underserved citizens, a rising population of older citizens, new health care environments such as managed care, and new practice models created by the explosion of communication technologies.

PA education will continue to prosper to the extent that it resists the temptation to become static and to simply provide an educational base for a profession. PA education must look for future direction in the place where it has found direction in the past, namely, in the needs of society. It must continue to dream dreams and see visions. It must actualize the dreams with energy, innovation, and determination.

CLINICAL APPLICATIONS

1. Explore the history of your PA program.
   - ➤ Who were the founders?
   - ➤ What was the founding mission of the program?
   - ➤ If your program was created within the past 5 years, find out the basis and assumptions for the curriculum design (both didactic and clinical). If your program has a long history, find out how the curriculum has changed across time in both the didactic and clinical phases.
2. Interview at least one graduate from your program's first class.
   - ➤ What were that person's motivations for enrolling in the initial class of a new program?
   - ➤ What were the selection criteria for the first class?
   - ➤ What were the barriers to practice and utilization for new graduates?

REFERENCES

1. Selected Training Programs for Physician Support Personnel, U.S. Department of Health, Education and Welfare. Bethesda, MD: National Institutes of Health, 1971.
2. American Medical Association Council on Medical Education. Essentials of an approved educational program for the assistant to the primary care physician. In: Sadler AM, Sadler BL, Bliss AA (eds). The Physician's Assistant Today and Tomorrow. New Haven, CT: Yale University, 1972.
3. Sadler AM, Sadler BL, Bliss AA. The Physician's Assistant Today and Tomorrow. New Haven, CT: Yale University, 1972.
4. Brindley D, Bennefield RM, Danyliw NQ. 20 hot job tracks. US News 1997;123(16):98.
5. Sixth Annual Report on Physician Assistant Education Programs in the United States, 1989-1990. Alexandria, VA: Association of Physician Assistant Programs, 1990.

6. Sixteenth Annual Report on Physician Assistant Educational Programs in the United States, 1999-2000. Alexandria, VA: Association of Physician Assistant Programs, 2000.

7. Twelfth Annual Report on Physician Assistant Educational Programs in the United States, 1995-1996. Alexandria, VA: Association of Physician Assistant Programs, 1996.

8. Commission on Accreditation of Allied Health Education Programs. Standards and Guidelines for an Accredited Educational Program for the Physician Assistant. Marshfield, WI: Accreditation Review Committee on Education for the Physician Assistant, 1997.

9. Fourth, 7th, 12th, 16th, 17th Annual Reports on Physician Assistant Education Programs in the United States. Alexandria, VA: Association of Physician Assistant Programs.

10. 2001 Physician Assistant Programs Directory. Alexandria, VA: Association of Physician Assistant Programs.

11. Miller AA. Proceedings: Defining the Future Characteristics of Physician Assistant Education. Alexandria, VA: Association of Physician Assistant Programs, 1996.

RESOURCES

Association of Physician Assistant Programs. Annual Report on Physician Assistant Educational Programs in the United States, 1984-1985 through 1996-1997. Alexandria, VA: APAP. *The Association of Physician Assistant Programs annually surveys its member programs on a wide range of characteristics of PA education. These include financial resources and costs, personnel, applicant and student characteristics, and information on graduates. Periodically and most recently in the 1994-1995 edition, the report includes information on the curricula of PA programs.*

U.S. Department of Health and Human Services, Public Health Service, Health Resources and Services Administration, Bureau of Health Professions, Division of Medicine, Special Projects and Data Branch. Physician Assistants in the Health Workforce 1994: Final Report of the Advisory Group on Physician Assistants and the Workforce, Council on Graduate Medical Education. Washington, DC: Health Resources and Services Administration. *This report examines the place of the physician assistant in the nation's force of health care workers. It comments on the economic aspects of using PAs and attempts to project the future need for PAs.*

Association of Physician Assistant Programs. Physician Assistant Programs Directory. Alexandria, VA: APAP. *This annual publication profiles each of the PA educational programs in the nation. It provides information on characteristics particular to each program, the cost of education, entrance requirements, the curriculum, and credentials awarded.*

Association of Physician Assistant Programs. Physician Assistants for the Future: An In-Depth Study of PA Education and Practice in the Year 2000. Alexandria, VA: APAP. *Written in 1989, this study sought to envision the status of PA education in the year 2000. Many of its recommendations have proved to be pertinent.*

CHAPTER 3

Credentialing: Accreditation, Certification, and Licensing

Donald M. Pedersen

INTRODUCTION

Credentialing is a process that gives a title or credit showing that a person is entitled to, or has a right to exercise, official power. Credentialing affects PA students initially while they are enrolled in their programs of education, and subsequently when they are graduates entering the health care marketplace. The right to exercise the official power identified in the definition of credentialing is a significant responsibility that must be understood and accepted by both PA students and the institutions charged with educating them. This chapter discusses two separate and distinct credentialing procedures: the credentialing of PA programs and the credentialing of individual PAs on the state and national levels.

PROGRAM CREDENTIALING

The process of credentialing PA programs takes the form of accreditation, which is defined as putting into

a reputable category, vouching for as in conformity with a standard, recognizing as maintaining standards that qualify the graduates for professional practice, and providing with credentials. PAs have made remarkable professional growth that belies the relatively short history (35 years) of the profession. In terms of acceptance and privilege to practice, the accreditation process by which PA programs are evaluated is fundamental to the profession's success.

Accreditation Review Commission on Education of the Physician Assistant (ARC-PA)

On January 1, 2002, the Accreditation Review *Committee* on Education for the Physician Assistant became the Accreditation Review *Commission* on Education for the Physician Assistant. This was a small name change but a monumental step forward as this organization became a freestanding accrediting agency for the evaluation and accreditation of physician assistant educational programs in the United States. Table 3-1 contains a chronological timeline of events leading up to this most recent process change. The ARC-PA is now the sole authority for PA program accreditation, no longer needing to rely on a third party. The goals of the ARC-PA are as follows:

➤ To foster excellence in PA education through the development of uniform national standards for assessing educational effectiveness.

➤ To foster excellence in PA programs by requiring continuous self-study and review.

➤ To assure the public as well as professional, educational, and licensing agencies and organizations that accredited programs have met defined educational standards for preparing PAs for practice.

➤ To provide information and guidance to individuals, groups, and organizations regarding PA program accreditation.

The predecessor to the accreditation review commission on education for the physician assistant was the Commission on Accreditation of Allied Health Education Programs (CAAHEP), which was incorporated in June of 1994 and was a national, voluntary, specialized accreditation agency. CAAHEP was independent of any single professional organization or agency and represented a broad range of health care disciplines. CAAHEP was recognized by the Commission on Recognition of Postsecondary Accreditation and by the U.S. Department of Education. CAAHEP represented the present-day expression of the American Medical Association's (AMA's) long history of collaboration and leadership in education and accreditation.

The predecessor to CAAHEP was the Committee on Allied Health Education and Accreditation (CAHEA), which was organized in 1977. Through its long and successful history, CAHEA accredited programs in some 26 allied health occupational areas. During its sponsorship of CAHEA, the AMA collaborated with more than 50 national allied health professional organizations and medical specialty societies having interests in allied health education.

While operational, CAHEA and its affiliates constituted the largest accrediting consortium in the United States, both in the number of professional organizations involved and in the number of programs accredited.[1] In 1992, CAHEA had 20 review committees evaluating approximately 2800 accredited programs in more than 1500 institutions of higher learning. General public and governmental acceptance of the CAHEA system was evidenced by the fact that federal agencies and nongovernmental foundations used the lists of CAHEA-accredited programs to determine eligibility for special institutional grants, student grants, and other financial aid awards. The Council on Postsecondary Accreditation and the U.S. Department of Education recognized CAHEA as *the* accreditation agency for physician assistant programs.[2]

Although accreditation of physician assistant programs no longer takes place under the auspices of the AMA, the same standards of excellence and operating procedures remain intact under the ARC-PA umbrella.

The ARC-PA accreditation review process for the physician assistant is driven by a set of generic guidelines, or *Standards,* that guide programs in developing and maintaining acceptable quality in their educational offerings. Endorsed by a broad consensus within the medical community, the *Standards* represent current, nationally accepted guidelines for all aspects of program operation. The process reviews curriculum and instructional objectives, classroom laboratory and library facilities, clinical affiliations, faculty qualifications, admissions processes, student issues, fiscal stability, program publications, record-keeping systems, and administration. Programs must provide evidence of an ongoing critical self-study process and must undergo an on-site evaluation. Graduation from an ARC-PA–accredited program benefits students by providing the following:

1. Assurance that the program meets nationally accepted standards.

2. Recognition of their education by their professional peers.

3. Eligibility for professional certification, registration, and state licensure.

The ARC-PA specifically monitors the accreditation status of physician assistant programs, conducts on-site visits to sponsoring institutions, and determines programs' compliance with the *Standards.* Composed of representatives from the American

Table 3-1 Chronological Timeline for Accreditation of Physician Assistants	
Date	**Action**
May 28, 1971	The development of the *Essentials of an Accredited Educational Program for the Assistant to the Primary Care Physician* was undertaken by the American Medical Association (AMA) subcommittee of the Council on Medical Education's Advisory Committee on Education for Allied Health Professions and Services. The subcommittee included representatives from the American Academy of Family Physicians (AAFP), American Academy of Pediatrics (AAP), American College of Physicians (ACP), American Society of Internal Medicine (ASIM), American Medical Association (AMA), and Association of American Medical Colleges (AAMC). The *Essentials* prepared by the subcommittee were approved by those organizations, except for the AAMC, which declined to approve or endorse the *Essentials*.
November 30, 1971	The AMA House of Delegates, with the endorsements noted and on recommendation of the Committee on Medical Education, adopted the *Essentials,* clearing the way for the approval of educational programs that met or exceeded *Essential* requirements.
December 18, 1971	Organizational meeting of the then-titled "Joint Review Committee for Educational Programs for the Assistant to Primary Care Physician" (JRC-PA).
February 7, 1972	The first formal meeting of the JRC-PA was convened. Dr. Malcolm L. Peterson, representative of the American College of Physicians, was elected the first Chairman of the JRC-PA.
June 1972	The JRC-PA made its first accreditation recommendations.
1973	American College of Surgeons (ACS) adopted *Essentials for an Educational Program for the Surgeon's Assistant.* Originally, the ACS Committee on Allied Health Personnel reviewed applicant programs' compliance with the *Essentials.* In April, the JRC-PA appointed three graduate PAs to serve as members-at-large for 1-year terms.
March 1974	The sponsors of the JRC-PA and the AMA recognized the American Academy of Physician Assistants (AAPA) as the fifth sponsor of the review committee.
September 1975	The ACS became part of the JRC-PA.
1976	The review committees for the Assistant to the Primary Care Physician and the Surgeon's Assistant were merged.
December 1976	The AMA House of Delegates voted to delegate its responsibility for adoption of proposed *Educational Standards (Essentials)* to the AMA Council on Medical Education and authorized the transfer of responsibility for accreditation from the AMA Council on Medical Education to its Committee on Allied Health Education Accreditation (CAHEA). This new committee was a modification of the council's former Advisory Committee on allied Health Education. These changes were instituted to effect complete compliance with the U.S. Office of Education Criteria for National Accrediting Agencies. CAHEA was designed to represent communities of interest for which accreditation actions were taken. The committee was composed of representatives of allied health professions, medicine, continuing medical education (CME), and the public.
1978	JRC-PA sponsors recognized the Association of Physician Assistant Programs (APAP) as the seventh sponsor to the committee.
December 1981	The ASIM withdrew its sponsorship of the JRC-PA.
September 1982	The sponsoring organizations reduced their representation from three to two members for each of the sponsors, except for the American Academy of Physician Assistants, which remained at three representatives.

Table 3-1	Chronological Timeline for Accreditation of Physician Assistants—cont'd
Date	**Action**
1988	The committee was renamed the Accreditation Review Committee on Education for the Physician Assistant (ARC-PA).
March 1991	The AMA requested the transfer of the administrative responsibility for the ARC-PA to another sponsoring organization of the committee.
September 1991	The AAPA accepted transfer of administrative responsibility. The corporate offices of the ARC-PA were established in Marshfield, Wisconsin.
1994	CAHEA was dissolved and accreditation activities were transferred to a new, independent agency—the Commission on Accreditation of Allied Health Education Programs (CAAHEP).
March 1995	The ARC-PA approved the addition of a third representative from the APAP.
September 1995	The ARC-PA was incorporated.
March 1996	A study was initiated to determine the feasibility of withdrawal of ARC-PA from the CAAHEP system and establishment of a freestanding accrediting agency.
March 2000	The members of the ARC-PA voted to "become a freestanding accrediting agency for the PA profession" with the implementation date of January 1, 2001.
January 1, 2001	The Accreditation Review Commission on Education for the Physician Assistant (ARC-PA) began operations.

From McCarthy John, Stuetzer Laura, Somers James. Perspective on Physician Assistant Education, Vol. 12. No. 1, Winter 2001, page 25.

Academy of Family Physicians, the American Academy of Pediatrics, the American Academy of Physician Assistants (AAPA), the American College of Surgeons, the American College of Physicians, and the Association of Physician Assistant Programs (APAP), the ARC-PA makes formal accreditation decisions. The extent to which a program complies with the *Standards* determines its accreditation status. The *Standards* therefore constitute the minimum requirements an accredited program must meet. Learning experiences and curriculum sequences in basic and clinical medical education must provide program graduates with the necessary knowledge and skills to perform accurately and reliably the functions described in and implied by the "Description of the Profession" in the ARC-PA *Standards.*[3]

As delineated in the *Standards,* the PA is academically and clinically prepared to provide health care services with the direction and responsible supervision of a doctor of medicine or osteopathy. Within the physician/PA relationship, physician assistants make clinical decisions and provide a broad range of diag-

nostic, therapeutic, preventive, and health maintenance services. The clinical role of physician assistants includes primary and specialty care in medical and surgical practice settings. Physician assistant practice is centered on patient care and may include educational, research, and administrative activities.

The role of the PA demands intelligence, sound judgment, intellectual honesty, appropriate interpersonal skills, and the capacity to react to emergencies in a calm and reasoned manner. An attitude of respect for self and others, adherence to the concepts of privilege and confidentiality in communicating with patients, and a commitment to the welfare of patients are essential attributes.

The specific tasks performed by individual physician assistants cannot be delineated precisely because of the variations in practice requirements mandated by geographic, political, economic, and social factors. At a minimum, however, PAs are educated in areas of basic medical science, clinical disciplines, and discipline-specific problem solving. Physician assistant practice is characterized by clinical knowledge and skills in areas traditionally defined by family medicine, internal medicine, pediatrics, obstetrics, gynecology, surgery, and psychiatry/behavioral medicine. Physician assistants practice in ambulatory, emergency, inpatient, and long-term care settings. Physician assistants deliver health care services to diverse patient populations of all ages with a range of acute and chronic medical and surgical conditions. They need knowledge and skills that allow them to function effectively in a dynamic health care environment.

Services performed by PAs while they practice with physician supervision include, but are not limited to, the following:

➤ **Evaluation.** Elicit a detailed and accurate history; perform an appropriate physical examination; order, perform, and interpret appropriate diagnostic studies; delineate problems; develop management plans; and record and present data.

➤ **Monitoring.** Implement patient management plans, record progress notes, and participate in the provision of continuity of care.

➤ **Therapy.** Perform therapeutic procedures and manage or assist in the management of medical and surgical conditions, which may include assisting surgeons in the conduct of operations and taking initiative in performing evaluative and therapeutic procedures in response to life-threatening situations.

➤ **Patient education.** Counsel patients regarding issues of health care management, including compliance with prescribed therapeutic regimens, normal growth and development, family planning, and emotional problems of daily living.

➤ **Referral.** Facilitate the referral of patients to other health care providers or agencies as appropriate.[3]

Once ARC-PA accreditation is granted, periodic reviews and on-site evaluations by an accreditation team are required for maintenance of accreditation. The ARC-PA meets semiannually to consider applications for provisional, initial, and continuing accreditation. The educational process is improved frequently as programs make modifications to maintain or exceed the accreditation *Standards* or to build upon insights gained from an on-site evaluation.

In summary, the process of accreditation by the ARC-PA involves four steps:

1. **Application for accreditation.** The chief executive officer of the sponsoring institution submits to CAAHEP an application for accreditation.
2. **Self-analysis.** The program members complete a self-analysis and submit a self-study report to the ARC-PA. The report examines the program's sponsorship, curriculum, resources, and operational and student policies and practices.
3. **On-site review.** A volunteer team of individuals knowledgeable about the education and practice of PAs reviews the program on site.
4. **Review committee evaluation.** After consideration of the application, the self-study report, and the report of the on-site review, the ARC-PA formulates an accreditation decision.

A formal notice of accreditation status is sent to the chief executive officer of the institution and to the program director.

Further information on PA program accreditation can be obtained by contacting ARC-PA, 100 North Oak Avenue, Marshfield, WI 54449-5788, (715)389-3785.

Association of Physician Assistant Programs

Although not a credentialing body, the Association of Physician Assistant Programs (APAP) is involved in continuing quality control of the educational experience for physician assistant students. APAP was founded in 1972 by a group of concerned program faculty who saw a need to address the important issues of accreditation, certification, continuing education, role delineation for PAs, and the overall goal of improving the quality and accessibility of health care through the selection, education, and deployment of PAs.[4] In 1973, APAP established a national office with the AAPA in Washington, D.C. Currently, APAP continues to share a national headquarters and staff with the AAPA in Alexandria, Virginia.

Throughout the United States, more than 130 ARC-PA–accredited programs are members of APAP. The mission of APAP is to assist physician assistant educational programs in the instruction of highly educated PAs in numbers adequate to meet society's needs. The specific goals of the organization are as follows:

➤ To foster faculty development.

➤ To promote excellence within PA programs.

➤ To facilitate research and scholarly activities.

➤ To advocate for PA education.

➤ To maintain and sustain the organization.

APAP ensures quality PA education through the development and distribution of educational services and products specifically geared toward meeting the emerging needs of PA programs. This provision of quality physician assistant education strengthens the PA profession, the health care industry, and ultimately, the care provided to patients.

APAP's Board of Directors is elected by its member programs, and individuals from member programs make up committees assigned to specific activities. The association participates in the activities of the ARC-PA through the appointment of a faculty representative to the ARC-PA Commissioners. Additionally, collaboration with and representation on the ARC-PA give APAP the privilege to affect the policies and procedures. APAP also enjoys representation on the National Commission on Certification of Physician Assistants (NCCPA), the body that administers the PA National Certifying Examination and National Re-certifying Examination.

The organization's monthly publication, *APAP Update,* reports on issues of importance to PA program faculty and affiliated agencies, including legislation, educational technology, professional news, and faculty employment opportunities. In conjunction with Saint Francis University PA Program in Loretto, PA, APAP publishes the *Annual Report on Physician Assistant Educational Programs in the United States,* which contains information on faculty, programs, student characteristics, practice specialties and settings, and geographic distribution of PA graduates. APAP also generated *Physician Assistants for the Future,* an in-depth study conducted in the mid-1980s that projected PA education practice in the year 2000. It included a vision statement that describes the future PA and provides recommendations for programs for use in formulating future educational plans. Supported by a grant from the Health Resources and Services Administration, APAP revisited this theme

and produced the 1996 document, *Defining the Future Characteristics of Physician Assistant Education.* A panel of experts as well as multiple focus groups explored the future of PA education, and recommendations were offered for use by PA program faculty and others.

Each year, APAP publishes the *Physician Assistant Programs Directory,*[4] which provides information on individual association member programs for potential students, guidance counselors, teachers, and librarians. APAP's research priorities are evaluating the functional performance of physician assistants, learning which curriculum efforts are effective, and studying the various health care delivery systems in which PAs work most efficiently. The research results are published and provided to federal officials and funding agencies interested in PAs. Research results also help member programs to evaluate and refine their curricula so that they can continue to provide quality education to their students.[4]

To facilitate the research goals of the APAP, the organization created the APAP Research Institute in 1996, with the purpose of coordinating an endowed Research Grants Program. The APAP Research Endowment Fund awards APAP member faculty multiple small grants on an annual basis for research related to physician assistant education. In 1997, the first three grant awards were made for $5000 each and addressed the following topics:

1. A survey to assess medical market demand for PA program graduates.

2. An analysis of PA postgraduate residency training in the United States.

3. PA preparation for patient education.

In conjunction with the University of Utah PA Program, APAP also publishes a peer-reviewed journal, *Perspective on Physician Assistant Education,* as part of its Research Institute activities.

Another important area of interest for APAP has been faculty development. APAP is conducting several ongoing activities to promote the development of PA program faculty. In 1996, APAP was awarded a federal PA Workforce and Faculty Development contract, funded by the Bureau of Health Professions, Health Resources and Services Administration, U.S. Department of Health and Human Services. Part of this contract provided for intensive faculty development in the areas of basic faculty skills, senior faculty skills, and minority issues. Also in 1996, APAP held its third annual Leadership Training Institute. This faculty development initiative was also funded by the Bureau of Health Professions. During APAP's two national conferences, in May and October of each year, additional educational sessions are offered for faculty functioning at all levels, including administrators, junior and senior faculty, and clinical coordinators (see Box).

FACULTY ROLES

Although students frequently see PA program faculty members as primarily involved with their specific program's educational activities, most faculty members also have major investments in state and national PA educational activities. All these activities are viewed not only as opportunities to represent the program but also as personal growth and networking opportunities for the individual faculty member. Typical volunteer assignments and activities of PA program faculty members might include the following:

- Site visitor or evaluator for the Accreditation Review Committee.
- Test item writer for the NCCPA test item committees for the PANCE or re-certification examination.
- Test item writer for the APAP PACKRAT project.
- Elected officer, committee chair, or committee member for APAP activities.
- Member of the Accreditation Review Committee.
- Grant reviewer for the division of medicine (PA training grants or other federal primary care initiatives).
- Elected officer, committee chair, committee member, or House of Delegates representative for state PA academies.
- Nationally elected AAPA officer or appointee to councils, committees, or task forces.
- Special appointments to federal and state councils and boards.

These activities are developed and coordinated by the APAP Faculty Development Institute. Two self-assessing examinations have been initiated by APAP: the Physician Assistant Clinical Knowledge and Assessment Tool (PACKRAT) and the Graduate Rating and Assessment Tool (GRADRAT). PACKRAT is a self-assessment examination designed and developed to assess PA student clinical knowledge and to identify areas of strength and weakness. In its first year, the examination was distributed to more than 1500 PA students nationwide. GRADRAT is also a self-assessment examination designed for the practicing PA. Another member service is the Program Assistance and Technical Help (PATH) program. PATH is a confidential consultation service designed to assist established and developing programs in achieving and maintaining quality in PA education. Trained, experienced consultants provide a variety of services ranging from national workshops to general consultations, as well as more focused consultations that deal with a single issue. For further information, contact APAP, 950 N. Washington Street, Alexandria, VA 22314, (703)836-2272.

GRADUATE CREDENTIALING

Credentialing of graduate PAs has two components, both of which the new PA must understand in order to obtain the right to practice:

1. A national system of certification available to graduates of ARC-PA–accredited programs.
2. A myriad of individual state credentialing procedures.

National Certification and Re-certification

In contrast to accreditation, a process applied to educational programs, certification is a process involving individuals. Typically, certification involves a nongovernmental agency or association that grants recognition to an individual who has met certain predetermined qualifications specified by that agency or association. In 1971, the AMA House of Delegates directed its Council on Health Manpower to assume a leadership role in sponsoring a national program for certification of the Assistant to the Primary Care Physician. National certification was favored to give

PAs geographic mobility, provide the physician employer with some evidence of employment transitions competency, and permit greater flexibility in employment transition.[5]

National Board of Medical Examiners

Following endorsement by the Federation of State Medical Boards, the AMA's Council of Health Manpower and the National Board of Medical Examiners (NBME) began a collaborative effort to develop a national certification process for PAs. The NBME, with its long history of evaluating the competency of medical providers, was a logical choice for the task, and in 1972, it accepted responsibility for developing a national certifying examination. The Physician Assistant National Certifying Examination was developed to ensure that individuals achieved minimum standards of proficiency in primary health care delivery. The examination was administered in 1973 and 1974 by the NBME. Subsequent annual examinations have been administered by the NCCPA.

National Commission on Certification of Physician Assistants

The NCCPA was established in 1974 by the federal government, the AMA, and various medical specialty groups. The board of directors of the NCCPA includes representation from the following organizations: American Academy of Family Physicians, American Academy of Pediatrics, American Academy of Physician Assistants, American College of Physicians, American Society of Internal Medicine, American College of Surgeons, American Hospital Association, American Osteopathic Association, American Medical Association, Association of American Medical Colleges, Association of Physician Assistant Programs, Federation of State Medical Boards of the United States, National Medical Association, and U.S. Department of Defense.

The NCCPA has responsibility for the following functions[5]:

➤ Determining eligibility criteria for the entry-level examination.
➤ Reviewing applications to take the examination, then registering candidates.

➤ Administering the examination under contract to the NBME.
➤ Determining the standards for the entry-level examination.
➤ Issuing and verifying certificates.
➤ Re-certifying physician assistants through periodic administration of an examination.
➤ Publishing lists, by state, of physician assistants certified each year.
➤ Serving as a resource to assist state medical boards, at their request, in establishing and modifying physician assistant legislation, rules, and regulations as they pertain to national certification.
➤ Conducting research activities to disseminate information regarding the physician assistant's responsibilities to the government, professional organizations, the general public, and others.

This list of responsibilities grew out of the two tasks with which the NCCPA was charged. First, it was to certify and re-certify people who would be called physician assistants to assure the public that the quality of practitioners met a national standard. Second, the NCCPA needed to ensure the relevance of the examination to the practice engaged in by the physician assistant.[2]

A system of mandated continuing medical education (CME) to maintain national certification began in 1975. Those certified are required to log 100 hours of CME every 2 years. The use of the designation "C" (for "certified") after the initials "PA" indicates that the individual so designated has taken and passed the initial examination and adheres to the CME requirement set forth by the NCCPA. The title "PA-C" is a registered service mark, and its use is strictly limited to individuals who have met the listed requirements. For further information regarding any NCCPA activities, contact NCCPA, 6849-B2 Peachtree Dunwoody Road NE, Atlanta, GA 30328-1610, (707)399-9971.

Examinations

Initially, the annual certifying examinations had a primary care orientation and included a multiple-choice question component, a patient management problems component, and a clinical skills component. The patient management problems were discontinued in

1990, and the clinical skills portion, which allowed for direct observation of the examinee's physical examination technique and decision-making skills, was discontinued in 1997.

Currently, the Physician Assistant National Certifying Examination (PANCE) is administered multiple times throughout the year and consists of 360 multiple-choice questions. The examination is administered by computer and consists of three test sections of 120 questions each. Examinees are allotted 2 hours for each session, for a total of 6 hours of testing time. The present cost of the examination is $425. The historic surgery specialty examination is no longer one of the PANCE requirements. It has become a separate special recognition examination and is administered in a testing session near the PANCE testing. This special recognition examination consists of 180 multiple-choice questions. Both examinations are administered through Prometric (Sylvan) Testing Centers throughout the United States.

In response to actions approved by the NCCPA Board of Directors in late 1995 and early 1996, a Content-Based Standard Steering Committee was created and charged with establishing pass/fail standards for the NCCPA examination that are based on the content and difficulty of questions contained in the examination forms, rather than on the relative performance of other candidates. Historically, passing standards for NCCPA examination have been normative (grading on the curve). As of the 1997 scoring of the PANCE, examiners used a criterion-referenced passing-point strategy. This content-based strategy is characterized by the selection of an absolute standard; for example, if 50% of examinees meet that standard, then 50% will pass, or if 100% of examinees meet the standard, then 100% will pass.[6]

Since 1985, only those individuals graduating from a program accredited by CAHEA or its successors, CAAHEP and ARC-PA, are eligible to sit for the examination. Before 1985, however, the examination was also open to informally trained individuals and nurse practitioners. For this reason, individuals who have previously taken this examination are eligible to re-register to sit for it again.

Maintaining certification with the NCCPA is an ongoing process, beginning with successful completion of the PANCE and continuing throughout a career with the periodic passage of a re-certifying examination and the logging of CME credits. Individuals who pass the PANCE receive a time-limited NCCPA certificate, valid for 2 years. To maintain certification beyond the initial expiration date, a PA is required to reregister every 2 years and document 100 hours of CME. In addition, as a part of the process, the PA is required to take a re-certifying examination every 6 years. The Physician Assistant National Re-certifying Examination (PANRE) is administered once a year by the NCCPA in the spring.[6] Case Study 3-1 presents the dilemma of several PAs concerning certification and re-certification.

CASE STUDY 3-1

The following situations reflect some of the difficult issues facing practicing PAs concerning certification and re-certification.

Richard has just received notification that he did not pass his entry-level NCCPA examination. Fortunately, his state's temporary licensure provision gives him two additional chances to pass the exam because it is now given multiple times a year. Richard is struggling with the decision of when to retake the exam. If he takes the exam sooner (which would still give him the opportunity to retake it one more time), he might pass, but he also feels he will be less well prepared. If he waits until the second administration of the exam, he feels he will be better prepared, but he won't have another chance.

Susan is not planning to practice for several years, during which time she plans two pregnancies. During this family time, she would normally be scheduled for her second re-certification exam. The state in which she practices requires successful completion of the re-certification exam as well as documentation of CME hours. Susan is concerned that she will not do well on the exam because she will not be practicing; however, she does not want to retake the entry-level exam in order to return to practice. What should she do?

James is a physician assistant in a midwestern state who has been practicing for 23 years and is now preparing to take his third NCCPA re-certification exam. Although he worked in primary care for 19 years, he is now working in the subspecialty of pediatric neurology. The state in which he practices does not require the re-certification exam, although it does require documentation of CME. If he chooses not to take the re-certification exam, he will no longer be able to use the title "PA-C" after his name. He is uncertain what to do.

Alternative Pathway to Re-certification

A consensus about the need for the re-certification examination has never developed among physician assistants. Many PAs become quite specialized after 6 years of practice, and some believe that the primary care focus of the re-certification examination is an inaccurate measure of ongoing clinical competence in their practice area.[2] This dilemma has led to a cooperative agreement between the NCCPA and the AAPA about developing a pathway for continued certification that would circumvent the national re-certification examination. Currently, a Pathway II exists for re-certification. Established in 1998, Pathway II looks at a combination of activities: continuing medical education, formal coursework, teaching, and a self-assessment test. These activities have variable numbers of possible points attached to them, and the individual desiring to adopt this approach to continued certification needs to garner a specified number of points within a certain time frame to remain current. Academy leaders are hopeful that Pathway II will become a valid process that will resolve many of the controversial issues surrounding re-certification.[7]

At the core of these re-certification requirements are the goals established by the NCCPA to implement a system that encourages continued scholarship among PAs, and to assure the public that there is a standard with which to measure clinical skills and current medical concepts within the physician assistant profession. In the past, PAs who were not successful in completing a re-certifying examination received an updated certificate that was valid for 2 additional years and were required to attempt to pass an examination again within those 2 years. Beginning in 1998, with the implementation of an end point, these interim allowances are no longer permitted, and PAs are required to log CME hours and re-register within an established period of time. Furthermore, PAs are required to pass one of the two available re-certifying examinations, either the PANRE or the examination that is part of the Pathway II program. These revised requirements must be met in order for a PA to maintain national certification from the NCCPA.

State Credentialing

Greater recognition of physician assistants as health care providers has led to the development of state laws and regulations governing their practice. Recognition of PAs in state law and delegation of authority to a state regulatory body that oversees their practice serve two main purposes: to protect the public from incompetent performance by unqualified nonphysicians, and to promote appropriate expanded delegation within the scope of PA practice by assuring consumers, physicians, and others that PAs are competent.[8] In the late 1960s and early 1970s, while the PA concept was beginning to blossom, there was pervasive dissatisfaction with the prevailing method of credentialing health professionals. Sadler and colleagues[5] summed up the mood of the time:

> *"At a time when the entire licensure scheme for regulating health personnel is under widespread attack as being archaic, inefficient, and destructive of change, a variety of delegation amendments to state medical practice acts have been enacted as a direct result of the physician assistant movement."*

Through their willingness to remain legally dependent, to accept delegation from physicians, and to work under the supervision and control of the physician, PAs are able to function under broad and flexible legal umbrellas that allow them to perform to their capacity.[5]

During that time, a patchwork of approaches was initiated, and many states put forth amendments to state medical practice acts that allowed for the delegation of tasks by the physician to an assistant. Such initial amendments typically consisted of a brief paragraph allowing PAs to function. Most states also identified an agency that would assume the responsibility for regulation of this fledgling profession.

Despite the flexibility of the delegation amendments, it became increasingly clear to many state regulatory agencies that they were inadequate to deal with the tremendous growth in responsibility of the PA profession. Today, most states realize the need to reexamine the definition of the scope of physician assistant practice, and most recognize that PAs must engage in clinical decision making in order to practice effectively. As they rework legislation relative to physician assistant practice, some states continue to register PAs, thus giving rise to the designation "RPA-C" (the "R" indicating registration in the particular state), whereas other states have adopted licensure laws to govern PAs.

Statutory authority to promulgate rules and regulations to accompany such laws is typically given to an agency, such as a state medical board. Through the Administrative Rule Making Act, the rules and regulations that are developed, although easier to change than statutes, carry the same weight as laws. State statutes, rules, and regulations are as varied as the states they represent. Whatever the arrangement, the two most consistent criteria for practice in a particular state remain successful completion of the NCCPA national certifying examination and graduation from an ARC-PA–accredited physician assistant training program.

Physician assistants are playing an ever-increasing role in the regulation of their own profession. Eight states have regulatory bodies strictly for PAs (Arizona, California, Iowa, Massachusetts, Michigan, Rhode Island, Tennessee, and Utah). Approximately 25 state medical boards have PA committees. Some of the committees are advisory, but others have significant responsibilities in rule making, review of applications, and discipline. There are seats for physician assistants on 11 other medical, osteopathic, or disciplinary boards.[8] The AAPA strongly endorses the authority of designated state regulatory agencies in accordance with due process to discipline PAs who have committed acts in violation of state law. Disciplinary actions include, but are not limited to, suspension and revocation of an individual's license or certificate of registration. The Academy also endorses the sharing of information among the state regulatory agencies regarding the disposition of adjudicated actions against physician assistants.[8]

Registration

In most states where PAs are registered, issues related to PA practice are addressed either by a subcommittee to a state medical board that has been formed to deal with physician assistant practice, or by a state medical board that includes a seat (or seats) for PA representation. The medical board most often functions in an advisory capacity to a state governmental agency, such as a department of commerce or department of business regulation. In rare instances, physicians are regulated by a nongovernmental agency, and in such cases, PAs are generally covered by the same arrangement.

Licensure

An increasing number of states are creating separate PA licensing boards as a result of new physician assistant practice acts that replace the initial delegation amendments to medical practice acts. Such boards are usually composed of practicing PAs and practicing physicians who employ or work with PAs. The boards are typically advisory to a governmental agency, which has ultimate authority in the regulation of physician assistants.

CONCLUSION

Presently, all states have enacted laws or regulations recognizing physician assistants. The AAPA provides up-to-date summary information on state requirements for PA practice. For further information on a specific state's statutes and regulations, the reader is advised to contact the appropriate state agency.

CLINICAL APPLICATIONS

1. Interview the director of your physician assistant program to review the program's accreditation history.
   - ➤ When was it first accredited?
   - ➤ What are the current evaluation and growth issues for the program?
   - ➤ What experience do the director and other faculty members have as evaluators and site visitors for other PA programs?

➤ What changes does your program director foresee in the future accreditation of PA programs in general and your program specifically?

2. Review the past and present PA literature on the issues of initial certification and re-certification.

➤ What are the commonly held views regarding the advantages and disadvantages of each examination?

➤ What has been the history of certification requirements in your state?

➤ Would you recommend any changes in your state licensing act regarding certification?

➤ Why or why not?

REFERENCES

1. Committee on Allied Health Education and Accreditation. Accredited Allied Health Education Programs Facts and Figures. Chicago: American Medical Association, 1991.
2. Schafft GE, Cawley JF. The Physician Assistant in a Changing Health Care Environment. Rockville, MD: Aspen Publications, 1987.
3. Accreditation Review Commission of Education for the Physician Assistant Accreditation. Standards for Physician Assistant Education, 2001.
4. Physician Assistant Programs Directory, ed 11. Alexandria, VA: Association of Physician Assistant Programs, 1992.
5. Sadler AM, Sadler BL, Bliss AA. The Physician's Assistant Today, and Tomorrow: Issues Confronting New Health Practitioners, ed 2. New Haven, CT: Yale University Press, 1972.
6. New Pass/Fail Standard-Setting Procedures Implemented. Commission Update. Atlanta, GA: Newsletter of the NCCPA, Summer/Fall 1997;1:2, 6.
7. Fichandler B. Alternative pathways to recertification (letter to the editor). Physician Assist 1992;16:15.
8. Physician Assistant State Laws and Regulations, ed 6. Alexandria, VA: American Academy of Physician Assistants, 1992.

RESOURCES

Annual Report on Physician Assistant Educational Programs in the United States, Association of Physician Assistant Programs, 950 N. Washington St., Alexandria, VA. *This report, prepared and published annually, provides detailed data on all aspects of PA education. Information includes characteristics of PA program personnel, class size and current enrollment for specific PA programs, tuition and expenses of PA students, employment characteristics of recent graduates, and trends in starting salaries.*

Allied Health Education Directory, American Medical Association, Chicago. *This annually updated report includes information on all currently accredited allied health programs, including physician assistants. The report provides a history of the profession, an occupational description, information on licensure and employment characteristics, and a list of currently accredited PA programs.*

Annual Directory, Physician Assistants-Certified, National Commission on Certification of Physician Assistants (NCCPA) Atlanta, GA. *Updated and published annually, this publication includes lists and addresses of PAs holding current certification from the NCCPA.*

Physicians Assistants in the Health Workforce, 1994. Final Report of the Advisory Group on Physician Assistants and the Workforce submitted to the Council on Graduate Medical Education (COGME). Health Resources and Services Administration, Division of Medicine, Rockville, MD. *This report contains the deliberations and decisions of a federal work group convened as one component of the federal health reform activities in 1993-94. The document projects future needs for physician assistants and recommends policy directions for the PA profession.*

CHAPTER 4

The Political Process

Nicole Gara and Ann Davis

INTRODUCTION

Please do not skip this chapter just because you never intend to become involved in politics. You have entered medicine during a period that will see rapid and profound changes in health care delivery. Where there is change, there is politics. You *are* involved in politics. Being involved in politics is nothing to be ashamed of because, in its truest sense, politics is merely the art of getting things done—and PAs are masters at getting things done!

This chapter is not written for professional lobbyists. It is written for the rest of us. Because it deals with the political process of making laws and regulations, you will find frequent use of words such as *most* and *usually*. Just as there is a good deal of ambiguity in law, there can be a good deal of it in the making of laws. This lack of predictability can be difficult for PAs because it seems unscientific. After you work with lawmakers for a while, however, you will become comfortable with this level of uncertainty.

The chapter is divided into five parts: individual responsibilities, the structure and function of

professional organizations, the legislative process, the regulatory process, and case studies. Because state processes generally are structured along the lines of federal processes, the description of the federal system precedes the description of state mechanisms. In the discussion of state activities, where and how you can exert influence is integrated into the text.

The word *you* is used frequently. Please do not interpret this to mean that anyone expects or wants you to take on the entire government single-handedly. Although individualism is highly valued in our society, the fact is that government responds best to group pressure. You can be an important part of the PA group.

INDIVIDUAL RESPONSIBILITIES

Like every other physician assistant, you have a personal responsibility to understand the political process and to use that knowledge to advance the interests of your patients and your profession. There are many levels of involvement. You can stay abreast of current issues and trends in health care by reading journals, newspapers, and professional publications. You can provide moral or financial support for the efforts of others who work on your behalf. You can become one of those workers yourself, participating in the government-related activities of PA and other health care organizations. You can seek appointment to a licensing board or run for public office at the local, state, or national level.

If running for public office is not for you, consider supporting a candidate whose positions on health care and other issues are compatible with your own. There are dozens of ways to support a candidate: becoming a campaign manager or an issues coordinator, hosting a fundraiser, canvassing for votes, working on a phone bank to solicit supporters, organizing a committee of "Physician Assistants for Candidate N," speaking at community functions in support of the candidate, distributing campaign materials, working to "get out the vote" on election day, and, most important, voting.

If campaign work is not attractive or feasible, consider volunteering your services to individuals already elected to federal or state office. One valuable function you can perform is to advise elected officials about health care issues affecting your community. All legislators are called upon to make decisions on a wide variety of topics. Having a constituent health care expert as a resource can be a great asset.

Make friends before you need them. If legislators and others in government know you and understand the valuable role that PAs play in health care delivery, they will be more likely to come to your assistance when you need help. Your credibility will have been enhanced if, in the past, you were involved with issues that were not self-serving, such as bicycle safety measures, prenatal care, and health care for the homeless. If you know someone has introduced legislation in one of these areas, offer your personal support. Historically, physician assistants have been interested in the broader health care issues because resolving these issues has benefited patients. If you maintain a genuine interest in patient welfare, rather than speaking up only when someone threatens your professional "turf," you will earn genuine respect.

You can do several things to influence the legislative and regulatory processes, even when no issues in which you are interested are awaiting legislation. In fact, if you do these things routinely, you will enhance your credibility—and that is like money in the bank.

The first thing to do is to maintain contact with your elected representatives. The idea is to have them smile, instead of groan, when they see you coming. When you visit, it is best to make an appointment and to be prepared to discuss a specific issue. Of course, you will not wait until the busiest days of the legislative session, when everything is in turmoil, to make your visit. A personal visit is not the only option. You may read something about your representative's pet project and write him or her a letter of support (if, in fact, you do support it). Such letters are read and often remembered. If you receive an interesting piece of information on health care that you think might be useful, pass it along.

You may also do this with regulators. Remember, regulators are all people who are trying to develop or maintain a level of expertise. They need information—provide it. A good relationship with a legislator, a legislator's staff person, or a regulator is invaluable.

Finally, support your state and national PA organizations. This suggestion is not just another pitch for membership; it is a tactical imperative. When any organization testifies before a governmental body, one of the first questions asked is, "How many people does your society represent?" The larger the number, the more credibility the organization is given. It is also important to know where your professional organizations stand on an issue before you go to your representative's office to voice your opinion. If you are an active member, you may have already influenced the organization's policy-making process. Even if you disagree with the group's final determination, at least you will understand how and why it reached its decision, and you may choose to remain silent rather than undercut its efforts.

Remember the value of belonging to a professional organization. There is a symbiotic relationship between an organization and its members. Organizations need you and you need them. They know the legislative and regulatory processes, as well as what issues are under consideration. You know the issues from a personal perspective, because you confront them daily. Your personal perspective is essential and should be conveyed to lawmakers or regulators, particularly when your association says it is time to call, write, or visit them.

One of the first things you must know about government is that it regulates almost every aspect of your professional life. The most important law affecting you as a physician assistant is one passed by the state and implemented by a state licensing board or agency—the PA practice act.

PRACTICE LAWS

Occupational regulation is the prerogative of the state, rather than the federal government. Each state licenses, certifies, or registers a number of different professions and occupations—everyone from physicians and architects to barbers and plumbers. The goal of occupational regulation is to protect public health and safety. This is done by granting licenses only to individuals who meet minimum standards of education and skill; by defining a scope of practice; and by disciplining those who break the law or fail to uphold certain professional standards. A licensing or regulatory agency can seek an injunction and ultimately revoke a license in order to prevent the public from being harmed by a negligent or incompetent practitioner. Lawbreakers may also face civil or criminal penalties.

Physician assistants belong to a regulated profession. In broad terms, this means that an individual seeking to work as a PA must first obtain permission from the state and then abide by any conditions of practice that the state has established. The requirements for securing this permission, which is called licensure, state certification, or registration, vary from state to state. As a result of efforts by the American Academy of Physician Assistants (AAPA) and state PA associations, there is growing uniformity in the laws that govern PAs. Total uniformity is an unrealistic goal because each state writes its laws slightly differently and cherishes its prerogative to do so. The differences in style and content are problems with which every regulated occupation and profession must cope.

The basis for regulation of physician assistants is found in the language of the PA practice act. The law may be included in the medical practice act, which governs doctors, or it may be a separate section of the state statutes. The law is further amplified by regulations issued by the licensing board. Every PA should have a copy of the current state law and regulations governing his or her practice, which may be obtained from the licensing board or found on the licensing board's web site. Ignorance is no excuse if you are ever accused of breaking the law.

Who is responsible for licensing and regulating physician assistants? In most cases, the regulatory agency is the Board of Medical Examiners, the same entity that licenses physicians. A small number of states have separate PA boards. A handful of states have departments of education or professional regulation that register all health practitioners. A list of PA state regulatory agencies is available on the AAPA web site at www.aapa.org.

In the law and regulations, you will find details about qualifications; applications and fees for licensure; scope of practice, or what physicians may delegate to PAs; supervision requirements; prescribing and dispensing privileges; criteria for license renewals, changes in employment, and identification; protection of the title "physician assistant"; and what constitutes a violation of the law and the disciplinary measures that can be invoked; as well as information about administrative procedures and due process. You may also find information on the composition, terms of appointment, and other powers of the regulatory board, allowing you to determine what role, if any, PAs play in the state's regulatory system. Most medical boards have PA advisory committees that provide physician assistants with a way to participate in, and contribute to, the regulatory process.

The two most basic requirements for obtaining state credentials as a PA are:
1. Graduation from an accredited physician assistant educational program.
2. Passage of the Physician Assistant National Certifying Examination (PANCE), administered by the National Commission on Certification of Physician Assistants (NCCPA).

The NCCPA examination, though part of a voluntary, private sector certification process, can be viewed as a national licensing examination. Every state requires that potential licensees have passed it. Although a few states may test PAs on their familiarity with state law, none of them administers its own examination to test clinical knowledge.

Nearly all states will grant a graduate or temporary license to new graduates who are awaiting administration of the PANCE or who have taken the exam and are waiting for the results. A temporary license generally requires you to work with closer supervision and fewer privileges than fully licensed PAs. It expires upon receipt by the state agency of your examination scores and can be converted to a permanent license if you have passed the examination.

Your state license, certificate, or registration must be renewed on a regular cycle—every 1, 2, or 3 years. There is usually a renewal fee. Some jurisdictions require that you provide evidence that you have maintained your NCCPA certification or that you have completed a minimum number of continuing medical education (CME) credits. Keep in mind that the NCCPA certification system must be dealt with separately; do not confuse it with your state license, certification, or registration. To maintain *national* certification, you must pay NCCPA a fee and register 100 hours of CME every 2 years. It is also necessary to re-certify every 6 years, traditionally by taking an examination. You may use the letters "PA-C" after your name only if you are currently certified by the NCCPA.

The PA law and regulations also include criteria for physician supervision. It is rare to find a requirement that the supervising physician be present at the site of your practice 100% of the time. Most states include in their definition of supervision the ability of the physician and the PA to be in contact with each other by telephone, radio, or telecommunication. More details may be specified if the PA will be practicing in an office or clinic separate from the supervising physician. Although no state allows a PA to work independently (i.e., without a supervising physician), the necessity for supervision does not generally mean that the PA and physician must work at the same location.

All but a few states have authorized physician assistants to sign prescriptions if the supervising physician agrees to delegate this responsibility. The law or regulations may specify which kinds of medications a PA may prescribe—controlled or noncontrolled substances, or only those medications listed on a formulary approved by the licensing board—or it may be the physician's decision. The authority to dispense medications is also regulated by the state. Pharmacists vigorously protect this privilege and make good arguments for a separation of the prescribing and dispensing functions. Therefore, a physician's or PA's ability to provide patients with medications from a supply maintained in the office or clinic is often more easily justified in rural areas or other locations without pharmacy services. Some states do not permit anyone other than a pharmacist to dispense drugs. In most jurisdictions, giving patients drug samples that have been supplied by a pharmaceutical company is not the same as dispensing.

Regulation of the PA profession has been evolving since the first practice act was passed in the late 1960s. The founders of the profession made a conscious, political decision to establish a system in which PAs were recognized under the licenses of their employing physicians. Changes in health care delivery and greater numbers of PAs, as well as the need for administrative efficiency, have persuaded many states to modify this approach. The more modern system, advocated by the AAPA, is one in which licensure is granted to a PA on the basis of his or her credentials; that is, upon proof of meeting the educational and examination requirements of the law. In states that have made this adjustment, employment and physician supervisors are handled as separate parts of the application process. Such systems greatly facilitate a PA's ability to continue working despite a change in supervisors or employers. However, some states still require the resubmission of all original application materials each time a PA changes jobs or supervisors.

A good state law is one that allows physicians to delegate to PAs any task or responsibility within their scope of practice that the PA is competent to perform. However, a PA's scope of practice can be limited by a law, a regulation, or even a licensure application that contains a list of tasks that physicians may delegate. It can be limited by a system in which licensing board members are allowed, when reviewing PA job descriptions, to arbitrarily delete certain procedures on the basis of their personal biases. It can also be limited by legislators who do not understand the depth and breadth of PA skills and training. That is why this chapter was written; so you can begin to appreciate the importance of actively protecting and advancing PA practice through the political process.

INDIVIDUALS: PART OF THE WHOLE

This section provides you with information on the structure and mission of your professional organizations—the American Academy of Physician Assistants and the state PA academies.

The American Academy of Physician Assistants, established in 1968, is the national professional society for PAs. At the headquarters building in Alexandria, Virginia, a full-time staff carries out the organization's major activities: government relations, research and data collection, public education, publications, continuing medical education, employment, and other member services. One of the Academy's most important functions is to speak for the profession before the U.S. Congress and federal agencies. Even in a representative democracy such as the United States, it is difficult for one person to single-handedly affect the shape of laws and regulations. It is generally true, although perhaps regrettable, that legislators and bureaucrats are more responsive to organizations that convey the interests of a large group than they are to individuals (except when many individuals are acting in concert). Efficiency, accountability, and credibility come into play here. Therefore, the Academy performs an important role when it voices the PA profession's views on federal legislation and regulations.

Lobbying is done daily by the professional staff of the AAPA. At congressional hearings or during appointments with lawmakers and their aides, the staff may be accompanied by PAs who are elected officers of the Academy or who have special expertise or established relationships with the legislators. Legislative alerts and Academy publications are used to inform AAPA members about important issues or to request that they contact their congressional representatives or a federal agency about a particular subject. Each fall, more than 200 physician assistants from across the country spend a day on Capitol Hill, discussing health issues, as well as legislation that affects the profession, with their senators and representatives.

On the state level, PA interests are represented by state PA associations. These associations are chartered constituent chapters of the AAPA. Among its other projects, each state Academy must advance the interests of the profession before the legislature, the licensing board, and other state agencies. A growing number of PA state societies employ professional association management staff. However, even in the chapters with paid employees, the most substantive work is done by the members themselves. The AAPA government affairs staff members help chapter leaders with these projects by providing information, technical and financial resources, and consultation services. For example, the AAPA can supply copies of other state laws, model language, sample fact sheets, and demographic data, as well as analyses of proposed rules and legislation. The Academy's goal is to promote uniformity and maximize the ability of PAs to use their skills.

FEDERAL LEGISLATIVE PROCESS: HOW A BILL BECOMES LAW

The legislative processes in the U.S. Senate and the House of Representatives are similar, although each chamber has its own rules and traditions. With only 100 members, the Senate seems flexible and informal compared with the 435-member House, in which a strict hierarchy and rigid system of rules are necessary to expedite business.[1]

Approximately 10% of the legislation introduced during each 2-year Congress is related to health issues.[2] For example, Congress authorizes and appropriates money for grants to physician assistant educational programs; National Health Service Corps loans and scholarships; Medicare; rural health; research at the National Institutes of Health; and hundreds of other programs. Because laws passed by Congress affect each of us, directly or indirectly, in our personal and professional lives, it is important to understand the federal lawmaking process and how it can be influenced.

Legislative proposals may be introduced by senators or representatives when Congress is in session.

The bill—prefixed with *HR* when introduced in the House of Representatives and *S* when introduced in the Senate—is given a number that is based on the order of introduction. It is then referred to a committee that has jurisdiction over the bill's subject matter.

The committee is the heart of the legislative process because it is here that a bill receives its sharpest scrutiny. Professional staff expedite the committee's business by researching issues, identifying supporters and opponents, and designing politically acceptable options and compromises. When a committee decides to act on a legislative proposal, it generally conducts hearings to provide the executive branch, interested groups, and individuals an opportunity to formally present their views on the issue.[2] After hearings have ended, the committee meets to "mark up" the bill—that is, to decide on the language of amendments. When a committee votes to approve a measure and send it to the floor, it justifies its actions in a written statement called a *report,* which accompanies the bill. The committee report is useful because it describes the purpose and scope of the bill, explains the committee amendments, indicates proposed changes in existing law, and frequently includes instructions to government agencies on how the language of the new law should be interpreted and implemented.[1]

Most bills never make it out of committee. The enormous volume of legislation (approximately 25,000 measures in each 2-year Congress) makes it impossible for every bill to be considered. In addition, many are duplicative, lack sufficient support, or are purposefully ignored in order to "kill" them. Only about 2% of all bills introduced are enacted into law.[2]

The route to a vote by the full House of Representatives usually lies through the Rules Committee, which sets guidelines for the length and form of the debate. The Senate, on the other hand, calls up a bill by voting on a motion to consider it or by "unanimous consent," in which the bill comes up for a vote if no one objects. In both houses, bills may be further amended on the floor prior to the vote on passage. However, because lawmakers rely heavily on the committee system to ensure that issues are carefully and expertly assessed, amendments on the floor need considerable support in order to be approved.

When a bill has been passed, it is sent to the other chamber for action, where the entire legislative process starts over. Often, the House and Senate consider similar bills. If the measures passed by the two bodies are identical, the resultant bill is sent to the White House for the President's signature. Usually, the measures are not identical, and unless the chamber that first passed the bill agrees to the changes made by the second, a House–Senate conference is arranged to resolve the differences.

Conference committees are composed of members of the committees that originally considered the bills. Theoretically, the conferees are not authorized to delete provisions or language that both the House and the Senate have agreed to, nor are they supposed to draft or insert entirely new provisions. In practice, however, they have wide latitude. When agreement is reached, a conference report is written that includes a final version of the bill with the conferees' recommendations. Each chamber must then vote on the report. If no agreement is reached by the conferees, or if either chamber does not accept the conference report, the bill dies.

A bill that has been approved by both chambers of Congress is sent to the White House. If Congress is in session and the President does not sign the bill within 10 days, it becomes law automatically. If the president favors the bill, he may sign it into law. If he does not like it, he may veto it by returning it to Congress without signature. To override the President's veto requires a two-thirds vote in both the House and the Senate.[1]

Interested individuals can monitor congressional activity by watching televised floor proceedings or by reading various government documents. Copies of bills, as introduced, reported, and passed, are available from the House and Senate document rooms and may be accessed electronically at http://thomas.loc.gov. The document rooms also have the committee reports that accompany the bills and copies of "slip laws," the first official publication of newly enacted statutes. Hearing transcripts are frequently published by committees. Proceedings on the floor of both chambers are reported daily in the *Congressional Record,* which is available electronically at http://www.access.gpo.gov.

STATE LEGISLATIVE PROCESS

Like the federal legislative process, the state process is set into motion when someone defines a condition that they perceive requires change. For example, in a state that lacks legislation to authorize physician-delegated prescriptive authority for PAs, the need for change would be great. As the solution to the problem or to a situation requiring change begins to crystallize, it is put down in writing and becomes a bill or, in some states, a resolution (Fig. 4-1). Although writing a bill is usually considered the legislator's job, sometimes the best way to get what you need is for your state chapter to work closely with the legislative staff in this initial phase. Most legislatures employ professional staff to draft bills requested by senators and representatives.

The next step is sponsorship. If a representative has written the bill, he or she will usually sponsor it. If your state chapter has written the bill, a sponsor will have to be found. You may select your personal representative, one who is known to be sympathetic to your cause, or a member or chairperson of the committee to which you expect the bill will be referred. Bipartisan sponsorship is a good idea, particularly if different political parties control the state house, the state senate, or the governorship.

Once the bill is printed, it is placed on the legislative calendar and "introduced." The introduction is a reading of the bill before all the members of the chamber in which it is introduced (all states except Nebraska have bicameral legislatures, that is, two chambers). In most states, there is a gatekeeper committee, usually the rules or finance committee. If you want to influence when (or whether) a bill is introduced, you need to know which committee performs this function and, ideally, you must know someone who is assigned to the committee. Alternatively, having a good relationship with the clerk or staff of the committee is invaluable if you want to know when a particular bill is to be introduced.

Once a bill has been introduced, it is referred to committee for study. It is here that you and your state chapter become a crucial part of the process. Given the diversity of issues with which legislators are faced, it is impossible for them to know everything about every subject. In the area of medicine, you know more about PAs than your legislator does. So when your bill is referred to committee, write to or visit your personal representative, the members of the committee to which it has been referred, and the chair of that committee. Do not wait for the actual committee meeting at which your bill will be considered because that may be too late! Committees often publish calendars, but frequently, if you receive a calendar in the morning mail, it is impossible to rearrange your schedule so that you can make a 1 PM meeting the same day in a city 3 hours away. Even if you do get there, the rules of the committee may preclude your speaking. Once again, regular contact with a legislative staff person can be vital.

If you go to the Capitol, you may not meet with the actual representative, but with one of the staff instead. Do not feel slighted. Staff members usually concentrate their activities in particular subject areas in order to develop considerable specific expertise. The staff member will have some knowledge about the issue and will welcome an opportunity to learn more.

You should remember a few things about making legislative visits. First, they are only the first step. Rarely does one isolated visit send a bill sailing through the legislature. Do not feel compelled to "win the battle" here. Keep your visit short and to the point. Second, keep it pleasant. This does not necessarily mean you will agree on everything. That's all right. Offer to send additional information to clarify your position. You may want to leave a one-page statement or data sheet behind. Make sure it is a good-quality reproduction. Also, leave your name, address, and phone number. Finally, remember to follow up. Always send a prompt note thanking the legislator or staff person for his or her time. Emphasize your areas of agreement, and send along any material you promised. If you met with a staff person whom you found particularly pleasant or well informed, a note to the boss never hurts.

Going to visit a legislator requires preparation. Even the best professional lobbyists rarely walk into an office and start talking "off the cuff." Sit down and do your homework. What are the pros and cons of the bill? Too many people go into a legislative visit without considering both sides of an issue. That is fine if

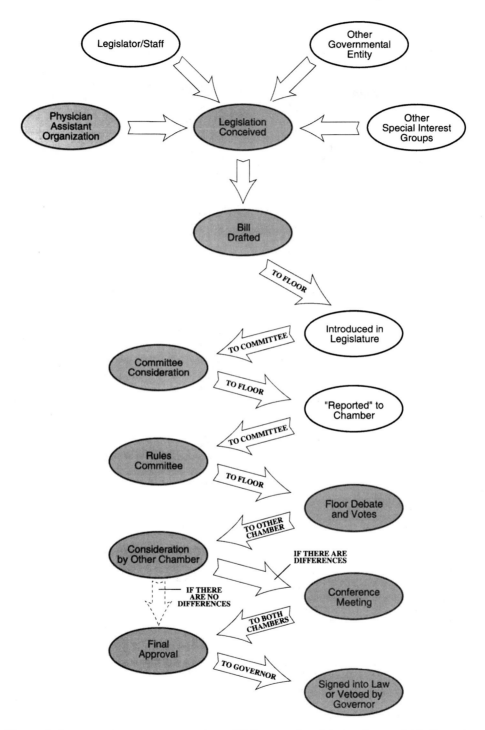

Figure 4-1 The legislative process, or "How a Bill Becomes Law," designates a point in the process at which your involvement is needed.

the legislator agrees with you, but it leaves you in a fix if he or she doesn't. Think of the questions the opposition might raise, and have non-confrontational answers ready. Consider how this bill is going to affect the legislator's constituents. Does the legislator represent a medically underserved area in which allowing PAs to write prescriptions, for example, would improve the quality of health care the constituents are receiving? How does the bill fit into the legislator's own health care agenda?

Attending a committee meeting can be a revealing experience. Find out in advance whether you and other PA association representatives will be allowed to speak while the meeting is in session. Often you will not, but by watching the give and take during the meeting, you can decide who needs to be targeted for a special visit. In some committees, there is no give and take. The clerk reads off the bill numbers and the committee members vote. All discussions have been held and all decisions made prior to the meeting, which is why it was so important to visit all the committee members as soon as you found out which committee was going to handle your bill.

Once a committee approves a bill, it goes to the full chamber. Again, you must maintain staff contact to know when it will be on the legislative calendar. Another series of visits may be needed prior to that vote. You recall that when the bill was introduced, that was its first "reading." Although most states require three separate readings on three separate days, some do not. In some states, the only requirement is that the legislators have possession of the bill for a given number of days, commonly as few as three. This is particularly important to remember at the end of the legislative session, when everything is quite chaotic and a bill that legislators have had in hand for months may advance from the first to the third reading and a final vote in 30 seconds. In states in which many bills are introduced each session, it is important to remember that the legislative calendar is dynamic. It is often perfectly acceptable to do tomorrow's bills in addition to today's.

Fortunately, most states now post legislative calendars and bill scheduling information on the state legislature's web site. The address for state web sites includes the two-letter abbreviation for the state, and "us." For example, the Virginia state web address is http://www.va.us.

For the most part, the full House follows a committee's recommendation on a particular bill. If you do not consider that recommendation wise, then you can contact everyone again and express your concerns. You may be able to get two or three sympathetic legislators to orchestrate the floor debate so that those concerns are brought to the attention of the full body.

A bill that passes the first chamber must then be introduced in the second chamber. Everything you did in the first chamber must be repeated—visits, thank you notes, committee meetings, more visits. The process may be conducted slightly differently in the two chambers, so be sure you learn the rules.

Once a bill has passed both chambers, it must be signed by the governor before it becomes effective. It is perfectly legitimate to attempt to influence the executive chamber. Action here must be planned in advance because the governor may sign the bill the moment it crosses his or her desk. In some states, agencies that will be implementing the bill—the Health Department, for example—may write memoranda to the governor recommending signature or veto of a particular bill. If you can talk to the person who will be writing the memorandum, you may be able to influence its content. Know what the "vest-pocket veto" provisions are in your state. In some states, if the governor does not sign the bill within a fixed period, it is automatically vetoed.

If your bill is vetoed, there is always the outside chance that two thirds of the members of each House can be persuaded to override the veto. It is a long shot, but it may work. If you have not yet prevailed, however, do not dismay. You may still have an opportunity to make some changes during the regulatory process.

FEDERAL REGULATORY PROCESS

The legislative branch of government makes laws that typically contain policy statements and directives. It then delegates to the executive branch—the agencies of the federal government—the authority to implement them. This has been a normal feature of American government since 1790, when the first Congress declared that traders with the Indians should observe "such rules and regulations as the President shall prescribe."[3]

Federal regulations generally describe how a program is to be administered. For example, for longer than two decades, Congress has authorized grants to physician assistant educational programs. The law specifies the total spending for PA program grants but does not provide details on the application process, the basis for determining the recipients, the schedule for awarding the grants, and so on. These details are covered in the regulations.

The federal Administrative Procedures Act (APA) guides agencies in their rule making. The APA procedure has four fundamental elements. First, it guarantees that notice of proposed rule making is published in the *Federal Register*. Second, it gives "interested persons," which really means everyone, the opportunity to comment on the proposal through at least written submissions. Third, it requires the agency to create a "statement of basis and purpose," justifying and explaining the final rule. Last, it requires publication of the final rule and creates a 30-day gap between publication and the effective date.[3]

Therefore, when a new law is passed, an existing law is amended, or a policy requires clarification, the affected federal agency publishes a notice of proposed rule making in the *Federal Register*. The notice includes the proposed rules and their statutory basis; provides background on their content; invites participation from the public through the submission of written comments, data, or arguments; and sets a deadline for the receipt of such comments. Comments must generally be submitted within 30, 60, or 90 days. On the federal level, hearings are seldom held.

Federal agency staff members analyze the comments and may make revisions in the rules on the basis of the information received. When final rules are published in the *Federal Register,* they are prefaced by a discussion of the comments, accompanied by the agency's response to them. For example, in 1989, the Health Care Financing Administration published final rules that changed the Medicare system for certification of nursing homes.[4] The preamble to the rules contained the following discussion:

Paragraph (e): Physician Delegation of Tasks

Comment: In proposed section 483.40(e), we would permit physician delegation to physician extenders, that is, physician assistants and nurse practitioners, of tasks that the regulations do not otherwise require to be performed by the physician personally. An overwhelming majority of commenters expressed general support for permitting the delegation of tasks to physician extenders.

Response: We believe that, to the extent feasible, the regulations should be written in a manner that allows for the effective utilization of physician extenders in the nursing home setting. For this reason, we are withdrawing our proposed requirement in section 483.40(b) that all orders be signed by the physician personally. This means that under sec. 483.40(e)(2), requirements concerning physician signature or countersignature of orders are determined by individual State law and facility policy. . . .

We also believe that the regulations should be revised to permit at least some measure of delegation to physician extenders of the physician visit function. We remain concerned, however, that at least a minimal degree of direct personal contact between physician and patient should be maintained.

Therefore, in sec. 483.40(c)(4), we require that the physician perform the initial visit personally and in sec. 483.40(c)(5), allow the physician the option of alternating with the physician extender in making subsequent required visits.

There are exceptions to this procedure—some based in law, others in politics—but it represents the most common method of federal rule making.

General and permanent rules published in the *Federal Register* by the executive departments and agencies of the federal government are codified in the *Code of Federal Regulations*. The *Code* is divided into 50 titles that represent broad areas subject to federal regulation, such as "public health." Each title is further divided into chapters, and the chapters into parts covering specific agencies and regulatory areas.[5] The *Code* is always changing, in response to either acts of Congress or agency revisions of regulations. The *Federal Register,* published daily, is available in most public libraries, by subscription, and on the Internet at http://www.access.gpo.gov. The *Code of Federal Regulations* is sold by the Superintendent of Documents, U.S. Government Printing Office, Washington, D.C., and may be viewed at the same Internet address listed above.

STATE REGULATORY PROCESS

Agencies, boards, and departments are the regulators at the state level, and they touch what every citizen does every day. They are responsible for inspecting food, keeping the costs of utilities at a given rate, and of course, governing the practice of medicine.[6] Although almost everyone knows when it is time to write to elected representatives, few know when, let alone how, to interact with agencies. This is crucial because "the rise of administrative bodies has probably been the most significant legal trend of the last century and perhaps more values are affected by their decisions than by those of all the courts. . . . They have become a veritable fourth branch of the Government, which has deranged our three-branch legal theories as much as the concept of a fourth dimension unsettles our three-dimensional thinking."[7] Agencies are here to stay, and it behooves us to learn how to deal with them.

Agencies (the inclusive term used in this chapter for regulatory bodies) are set forth in the Constitution, are created by legislatures, or are created by executive order and sanctioned by the legislature. The powers of the agency come from the body that creates it.[6] The work of agencies and legislatures is intertwined, but the players and the processes are very different.

First, the players. Legislators are elected by the people of the state and stay in office only as long as their work satisfies the voters, unless the length of time they may serve is limited by the law. Top-level agency personnel are usually appointed by the governor (with confirmation by one or both houses of the legislature) and serve at the pleasure of the governor. Mid-level agency employees are generally civil service employees, although some political appointments exist at this level as well. Many of these people are career civil servants; they intend to make the government their life's work. Contrast this time frame with that of a legislator, who must think in terms of 2 or 4 years, depending on when he or she is up for re-election. Commissioners or department secretaries, the top-level personnel, may be career civil servants or they may have aspirations for elected office. As such, their thinking is hybrid: They need to think of the long-term policy implications of their actions, as well as how such actions may influence

the governor's re-election a few years hence. So legislators and agency personnel think in different time frames and at different paces.

Legislators and bureaucrats also think differently in terms of content. A legislator is elected to represent all the interests of his or her district—the schools, the environment, the businesses. Legislators must also keep overall interests of the state in mind when involved in policy matters or budget negotiations. It is somewhat unrealistic to expect any one person to become expert in all these areas, particularly within 2 or 4 years. Add to that the need to balance the competing interests, and you have an almost impossible task. Contrast this situation with agencies. The subject matter is limited and specific—education, environment, *or* business, not all three. Agency personnel who work with an agency over a long period become quite expert in their specific subject areas. Because of their expertise and the fact that they do not depend on your good will to keep their jobs, agency personnel may be the people who can answer your questions correctly—even if they do not give you the answers you want to hear.

But what is it that agencies do? For this discussion, let us focus on the agency's function in creating rules and regulations. Like Congress, state legislatures pass laws (also known as statutes), whose language provides only a skeleton for a given policy. It is the agency's job to flesh out this skeleton by promulgating detailed rules and regulations.[8] The legislature may pass enabling legislation for physician assistants that says, "A physician assistant is anyone who is licensed by the State Board of Medicine as a physician assistant." But how does one get licensed? This is the sort of thing that will be detailed in state regulations. For example, to be licensed as a PA, one must be a graduate of a physician assistant program, pass an examination, and be of good moral character. Regulations, in most cases, have the force of law.

Just as you can influence the legislative process, you can affect the regulatory process. The process is quite well defined in most states, and regulations are not drafted in smoke-filled rooms. With a few exceptions, states follow the 1981 modifications of the Model State Administrative Procedures Act (MSAPA), which sets forth a specific rule-making process that includes public notification and public comment. Your elected representative should be able to refer you to the agency in your state that is charged with enforcing your state Administrative Procedures Act. If you anticipate a protracted exchange on a regulatory level, it is wise to review the provisions of this act with the help of an attorney conversant in administrative law.

Once a law has been passed, an agency (or agencies) is charged with developing the regulations necessary to implement it (Fig. 4-2). Usually, the staff of a bill's sponsor can tell you who is going to be writing the regulations. This is the time to get involved because it is much easier to influence what gets written than it is to change what *has* been written. Your initial contact with the regulator should focus on gathering and giving information. Are there any special concerns the agency needs to address in writing these regulations? What outside pressures might be brought to bear on the drafting? When does the agency intend to promulgate the regulations?

Unless you know the political atmosphere in which the regulator is operating, you cannot supply really useful information. You know the language of PA practice, and the regulator knows the language of regulation. You need to work together. If the regulator has never worked with PAs before and regards you as just another professional trying to protect your own turf while he or she is trying to tend to the needs of the people of the state (and make the agency look good in the process), the two of you are bound to be in conflict. You must know at the outset what your bottom line is and be frank about it. If you disagree with the regulator, fine; there are ways to deal with that. Over time, you will find that the more realistic you are with regulators, the more realistic they will be with you. Just as you would never give inaccurate information to a legislator, do not give inaccurate information to a regulator. Such people are going to be around for a long time and they have very, very good memories.

Once the initial regulations are written, the MSAPA requires that interested parties be notified. Notification can take many forms. In larger states, the proposed regulations can be published in a register or some other regular publication that includes nothing

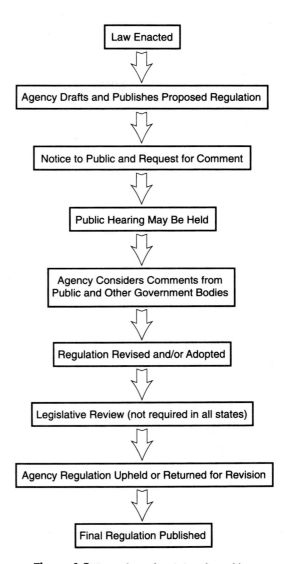

Figure 4-2 Procedures for state rule making.

but proposed regulations. In smaller states, they might be published in a newspaper that has statewide circulation. In states that have adopted MSAPA, if you have notified the agency in advance that you want to know about any rules it promulgates, your name is added to its mailing list. If you have not made such a written request, do not assume that just because the agency personnel know that you are interested in PA issues, they will notify you. Although it is the agency's responsibility to notify the public, that responsibility does not extend to personal notification. It is also unwise to rely on your agency "contacts" to inform you of a proposed rule. Their primary responsibility is to the agency. If they know your organization is going to make the rule-making process difficult, they might not notify you in advance.

A comment period follows notification, during which anyone may submit written suggestions to the agency as to how the regulation might be improved. Like all other written communication with government, your comments should be succinct and unemotional. Your state PA organization may also be submitting comments, so you should try to express your ideas in concert with theirs. "In concert" does not mean using a form letter or parroting what the organization says. Your own thoughts and insights will be more persuasive than someone else's.

Depending on the statute that was passed and on the particular state administrative procedure act, public hearings may be required. Individual testimony is usually limited to 5 or 10 minutes, including questions and answers. The agency will ask you to submit a written copy of your testimony. When you testify, it is best not to read from your written copy. Paraphrase what you have written and answer any questions the regulators may have. Some people find public testimony intimidating. You might find it useful to watch testimony before state or federal agencies on your public access television channel. It is much easier if you are well prepared and remember that the regulators work for you. In some cases, you may wish to bring in experts from the AAPA or another organization that has had experience with the issue. Many states, however, believe they know how to do things perfectly and may not be interested in how someone else approaches the problem.

After the comment period and hearings, a modification of the proposed regulation is published and subsequently adopted. Some states have a time frame within which a regulation must be adopted or the process terminated.

In many states, the legislatures have not welcomed the rise of the administrative agencies just described. In an effort to curb what they saw as usurping of legislative mandates, they have adopted sunset laws and legislative oversight procedures. In a sunset law, the statute authorizing the existence of a regulatory agency expires in a fixed number of years unless it is reviewed and reauthorized by the legislature. In states with legislative oversight provisions, a committee of the legislature reviews all proposed regulations. State PA organizations have used these opportunities successfully to achieve needed change.

As you might expect, the regulatory process just described is somewhat neater than the reality. Some variations on the theme follow. All of the steps in the process have time limits. Perhaps the proposed rule needs to be published in only two consecutive weekly issues of the newspaper. Any PA group should make sure that one of its members is reading proposed rules all the time. Most states have emergency adoption provisions that allow an agency to circumvent the time limits.[6] It only makes sense that if the state health department detects an increase in tuberculosis (TB) cases in August, it is not going to want to wade through the entire process, which may take 90 days, before requiring TB skin testing in selected students entering preschool. Usually, emergency rules are effective for only 120 days with the option of one extension, after which time the agency must go through the notification and comment process. Another variation from the norm would be one in which reality is what the agency says it is. In some states, for example, with all proposed rules, regulators must submit an analysis of the regulation's impact on small businesses. A common comment in this section is, "There is no impact on small businesses, therefore no analysis was conducted." In regulations pertaining to PAs, it can be argued that a physician's office is a small business and physicians employ PAs, thereby forcing an analysis. Of course, such an argument would be made only if the rule were going to have a dire effect on PA practice.

CASE STUDIES

Examples of the legal and regulatory processes are presented in the following case studies of actual occurrences.

CASE STUDY 4-1

Practice act for Mississippi

Over a 20-year period, starting in the 1970s, every state except Mississippi successfully enacted legislation authorizing legal practice by physician assistants. In Mississippi, efforts to pass a PA practice act were met by very strong opposition from organized nursing. In the 1970s and 1980s, many bills were introduced in the legislature, but concerted lobbying by nurses overcame whatever support the Mississippi PAs could mount. As time passed, a serious dilemma developed. Without a law making it legal to practice as a PA, jobs became scarce, the number of PAs in the state shrank, and the Mississippi Academy of PAs (MAPA) lost its ability to pursue a vigorous legislative campaign.

In the 1990s, things began to change. The core of the Mississippi Academy for many years had been PAs stationed at a U.S. Air Force base near Biloxi. Their exemption from state law and periodic transfers, however, made it difficult for them to pursue legislation. In 1992, several Air Force PAs were thinking seriously about retiring and staying in Mississippi, and another PA, born in the state and now an educator, returned to teach at a state university. Another PA educator and a PA who worked with a respected cardiothoracic surgery group had renewed enthusiasm for a legislative effort. Several PAs joined the staff of the Veterans Administration Hospitals in Jackson and on the Gulf coast and became committed leaders of the state PA association. With this revitalized core of members, MAPA contacted the American Academy of Physician Assistants for assistance and began to plan both revitalization of the chapter and another legislative effort. The first steps toward a lobbying campaign included identifying physician supporters, potential employers, and rural health advocates.

In 1994, MAPA, with the help of AAPA staff, began serious work on a comprehensive legislative campaign. The plan included opening a dialog with both the state medical society and the Mississippi Nurses Association (MNA). MAPA and AAPA representatives met with the medical licensing board, the medical society, and the nurses association. As a result of these meetings and continued communication, the licensing board agreed to support PA legislation, and the medical society withdrew its opposition. In fact, the medical society published an excellent article, "Physician Assistants in Mississippi," as a lead story in its journal.

The meeting with the Mississippi Nurses Association was also productive. The PAs made a presentation on physician assistant education and practice and answered questions for longer than an hour. At the end of the meeting, the MNA board of directors agreed to reevaluate its opposition and to keep open the lines of communication. The following month, MNA decided to remain neutral on PA legislation in the 1995 legislative session.

MNA opposition resurfaced early in 1995, however. According to MNA leaders, it was the direct result of rules drafted by the medical licensing board, which if adopted, would have imposed new restrictions on physicians who work in collaborative roles with nurse practitioners (NPs). In a letter to the chairman of the public health committee in the Mississippi House of Representatives, MNA stated, "until recent issues have been settled and there is some assurance that nurse practitioners will not be squeezed out of the health care picture, we find it impossible not to oppose a bill that will give physicians complete control over one provider while enacting rules and regulations that will greatly inhibit the practice of another." Because of the letter from the nurses association, the chairman refused to schedule a hearing on the PA bill, thus killing the measure in the 1995 legislative session.

Determined to persevere, MAPA and AAPA, again acting in concert, started preparing for the 1996 session. A lobbyist was hired who had previously worked for the medical society, and the process of lining up additional supporters was begun. By the start of the 1996 session, the list of supporters had grown to include the Mississippi State Medical Association, the Mississippi Academy of Family Physicians, the Mississippi Primary Care Association, and the medical licensing board. The bill was sponsored by the only physician and the only nurse serving in the House of Representatives.

Although the nurses association had promised to maintain an open dialog, it failed to respond to overtures from the PAs. MAPA's lobbyist made numerous appointments with her counterpart at the nurses association, all of which were canceled by MNA at the last minute. At the start of the 1996 session, MNA announced that it would once again oppose PA licensure.

A hearing on the PA bill was held at the Mississippi Capitol Building in late January 1996. Ten physician assistants, the MAPA lobbyist, and a representative from the primary care association were present to support the measure. In addition, a physician representing the medical society gave very compelling testimony in favor of the legislation. The only opposition came from nursing.

The nurses' opposition focused on the following three points:

1. Nurse practitioners, they said, could fill all the unmet health needs in the state.
2. The scope of PA practice would be too broad because of regulation by the medical licensing board.
3. Licensing PAs would lead to the establishment of a PA training program that would compete with NP programs for state funds.

Despite testimony refuting these points, the subcommittee chairman refused to call for a vote, again letting the bill die in subcommittee. Undeterred, the PAs in Mississippi and their supporters began plans for the 1997 session. Prior to the opening of the legislature, MAPA again invited MNA to discuss the nurses' concerns. In mid-December 1996, representatives from MAPA, AAPA, and MNA met in Jackson.

Following the meeting and after further discussions involving nursing leadership and nurse practitioners in the state, MNA submitted a list of five proposed changes to the PA bill. The PA negotiating team made numerous counterproposals, and eventually all but one issue were resolved. The nurses association refused to negotiate on its demand that PAs must hold a master's degree in order to be licensed in Mississippi. "The nursing community supports strongly that a provider who will be practicing in the same arena should hold to these same standards," they wrote. It is important to note that when this letter was written, there was no statutory or regulatory requirement for NPs in Mississippi to hold a master's degree, although the state nursing board was said to be considering regulatory changes to add this requirement.

The PAs rejected the demand. MAPA went forward with a bill requiring only that PAs be graduates of accredited PA educational programs and that they pass the NCCPA certification examination. Materials were prepared for legislators that explained the intensive clinical training that PAs receive, as well as the concept of competency-based (as opposed to academic degree–based) professional education.

With the start of the 1997 session, legislators were greeted with three bills that would regulate the practice of PAs in Mississippi. New additions to the list of supporters included the Mississippi chapter of the American College of Emergency Physicians, the National Association of Community Health Centers, the National Association of Rural Health Clinics, and the Southern Regional Project on Infant Mortality. The nurses association was once again the only group opposing PA legislation.

A hearing was held in a House subcommittee, and just as in the previous year, the chairman refused to call for a vote. He promised, however, that the PA licensing bill would not die for lack of a vote in his subcommittee again. He said that a vote would be taken in the 1998 session.

The Mississippi PAs and their supporters immediately began planning for the coming year. The National Rural Health Association signed on as a supporting organization. MAPA representatives booked professional exhibit space at meetings of the Mississippi State Medical Association, the Mississippi Academy of Family Physicians, the Mississippi Hospital Association, and the Mississippi Rural Health Association. The Southern Regional Project on Infant Mortality concluded a study on the use of PAs, NPs, and nurse midwives in the South and, in its published report, called for licensure of PAs in Mississippi.

In December 1997, a Senate subcommittee held a special hearing on the PA issue. The immediate past president of the Mississippi Academy of Family Physicians spoke on behalf of PA licensure. Senators asked questions that indicated their increased understanding of the issue, and one of them subsequently introduced a bill for the 1998 session. On the House side, a bill sponsored by four lawmakers was introduced. The Mississippi Academy of Family Physicians declared that passage of a PA licensing law was one of its legislative priorities for the year. Continued full opposition by the nurses association, however, made passage of a bill in 1998 impossible.

By the end of the 1998 legislative session, it became apparent that an upgrade in strategy was required. The MAPA-AAPA team made four major changes. First, because 1999 was an election year for Mississippi legislators, a political action committee was established and contributions were made to approximately 70 candidates. Second, a biweekly newsletter, *The Inside Scoop,* was started, to keep supporters up-to-date on developments as they occurred. Third, the grassroots network was expanded to include more PA students, family members, physicians, business leaders, and health care advocates. And last but not least, the public education campaign was expanded. Editorial boards, reporters, and radio and TV stations were contacted in order to increase coverage of the issue.

The 1999 session brought continued opposition from the nurses and no success for the PA legislation. However, momentum was clearly building, and the MAPA-AAPA team sought additional channels for advocacy. A second lobbyist was added, and meetings were held with key legislators and opinion leaders throughout the state. To maintain open communication, meetings were also held with the medical licensing board.

Near the end of 1999, the team met once again with the nurses association. The nurses were still insisting on a master's degree as a prerequisite for PA licensure. This idea had been unthinkable 5 years earlier, but the PAs recognized that events had overtaken them. The PA academic environment had changed. More and more PA programs were offering master's degrees, and the profession was actively discussing whether master's degrees were not, in fact, an appropriate reflection of the rigor of PA education. Thus, the PA negotiating team proposed that there be a requirement for a master's degree at a future date and immediate licensure eligibility for all PAs currently in the state regardless of their academic degrees. The nurse negotiating team accepted the proposal. The MAPA-AAPA team then traveled the state to discuss this concept with nearly every PA in Mississippi. Everyone agreed to support the compromise, and the stage was set for success.

The chairmen of the House and Senate health and welfare committees agreed to sponsor legislation, and because there was no opposition, the bill moved quickly through the legislature. It passed the House by a vote of 118-1 on March 1, 2000, and sailed unanimously through the Senate. The governor signed the bill on April 24, 2000.

A Mississippi political observer described the victory as a textbook case of how to get legislation passed over strong opposition: "Marshall the facts, make the case in human rather than policy terms, put together a team of active volunteers and professionals, think long term, be willing to compromise, and exhibit the patience of Job."

And the icing on the cake? Because the medical board had been in the loop and thus had developed a good understanding of the physician/PA team concept, they quickly issued rational and workable regulations. Adopted less than 5 months after enactment of the law, the regulations define PA scope of practice as recommended by the AAPA; that is, as any medical service delegated by a supervising physician, including prescribing.

CASE STUDY 4-2

Swimming upstream in Louisiana

Louisiana has a set of political circumstances that make changing the law and rules a true challenge. The state legislature meets for 60 legislative days in odd-numbered years. (Thirty-day sessions are held in even-numbered years, but they are limited to specific fiscal business.) Prior to 1999, medical board members were appointed for life and as a result were not very responsive to public pressure.

The initial legislation recognizing PAs was passed in 1977 and, as with many of the early practice acts, was quite restrictive. It barred PAs from using independent medical judgment except in emergencies and prohibited physician-delegated prescribing. Despite the difficult political environment, the Louisiana Academy of PAs (LAPA) knew that improvements had to be pursued.

Incremental changes began in 1992. LAPA leaders began by convincing the medical board to use PAs as reviewers of PA applications for state certification. The following year, LAPA retained a very old and respected law firm for advice on potential statutory and regulatory changes. By mid-1993, a bill had been drafted that modernized many aspects of PA practice. Most PAs in the state thought prescriptive authority should be the primary goal of the legislation, but LAPA leaders knew that including prescribing in the bill would lessen its chances of success. The legislation, without prescribing language, was passed. It mandated the establishment of a PA advisory committee to the medical board, eliminated burdensome paperwork, and clearly designated PAs as agents of their supervising physicians. This was a significant step forward, but much remained to be done.

In 1995, LAPA was back at the legislature with a bill designed to authorize institutional employment for PAs. It also allowed hospital-employed physicians to supervise PAs and marked the beginning of an alliance between LAPA and the hospital association.

More success came in the 1997 and 1999 legislative sessions, when a ban on PA use of "independent medical judgment" was repealed, supervision requirements were significantly improved, and state certification was changed to state licensure. But a provision authorizing physician-delegated prescriptive authority, strongly opposed by the medical society, had to be dropped from the 1999 legislative proposal.

Faced with continued medical society opposition to prescriptive privileges, LAPA leaders decided to regroup and focus on building liaisons within the state. They began a series of substantive meetings with physician organizations. At the same time, a change in legislative leadership made lawmakers more receptive to PA issues. The state was faced with a crisis in funding its low-income and charity care programs, and legislators began to talk about ways to cut health expenditures. Although LAPA leaders had planned to sit out the 2001 session, legislators came to them asking if authorizing PAs to prescribe would encourage them to move to rural areas where Medicaid patients were in need of care. The answer, of course, was "yes."

As legislators moved to support PA prescribing, the state society of family physicians also voted to lend its support. Just prior to the start of the 2001 legislative session, the medical society agreed to remain neutral on the prescribing bill. LAPA leaders were optimistic about the bill's chances, and their optimism appeared to be justified. The bill was passed by the Senate. But then the physicians in Shreveport broke with the state medical society and voted to oppose the PA prescribing bill. Their vocal opposition slowed its progress in the House.

LAPA activated its grassroots network. PAs throughout the state contacted their legislators, urging support for the measure. Based on a vote count, it looked like the bill would pass the House. But it was not to be. On the House floor, a legislator with family connections to physicians and pharmacists voiced loud opposition to the bill. No legislators spoke passionately in support of the legislation, and the opponent was able to sway those lawmakers who had reservations. The bill died by a vote of 40 in favor, 60 opposed.

As the session ended, LAPA leaders received a letter from a friendly legislator. He told them that because physicians appeared to be split on the issue, legislators just weren't sure it was the right thing to do.

CASE STUDY 4-3
Sequential improvement in Texas

In 1989, an amendment to the Texas medical practice act was passed that permitted physicians at sites serving medically underserved populations to delegate to PAs the authority to prescribe. Six years later, another amendment was enacted that allowed physicians to delegate prescribing to PAs at each physician's primary practice site, and at hospitals and long-term care facilities. This case study is based on a taped interview with Justine Strand, PA-C, chair of the Texas Academy of PAs (TAPA) government affairs committee during 1989, and Tim King, PA-C, legislative coordinator for TAPA during 1995.

Strand: In 1989, we knew we had a golden opportunity to make a change as part of a legislative initiative known as the "Rural Health Rescue Act." Before that time, PAs couldn't really be effective in rural areas because they could not prescribe. The rural health legislation served as a vehicle for changes we had been waiting to make. It was a natural opportunity for us to jump in as part of the rural health solution.

King: It wasn't quite so obvious a window in 1995, but the point that timing is key really is crucial. By 1995, we had a track record with PA prescribing in rural areas, we had built some lines of communication with the appropriate players, and it looked as if we could create an opportunity. I think people should watch for windows of opportunity and also be sensitive to times when it is prudent just to wait.

Strand: I think that's right. In 1989, we didn't have all of those alliances. We needed to start by educating ourselves. Leading up to and during the legislative session, I read two newspapers every day just to get the "lay of the land." I also made it a point to meet lobbyists for a variety of causes and issues. Their insights were invaluable. They taught me how the state legislature works in Texas.

King: We also have been very fortunate to have an attorney who is also a lobbyist who has worked for TAPA for a very long time. Justine, in 1989, you actually registered as a lobbyist yourself, right?

Strand: That's right. I lived in Austin, and my employer gave me some time off, so I spent a lot of time at the Capitol Building, representing TAPA. Even then, our attorney was very helpful. He would tell me who to stay away from, and he handled some of the most opinionated legislators without me.

King: In 1995, we called on him, too. We really learned just how important it is to have PAs watching all of the minutiae. Our attorney missed a key issue just because he couldn't see it as a PA. I think it really is important when you have professional representation to work just as hard as if you didn't.

Strand: We also got lots of help from the AAPA government affairs staff. Frequently, I would call just to get feedback on an idea. That was incredibly helpful.

King: By 1995, we had some key lines of communication. At that point, I wouldn't have called them allies, but at least we had people we could talk to at the Texas Medical Association, the Texas Academy of Family Physicians, the Texas Osteopathic Medical Association, and the Texas Department of Health.

We needed to take in a bill that had everyone's agreement. You know, state legislators don't want to have to make tough choices or to choose between competing forces. They prefer to pass a bill that contains pre-negotiated agreements. Even though we didn't get everything we wanted, we were able to craft a bill that everyone could sign on to. That was critical.

By the way, I would call those groups our allies now. Through the years, they have really learned to understand PAs. They understand how passing good laws for PAs is important for physicians.

Strand: We needed those lines of communication within our own organization, too. During the legislative session, I frequently sent a written "insider update" to key members of the TAPA leadership. This made it easy to get quick decisions because everyone had most of the background information.

King: In 1995, the TAPA board made a decision to invest a small group with the authority to make the sort of split-second decisions that are sometimes required during legislative negotiations.

Strand: Did you have good success in getting grassroots PAs to contact their legislators?

King: I would say yes and no. There is never enough grassroots lobbying. You can always use more. But we made a real effort to use every single

Texas PA in our effort, and in many instances, they were very effective.

The organizational structure, lessons learned, and liaisons described by Justine and Tim were used as a foundation for TAPA leaders in the legislative sessions that followed. Key alliances have formed a strong base of support. The law has been fine-tuned to update the prescribing provisions, improve requirements for physician/PA teams caring for patients in hospitals, and clarify that PAs are the agents of their supervising physicians. Future improvements are being planned.

CONCLUSION

The preceding cases are diverse in terms of time and geography, but they do have common threads. What lessons can be learned from these cases?

1. You do not need a huge number of people or a large war chest to win a legislative battle. What was crucial in all cases was that each individual considered it a personal responsibility to work with the state chapter to effect a legislative change. Likewise, none of these state chapters was exactly rich. Rather than letting lack of money deter their efforts, they made creative use of the resources they had.

2. You need to mobilize the membership. Although in each case only a small number of people were actually "working" the legislature, the membership was behind them. They wrote letters and made telephone calls. Membership input is crucial. If you choose to be a chapter leader, give the membership the information they need to write an intelligent letter. If you choose not to be a chapter leader, write intelligent letters when asked.

3. You do not have to be a professional lobbyist to win. Professional lobbyists are great—they know the system and when to pull which strings—but you can do much of what they do. Legislators want honest information. Deliver it with enthusiasm, and you are halfway home.

4. Look for windows of opportunity in both timing and alliances. Sometimes the best strategy is to wait until a powerful opposing force is neutralized by an election or expiration of a term of office.

5. There is no need to "go it alone." All three state organizations used, to a greater or lesser degree, the AAPA. You may need financial assistance or technical assistance. If your state organization does not ask for it, you will get neither. Alliances with physician organizations can be extremely helpful in making both legislative and regulatory changes.

6. You must be persistent. In "government time," all three of these state chapters far surpassed the 3-minute mile. Do not be discouraged if your efforts require two or three legislative sessions to complete. Keep at it.

7. The most important lesson: Keep patients first. It is not novel, it is not clever, it is just PAs expressing what they truly believe.

Contrary to what we hear every day about the failure of government, the system does work. It works because individuals and organizations keep doing their part to make it work. We hope this chapter will make it easier for you to be effective and even excited about your part in the political process.

CLINICAL APPLICATIONS

1. You are a PA living in a state that does not have prescriptive privileges for PAs. You have been asked by the state chapter to become politically active on behalf of your profession to improve health care in the state. Compose a sample letter that could be directed to a state legislator, expressing your support of prescriptive privileges for PAs. Prepare information and handouts that you might use in visiting a state legislator's office. Discuss other activities that you might propose to the state chapter leadership that could help in this legislative effort.

2. Examine the health care needs of your local community. Discuss ways in which legislation and regulations could improve the health status of your community.

REFERENCES

1. Congressional Quarterly's Guide to Congress, ed 3. Washington, DC: Congressional Quarterly, 1982.
2. Congress and Health: An Introduction to the Legislative Process and Its Key Participants, ed 3. New York: National Health Council, 1979.

3. Koch CH Jr. Administrative Law and Practice. St. Paul, MN: West, 1985.
4. 54 Federal Register 5342. Washington, DC: U.S. Government Printing Office.
5. 42 CFR § 61.1. Washington, DC: U.S. Government Printing Office.
6. Davis KC. Administrative Law: Cases, Text, Problems. St. Paul, MN: American Casebook Series, 1977.
7. Jackson JR (dissenting). Federal Trade Commission v Rubberoid. 343 US 470 487 (1952).
8. Christoffel T. Health and the Law: A Handbook for Health Professionals. New York: Macmillan, 1982.

RESOURCES

American Academy of Physician Assistants. Physician Assistants: State Laws and Regulations. Alexandria, VA: AAPA, 2002. *Contains detailed summaries of more than 25 key provisions of the PA laws and regulations, state by state. Includes an address list of PA licensing authorities and other information on regulation and the profession. New editions are published regularly.*

American Academy of Physician Assistants. Physician Assistants: Prescribing and Dispensing. Alexandria, VA: AAPA, 2001. *Provides a summary of legal provisions in states that authorize physicians to delegate prescriptive authority to physician assistants. Updated as changes occur.*

American Academy of Physician Assistants. Legal Opinions on Physician Assistant Orders. Alexandria, VA: AAPA, 2002. *Attorneys general and other legal authorities in many states have clarified the authority of physician assistants to issue patient care orders to nurses. This document summarizes these legal rulings and advisory opinions and is updated as changes occur.*

American Academy of Physician Assistants. Taking Charge: State Government Affairs Handbook. Alexandria, VA: AAPA, 2001. *Written for state PA associations to explain the legislative and regulatory processes and describe the fundamentals of a good state government affairs program. Includes guidelines for writing PA laws and regulations.*

American Academy of Physician Assistants. Team Building: Developing Effective Organizational Relationships. Alexandria, VA: AAPA, 2001. *A handbook full of ideas about organizational liaison and coalition building. Gives PA organizations a step-by-step guide for working with companion groups.*

www.aapa.org *The AAPA's web site provides information about the PA profession and key governmental issues.*

Guyer RL. Guide to State Legislative Lobbying. Gainesville, FL. Engineering THE LAW, Inc, 2000. *A skill-building guide for individuals and organizations that want to influence their state legislatures.*

Meredith J, Myer L. Lobbying on a Shoestring: How to Win in Massachusetts . . . and Other Places, Too. Boston: Massachusetts Poverty Law Center, 2000. *A guide through the legislative process for individuals or organizations that want to change a law.*

CHAPTER 5

Public Health Perspectives

Jeffrey Hummel

INTRODUCTION

It is common for students of clinical medicine, whether in medical schools or in physician assistant (PA) training programs, to be impatient with material that does not relate directly to pathophysiology. This is partly because of the power and status of curative medicine—not just in the United States but also in all cultures—and partly because of the overwhelming complexity of the material for which students are responsible as they strive to become competent clinicians. Students often feel that they do not have time to worry about issues such as prevention because they need to concentrate on learning treatment—already sick patients might die if students don't know the right antibiotic for an infection or the right test for abdominal pain.

In reality, students must know clinical material well in order to be competent clinicians, and they must become competent clinicians to have any credibility as health care professionals. In terms of actual reduction of suffering and avoidable death, however, it is the prevention of infections through immunizations, the prevention of injuries through the use of bicycle helmets and seat belts, the reduction of child abuse through treatment of family dysfunction and alcohol dependency, and the prevention of cardiopulmonary disease and cancer through smoking cessation programs that will have the greatest impact on the quality of life of their patients.

There are several reasons to specifically teach public health and community medicine to physician assistant students. First, mid-level practitioners in primary care were intended to work in health personnel shortage areas (HPSAs). In rural communities and impoverished urban neighborhoods, health services must rely heavily on prevention and treatments aimed at the community as a whole because there may be inadequate numbers of providers, and because the cost of medical care is often greater than many people can afford.

Second, in urban areas, it is common to find physician assistants in emergency departments and other settings where trauma is a major part of their work. To be a complete clinician, one must understand that injuries are not "accidental," but rather are preventable. To really save lives, one must be able to educate patients about the things in their lives over which they have control that place them at increased risk for injuries. Third, given an increasingly sophisticated public, all clinicians have an obligation to understand the basic concepts of public health, such as probability theory and screening programs, in order to be able to explain diseases and the meaning of test results to their patients and to the public.

DIAGNOSIS AND TREATMENT IN COMMUNITY MEDICINE

The primary role of the clinical practitioner is to make a diagnosis and then treat appropriately. The clinician has various tools at his or her disposal for these tasks, and the process is highly structured to ensure that as little as possible is left to chance. Gathering and integrating information is the process by which a diagnosis is made. The clinician gathers information from a medical history, which is usually obtained from the patient but is often supplemented by interviewing family members or friends, and through review of old records. The clinical database, built from historical information, is supplemented by performing a physical examination; then a diagnosis is confirmed by appropriate use of the increasingly complex array of available laboratory tests and diagnostic procedures. Treatment may take the form of medications, surgical procedures, therapy sessions, or perhaps just listening in a supportive manner and providing information or reassurance.

Public health and community medicine are also practiced according to the model of diagnosis and treatment. Many of the procedures for gathering the information needed to make a diagnosis or formulate a treatment plan are also highly structured, although the tools are usually quite different from those used in clinical practice. The information-gathering tools are those needed to assess the health status of a community or a large population. They rely heavily on *epidemiology,* which is defined as the "study of the amount and distribution of disease within a population by person, place, and time."[1] The student of community medicine must learn to think in terms of rates of death or disease and must learn how to evaluate reports that compare rates in different populations or at different times. He or she must also learn to evaluate studies that attempt to define the role of various factors influencing the morbidity and mortality of a disease. Treatment in community medicine involves strategies to decrease the negative impact of a disease on the community. There is a major emphasis on prevention, education, and community involvement in programs for lowering the morbidity or mortality associated with a given disease. As in clinical medicine, the treatment must be tailored to the patient. What works in one community may not work in another.

Before the specific tools used in the diagnosis and treatment of community pathology are discussed, it is useful to briefly survey the historical and philosophical context in which all clinicians today are working, whether they choose to pay attention to it or not.

THE STORY SO FAR

Health conditions affecting the public have changed dramatically in this country during the past century, and likewise, our models for thinking about public health have evolved. At the turn of the last century, the United States was essentially a developing nation, in which much of the rural population lacked access to running water, flush toilets, and universal education. The mortality in children younger than 5 years, largely due to infectious diseases, accounted for 34% of all deaths. Only 3% of the population was over age 65 years, and 52% of the population was under age 21.[2] Public health policy focused largely on tracking infectious diseases and enforcing sanitation codes.

By 1970, death from infection in children had become a rarity, owing primarily to improvement in the standard of living, but also as a consequence of technological advances such as antibiotics and immunization. During the remainder of the 20th century, the health problems of greatest concern to the country became chronic diseases (such as cardiovascular disease), cancer, and injuries. The major focus of public health planners comprised the creation of programs for disease prevention, access to health care for underserved populations, and ways to limit the cost of a health care system built around the use of high technology.

PUBLIC HEALTH GOALS

The 1990s witnessed a change in public health priorities as the country transformed into a society based on information transfer and service industries. Many chronic diseases have become manageable to the point that further technological advances are producing less and less benefit in terms of extended life span. We have come to see the causes of illness in our society not as shortcomings of the medical system, but rather as the result of unhealthy lifestyle, stress, dysfunctional behavior, and alienation of large segments of the population, both young and old, from a sense of common societal purpose. Goals such as "health for all by the year 2000," which may have

been within reach on a technological level, have remained distant at the turn of the millennium owing to forces in the physical, social, and cultural environment over which health planners have little control. The most important and most poorly controlled current epidemics are obesity, drug abuse, alcoholism, depression, human immunodeficiency virus (HIV) infection, violence, and family dysfunction. Whereas public health policy in the past concentrated on changing health services to meet the changing needs of the public, authors such as Alan Dever[2] have called for a new strategy, called a "healthy public policy," which seeks to focus health planning on the whole panorama of environmental, behavioral, biological, and health service factors that influence the major illnesses of our times.

Blum,[3] LaLonde,[4] and Dever[5] have argued that analysis of any community health problem must specifically look at the roles played by the environment, lifestyle, human biology, and health services in maintaining a disease dynamic and must address how factors in each of these areas may be altered to reduce the impact of the disease on the community. A graphic representation of this concept is shown in Figure 5-1.

WHOLE SYSTEMS VIEW OF HUMAN HEALTH
Environment

The environment of an individual has a more profound effect on all aspects of a person's health behaviors than has often been attributed in the usual scope of clinical medicine.

Physical Environment   The fetus may be irreparably damaged before birth by chemicals, radiation, or viruses. The environment of a child may include risks from lead or asbestos, busy streets, and neighborhood violence. As adults, we must survive in a world beset by global warming, reduction of the atmosphere's protective ozone layer, and threatened loss of vital portions of the ecosystem.

Social Environment   Children are highly vulnerable to role models in every aspect of behavior, from cigarette smoking to attitudes toward education and career choices. Primary role modeling usually occurs within the family. When the family structure is intact,

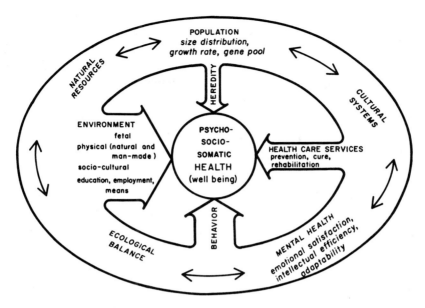

Figure 5-1 The Environment of Health model. (From Blum HL. Planning for health: developmental application of social change theory. Human Science Press 1974;3.)

socialization becomes part of normal child development. The social environment for the child of a fragmented or dysfunctional family may increase the child's risk for disease throughout his or her life. School and work are social environments that either can serve as part of a person's support system or may be major sources of stress and risk for unhealthy interactions.

Psychological Environment Self-esteem is the first casualty for a victim of child abuse, particularly sexual abuse. Low self-esteem, in turn, places the victim at risk for drug and alcohol dependency and for becoming an adult participant in a dysfunctional family in which the risk of child abuse is high.

Lifestyle

Leisure Activities Many Americans face an increased risk of cardiovascular disease because of lack of regular exercise. On the other hand, some forms of exercise can result in avoidable injury. Bicycling without a helmet, for example, places a person at a greatly increased risk for a debilitating head injury,

and other sports, from jogging to skiing, may result in injuries that increase the risk of degenerative joint disease.

Consumption Patterns Smoking cigarettes predisposes a person and those in his or her immediate environment to lung disease, heart disease, cancer, and giving birth to babies with birth defects. Alcohol consumption places a person and friends or immediate family members at risk for motor vehicle accidents and other injuries, family dysfunction, domestic violence, and child abuse. The drinker is also at risk for the medical complications of alcohol abuse, including liver and pancreatic disease, peptic ulcers, neuropathy, hypertension, and malnutrition.

Employment and Occupational Risks Many occupations, such as deep rock mining and farming, carry a high risk of acute and chronic injury as well as death, whereas occupationally related cancers have been directly linked to such jobs as roofing and tire manufacturing. As the United States moves to a service-based and information transfer–based industry, the occupational risks are changing to include more syndromes related to overuse and stress. Low-paying service industry jobs also carry a high risk of inadequate or nonexistent medical insurance.

Human Biology

Many physical and emotional characteristics of an individual are present at birth, and these attributes may either protect someone from or predispose a person to certain disease states.

Genetic Inheritance   Susceptibility to disease and individual reaction to external stresses are determined in many ways by our genetic endowment. For example, some individuals carry human leukocyte antigen (HLA) markers for genetic predisposition to develop diabetes if they are exposed to certain viral infections.

Maturation and Aging   Even when people are protected from preventable disease, the human body tends to deteriorate on multiple levels somewhere between the ages of 75 and 95 years. Yet different organ systems may deteriorate prematurely in patterns that tend to run in families, placing their members at increased risk for dementia, coronary disease, or osteoporosis.

Complex Internal Systems   Different people respond to stress in different manners, which remain characteristic throughout their lives. Some get ulcers and others have asthma attacks, and still others have dermatitis, headaches, or diarrhea, when stress levels exceed their personal thresholds.

System of Medical Care Organization

The medical system is composed of all the facilities and delivery systems available for acute, chronic, and preventive care. This includes all clinics, hospitals, long-term care facilities, and home health care systems.

Fee-for-Service Model   The medical system in the United States has traditionally been built on a fee-for-service (FFS) model, which over the past 40 years has been transformed from a network of individual physicians into a highly competitive arena in which health corporations and large multi-specialty groups

employ a wide spectrum of health providers and market their services to the medically insured. Currently, most Americans are insured through their workplace by third party payers, which in turn contract with large groups of providers to provide services to their patients on a discounted fee-for-service basis. Insurance companies have historically attempted to limit costs by placing restrictions on which providers a patient could see, which tests they would authorize, and which drugs were on the formulary. A new generation of insurance products is now being developed that give patients greater choice in providers but transfer to them a portion of the increased cost associated with particular choices. Insurance companies now offer many different insurance products with co-pays, deductibles, and co-insurance, all of which may vary depending on which provider the patient chooses to see and which drugs the provider chooses to prescribe.[6]

HMOs   Health maintenance organizations (HMOs) contract with groups of patients who prepay for their medical care, usually as an employment benefit or under contract from Medicare. Some HMOs are staff or group model systems in which the providers are paid a salary by the integrated delivery system in which they are employed; however, most HMOs in the early 21st century are merely insurance companies that offer a set of prepaid medical benefits to their enrollees. The HMOs then contract with groups of physicians, who are paid a set fee per member per month to provide whatever services their contract specifies. Although HMOs succeeded in reducing the cost of medical care by reducing the incentive for physicians to provide services for which there may be little proven benefit, in the process they alienated large segments of society by restricting access to care at a time of economic prosperity. In general, staff model HMOs (i.e., integrated delivery systems that receive a global capitation payment for all services that a patient may need) have the strongest motivation to invest in services that have been shown to promote wellness and keep patients healthy.

Community Clinics   For the rising number of uninsured people (many of whom are children), the only place to obtain health care is in the understaffed and underfunded system of community clinics. Health care is usually provided on a sliding fee scale, and services may be limited.

HEALTH CARE SYSTEM ISSUES
Access to Services

All of the preceding systems restrict access and resources. The fee-for-service system restricts access to those with the resources to pay, whereas access to care in HMOs and community clinics is restricted by waiting times for appointments, referrals, and procedures, or by sliding fee scales and co-pay requirements.

Quality Assurance

There are no detectable differences in quality between HMO and FFS medicine. In the 1970s, HMOs had shorter hospitalization times, but federal reimbursement guidelines have put equal pressure on the two systems, eliminating many cost advantages of HMOs.[7]

Cost Containment

Many powerful forces are driving the ever-increasing cost of providing health care in this country:

➤ Although access to health care has not improved since Medicare and Medicaid were enacted in the 1960s, health insurance benefits have been extended to include such services as prescription drugs, mental health care, and alcohol and substance abuse treatment programs. The changing demographic picture of the U.S. population will lead to greater utilization of health care in the future because the increase in the number of elderly will continue well into the next century, pushing overall medical expenditures higher.

➤ Health insurance is, by nature, inflationary, because the cost is not borne directly by the consumer, and both the patient and the provider have an incentive to order more tests and use more resources. Even if the patient is cost and quality conscious, patients have only limited ability to shop for lower prices and to gauge differences in quality.

➤ The technology on which modern medicine is based is very expensive, and it requires the use of highly skilled technicians. A highly paid workforce of allied health professions has proliferated in the wake of each technological advance.

➤ Physicians function in a social context in which both the patients and the medical peer culture expect the high-technology equipment to be used. The incentive for ordering tests is based in part on the widespread practice of defensive medicine, arising from the fear of malpractice suits brought for late or missed diagnoses. All clinicians make decisions with incomplete information because information is expensive and sometimes is obtained at considerable risk to the patient. The number of data points needed to manage an illness depends to an extent on how "risk averse" the clinician is. The higher the clinician perceives the risk to be, the more tests he or she tends to order, regardless of whether the perceived risk is due to the severity of the illness or to lack of rapport with the patient and family. In an environment where fear of litigation is high, more tests are ordered.

➤ In our culture, specialists have a higher status than people with a wide range of skills. In addition, the reimbursement for high-technology procedures (which are almost exclusively the domain of subspecialties) is so high compared with reimbursement for cognitive functions that most medical students currently choose specialty training over primary care fields. Medical training programs are therefore producing an inadequate number of primary care providers. At the same time, there is already an excess number of physicians in many highly paid specialties, some of whom, because of competition, are treating patients and being reimbursed at specialty fee scales for problems that could be treated with equal or greater competence by a primary care provider.

➤ Pharmaceutical companies are insulated from true market competition. Although some pharmacies list prices of common drugs, the ability of most patients to find the lowest price for a given drug is limited, and patients usually play almost no role in the selection of specific medications or brands. Commonly, physicians do not know the prices of the drugs they prescribe. New innovations, such as ePocrates software (available on palm-top computers), allow the prescribing provider to compare costs in the exam room while choosing a medication to prescribe.

➤ The multiple-payer insurance system in the United States is estimated to spend as much as 25 cents of each health care dollar collected on marketing insurance contracts, billing, and other activities not directly related to health care delivery. Countries with national health insurance and a single-payer system have been able to keep analogous costs to less than 10 cents of every dollar.[8]

Several other less powerful forces are operating to keep health costs down. First, prepaid health plans (HMOs) that pay the provider on a capitation basis tend to keep costs down, although the trend appears to be away from capitation. There is some evidence that HMO patients may be more likely than FFS patients to seek preventive services.[9] Second, hospital utilization review departments that have targeted unnecessary hospitalization days have managed to reduce health care costs. Third, diagnosis-related guidelines (DRGs) are a federal reimbursement policy, implemented in the mid-1980s, that sets the Medicare payment for a patient hospitalized with a given diagnosis at the level of the average cost for a patient with that diagnosis, rather than on the basis of costs actually incurred for the particular hospitalization. This policy places the hospital or HMO at risk for any cost overruns, regardless of whether they are due to case complexity or health service inefficiencies.

There is a growing movement in the United States and Europe for patients to carefully examine every aspect of medical care to be sure that it is founded on solid evidence for effectiveness. The standards for evidence-based practice include several grades of evidence, the highest of which is the randomized controlled trial. Many of the diagnostic tests and treatments used in modern medicine make sense physiologically and are based on the experience of experts who may have a subtle bias for high-technology tests and treatments. Yet these characteristics do not necessarily mean that such practices can be shown to be effective.

When randomized controlled trials are conducted, many practices, such as screening for prostate cancer,[10] cannot be shown to make any improvement in the outcomes of patients who undergo them. Evidence-based medicine has provided a framework for evaluating effective practice in medicine, called the number needed to treat (NNT). Using risk ratios obtained from well-designed randomized controlled trials, it is possible to determine the number of people who would have to have their low-density lipoprotein (LDL) cholesterol lowered by a given amount for one life to be saved during the same time frame.[11]

The tools for an evidence-based approach to clinical practice are readily available through such journals as the *New England Journal of Medicine's Journal Watch* or the American College of Physicians' *Journal Club*. One way to obtain the number needed to treat for a practice in question is to use one of the British evidence-based web sites such as Bandolier at http://www.jr2.ox.ac.uk:80/bandolier/. Such resources provide crucial support to many primary care groups seeking to improve outcomes and lower the cost to patients by restricting diagnostic and treatment strategies to evidence-based practices whenever possible.

It must be remembered that the bulk of the expenditures for health care in the United States is used to provide the salaries for people who work in the health industry. If costs are reduced, people in the health industry will be laid off, whether they are insurance clerks, health administrators, or health professionals. Any effective plan for reduction of health care costs must consider the complex interaction between the health industry and the U.S. economy as a whole.

DIAGNOSTIC TOOLS IN COMMUNITY MEDICINE

All the diagnostic tools of community medicine are based on observations. Observations by individuals are important in forming impressions about patterns of disease. Because each clinician encounters a relatively small number of cases, whether of injuries or of a particular illness, one must be careful to confirm one's observations using information derived from the surveillance of large segments of the population. Much of the information on which community diagnoses are based comes from regular publications of federal, state, and local government agencies that constantly monitor and distribute their observations to anyone who is interested. Such reports are usually available not in journals, but rather from the source agency, and the existence of reports on specific subjects can often be determined through a phone call to the agency. People who work in public health departments, especially at the state or local level, are usually delighted that a practitioner is interested in their reports, and many times, a single phone call uncovers several new local sources of information. Examples of relevant information sources include the following:

➤ *Morbidity and Mortality Weekly Report,* a publication prepared by the U.S. Public Health Service Centers for Disease Control and Prevention and printed by the *New England Journal of Medicine.*

➤ State department of health bulletins and reports.

➤ County department of public health bulletins and reports.

➤ Tribal health boards, native health corporations, migrant health boards, and other agencies dealing with minority populations.

➤ Research and policy groups, commonly comprising university-based researchers and state or county health planners.

➤ Departments of public health in state universities

Often, relevant observation for community diagnosis consists of noticing occurrences in one's own community that might be ignored by most people but to the observant practitioner may lead to an important diagnosis. Thus, a clinician may find himself or herself in a position to work with community leaders to point out a pattern of preventable disease that was previously overlooked, as is demonstrated in Case Study 5-1.

CASE STUDY 5-1

In the mid-1970s, an observant pediatrician working in a community clinic in Seattle became concerned about the number of children he was seeing with tap-water scalding burns. The first question he had to answer was, "How big a problem is this?" He went to two sources. The first was the National Electronic Injury Surveillance System, which is maintained by the U.S. Consumer Product Safety Commission and monitors product-related injuries in 119 hospital emergency rooms throughout the country. The pediatrician discovered that in 1975, there were an estimated 543 tap-water scalds in children under 15 years of age in the United States that were serious enough to be seen in an emergency room. Of these, 32% required hospitalization. The second source was a chart review of Children's Orthopedic Hospital and the regional burn unit at Harborview Hospital to determine the severity and circumstances of the scalding requiring hospitalization. The review revealed that tap-water scalding in children tended to be more extensive than other scalding, and it was associated with a mortality rate of 12.5%. In 45% of tap-water scalds, the victim or a peer turned on the tap, and of those cases in which an adult turned on the tap, 60% involved child abuse. The pediatrician and his colleagues also performed a home survey to determine the average temperature of water heaters in the homes of the community. They found that the average temperature was 142° F, which is sufficient to cause a full-thickness scald in an adult in less than 6 seconds.

This group began working with the local utility and the media to increase public awareness of the importance of reducing water heater temperature in order to prevent scalds. They were able to work with child safety groups to help legislators in Washington and other states enact laws to require that new water heaters be preset at 120° F.

A follow-up study done in 1991 showed that the average temperature of hot water in homes had been reduced to 122° F. (At this temperature, it takes more than 2 minutes to cause a full-thickness scald.) Meanwhile, the admission rate for tap-water scalds in children at Children's Hospital and the Harborview Burn Unit had fallen by 56%, and no children had been admitted with full-thickness burns.[12, 13]

The key to success in the preceding example lies in demonstrating that the observed pattern of injury was due to specific factors that were elevating risk; it was not simply a random variation or bad luck. This meant that the risk factors could be identified and altered. In the following discussion, several basic tools are described that are used in community medicine to compare observations so that we can draw meaningful conclusions.

Basic Statistical Measures

The sophisticated, if somewhat jaded, U.S. consumer has come to view statistics as a tool for supporting or distorting nearly any point of view. There is no question that statistical data can be misused to give erroneous impressions, but in community health, there is usually no better tool for measuring the health status of a large group of people or for documenting baseline conditions and measuring change. For this reason, statistics is the cornerstone of modern epidemiology. Any practitioner with a basic understanding of measures of disease and awareness of some of the common pitfalls for misinterpretation can learn to evaluate the deluge of articles, studies, and reports at his or her disposal.

The statistical tools discussed here are descriptive. Much of what a community health practitioner does is compare descriptive data from two or more groups and apply statistical tests to determine whether the differences are statistically significant, that is, whether the differences observed are greater than could have reasonably occurred by chance alone. In this chapter, statistical analysis is not discussed. The student interested in a greater understanding of biostatistics is encouraged to pursue the subject through other sources.

Descriptions of a Population   When one describes a population of people, measures of continuous variables, such as age, income, and test scores, can be divided into indices of central tendency (the middle value) and indices of variation (how closely the values are clustered around the central value).

Indices of Central Tendency   The most useful indices of central tendency are the mean (the average value), the median (the 50th percentile), and the mode (the most common value). When a population is distributed in a symmetrical or bell-shaped curve, the mean, the median, and the mode are all the same, as is shown in Figure 5-2. An example of such a distribution is serum calcium values for a population of normal people. When a population of values is not a bell-shaped curve as shown in Figure 5-2, the mean, median, and mode are different. This is so because outlying values at either end of the range pull the mean, but exert no corresponding influence on the median or the mode.

Indices of Variation   Commonly used indices of variation are range (the difference between the highest and lowest values) and standard deviation (the average distance all the measured values are from the mean). The range tells only the highest and lowest values and tells nothing about how closely the

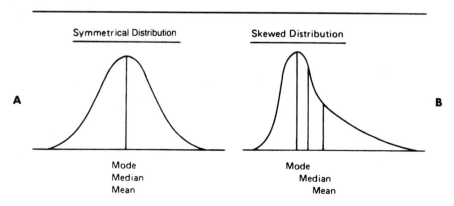

Figure 5-2 Bell-shaped curve *(A)* and skewed distribution *(B)*. *(From Morton RF, Hebel JR, McCarter RJ: A Study Guide to Epidemiology and Biostatistics, ed 4. Gaithersburg, MD: Aspen Publishers, 1996;50. Reprinted with permission from Aspen Publishers, Inc., ©1996.)*

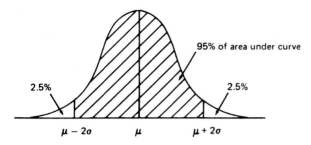

Figure 5-3 Normal distribution with standard deviations. *(From Morton RF, Hebel JR, McCarter RJ. A Study Guide to Epidemiology and Biostatistics, ed 4. Gaithersburg, MD: Aspen Publishers, Inc., ©1996.)*

values are clustered around the mean, although it is easy to measure. Standard deviation is not a number that is easily calculated without a computer, but it is important to understand. A small standard deviation means that the values are tightly clustered around the mean, and a large standard deviation means that the values are spread out. When the distribution is a bell-shaped curve, 95.4% of the values are within two standard deviations (2SD) of the mean, as is shown in Figure 5-3.

Use of Indices   Using these indices, one can give a meaningful description of a population, such as is provided in Case Study 5-2.

CASE STUDY 5-2

If we wish to describe a small Alaskan village with a population of 125, we might find that the mean age is 20, the median is 15, and the mode is 8, with a range of 3 months to 75 years. This says that there are more 8-year-olds than any other age group, half of the people are age 15 or younger, the average age is 20, the youngest person is 3 months, and the oldest is 75 years of age.

Rates and Ratios

Measures of Mortality One of the ways used to describe the health of a group of people is to count the number of deaths during a given period of time, usually 1 year. In order to compare groups, it is essential to standardize the size of the denominator and speak, for example, of the number of deaths per 1000

people. This is called the *crude mortality rate* (CMR). It is calculated as follows:

$$CMR = \frac{\text{All deaths in a calendar year}}{\text{Population at mid-year} \times 1000}$$

$$= \text{deaths per 1000}$$

The CMR depends heavily on the age composition of the population. The CMR in a wealthy retirement community may be very high compared with that of a poor inner city population composed mostly of young people.

A much clearer picture of the health status of a population may be obtained by examining the *age-specific mortality rate* (i.e., the mortality rate for each age group). The crude mortality rate may obscure the health status of certain age groups that are doing better or worse than the population as a whole. An extreme example is shown in Table 5-1. It is apparent that although the CMR for whites is higher than that for blacks, the age-specific mortality for blacks is higher for each age group. The answer to this puzzle lies in the fact that the white population is old and the black population is relatively young. Therefore, a death rate of 59.7 per 1000 among whites older than 65 years is equivalent to a large total number of deaths because the elderly white population is large. The black population is mostly young, so the total number of blacks who die each year adds up to fewer deaths per thousand; because the death rates for younger people are usually considerably lower than those for the elderly, within each age stratum, blacks are more likely to die than whites.

It is usually useful to break down (stratify) mortality rates by sex to obtain the *sex-specific mortality rate* because males often have higher mortality rates than females.

Mortality rates may also be stratified by cause. *Cause-specific mortality rate* is defined as follows:

$$\frac{\text{Deaths due to a certain cause in a calendar year}}{\text{Population at mid-year}} \times 1000$$

Thus, one can talk about the mortality rate for sudden infant death syndrome (SIDS), which in Washington State, was 24 per 1000 in white children, 48 per 1000

Table 5-1	Mortality Rates per 1000 People by Age and Race in Baltimore, 1972						
Race	**All Ages**	**<1 Yr**	**1-4 Yr**	**5-17 Yr**	**18-44 Yr**	**45-65 Yr**	**>65 Yr**
White	15.2	13.5	0.6	0.4	1.5	10.7	59.7
Black	9.8	22.6	1.0	0.5	3.6	18.8	61.4

From Morton RF, Hebel JR, McCarter RJ. A Study Guide to Epidemiology and Statistics, ed 4. Gaithersburg, MD: Aspen Publishers, 1996:22. Reprinted with permission from Aspen Publishers, Inc., ©1996.

in Native American children, and 53 per 1000 in African-American children in 1988.[14]

Because not all cases of a disease result in death, it is often useful to describe mortality in terms of the *case fatality ratio,* which is defined as

$$\frac{\text{Number of deaths due to a disease in a specified period}}{\text{Number of cases of the disease in the same period}} \times 100$$

This is a useful measure for describing infectious disease. For example, the case fatality ratio for rabies is quite high. Whether it constitutes a major public health issue depends on the incidence of the disease.

Incidence and Prevalence

Incidence is the number of new cases that occur during a given time. It is expressed as a rate, such as the number of cases per 1000 people at risk for the disease. Incidence says nothing about either how long a person has the disease or the outcome of the disease.

An estimated total of 343 cases of newly diagnosed acquired immune deficiency syndrome (AIDS) were reported in King County, Washington, during 1997.[15] If the total population at risk during the year was 1,652,775, the incidence would be calculated as follows:

$$343/1,652,775 \times 100,000 = 20.8 \text{ per } 100,000$$

Incidence does not tell how many people have the disease at any point because it doesn't count those who were alive with previously diagnosed disease, nor does it tell how long any affected person has had the disease.

Prevalence refers to the number of people with a disease at a given point in time *(point prevalence).*

Prevalence can also be used to refer to the number of people with a disease during a certain period *(period prevalence).* In both cases, prevalence is expressed as the number of cases over the population at risk for the disease. Prevalence cases include both cases that begin during the measurement period and those already present when the measurement period began.

At the end of 1997, there were 2095 people with AIDS living in King County. The prevalence of AIDS in 1997 was therefore

$$2095/1,652,775 = 126.8 \text{ per } 100,000$$

Incidence and prevalence are related because the number of people with a disease is a function of how many people acquire the disease and how long they have it:

$$\text{Prevalence} = \text{Incidence} \times \text{Duration}$$

It is convenient to think in terms of a "prevalence pot." A member of the population goes into the pot by becoming an incident case (i.e., getting the disease) and is removed from the pot either by dying or by recovering from the disease. In many situations, if one knows the incidence and average duration of the disease, one can calculate the disease prevalence. Because both the prevalence and the incidence are given in our example of AIDS cases in King County, the duration of illness can be calculated. People do not recover from AIDS, so the average time from diagnosis to death is calculated as follows:

$$\begin{aligned} \text{Duration} &= \frac{\text{Prevalence}}{\text{Incidence}} \\ &= \frac{126.8/100,000}{20.8/100,000} \\ &= 6.1 \text{ years} \end{aligned}$$

Risk Factors, Relative Risk, and Attributable Risk

To know the average risk of acquiring a particular illness, it is necessary to look no farther than the incidence of the disease. Many times, however, a clinician may wish to explain how a particular behavior, such as smoking, places the patient at increased risk for a disease, such as cardiovascular disease. The medical literature is full of estimates of how exposure to such risk factors may increase one's risk. The clinician's job is to understand what these measures of risk mean and to be able to explain them intelligently to patients.

If a man is at twice the risk of having a heart attack because of smoking cigarettes, he has a *relative risk* of 2. Thus

$$\text{Relative risk} = \frac{\text{Incidence among exposed}}{\text{Incidence among non-exposed}}$$

Table 5-2 illustrates this concept by showing the death rate among men from coronary disease for smokers and nonsmokers. The relative risk for smokers is 4.45/2.22 = 2.[16] The risk for male nonsmokers depends on other risk factors, such as age, hypertension, cholesterol level, and family history. The risk from smoking multiplies the risk from other risk factors. A man with a positive family history of cardiovascular disease and hypertension who smokes is multiplying his risk of death from coronary disease by 2; the smoker without other risk factors is multiplying his lower risk by the same relative risk.

Table 5-2   Death Rates for Smokers, Ex-Smokers, and Nonsmokers

Risk Category	Death Rate, 1000 Person-Years
Nonsmokers	2.22
1-2 pack/day smokers	4.45
Ex-smokers	2.44

From Ockene JK, Kuller LH, Svendsen KH, Meilahn E. The relationship of smoking cessation to coronary heart disease and lung cancer in the multiple risk factor intervention trial [MRFIT]. Am J Public Health 1990;80:954.

If, however, the question is how much of the risk is due to smoking, it is important to understand the *attributable risk*, which can be defined as follows:

$$\text{Attributable Risk} =$$
$$\text{Incidence among exposed} - \text{Incidence among non-exposed}$$

If a smoking cessation program is successful and a group of men reduce their risk from 4.45/1000 to 2.44/1000 by quitting, the Attributable Risk of continuing to smoke is 4.45 − 2.44, or 2.01. This means that 2.01 deaths per 1000 men per year can be prevented if they all quit smoking. The Attributable Risk of starting to smoke in the first place is 4.45 − 2.22, or 2.23 deaths per 1000 men per year.

Basic Epidemiological Methods

When gathering data for making a diagnosis of pathology in a community, one must describe the characteristics of morbidity just as one would describe a clinical case when presenting it to an attending physician. The basic parameters by which the distribution of a disease within a population is described are person, place, and time. This is true for an acute outbreak of an infectious disease, as well as for chronic diseases such as AIDS, diabetes, and coronary insufficiency.

Demographics: Who Is Affected?

Just as a clinical presentation begins with the age and sex of the patient, in community medicine, it is important to define whom one is speaking about. The most commonly used variables for describing a population are age, sex, ethnic background, and socioeconomic status. For example, Figure 5-4 shows the age and sex distribution for people with AIDS in the United States in 1990.

It may be useful, depending on the context, to use other characteristics to describe who is affected once the risk factors for the disease are known. For example, Figure 5-5 categorizes who is affected with AIDS according to the factors that placed them at risk for the disease.

Location: Where Are the Affected People?

Maps are one of the most efficient methods for showing location. In the case of a common disease such as

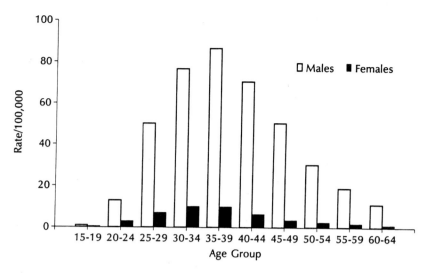

Figure 5-4 Acquired immune deficiency syndrome (AIDS): annual rates per 100,000 adult population, by selected age group and sex for reported cases, United States, 1990. *(From MMWR 1991;39:16.)*

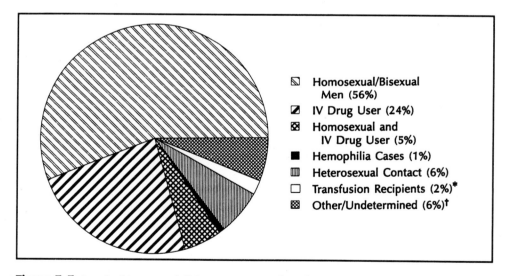

Figure 5-5 Acquired immune deficiency syndrome (AIDS): reported adult/adolescent cases, by exposure category, United States, 1990.

*This category includes 14 transfusion recipients who received blood screened for HIV antibody and one tissue recipient.

† "Other" refers to four persons who developed AIDS after exposure to HIV-infected blood within the health care setting, as documented by evidence of seroconversion or other laboratory studies. "Undetermined" refers to patients whose mode of exposure to HIV is unknown. This category includes patients under investigation; patients who died, were lost to follow-up, or refused interview; and patients whose mode of exposure to HIV remains undetermined after investigation. *(From MMWR 1991;39:16.)*

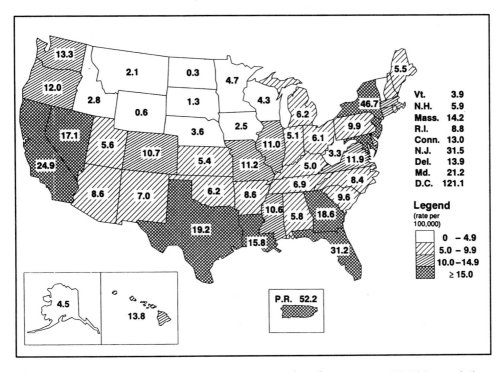

Figure 5-6 Acquired immune deficiency syndrome (AIDS): cases per 100,000 population, reported to the Centers for Disease Control by state, United States, 1990. *(From MMWR 1991;39:17.)*

AIDS, it may be useful to display the rates by state, as shown in Figure 5-6. For rare diseases, however, it may be more informative to use a smaller unit of area, such as in Figure 5-7, where the number of cases (in this instance, it is not a rate) for Rocky Mountain Spotted Fever is shown by county.

Time: When Does the Disease Occur?   The pattern by which the incidence or prevalence of a disease varies over time may give a considerable amount of information about how well controlled the disease is. Figure 5-8 shows the steady increase in incidence of AIDS. The lower number of "known dead" in 1989 and 1990 is the result of:

1. The fact that the persons reported for these years have not had the disease as long as those reported for earlier years.
2. The availability of aggressive treatment of opportunistic infections and prophylaxis regimens for

prevention of *Pneumocystis carinii* pneumonia that have extended the life expectancy of people infected with HIV.

Other diseases have temporal patterns that reflect the dynamics of risk factors for the disease. Arboviral encephalitis rates rise during the late summer months because of the life cycle of the mosquito, which serves as the vector for disease transmission. Small-plane crashes in Alaska are more common in September because of risks associated with overloading small floatplanes on hunting trips.

Looking for Disease: Screening Programs

Criteria for Screening   Screening programs are used to identify asymptomatic individuals with a specific disease who are otherwise indistinguishable from normal healthy people. Screening tests are not designed to be diagnostic, but rather to identify people on whom diagnostic testing should be done. Mass

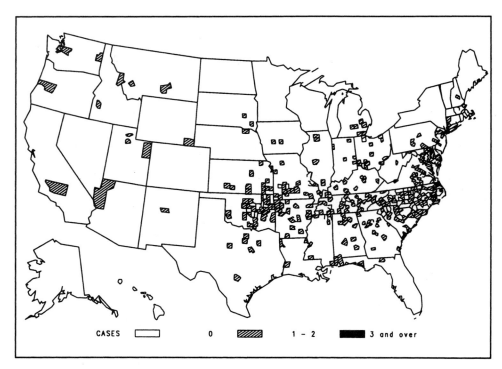

Figure 5-7 Typhus fever, tick-borne (Rocky Mountain spotted fever): reported cases by county, United States, 1990. *(From MMWR 1991;39:50.)*

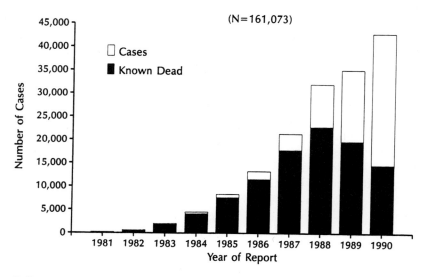

Figure 5-8 Acquired immune deficiency syndrome (AIDS): cases and known deaths, by year of report to the Centers for Disease Control, United States, 1981-1990. *(From MMWR 1991;39.)*

screening is done on a large general population, such as when cholesterol testing is performed in shopping malls, or it can be done by a clinician on the patients who come in for a physical examination, in which case it is often referred to as "case finding."[17] In either situation, screening is appropriate only when the following three conditions are met:

1. The disease being screened for should be an important cause of morbidity or mortality.
2. A relatively safe screening test or procedure should be available at a reasonable cost that can detect the disease at an early stage.
3. A treatment for the screened condition must be available that is acceptable to patients and more effective when the disease is identified at an asymptomatic stage.

Examples of diseases for which screening programs have been established are breast examination and mammography for breast cancer, Pap smears for cervical cancer, and Hemoccult screening for colon cancer. On the other hand, screening for lung cancer with periodic chest radiographs has been abandoned because early detection was found to make no difference in survival.

Sensitivity and Specificity   The utility of a screening test is determined by comparing it with some definitive, more costly or more risky diagnostic test (such as a biopsy), called a "gold standard," which is used to determine whether the patient has the disease. The ability of a screening test to identify a person who actually has the disease is called its *sensitivity.* Sensitivity is defined as follows:

$$\frac{\text{Number of people with the disease detected by the screening test}}{\text{Number of people with the disease who were tested}} \times 100$$

If the sensitivity of a test is high, it can detect most cases of the disease. If, for example, the enzyme-linked immunosorbent assay (ELISA) test for HIV antibody has a sensitivity of 99.5% for every 1000 people screened who are infected with the virus, 995 will be detected using this test. It is important to note that sensitivity tells nothing about the false-positive

results, that is, the number of times a test is positive in people who do not have the disease.

Specificity, on the other hand, refers to the ability of a test to determine that a person does not have the disease. Specificity is defined as follows:

$$\frac{\text{Number of people without the disease detected by the screening test}}{\text{Number of people without the disease who were tested}} \times 100$$

If the specificity of a test is high, a large percentage of patients with a negative test result do not, in fact, have the disease. It is important to note that specificity says nothing about the number of false-negative results, that is, the number of times a test is negative in people who actually have the disease.

For example, if the specificity of the ELISA test for HIV is at least 99%, as many as 10 of every 1000 patients screened will have positive test results, owing in all likelihood to cross-reactivity with antibodies to other antigens, even though they do not have HIV. In order to identify these people with false-positive results (those without the virus), who at this point cannot be distinguished from those with true-positive results (those with the virus), it is necessary to run a confirmatory test called the Western blot analysis. The Western blot by itself is no more specific than the ELISA, but it tests for different antigens. Positive results on both tests constitute virtual certainty of HIV infection. In general, the more specific a test is, the less sensitive it becomes. The more confident one is that someone with a negative test result does not have the disease, the greater will be the chance that the test missed someone with the disease. The opposite is also true. The more confident one is that a test has identified a person who truly has the disease, the greater will be the chance that the test has also falsely identified people who do not have the disease.

Predictive Value   What a clinician really wants to know about a test is, if the result is positive (or negative), what is the probability that the patient does (or does not) have the disease? In other words, what is the predictive value of a positive or negative test result? If a test is very sensitive, the predictive value of a negative result is high because the test has a high percentage of true-positive results and, presumably, a relatively large number of false-positive results. People who test negative are quite unlikely to have the disease, so the predictive value of a negative result is high. It is analogous to wanting to catch all fish down to a certain size with a net. If you make the holes in the net smaller than the size of the desired fish, you can be relatively confident that very few fish of the proper size will get away, but the net will also catch a number of fish that are too small (false-positive). If a fish has made it through the net, you can predict with a high degree of certainty that the fish was smaller than you wanted.

If the specificity of a test is high, the predictive value of a positive result is high. In this case, the holes in the fish net are set larger than the desired size of the fish. The net therefore misses some of the acceptable fish, but you can predict with a high degree of certainty that any fish that is caught will be of adequate size.

Still, the predictive value of a test depends on more than simply its sensitivity and specificity. It also depends on the prevalence of the disease in the population being screened. In the simplest example, if one were to screen a population in which no one had the disease, all the positive results would be false-positive, and the predictive value of a positive result would be zero, regardless of the test's sensitivity or specificity. On the other hand, if one were to screen a population in which everyone had the disease, all the negative results would be false-negatives. The higher the prevalence of a disease in a population, the higher the predictive value of a positive screening test result. The lower the prevalence of a disease, the greater the predictive value of a negative result.

This is the reason that exercise electrocardiogram (ECG) (treadmill) testing is of value in the workup of middle-aged men with exertional chest pain, in whom the prevalence of coronary artery disease is between 80% and 90%.[18] On the other hand, exercise ECG testing is not useful as a screening test in asymptomatic middle-aged men, such as airline pilots, in whom the prevalence of coronary artery disease is relatively low, perhaps 1%. In the symptomatic man,

the predictive value of a positive result is 98%, and that of a negative result is more than 80%. In the asymptomatic airline pilot, although the predictive value of a negative result is 99%, the positive predictive value of a positive result is only 16%, that is, a positive result is right only 16% of the time.[19]

Probability Theory and Normal Laboratory Tests Laboratory test results are usually expressed in relation to a normal range of values. This normal range is usually agreed upon as that range in which 95% of normal values fall. If the normal range were set to include 99% of normal values, it would also be more likely to include some values that indicate the presence of a disease. Agreeing on a 95% range for normal values assumes that 5% of results in normal people for any given laboratory test will fall outside the normal range. This means that when a panel of 12 or 24 tests is run on a single patient, very commonly at least one result falls slightly outside the normal range just by chance alone. The first step in following up an abnormal laboratory test result is usually simply to repeat the test.

The same situation applies to blood pressure monitoring. The values that have been set as the upper limit of normal are probably exceeded in most people at various times during the day. Probability alone produces a chance of an abnormal value when a person's blood pressure is tested. This is one of the reasons it is necessary, after obtaining a high blood pressure reading, to repeat the test using a sphygmomanometer on at least three separate occasions before subjecting the patient to the expense, inconvenience, and risk of antihypertensive medication.

TREATMENT IN COMMUNITY MEDICINE

As was stated in the beginning of this chapter, the paradigm of data gathering, making a diagnosis, and then formulating a treatment plan is applied to community medicine, just as it is to the treatment of individual patients. The diagnosis must be correct for the treatment to be effective, but without an emphasis on treatment, studies of disease and injury patterns are nothing more than intellectual exercises that have little to do with improving the health of the community. The optimal treatment strategy for a given condition depends not only on the problems, but also on the available individual and community resources. Community health care treatment can be divided into three general categories:

1. Micro-level treatment, that is, interventions that are carried out through the one-on-one interaction between a health care provider and his or her patients.
2. Community-level treatment, in which an entire community is stimulated to mobilize its local resources in order to change the local environment in a way that reduces morbidity and mortality.
3. Macro-level treatment, in which public policy decisions are made and legislation is enacted in response to a perceived health threat.

Each of these strategies is important. Different people have different skills and therefore tend to focus their efforts in one or two of these categories, but all three categories are important and must be used if a community is to benefit from an intervention.

Public Health Treatment on a "Micro" Level

Talking With Patients   The way a practitioner talks with his or her patients, and what is talked about, is one of the most valuable tools available for public health intervention by clinicians. Clinicians are used to thinking in terms of telling patients what they should do to get better: take this medication, stop smoking, drink less, lose weight, and get more exercise. This approach may be effective for some people who are waiting for their health care provider to tell them, but usually, being told what to do one more time is not sufficient to successfully change a dysfunctional lifestyle issue with which the patient has been struggling unsuccessfully for years.

Several strategies may be more effective. First, the best way to be heard is to listen. The practitioner should ask a patient first what he or she thinks is the problem and then about what has worked and what has not worked. It is surprising what one may learn. Most patients can be talked to as one might talk to a highly educated brother or sister with expertise in a nonmedical field. One should use common words and explain in detail using pictures and visual images.

Second, when discussing an illness, the practitioner should think of the factors in the environment that made the illness or the injury more likely to happen. He or she should then explain how these factors work and what the patient could do to reduce the risk. As the saying in Iowa goes, "If you plant corn, what you get is corn." If children are sent out in the sun to play without sun protection, they become adults with sun-damaged skin who are at high risk for skin cancers.

Third, it is important to appreciate and communicate the importance of the appropriate timing for an intervention. The Iowa corn saying continues, ". . . but you don't get corn tomorrow." The sunburned children will not have skin cancer tomorrow, but rather after they grow to be adults. Likewise, a clinician may struggle to think of creative ways to discuss HIV and safe sex with teenagers who come to the office for treatment of acne. He or she may tell parents that they need to discuss sexuality and AIDS with their teenagers at home. All of that is important, but clinicians also need to be discussing with parents of an infant how to establish patterns of communication with their child at an early age, so that the child learns that his or her own thoughts, questions, and fears are taken seriously by the parents and that he or she is respected as an individual. The parents need to be helped to see that by starting in the child's infancy, they are building the micro-environment that will determine how their child makes decisions when he or she does not have an adult to turn to for guidance.

Most of what effective clinicians do on a micro-level involves planting seeds and trying to encourage their patients to think globally about the health issues that concern them and their families on a local level. This is much better done in a personal style than by lecturing (e.g., by asking parents how they deal with their children's television watching rather than lecturing them on how TV is bad for children). It is possible to talk about research that demonstrates a clear relationship between the amount of violence watched on TV and violent behavior in susceptible adolescent males, particularly in households without a nurturing male adult role model.[20] Ideas can be shared, such as saying that some parents have tried setting a limit on the amount of TV watching equal to the amount of time the child is read to aloud by a parent. This type of information needs to be offered as ideas rather than dogma for it to have a chance to grow.

Occasionally, there are potential emergencies, such as a depressed teenager living in a house in which guns are present. Situations like this need to be handled carefully, with respect for all people involved and all points of view, but with a clear understanding of the magnitude of the risk.

Working preventively one-on-one with patients can be highly effective on a small scale and, when amplified by many practitioners, can have a tremendous cumulative effect. It is a treatment method in which all clinicians can participate, and it has the added advantage of improving the relationship between clinicians and their patients.

The Importance of Being a Role Model   Health care providers are role models. This is most obvious in a small community, where people may wait to see how much the new provider drinks before deciding how much he or she can be trusted. This type of scrutiny makes many health care workers uncomfortable, and anonymity is part of the attraction of an urban practice. Yet even in a large city, the PA or physician is a role model, either a good one or a bad one. This fact can play an important part in creating an environment in which the norm is for bicycle riders to wear helmets and for adults to discourage children from smoking.

Public Health Treatment on a Community Level

It is common for a health care provider to begin as an outsider in the community in which he or she works. Whether to an Alaskan Native village, a rural small town, or a suburban clinic, most physicians and mid-level practitioners move to a new community to take a job. The position as an outsider is an excellent opportunity to see things that might be taken for granted by residents, but it also raises the issue of community ownership of a problem.

What is seen as a problem by the outsider, however, may be more complex from the perspective of community members, and the politics of the community may not be immediately understandable to the newcomer, as is shown in Case Study 5-3.

CASE STUDY 5-3

A new physician assistant is concerned about the rate of alcohol use in an Alaskan village and its effect on child neglect and domestic violence. She decides to devote her energy to building a coalition in the town to help the town "go dry," that is, outlaw the possession of alcohol in town. She is successful, and during the next year, the consumption of alcohol drops. However, during the same period, three young people die from drowning and hypothermia while smuggling liquor from a town 50 miles upriver. The PA learns that similar "accidents" also occurred the last time the town was "dry." Members of the community council owned the town liquor store. Liquor sales accounted for a large percentage of the money used to fund several important social services, including home health for senior citizens. After the town goes dry, the balance of power and cooperation is altered. Social services are reduced, and the community council becomes more polarized than it had been in the past.

Solutions that come from within the community are generally better than those imposed from outside. In the United States, the Lone Ranger represents an archetypal figure for problem solving, and Americans from all points on the political spectrum tend to create situations in which they want to ride into town, shoot the bad guys, and then ride out on a white horse, expecting everyone to thank them. This scenario presents several generic difficulties. Even if a solution is just what everyone agrees was needed, reliance on an outside hero figure encourages dependency, rather than fostering a sense in the community of an ability to solve problems. In addition, the community members have to continue living there with the side effects of the treatment, to which an outsider is often oblivious. A constructive process for a health care provider to follow can be divided into the following steps:
1.   Observe and verify the existence of important patterns of disease and injury.
2.   Using as many community sources of information as possible, construct a model of the disease

dynamic that includes the environmental, lifestyle, biological, and health service factors that may influence the impact the problem is having on the community.

3. Make a list of all the community groups that must participate in any workable solution. Omissions at this stage can spell political disaster for otherwise well-intentioned projects. The list usually includes many of the following components, and almost certainly others as well, depending on the nature of the problem being addressed and the characteristics of the community:

   a. *Federal, state, and local health departments.* Not only are these agencies often reliable sources of preexisting health information, but they may also be able to describe what efforts have already been made to solve a given health problem.

   b. *Service organizations.* Groups like the Elks, the Veterans of Foreign Wars, and the Chamber of Commerce often have considerable power in a community regardless of its size, and they are usually interested in health-related issues. Their members may have ideas about how to fit a health intervention project to the town. If there is political opposition to your ideas, you need to maintain a cordial alliance with the service organizations and attempt to find solutions that meet their needs.

   c. *Community groups.* Church groups, parent and teacher organizations, neighborhood councils, and consumer groups are similar to service organizations in their importance in designing a community health intervention. Most such groups can offer insight into the problem and can envision the right solution for the community.

   d. *Media.* In small communities, the media consist of newspapers and perhaps radio. In large communities, they may also include television. All are important in gaining the confidence of the community once a plan is formulated that meets the needs of all concerned.

   e. *Key individuals exist in every community.* These are people to whom community members and leaders listen because they have credibility. They may or may not be included in the groups already described, but they often need to be specifically sought out.

4. Serve as a facilitator for the communication of ideas. The job of a health care provider may be less one of offering a treatment than of persuading community members to think about the problem and begin working together to solve it. The mark of the expert facilitator in this situation may be that when the project is completed, the community members believe that they did it themselves, without anyone's help.

Public Health Treatment on a "Macro" Level

If health care providers are to broaden their purpose to include the creation of a healthy public policy, they must begin to view the arena in which public policy is made as an appropriate forum for implementation of preventive health strategies. The major components of this involve helping to change public opinion and influencing the decisions of policymakers. In general, public opinion drives policy decision making, and any effort to change public policy must be based on widespread public support. Public opinion is not, however, automatically translated into public policy because decision makers tend to respond to the wishes of the voting electorate less often than to the financial contributions of election financiers, who may view their own interests as a higher priority than the health of the public. An example of such a dynamic can be seen in the legislative resistance to gun control in the United States despite strong epidemiological evidence that the availability of handguns is a key factor in high homicide and suicide rates and the fact that nearly 70% of the U.S. public favors some form of control on handguns and automatic assault rifles.[21]

Any health problem for which risk factors can be identified, and that is amenable to prevention, can be approached from a number of possible directions. To reduce the mortality from house fires, for example, one might decide to invest the resources of the community in more firefighting crews or to require smoke detectors in all homes and sprinklers in all new homes. Before deciding how to commit limited resources, it is important to be able to evaluate the effectiveness of different strategies.

The study of injuries that follows here serves as a useful illustration of how thinking about preventive health strategies can be organized. The same principles can be applied to other situations in which public policies affect disease.

Automobile injuries, for instance, can be thought of as consisting of three phases, as shown in Table 5-3:
1. Pre-crash phase.
2. Crash phase.
3. Post-crash phase.

In each of these phases, four elements are at work:
1. Host (human) factors.
2. Vector (vehicle).
3. Physical environment.
4. Socioeconomic environment.

The examples given in the table for each of these categories are far from exhaustive but serve as an illustration. It can be appreciated that a campaign to reduce death and injury from motor vehicle crashes must be carried out on multiple levels simultaneously, and that many of the factors affecting each phase of the crash are best dealt with by legislative bodies. Money must be appropriated to improve road condi-

tions, to install adequate traffic signals, and to enforce speed limits and drunk-driving laws. The costs of passive restraints, antilock brake systems, and gas tanks that will not rupture must be borne by the buyers of new cars, or else the costs of death and injury fall on society as a whole and disproportionately on the victims of preventable mishaps.

Just as in the example of preventing tap-water scald injuries in infants, interventions that need only passive involvement of people, such as requiring that manufacturers of hot water heaters preset them at a lower temperature, are more dependable than measures that necessitate active involvement, for the simple reason that compliance with passive-type measures is automatic. For example, air bags and antilock brake systems require no driver involvement in order to work, but they are expensive. On the other hand, seat belts are inexpensive, yet to be effective they must be attached each time a person gets into a car; use of seat belts varies greatly, depending on local laws and public attitudes.

There is at times a clear conflict between individual choice and public health. The laws that may be required to reduce injuries and their associated costs to society often infringe upon the individual liberties of citizens.[22] This concept is illustrated in Case Study 5-4.

Table 5-3	Injury Matrix			
Phase	**Host Factors**	**Vector**	**Physical Environment**	**Socioeconomic Environment**
Pre-crash	Experience ETOH/Drugs Vision	Brakes, tires, speed, load, controllability	Visibility Road condition Signals	Alcohol laws Speed limits Safe driving
Crash	Safety belt Osteoporosis	Speed and weight Restraints Contact surface Load containment	Guard rails Embankments Median barriers	Attitude enforcement about seat belts and child seats
Post-crash	Age Physical condition	Fuel system integrity	EMS distance and quality Rehabilitation	Support for trauma center, EMS personnel

From National Committee for Injury Prevention and Control. Injury prevention: meeting the challenge. Am J Prev Med Suppl 1989;5:8.
EMS, Emergency medical services; *ETOH,* ethyl alcohol.

Between 1966 and 1975, all states except California, Illinois, and Utah adopted laws mandating that motorcyclists wear helmets, on the basis of overwhelming evidence that helmets reduce the risk of death and serious injury in a crash. When the federal government in 1975 tried to withhold highway safety funds from the non-compliant states, Congress prohibited the use of such methods of ensuring that states enforce helmet use, and as a result, many states rescinded their helmet laws. Opponents of helmet laws argued that the State has no right to force "responsible behavior" on a citizen if the behavior affects no one else. Proponents of helmet laws point to statistics such as a $107 billion national price tag for injuries during the year 1985, a cost that is borne by society as a whole through increased insurance rates and use of Medicare and Medicaid funds. The cost of lost productivity as a result of injuries and death is not included in this figure.

Solutions to this and other complex problems can be very difficult for all members of society to agree upon. For this reason, it is useful to ask, "What would be the healthy public policy regarding the issue?" In many cases, this question is not asked. The community health care practitioner can play many roles in formulating a healthy public policy, and most of them involve asking the right questions in an effort to educate the public and the policymakers.

POPULATION-BASED MANAGEMENT OF CHRONIC DISEASE

Occasionally, one encounters an aspect of medical practice in which the economic interests of patients, providers, third party payers, employers, and pharmaceutical companies all appear to be aligned. In contrast to the more common scenario in which (due to shrinking resources) innovations such as new medications or new methods for payment tend to pit one part of the medical community against the others, disease management, at first glance, would appear to be a winning concept for everyone. Take diabetes, for example. If an innovative way of providing care to a defined population of patients with diabetes were to result in improved outcomes, everyone would appear to benefit. The delivery system would be reimbursed for providing additional services to achieve lower average blood sugars, blood pressures, and lipids; patients would experience lower rates of heart attack and kidney failure; employers would experience less sick leave; third party payers would have lower expenses for hospitalization and dialysis to offset the additional payments to primary care; and pharmaceutical companies would sell more drugs for glycemic control, hypertension, and hyperlipidemia. The same concept should apply to patients with heart disease, patients with asthma, and those with other chronic conditions.

Because of the attractiveness of these arguments to purchasers, payers, and federal policy agencies, disease management has become a popular concept in many parts of the health care system. Most disease management work has been focused on chronic illness. The basic concept involves an organized approach to a large number of patients (a population) with a particular medical (usually chronic) condition. The goal of disease management efforts is to develop systems for delivering health services that bring interventions supported by medical evidence to all members of the population, while monitoring outcome measures in order to track improvement within the population.

Needs That Must Be Addressed in Caring for Patients With Chronic Illness

The needs of patients with chronic illness, who by definition cannot expect to be cured, are as follows:

1. They must engage in activities that promote health and build physiologic reserve, including exercise, nutrition, social activities, and sleep.
2. They must interact with health care providers and systems, and must understand and adhere to recommended treatment protocols.
3. They must monitor their own physical and emotional status, and make appropriate management decisions on the basis of symptoms and signs.
4. They must manage the impact of their illness on their own ability to function in important roles,

on their emotions and self-esteem, and on their relationships with others.

At the same time, the medical delivery system needs to:

1. Assure delivery of those interventions (evaluations and treatments, both medical and psychosocial) that have been shown by rigorous evidence to be effective.
2. Empower patients to take responsibility for the management of their conditions.
3. Provide information, support, and resources to assist patients in self-management tasks.[23]

The greatest challenge for providers is to keep track of all the patients and to make sure that they are regularly monitored over long time intervals so that changes in their health status can be detected.

Population-based disease management began in single-payer systems in Europe and in staff model HMOs in the United States, where the concept of investing in organized systems of care for high-risk populations in order to prevent expensive treatments later made obvious economic sense.[24] During the 1990s, after years of evaluating successes and failures of efforts to manage different chronic illnesses, researchers in the United States developed a conceptual framework that identified the components of a program that need to be in place for disease management efforts to be effective.[25] The goal in chronic illness care is to ensure that planned productive interactions take place between activated patients and a proactive medical team so that patients receive the medical care and self-management support they need to slow disease progression and minimize preventable complications.

The Model

There are four essential components of programs for chronic illness care. The first is an information system in the form of a registry of all patients with the chronic condition so that patients who may have fallen through the cracks and are overdue for monitoring or intervention can be easily identified. The second is a system of decision support, including evidence-based guidelines for all providers to follow, and point-of-care reminders to help providers remember chronic illness tasks that need to be done when patients come into the clinic for any reason. The third

is people whose job it is to follow through on the important clinical tasks identified by the guidelines and the information system. These include bringing patients in for tests that are overdue, changing medications regimens when necessary, and working with patients to support them in addressing the four needs identified previously. It has become clear that physicians are simply too busy trying to keep up with the demands of ambulatory care to be expected to take on the complex task of chronic illness care. The fourth component is linkage to community-based organizations that provide support to patients with chronic illness such as the American Diabetes Association, State and County Health Departments, religious organizations, and so forth.[26]

The Challenge

Most delivery systems don't have a registry, and in a mixed-payer environment, most office practices find that there is no way to be reimbursed for many of the tasks involved in chronic disease management. Consequently, many medical practices are lacking in functional programs for chronic illness care and disease management. As a result, third party payers have begun to move into the vacuum by starting disease management activities of their own. Although it is true that insurance companies are under pressure to reduce costs by preventing hospitalizations, it is not clear which types of disease management efforts actually reduce cost. Pressure on third party payers comes in the form of increasing scrutiny from purchasers (employers), which use published performance measure report cards, including clinical outcomes, over which the insurers have limited control.[27] Increasingly, third party payers are concluding that they cannot wait for the countless small practices with which they contract to develop systems to better manage chronic illness outcomes. The net effect is that health insurance companies have started to become involved in providing medical care directly to patients outside of the medical groups with which they have contracted to provide care.

The insurance companies attempt to improve chronic illness care in several ways. First, by using claims data, they create and send reports to physicians listing the patients in the physician's practice covered by the particular insurance company. These reports show the physician how he or she is doing in caring for the insurance company's patients who have a specific chronic illness, which is usually only a fraction of the total number of patients a physician has with that disease. Second, third party payers often contract with national disease management companies, which employ nationally centralized nurses who contact patients by telephone in an effort to help them manage their chronic illness. This creates a number of inefficiencies and often tends to undermine the efforts of provider groups to develop and run quality improvement programs for their own patients because it diverts resources for medical care away from medical practices. These practices negatively impact chronic illness care in the following ways:

1. The claims data on which insurance company information is based are 2 to 3 months old and are severely limited in clinical detail. Although these reports may be better than having no data at all, they are inferior in both timeliness and accuracy to clinical reports that could be generated from within a delivery system.
2. Clinical reports provided by payers are by nature fragmented from the perspective of the provider because they discuss only the patients of a particular insurance company. Providers may be given a list of two or three patients from one insurance company but have no total list of all their patients with a chronic illness. Physicians often throw these reports away because of their limited utility.
3. When payers contract with one or more national disease management companies (many patients have more than one chronic disease), the patient will have multiple health care personnel, giving often mixed messages in efforts to manage overlapping medical conditions, thereby leading to fragmentation of medical care.
4. Carve-outs to disease management companies reduce the money the payer has to support primary care, which undermines the already precarious economic base for the primary care system. At worst, this could lead to a situation in which, much like some mental health plans, a primary care provider will not be reimbursed for treating the carved-out illness because the resources for that aspect of medicine have already been paid to a national disease management company.

In many ways, population management of chronic illness within a medical practice is a perfect example of applying public health principles to clinical medicine; so it is ironic that public health principles, which have been ignored by much of the medical profession for so many years should be brought to clinical medicine as part of the corporate takeover of health care in the United States. One solution is for delivery systems to rapidly develop their own internal disease management programs and contract with third party payers to provide disease management activities that include all of the essential components of the model described earlier.[28] Because clinical data from within the delivery system will be more accurate than claims data, and because the clinical follow-through will be an integral part of primary care instead of competing with it, such "carve-in" programs will be more efficient and will lead to better outcomes than "carve-outs." Reimbursement for this work is generally tied to measurable clinical outcomes; therefore, chronic illness care programs, in order to be financially viable, will have to be clinically effective.

The Roles of PAs

Some physician assistants confuse disease management with case management and mistakenly assume that participation in chronic illness care is nursing work that physician assistants should not be asked to do. Physician assistants have always brought a wide array of backgrounds, interests, and skills to their profession, and they have used their flexibility to respond to opportunities throughout the health care system. There are many ways in which physician assistants can play major roles in disease management, and there are just as many reasons why PAs might find this area of medical care to be rewarding.

1. PAs often have highly developed computer skills and are able to participate in the medical informatics side of population medicine by helping to design and run the databases, disease registries, and clinical reports on which a disease management program is based.
2. Many of the follow-up clinical tasks needed by patients with heart disease, diabetes, or asthma

require changing medications to get lipids, blood pressure, or bronchospasm under better control. Unlike registered nurses (RNs), to whom this work has often been given, PAs have authority to change medications to bring physiological outcomes under better control. Also unlike RNs, PAs can be reimbursed for counseling patients in all aspects of self-management support.

3. Much of this work can be done in a way that augments the productivity of physician assistants and increases their value to the delivery system. When visit volumes are down, an up-to-date list of patients who need to be reminded to come in for better control of blood sugar, blood pressure, or lipids can serve as a way to fill appointments with patients who will clearly benefit from the visit.

4. Medical practice is rewarding and challenging in many ways, but it not usually a place to express one's need for creativity. Designing new ways to deliver care to entire populations of patients with common conditions such as diabetes, asthma, heart disease, osteoarthritis, osteoporosis, HIV/AIDS, frailty, or depression can serve as a creative outlet that many PAs may find to be a "big picture" counterbalance to the one-on-one rapid pace of ambulatory care.

5. Although there is little evidence to show that physicians or physician assistants change their clinical practice based on what is presented in formal continuing medical education (CME) lectures, there is growing evidence that clinicians really learn and change their behavior when they become involved in clinical quality improvement programs on a local level.[29,30] Chronic illness care programs use clinical improvement methodology that monitors outcomes, tests new ways of delivering care, and makes better clinicians out of those who are doing the work.

INTERDISCIPLINARY TEAMS

It has long been appreciated that physicians and other providers working in clinical isolation face extraordinary challenges in maintaining current medical standards of practice and preventing career burnout.[31,32] The most striking examples of this are seen in rural settings, yet even in most group practices and large clinics, physicians often remain in significant clinical isolation, usually working with a single nurse or medical assistant. Even in settings where there is a high degree of clinical communication between providers, individual physician practices are at a major disadvantage in the simultaneous management of multiple, complex workload streams.

Primary Care Workload Streams

It is useful to think of the work of primary care as occurring in three different workload streams, all of which compete for the busy clinician's time and energy, and all of which must be carefully managed if patients are to receive the highest quality of care. The three streams are acute episodic care, chronic care, and preventive care. *Acute care* refers to the approximately 60% of primary care situations in which a patient seeks an office visit, the sooner the better, for assistance with a new or recurrent problem that requires diagnosis and treatment, which either resolves or stabilizes over a finite period of time and sometimes results in death. *Chronic care* pertains to the ongoing management of conditions for which there is no cure, often involving a common final pathway for organ system malfunction, and for which complications arise over time. *Preventive care* is the proactive effort to reduce morbidity and mortality outcomes in conditions for which the periodic use of screening, vaccination, education, and behavior change techniques has been shown to be effective.

In the office setting, the work of these three streams is occurring simultaneously on any given day in any given patient, and as such, they compete for the attention of the busy provider. Some of this work, particularly the preventive care stream, can be automated. Computers have increased the ease with which it is possible to send reminders to patients when screening tests and vaccinations are due. Physician accountability for specific quality of care, service, and cost outcomes may increase motivation to improve performance in managing the three workload streams simultaneously, but it does not make the job any more possible to do in a busy office practice.

Five Characteristics of Successful Interdisciplinary Teams

In 1994, the Bureau of Health Professions released the findings of a task force that studied the use of interdisciplinary teams in health care. Task force members identified five characteristics of successful interdisciplinary teams[33]:

1. Team members provide care to a common group of patients.
2. Team members develop common goals for performance outcomes and work together toward these goals.
3. Appropriate roles and functions are assigned to each team member. Members understand and respect the roles of others.
4. All members contribute and share essential information about both tasks and group process.
5. The team has a mechanism to assure that plans are implemented, services are coordinated, and performance of the team is evaluated.

Experience from other industries suggests that certain conditions in a work environment can move an organization from simply talking about teams to actually promoting high-performance teams (wisdom of teams):

1. Significant performance challenges energize teams, regardless of where they are in an organization.
2. A strong performance ethic promotes teams more effectively than does a team-promoting environment alone.
3. Biases toward individualism need not get in the way of team performance.
4. Discipline within the team and across an organization creates optimal conditions for team performance.

Team Structure and Function

There is no universal structure for a primary care team. The structure of a team should match not only the functions that the team must perform but also the time commitment and skill level of individuals on the team. An example of a simple team structure might be one physician, one PA, one licensed practical nurse (LPN), and one medical assistant (MA). At the small end, teams start to become indistinguishable from individual physician practices and therefore achieve none of the efficiency of teams. An example of a complex team might be two physicians, two PAs, one registered nurse, two LPNs, and two MAs. Teams larger than 8 to 10 individuals start to encounter limitations imposed by group dynamics, which may make communication, agreement on norms, and decision making less efficient than for smaller-sized teams. Regardless of the configuration, a team's success in meeting performance goals will depend on how clearly those performance goals are defined and how well team members internalize the previously listed five characteristics of successful teams.

One of the crucial functions that a team must perform is to meet regularly, usually weekly. This requires physician leadership in the setting of priorities and delegation of tasks. The team meeting is where the work of the team is planned. Someone, and not necessarily a physician, must keep the agenda and run the meetings. Although some variation is to be expected, there is a natural progression of priorities as a new team forms. The first task for a team is to establish norms for such things as meeting times, work schedule, interpersonal communication, time off, and other ground rules for working together. In general, the stronger the physician leadership and the more explicit the agreements on norms at the beginning of a team's existence, the easier it will be for the team to devote its full combined energy to the work of providing high-quality health care to its patients.

Once a team has defined itself and established its norms, the overriding priority becomes getting control of the acute episodic care workload stream. Until a team becomes adept at managing the work of providing high-quality acute care with excellent service, any major efforts to organize the chronic care work will be wasted. The task of providing access for acute care is complicated by economic demands of the health care environment to reduce costs in order to remain price competitive. For a primary care team, the demand to keep costs down translates directly into a greater patient load with increased demand for acute episodic care, regardless of whether a team is working in a totally managed care system or in a mixed fee-for-services/capitated network model. One of the greatest challenges for physicians in an interdisciplinary team, therefore, is to learn how to delegate clinical tasks to other team members and then be readily available for clinical supervision, teaching, and backup for those team members to whom clinical tasks are delegated.[34]

The team's work of delivering medical services to a large group of patients can be understood as a number of highly organized processes involving multiple team members. These work processes lend themselves to methods for process improvement that have been developed in other industries and adapted to health services by Berwick and others.[35,36] For example, a team in which each provider works with his or her "own" medical assistant may find that there is less overall wasted time (and therefore a potential for improved performance) when one medical assistant rooms patients for two providers. This may require synchronizing the two providers' schedules so that two patients are less likely to arrive simultaneously. Once this change is made, the second MA may have time to perform tasks for which previously there was no time, such as reviewing records to see which patients are not up-to-date with immunizations or screening tests. In order for this change in work process to succeed, the team may find it necessary for both providers to agree on common ways of rooming patients because reducing variation in provider styles will make the work of the medical assistant more efficient. In fact, without reducing variation of provider style, it may not be possible for the MA to room patients for both physicians without an increase in wait times and reduced service quality.

At each step in a process improvement change, it is essential that the team keep clearly in mind the goal it is trying to accomplish, seek out innovations that have a good chance of resulting in improvement, and then find simple objective ways of measuring the improvement.[37] The interdisciplinary primary care team has as its challenge the task of learning new skills necessary to become a cohesive working unit while improving the processes of health service delivery, and doing so with a significantly larger population of patients than physicians have historically managed by themselves.

Interdisciplinary Primary Care Teams

Physician assistants play a crucial role in establishing and maintaining a smooth flow of acute episodic care for a team, without which any major work on chronic disease management is premature. Of major importance then is the understanding by PAs of several key aspects of the relationship of physician assistants to the physician and other team members. The relationship between physician assistants and physicians in an interdisciplinary team involves the simultaneous use of three specific roles on the part of the PA: the substitution role, the supplementary role, and the complementary role.[38]

Substitution Role   Research over the past 30 years has established that physician assistants can diagnose and treat somewhere between 80% and 90% of medical problems that present to a primary care practice without concurrent supervision. Furthermore, PAs can achieve levels of clinical quality and service outcomes that are indistinguishable from those of a physician and can substitute for a physician in providing the majority of acute episodic care.[39] That is not to say that PAs can replace physicians at a 5:1 ratio. Rather, unless the team elects to triage only a limited scope of practice to the physician assistant, it must plan for up to 20% of cases seen by a PA to require some presentation of the case to the team physician while the patient is in the clinic. This is called concurrent supervision and does not usually require more than 2 or 3 minutes of physician time, but the skills necessary for this kind of supervision must be perfected as a team process.[40] In addition to concurrent supervision, the team must have a mechanism for retrospective supervision by which certain types of cases seen by a physician assistant are reviewed at specified intervals by a team physician. Lastly, team discussion of clinical cases should provide a forum for review of evidence supporting different types of diagnostic and therapeutic strategies; this approach guides the PA in a form of prospective supervision, as the different providers on a team converge on a common, evidence-based practice style.

Supplementary Role   Although there may be some advantages to having a PA manage "easier cases" while a physician has more time for "difficult cases," there are reasons why this type of supplementation should be kept to a minimum. First of all, it is not usually possible to accurately triage patients by disease complexity, and efforts to do so commonly result in conflict between providers and the person doing the triage. In addition, efforts to give physicians more time for more difficult cases often work better in theory than in practice and may lead to inadequate time for concurrent supervision. The increase in perceived workload on the part of physicians has the potential to increase tensions between team members.

A more flexible type of supplementary role involves establishing a team norm. If any provider is involved with a time-consuming complex case, the other providers on the team will support the team practice by providing clinical backup and by seeing patients on the schedule of the provider who is running late. This keeps the impact of complex cases on the team's service quality at a minimum. By supplementing each other's access capacity, the team members can reduce the variation in service quality that is common in any medical practice. In order for this approach to work, all team members must fully understand the attributes of highly functioning teams, spelled out by the Bureau of Health Professions Task Force, which were discussed previously.

Complementary Role

It is entirely natural for different providers to develop different areas of interest and expertise. Physician assistants who pursue clinical skills that complement those of the physicians on their team become a resource that increases the team's collective value. The successful team will learn to encourage and then rely on a PA who spends time learning skills and gaining knowledge in specialty areas in which the physicians on the team may feel particularly weak. Physician assistants have traditionally performed this role in orthopedics, but in any given team, the areas of greatest physician discomfort, often seen in high levels of specialty referral, are particularly fruitful places for PAs to develop complementary roles.

Coming Full Circle—Back to Chronic Care

As a team begins to perfect the job of managing the acute care workload stream and to achieve the kind of service quality outcomes that patients are now demanding of their providers, the opportunity will present itself for the team to expand its attention to include management of chronic disease. This is understood as the most efficient way to improve clinical quality outcomes. Many of the nationally recognized quality indicators are directly tied to chronic disease outcomes,[41] and providers almost universally are easily enthused about medical advances that have been shown to result in improved outcomes for their patients.

Team Approach   The work of chronic care management belongs to the team as a whole and requires the understanding and involvement of all team members. Individual tasks may lend themselves to one team member or another with skills such as database management or teaching. One of the crucial steps in managing a chronically ill population is building a computerized registry to hold information the team uses to identify which patients have met specific criteria for optimal medical management and which have not. Maintaining the registry and searching it for patients to bring in for specific tests or treatments can be done by nursing staff with computer skills.[42]

Deciding on the diagnostic and therapeutic criteria that must be met for patients to be optimally managed is a job that falls to experts in the evaluation of evidence-based guidelines. The team physicians and physician assistants may participate in such planning, but even if they do not, they need to lead the team's efforts to implement those standards. For example, a team physician should review all patients with heart failure to see which should have a cardiac echocardiogram.

Much of the work in chronic disease management involves teaching patients disease management skills and coaching them in behavior modification, such as weight loss, smoking cessation, and regular exercise. Nurses have usually received extensive training in this type of work, and teams may find it a natural nursing role. On the other hand, group visits for patients with specific conditions, such as frail elderly at highest risk for falls and hip fractures, may reflect a multidisciplinary effort involving physical therapists and pharmacists, as well as the team nurse and physician or PA.[43]

Threats to Team Performance   Efforts to introduce programs for organized chronic disease management can be undermined by rewarding efficiency with more work, such as giving a team more patients as a reward for managing many patients well. The most powerful driver for this dynamic is the tremendous pressure for competition solely on the basis of cost because many of the cost reduction benefits of chronic disease management in most cases will be realized only several years in the future. For this reason, the leadership of an organization must ensure that the "significant performance challenges" it provides for its teams include not only those related to short-term cost performance. The leadership must also ensure that adequate emphasis is given to the creation of high-quality clinical performance challenges to reward teams that manage chronic diseases in a way that is likely to reduce future costs.

An example of this is a performance challenge to have all patients with diabetes screened for microalbuminuria as an early marker for diabetic renal disease. Renal failure can be prevented in such patients by initiation of low-dose angiotensin-converting enzyme (ACE) inhibitors or alternative medication. The effort invested by teams in perfecting processes that result in 100% of appropriate diabetics being screened will lead to major reductions in cost for end-stage renal disease; yet the savings from the additional work may be evident only years after the screening and preventive treatment are begun.

Instability within a team is another threat to the management of multiple workload streams. Whenever one team member is replaced, or the team is reconstituted, there is a natural consolidation of effort to get the acute care work back in control. During this phase, chronic care may slow considerably or even stop. A team should plan for a change in performance when such a personnel change occurs, but it is in the interest of all parties for instability in primary care teams to be reduced to a minimum. The leadership of a health care delivery system must do everything in its power to protect highly functioning teams from avoidable turmoil.

THE FUTURE OF PUBLIC HEALTH PERSPECTIVES IN MEDICINE

The emergence of terrorism as a significant threat to the health of the U.S. public has created a new role for public health in modern medicine, one that is at the center of plans for improving the security of citizens of this country. The threat of bio-terrorism, which emerged in the wake of September 11, 2001, represents a major challenge to public health officials across the country. The list of organisms that could be used for bio-terrorist attacks includes bacteria such as anthrax, which historically caused limited albeit often lethal outbreaks in agricultural communities, and other viruses or bacteria such as rubella and *Yersinia pestis,* which historically were responsible for pandemics that shaped human history over thousands of years. What these diseases have in common is that they can be easily spread to humans in the crowded conditions of today's urban environments, and they are diseases for which effective vaccinations either have not been developed or have been allowed to lapse owing to a sense of complacency following a general improvement in health due to socioeconomic growth over the past century.

Although a bio-terrorist attack will usually unfold at a significantly slower pace than say a truck bomb or a passenger airplane flying into a crowded office building, there is in both cases an early phase of the attack if it is recognized, during which damage and mortality can be greatly reduced in much the same way that the passengers who stormed the cockpit of the hijacked airplane heading for Washington D.C. on September 11th reduced the potential mortality of that attack. In the case of bio-terrorism, the challenge is to be able to identify an act of bio-terrorism as early as possible, and before the organism has been widely disseminated in the public. Unfortunately, the prodromal symptoms of most organisms of use to bio-terrorists are similar to those of common viral infections. The first clue that a bio-terrorist attack has occurred may be the deaths of multiple individuals in a suspicious clustering. By then, if a highly contagious organism such as smallpox or Ebola virus has been used as a weapon, the infection may already have been spread to thousands of other people.

The growing use of electronic medical records around the country offers the potential for a symptom surveillance system, which would use data mining techniques that have been developed in the nuclear industry and the airline industry to identify patterns that represent aberrations in the normal background activity of highly complex enterprises. Data mining applied to data streams from primary care and emergency facilities across the country should allow researchers to describe the normal patterns of respiratory illness throughout the year, with predictable peaks due to known epidemics such as influenza and respiratory syncytial virus. Against the backdrop of a normal pattern, a cluster of symptoms occurring in a dozen different clinics in different health care organizations situated within 5 miles of an international airport in a major metropolitan area could be identified as a potential act of bio-terrorism within hours, instead of taking days to suspect an abnormal illness pattern, as would probably be the case today.

One added benefit of such a surveillance system would be the ability of public health researchers to look for unexplained patterns of such things as child vehicular injuries associated with certain home address zip codes, rather than waiting for an alert emergency room physician to identify a pattern and then perform the detective work described in Case Study 5-1. It is entirely possible that new patterns of injury and illness that we have not yet considered may emerge from such a surveillance system of the health of the public.

CONCLUSION

The transition of medicine to a world in which there are major financial incentives for keeping patients well has occurred at a time when computerized information systems are making possible new approaches for the optimal management of chronic diseases. To take full advantage of this new environment, primary care professionals will need to restructure how medical services are delivered. Gradually, the world of health services appears to be changing from one in which individual doctors provide care one-on-one to a limited number of patients, to a world in which physician-led interdisciplinary teams will provide a wide array of services to populations of patients. To the fullest extent possible, the activities of teams of the future will be founded on evidence-based interventions, while their performance will be closely monitored by team members themselves as they seek to constantly improve their outcomes as measured by clinical quality, service quality, and cost.

CLINICAL APPLICATIONS

1. Contact your local health department officials (city or county), and ask them to provide you with information about their process for handling "reportable diseases." Obtain the list of reportable diseases for your state. Discuss with the health department staff the compliance of health care professionals in reporting these diseases and the issues of maintaining patient confidentiality in dealing with these cases.

2. Design a PA job description that incorporates the concepts of population-based care for specific populations (e.g., the frail elderly, pediatric diabetic patients, high-risk athletes with recurrent injuries). Include in your job description the appropriate clinical and technological skills that are needed to efficiently and effectively manage the population.

3. Think about the parts of your medical practice that are computerized that could be used as data sources for a registry of all the patients in your clinic who have diabetes. Is the billing system computerized? What about laboratories? If you were to create an Excel spreadsheet to follow these patients to make sure that all of them had had all of the tests for diabetes that are recommended by the American Diabetes Association guidelines, what additional data would you need besides things that are already in electronic format. Can you think of a way to get that information into a registry?

REFERENCES

1. Mausner JS, Bahn AK. Epidemiology: An Introductory Text. Philadelphia: WB Saunders, 1974.
2. Dever GEA. The pursuit of health. Soc Indicators Res 1977;4:475.
3. Blum HL. Planning for Health: Developmental Application of Social Change Theory. New York: Human Sciences Press, 1974.

4. LaLonde M. A New Perspective on the Health of Canadians. Ottawa: Office of the Canadian Minister of National Health and Welfare, 1974.

5. Dever GEA. Community Health Analysis: Global Awareness at the Local Level. Gaithersburg, MD: Aspen Publishers, 1991.

6. Robinson JC. Renewed Emphasis on Consumer Cost Sharing in Health Insurance Benefit Design. *Employers are demanding and insurers are offering insurance products with higher deductibles and co-payments, to offset premium increases.* Health Affairs 2002; March 20.

7. Stern RS, Juhn PI, Gertler PJ, Epstein AM. A comparison of length of stay and costs for health maintenance. Arch Intern Med 1989;149:1185.

8. Woolhandler S, Himmelstein DU. The deteriorating administrative efficiency of the U.S. health care system. N Engl J Med 1991;325:1316.

9. Retchin SM, Brown B. The quality of ambulatory care in Medicare health maintenance organizations. Am J Public Health 1990;80:411.

10. Selley S, Donovan J, Faulkner A, et al. Diagnosis, management, and screening of early localized prostate cancer. Health Technol Assess 1997;1:1.

11. Rembold CM. Number-needed-to-treat analysis of the prevention of myocardial infarction and death by antidyslipidemic therapy. J Fam Pract 1996;42:577.

12. Feldman KW, Schaller RT, Feldman JA, McMillon M. Tap water scald burns in children. Pediatrics 1978;62:1.

13. Erdmann TC, Feldman KW, Rivara FP, Heimbach DM, Wall HA. Tap water burn prevention: the effect of legislation. Pediatrics 1991;88:572.

14. The State of Washington's Children: June 1991 Report. Washington Child Health Research and Policy Group.

15. Washington State/Seattle-King County HIV/AIDS Epidemiology Report: December 19, 1997. Seattle, WA: Seattle-King County Health Dept, 1997.

16. Ockene JK, Kuller LH, Svendsen KH, Meilahn E. The relationship of smoking cessation to coronary heart disease and lung cancer in the multiple risk factor intervention trial (MRFIT). Am J Public Health 1990;80:954.

17. Fletcher RH, Fletcher SW, Wagner EH. Clinical Epidemiology. Baltimore: Williams & Wilkins, 1988.

18. Diamond GA, Forrester JS. Analysis of probability as an aid in the clinical diagnosis of coronary artery disease. N Engl J Med 1979;300:1350.

19. Ellestad MH. Stress Testing: Principles and Practice, ed 3. Philadelphia: FA Davis, 1986.

20. Comstock G, Strasburger VC. Deceptive appearances: television violence and aggressive behavior. J Adolesc Health Care 1990;11:31.

21. Luftin C, McDowall D, Wiersema B, Cottey TJ. Effects of restrictive licensing of handguns on homicide and suicide in the District of Columbia. N Engl J Med 1991;325:1615.

22. The National Committee for Injury Prevention and Control. Injury prevention: meeting the challenge. Am J Prev Med Suppl 1989;5:8.

23. Wagner EH, Austin BT, Von Korff M. Organizing care for patients with chronic illness. Mil Quarterly 1996;74:511.

24. Lasker RD, et al. Improving the Quality and Cost-Effectiveness of Care by Applying a Population Perspective to Medical Practice. Medicine and Public Health: The Power of Collaboration. The New York Academy of Medicine, 1997, pp 77-89.

25. Wagner EH. Chronic disease management: what will it take to improve care for chronic illness? Eff Clin Pract 1998 Aug-Sep;1:2.

26. VonKorff M, Gruman J, Schaefer JK, Curry SJ, Wagner EH. Collaborative management of chronic illness. Annals of Internal Medicine 1997;127:1097.

27. Schauffler HH, Brown C, Milstein A. Raising the bar: the use of performance guarantees by the Pacific Business Group on Health. Health Affairs 1999;18:134.

28. Staker LV. Changing clinical practice by improving systems: the pursuit of clinical excellence through practice-based measurement for learning and improvement. Quality Management in Health Care. 2000;9:1.

29. Parochka J, Paprockas K. A continuing medical education lecture and workshop, physician behavior, and barriers to change. J Contin Educ Health Prof 2001 Spring;21:110.

30. Goldberg HI, Wagner EH, Fihn SD, Martin DP, Horowitz CR, Christensen DB, Cheadle AD, Diehr P, Simon G. A randomized controlled trial of CQI teams and academic detailing: can they alter compliance with guidelines? Jt Comm J Qual Improv 1998 Mar;24:130.

31. Forti EM, Martin KE, Jones RL, et al. Factors influencing retention of rural Pennsylvania family physicians. J Am Board Fam Pract 1995;8:469.

32. Dunlap DA. Resource networking in rural health education: strategies to reduce professional isolation and promote collaboration in health education. Health Educ 1984;15:40.

33. Interdisciplinary Health Care Teams in Practice. Washington: U.S. Department of Health and Human Services, 1995.

34. Stuart ME. Changing clinical practice: messages, messengers, and methods. HMO Pract 1996;10:100.

35. Berwick DM. Eleven worthy aims for clinical leadership of health system reform. JAMA 1994;272:797.

36. Berwick DM. A primer on leading the improvement of systems. Br Med J 1996;312:619.

37. Langley G, Nolan K, Norman C, et al. The Improvement Guide: A Practical Approach to Enhancing Organizational Performance. San Francisco: Jossey-Bass Publishers, 1996.

38. Starfield B. Primary Care: Concept, Evaluation, Policy. New York: Oxford University Press, 1992.

39. Health Technology Case Study: Nurse Practitioners, Physicians, and Certified Nurse-Midwives: A Policy Analysis. Washington: Congress of the United States, Office of Technology Assessment, 1986.

40. Usatine RP, Nguyen K, Randall J, et al. Four exemplary preceptors' strategies for efficient teaching in managed care settings. Acad Med 1997;72:766.

41. Toward the development of uniform reporting standards for managed care organizations: the Health Plan Employer Data and Information Set (Version 2.0). Jt Comm J Qual Improv 1993;19:566.

42. Griffin S, Kinmonth AL. Diabetes care: the effectiveness of systems for routine surveillance for people with diabetes. In: Williams R, Bennett P, Nicolucci A, et al (eds). Diabetes Module of the Cochrane Database of Systematic Reviews [database on disk, CD-ROM, and online; updated 01 December 1997]. The Cochrane Collaboration; Issue 1. Oxford: Update Software, 1998. [Updated quarterly.]

43. Province MA, Hadley EC, Hornbrook MC, et al. The effects of exercise on falls in elderly patients: a preplanned meta-analysis of the FICSIT trials. Frailty and injuries: cooperative studies of intervention techniques. JAMA 1995;273:1341.

RESOURCES

Dever A. Community Health Analysis: Global Awareness at the Local Level. Gaithersburg, MD: Aspen Publishers, 1991. *Dever's book on community health analysis brings to life many of the statistical principles on which epidemiology is founded, by presenting these tools in the context of improving the lives of people in communities around us. His new book,* Improving Outcomes in Public Health, *also from Aspen Publishers, is an updated version that includes new concepts such as evidence-based medicine and the latest quality improvement techniques from clinical medicine. He does this from a public health point of view, which is a unique and valuable perspective.*

Von Korff M, Grumman J, Schaefer J, Curry SJ, Wagner JJ. Collaborative management of chronic illness. Ann Intern Med 1997;127:1097. *The work that these pioneers in population-based medicine are doing at the Group Health Center for Health Studies is reshaping the way we think about the structure and function of primary care practice. This is one of many articles by these authors that spell out the principles by which patients can be encouraged to participate in the management of their own diseases, in ways that help providers improve the quality of outcomes at lower costs.*

Sackett D, Richardson S, Rosenberg W, Haynes B. Evidence-Based Medicine: How to Practice and Teach EBM. London: Churchill-Livingstone, 1997. *This is the best practical book on the theory and practice of evidence-based medicine for the busy clinician, particularly when there is an opportunity to teach. It makes understandable the basic tenets of applied epidemiology such as NNT and risk ratio in a way that leaves the reader inspired and enthused. The book also provides an introduction to finding evidence-based resources at the fingertip of any clinician with access to the worldwide web.*

The Improvement Guide: A Practical Approach to Enhancing Organizational Performance. Langley, Nolan, Nolan, Norman and Provost. San Francisco: Jossey-Bass Publishers, 1996. *Nolan and others have taken some of the most important principles of quality improvement from many industries and distilled their lessons in a way that can be of tremendous value to leaders in health care who are seeking positive change from within the health profession.*

CHAPTER 6

Ethical Issues

Martin L. Smith

INTRODUCTION

The provision of health care during the second half of the 20th century and now into the 21st century has undergone significant changes. Medical discovery and technology have created new opportunities to extend human life both at its beginning and at its end. A greater emphasis on patient autonomy and participation in health care decision making has caused a shift in the professional/patient relationship from a dominant model of paternalism to one of partnership. At the same time, malpractice suits and fear of legal liability have contributed to greater suspicion and mistrust between health care profession-

als and their patients. Escalating costs and decreasing reimbursement for care have made finances a major consideration, not only in administrative offices but also in patient rooms. Diseases such as acquired immune deficiency syndrome (AIDS) have dramatically changed the way health care professionals relate to their patients and perform routine procedures such as physical examinations and blood tests. Debates about human cloning for therapeutic purposes, tissue banking, and the potential uses of embryonic stem cells have created additional ethical complexities in research endeavors aimed at clinical applications.

For any health care professional, including the physician assistant (PA), this changed landscape of health care delivery has produced a multitude of challenging and sometimes puzzling ethical situations and dilemmas. Some of these dilemmas are as ancient as the Hippocratic oath ("What I may see or hear in the course of the treatment . . ., I will keep to myself. . . ."). Others are as new as the latest technological innovation or research protocol that created the dilemma (e.g., should a patient with Parkinson's disease be treated with stem cells taken from cryo-preserved embryos?). Some ethical issues may arise because working relationships have gone wrong (e.g., the PA's physician-supervisor may be impaired or may ask the PA to do something illegal). Others may arise because of personal and deeply held moral convictions and beliefs (e.g., the PA who is opposed to abortion or sterilization yet is asked to participate in patient counseling leading to these procedures).

The kinds of ethical issues and questions encountered by the PA can range from the routine and common to the extraordinary and infrequent. When patients pursue the restoration of health or the prevention of illness through routine appointments and practices, they develop a moral relationship with the PA and regularly expect this relationship to be characterized by respect, courtesy, truthfulness, and understanding. This *relational ethic*,[1] exercised regularly but not exclusively in the outpatient clinic office and when the PA is engaged with patients and families in long-term relationships, aims to create a favorable context within which the PA can respond to patients' needs and their experiences of illness. The development and maintenance of the relationship may be just as important as or even more important than the individual decisions and behaviors of the participants.

In contrast but not in contradiction, the PA less commonly may be engaged in a *decisional ethic* with patients. Tough decisions, sometimes with a human life in the balance, must be made. When is it appropriate for a "Do Not Resuscitate" order to be written for a patient? At a family's request, can artificial nutrition and hydration be withdrawn from a comatose patient? After a 14-year-old patient has been diagnosed with cancer, should the PA honor parental wishes that the patient not be told of the diagnosis? Such decisions become even more complex and difficult when the participants have no previous experience with each other and will part company once decisions have been made and carried out.

The Code of Ethics of the Physician Assistant Profession (see Box) provides an ethical framework for the PA facing relational and decisional issues.[2] Through this code, standards for governing the conduct of PAs in their interactions with patients, colleagues, other health care professionals, and the general public are articulated. Yet, as the introduction to the code states, no professional code can encompass all ethical responsibilities or be comprehensive in enumerating all obligations. The conscientious PA, striving to provide competent and committed service, needs more than a copy of the Code of Ethics in hand to deal adequately with the complexities and realities of contemporary health care.

Like a code of ethics, a single book chapter on clinical ethics cannot adequately address all or even most of the issues, questions, and dilemmas that PAs will encounter as they strive to carry out their ethical duties and responsibilities. This chapter therefore does not attempt to do the impossible. After a brief description of some recent historical events that have contributed to the current context of clinical ethics, core ethical concepts and definitions are discussed, and a limited number of specific ethical issues are addressed. Ethics resources are recommended for handling more difficult and complex situations. This chapter's ultimate goal is to help the PA to become a better practitioner, colleague, and professional.

HISTORICAL CONTEXT OF CLINICAL ETHICS

The preceding section reviewed in general terms a few of the forces and factors that have changed health care over the past few decades. A brief discussion of some specific historical events that occurred during this period provides a context and rationale for some of the ethical values and principles that have emerged and that are emphasized in contemporary health care, especially in the United States.

CODE OF ETHICS OF THE PHYSICIAN ASSISTANT PROFESSION

The American Academy of Physician Assistants recognizes its responsibility to aid the profession in maintaining high standards in the provision of quality and accessible health care services. The following principles delineate the standards governing the conduct of physician assistants in their professional interactions with patients, colleagues, other health professionals and the general public. Realizing that no code can encompass all ethical responsibilities of the physician assistant, this enumeration of obligations in the Code of Ethics is not comprehensive and does not constitute a denial of the existence of other obligations, equally imperative, though not specifically mentioned.

Physician Assistants shall be committed to providing competent medical care, assuming as their primary responsibility the health, safety, welfare, and dignity of humans.

Physician Assistants shall extend to each patient the full measure of their ability as dedicated, empathetic health care providers and shall assume responsibility for the skillful and proficient transactions of their professional duties.

Physician Assistants shall deliver needed health care services to health consumers without regard to sex, age, race, creed, socio-economic and political status.

Physician Assistants shall adhere to all state and federal laws governing informed consent concerning the patient's health care.

Physician Assistants shall seek consultation with their supervising physician, other health providers, or qualified professionals having special skills, knowledge or experience whenever the welfare of the patient will be safeguarded or advanced by such consultation. Supervision should include ongoing communication between the physician and the physician assistant regarding the care of all patients.

Physician Assistants shall take personal responsibility for being familiar with and adhering to all federal/state laws applicable to the practice of their profession.

Physician Assistants shall provide only those services for which they are qualified via education and/or experiences and by pertinent legal regulatory process.

Physician Assistants shall not misrepresent in any manner, either directly or indirectly, their skills, training, professional credentials, identity, or services.

Physician Assistants shall uphold the doctrine of confidentiality regarding privileged patient information, unless required to release such information by law or such information becomes necessary to protect the welfare of the patient or the community.

Physician Assistants shall strive to maintain and increase the quality of individual health care service through individual study and continuing education.

Physician Assistants shall have the duty to respect the law, to uphold the dignity of the physician assistant profession, and to accept its ethical principles. The physician assistant shall not participate in or conceal any activity that will bring discredit or dishonor to the physician assistant profession and shall expose, without fear or favor, any illegal or unethical conduct in the medical profession.

Physician Assistants, ever cognizant of the needs of the community, shall use the knowledge and experience acquired as professionals to contribute to an improved community.

Physician Assistants shall place service before material gain and must carefully guard against conflicts of professional interest.

Physician Assistants shall strive to maintain a spirit of cooperation with their professional organizations and the general public.

Reprinted by permission of the American Academy of Physician Assistants.

The Nuremberg Code

Immediately after World War II, the inhumanities and cruelties of Nazi Germany and Adolf Hitler's Third Reich became known to the world. During the Nuremberg war crime trials, the world also learned of the atrocities committed by Nazi physicians in the name of medical research.[3] Hundreds of thousands of death camp prisoners were the unwilling subjects of excruciating, generally fatal, and often frivolous experiments.[4] Extensive sterilization experiments were carried out, designed to determine the most efficient means of rendering infertile large numbers of racial "inferiors." The eyes of children were injected with the chemical methylene blue in an attempt to change their eye color to a more Aryan blue. Prisoners were injected with typhus, hepatitis, tuberculosis, and malaria organisms to provide data that might prevent epidemics in the military. At the Dachau concentration camp, male civilian prisoners (often naked) were immersed in a tank of ice water and then subjected to different methods of rewarming; the purpose was to establish the most effective treatment for victims of immersion hypothermia, particularly crew members of the German Air Force who had been shot down into the cold waters of the North Sea.[5] Part of the tragedy of these and the many other "medical experiments" conducted under the Nazi regime was that many esteemed physicians, sworn to be healers, turned to murder and torture.

In the United States during World War II, because of an all-out effort to defeat German and Japanese military advances, medical research was conducted to find preventives to dysentery, influenza, venereal diseases, and malaria.[6] Experiments were designed to counter these diseases in order to benefit vulnerable U.S. soldiers. Prisoners in state penitentiaries, institutionalized persons with mental retardation, and residents of asylum wards became research subjects. In this wartime environment, individual consent and voluntary participation were regarded as secondary to the sacrifices required of all citizens, whether they were on the battlefield or on the home front.

From 1946 to 1949, the trials of Nazi war criminals took place before the Nuremberg military tribunal. Largely as a reaction to the Nazis' outrageous treatment of prisoners in the name of research, the Nuremberg Code of Ethics in Medical Research was developed.[7] This code contains ten articles, the first of which discusses voluntary consent in great detail. The code also sets forth other criteria that must be met before an experiment using human subjects can be judged ethically acceptable. Through the Nuremberg Code (and other research codes written since that time, for example, the Declaration of Helsinki[8]), the welfare of the individual subject has been established as the highest value, above any other consideration of what might benefit humanity or medical science.

The National Research Act

Further events and revelations during the next few decades made it clear that more than a general code for research ethics was needed if the welfare of individual research subjects was to be protected. Three notorious research projects in the United States contributed to the growing awareness of the need for additional action.

The first project was conducted at the Jewish Chronic Disease Hospital in Brooklyn (New York) in 1963. Twenty-two elderly patients, including several who were senile, one who was deaf, and another with advanced parkinsonism, were injected with live cancer cells in an effort to discover whether the cells would survive in a person who was ill but did not have cancer. The chief researcher did not seek the participants' informed consent because he was afraid the word "cancer" might discourage them from participating in the research project.[4]

The second project was initiated by the U.S. Public Health Service. The study involved poor, uneducated black men with syphilis in Tuskegee, Alabama, and lasted from 1932 until 1972.[9] The original study population consisted of 399 males with syphilis and 201 without. The study was originally intended to last for 6 to 9 months, and its goal was the study of the effect of untreated syphilis. Although in the 1940s penicillin became available, the researchers did not tell the subjects that their syphilis could be treated, nor did they provide treatment. A panel convened in 1969 by the

U.S. Centers for Disease Control reviewed the experiment and decided against treating the men. Only in 1972, after great publicity about the study, did the U.S. Department of Health, Education, and Welfare put an end to the study. In 1997, at a White House ceremony attended by the eight surviving victims of the study, President Bill Clinton apologized to all those hurt by the experiment, saying: "We can end the silence. We can look you in the eye and finally say on behalf of the American people, what the United States government did was shameful, and I am sorry."[10]

The third project was administered in 1967 at the Willowbrook State School, New York.[11] Children who were mentally retarded were injected with hepatitis in the hope of finding a way to reduce the damage done by the disease. The parental permission obtained for the study had an element of coercion: it was difficult to gain admission to the institution, and if parents granted permission for research participation, their children were admitted both to the project and to the school.

As a response to these events and other situations of research abuse, in 1974, the U.S. Congress passed the National Research Act, establishing the National Commission for the Protection of Human Subjects of Biomedical and Behavioral Research. In 1978, this commission issued an ethical policy statement known as the Belmont Report.[12] The fundamental principles set forth by the report are respect for persons, beneficence, and justice. Regarding respect for persons, researchers are to acknowledge and respect people's autonomy through informed consent, and they must protect those with diminished autonomy. The report's articulation of the principle of beneficence directed researchers toward the following two complementary duties:

1. Do no harm.
2. Maximize possible benefits and minimize possible harms.

The principle of justice addressed the fair distribution of both the burdens and the benefits of human research.

A second tangible effect of the National Research Act was its recommendation that every institution receiving research funds from the federal government should establish an institutional review board (IRB).

As defined by the National Commission in 1974, IRBs are to be standing committees of both professionals and laypersons who must review all biomedical and behavioral research proposals to ensure that they conform to ethical standards for protecting the rights of potential research subjects. Today in the United States, any research proposal involving human research subjects must be reviewed by an IRB before the study can begin.

Medical Discovery and Technology

In 1900, the life expectancy at birth of the average person in the United States was 47.3 years. A child born in the year 2000 in the United States can expect to live to the age of 76.9 years.[13] This dramatic statistical change can be attributed to many factors, including better treatment of acute and infectious diseases (e.g., pneumonia, tuberculosis), a heightened awareness of health for many Americans,[14] preventive measures such as immunizations, and a cleaner and safer water supply. Appropriately included on a list of such factors are advances in medical knowledge, treatments, and technologies. Ventilators, medically supplied nutrition and hydration via various modalities, blood transfusions, antibiotics, and cholesterol-lowering and blood pressure medications make up only a partial list of the discoveries and treatments that have contributed to both the quantity and quality of life for many people. Hemodialysis, cardiopulmonary resuscitation (CPR), solid organ transplantation, and genetics, all of which also belong on any such list, deserve special comment because of the ethical issues each has generated and continues to generate.

In 1960, the hemodialysis procedure was improved sufficiently to make long-term dialysis possible. This new "artificial kidney" was the first life-prolonging, highly technological treatment to capture the public's attention.[15] Part of the interest resulted from the treatment's high monetary cost and the shortage of dialysis machines. A critical question became which patients should receive the treatment because those not treated would likely die of renal failure. At University Hospital in Seattle, Washington, a committee was created to select the patients who would receive dialysis. This committee was dubbed "the God Committee" because in essence, it was deciding who would live and who would die. The rationing of dialysis and its accompanying controversy ended in 1972, when the federal government amended the Social Security Act to include medical coverage for all patients with end-stage renal disease. With dialysis techniques and machines now more readily available, a new set of ethical issues has emerged, especially concerning discontinuation of dialysis for patients whose quality of life is significantly diminished in comparison to their quality of life when dialysis was initiated.

The year 1960 was also the year of the first published study reporting the relative success of closed-chest compression and CPR.[16] The earliest successful uses of CPR involved healthy persons who were experiencing unexpected cessation of cardiac or respiratory functions (e.g., victims of electrocution, drowning, suffocation, automobile accidents). A 1974 statement by the American Heart Association and the National Academy of Sciences emphasized this point: "The purpose of cardiopulmonary resuscitation is the prevention of sudden, unexpected death. Cardiopulmonary resuscitation is not indicated in certain situations, such as in cases of terminal irreversible illness where death is not unexpected. . . . Resuscitation in these circumstances may represent a positive violation of an individual's right to die with dignity."[17] For many persons experiencing sudden and unexpected death, CPR has been a significant life-saving discovery. But during the intervening decades, a societal and medical expectation has emerged that all persons should receive CPR in the event of cardiac or respiratory arrest, even patients who are terminally or irreversibly ill—unless a DNR order has been written. This evolving expectation has resulted in part from the proliferation of Emergency Medical Services, public awareness campaigns and training about mouth-to-mouth resuscitation, and now more recently, the placement of automatic external defibrillators in shopping malls and in airplanes. As a result, a new set of ethical issues has emerged, including the "medical futility" of performing CPR on some patients (e.g., critically and terminally ill patients with widespread metastatic cancer), and whether for such situations, a Do-Not-Resuscitate order can be written without patient or surrogate consent.

The first successful transplant of a major human organ occurred in 1954, when a kidney was transplanted between identical twins. Advances in transplant technology, including improved surgical techniques and the development of anti-rejection therapy, have led to routine transplantation of the kidney, heart, liver, lung, and pancreas. Along this path of progress, difficult ethical and societal questions have been raised. For cadaveric donation, determination of death needed to be clarified because cardiopulmonary resuscitation and the use of ventilators made cardiac and respiratory arrest less decisive as the markers of death. Brain-death criteria, first delineated by an ad hoc committee at Harvard Medical School in 1968, became generally accepted in the United States, especially through the passage of brain-death statutes in many states. Prior to establishment of these criteria, many physicians had believed that they risked prosecution for murder if they harvested needed organs. The Uniform Anatomical Gift Act, passed in the late 1960s and early 1970s in all 50 states and the District of Columbia, clarified the right of individuals to determine how their organs would be used after death. The significant shortage of organs for transplantation and the accompanying issue of how to increase the supply of organs are among the unresolved ethical and social questions related to transplantation. Living donors for kidney transplantation, and more recently, living segmental donations of lung and liver lobes have increased the supply of organs, but have not eliminated accompanying ethical concerns, such as donor safety and the acceptable amount of risk for healthy donors, as well as donors' psychosocial assessment.[18]

The human genome project is a large international effort to elucidate the genetic makeup of several living organisms, including that of humans. The aim of this project is to establish a complete working knowledge of the organization of deoxyribonucleic acid (DNA) in both humans and the model organisms. This knowledge will provide an unprecedented resource to form the basis for further, even more sophisticated research. For clinical practice, this information will aid in the identification, characterization, and understanding of genes that directly and indirectly lead to human disease. As genetic diagnostic testing becomes more commonplace, and as research protocols for gene transfer are proposed in increasing numbers, ethical issues already are emerging. For example, the results of genetic tests can be both welcome and disturbing, so issues such as informed consent and pre-test and post-test genetic counseling are extremely important. Because of the gap between genetic information and known therapies, few treatments are now available for discovered genetic conditions. If treatments are not available, should the tests even be done? Once tests are performed, who should have access to the information about particular patients? What safeguards are in place to protect the confidentiality of this information and to prevent persons from losing their jobs or health insurance or protect them from discrimination based on their genetic predispositions? As the science of genetics develops, the ethical and social concerns will increase.[19]

The President's Commission

In November of 1978, the President's Commission for the Study of Ethical Problems in Medicine and Medical and Behavioral Research was created; its members began work in January 1980.[20] The charge to the Commission from the U.S. Congress was to conduct studies and to report on relevant topics, including the definition of death, informed consent, and access to health care. By early 1984, the Commission had published nine reports, the proceedings of a workshop on "whistle-blowing" in research, and a guidebook for local IRBs. Additional issues addressed during the 3-year existence of the Commission were genetic screening and counseling, life-sustaining treatment, and privacy and confidentiality. The studies and reports of the President's Commission provoked great interest and established a model for finding consensus where it existed and for articulating ethical conflicts when consensus could not be found. These reports present a significant synthesis and a valuable resource for the topics taken up by the Commission. The Commission's statutory authority expired in March 1983 and was not renewed.

CORE CONCEPTS IN CLINICAL ETHICS

As the field of clinical ethics has taken shape over the past few decades, some foundational or core concepts

as well as terminology and definitions have emerged. Many of the ethics terms are taken from the discipline of philosophy; therefore, they may seem like a foreign language to those whose training and careers are focused on clinical knowledge and expression. A familiarity and comfort with the core concepts and terms will help the PA reflect on, discuss, and read with understanding about the ethical aspects of clinical care.

Ethical Theories

In the business of daily living, both within and outside clinical practice, PAs frequently encounter situations in which they ask themselves, "What should I do?" For example, the question arises when a store clerk mistakenly gives too much change after a purchase, or in the examining room, when a patient refuses recommended and likely beneficial treatment. In such situations, what should be done? A decision leading to action must be made.

In general, an *ethical theory* is the process by which particular ethical decisions are justified.[21] It is the means by which information, competing values, and interests are organized and by which an answer is formulated to that basic question, "What should I do?" The main purpose of a theory is to provide consistency and coherence for decision making. With a particular ethical theory as a framework for decision making, a person does not have to figure out where to begin each time a new problem is faced, and the person may be able to state a position more clearly and accept responsibility for decisions.

Two major ethical theories are consequentialism (sometimes referred to as teleology, or utilitarianism) and deontology.[22] *Consequentialism* answers the question "What should I do?" by considering the consequences or results of the various options. The goal is to ensure that an action provides the greatest amount of good or happiness, or the least amount of harm, to the greatest number of people. According to a strict application of this theory, no action in and of itself is wrong. The rightness or wrongness of an action is determined by the action's consequences. Lying, breaking a promise, or even killing, in some situations and depending on the consequences, could be the right action. Consequentialism is attuned to the nuances of life and the specific circumstances of each situation.

Deontology (*deon* in Greek means "duty") looks to formally established rules and principles governing human behavior in order to answer the question "What should I do?" Rules such as the Ten Commandments and even a professional code of ethics are viewed as primary determinations of duty. Deontology focuses on the nature of actions themselves rather than on their consequences. Certain actions are right; certain actions are wrong. Once the rules are known or the duties are determined, then what is ethical or unethical can be fairly evident. The German philosopher Immanuel Kant is frequently associated with deontology. As a fundamental principle for deontological thinking, he referred to the *categorical imperative,* which holds that a person should act only on that rule or maxim that can be universal or applied to most situations.

These two theories obviously view decision making and evaluation of human behavior from two different perspectives. That does not mean that when one is considering a specific ethical issue, the two theories must lead to contradictory conclusions. Two persons, one with a deontological perspective and the other with a consequentialist perspective, can agree on the ethical evaluation of a particular situation. For example, both could be opposed to medically assisted suicide, but for different reasons. The deontologist might start with the general rule, "Thou shalt not kill," or "Innocent life should be protected." The consequentialist might be concerned about the adverse effects of assisted suicide on health care professionals or society. Despite different ways of making moral decisions, their conclusion is the same: assisted suicide is wrong.

In thinking through various ethical issues, people sometimes move from one theory to another. Attention to which theories are being used by the participants in discussions or debates about ethical dilemmas may give clarity to the reasons for agreement or disagreement among them.

Basic Ethical Principles and Values

As a result of clinical experiences and reflection on those experiences, some common ethical principles and values have been identified that most people are able to agree with, regardless of theoretical, philosophical, or religious positions. These generalized and abstract articulations of important values are regularly woven into codes of ethics and ethics policies and guidelines. Authors of clinical ethics literature consistently identify four principles and values:

1. Respect for persons, including their autonomy.
2. Beneficence.
3. Nonmaleficence.
4. Justice.[22]

Respect for Persons   Respect for persons and their autonomy incorporates a diverse set of ideas, including self-determination, freedom of choice, and privacy. These are major values in countries such as the United States, where democracy has flourished and "life, liberty, and the pursuit of happiness" are protected by constitutional law. The practical application for clinical offices and hospital rooms is that each patient should be viewed and treated as an autonomous or self-determining person who is allowed to act in accord with freely self-chosen and informed goals, as long as those actions do not interfere with or infringe upon the autonomous actions of others. An adult person's choice to use tobacco in the privacy of his or her own home or automobile can be used to illustrate respect for persons and their autonomy. The conscientious PA will encourage a patient's abstinence from tobacco use, will educate the patient about the known harms and risks of using tobacco, and will provide referral information for smoking cessation programs. Ultimately, however, if the value of respect for persons and their autonomy is to be upheld, adult patients must be left free to make their own decisions about smoking.

Beneficence   The principle of beneficence affirms the duty to help secure the well-being of others. In the clinical setting, this principle emphasizes the responsibility of the PA and other health care professionals to *benefit* their patients. Patient benefit certainly includes physical health, but it can also incorporate other patient interests resulting from good health, such as pursuing employment, maintaining meaningful relationships, and participating in hobbies. The principle of beneficence is a partial if not dominant motivator for most people who choose health care careers; they wish to provide benefit to people by helping them achieve a better quality of life through better physical health.

Nonmaleficence   A complementary principle to beneficence is the principle of nonmaleficence, which is the technical way of stating the obligation not to harm people. "Above all, do no harm" is an ancient expression of this basic principle. The duty of nonmaleficence imposes the obligation not to harm someone intentionally and directly. In the arena of health care, the "do no harm" principle can be actualized only in relationship and in proportion to the principle of beneficence. This is so because there are very few situations in which clinicians do not harm, cause pain or discomfort, or at least expose their patients to a risk of harm. A patient undergoing radiographic examination is exposed to risk of harm from this diagnostic procedure. Routine blood sampling for laboratory tests carries the risk (although small) of infection and bruising and can be uncomfortable. Medications with their side effects, surgical procedures, and invasive diagnostic tests do harm to patients. In most cases, the harm or risk of harm is justified by the benefits of the procedures and treatments. When one is balancing burdens or harms with benefits, a basic guideline is to maximize possible benefits while minimizing possible harms. In other words, nonmaleficence should be balanced with beneficence.

Justice   The fourth and final principle, justice or fairness, deals with patient access to resources, which in health care are becoming more and more scarce. The principle of justice requires that the benefits and burdens associated with health care be distributed or allocated fairly. Another way of expressing the principle of justice is that equals ought to be treated equally. Dilemmas of distributive justice arise most frequently when resources are scarce and therefore insufficient to meet the needs of everyone. How do we decide fairly who gets what in such situations?

On a lower or micro-allocation level, questions of justice arise when two patients with similar medical acuity are both in need of one available bed in an already crowded intensive care unit (ICU). On a higher or macro-allocation level, is it just or fair that millions of citizens in the United States have no health insurance for even basic or preventive care, while others have full coverage for expensive and long-term hospitalizations? Like autonomy and respect for persons, justice is a culturally comfortable principle in countries such as the United States. Although the principle is comfortable and familiar, however, the actualization of justice is complex and problematic.

Ethical Dilemmas   One interpretation of an *ethical dilemma* is that it is a situation in which two or more of the four principles just described are in conflict with one another. For example, in reference to the tobacco-using patients mentioned earlier, the PA desires to benefit and reduce harm to the patient through encouragement, education, and referral. These efforts can be thwarted, however, if patients, exercising their self-determination, still choose to smoke.

There is general agreement among ethicists that none of the four principles is absolute (i.e., must be upheld always, regardless of the situation). In fact, in many ethical dilemmas, upholding all the principles would be impossible because a choice must ultimately be made as to which principle will be upheld in situations of unresolved conflict between or among principles. Each principle can be limited and conditioned by the circumstances of the situation and by the other principles that may be at stake. Already, it has been shown that nonmaleficence is not absolute: directly harming patients (e.g., by an amputation) could be conditioned and justified by the prospects of benefit and by patient wishes (i.e., autonomy). As another example, justice should prevail over autonomy when a patient whose condition does not meet standard medical criteria for ICU admission demands admission nonetheless.

Models for Decision Making

The resolution of ethical questions and dilemmas requires more than a knowledge and an understanding of ethical theories, principles, and values. To ensure that good decisions are made, the PA and other members of the health care team also should adopt and try to follow a process or model for decision making. Most suggested decision-making models include the following[23] or similar steps:

1. Data collection, including background information on the situation and identification of those persons involved in the decision.
2. Identification and evaluation of all possible options and their projected outcomes through the application of ethical principles and theories and through a consideration of known cases similar to the new case at hand.
3. Resolution and decision through selection of an ethically justified option.
4. Action to carry out the decision.
5. Reflection after the fact to reinforce the process and to learn and prepare for future dilemmas.

The goal of this and any other decision-making process is to arrive at a good, ethically justified choice rather than a perfect solution that upholds all the values and principles at stake. If perfection without some regret is the ultimate goal, participants in ethical dilemmas will be regularly frustrated and will set themselves up for failure.

A complementary model for ethical decisions that has emerged in the field of clinical ethics in recent years is based on *casuistry*.[24] To gain an understanding of this word, readers should view the word *case* as a root to the word *casuistry*. As a complement to a rigorous theory-based or principle-based model, casuistry is a method of moral reasoning based on practical judgments about the similarities and differences between cases. According to the method of casuistry, attention must first be given to the details and specific features and circumstances of the case or situation at hand. Then, an attempt is made to identify previous and known cases that are analogous to the new case. If such previous or *paradigm* cases can be identified for which strong consensus already exists as to right and wrong conduct, then light may be shed on the ethical and unethical options for the new case. In the process of identifying similarities and differences between cases, the moral maxims or rules of thumb functioning in the paradigm cases are determined. Examples of moral maxims include the following:

➤ A patient's refusal of treatment should not be accepted without discussion with the patient.

➤ Physicians should not be required to provide care that they consider to be medically futile.

➤ A lesser harm can be tolerated to prevent a greater harm.

For the new case, a determination must be made as to which maxims should rule the case and to what extent. Finally, a resolution for the case can occur through accumulation of arguments for one option or another. In the previous five-step decision-making process, the use of casuistry fits into step number two.

THE PROFESSIONAL MORAL AGENT

Although there is no universally accepted definition of what it means to be a *professional,* features that usually characterize the professions include extensive training, a significant intellectual component, provision of an important service to society, certification, organization of members, and individual exercise of autonomy and judgment.[25] PAs individually and as a group fulfill these criteria and so appropriately are viewed as professionals.

Like other health care professionals, conscientious PAs should be attentive to a 2-fold process of professional growth:

1. The development of technical skills and medical knowledge through study, instruction, and education.
2. An inner-directed process that develops relevant attitudes, character traits, and virtues.

The goal of this professional growth is to enable the PA to act consistently and responsibly for the patient's welfare and best interests, that is, to be a good *moral agent.*

Patients come to clinics and hospitals because they have certain physiological needs that require the PA to act or to be an *agent.* The interpersonal nature of the PA/patient relationship gives the PA's agency its *moral* dimension. As a professional, the PA is expected to act within the bounds of acceptable standard practice and to exercise responsibly a considerable degree of autonomy and personal judgment when interacting with and for patients.

Technical Skills and Competence

The proper exercise of the professional moral agency of the PA depends on technical proficiency and competence, that is, the general knowledge and skills required for performing PA duties for the benefit of patients. There may be a tendency to view this knowledge and these skills as simply clinical requirements and to be inattentive to their moral dimension. Professional tools such as history taking, physical examination techniques, and interviewing and communication skills are moral as well as clinical interventions because they potentially contribute to the health, safety, welfare, and dignity of patients.

The knowledge, technical competence, and skills of the PA must be continually updated through training. Continuing education of the PA is not a luxury or peripheral to the PA's moral agency but is essential to its proper exercise. As stated in the Code of Ethics of the PA Profession, the PA "shall strive to maintain and increase the quality of individual health care service through individual study and continuing education."[2] What this means practically, for example, is that time and resources must be designated for attendance at professional conferences and workshops and for reading and study of relevant clinical, ethical, and legal literature. From the point of view of the PA's professional moral agency, certification and re-certification are not bureaucratic roadblocks intended to aggravate and frustrate, but are declarations of competence: they indicate that an individual PA has kept up with the rapidly changing field of medicine and that he or she is worthy of trust.

Possessing and developing technical competence for enhancing a patient's health and well-being should not negate the honest acknowledgment of personal or professional limitations and uncertainties. Maximizing possible benefits while minimizing possible harms to the patient may require saying to a patient, "I don't know the answer to that question," or even referring a patient to another professional with different or better skills.

Personal Attitudes and Virtues

The exercise of moral agency for the good of patients is not identical with or reducible to the clinical competency and command of the technical skills as just discussed. PAs must also integrate and infuse their technical expertise with personal character traits and attitudes such as empathy, respect, honesty, friendliness, and fairness. In other words, PAs (as well as other health care professionals) should have as a goal to act consistently in good ways with a commitment to being a good person in private, professional, and social life.[26] What is proposed here is that the PA should be a virtuous person, that is, someone who is continually attentive to developing good personal habits for relating to others.

One way of giving greater clarity to this "humanistic" side of PA practice and moral agency is to focus on character traits and habits that correspond to the particular needs of patients. How illness is experienced by people and the needs it creates in them can serve as an objective guide for professional character development.[27] People with medical problems who present to the clinic or the hospital seek relief and the restoration of health through personal attention, diagnosis, and treatments. They need and expect clear and caring communication, including an understanding of their doubts and fears. They desire patience and respect for the sometimes difficult decisions they must make, in accord with their own reasons, values, and goals. Most patients want to be partners in their own health care and in the prevention of future problems, and they hope for patience with their efforts to be educated and to understand medical information. They desire to be moral equals in the PA/patient relationship, bringing to the relationship their own expertise about their histories and hopes. They expect courtesy, friendliness, and confidentiality regarding disclosed information. They hope for unprejudiced, equal access to the PA's time, experience, and talents.

On occasion, because of acute or chronic debilities and diseases that assault patients' self-image and identity, they may even raise with the PA questions about the meaning of their lives, their pain and suffering, or their losses and grief. The moral agency of the PA does not necessarily include expertise in such "spiritual" issues but does require openness to discussing spiritual concerns with patients; addressing these issues in a respectful and careful way; and knowing how and when to refer patients to others (such as chaplains) for spiritual support.[28]

The appropriate attitudes and virtues corresponding to patient needs and expectations should be given continual attention and development, just as technical skills and competence are. Long hours, stress, "difficult" patients, and lack of appreciation can wear down virtuous patterns of behavior in the professional. The PA periodically may need to be reminded about the experiences of illness from the patient's perspective, so that detachment and scientific expertise do not eliminate empathy and caring.

One current proposal for health care professionals to participate imaginatively in the experiences of patients and to be sensitized to their needs is the reading of contemporary and classical literature (e.g., poetry, novels, short stories) with medical themes.[29-31] The reading of artfully told renditions of the inherent drama of sickness and its deprivations and lessons can offer a fresh and renewing way of looking at the medical encounter.[32] The premise is that empathy for patients' situations can be developed through a consideration of human life and experience inspired by reading stories and novels and by discussing narratives, paintings, and even role models.[33]

PATIENT COMMUNICATION

As indicated in an earlier section of this chapter, the second half of the 20th century witnessed a radical revolution and transformation of the clinical encounter between health care professionals and patients.[34] Regarding patient/professional interactions, the "parentalism" or paternalism that characterized the relationship in former days has been replaced by a new model that emphasizes a partnership between the professional and the patient in a process of shared decision making.

Generally, most patients do not want to be treated as child-like, passive, obedient recipients of care; rather, they want to be seen and heard as equal and full moral agents in their pursuit of health care.

For this new model to be realized in individual situations, clear and open communication between the professional and the patient is essential. Patients have a personal, experiential knowledge about themselves and their illnesses that should be combined with the general scientific knowledge of human health and disease that the PA can be expected to possess. The meeting of these two worlds of expertise can occur only in a context of respectful and mutual communication.

Patient-Centered Encounters

History taking and interviews, especially when they are part of initial and early encounters between the PA and the patient, should be patient centered.[35] This aim can be problematic because patients may perceive themselves as being in the "foreign land" of medicine, may be intimidated by the PA's authority and status, and may have only vague and imprecise language to describe their symptoms and ailments. Motivated by the goals of establishing a therapeutic relationship with the patient and of discovering and helping to relieve the patient's concerns and discomforts, the PA can facilitate an atmosphere and setting that is conducive for patients to tell their stories. Ordinary courtesies contribute to this patient-centered approach, for example, the PA's introducing himself or herself, welcoming the patient, using the patient's name, ensuring privacy and comfort, and helping to put the patient at ease with conversation about non–health-related topics.

Asking open-ended questions can encourage patients to reveal their personal goals and values. The PA may need to use imagination, metaphors, and images to solicit patient responses. In the larger context of a *relational ethic,* these suggestions and skills are more than creative clinical tools; they are affirmations of and encouragement to patients as partners in the pursuit of their own health care. Chapter 10 presents additional information about both interviewing and communication skills.

Informed Consent

Repeated clinical encounters between the patient and the PA can be interpreted as cumulative steps in a process of informed consent to treatment and the health care plan.[36,37] A presupposition here is that informed consent should not be reduced to a single event occurring at a specific moment in time, characterized by a one-way giving of information to the patient, and concluding with the patient's witnessed signature at the end of a consent form. Rather, informed consent is better understood as a process of shared decision making, achieved whenever possible by multiple encounters over time in a context of communication, partnership, and even negotiation.[38] One important outcome of this process and partnership model is an increased likelihood that particular treatments will be understood by patients in the wider context of treatment goals, that is, that patients will come to know what the specific treatment is ultimately meant to do.[39]

During repeated and routine encounters and appointments, patients can come to better understand their treatment plan, self-care and preventive techniques, expected medical regimens, prognosis, and even financial obligations. Routine visits are also opportunities for patients to speak about their goals, values, frustrations, expectations, and any reasons for difficulty in complying with treatment. Medical record notations should reflect these patient self-disclosures. Acute complications, whether handled over the telephone or in person, can also contribute to this mutually respectful and trust-building process of informed consent.

Barriers to informed consent and communication can arise owing to a patient's dementia, age, mental retardation, or emotional distress or immaturity; acuity of the medical condition; deficits in attention span and memory; or fatigue, anxiety, or passivity. Assessment of the patient's ability to make health care decisions and to carry out the treatment plan may be needed.[40] If a patient clearly cannot communicate a choice, understand relevant information, appreciate the current medical situation and its consequences, and manipulate information rationally, an alternate or surrogate decision maker (usually a family member or friend) should be identified to speak on behalf of the patient's best interests or previously expressed wishes. Even when a surrogate is needed, inclusion of the patient in conversation, communication, and education should occur to the greatest extent possible.

The ethical value of respect for persons supports giving children and adolescents as much opportunity as possible to participate in decisions about their health care. Some cautions are certainly appropriate. The personal values of children and adolescents are more likely to change with time than are those of an older individual, owing to lack of experience, being less reflective about choices, and being more interested in the present.[41] Nevertheless, decisional capacity and freedom can be viewed as developmental and

individual, with many older children and adolescents possessing these characteristics to some degree. Weithorn and Campbell[42] have concluded that children around the age of 7 years usually are capable of *assenting* to treatment (i.e., agreement), and that adolescents at about age 14 years usually can voluntarily *consent* to treatment.

Confidentiality

In the history of philosophical ethics, there has been debate about whether *privacy* is a value derived from the value of respect for persons and their autonomy, or a fundamental, universal value and need, with its own nature and importance.[22] Regardless of one's conclusions about this question, privacy and the correlate of *confidentiality* are generally accepted as essential for a therapeutic relationship between health care professionals and patients.

The purpose of confidentiality is to prevent unauthorized people from learning information shared in confidence.[43] Stated more positively, confidentiality promotes the free flow of information between professional and patient, thereby encouraging patient disclosure, which in turn should lead to more accurate diagnosis, better patient education, and more effective treatment.[44] A working principle regarding confidentiality is that professionals should not disclose privileged information about a patient without the patient's informed consent.

Within the complexities of clinical care, however, dilemmas about disclosing confidential information can arise. Although the World Medical Association in both its original (1949) and amended (1968, 1983) International Code of Medical Ethics asserted that confidentiality should never be breached under any circumstances,[44] more recent professional codes of ethics (including that of the PA profession) acknowledge that in some situations, the value of confidentiality may have to be overriden for the sake of more important values at stake in a particular clinical situation. For example, the Code of Ethics of the PA Profession mandates the PA to uphold the doctrine of confidentiality "unless required to release such information by law or such information becomes necessary to protect the welfare of the patient or the community."

A patient's positive test for human immunodeficiency virus (HIV) could create such a situation for a justified breach of confidentiality. Most legal jurisdictions mandate a duty for the professional to report to public health authorities cases of HIV positivity. Further, many professional associations foresee the possibility of a "duty to warn," through discrete disclosure, any identified individuals who are in clear and imminent danger if an HIV-positive patient cannot be persuaded to change behaviors or to notify those at risk of exposure.[45-48] A conclusion to be drawn from this example is that although confidentiality is significant for the therapeutic relationship and in most situations should be upheld, it is nevertheless not an absolute and unconditional value, and it can and even should be overridden in some narrow conditions.

The PA's role in relationship to a supervising physician frequently creates situations that further exemplify the limits of patient confidentiality. The PA and supervising physician should have regular and ongoing communication regarding the care of each patient. Part of this communication may include the sharing of confidential, medically relevant information. For the medical benefit of the patient, this sharing of information between PA and physician is justified and appropriate. What should be done if the patient discloses information to the PA and then asks that no one be told, not even the physician? In order to avoid this kind of conflict, the PA should routinely inform patients at the time of initial interviews that he or she has a responsibility to discuss with the supervising physician whatever is disclosed during the patient interview.

Finally, the "electronic age" of instant communication has created additional challenges and even threats to patient confidentiality.[49,50] The routine use of fax machines and the computerization of medical records in outpatient clinics and in hospitals demand additional safeguards to prevent inappropriate or unauthorized access to patient information. The requirements of the Health Insurance Portability and Accountability Act (HIPAA) will most certainly add "legal teeth" to the need to safeguard patients' protected health information.[51]

The obligation to respect patient confidentiality needs to be instilled in all those who have access to patient information. In the end, the most important safeguard will continue to be individual and personal commitment to a virtue that goes back as far as the Hippocratic oath, that is, to show respect for patients by respecting the privacy of their medical information.

CASE STUDY 6-1

Ms. P is a 42-year-old secretary diagnosed with breast cancer. She has had a lumpectomy and is currently undergoing chemotherapy. The primary care PA receives a telephone call from Ms. P's employer, who expresses his concern for Ms. P in a sympathetic tone of voice and asks when she can be expected to come back to work. He states that he wants to have an office party for her on her return. The PA states that he appreciates the employer's concern, but he does not know when Ms. P will return to work.

During Ms. P's next visit, the PA mentions that the employer had called expressing his concern. Ms. P says, "I hope you didn't tell him anything. He's been on my case for a long time, and he would love to have an excuse to fire me. I've been worried about my absences for chemo." The PA replies that he did not reveal any information to the employer and silently breathes a sigh of relief.

The PA realized that he might have released confidential information inappropriately because of the employer's tone of concern. Fortunately, the PA did not know the answer to the employer's question and did not divulge information about the patient. The PA learned from this experience to be sure to ask a patient's permission before discussing any confidential information, even with people who appear to be concerned about the patient's welfare.

Patient Compliance

One of the challenges of PA/patient communication is for the PA to encourage and motivate patients to accept and follow recommended treatment but to avoid any semblance of coercion, manipulation, or deception. The temptation to manipulate, deceive, or coerce to attain a good end (e.g., what the PA believes to be in the best interests of the patient) may be strongest if the patient is noncompliant, that is, fails to cooperate in carrying out that portion of the medical care plan under his or her control.

A possible explanation for incidences of noncompliance is that they are simply a natural result of the greater emphasis on patient self-determination. Patients have greater control and power, and so for their own reasons, some patients will choose not to follow recommended treatment. Although there may be an element of truth in this explanation, the reverse may also be true. If patients are approached paternalistically and their role in forging their own treatment plan is not honored, they may be less cooperative and compliant.

In situations of patient noncompliance, there is a tendency to find fault with or to blame the patient. The PA and other health professionals should first, however, explore practical reasons for a patient's lack of compliance. They would do well to seek answers to some of the following questions[52]:

➤ Has the communication with the patient been clear, effective, and consistent?
➤ Have differing or confusing messages been given?
➤ Is the patient able to comply physically or mentally; for example, are there auditory, visual, or dexterity deficits, or memory, organizational, or psychological problems?
➤ Is the patient able to read?
➤ Does the patient have the transportation necessary for making clinic visits or for purchasing prescription medications?
➤ Are there financial, social, cultural, or employment issues that contribute to the noncompliance?
➤ Is the noncompliance a sign of patient denial about an illness or disease?

If the answer to some of these or similar questions is affirmative, solutions and strategies for the specific barrier to compliance should be sought in cooperation with the patient.

All barriers to compliance are not discovered for every case, nor do all situations of noncompliance give way to creative solutions. A PA has fulfilled the obligation to patients after having made reasonable and genuine efforts to counter the noncompliance while respecting the freedom and autonomy of patients. In a partnership model of health care, each party must contribute to the process. Even when one party does not contribute or respond, the other party can have fulfilled his or her respective responsibilities.

CASE STUDY 6-2

Mr. J is a 35-year-old HIV-positive patient with a history of intravenous (IV) drug use and needle sharing for 10 years. He is being treated and is having a good response. Mr. J has been in drug treatment several times, and each time he was able to stop his drug use for 6 months to a year, with his wife's encouragement and support. His last relapse was 8 months ago. He entered a treatment program and has been drug free for 2 months. The PA caring for Mr. J knows of the importance of Mrs. J in her husband's recovery process and is also aware of Mrs. J's frustration about Mr. J's behavior during relapses. He takes his HIV medicine only sporadically while using street drugs. The couple has declared bankruptcy because of debts incurred by his drug habit. Mrs. J works two jobs, and Mr. J is unable to work.

Mr. and Mrs. J visit the PA together and announce that they want to have a child. Mrs. J is aware of her husband's HIV status. She tested negative 2 years ago, and they have had unprotected sex since then.

The PA spends time with the couple, educating them about the potential risk to a child, as well as the research on potential fetal protection from HIV if the mother takes AZT (zidovudine) during pregnancy. The PA encourages Mrs. J to be retested for HIV. Through asking questions and listening carefully, the PA gets the impression that Mrs. J wants to have a child to save the marriage, and that Mr. J is willing to agree but is not enthusiastic.

The PA's discussions with the couple and patient education take place during clinic visits over several weeks. Mr. J misses two appointments and returns to the clinic 3 months later. He reports that Mrs. J has filed for divorce and that her HIV test last month was negative. Mr. J appears to be relieved and says that he did not want to have a child.

This case raised several ethical issues for the PA, including compliance and patient autonomy.

Mr. J's drug addiction threatened his health and compromised his compliance with his HIV care. The PA had been frustrated about Mr. J's compliance during addiction relapses but realized Mr. J did his best to comply when he was drug free. The principle of patient autonomy holds that Mr. J (and Mrs. J) can make decisions affecting his own health and the health of a potential child, including having unprotected sex. The PA worried about Mrs. J's HIV status, the potential risk to a child, and the fragility of the couple's relationship, while recognizing that Mr. J was her patient and Mrs. J was not. The PA chose to educate both parties, with Mr. J's permission, creating a climate for the couple to explore their feelings about their marriage and pregnancy and to make informed choices.

END-OF-LIFE CHOICES

The best efforts and achievements of modern medicine ultimately cannot prevent death for individual patients. This unavoidable reality that someday will confront all patients (and their families and friends) creates a special responsibility for the PA to initiate advance care planning through conversations with patients about their wishes regarding end-of-life options and preferences.

Such conversations are not easy. In addition to sensitivity to patient feelings and beliefs, these conversations require a familiarity with the ethical and legal consensus concerning forgoing life-sustaining treatment, skills in providing palliative care and hospice, and an ability to educate patients about advance directives (e.g., living will, medical power of attorney for health care, out-of-hospital DNR orders). Chapter 46 discusses in greater detail clinical issues of dying and death.

Forgoing Life-Sustaining Treatment

In 1976, the New Jersey Supreme Court decided in the case of Karen Ann Quinlan that a respirator could be removed from this young adult woman who was in a persistent vegetative state.[53] Since that time, an ethical and legal consensus has emerged in the United States concerning the forgoing (i.e., withdrawing or withholding) of life-sustaining treatment, especially

for patients who are terminally ill or whose medical condition is irreversible. In this context, a life-sustaining treatment can be any medical intervention, technology, procedure, or medication that forestalls the moment of death. Examples include mechanical ventilation, dialysis, cardiopulmonary resuscitation, antibiotics, blood transfusions, vasopressors, and medically supplied nutrition and hydration.

Clinical ethics, legislative enactments, and court case decisions generally have affirmed the right of adult, informed, competent patients to refuse recommended treatments, including those that could sustain life or forestall death. Likewise, when a terminally ill patient is experiencing pain, medication and other medical interventions may be used to give relief, even if the relief potentially leads to an earlier death.[54,55] The termination of a life support regimen in these situations is not murder, killing, or assisted suicide, but is viewed as "allowing nature to take its course." When a decision is made to forgo a life-sustaining treatment, abandonment of the patient or any perception of abandonment is to be avoided; the patient should continue to receive all appropriate medical and nursing care to relieve pain and suffering.

These affirmations must be balanced with a consideration of the claims and responsibilities of health care professionals. Physicians, PAs, nurses, and other health professionals have a right to remain true to their own consciences and moral beliefs. If, for reasons of conscience, any of these professionals cannot participate in the forgoing of a life-sustaining treatment, allowance should be made for the professional to withdraw from the case, and for the orderly transfer of the patient to the care of others who have the same level of clinical expertise.

A secondary issue often raised in relation to end-of-life choices is whether there is an ethical difference between withholding and withdrawing a treatment. Some people have argued that there is a difference, such that in a particular situation, withholding a treatment might be viewed as ethical but withdrawing that treatment (once it is started) is always unethical. Therefore, for example, a patient might be counseled to make a good decision about whether to go on a ventilator for an unexplained acute breathing complication because once the ventilator is started, it could never be ethically or legally withdrawn while the patient is alive. In other words, the ventilator could be withheld, but not withdrawn. This argument and distinction have been generally rejected.[54,56,57] Although it may be psychologically more difficult for health care professionals to stop or withdraw a life-sustaining treatment from a critically ill patient, there is no ethical or legal obligation to continue if it is properly refused and no longer beneficial. In fact, it is ethically preferable to try a treatment and then withdraw it if it fails than not to try it at all.

An additional issue pertaining to end-of-life choices focuses on the terms *ordinary means* and *extraordinary means,* which are often used in an attempt to distinguish treatments that may be ethically withheld or withdrawn from those that may not. On the basis of this proposed distinction, the argument would be that any treatment or therapy that is extraordinary is not obligatory and therefore can be forgone; what is ordinary must always be provided. A problem with these terms is that they can often be a great source of confusion.

The distinction between ordinary means and extraordinary means is sometimes made by appealing to the prevalence of a treatment or its level of technological complexity. This can be misleading because it focuses attention on factors that are not ethically relevant to the decision to forgo treatment.[54] What is more important is whether the treatment provides sufficient benefit to the patient in relationship or in proportion to the burdens that the treatment may impose. Proportion of burden to benefit is a more appropriate issue than trying to label a treatment as ordinary or extraordinary.

Assisted Suicide and Euthanasia

The issues of assisted suicide and euthanasia cannot be ignored within a general discussion about end-of-life choices. Assisted suicide has usually been distinguished from decisions to forgo life-sustaining treatments (as discussed previously). In situations of assisted suicide, death is caused by the person who intentionally and directly takes his or her own life (thus, it is properly called *suicide,* or *self-killing*): the means (such as a prescription drug) or information (such as how many pills to take) is knowingly supplied by someone else (thus, the "assisted" part of the suicide). Some major medical societies such as the American Medical Association recognize the ethical justification for allowing the death of terminally ill patients to occur by forgoing life-sustaining treatments, but they oppose assisted suicide. In the United States, physician-assisted suicide has been a legal option for terminally ill residents of Oregon since 1997.[58] During the first 4 years of the Oregon legislation (1998-2001), 91 persons died after ingesting lethal doses of medications prescribed by their physicians.[59]

Euthanasia literally means a "good death" or "happy death." Euthanasia is commonly differentiated from suicide and assisted suicide because the person who actually does the killing is not the patient but someone else. Usually, the motive for ending the life of someone through euthanasia is one of mercy, that is, to end the patient's pain and suffering. If a physician (or a PA) ended the life of a patient by injecting the patient with an overdose of a powerful medication, the professional would be committing an act of euthanasia, and not assisted suicide. Euthanasia continues to be illegal everywhere in the world, with the exception of the Netherlands, where euthanasia was legalized in April of 2001. In 1995, the Northern Territory of Australia passed a law to permit euthanasia, but the law was overridden by the Australian national parliament.

For adult patients with the ability to make their own health care decisions, a primary argument for assisted suicide and euthanasia is based on patient autonomy; that is, that patients should be allowed to decide to end their lives in this way if their decisions are free and informed. Other arguments in favor of assisted suicide and euthanasia include the benefit for dying patients to have their pain and suffering mercifully ended; the claim that assisted suicide and euthanasia already occur secretly but are available only to those who know where to go; and that these ways of ending life should be made available equally to all suffering patients. An argument for the involvement of health care professionals in these decisions and actions is that they know the human body best and therefore have the expertise to bring about a quick and painless death for dying patients.

Persons who oppose assisted suicide and euthanasia often refer to the "slippery slope" that they fear society will slide down if these ways of ending life are permitted. The fear is that if competent adult patients are allowed to receive such direct assistance to have their lives ended, then it will only be a matter of time before patients who do not make such requests will have their lives ended too. The assumption is that society will begin to exert pressure on vulnerable persons (e.g., the frail elderly) to "get out of the way" by having their lives ended. The "right to die" could become a "duty to die." Other arguments against assisted suicide and euthanasia include the claim that what dying patients need is better pain management, not to have their lives ended, and (from more of a religious perspective) the assertion that life is sacred and is a gift and that religious commandments such as "Thou shalt not kill" apply to sick people as well as the healthy. Regarding the involvement of health care professionals in these decisions and actions, the argument is made that to kill patients, no matter what the circumstances, is a betrayal of what it means to be a health professional committed to the promotion of health and life.

Advance Directives

The Patient Self-Determination Act of 1990 (PSDA) mandated, as part of a health care provider's agreement with Medicare, that during the admissions process, hospitals, health maintenance organizations, skilled nursing facilities, home health agencies, and hospice programs provide written information to patients about advance directives and inquire whether a patient has executed such a directive.[60-62] If an advance directive has been made in writing by the patient, this fact is to be noted in the patient's medical record.

Four types of written advance directives have been identified:
➤ Living will.[63]
➤ Medical power of attorney for health care.[64]
➤ Patient values history.[65]
➤ Medical directive.[66]

Living wills commonly anticipate two medical situations: terminal illness and permanent unconsciousness (or an irreversible condition). In advance of either of these two prognoses, patients (through living wills) direct physicians and family about their wishes regarding life-sustaining or death-forestalling treatments. The *medical power of attorney for health care* allows a patient to designate a proxy or surrogate to make health care decisions when the patient is unable to do so. Most states in the United States have legislatively approved the validity of at least one of these two types of written advance directives. PAs and other health care professionals should seek information about their own state laws regarding these two advance directives.

Because living wills tend to be fairly vague about medical eventualities, other advance directive tools have been developed. One is a *patient values history,* which proposes, through a series of structured interviews with the patient, to identify the patient's values that can be used as guides by surrogates and physicians when decisions must be made for the patient. Examples of proposed interview questions include the following:
➤ How important is it for you to be independent and self-sufficient?
➤ What goals do you have for the future?
➤ What will be important to you when you are dying (e.g., physical comfort, no pain, family members present)?

Another advance directive tool aimed at specifying patient wishes about end-of-life choices is the *medical directive.* Through interviews or by filling out a form, patients are asked to imagine themselves in situations of coma, unconsciousness, or brain damage with various prognoses and then to indicate their wishes about life-sustaining treatments such as cardiopulmonary resuscitation, a ventilator, medically supplied nutrition and hydration, and major and minor surgery. Neither the medical directive nor the patient values history has been legislatively recognized in any state.

The PSDA has increased public awareness about patients' rights to give informed consent or to refuse recommended treatment, and the rightful role patients have in their own end-of-life decisions. Nonetheless, there is general agreement that the time of hospital or nursing home admission is not the best time for proper and substantive discussion about such issues.

During the admission process, patients commonly are seriously or acutely ill, mentally debilitated, or even unconscious. Regularly, these discussions upon admission are carried out as an administrative task (e.g., between admissions personnel and patient) rather than as a part of a clinical process (e.g., in the context of the professional/patient relationship and/or the taking of a history and physical).

The context of a PA/patient discussion and identification of general health care goals, values, and patient perception of quality of life (usually in the outpatient setting) is better suited for soliciting patient wishes regarding life-sustaining or death-forestalling therapies.[67] In this less stressful setting, patients can be engaged in a process of advance care planning,[68,69] and they can be educated about the various options and therapies that may be considered for them when they have experienced a loss of decisional capacity in the situation of a life-threatening illness. Through a series of office visits and interviews with the PA, patients have the opportunity to reflect on these issues and raise their questions. Confusion, fears, and misunderstandings can be addressed. If necessary, referrals to other professionals such as social workers, clergy, or lawyers can be made. Actual documents written in accordance with state law can be provided or reviewed, discussed, and then incorporated into the patient's medical record.

PAs and other professionals may be reluctant to initiate conversations with patients about end-of-life choices, especially with young adults and generally healthy individuals, for fear of scaring or upsetting them needlessly. However, the opposite may be true: many patients wait for the health care professional to initiate these discussions, welcome the opportunity, and are even relieved when such discussions occur.[70]

PROFESSIONAL AND INSTITUTIONAL RELATIONSHIPS

The PA's relationships with colleagues, supervising physicians, other co-workers, and employers are regularly characterized by harmony and compatibility. At times, though, these various relationships may entail circumstances that create ethical concerns and dilemmas for the PA. Impairment of a colleague or supervisor,[71] personality clashes, prejudices, and differences

of opinion regarding appropriate patient volume and what constitutes quality of care are a few factors that can create tensions and dilemmas in the PA's work environment.

Additional ethical questions can arise because of the commercialization of health care during recent decades. Frequently, the various concerns, questions, and dilemmas for the PA involve conflicts of obligation and loyalty.

Intraprofessional and Interprofessional Conflicts

Some conflicts of obligation and interest result from a sense of loyalty to one's profession and other PAs, and because some colleagues in the workplace may be friends. Having observed that a colleague's personal problems (e.g., substance abuse, mental health problems such as stress or depression) are interfering with the proper care of patients, the PA may be tempted to cover up the resultant behaviors or to protect the colleague from disciplinary action. The professional responsibility to benefit patients (beneficence) and protect them from harm (nonmaleficence) may be compromised. Privately confronting the impaired individual may lead to betterment of behavior, but in cases of substance abuse or emotional problems, referral and professional assistance may be needed. Sharing the dilemma, in confidence, with another colleague or superior could lead to the formulation of an action plan that ultimately benefits patients as well as the impaired professional. A state medical or PA association might be a valuable resource for formulating a plan of action.

Educational achievement, status in the organization, and even cultural and religious background can place the PA in a powerful position vis-à-vis other health care professionals and personnel, such as laboratory technicians and receptionists. Such social distance can lead to an irresponsible use of power in medicine. Verbal and even physical abuse can occur as a result of perceiving others as lower in the traditional hierarchical relationships within medicine. Additionally, during high-stress periods in busy outpatient clinics or hospital rounds, the PA may be tempted to blame subordinates or direct at them misplaced feelings of anger and frustration. A failure to recognize these behaviors as inappropriate and unethical can lead to tolerance of the behaviors and even complacency about them. The ethical value of respect for persons should be primary, and problems in relationships with co-workers that routinely cause stress owing to expressed or repressed emotions should be dealt with directly or through the use of an outside consultant.

Of special interest to the PA is the relationship with the supervising physician.[72,73] For the good of patients, a mutually respectful relationship between PA and physician is essential and should be fostered. Conflicts that interfere with and detract from high-quality patient care need to be identified and addressed. Mediation by a skilled professional (e.g., liaison psychiatrist, social worker) may be necessary. More extreme responses to serious conflicts include the PA's leaving a practice to begin in another and "whistle-blowing"[74]—the disclosure or reporting of perceived unprofessional behavior and practices, with the disclosure being either internal or external to the organization and done either anonymously or by identifying oneself as the whistle-blower.

Business Concerns and Conflicts

In the current competitive climate of health care delivery, the PA may face a variety of situations in which conflicts of interest occur because of economic or business concerns. This is increasingly likely as managed care strategies continue to dominate health care delivery, and as physicians, group practices, institutions, and agencies are forced to abandon financial reimbursement through fee-for-service and enter into contracts with managed care organizations (MCOs). The PA's sense of responsibility and the policies and practices of the employing clinic or hospital or physician influence how such conflicts of interest are handled. Examples of conflicts of interest in this arena change as the business climate of health care changes, but following are a few illustrations of what the PA may face.[75]

The supervising physician or PA may have a monetary investment in a radiology center where patients could be sent for unnecessary x-rays. Free drug samples given to the PA from a pharmaceutical company could be sold to patients. Deals could be worked out with pharmaceutical representatives so that monetary "gifts" or kickbacks are given to the PA for the volume of prescriptions written for particular medications. The PA may hold stock in a drug company and then make sure that prescriptions are written for a drug sold by that company, even if another drug has proven to be more effective or is simply less expensive for a particular illness. "Finder's fees" could be offered by a pharmaceutical company to a PA for every research subject successfully enrolled in a research protocol sponsored by the pharmaceutical company.

Additional conflicts of interest can arise for PAs in promoting the best interests of their patients if a managed care contract impedes referrals to specialists; if a contract forbids the PA or physician from informing patients about needed services available outside the plan but not covered by the plan (so-called "gag clauses," now outlawed in some states); or if a resource utilization manager, following the MCO's practice guidelines, denies the patient medically recommended diagnostic tests or treatments. In a new role for some PAs, they may need to assist patients through the MCO's appeals process in order for the patient to gain access to needed and recommended medical procedures.

As a general guide, the Code of Ethics of the PA Profession states, "PAs shall place service before material gain and must carefully guard against conflicts of professional interest."[2] In trying to apply this general rule to specific situations, the PA should have the patient's welfare foremost in mind. PAs are not simply business people with a code of ethics. Part and parcel of the PA profession is to establish caring, trusting, and healing relationships with patients.

PAs are not the only health care professionals who face such situations. Most notably, the American Medical Association has addressed some of these questions and has issued guidelines for its membership.[76-78] Familiarity with the official statements, guidelines, and suggestions of other professional organizations may help the PA avoid as well as appropriately manage conflicts of interest.

ETHICS RESOURCES

The conscientious PA may at times feel overwhelmed by the demands of the profession. Clinical expertise must be maintained in accord with continuous scientific and technological developments. Patients' expectations and demands change and increase. Ethical questions and quandaries may seem to arise at every turn. For ethical issues, at least, the PA need not struggle alone and without guidance. The American Academy of Physician Assistants' "Guidelines for Ethical Conduct for the Physician Assistant Profession," a document that describes the application of ethical tenets to the clinical arena, is available on the AAPA web site at http://www.aapa.org/policy/ethical-conduct.html. Other ethical resources are increasingly available, as discussed in the following paragraphs.

Ethics Consultants and Committees

Clinical ethics consultants and health care ethics committees (HECs) are frequently available to assist PAs and other health care professionals in making decisions when duties and values seem contradictory or confused. Clinical ethics consultants generally have received professional training in philosophy, theology, law, medicine, ethics, religion, or nursing, with specialized education and experience in clinical ethics.[79-82] Two primary areas of their activity are ethics education and case consultation. In the latter function, the role of the ethics consultant is not to make decisions for the parties involved, but to help analyze the case at hand, using knowledge of a moral reasoning process and of relevant cases from the literature and personal experience, and then to recommend appropriate, ethically supportable options for action.

Ethics consultants can provide timely, reasoned insight, guidance, and advice. For the PA interested in pursuing a greater understanding of particular ethical issues (e.g., patient confidentiality, informed consent, conflict of interest), ethics consultants can provide bibliographies and suggested readings and can facilitate educational experiences.

HECs exist in more than 90% of hospitals in the United States.[83] These committees usually have a diverse and multidisciplinary membership, and have three basic functions:

1. Promotion and provision of ethics educational efforts for the institution and the local community.

2. Ethics case consultation, both prospective and retrospective.

3. Policy formulation, recommendation, and review.[15,84,85]

When consulted on a particular issue, an HEC can provide a broad range of viewpoints. Commonly, a clinical ethics consultant is a member of the HEC. Availability and access to the committee are usually determined by the committee's mandate from the administration of a particular institution. The PA who is especially interested in the ethics of clinical care might wish to seek membership on an HEC.

Ethics Literature

Professional journals (including those for PAs) routinely publish articles on clinical ethics topics and on case studies. Attention to this literature can offer the PA creative approaches to problems and ways to enhance and enrich relationships with patients.

Journals, newsletters, and publications entirely devoted to clinical ethics are available. Ethics consultants or members of HECs who are familiar with this literature can direct PAs regarding subscription information and choices according to interests and needs.

On-line Internet Resources

A growing number of web sites now exist for clinical ethics information and continuing education. Useful web sites include Georgetown University's Kennedy Institute of Ethics, the Center for Biomedical Ethics at the University of Pennsylvania, the Joint Center for Bioethics at the University of Toronto, and the National Institutes of Health Bioethics Resources. More specific concerns and topics (e.g., end-of-life decisions, hospice) are often addressed on the web pages of corresponding organizations dedicated to particular issues (e.g., Choice in Dying, the American Hospice Foundation). See the Resources section at the conclusion of this chapter for selected web addresses.

CONCLUSION

In contemporary ethical analysis and decision making, respecting persons and their autonomy, benefiting the patient, avoiding direct harm to the patient, and promoting justice are basic ethical values that guide health care professionals. These values are also the foundation for the relational and decisional ethics proposed here for the PA.

The relatively recent growth of interest in clinical ethical issues and the development of clinical ethics as a field of study need not produce in a PA a sense of insecurity regarding his or her ability to deal with ethical issues. The individual PA's moral upbringing and the process of professional training provide a wealth of moral knowledge and insight. The PA may not always be familiar with particular ethical issues or with the language of ethics, however. Reading, attending conferences, talking to colleagues, "surfing the Internet," and consulting with clinical ethicists can help to expand one's interest, knowledge, and comfort in recognizing and addressing ethical issues in everyday clinical practice. Ethical knowledge, together with an ever-present focus on the best interests of patients, will serve to promote the humanistic practice of the PA.

CLINICAL APPLICATIONS

1. Two of your colleagues are discussing a situation involving a surgeon at the local hospital. They describe the surgeon as a "heavy drinker who hasn't hurt anyone yet, but it's just a matter of time." One colleague states, "Think of the harm he might do if he doesn't stop drinking." The other colleague replies, "It's just wrong, what he's doing. Health professionals shouldn't act that way."
   ➤ Which colleague has a deontological perspective, and which has a consequentialist perspective?
   ➤ Assuming that you enter the conversation, which perspective would you be more likely to articulate?
   ➤ Assuming that you work with this surgeon, how would you handle the situation?
   ➤ Can you think of other similar cases that were handled in an ethically supportable manner?
   ➤ What are your options and responsibilities if he is impaired?

2. You are the PA in Case Study 6-1.
   ➤ What would you say in response to the employer's phone call?
   ➤ What would you say if Ms. P's aunt called and asked for information about her niece's prognosis?

3. Mrs. M is an 80-year-old widow who was admitted to the hospital unconscious from a motor vehicle accident. She is in a coma, and it appears very unlikely that she will regain consciousness. Her closest relatives, a 55-year-old daughter and a 50-year-old son, have gathered at the bedside. Mrs. M has lived with her son and his family for the past 10 years. The daughter lives in another state with her family and has seen her mother three or four times a year. There is no advance directive, living will, or medical power of attorney. The daughter insists that you "do everything for my mother." The son states that his mother had told him that she didn't want "heroic measures—don't make me live as a vegetable."
   ➤ What further information would you elicit about Mrs. M and her family?
   ➤ What resources would you use to work toward an ethical solution?
   ➤ What is your approach for handling this situation?

REFERENCES

1. Brody H. Stories of Sickness. New Haven: Yale University Press, 1987.
2. American Academy of Physician Assistants. Code of Ethics of the Physician Assistant Profession. Alexandria, VA: American Academy of Physician Assistants (Adopted 1983, House of Delegates; Amended 1985, House of Delegates).
3. Lifton RJ. The Nazi Doctors: Medical Killing and the Psychology of Genocide. New York: Basic Books, 1986.
4. Lyon J. Experimenting with humans. Part I: history and context. Second Opin 1987;6:62.
5. Berger RL. Nazi science: the Dachau hypothermia experiments. N Engl J Med 1990;322:1435.
6. Rothman DJ. Ethics and human experimentation: Henry Beecher revisited. N Engl J Med 1987;317:1195.
7. Mappes TA, Zembaty JS. Biomedical Ethics. New York: McGraw-Hill, 1986.
8. Declaration of Helsinki. Bull Med Ethics 1997;130:8.
9. Jones J. Bad Blood: The Tuskegee Study of Untreated Syphilis in the Negro Male. New York: Free Press, 1981.
10. Davis D. Legal trends in bioethics. J Clin Ethics 1997;8:319.

11. Krugman S. Experiments at the Willowbrook State School. Lancet 1971;1:966.

12. U.S. Department of Health, Education and Welfare. Ethical Principles and Guidelines for the Protection of Human Subjects of Research (Belmont Report). DHEW publication no. (OS)78-0012. Washington, DC: Government Printing Office, 1978; vol 1, appendix:2-4.

13. U.S. Department of Health and Human Services' Centers for Disease Control and Prevention. Deaths: Preliminary Data for 2000. Available at http://www.cdc.gov/nchs.

14. Barsky AJ. The paradox of health. N Engl J Med 1988;318:414.

15. Ross JW, Bayley C, Michel V, Pugh D. Handbook for Hospital Ethics Committees. Chicago: American Hospital Publishing, 1986.

16. Kouwenhoven WB, Jude JR, Knickenbocker GG, Baltimore MSE. Closed-chest cardiac massage. JAMA 1960;173:94.

17. The American Heart Association and the National Academy of Sciences—National Research Council. Standards for Cardiopulmonary Resuscitation (CPR) and Emergency Cardiac Care (ECC). JAMA 1974;227(suppl):833.

18. Cronin DC, Millis JM, Siegler M. Transplantation of liver grafts from living donors into adults—too much, too soon. N Eng J Med 2001;334:1633.

19. Green ED, Waterston RH. The human genome project. JAMA 1991;266:1966.

20. President's Commission for the Study of Ethical Problems in Medicine and Biomedical and Behavioral Research. Summing Up, The Ethical and Legal Problems in Medicine and Biomedical and Behavioral Research. Washington, DC: U.S. Department of Commerce, 1983.

21. Shannon T. Bioethics, ed 3. Mahwah, NJ: Paulist Press, 1987.

22. Beauchamp TL, Childress JF. Principles of Biomedical Ethics, ed 5. New York: Oxford University Press, 2001.

23. Kanoti G. Ethics and medical-ethical decisions. Crit Care Clin 1986;2:3.

24. Jonsen AR, Toulmin S. The Abuse of Casuistry: A History of Moral Reasoning. Los Angeles: University of California Press, 1988.

25. Bayles MD. Professional Ethics. Belmont, CA: Wadsworth Publishing, 1981.

26. Pellegrino ED. The virtuous physician and the ethics of medicine. In: Shelp EE (ed). Virtue and Medicine: Exploration in the Character of Medicine. Dordrecht, Holland: D Reidel, 1985;237.

27. Drane FJ. Becoming a Good Doctor: The Place of Virtue and Character in Medical Ethics. Kansas City, MO: Sheed and Ward, 1988.

28. Astrow AB, Puchalski CM, Sulmasy DP. Religion, spirituality, and health care: social, ethical, and practical considerations. Am J Med 2001;110:283.

29. Downie RS. Literature and medicine. J Med Ethics 1991;17:93.

30. Radwany SM, Adelson BH. The use of literary classics in teaching medical ethics to physicians. JAMA 1987;257:1629.

31. Nixon LL. Patients are more than their illnesses: the use of story in medical education. Law Med Health Care 1990;18:419.

32. Radey C. Telling stories: creative literature and ethics. Hastings Cent Rep 1990;20:25.

33. Spiro H. What is empathy and can it be taught? Ann Intern Med 1992;116:843.

34. Bartholome WG. A revolution in understanding: how ethics has transformed health care decision making. Q Rev Bull 1992;18:6.

35. Smith RC, Hoppe RB. The patient's story: integrating the patient- and physician-centered approaches to interviewing. Ann Intern Med 1989;111:51.

36. Connelly JE. Informed consent: an improved perspective. Arch Intern Med 1988;148:1266.

37. Faden RR, Beauchamp R, King NMP. A History and Theory of Informed Consent. New York: Oxford University Press, 1986.

38. Lidz CW, Appelbaum PS, Meisel A. Two models of implementing informed consent. Arch Intern Med 1988;148:1385.

39. Meisel A, Kuczewski M. Legal and ethical myths about informed consent. Arch Intern Med 1996;156:2521.

40. Grisso T, Appelbaum PS. Assessing Competence to Consent to Treatment, A Guide for Physicians and Other Health Professionals. New York: Oxford University Press, 1998.

41. Leiken SL. Minors' assent or dissent to medical treatment. J Pediatr 1983;102:169.

42. Weithorn L, Campbell S. The competency of children and adolescents to make informed treatment decisions. Child Dev 1982;53:1589.

43. Winslade WJ. Confidentiality. In: Reich WT (ed). Encyclopedia of Bioethics, rev ed. New York: Simon & Schuster Macmillan, 1995.

44. Walters L. Ethical aspects of medical confidentiality. In: Beauchamp TL, Walters L (eds). Contemporary Issues in Bioethics, ed 3. Belmont, CA: Wadsworth Publishing, 1989.

45. International Code of Medical Ethics, 1949 World Medical Association. In: Reich WT (ed). Encyclopedia of Bioethics, rev ed. New York: Simon & Schuster Macmillan, 1995.

46. Council on Ethical and Judicial Affairs of the American Medical Association. Report on Ethical Issues Involved in the Growing AIDS Crisis. JAMA 1988;259:1360.

47. American Psychiatry Association. AIDS policy: confidentiality and disclosure. Am J Psychiatry 1988;145:541.

48. Health and Public Policy Committee, American College of Physicians, and the Infectious Diseases Society of America. Acquired immunodeficiency syndrome. Ann Intern Med 1986;104:575.

49. Mandl KD, Kohane IS, Brandt AM. Electronic patient-physician communication: problems and promise. Ann Intern Med 1998;129:495.

50. Woodward B. The computer-based patient record and confidentiality. N Engl J Med 1995;333:1419.

51. Fleisher LD, Cole LJ. Health Insurance Portability and Accountability Act is here: what price privacy? Genet Med 2001;3:286.

52. Scofield GR. The problem of (non)compliance: is it patients or patience? HEC Forum 1995;7:150.

53. In re Quinlan, 70 NJ 10, 1976.

54. The Hastings Center. Guidelines on the Termination of Life-Sustaining Treatment and the Care of the Dying. Bloomington, IN: Indiana University Press, 1987.

55. Sulmasy DP, Pellegrino ED. The rule of double effect, clearing up the double talk. Arch Intern Med 1999;159:545.

56. Meisel A. Legal myths about terminating life support. Arch Intern Med 1991;151:1497.

57. American College of Physicians. Ethics Manual, Fourth Edition. Ann Intern Med 1998;128:576.

58. Chin AE, Hedberg K, Higgenson GK, Fleming DW. Legalized physician-assisted suicide in Oregon—the first year's experience. N Engl J Med 1999;340:577.

59. Hedberg K, Hopkins D, Southwick K. Legalized physician-assisted suicide in Oregon, 2001. N Engl J Med 2002;346:450.

60. LaPuma J, Orentlicher D, Moss RJ. Advance directives on admission: clinical implications and analysis of the Patient Self-Determination Act of 1990. JAMA 1991;266:402.

61. McCloskey EI. The Patient Self-Determination Act. Kennedy Inst Ethics J 1991;1:163.

62. Greco PJ, Schulman KA, Lavizzo-Mourey R, Hansen-Flaschen J. The Patient Self-Determination Act and the future of advance directives. Ann Intern Med 1991;115:639.

63. Emanuel EJ, Emanuel LL. Living wills: past, present and future. J Clin Ethics 1990;1:9.

64. Annas GJ. The health care proxy and the living will. N Engl J Med 1991;324:1210.

65. Lambert P, Gibson JM, Nathanson P. The values history: an innovation in surrogate medical decision-making. Law Med Health Care 1990;18:202.

66. Emanuel LL, Emanuel EJ. The medical directive: a new comprehensive advance care document. JAMA 1989;261:3288.

67. Emanuel LL. PSDA in the clinic. Hastings Cent Rep 1991;21:S6.

68. Teno JM, Lynn J. Putting advance-care planning into action. J Clin Ethics 1996;7:205.

69. Prendergast TJ. Advance care planning: pitfalls, progress, promise. Crit Care Med 2001;29(suppl):N34.

70. Wolf SM, Boyle P, Callahan D, et al. Sources of concern about the Patient Self-Determination Act. N Engl J Med 1991;325:1666.

71. Mott JS. Dealing with the impaired supervisor. Physician Assist 1990;14:93, 99.

72. Stolberg S, McElhinney TK. Conflict between physician and physician assistant. Physician Assist Newsletter Ethics 1991;1:1.

73. Cerrato PL. What to do when you suspect incompetence. RN 1988;51:36.

74. Dougherty CJ. Whistleblowing in health care. In: Reich WT (ed). Encyclopedia of Bioethics, rev ed. New York: Simon & Schuster Macmillan, 1995.

75. Stuetz B. Pharmaceutical companies and PA's: a conflict of interest? Physician Assist Newsletter Ethics 1991;1:3.

76. Council on Ethical and Judicial Affairs of the American Medical Association. Gifts to physicians from industry. JAMA 1991;265:501.

77. Council on Ethical and Judicial Affairs of the American Medical Association. Conflicts of interest: physician ownership of medical facilities. JAMA 1992;267:2366.

78. Council of Ethical and Judicial Affairs. Ethical issues in managed care. JAMA 1995; 273:330.

79. Fletcher JC, Quist N, Jonsen AR. Ethics Consultation in Health Care. Ann Arbor: Health Administration Press, 1989.

80. Glover JJ, Ozar DT, Thomasma DC. Teaching ethics on rounds: the ethicist as teacher, consultant, and decision-maker. Theor Med 1986;7:13.

81. Pellegrino ED. Clinical ethics: biomedical ethics at the bedside. JAMA 1988;260:837.

82. Purtilo RB. Ethics consultations in the hospital. N Engl J Med 1984;311:983.

83. McGee G, Caplan AL, Spanogle JP, Asch DA. A national study of ethics committees. Am J Bioethics 2001;1:60.

84. Fleetwood JE, Arnold RM, Baron RJ. Giving answers or raising questions? The problematic role of institutional ethics committees. J Med Ethics 1989;15:137.

85. LaPuma J, Toulmin S. Ethics consultants and ethics committees. Arch Intern Med 1989;149:1109.

RESOURCES

Beauchamp TL, Childress JF. Principles of Biomedical Ethics, ed 5. New York: Oxford University Press, 2001 (454 pp). *Presents basic ethical principles and theories, as well as duties within professional/patient relationships. Ten case studies for reflection and discussion are included in an appendix.*

Coutts MD. Basic resources in bioethics. Kennedy Inst Ethics J 1991;1:75. *Provides partial but useful listing of bioethics organizations, books, journals, newsletters, and articles. Subsequent issues of this journal have included bibliographies on specific ethics topics.*

Dubler N, Nimmons D. Ethics on Call: A Medical Ethicist Shows How to Take Charge of Life-and-Death Choices. New York: Harmony Books, 1992 (403 pp). *Writing for laypeople, the authors aim to empower patients and families to take charge of their critical care decisions. Cases are used to illustrate the special issues as well as the universal needs of such patient populations as infants, children, teenagers, and senior citizens.*

The Hastings Center. Guidelines on the Termination of Life-Sustaining Treatment and the Care of the Dying. Bloomington, IN: Indiana University Press, 1987 (159 pp). *Practical guidebook that includes a model for ethical decision making at the end of life, as well as specific discussions of the ethical use of ventilators, dialysis, cardiopulmonary resuscitation (CPR), blood transfusions, artificial nutrition and hydration, antibiotics, and pain medications.*

Kuczewski MG, Pinkus RLB. An Ethics Casebook for Hospitals, Practical Approaches to Everyday Cases. Washington, DC: Georgetown University Press, 1999 (219 pp). *This book is a collection of 31 cases with commentaries and bibliographical listings designed for ethics educational efforts in hospitals. Each chapter and case presentation includes a narrative of facts, identification of issues, consideration of key points of view, a commentary, and references.*

Lo B. Resolving Ethical Dilemmas, A Guide for Clinicians, ed 2. Philadelphia: Lippincott Williams & Wilkins, 2000 (369 pp). *Using realistic introductory case illustrations for each of the book's 45 chapters, the author addresses a wide range of clinical ethics issues. The author is a physician-ethicist who combines appropriate amounts of foundational material with practical and useful applications.*

Mukand J (ed). Vital Lines: Contemporary Fiction About Medicine. New York: St Martin's Press, 1990 (436 pp). *A collection of 56 literary short stories about patients, illness, and health care professionals. Medical topics include artificial insemination, AIDS, burn units, CPR, rape, mental illness, and disability.*

Pence GE (ed). Classic Works in Medical Ethics. Boston: McGraw-Hill, 1998 (399 pp). *An anthology of contemporary articles written by leaders in the field of clinical ethics. Topics include death and dying, reproduction, abortion, allocation of resources, genetics, and AIDS.*

Ross JW, Glaser JW, Rasinski-Gregory D, Bayley C. Health Care Ethics Committees, The Next Generation. Chicago: American Hospital Publishing, 1993 (188 pp). *Provides practical direction for persons serving on health care ethics committees. Sample policies, procedures, and assessment tools are provided.*

Veatch RM, Flack HE. Case Studies in Allied Health Ethics. Upper Saddle River, NJ: Prentice Hall, 1997 (290 pp). *A collection of 81 cases, each one focused on an ethical principle or a special problem area. Each case is followed by a commentary and analysis.*

WEB SITES

American Academy of Physician Assistants, "Guidelines for Ethical Conduct for the Physician Assistant Profession." Available at http://www.aapa.org/policy/ethical-conduct.html.

Georgetown University's Kennedy Institute of Ethics. Available at http://www.georgetown.edu/research/kie/.

University of Toronto's Joint Centre for Bioethics. Available at http://www.utoronto.ca/jcb/.

National Institutes of Health—Bioethics Resources on the Web. Available at http://www.nih.gov/sigs/bioethics/.

Partnership for Caring: America's Voices for the Dying (formerly Choice in Dying). Available at http://www.partnershipfor-caring/org/.

CHAPTER 7

Medical Legal Issues

John M. Schroeder

INTRODUCTION

Since the Norman Conquest of England in 1066 C.E., a body of law has evolved on how to resolve situations in which one person has injured another. Individual situations were brought before judges, who recorded the facts of the case and the reasoning applied in their decisions. Over time, certain common fact situations became apparent, and certain principles of law evolved. The body of evolving law regarding personal injury, or negligence, became known as *tort law*. Medical negligence law is a subset of tort law. Under tort law, the courts try to resolve situations in which a health care provider is accused of injuring a patient. This chapter presents an overview of the stages of a medical malpractice suit.

HISTORY OF MEDICAL MALPRACTICE LAW

Following its independence in 1776, the United States adopted much of the English legal system, including that body of law dealing with personal injury. English legal precedents became part of the foundation of the American legal system. Over the past 1,000 years, through many thousands of legal decisions in individual personal injury cases, certain legal principles and procedures developed that govern medical malpractice law. Legal principles and procedures evolving from decisions in individual cases are referred to as the *common law*.

Paralleling the evolution of the common law in the courts, legislative bodies periodically have written laws that have either codified principles from existing common law decisions or initiated changes from the common law. These laws passed by legislatures are referred to as *statutes* or *statutory law*.

In some situations, legislatures may delegate to other organizations or agencies the right to create *rules and regulations*. For example, state legislatures frequently delegate rule-making authority as regards PA practice to state boards of medicine. PA practice rules and regulations promulgated by the state board of medicine carry the weight of law. Implementing, or administering, the rules and regulations developed by regulatory agencies involves the application of *administrative law*.

Each state and the federal government has evolved its own mix of common law decisions, statutes, regulations, and administrative laws that control medical malpractice litigation within its particular jurisdiction. Even though there are 50 different state legal systems

127

as well as a federal system in the United States, there are many legal concepts and procedures that are common to all these systems.

(A)

A potential plaintiff, Mrs. Jones, presents herself to the office of an attorney, Mr. Gonzalez. Mr. Gonzalez is an experienced medical malpractice attorney. Mrs. Jones is angry with her husband's health care providers, Dr. M. Smythe and Mr. B. Thatcher, PA-C, and wants to know if she can sue them over the care they gave her late husband.

Mr. Gonzalez realizes that several conditions must be present if a viable case is to be made against the health care providers. One of those conditions is that the events that constituted malpractice must not have happened too long ago. He therefore asks Mrs. Jones when she thinks the negligence occurred.

(B)

Mr. Gonzalez realizes that in order to be successful in any medical negligence lawsuit, he has the burden of proving, on behalf of his client, certain essential elements.

(C)

Mr. Gonzalez questions Mrs. Jones about the nature and duration of the relationship that existed between her husband and the clinicians, Dr. Smythe and Mr. Thatcher. He also inquires about her husband's health history.

(D)

Mr. Gonzalez asks Mrs. Jones to sign a record release form so that he can obtain copies of her husband's medical records. It is Mr. Gonzalez' intent to have these records reviewed by a medical expert to determine (1) what was the standard of care, (2) whether the standard of care was breached, and (3) whether any breach of standards of care resulted in injury to Mr. Jones. Mr. Gonzalez will select experts with the same or similar training as the defendant clinicians.

(E)

Mr. Gonzalez will ask the expert he has hired to review the medical records to determine whether the defendant clinicians did something they should not have done, or failed to do something that they should have done.

(F)

Mr. Gonzalez realizes that inappropriate acts and omissions do not constitute negligence unless those acts or omissions result in injury to the patient. Mr. Gonzalez has the burden of proving that the acts or omissions of the defendants caused the patient's injuries.

(G)

If acts of negligence occurred, Mr. Gonzalez must determine what those acts were, who participated in those acts of negligence, and who was responsible for those acts being committed. Sometimes it is not clear who is responsible for the negligent acts until a lawsuit has been filed and testimony taken from witnesses. Mr. Gonzalez knows that he must understand the business and contractual relationships that exist among all those who cared for Mr. Jones. Mr. Gonzalez is particularly interested in finding out the employment status of Mr. Thatcher, PA-C. If he fails to list all the appropriate defendants when he files a case, the statute of limitations may run out on one or more potential defendants and expose Mr. Gonzalez to a legal malpractice claim.

(H)

Mr. Gonzalez will try to determine whether or not Mr. Jones was a compliant patient.

(I)

Mr. Gonzalez must determine whether or not Mr. Jones consented to the treatment that he received. He must also determine whether or not Mr. Jones was given adequate and accurate information upon which to base his consent to treatment.

(J)

Mr. Gonzalez must determine all of the injuries that Mr. Jones suffered as a result of negligence by the defendants, so that he can determine how much in money damages the defendants should reasonably have to pay. Because Mr. Jones is dead, any lawsuit for his injuries must be brought on behalf of his estate.

(K)

Mr. Gonzalez must also determine if, as a result of the defendants' negligence, the wife, Mrs. Jones, has been "injured." If she has been injured by the negligence, she may have a claim against the defendants also.

(L)

Mr. Gonzalez must determine whether the acts of negligence are so egregious as to warrant a request for punitive damages.

(M)

Having satisfied himself that Mr. Jones was injured because of negligent care, feeling confident that he can prove all the necessary elements in this medical negligence case, and believing that the time and money expended on this case are worth the risk, Mr. Gonzalez files a lawsuit.

(N)

Dr. Smythe and Mr. Thatcher, PA-C, having received the petition and summons, contact their malpractice insurance carrier who, in turn, arranges for Ms. Sikorski, a malpractice defense attorney, to defend against the claim filed by Mr. Gonzalez.

(O)

Ms. Sikorski files an official response to the petition, denying that her clients have committed any negligent acts that resulted in injury to Mr. Jones.

(P)

Mr. Gonzalez and Ms. Sikorski enter into a period of discovery, during which each side is able to gather facts and information from the other side.

(Q)

At some point during discovery, Ms. Sikorski and Mr. Gonzalez appear before the judge assigned to the case to arrange for a trial date and narrow the issues to be addressed at trial.

(R)

At trial, both attorneys present the evidence they feel best explains the facts in the case. Mr. Gonzalez presents evidence that he feels establishes the negligence of the defendants and the injuries resulting therefrom. Ms. Sikorski presents evidence that she feels exonerates the defendants.

STATUTES OF LIMITATIONS

Courts and legislatures do not like individuals to delay bringing their lawsuits, including medical malpractice actions. Undue delays in filing a lawsuit permit evidence to be lost, witnesses to die or be lost, and witnesses' memories to become obscured. Delays in bringing actions create a burden on the courts and society, both of which want early and prompt resolution of legal claims. As a result, all jurisdictions have created *statutes of limitations*. Statutes of limitation set time limits within which lawsuits must be initiated. Statutes of limitations vary in each jurisdiction but generally allow 2 years from the time the plaintiff *knew or should have known* that he was the victim of malpractice to file his lawsuit. If the plaintiff does not file an action within the period allowed by the statute, the action will be forever barred.

The phrase *knew or should have known* can create seemingly unfair results. For instance, one plaintiff may *know* that her surgeon operated on the wrong lumbar disk (not the one intended to be removed by the surgeon, or the one agreed upon in the patient's operative permit after informed consent) immediately following surgery. If she fails to file a lawsuit until 2 years and 1 day after she knew of the negligent surgery, she will have lost her right to sue.

Another patient may not have been told by his surgeon that the wrong disc was removed. After 5 years has passed, a magnetic resonance imaging (MRI) ordered by another practitioner reveals the mistake. The MRI gives the patient knowledge that the wrong disc was removed, and now the patient *should know* that malpractice may have occurred. For this patient, the statute of limitations begins to run on the day he receives the MRI results. This patient now has 2 years within which to file an action, giving him a total of 7 years to initiate his lawsuit.

Sometimes, information about negligent care may not be available or may be intentionally kept from a patient. In that case, the statute is tolled, or does not begin running, until the patient is given that knowledge. Therefore, health care providers cannot benefit from keeping information from the patient in hopes that the statute of limitations will run out. Despite the apparent disparity in the previous examples, both patients have 2 years to file after they learn of the negligent treatment (see Case 7-1 [A]).

ELEMENTS OF MEDICAL NEGLIGENCE

The following elements must be present and proven before a successful medical negligence lawsuit can be brought:

➤ Duty.
➤ Breach of duty.
➤ Causation.
➤ Injury/Damages.

The burden of proving that negligence occurred falls on the plaintiff (patient). Each of the previously listed elements must be proved by the plaintiff, and the jury must be convinced of the plaintiff's proof by a "preponderance of the evidence." Preponderance of the evidence means that the plaintiff's evidence must be more likely true than the defendant's evidence. Preponderance of the evidence refers to the quality and believability of the evidence, and not to the quantity of evidence presented. The "preponderance" standard of proof is a lesser standard than the "beyond a reasonable doubt" standard that is applied in criminal cases. Medical negligence cases are not criminal cases. They are civil, not criminal, causes of action that do not threaten the defendant's life or liberty, and therefore, the lesser standard is applied (see Cases 7-1 [B and C]).

Duty

To owe a *duty* to another person implies that there is some relationship between the individual parties. In medicine, that relationship is the patient/clinician relationship. In order for a duty to be owed to a patient, a patient/clinician relationship must exist. At trial, the plaintiff must always prove the existence of that relationship. The patient/clinician relationship may be either express or implied. An express relationship occurs when the clinician formally agrees to treat the patient. An implied relationship occurs when there is no formal agreement, but the facts and circumstances indicate that a relationship exists.

The existence of a patient/clinician relationship gives rise to certain obligations for both the clinician and the patient. The scope of the obligations that the clinician owes to the patient is defined as the *standard of care*. The standard of care for clinicians is generally defined as that level of care that would be provided by a reasonably prudent clinician under

similar circumstances. The reasonably prudent PA has the knowledge and skills that are possessed normally or ordinarily in the profession. Thus, the actions of the clinician are not compared with what would be done by the most astute or best clinician. They are compared with actions that would be normal and ordinary under the circumstances of the case (see Case 7-1 [D]).

The standard of care varies from case to case, based on the facts and circumstances in the particular case. The standard of care, or how a particular patient should have been treated, can be established by the testimony of expert witnesses, practice guidelines, textbooks, statutes, rules and regulations, and other sources that demonstrate appropriate care in the circumstances of the case. Both the plaintiff and the defendant clinician will put on evidence of what they believe the standard to be. The jury will review the evidence and determine, by a preponderance of the evidence, the standard of care to be applied.

Most states hold clinicians in their jurisdiction to a *national standard* of medical care. A national standard implies that the quality of medical care should be the same regardless of geographic location. Proponents of a national standard of care make the point that medical education is standardized, continuing medical education is accessible, and modern communication systems make consultation readily available. For example, if a new drug is being used nationwide as the most appropriate treatment for a condition, all clinicians should be using that drug for that condition. Under the national standard, expert witnesses from across the country may testify.

Some states, however, hold their clinicians to a *local standard*, or *locality rule*. The local standard of care holds the clinician to a standard of reasonable prudence as practiced in the same or similar location. For instance, if a rural community has four physicians and all of them fail to prescribe the newer, but available, medication when it is indicated, there would be no malpractice because nonuse of the drug was the local standard. The local standard implies that there are different standards of care for different states, and among rural, suburban, and urban clinicians. Under the locality rule, the expert witness must be from the same community or from a community that is similar in size and resources. The law is evolving away from the locality rule and is slowly embracing the national standard.

To succeed in a medical negligence action, the plaintiff must convince the jury that her interpretation of the standard of care is the correct one. The jury determines the standard of care by weighing evidence presented by both sides. In virtually every case, a medical expert will be called who must state that the specific acts of the defendant clinician did not meet the applicable standard, whether national or local.

However, sometimes the fact that negligence occurred is so obvious that the patient's injury "speaks for itself," and expert testimony may not be necessary. The legal doctrine of "res ipsa loquitur" ("the thing speaks for itself") can be applied in circumstances where the facts show that even though the specific act of negligence is not known:

➤ The patient's injury was most likely due to negligence.
➤ The only one who could have committed the negligent act was the clinician.

In such a case, an expert witness may not be necessary.

For example, assume that while you sit in the waiting room, your unscratched car is rolled into one end of a carwash and comes out the other end with multiple scratches and dents. You do not know exactly what happened in the carwash, but it is obvious that:

➤ Scratches and dents usually do not happen in a carwash unless some negligence has occurred.
➤ The operator of the carwash was, at all times, in control of your car and the carwash equipment while your vehicle was in the carwash.

The jury can presume the operator's negligence without the necessity of presenting expert testimony about how the scratches and dents actually occurred. Once the jury is allowed to presume negligence, the burden shifts to the defendant to prove that he was not negligent.

In a medical context, assume a patient undergoes laparoscopic fulguration of endometriosis. The patient is anesthetized and is not a witness to the actual surgery. Following the surgery, it becomes apparent that the pelvic organs were severely and extensively burned, necessitating bowel resection, hysterectomy, and oophorectomy. The jury can conclude that negligence occurred if:

➤ Severe, extensive burns of the bowel, uterus, and ovaries do not usually occur in the absence of negligence.
➤ The only one who controlled the equipment and could have created the extensive burns was the surgeon.

The doctrine of res ipsa loquitur can also be helpful to the patient in those cases wherein there is a "conspiracy of silence." Assume in the previous scenario that there were two surgeons involved in the above procedure, and neither will point a finger at the other to determine the negligent party. If the jury presumes negligence under the doctrine of res ipsa loquitur, the burden shifts to each silent co-surgeon to prove he was not negligent (see Case 7-1 [E]).

Breach of Duty

The plaintiff must convince the jury that the defendant clinicians did not meet, or that they breached, the standard of care. A *breach of duty* can be an act of either omission or commission. The defendant may have failed to do something she should have done (act of omission), or she may have done something she should not have done (act of commission). Evidence of a breach of duty may be presented by expert testimony, admissions or testimony of clinicians involved in the case, medical records, witness testimony, and other information presented for consideration (see Case 7-1 [F]).

Causation

The burden falls on the plaintiff to prove that the defendant clinician's breach of duty actually "caused" the bad outcome experienced by the patient. Because medical care is sometimes complex and an individual's physiology is dynamic and idiosyncratic, causation is often the most difficult aspect of a case to prove. Often, there are plausible explanations or intervening events, other than negligence, that may have caused or contributed to the patient's bad outcome. Thus, the plaintiff must establish that the breach of duty by the clinician is the direct or "proximate" cause of the injuries experienced by the patient. *Proximate* cause means that the acts of the defendant were a substantial factor in producing the injury to the patient. As with the other elements of negligence, evidence of causation may be presented by expert testimony, admissions or testimony of clinicians involved in the case, medical records, witness testimony, and other information presented for consideration (see Case 7-1 [G]).

Many factors may have contributed to the injury of a patient. Other clinicians may have participated in the care of the patient, and their acts or omissions may have intervened and caused or contributed to the patient's injuries. Other clinicians, whose acts or omissions do contribute to the patient's injuries, are called *joint tortfeasors*. Practitioners who come together only to care for a specific patient, and otherwise have no business or contractual relationship with each other, may be considered independent contractors who are responsible only for their own acts of negligence. The negligence of one independent contractor will not, by vicarious liability, be imputed to another person. Lawsuits for negligent acts by independent contractors are filed against the specific independent contractor named.

Some practitioners, however, may be agents or employees, and they may be acting on behalf of a partnership, professional corporation, group, clinic, or hospital. Furthermore, some of the care provided to the patient may be given by technicians and other medical personnel, who may also be employees of a physician, group, clinic, hospital, or other health care organization. Under the legal theory of *vicarious liability,* an employer or supervisor may be held liable for the negligent acts of her employees or agents. This legal theory evolved from the principle that the master had the right to control his servant and was therefore responsible for the servant's negligent acts. Lawsuits for negligent acts by agents or employees will generally list both the employee and the employer as defendants.

Physician assistants may be either *independent contractors* or *employees* of a health care organization or practitioner. The greater the degree of control that an organization has over the acts of the PA, the more likely it is that the court will find that the PA is an employee, and will attribute vicarious liability to the employer. If the organization or practitioner pays the PA for her services, but does not control her specific day-to-day activities, it is more likely that she is an independent contractor.

A PA who is an independent contractor is responsible for his own acts, and his acts will not be attributed to the organization or practitioner with whom he has contracted. Vicarious liability, on the other hand, can be imputed to employers of physician assistants if the PA is acting within the *scope of employment*. Scope of employment generally means doing those activities that the PA normally performs for the employer. Intentional injuries, such as assault or battery of a patient, and other activities unrelated to one's job duties are not considered within the scope of employment. Vicarious liability can also be imputed to the supervising physician of a PA, even if the supervising physician is not the employer of the PA. Virtually every state law regulating the duties of supervising physicians indicates that the supervising physician assumes liability for the negligent acts of the PA (see Case 7-1 [G]).

Acts of noncompliance by the patient may have been factors that contributed to the injuries received by the patient *(contributory negligence)*. In some jurisdictions, the patient must not have contributed in any way to his injuries, or the case will be barred. This legal precept is rarely employed in medical negligence cases. More common is the theory of *comparative negligence,* whereby the negligence of the patient is compared with the negligence of the defendant. The patient's comparative negligence causes a reduction in the liability of, and damages paid by, the defendant. There are several forms of comparative negligence. In one example, assume that the jury finds that the defendant clinician is 90% at fault for the patient's injuries, and that the patient is 10% negligent in causing his own injuries. If the jury finds the total damages suffered by the patient to be $100,000, the defendant clinician will have to pay only 90%, or $90,000.

The fact that the patient came to you in an already weakened condition is not an excuse or defense for treating him negligently. You should not drop patients on their heads under any circumstances. If you do so, and they are injured, you cannot defend yourself by saying that the patient's skull was abnormally thin.

This legal concept is often referred to as the *thin skull doctrine*. You take the patient as you find them. In other words, even if the patient has some preexisting condition that predisposes her to injury, you are not excused from your negligent treatment of the patient. A preexisting condition is not a form of comparative negligence. The same doctrine holds true for other preexisting conditions such as diabetes mellitus (see Case 7-1 [H]).

The ethical principles of autonomy and self-determination hold that an individual's body is inviolable. Under legal principles, if someone threatens to hit you with a stick, and he has the stick and the apparent ability to hit you with it, he has probably committed an assault. If that person actually touches you with the stick, without your consent, he has committed a battery. Battery is a nonconsensual touching. In the medical context, patients have a right to refuse to be touched, and therefore, they have the right to refuse treatments and therapies, no matter how necessary those procedures may seem to clinicians. The only way a clinician can "touch" a patient is by obtaining the patient's consent to do so. From these fundamental ethical and legal concepts has developed the legal theory of *informed consent*.

Consent can be either *express* or *implied* by the circumstances. An express consent is usually written and occasionally verbal. An implied consent to treat is implied from the circumstances. For instance, if someone appears at the emergency room door and collapses before she is able to sign a consent form, consent to treatment may be implied by the fact that the patient was on her way to the ER, presumably for treatment. Implied consent fosters society's desire to have its health care providers, and others, render assistance in emergencies without fear of incurring liability. As a result, implied consent has led most states to create statutes *(Good Samaritan Laws)* that allow for emergency treatment when consent cannot be obtained. In addition to express and implied consent, consent can also be substituted.

Substituted consent occurs with children or incompetent adults, when treatment decisions are made by someone acting on behalf of the patient. An extension of the substitute consent doctrine occurs with guardians, living wills, advance directives, and "power of attorney," whereby the patient or court designates someone to make health care decisions on the patient's behalf in the event that the patient is unable to do so.

For consent to be *informed,* the patient must be given sufficient information such that she can make a reasoned decision. It is rare today for patients to receive no information about their health care options, so most litigation for lack of informed consent is over the sufficiency, that is, quantity and quality, of the information provided. Depending on the jurisdiction, three different standards are used to determine the sufficiency of the information that was actually provided.

One standard attempts to determine what the *reasonable clinician* would reveal under the circumstances. This standard is opposed by those who feel the patient loses self-determination over his body if the clinician can control the quantity or quality of information provided.

The second standard is subjective, and it consists of merely asking the injured patient if the information turned out to be adequate for her to make an informed decision. This standard is opposed by those who feel the injured patient will always say the information provided was inadequate, just to get her case to the jury.

Under the third standard, the jury is asked to determine what information the *reasonable patient* would have required under the circumstances. This third standard is considered more objective. Regardless of the standard applied, the important question for the clinician is, how much information is enough? At a minimum, the information should include the risks (inherent and potential) and benefits (including likely outcomes) of the proposed procedure and all of the available alternative treatments, including no treatment at all (see Case 7-1 [I]).

Injury/Damages

If your car is destroyed by a negligent driver, the court can "make you whole" by having the defendant replace your car. But if someone has lost a leg, an ability, or a life, there is no way that the court can replace what has been lost. The only thing the court can do is offer money as compensation. Injuries to patients can be physical, mental, or financial, and include pain and suffering, past and future medical expenses, and financial losses such as lost wages, both past and future. One goal of a negligence trial is to determine the nature and extent of the injuries received, and to fashion a method of compensating the patient for those injuries. Injured patients can be compensated for economic losses such as medical expenses incurred as a result of the injuries and lost wages due to time off work. These measurable injuries are easily calculated from bills and pay stubs.

The plaintiff can also receive monetary compensation for intangible injuries such as pain and suffering. The plaintiff's attorney must put on evidence regarding the nature and duration of the plaintiff's pain and suffering to convince the jury that compensation is due. Among these intangible injuries are loss of mobility, loss of intimacy with a spouse, loss of fertility, loss of cognitive abilities, and loss of the enjoyment of life. Certainly, these are significant personal losses, but how can they be fairly and reasonably compensated?

High damage payment awards for tangible and intangible injuries seem unfair to some people, are implicated in high malpractice insurance costs, and have resulted in legislatures placing *damage caps* on the amount of compensation that can be paid to the plaintiff. Damage caps set an upper limit on the amount of damages a defendant clinician must pay, but they can also prevent the injured patient from being fully compensated for his injuries (see Case 7-1 [J]).

The spouse and family of an injured or dead patient suffer losses as a result of the defendant clinician's negligence. These losses may give rise to a separate but related claim against the defendant for such loss of spousal consortium. *Loss of consortium* claims are designed for the loss of companionship, love, comfort, and support of the injured or dead spouse. Though separate and distinct from the claims of the injured patient, these claims are almost always attached to, and tried at the same time as, the patient's claim (see Case 7-1 [K]).

Not every case of medical negligence warrants *punitive damages*. Punitive damages are not meant to compensate the injured plaintiff, they are meant to punish the defendant. Punitive damages are special damages that are permitted only if the negligent acts were so outrageous as to warrant a financial punishment of the defendant. The outrageousness of the negligent acts may not be apparent until after the case has been filed and evidence gathered, so punitive damages are often requested initially but may be dropped later in the case, if inappropriate. The court or jury must determine whether punitive damages are warranted in a particular case. Legislatures have placed caps on punitive damage awards in some jurisdictions (see Case 7-1 [L]).

Medical malpractice lawsuits can be expensive to pursue, and they can take 9 to 24 months, or longer, to get to trial. This is a large investment in time and money. It is not unusual for a case to cost the plaintiff in excess of $50,000 to $100,000 from the time of filing the case through trial. The defense has similar costs. These costs consist of fees for filing, depositions and court reporters, expert witness reports and testimony, travel, and other sundry expenses. If the plaintiff had to pay $50,000 up front, there would be very few people who could afford redress in the courts. Therefore, most medical malpractice cases are taken on a *contingency fee*. Typically, the plaintiff's attorney will pay the costs of litigation contingent on the agreement that these costs will be paid back to the attorney out of any award given by the jury. If the case is lost, the plaintiff's attorney will typically absorb the loss, and will not try to collect the costs from the plaintiff. In addition to reimbursement for the costs of litigation, the plaintiff's attorney will receive some part of the jury award for his time and efforts. If the plaintiff's attorney has been cautious and objective in evaluating and preparing a case, she can have some confidence about being successful, thus reducing the risk of loss.

The defense attorney incurs costs similar to those of the plaintiff. She is typically paid an hourly fee for her work. The defense attorney is most often paid by the medical malpractice insurance carrier that was covering the clinician at the time of the incident.

PRETRIAL PROCEDURES

In order to file a case, the plaintiff's attorney will draft a document called a *petition* or *complaint* and will file this document at the courthouse. The petition is a notice to the defendant clinician that he is being sued for negligence. Some jurisdictions require the petition to be very specific about the claims against the clinician; others allow a general statement of the facts. The petition is conveyed to the clinician along with a *summons*. The summons announces to the defendant that he is under the jurisdiction of the court, and that he must respond to the plaintiff's petition (see Case 7-1 [M]).

PAs may be insured under the same policy as their supervising physicians, or they may have their own policy. If all defendants are covered by one insurer, there will usually be one defense attorney working on the case. If there are separate insurance policies, each clinician will typically have his own defense attorney. Defense attorneys will look out for the interests of their client, but frequently they are able to work together in a unified defense of all defendant clinicians (see Case 7-1 [N]).

After meeting with her clients, reviewing the medical records, and often talking with expert witnesses, the defense attorney must file an *answer* to the petition of the plaintiff. The answer must either admit certain facts alleged in the petition or deny those facts. The petition and the answer are the first effort to define the issues and facts in the case (see Case 7-1 [O]).

Courts have tried to eliminate "trial by ambush," in which facts and information are not available to both sides in advance of the trial. To do this, courts oversee the exchange of information through various mechanisms. This period of information exchange is called *discovery*. Discovery is often a long, drawn-out process that may last a year or longer. Each side may send the other a *request for production* of documents and other "things" from the opposing side. These requests may be for production of medical records, certain correspondence and reports from expert witnesses, instruments and devices, and other evidence that may be relevant to the case. Failure to comply with a legitimate request may result in a contempt of court citation or other sanctions for the noncompliant attorney.

Each side may also request information regarding the testimony of all potential witnesses. To facilitate this, each side must supply the other with a list of witnesses that it intends to call. Surprise witnesses are rarely allowed. Each side may request information on the testimony of the other's witnesses by *written interrogatories* to which the witness must respond. Furthermore, each side may also take the oral *deposition* of any witness. This deposition testimony is taken down word for word by a court reporter and then is transcribed into book form. If witnesses change their testimony at trial, their deposition testimony may be used in an attempt to impeach the credibility of the witnesses and their testimony. In a deposition, the attorneys are allowed wide latitude in questioning the witness, often asking questions that would never be allowed at trial. Discovery, when appropriately carried out, prevents surprises at trial.

Effective discovery also facilitates settlement of many cases. Once the strength and weakness of the facts and evidence are clear to both plaintiff and defense, one or both sides may wish to avoid trial. A weak plaintiff's case (or strong defense case) may necessitate dropping the lawsuit altogether, or make a low settlement offer seem appealing. A strong plaintiff's case (or weak defendant's case) may cause the defendant to recognize the risk of going before a jury that may award a large sum to the injured patient. A settlement takes away the uncertainty and idiosyncrasy of jury decisions. The majority of medical negligence cases settle, and they do so toward the end of discovery and before trial (see Case 7-1 [P]).

Scheduling conferences and other *pretrial conferences* take place between the attorneys and the judge. These conferences facilitate moving the lawsuit toward trial and also narrow the issues in the case. Discovery often exposes areas where there is no controversy. For example, the defendant clinician may agree that a patient/clinician relationship did exist, eliminating the need for plaintiff to present evidence on this subject to the jury. The parties may *stipulate* to those facts that are not in controversy, expediting the trial. The judge will meet with the attorneys to determine how much time the trial will require, including the permitted length of time that attorneys may spend doing opening statements and closing arguments to the jury. Conflicts regarding the admissibility of certain evidence will often be resolved during these meetings (see Case 7-1 [Q]).

TRIAL PROCEDURES

The judge will call a group of citizens to the courthouse from which the attorneys must select a jury. The number of jurors needed differs with the jurisdiction. The attorneys are allowed to question, or *voir dire,* potential jurors to determine if they have some bias in the case. Each side, along with the judge, is allowed to eliminate, or *strike,* some potential jurors from consideration. After the jury has been selected, the judge will seat the jury and the trial will begin.

Each attorney is allowed a prescribed amount of time to make an *opening statement* to the jury. The plaintiff's attorney gives the first opening statement, followed by the defense attorney. The opening statement is not evidence in the case. It is the attorneys' chance to give the jury an overview of the case, pointing out issues and witnesses that will appear. If skillfully done, the opening statement can be a persuasive framework from which a juror may view the evidence.

Since the burden of proving that the clinician was negligent falls on the plaintiff, the plaintiff presents her evidence first. The plaintiff will call all of her witnesses to the stand to testify, enter all of her evidence, and "prove" all the necessary elements of a medical negligence case. After the plaintiff's attorney presents and questions a witness, the defense attorney may cross-examine that witness. At the completion of the plaintiff's case, the plaintiff will "rest," and the defendant then puts on his case. The defense will then call his witnesses and enter evidence that would tend to exonerate the defendant. The plaintiff's attorney will be permitted to cross-examine each defense witness.

Because depositions have usually been taken, the testimony of the witnesses is already known to the attorneys. There are, therefore, few surprise statements by witnesses if the depositions were done well. The art of trial law is to present the evidence and testimony of witnesses in a logical, effective, and believable way in order to convince the jury of a point of view.

After both the plaintiff and the defendant have presented their cases, the judge will instruct the jury on the law that should be applied to the facts of the case. Both the plaintiff's attorney and the defense attorney have an opportunity to advise the judge as to the law that they feel should be applied to the case and given to the jury. The judge makes the final determination of what the *jury instructions* will be, followed by jury deliberation and the jury's decision (see Case 7-1 [R]).

CONCLUSION

It is important to recognize that bad medical outcomes do not necessarily constitute medical malpractice. Although PAs' communication skills are often regarded as reducing the risk of malpractice suits, nevertheless PAs do become involved in legal actions by patients.

Strategies to prevent malpractice suits include knowing and following the laws in your state, practicing within ethical standards, always identifying yourself as a PA, and following guidelines for medical record documentation. See Chapter 9 for information on patient records and preventing medical errors.

The hallmarks of the PA profession—knowing one's limitations and working with physician supervision—form the basis of quality medical practice, as well as effective risk management.

RESOURCES

Boumil MM, Elias CE. The Law of Medical Liability in a Nutshell. St. Paul, MN: West Publishing Company, 1995. *A very good but brief overview of medical liability issues and law for the novice or student. Content areas include the following: Establishing the professional relationship, negligence-based claims, informed decision making, vicarious liability and multiple defendants, reforming the litigation system, hospital liability, contract, warranty and strict liability, and intentional torts.*

Younger P, Conner C, Cartwright KK, Kile S, Forsyth JC. Physician Assistant Legal Handbook, Aspen Health Law Center. Gaithersburg, MD: Aspen Publishers, Inc., 1997. *This excellent resource relates specifically to legal issues involving physician assistants. Content areas include the following: PA education, licensure and scope of practice, prescribing and dispensing, employment law, and third-party reimbursement.*

Restatement of the Law: Torts (2nd ed). American Law Institute: American Law Institute Publishers, 1979 (annually updated). *This updated tome is for the truly interested reader who wants greater depth of information. The restatement is an attempt to organize (restate) common law court rulings into related and coherent blocks of information. Restatements do not reflect statutes, which can alter common law rules and principles. The Restatements are drafted by respected scholars, attorneys, and jurists. They are useful as a fundamental legal research tool and study aid.*

CHAPTER 8

Cross-Cultural Perspectives

Ronald D. Garcia and Mary Em Wallace

INTRODUCTION

This chapter attempts to provide a framework for approaching patients from diverse cultural backgrounds. It is beyond the scope of the chapter to cover adequately the specific information for each cultural group. Attempts to do so would probably only contribute to stereotyping of people. No attempt has been made to include specific information about special groups of people who share subcultures. For example, many people who are hearing impaired communicate through sign language and share customs and understandings that can be regarded as a subculture. Similarly, people involved in gay and lesbian lifestyles are often considered to be members of subcultures.

It is difficult to classify all of the ethnic groups in the United States. The Asian/Pacific Islander subgroups, for example, encompass more than 20 separate ethnicities, representing people who have ties to such diverse places as China, Japan, Polynesia, Southeast Asia, and the Indian subcontinent. Hispanic subgroups can be identified by their multiple countries of origin in Central and South America and islands such as Puerto Rico and Cuba. Thus, a global category such as "Asian" or "Hispanic" can mask important differences. Religion has a significant effect on beliefs and practices and thus is a determining factor in the concept of ethnicity. Health care practices among African-Americans are greatly influenced by the area of the United States in which they reside. It is beyond the scope of this chapter to list all of the pertinent patient beliefs that practicing PAs will encounter.

This chapter is intended to serve as an introduction to cultural differences. Excellent data are available elsewhere regarding cultural practices for specific groups. The resources listed at the end of the chapter offer further information.

ASSUMPTIONS

The concepts of culture and ethnicity are intertwined and are subject to many different definitions. This chapter has been written with certain assumptions in an attempt to avoid semantic difficulties; these assumptions are as follows:

➤ *Ethnicity* can include race, country of origin, religion, and, in many cases, specific subgroup identification—for example, identifying the Sioux as a specific group of Native Americans. The United Nations has advocated the use of *ethnic group* as a more comprehensive term than *race*.[1] This decision probably reflects the reality of the complex biological, historical, racial, and religious factors that make up a group identity.

➤ *Culture* consists of all the assumptions, beliefs, and expectations that influence behaviors and decision making.

➤ Income, socioeconomic status, and age can have significant influence on the cultural assumptions of an individual or family.

➤ *Acculturation,* or the extent to which an individual or family is familiar and comfortable with the expectations of the majority or host culture, greatly influences patients' health-oriented beliefs, assumptions, and practices.

➤ The length of time people have been in the country, their socioeconomic status, and the amount of control they feel they have over their society (e.g., voting, intermarriage, political decision making) have a big impact on health care assumptions and decision making, as well as on how comfortable they are with a health care provider and the extent to which they interact as equals with a health care professional.

➤ The wide range of differences among individuals within a specific ethnic group is likely to have an equal or greater influence on health care decision making than the differences among separate groups.

➤ In the United States, the idea of a "melting pot" was previously regarded as an ideal.[2] In the 1990s, there appeared to be a growing emphasis on recognizing and celebrating cultural differences.[3]

➤ Respect is the key to establishing a beneficial relationship with people who have different backgrounds and assumptions.

➤ The most important information about ethnicity is based on details received from patient interactions. The *real* teaching moments come from what patients say, or perhaps do not say, during a clinical visit.

➤ Probably the most comfortable patient care situation is one in which a patient and a provider share the same ethnic background and life experiences because this makes it easier for both of them to feel understood and valued.

This chapter contains many brief case presentations to make the material clinically relevant. However, even with the use of examples, it is difficult to arrive at an approach to cultural differences that accentuates individual sensitivity without creating or reinforcing stereotypes. After reviewing this chapter, the reader should be able (1) to identify assumptions that can hinder communication and (2) to spot potential mistakes, which are highlighted by the different examples. This will help the reader to become more aware of his or her own assumptions and to start to evaluate his or her approach to cultural differences in the clinical situation.

DEMOGRAPHIC FOUNDATIONS

Before an attempt is made to develop a framework for a cross-cultural clinical encounter, it is important for the reader to look at some of the data that demonstrate health and illness outcomes in the United States for different racial and ethnic groups. The significant differences in outcomes emphasize how important it is that physician assistants (PAs) and other health care providers develop knowledge and competence in caring for racially and ethnically diverse patients.

MORTALITY

Race and ethnicity affect morbidity and mortality. In the United States, the overall life expectancy in 2000 was 76.9 years. For black males, it was 68.3 years, and for black females, 75.0 years, both record high figures. It is important to note that during the 1980s, the difference between blacks and whites in life expectancy had increased. In women, the difference had grown from 5.0 to 5.5 years, but it is currently at 5.0 again. In men, the change in difference was even more striking—from 6.2 to 7.4 years; a figure that has dropped back to 6.5.[4,5] Part of the change in life expectancy for black males resulted from a rise in death rates from homicide and human immunodeficiency virus (HIV) infection in men younger than 45 years of age. Nonetheless, 60% of the difference in life expectancies for black and white males and females at birth can be attributed to infant mortality, cardiovascular diseases, malignant neoplasms, and homicide.[4]

Specific mortality data clearly indicate that blacks have a higher death rate for many different types of disease entities. The data in Table 8-1 are limited to blacks, whites, and "other." These categories reflect collection and reporting procedures of the National Center for Health Statistics.

Tuberculosis persists as an important disease. The mortality differences shown in Table 8-1 are more pronounced when one looks at different age groups. For example, in people 55 to 64 years old, the death rate per 100,000 from tuberculosis in 1999 was 0.5 in white males, 3.2 in black males, and 3.1 in the "other" male category.[6]

The prevalence of diabetes differs among ethnic groups. Native Americans and Mexican Americans are at higher risk than whites for diabetes.[1] From the data in Table 8-2, it is apparent that diabetes has deadly effects many years earlier in blacks and other minority populations than in whites. This is an important disease to examine because of its chronic nature and the need for ongoing treatment. In addition to possible genetic factors, access to health care, patient education, and the quality of long-term care affect the course and outcome of diabetes. These differences are more pronounced when the data are broken down by age, as shown in Table 8-2.

Table 8-1 Mortality Rates Per 100,000 for Selected Diseases (1999)

Disease	Total	Black	White	Other
Tuberculosis	0.3	0.7	0.3	0.8
Diabetes	25.1	34.2	24.3	28.7
HIV infection	5.4	22.6	3.0	16.7
Conditions originating in perinatal period	5.2	14.8	3.9	11.7

Data from National Vital Statistics Report, 1999. Washington, DC: National Center for Health Statistics, 2000.

Table 8-2 Death Rates for Diabetes Mellitus by 10-Year Age Groups and Race (1999)

Race	25-34 Years	35-44 Years	45-54 Years	55-64 Years	65-74 Years
Black	3.1	9.0	31.3	91.7	186.9
White	1.3	3.7	11.1	32.8	82.9
Other	2.3	7.1	24.9	76.4	162.8

These figures represent death rates per 100,000 population in the specified group.
Data from National Vital Statistics Report, 1999. Washington, DC: National Center for Health Statistics, 2000.

Between the ages of 45 and 54, the rate at which African-Americans die from diabetes is nearly 300% higher than that for whites. This finding holds up despite the fact that insulin-dependent diabetes mellitus (IDDM) is more common among white Americans.[1]

Although information is limited, there has been speculation regarding genetic differences about diabetes. Both IDDM and non–insulin-dependent diabetes mellitus (NIDDM) have very low prevalences in western Africa. However, a genetic link has been found for IDDM in both blacks and whites in the United States. One theory is that the higher incidence is due to genetic admixture of blacks with whites.[1]

Hidden in the "other" category in Tables 8-1 and 8-2 are the Hispanic populations. The prevalence of diabetes in Mexican Americans and Puerto Ricans 45 to 64 years of age between 1994 and 1997 was 100% higher than among non-Hispanic whites.[4]

One obvious impact of HIV infection is premature death. Table 8-3 clearly demonstrates differences in premature mortality for blacks and whites. HIV is another important disease related to a higher rate of premature death in minority populations than among whites.

In 1997, the United States ranked 27th in infant mortality among industrial countries.[5] Table 8-4 demonstrates that a minority American child is much more likely to die than a white one.

Table 8-3   Death Rates for HIV by Age, Race, and Year

Age (Years)	1988		1999	
	Black	**White**	**Black**	**White**
15-24	3.8	1.1	2.3	0.2
25-34	37.8	10.1	28.3	3.9
35-44	50.2	14.0	56.7	8.0
45-54	23.0	8.4	53.5	5.8

These figures represent death rates per 100,000 population in the specified group.
Data from National Vital Statistics Report, 1999. Washington, DC: National Center for Health Statistics, 2000; and from Health, United States, 1990. US Department of Health and Human Services publication PHS 91-1232. Washington, DC: National Center for Health Statistics, 1991.

Table 8-4   U.S. Infant Mortality Rates According to Race/Ethnicity of Mother (1996-1998)

Maternal Race/Ethnicity	Mortality Rate
Chinese	3.4
Japanese	4.3
Cuban	4.7
Central and South American	5.2
Mexican American	5.8
Filipino	5.9
White	6.0
Puerto Rican	8.1
Native American	9.3
Black	13.9

These figures represent death rates per 1,000 live births in the specified group.
Data from Health, United States, 2001. U.S. Dept of Health and Human Services. Washington, DC: National Center for Health Statistics, 2001.

Table 8-5   Five-Year Relative Cancer Survival Rates

Sex and Site	1986-88		1989-96	
	Black	White	Black	White
Male				
All sites	37.7	51.8	48.5	60.1
Prostate	69.3	82.7	86.7	94.1
Female				
All sites	47.8	61.5	49.3	63.0
Breast	69.4	83.9	71.4	86.3

Percentage rates are based on follow-up through 1997. Data from Health, United States, 2001. U.S. Dept of Health and Human Services. Washington, DC: National Center for Health Statistics, 2001.

Cancer is a leading cause of death in the United States. One measure of health care in two different racial groups is reflected in the 5-year survival rates, as shown in Table 8-5.

It is interesting to take a closer look at the data on breast cancer. Although the incidence of breast cancer is higher for white women than for all other groups, the 5-year survival rate is higher for whites than for Mexican Americans, Native Americans, Filipinos, and blacks.[4] Many reasons for this difference have been hypothesized. One reason may be a delay in seeking care, so that the disease is further advanced at diagnosis. Differences in access to health care for screening during the asymptomatic phase of the disease or treatment may also affect the outcome. Finally, a genetic link has not been ruled out, although it is not proposed as likely.[7]

In the preceding paragraphs and tables, it is discouraging to note that the incidences and outcomes of many diseases are negatively affected by minority status. One finding that has become evident in older age groups has been termed the "racial mortality crossover phenomenon." A switch occurs at approximately age 75, when life expectancy has been shown to be higher for blacks than for whites. It has been hypothesized that people who are less physically strong die at younger ages in the minority population, leading to a more robust pool of people to survive to age 75.[8]

CAUSES OF DIFFERENCES

The reasons for cross-cultural differences are multiple. One way to represent the differences is through a Venn diagram, in which each circle represents a factor. The degree of overlap of circles for the factors is different for each individual and family. The broad categories include biological factors, socioeconomic status, cultural beliefs and practices, and acculturation and assimilation.

Biological Factors

Biological factors are derived from genetic differences themselves, as well as from the interaction between genetic material and the environment (e.g., obesity and hypertension). In terms of blood types, some minor differences have been found among the major racial groups, yet the differences in individuals within the same ethnic group are seen to be more dramatic than the differences between racial and ethnic groups.[1]

Socioeconomic Status

In 1999, 9.8% of U.S. whites had incomes below the poverty level, compared with 10.7% of Asians, 23.6% of blacks, and 22.8% of Hispanics.[9] The most recent data for Native Americans were collected in 1989; in that year, 31.2% of Native Americans had incomes below the poverty level.[10] It is disturbing to examine poverty rates among children. In 1999, 32.7% of black children and 29.9% of Hispanic children younger than 18 years of age were living below the poverty line, compared with 12.9% of white children.[9] Poverty has widespread and important negative influences on disease and the ability to obtain health care. It leads to (1) crowded living conditions, which increase the spread of communicable diseases, (2) delay in seeking treatment because of the cost of care, and (3) increased difficulty in purchasing medications and diagnostic tests.

Cultural Beliefs and Practices

Every cultural group, over generations, develops beliefs and behaviors to cope with major life transitions such as marriage, birth, child-rearing, illness, and death. In addition, beliefs about health and how to maintain it, as well as about foods and celebrations, become part of the invisible set of assumptions and behaviors that can have both a positive and negative effect on health status.

Acculturation and Assimilation

Acculturation refers to the extent to which an individual or family from a minority culture is able to understand and negotiate successfully the rules and expectations of the majority or host culture. It has many implications for health care beliefs, practices, and delivery. Many standard procedures involved in using the health care system can be frustrating for someone familiar with the culture, but obscure for someone who does not know the rules. How to obtain and use insurance, how to make appointments, appropriate behavior in a clinic waiting room or examination room, privacy issues, acceptable things to tell the provider, and use of ancillary services such as physical therapy and social work all offer potential for confusion and misunderstanding.

The *assimilation* process usually follows increased familiarity with and commitment to remain a part of the dominant culture. The process generally involves adaptation of the native culture in ways that promote participation in mainstream institutions. At times, participation in mainstream institutions, such as hospitals, universities, and places of employment, leads to pressure on the person to reject his or her cultural identity. Part of cultural pride is the ability to retain ethnic identity and still be successful in the majority culture. If an individual's or family's native identity is eroded, then self-confidence and ability to interact with the majority culture are weakened.

How a person experiences assimilation has an important impact on identity and self-concept, as illustrated in the following passage.

> I am American and I am black. I live and travel with two cultural passports, the one very much stamped with European culture and sensibilities and history. The other was issued from the uniquely black experience, which is like no other, born of slavery and hardship and tied to a land we might call home but that we blacks do not know, and most have never seen—Africa.
>
> Black Americans are different from white Americans, different from Americans who are also Italian or French or Irish, different in our experience. Their distinctions are not racial but ethnic or regional. They share common histories and culture and color. Because they are not marked, they can hide inside American society in ways that we cannot. And they have access to their homelands in ways we have been denied. Proximity, money, cultural awareness. Africa is far away and expensive to reach. More than that, our education tends to be as European as the education of any white kid. We do not know about Africa, only learn about it in geography class. Place-names on a map. Climate.[11]

The four major groups of factors related to cross-cultural differences are presented in Table 8-6. The impact of these factors can be seen in the following example.

CASE STUDY 8-1

Mrs. R is a 55-year-old Mexican American woman with NIDDM. She came into the clinic with the chief complaint of fatigue. It was found that she had a blood glucose of 228. Upon examination, the physician assistant noted funduscopic changes and decreased sensation in both feet.

Table 8-6   Factors Related to Cross-Cultural Differences

Biology	Racial groupings
	Genetic markers for disease
Socioeconomic status	Poverty
	Insurance
	Living conditions
Cultural beliefs and practices	Birth
	Child-rearing
	Diet
	Death
	Traditional definitions
	Access to traditional healers
Acculturation and assimilation	Number of years in country
	Language(s) spoken
	Comfort with host culture
	Integration with decision-making process of dominant culture

Mrs. R was at risk for serious diabetes complications and death. According to Table 8-6, it is possible that many overlapping factors contributed to her dangerous condition.

Biological Factors As has been mentioned earlier, diabetes is more prominent in Mexican Americans than among other ethnic groups in the United States. As is true with Native Americans, even after adjustment for increased body fat, the prevalence rate of NIDDM in Hispanics is approximately twice as high as for non-Hispanic whites.[4] Another contributing factor to her condition was Mrs. R's obesity. She had been overweight since the birth of her first child. She was not concerned about this because she regarded it as a natural process associated with being a mother and grandmother. Because she was on her feet all day, running after her three grandchildren and taking care of her husband, she believed she was getting enough exercise. Mrs. R took great pride in her cooking and often prepared traditional Mexican meals, most of which were cooked with lard, were served with beans refried in lard, and included flour tortillas. She cooked more food than was required so everyone could have a second helping. She used her tortillas as "utensils" to scoop up her food and often ate two or three tortillas at a meal. Sweets and junk food were very available in her household, and she enjoyed eating Mexican sweet bread.

Cultural Beliefs and Practices Health for this patient meant the ability to care for her children and grandchildren. She did not want to deprive her family in order to do something for herself. She was responsible for caring for her three grandchildren so that her children could go to work. Although she was obese, she did not believe that this was undesirable because most other women friends with children were nice and round.

Socioeconomic Status The family lived on the $1000 a month earned by her husband, who worked for a gardening company. Mrs. R was concerned about the costs of pills, diagnostic tests, and special foods.

Acculturation Mrs. R emigrated from a small town in Mexico. There, she had had access to a *herbalista,* whom she had consulted for her disease a few times when she was very thirsty and drinking a lot. Her father was a farmer in Mexico who died at the age of 66 from a "heart problem." The orientation she had received about her diabetes was that it should be treated only when there were symptoms. Therefore, she went to the medical facility infrequently, not only because she did not speak English well and was ill at ease there, but also because it was difficult for her to understand the importance of treatment when she was not experiencing symptoms.

Other Factors Another contributing factor to Mrs. R's hesitation in seeking help may have been fear. One of her sisters died at the age of 60 from kidney failure. Families who have lost loved ones from diabetes complications at a young age, or who have lived many years with its tragic effects—blindness, amputation, and kidney failure—are understandably fearful of long-term effects but are not necessarily knowledgeable about how to prevent them.

DETERMINING ETHNICITY

In any clinical encounter, documentation of an individual's racial background is an expected part of the "identifying data." Questions about ethnicity can be interpreted as offensive by patients who do not see the relevance of the information, as in the following dialogue.

> PA: *What ethnic group are you from?*
> PATIENT (in an irritated voice): *I don't like that question. Some of my family are from the Hawaiian Islands, but my father's mother is from Ireland, and my mother was born in Puerto Rico. I'm an American.*

The patient's response is consistent with the reality found in many American families of racial and ethnic mixture. One way to avoid such a response is to refrain from asking the question and instead judge a patient's ethnicity on the basis of dominant physical characteristics. Often, simple observation is appropriate and adequate, but with each assumption comes the risk of error and the consequence of making decisions and assumptions that will not fit. An alternative for dealing with this issue is to wait until later in the interview for cues, and then ask specific questions to clarify information consistent with the reason for the interview. It is hoped that as readers proceed through the chapter, they will draw on their own experience and information and become more aware of when it is appropriate and worthwhile to clarify a racial or cultural difference.

IMMIGRATION AND ACCULTURATION ISSUES

People who belong to the same ethnic or cultural group can have many different beliefs, attitudes, and perceptions. Important factors that contribute to differences within groups are related to how long they have been in this country and how comfortable they are with the language and customs.

Many people who are from different cultures have immigrated to this country. It may be helpful to ask patients born and raised in other countries about their immigration experience. The information usually contains clues about strengths, struggles, hopes, and family relationships that may be useful in identifying current stressors as well as addressing the patient's health care needs. Here is a quotation from an immigrant who has been in the United States for 13 years: *"I'd like to bring to the Philippines my husband to enjoy his remaining life. Not here, nobody talking, only me. He's happy there. There's always someone to talk with."*

She and her husband came to this country with the idea of making some money and then bringing over their 5 children and more than 15 grandchildren. Unfortunately, her husband suffered a stroke at age 50 and, owing to the resulting aphasia, dementia, incontinence, and hemiplegia, became very dependent. She had almost the full responsibility for his care. The loss of her extended family has made her burden greater and has negatively affected her husband's quality of life. This background information would allow the PA to make more effective and efficient interventions. An initial step would be to find out how a planned intervention would affect the available support system. For instance, an otherwise appropriate suggestion to move to a low-cost housing unit far from the location of her only sister and good friend *(comadre)* would probably lead to a greater burden and frustration for the caregiver, who already feels distant from family support.

Emigration to another country is a major personal and family event. The decision and the changes associated with the event are greatly affected by the context in which they were made and may influence current stressors. Whether political upheaval, economic hardship, or a desire to be with family members, the motivations for emigration are many and do have an impact, as shown in the following example.

CASE STUDY 8-2

Mrs. S, a Filipino woman, has been under a PA's care for essential hypertension. An attempt at diet control was unsuccessful. Therefore, medication was given. At the next visit, Mrs. S's blood pressure was higher. When queried about her medication usage, Mrs. S looked down.

When the provider asked whether the cost of the medication was a problem, Mrs. S replied, "I feel okay. I need to send money to my daughters, sisters, and brothers. They are poor. I don't know this time if they are using slippers or shoes . . . Ohhh very poor people. They are barefoot. They've got no shoes. They've got no boots to work in the fields. They have not much food. They have not much money. Even though I'm working hard here, I still feel the pain of them having no money in the Philippines. I give some money (to family in the Philippines)."

After discovering the immediate financial problem Mr. and Mrs. S were experiencing, the PA chose to spend more time in the interview exploring the costs of different antihypertensives, as well as the possible use of alternative healing practitioners. The PA also talked with Mrs. S about the expensive effects of hypertension if it is left untreated.

ROLE OF RESPECT

The rules of respect are likely to be clear and mutually understood when two people are from the same culture and socioeconomic class. As the differences become greater, however, the chances of misunderstanding and the possibility of making insulting mistakes increase.

The importance of respect is illustrated by the following comment made by an elderly black woman with multiple chronic problems when she was asked what advice she would like to give to new health care providers to help them be effective with minority patients.

Always bear in mind that patients are still human. Because so often that person has been rejected. They have been sort of pushed around. So always bear in mind that they hurt just like you do. And above all, they want to feel loved, and that somebody cares for them.

An example of problems related to respect can be seen in the following case study.

CASE STUDY 8-3

Ms. Maude J was born in the early 1900s. Her grandmother was a slave. During her youth and into current times, the use of her first name was reserved for very close friends and family members. When she went into the HMO clinic for her first visit, she was greeted by a PA who called her from the waiting room as "Maude J." Then, when they came to the examination room, the PA introduced herself with, "Hi, Maude, my name is Sue."

The PA, a 35-year-old white woman, was not being malicious. She was only addressing the patient the way she herself would like to be addressed. Her intention was to try to make Ms. J feel relaxed by treating her as an equal. Also, the PA was talking to the patient in the same way that she talked to the other clinic personnel. For many people, especially African-American elders, the correct use of a formal name is a part of respectful treatment.

PREJUDICE AND DISCRIMINATION

Prejudice and discrimination persist in many American institutions, including the health care delivery system. Consider the following comment.

I will say this to you. In my experience—and I'm 72 years old—the minority person has to really fight to get what is available. Somehow, I don't know why, our system is set up that way. There has to be some kind of a drawback. If it's nothing but just nit-picking with society. When they look at your color, automatically they draw conclusions. I don't say all of them. I'm not naive enough to have

locked everybody into the same bag. But this is what I have found.

Often, providers are not aware that certain actions or statements contain offensive racial content. Yet for patients, the offense can be painful and real. A health care provider who has not experienced racial or religious prejudice may have difficulty understanding the impact that racially insensitive acts or language can have on an individual's willingness to trust or believe in an individual or a larger system.

A 70-year-old African-American woman described the following frustrating event, which increased her sense of alienation from the health care system.

My husband and I went to the hospital. After the visit, they called a taxi for us. When the driver came, I said, "Are you looking for the D's?" I was telling him so he wouldn't have to go looking for us.

He didn't say one word. He walked on in there and went into the hospital, and evidently they told him, and maybe he thought, "I'm not going to carry those black people on." I don't know what he was thinking. He came out and went on past us. He didn't have anybody. And in a few minutes, he came back and got us.

I said, "I asked you if you were looking for the D's," and he said, "We don't want to talk about that." I don't bother nobody, and I just don't like to be humiliated.

Prejudice can come from the provider directly. The following interchange occurred during an interview between a practitioner and a black man who was questioned about his rehabilitation shortly after he became blind.

PATIENT: *In the beginning, when I was supposed to go on and get my training, we had one doctor. He kept our papers in his office. Along eight or nine months—close to a year, maybe, around a year—he was supposed to sign the papers and send them on over to the other hospital for rehabilitation. He kept the doggone papers in his office—wouldn't send them, and I was a year late getting my training. He kept them—this so-called white doctor—kept the doggone papers—that sort of thing.*
INTERVIEWER: *Do you have any idea why?*
PATIENT (with emotion): *Hold on a minute, hear? Prejudice because my skin was black, and he was in the position to hold back.*

Both this man and Mrs. D were hurt and humiliated. The primary reason they both gave for the way they had been treated was the color of their skin. The accumulation of such life experiences can adversely affect such a patient's interactions with the unsuspecting practitioner. On occasion, a practitioner's insensitivity to cultural background can recall a patient's past experiences with racism, leading to an unsatisfactory interaction.

PATIENT/PROVIDER INTERACTIONS

The physician assistant is in a role of authority as a health care provider. He or she is caring for a patient who has certain expectations. When the expectations and beliefs about the roles of patient and practitioner are similar, misunderstandings are reduced. The following case illustrates what can happen when the provider and the patient unknowingly have different assumptions.

CASE STUDY 8-4

Hugh B is a PA working in a rural medical clinic. His personal experience with hypertension has affirmed for him the belief that patients need to be assertive regarding their health care. He expects the patients he sees to ask questions when they don't understand, and he welcomes the challenge of answering the questions and helping people gain more control over their disease. He has been following Mr. T, who has hypertension, for the past 6 months and appreciates his patient's respectful and friendly manner. Hugh B wonders why Mr. T doesn't need more refills for his daily antihypertensive and is naturally suspicious that Mr. T is not taking the medication. The situation according to Mr. and Mrs. T is revealed by the following interchange.

MR. T: *I always respect my doctor when I go to the doctor. I trust him to help make remedy for my sickness. It is no good not to do right. Because you can't escape from God. Don't you know that? If you are not doing right to the people it is no good. God will punish you.*
MRS. T: *So when you do not take medicine, you are relying on God?*
MR. T: *Sure.*

MRS. T: *Can He get you well without medicine?*
MR. T: *I trust Jesus, even if I don't take medicine.*

Health care providers often find it difficult to ask questions of people from a different culture. It is as if the provider, whether PA, nurse practitioner, nurse, or physician, knows that there is a gap in his or her own understanding and, to avoid the risk of offending a patient or because of his or her own unwitting stereotypes, he or she minimizes the potential importance of questions that would be easy to ask of someone who was just like him or her. Examples of this can be seen in the following two patient encounters.

CASE STUDY 8-5

A family nurse practitioner working in a neighborhood clinic was seeing a 78-year-old Hmong woman, and her middle-aged daughter was acting as a translator. The woman came in and sat very straight during the interview in her traditional headdress and costume. The chief complaints were fatigue and constipation. The provider was suspicious that the woman was depressed.

In order to get a better picture, he asked about her sleep, diet, and habits. He hesitated to ask about drug use, but after he did, to his amazement, a long discussion followed between the mother and her daughter. In the end, the daughter told him, with the mother's apparent agreement, that the mother smoked opium daily.

CASE STUDY 8-6

A Mexican American man with a significant alcohol history had received care both in Mexico and in the United States. The following interchange with his wife is very revealing.

HUSBAND: *Here they don't ask about the drinking.*
WIFE: *The complete story is poorly covered.*
HUSBAND: *No one has asked me the questions. In Mexico, the doctors have asked me about my work, my drinking—all of this . . . It could be because they are more committed* [in Mexico].

Perhaps the difference this man experienced was reflective of a cultural difference. If the provider had been Mexican American or a Spanish speaker, would the man have been more willing to tell his story?

Cultural assumptions affect decision making in ways not always obvious. They can also affect the clinical encounter because the provider may find it difficult to understand the rationale and motives for a particular decision a patient has made.

CASE STUDY 8-7

MaryAnn was a busy practicing PA with an invalid mother who had been living in a nursing home for the past 7 years. Although it was initially difficult to place her mother in the nursing home and then to visit her, MaryAnn felt comfortable about the quality of care her mother was receiving. Her mother reiterated many times that she didn't want "to be a burden," and that MaryAnn really needed to direct her attention to her current life, which included the care of her family (husband and two children) and her career.

One day, MaryAnn met Mrs. P, who had been taking care of her husband since his stroke 5 years previously. He required approximately 7 hours of care a day. After obtaining a history from Mrs. P regarding her recurrent abdominal pain, the PA realized that some of the stress experienced by the caregiver was possibly influencing her abdominal pain. She then discussed the positive aspects of the option of placing Mr. P in a skilled nursing home and urged Mrs. P to carefully consider it.

Mrs. P immediately appeared irritated, although she remained polite for the duration of the interview. She never returned for a follow-up visit.

When questioned later about the experience, Mrs. P replied, "I will do my best for my husband to my—I can't explain—it's the *tabulan* or obligation. I'll do everything until he dies. I will not leave my husband—no. If I am sick, I don't know. If I got sick, I can hire another lady, but I watch that."

It is likely that the two women were operating from different cultural assumptions. In the PA's family, independence and "expert care" appear to be important factors. Mrs. P's priorities appear to be very different, and her responsibility to take care of her husband outweighs her need for

independence and the need to depend on outside "expert" resources for his ongoing care.

In fact, Mrs. P was Filipino, and caregiving is a more integral part of her culture. It is expected that family members will take care of their own elderly. An experienced Filipino social worker reported that in the Philippines, there is one nursing home, and it is never full. Filipino people consider it a *shame* for a family not to take care of its own. Therefore, children are more likely to see caregiving as they grow up, making it easier for them to accept and learn the role, as well as to develop a sense of self-reliance. Mrs. P had emigrated from her country as an adult and appeared to be operating very much under these cultural mandates.

In such a situation, it is likely that a health care provider never would find out why a patient suddenly stopped coming for treatment because patients frequently have difficulty complaining and often address problems by merely withdrawing from the interaction or going to another provider or clinic. It is useful, then, for providers to become aware of cultural differences and develop ways to learn from their patients about these differences.

Major decisions and life changes are affected by culture. For example, the preparation for and expectations of death and funerals are associated with important beliefs and practices that need to be respected.

CASE STUDY 8-8

Mr. and Mrs. G emigrated to this country from Mexico during their adult life. Because of proximity to their homeland, they have been able to return to their village many times. When Mrs. G was found to have a terminal disease, her daughters and sons were upset that she wanted to return "home" with her husband, their father.

She was able to explain to her family, "I would like to be buried in my village. Funerals are very expensive here. There it is free. Here all I have is the family—children. It is a big family, but there I have the entire village. *Comadres* and *compadres*, friends—all have been known for years. The old ones are gone, but the children still know. There is not anyone there who we do not know."

EXPLANATORY MODELS

In caring for patients from a cross-cultural perspective, one must understand how a particular person thinks about illness. This has been described by Kleinman and co-workers[12] as the patient's *explanatory model*. The set of perceptions, attitudes, and responses to a given illness experience can be thought of as a belief system. A person's belief system includes his or her explanation of the illness experience and can be based on spiritual, religious, or social circumstances. A person's explanatory model answers such questions as the origin of the disease, the purpose or role of the illness or the role of the person with the illness, and acceptable treatments and procedures. Kleinman presents a series of questions designed for the clinician to use in tapping a person's explanatory model.

1. What do you think has caused your problem?
2. Why do you think it started when it did?
3. What do you think your sickness does to you? How does it work?
4. How severe is your sickness?
5. What kind of treatment do you think you should receive?

Notice the parallels of thought between these questions and the standard medical workup. In each approach, the goal is to understand the origin and course of the disease in order to develop an effective treatment plan. Eliciting a patient's explanatory model can be crucial to caring for people with a different orientation to illness and disease because it provides valuable information that would probably not come out in the traditional medical workup. The following example illustrates the importance of a patient's explanatory model in making an assessment and developing a plan. What are the management issues presented by the following vignette?

CASE STUDY 8-9

A 22-year-old Vietnamese woman, 2 days post partum, appeared distant and unable to bond with her healthy newborn son. Staff members were concerned about her lack of response to the child and suspected that she was clinically depressed because of her general listlessness and passivity. She refused to bathe or take cold fluids such as water with chipped ice.

This example illustrates several beliefs that may confuse practitioners. According to her cultural beliefs, her baby, a beautiful healthy child, is a gift from the gods. The woman was unable to risk the gods' wrath by displaying too much attachment to the child. In her traditional culture, family members would have assumed supportive roles in child care during this period. Childbirth also is seen as consuming tremendous energy, particularly hot energy. Bathing and taking cold fluids would not restore the lost "hot" energy, so they would be resisted.

The more the provider can understand the beliefs held by the patient, the more able the provider is to talk about the disease and illness in a manner easily understood by the patient.

Berlin and Fowkes[13] propose a framework by which practitioners can interact with patients that allows for the exchange of a patient's explanatory model and the practitioner's medical model. The framework is contained in the mnemonic LEARN.

L: Listen with sympathy and understanding to the patient's perception of the problem.
E: Explain your perceptions of the problem.
A: Acknowledge and discuss the differences and similarities.
R: Recommend treatment.
N: Negotiate agreement.

This is an interactional model designed to encourage patients to explain their conceptualization of their illness. This shift from the usual factual history taking helps the health care provider to elicit information about the patient's understanding, prior experience, expected treatments, or sense of causality about the presenting illness experience. This information does not replace the standard database contained in the history of present illness but augments it with information not generally obtained in the more traditional patient encounter. An expanded discussion of each element of the mnemonic helps explain the model.

Listen   This is an active process designed to ascertain the patient's knowledge, understanding, unique attributes, course, and expected treatment modalities associated with the illness experience. Some useful questions for clinicians are: "What might be causing your problem?" "What do you think might make you feel better?" "Who else have you talked to about this problem?" "Did they make any suggestions?" Notice the quality of permission and interest embedded in these questions. Responses provide clues about etiology, expected treatment, and alternate health consultations.

Explain   This part of the model contains the clinician's understanding of the medical problem. Typically, the explanation is based on the biomedical model of disease process. In many instances, the clinician may not know the precise diagnosis but pursues a treatment plan designed to manage the presenting symptoms. The critical aspect here is to convey the clinician's strategy to the patient in a meaningful interaction.

Acknowledge   This step allows for the integration of information presented in the two previous steps. The patient's and the clinician's conceptualizations and management plans have been expressed. The goal of this step is to acknowledge the differences and similarities. Frequently, differences can be similarities when purpose and function are examined.

For example, a Mexican American patient presented with a stomachache she or he considered *empacho* (thought to be caused by food caught somewhere in the digestive tract, or by a person's eating something because he or she was forced to).[4,13] After obtaining a history, the health care provider tentatively diagnosed the problem as "functional abdominal pain, rule out peptic ulcer disease." By finding out and acknowledging the patient's perception of the problem, the provider learned that a common treatment for *empacho* is massage or "tugging" of the abdomen.

This step allows for validation of the patient's perception of both the disease and its treatment. It also gives the clinician an opportunity to learn about any patient-generated treatment plans or practices that might be harmful.

Recommend   This step is designed to formulate a treatment plan that incorporates information obtained in previous steps. Culturally sensitive information can now be discussed in terms of the clinician's treatment plan. For example, the Vietnamese male who is reluctant to allow blood to be drawn because of energy loss at a time of illness might find it more acceptable with the clinician's assurances that only a small amount will be taken.

Negotiate   This step is the most important aspect of the model. The provider and the patient decide together on the treatment plan. Prior input provides the clinician with insights about relevant patient concerns and expectations that should be incorporated into the treatment plan. As is seen in the example of the patient with abdominal pain, the use of traditional cures could easily be seen to complement the biomedical approach. When this approach is used, treatment plans often blend modalities from traditional cultural practices with elements from the mainstream biomedical model.

The essence of the LEARN model is to offer a way for clinicians to access how their patients are thinking about a particular illness experience. This is important in cross-cultural medicine because patients from different perspectives may interpret common symptoms differently from the clinician. Although these differences are sometimes surprising and perhaps amusing, awareness of them provides an opportunity for the clinician to learn about rich cultural traditions. The model is also based on an approach of respectful treatment. The questions are designed to let patients express their thoughts, attitudes, and practices without imposing the provider's value judgments. Such an approach leads to a much higher level of patient adherence to treatment plans and a greater provider understanding of the patient's expectations.

ELICITING BELIEFS AND ASSUMPTIONS

The ability to elicit a patient's beliefs and experiences can benefit the clinical encounter in many ways. First, it allows patients to be the teachers about their own cultural ideas and assumptions. If patients perceive that the provider is willing to listen to and respect what they have to say, they feel more included in their care. The clinician also can pick up on important understandable words and concepts to use when explaining disease causation or treatment strategies, as in the following exchange.

> PA: *When you said before that you didn't go to school because you were sick, what kind of sick were you?*
> PATIENT'S WIFE: *My legs—I did not walk—the bones—in the bones my sick. I walk like* (demonstrates supporting weight on arms) *one year. But my grandma she bring me to the . . . faith healer* (laughter). *Yeah, she massaged me with bile. I don't know where she got that, but she rubbed me with that and I walked.*

Knowledge of this experience gave the PA an important way of explaining to the patient's wife the role of physical therapy in the care of the patient, who had had a stroke.

Every culture has its own way of explaining disease and has its own approach to coping with it. Knowledge of previous successful treatment interventions can help the clinician to provide support and direction for future interventions.

CASE STUDY 8-10

Mr. B was 70 years old and had acute gouty arthritis. The PA wanted to know how he was coping with the disease, in order to decide whether to add another pain medication.

Mr. B answered, "I ask the Lord to hear me now and sometime give me some health and strength. That's what I tell Jesus."

"So, does that seem to help?" the PA asked.

"Yeah. It help me sometimes, because sometime I not feel so painful." He looked at his swollen gouty hand. "It's getting better."

This response revealed the role of religion in helping some patients to cope with chronic disease. Eliciting the information gave the PA an opportunity to acknowledge and support Mr. B's coping mechanisms, as well as to ascertain that further pain medication was not necessary at that time.

WORKING WITH INTERPRETERS*

Providing health care to non–English-speaking patients may or may not involve working with an interpreter. In either case, several considerations can be helpful to the practitioner. When an interpreter is available, it is crucial to remember that the primary relationship remains between the patient and the provider. Therefore, verbal and nonverbal elements of communication must be monitored in terms of the patient's responses throughout the interaction, regardless of the interpreter's presence. In general, working with an interpreter results in longer encounters and requires patience.

Before seeing the patient, the provider should review with the interpreter how the provider would like to conduct the interaction. The provider should specify a seating arrangement that ensures direct eye contact and observation between the practitioner and the patient. The interpreter should be instructed to observe and identify facial expressions, nuances, or intonation patterns that may indicate the patient's responses, as appropriate during the interaction. Nonverbal cues can indicate fear, surprise, anxiousness, or other reactions that affect the history of the illness episode or the acceptability of the proposed treatment plan.

The following case illustrates the importance of such nuances. After the Vietnam War, there was a large immigration of Hmong, a specific Southeast Asian ethnic group.

CASE STUDY 8-11

A health care provider was working in a rural clinic and loved children. She had the experience of often calming children by touching their heads. One day, about halfway through the interview with a Hmong family, she noticed that the family appeared very uncomfortable and eager to leave. At first, she thought it was probably due to concern about their 13-month-old child, who had otitis

---

*The material in this section is adapted from a workshop on cross-cultural medicine conducted by Larry Li and Stephen Ratcliffe at the Western Regional APAP meeting, Salt Lake City, Utah, July 20, 1991.

media. But when the same thing occurred a few weeks later with another Hmong family, she became curious. She described the experience to an interpreter, who told her that the Hmong believe that the head has great significance as the seat of life and that only one's close relatives are permitted to touch it.[14]

Interpreters should be discouraged from offering personal advice or comments, making assumptions, or omitting information. Lengthy translations because of technical terms or other matters are inevitable; "yes" or "no" responses to unusually long interactions between the patient and the interpreter should still be questioned. The interpreter should be encouraged to translate the patient's own words directly as much as possible. This gives the practitioner a better sense of the patient's conceptualization and emotional response to the illness episode.

Once these basic guidelines have been established, it is time for the clinician and the interpreter to meet with the patient. The interpreter should first be given time to meet with the patient and establish rapport. Just because two people speak the same language does not ensure flawless communication. In fact, several types of mismatches between patients and interpreters must be approached carefully or avoided if possible. These are opposite-sex interpreters for sexually related problems or medical conditions, very young interpreters for geriatric patients, and, sometimes, extreme differences in socioeconomic backgrounds. All can lead to complications in the interview.

Patients who speak a different language from the clinician often use daughters or sons for translators. However, the clinician must realize the difficulties faced by the child in this position during the visit. The child may have greater language ability and knowledge of the majority culture, but within the family, the child still needs to be under the adult's control. It is important for the health care provider to be sensitive to possible role conflicts, as illustrated in the following case.

CASE STUDY 8-12

Mr. R, a 65-year-old Mexican man, was being followed for Parkinson's disease at an inner city clinic. He and his wife lived with their eldest daughter and her five children. He had stopped taking his medication because it caused him to vomit, but when the symptoms came back, he realized it was time to go back to see the doctor.

As always, the daughter went as a translator. The physician, probably frustrated with the man's lack of compliance, scolded the daughter for not making sure her father took the medication.

The unfortunate outcome of this intervention was that the father, who was having a difficult time accepting the chronic nature of the disease and the necessity of taking daily medication, did not have an opportunity to express his fears or questions. The daughter also was confused and could see that the clinician believed she was not doing a good enough job. Yet, because of the rules in her culture and family, she *knew* she could not tell her father what to do. Finally, because she did not wish to appear incapable again, she did not ask the clinician questions about the disease. She also did not ask for clarification about *altas palabras* (complicated English words that even her younger sister, the family English expert, could not understand).

The health care provider should direct questions to the patient, such as, "What have you done to relieve the pain?" The provider should maintain eye contact with the patient, as appropriate, as the interpreter translates each question. It is helpful to use short simple sentences and to avoid medical jargon and colloquial metaphors. The provider and the interpreter should seek to provide culturally meaningful translations rather than literal ones. For example, instead of "MRI," one might use "a machine that looks at the bones and nerves in your back." The provider should elicit culturally specific information, as described in the LEARN mnemonic. This is an invaluable opportunity to learn about the patient's belief system and expectations about treatment and any other healing modalities currently in use. The provider should frequently ascertain the patient's understanding of questions and any assessments and treatment plans. This provides permission and an opening for the patient to clarify any concerns. On occasion, the interpreter might hesitate to pursue a question. This may result from unfamiliarity with the medical term, fear that the patient might think the interpreter is wishing the disease on the patient, or concern that the provider is asking something inappropriate or harmful. If for any reason, the interpreter hesitates or refuses to proceed in a given area, the cause must be determined immediately and a solution to the difficulty must be found.

Nonverbal communication is an important part of interacting with patients from other cultures, even with an interpreter. Eye contact can send various messages. In some cultures, it is a sign of respect and confidence, whereas in others, it can be a sign of hostility or rudeness. Practitioners can learn about how their patients use or are comfortable with silence and eye contact. Observing how family members interact or how the interpreter interacts with the patient during different parts and contents of the interview may provide some cues. The provider should note whether pauses or interruptions are tolerated or become opportunities to move on to new areas of dialog. Physical distance between communicators is influenced by cultural background. Although great diversity can exist in physical comfort zones, it would be respectful to allow the patient some flexibility in choice of seat location. The expression of pain or discomfort can be influenced by culture and gender role. A detached affect during the history of a traumatic event may not convey a lack of caring or impact on the patient, but rather may represent a coping mechanism.

Sometimes, by combining nonverbal cues such as facial expression and body posture, the provider can gain a sense of the extent of the patient's discomfort, anxiety, or depression. Body gestures can be rich sources of information. The provider should note when the patient moves or just physically reacts to the content of the interview. The movement may indicate uncomfortable or emotionally laden content, and its meaning could be pursued through the interpreter. Some cultures, such as the Vietnamese, consider pointing with the finger or foot to be rude and inappropriate communication. Observing how patients interact and asking what is permissible allows the clinician to learn about other cultures.

The checklist for the use of interpreters shown in the accompanying box contains many of the points just described. A PA may find it helpful to include it in his or her clinical resources to assist in work with interpreters. The inclusion of these few points can take less than 5 minutes in the discussion with the interpreter, yet can save hours of frustration, improve compliance, and possibly prevent dangerous mistakes.

CULTURE-SPECIFIC DISEASE EXPLANATIONS

Some cultures have very clearly developed disease entities that do not fit into standard biomedical disease categories. Although it is impossible to list specific beliefs of all groups, some common ideas found in many cultures can serve as guides for clinicians to elicit specific beliefs.

Balance appears to be a concept common to many explanations of health and illness. Belief systems found in Chinese, Haitian, Mexican, and Puerto Rican cultures support the notion that disease results from the body's being thrown into an abnormally hot or cold state. These states may be brought on by external circumstances or by food.[15,16]

In many cultures, illness is regarded as a consequence of an imbalance between the individual or family and the physical, spiritual, or social world. Therefore, logical treatments might include burning incense, wearing amulets, and avoiding certain individuals.[15] Sometimes the concept of balance could be applied to a history of being out of balance, or having a history of a traumatic event or mistakes in life choices. One woman explained the reason she believed her husband ended up with Parkinson's disease as follows: "You see, he drank for many years starting when he was young. When he was 17, his father died and, I believe, he would get drunk on the ranches. He drank a lot of wine, and he was an alcoholic I believe. And the attack on his brain was the result of this wrong."

Another common idea is that some diseases are due to the entrance of bad air or drafts, especially during periods of extreme susceptibility.[16] Consider the following interchange.

CHECKLIST FOR THE USE OF AN INTERPRETER

Before the clinical encounter:
- Determine a seating arrangement that allows the clinician to observe verbal and nonverbal interactions.
- Request the interpreter to include the patient's words in translation when possible.
- Ask the interpreter to identify for the practitioner any apparent or suspected strong emotional reactions.
- Encourage the interpreter, if he or she gets stuck at any time, to discuss the nature of the problem.
- Give permission to the interpreter to identify provider behaviors or questions that may be confusing or offensive, and to explain to the provider any patient or family behaviors or interactions that may be unusual or confusing.

During the clinical encounter:
- Allow time for the interpreter to establish rapport.
- Direct questions to the patient, not the interpreter.
- Maintain verbal and appropriate nonverbal contact with the patient, for example, respectful eye contact and touch.
- Ask questions in direct and short sentences.
- Observe the family for cues to content and style of interactions.
- Seek the cultural content of the illness experience, that is, explanatory models and use of alternative healers and treatments.

Closing the encounter:
- Summarize and validate key findings with the patient and the interpreter. Be receptive to clarification.
- Give the patient permission to ask questions about treatment plans.
- Discuss ongoing education.
- Seek information from interpreters who are trusted about provider cultural mistakes or patients' assumptions or belief systems that may be influencing patient interactions or compliance issues.

PATIENT: *Oh, they were brought on by the "air." The first time was when I was putting in a door in San Diego with a lady who asked me to put up a door that had glass. I believe that air from the north— northwest—because I didn't feel anything but this: the earth shook, and then air—aire de la tierra—from the earth came inside. Later, I asked the woman, and she said that she didn't feel the earth shaking or an earthquake.*

PA: *And did you ever see a doctor to get an explanation?*

PATIENT: *Yes, they thought it was the beginning of epilepsy. There in Mexicali they gave me a tonic.*

On occasion, traditional explanations are combined with current medical concepts. One Mexican American husband and wife, using two different yet complementary explanatory models, described a specific event.

> WIFE: *I knew of someone in San Ramon; he died while having intercourse. He wasn't old. He had a sudden attack and then they couldn't pull them apart.*
> HUSBAND: *It could have been because of susto (illness brought on by severe fright).*
> WIFE: *Or perhaps a heart attack. He had angina.*

CULTURAL COMPETENCE

Cultural competence is the clinician's ability to work effectively with patients from differing cultures.

Many aspects of this competence have been described in this chapter. The Stanford Geriatric Education Center has developed guidelines for describing cultural competence. These guidelines have been adapted to form the self-evaluation tool in the accompanying box. The tool can be used to evaluate aspects of a patient encounter to determine whether one is providing culturally sensitive care.

CULTURAL COMPETENCE SELF-EVALUATION

After meeting with someone who is from a culture other than your own, try to answer the following questions.

1. Did the history include, as appropriate, the patient's unique life experiences and beliefs about disease?
2. What cultural rules for skin touching, eye contact, and opposite-sex examinations does this patient operate under?
3. Did I obtain permission or give adequate explanation for asking a potentially embarrassing history question or performing a potentially intrusive examination? In what way?
4. Did my assessment and plan include what I know about the patient's ideas regarding the causation of the problem and appropriate treatment? How?
5. Did I use the patient's words in patient education regarding the causation of the problem and treatment? Which concepts or words were used?
6. What did I learn from this encounter about my own values and assumptions?
7. What did I learn from this patient about his or her values and assumptions?
8. How does this compare with my previous knowledge about other people from the same ethnic background or group?
9. What historical (e.g., immigration history) or ethnically mediated (e.g., diet) factors are affecting this patient's individual or family health problems now?

Practitioners who work with a large number of people from a specific ethnic group can use responses to these questions to avoid being a cultural klutz (doing or saying things that are offensive and alienating). In addition, responses will yield basic information about words and concepts that can be helpful in eliciting an appropriate and efficient history, as well as in formulating a respectful treatment plan with better potential for compliance.

CONCLUSION

This chapter serves as an introduction to cross-cultural medicine. The emphasis on clinical applications is an attempt to provide a springboard for clinicians to venture into this rich world of information. The changing demographics of our society pose many challenges for those in the helping professions. First, clinicians must become aware of their own cultural assumptions and belief systems. Second, clinicians must be sensitive to socioeconomic issues that affect provider-patient interactions and patient compliance. Third, clinicians must expand the usual biomedical conceptualization of disease and illness to include unique cross-cultural perceptions of causation and cure.

Demographic information and knowledge of racial and ethnic groups are helpful to the clinician in caring for patients. However, the most important teachers of cross-cultural health care are the patients and families who come seeking care daily. They come to a health care system that often has its own subculture—language, clothing, status symbols, and a set of expected behaviors for patients as well as practitioners. PAs are brokers of that system and therefore have a unique opportunity to bridge the gap.

CLINICAL APPLICATIONS

1. Review your own experiences in using interpreters. What worked? What didn't work? What were your own internal struggles in terms of making this communication work effectively? Share these experiences with your classmates.
2. Using the questions described under the "Explanatory Models" section of this chapter, review a recent health care problem that you, a

family member, or a friend may have had. Ask yourself the five questions that are suggested. Compare your answers to these more complex questions with the answer you might give to the more specific history of present illness (HPI) questions that are asked as part of routine history taking.

REFERENCES

1. Polednak A. Racial and Ethnic Differences in Disease. New York: Oxford University Press, 1989.
2. Gordon M. Assimilation in American Life. New York: Oxford University Press, 1964.
3. Wing-Sue D. The challenge of multiculturism: the road less traveled. Am Counselor 1992;1:6.
4. Health, United States, 1990. U.S. Dept of Health and Human Services publication PHS 91-1232. Washington, DC: National Center for Health Statistics, 1991.
5. Health, United States, 2001. U.S. Dept of Health and Human Services. Washington, DC: National Center for Health Statistics, 2001.
6. National Vital Statistics Report, 2001. Vol 49, no. 8. Washington, DC: National Center for Health Statistics, 2001.
7. Vernon SW, Tilley BC, Neale AV, et al. Ethnicity, survival and delay in seeking treatment for symptoms of breast cancer. Cancer 1985;55:1563.
8. Harper MS. Introduction. In: Harper MS (ed). Minority Aging: Essential Curricula Content for Selected Health and Allied Health Professions. Washington, DC: Health Resources and Services Administration, 1990. U.S. Dept of Health and Human Services publication HRS-P-DV 90-4.
9. U.S. Census Bureau. Poverty 1999: poverty estimates by selected characteristics. Available at http://www.census.gov/hhes/poverty/poverty99/pv99est1.html. Accessed 3 July 2002.
10. National Center for Health Statistics web site. Available at http://www.cdc.gov/nchs. Accessed 12 July 2002.
11. Harris E. Native Stranger. New York: Simon & Schuster, 1992.
12. Kleinman A, Eisenberg L, Good B. Culture, illness and care: clinical lessons from anthropological and cross cultural research. Ann Intern Med 1978;88:251.
13. Berlin EA, Fowkes WC Jr. A teaching framework for cross-cultural health care. West J Med 1983;139:934.
14. Stoffels S. Culturally sensitive nursing: the Hmong child with measles. Nurseweek/North 1990;6:8.
15. Harwood A. Ethnicity and Medical Care. Cambridge, MA: Harvard University Press, 1981.
16. Henderson G, Pimeaux M (eds). Transcultural Health Care. Menlo Park, CA: Addison-Wesley, 1981.

RESOURCES

Berlin EA, Fowkes WC Jr. A teaching framework for cross-cultural health care. West J Med 1983;139:934. *Guidelines for interacting with patients from different cultures are presented in the mnemonic LEARN—listen, explain, acknowledge, recommend, and negotiate. Each guideline is explained through clinical vignettes of patient encounters.*

Cross-cultural medicine a decade later. West J Med 1992;157:213. *The special issue focuses on the emergence of cross-cultural medicine as a growing area of importance to clinicians. Excellent national and regional demographic data are presented. The articles are written by clinicians for clinicians. Topics focus on specific clinical issues such as interpreters, refugee health, sexuality, aging, and mental health.*

Harper MS. Introduction. In: Harper MS (ed). Minority Aging: Essential Curricula Content for Selected Health and Allied Health Professions. Washington, DC: Health Resources and Services Administration. Dept of US Health and Human Services publication HRS-P-DV 90-4. *Contains a series of papers identifying needs associated with a growing geriatric ethnic population. Specific profiles are presented for Native American and Alaskan Native, African-American, Asian American, and Hispanic elderly.*

Harwood A. Ethnicity and Medical Care. Cambridge, MA: Harvard University Press, 1981. *A comprehensive and scholarly work on the field of cross-cultural medicine. Includes numerous recommendations for the clinician regarding the role of culture in clinical care. Solid overviews of different cultural groups are presented along with a discussion of common culturally bound illnesses.*

Henderson G, Primeaux M (eds). Transcultural Health Care. Menlo Park, CA: Addison-Wesley, 1981. *The book is organized into three major sections related to transcultural medicine: sociocultural dimensions of health care, folk medicine, and clinical care. Excellent cultural backgrounds are presented for African, Hispanic, Pacific Islander, Asian, and Native American groups. Key health beliefs are reviewed for each group along with case vignettes of practical clinical examples in the clinical care section.*

Spector R. Cultural Diversity in Health and Illness. East Norwalk, CT: Appleton-Century-Crofts, 1985. *After providing an overview of different general concepts, this text provides chapters on health and illness in the Asian American, African-American, Hispanic American, Native American, and white ethnic communities.*

Mead M (ed). Special issue: cross cultural medicine. West J Med 1983;139:1. *Entire issue dedicated to cross-cultural medicine. It offers an informative survey of major ethnic groups—African-American, Hispanic, Chinese, Japanese, Native American, Southeast Asian, and Filipino—in terms of beliefs, immigration status, traditional healers and modalities, perception and definition of disease, and expected treatment. Excellent bibliographies are given for each cultural group.*

Polednak A. Racial and Ethnic Differences in Disease. New York: Oxford University Press, 1989. *Well-referenced book that carefully reviews what is currently known regarding differences among diseases in different ethnic and racial groups.*

Ethnographic Reviews: State of the Literature Summaries. Working Paper Series. Stanford, CA: Stanford Geriatric Education

Center, 1990. *These papers, available from the SGEC (703 Welch Rd, Suite H-1, Stanford, CA 94305), give comprehensive summaries of the current literature, including immigration issues when appropriate, folk medical illness, and traditional cures. Recommended working papers are as follows.*

#3: *Moriokas Douglas N, Yeo G. Aging and Health: Asian/Pacific Island American Elders.*

#4: *Richardson J. Aging and Health: Black American Elders.*

#5: *Cuellar J. Aging and Health: Hispanic American Elders.*

#6: *Cuellar J. Aging and Health: American Indian/Alaskan Native Elders.*

CHAPTER 9

Patient Record

Kimberly Suggs, Ann M. Meehan, and Richard R. Rahr

PURPOSES OF THE PATIENT RECORD

The primary reason for keeping a thorough, accurate record of a patient's encounter with health care professionals is to provide the best possible medical care to the patient. This is of importance to the person providing the care, to the patient, to others involved in that care, and to the payers who reimburse for the services. The well-documented patient record serves as a real-time documentation tool, a communication tool, a tool for quality assessment and reimbursement validation, a mechanism for minimizing the risk of malpractice litigation, and a source of information for use in research and the education of clinicians.

Real-Time Documentation Tool

By concurrently recording accurately and concisely the treatments given to a patient and the thought processes that were used in the decision making, a health care professional can easily review the infor-

mation needed to decide what further action is warranted in the care and treatment of that patient. In a busy practice, a physician assistant (PA) sees many patients. Memory alone cannot be expected to provide all the pertinent facts about each patient.

Communication Tool

Many people are involved in the care of a patient. Physician specialists, nurses, nurse practitioners, physical therapists, occupational therapists, and PAs are some of the individuals who may need to refer to the record to plan the best possible care for the patient.

In today's health care environment, more services have moved to the outpatient setting, where patients are more mobile. Patients move through the health care organizations, clinics, and hospital departments to access the care needed. Thus, many different departments, services, and health care providers are

157

involved in the care of one patient. It is important that the patient's record or the information contained in that record be accessible so that all caregivers can have the opportunity to understand the patient's current condition, history, and care plan.

Coordination of the services that a patient may need can be done only through complete communication of the assessments and interventions that have already become part of the patient's care. The record provides the necessary communication link among all these caregivers.

The communication provided by the record can be even more crucial in a society in which people commonly move from community to community. Patients want to carry their records with them so that the providers in their new community can give them the best care possible. This sharing of information can save the patient money because tests need not be repeated unnecessarily.

Quality Assessment Tool

Individuals who provide care need to evaluate the quality of that care. They most often do so by reviewing the patient record. The outcome of treatment is one way that quality of care is determined. For example, in obstetrical practices, the desired outcome could be a live newborn that weighs more than 5 lb. In cases in which this outcome is not achieved, the records can be reviewed to determine whether the appropriate and necessary care was provided.

Outside agencies often audit records for quality assessment. Traditionally, those audits were done in inpatient settings. Professional review organizations (PROs) are charged with this task for inpatients in the Medicare program. This review covers the completeness, adequacy, and quality of medical care. However, with the implementation of medical necessity requirements and of the Medicare outpatient prospective payment plan, the focus of medical review now has also moved to the outpatient setting. The Office of the Inspector General (OIG) provides oversight of the services provided to Medicare patients. Each year, the OIG publishes its Work Plan, which outlines the areas on which the agency will focus its review.

Quality assessment, both by providers themselves and by outside agencies, requires a record that is thorough, accurate, and concise. Such a record allows the reviewer to reach the same conclusion as the caregiver.

Reimbursement Validation Tool

The record is often used to prove to commercial insurance companies and federal agencies that medical necessity requirements for treatment were met and that services billed were actually performed. With the implementation of the Medicare prospective payment system, Diagnosis-Related Groups (DRGs) in 1982, and Ambulatory Payment Classification (APC) in 2000, the patient record has become more important for validating the services billed. Likewise, the implementation of Relative Value Units, or RVUs, for physician reimbursement, has also enhanced focus on the patient record.

Often, copies of patient records are requested by PROs and federal fiscal intermediaries and carriers so that services provided can be confirmed and information filed on the claim can be validated. Audits are performed, using the itemized bill and the patient record, to justify all charges. If a treatment or test is not recorded by those providing the care, charges for such services may be denied. Physicians and other health care providers should be following the Documentation Guidelines of Key Components of Evaluation and Management Services in documenting services provided to patients in their practice. Hospitals, physicians, and other health care providers have been required to return millions of dollars to the government either for services that were not performed or for services that were not supported by the documentation in the patient record.

Likewise, managed care payers have increased their requirements for delineating covered services, and the information in the patient record is often used for justifying services. With increasing frequency, pre-admission screening is used to determine whether services are required. The record must include consistent information that verifies the facts as provided at the time of admission.

With costs for health care rising so rapidly, the record will be brought under closer scrutiny by more and more third party payers. The caregivers who will survive financially are those who maintain a clear understanding of payer requirements and who provide a detailed and accurate account of the status of the patient that includes all procedures performed and the diagnoses for which those services were provided.

Risk Management Tool

The best defense against malpractice litigation is a detailed, concise, and accurate record that shows that the person providing the care is competent and credible. An organized record that includes details of the status of the patient, as well as the information that was used to make decisions about plans for further care, will serve the PA well in avoiding any potential litigation.[1]

Education and Research Resource

The data contained in individual patient records, when collected and analyzed along with data from a larger population of records, furnish valuable information for assessing the effectiveness of both current treatments and treatments under development, as well as other types of clinical research. The clinical abilities of future health care providers are in part determined by review of the records of the patients they see in training. The future of health care depends on this use of patient data both individually and in aggregate.

CONTENT OF THE PATIENT RECORD

The organization providing care, whether it be a hospital, an outpatient clinic, or a physician's office, determines the exact format of the information to be collected in a patient's record. The content of the patient record is determined by accrediting agencies, regulatory agencies, professional organizations, and others. Guidelines can be found in the following, to name a few:

➤ Medicare Hospital Manual (HIM-10).
➤ Medicare Conditions of Participation.
➤ Joint Commission on Accreditation of Hospitals Organization.
➤ Fiscal Intermediary and Carrier Manuals.
➤ Local Medical Review Policies (LMRPs).
➤ Documentation Guidelines for Evaluation & Management Services.
➤ Teaching Physician Guidelines.

Patient information may be described as administrative or clinical. Detailed discussions of each are included below.

Administrative Information

Patient identification and demographic data must be recorded to ensure that the patient is properly identified; such information is used for the treatment of that patient only. At a minimum, it should include the patient's name, address, sex, race, and date of birth. Usually, the immediate family is named also. Financial data about insurance coverage or who will be responsible for the bill are also considered administrative information and are important in reimbursement claims for the services provided.

Consent forms for specific procedures or release of information are another type of administrative information. Consents (authorizations) must be signed by the patient or by an individual legally qualified to sign for the patient. State laws vary as to who may legally consent to treatment; therefore, it is important for the health care professional to know the content of these laws for the geographical area in which the treatment is given.

CASE STUDY 9-1

John Jones is a 39-year-old male college teacher with a 2-month history of angina, who presents with crushing substernal chest pain radiating to the left shoulder and jaw, which awoke him from sleep this morning. Self-treatment with nitroglycerin did not relieve his pain. He has accompanying symptoms of nausea, vomiting, and dyspnea.

Mr. Jones smokes two packs of cigarettes daily and drinks six beers three times a week. He is under considerable stress from a recent divorce. Further details about Mr. Jones' care, including his hospitalization and discharge summary, follow in the samples of medical records in this chapter.

Clinical Information

The clinical information required for a hospitalized patient varies according to the nature of the illness and the treatment required. Outpatient records should include details for those items that are pertinent to each visit.

Admitting Diagnosis For inpatients, the admitting or provisional diagnosis is supplied by the physician who is admitting the patient, generally with the admission orders upon admission. Outpatient visits require a patient's reason for the visit. This information is provided by the patient to the physician, PA, nurse, or other caregiver and is documented in the patient record. The patient's reason for visit is important for the care of the patient because it identifies why the patient presented for treatment and is also important in justifying the outpatient services provided to the patient.

History A complete history is required for both the first outpatient visit and the inpatient admission. This history is to be completed at the time of the visit or as soon as possible, but no later than 24 hours, after admission. The parts of a complete history are listed here; an example of a complete history is shown in Figure 9-1 in a problem-oriented medical record format.

Chief Complaint Usually, the chief complaint is the exact reason the patient sought medical attention, stated in the patient's own words. Both the nature and the duration of the symptom are recorded.

Present Illness A detailed recording of the exact signs, symptoms, and reactions of the patient, the present illness information can be collected in the "serial 7s" format: quantity, quality, onset, duration, chronology, alleviation, and aggravation. Another way to collect this information is chronologically, from the first presence of the problem until the hospital admission or clinic visit. Regardless of the number of problems reported, each is detailed individually. The traditional format for recording is the use of paragraphs. An alternative format developed by Lawrence Weed is discussed later.

Past Medical History Past medical history consists of general health, childhood illnesses, allergies, medical hospitalizations, surgical procedures, accidents, psychiatric history, medications, immunizations, blood transfusions, and pregnancies.

Psychosocial or Personal History This section normally includes residence, education, marital status, dietary habits, typical day, stresses, sexual activity, use of drugs, alcohol and tobacco, occupation, religion, hobbies, and outlook on life.

Family History The diseases among the patient's relatives in which heredity or personal contact may play a role are noted here. Allergies, infections, neoplasms, and mental, metabolic, endocrine, cardiovascular, and renal diseases are considered. The health status, ages, ages at death, and causes of death should be recorded for grandparents, parents, siblings, spouse, and children.

Review of Systems A review of the common symptoms of each body system is completed both to jog the patient's memory and to further define the present illness. A format for the common parts of a review of systems is as follows:
1. *General:* Weight changes, fatigue, weakness, fever, chills, heat or cold intolerance, fainting.
2. *Integumentary:* Ecchymosis, rashes, lesions, wheals, cyanosis, jaundice, erythema, changes in hair, nails, or skin.
3. *HEENT:* Cephalgia, blurred or double vision, blindness, glaucoma, cataract, hearing loss, otalgia, tinnitus, roaring in ears, vertigo, discharge from ear or eye, epistaxis, rhinorrhea, deviated septum, postnasal drainage, sinus pain, bleeding of teeth or gums, hoarseness, trouble swallowing, sore throat, bad taste in mouth, frequent tonsillitis.
4. *Respiratory:* Shortness of breath, wheezing, sputum production, repeated respiratory infections, cough, hemoptysis, asthma, bronchitis, emphysema, tuberculosis or fungal infection, abnormal chest x-ray, history of lung cancer, radiation therapy.
5. *Cardiovascular:* Chest pain, syncope, shortness of breath, orthopnea, paroxysmal nocturnal dyspnea, dyspnea on exertion, edema, abnormal electrocardiogram or echocardiogram, previous stress testing, rheumatic fever, scarlet fever, palpitations, thrombophlebitis, varicose veins, history of hypertension.

Text continued on p. 164.

HISTORY   John J. Jones   #12-12-12

Patient Data:
    Name: John J. Jones, Ph.D.
    Record Number: 12-12-12
    DOB: December 1, 1963
    Date: May 15, 2002
    Address: 2568 Campeche Cove
                             Galveston, TX   77553
    Marital Status: Divorced
    Informant: Self
    Occupation: Biologist

Patient Profile: This is a 39-year-old divorced white
    male who is a faculty member in graduate school at the
    University of Texas Medical Branch in Galveston. The
    patient is under stress due to a recent divorce and the
    custody of two children, ages 5 and 7. The patient
    smokes two packages of Camel cigarettes each day and
    drinks a six-pack of beer three times a week.

Chief Complaint: "I awoke at 5:30 this morning with a
    feeling like an elephant was sitting on my chest."

Problem #1: Acute Myocardial Infarction with Previous
    Angina Pectoris

Subjective: This is a 39-year-old white male biologist who
    presented to the emergency room at John Sealy Hospital
    at 6:30 AM with severe substernal chest pain. The
    patient awoke with a crushing substernal pain that
    radiated to his left shoulder and jaw. He took three
    0.4 mg nitroglycerin tablets five minutes apart
    without relief. The patient has nausea and vomited X 1
    with the vomitus being a yellow bile color with a
    bitter taste. He had hyperhidrosis, fatigue, weakness,
    vertigo, palpitation, and shortness of breath. Dr.
    Jones had been up late working on a grant proposal that
    is due Monday.
His angina pectoris has been treated for two months
    with isosorbide dinitrate 20 mg q.i.d., Inderal 20 mg
    q.i.d., and nitroglycerin 0.4 mg PRN, and has remained
    stable. The patient admits to smoking two packs of
    cigarettes per day for 20 years. He has a positive
    family history for MIs, CVAs, and hypertension. The
    patient is under a great deal of stress, with pressure
    at work to get his research funded as well as going
    through a recent separation and divorce with sole
    custody of two children, ages 5 and 7. A lipogram in
    July, 1996, showed a normal cholesterol level.

Figure 9-1 Sample patient history.

HISTORY   John J. Jones   #12-12-12

Problem #2:   **Reactive Depression**

Subjective: Dr. Jones has been having a feeling of sadness,
     sleep disturbance, crying, and suicide thoughts since
     October, when his wife left him for another man. She
     went to California with her new significant other
     without a desire to see him or the children. The
     patient and his wife had been married for 18 years
     without many marital problems. In September, he
     discovered his wife was seeing another man. In October,
     they agreed to separate, with Dr. Jones having sole
     custody of the children. The patient has terminal
     sleep disturbance with awakening at 5 AM each day,
     often in a cold sweat. He has no plans of suicide, but
     he has suicide thoughts often. He has not seen a
     psychiatrist because he has been too busy taking care
     of the children. He admits to poor appetite, twenty
     pound weight loss, with frequent bouts of nausea,
     diarrhea, and abdominal cramping.

Problem #3:   **Recent Divorce**

Subjective: Dr. Jones has been separated from his wife
     since October, 1991, when she left for California with
     another man. She has had only a few conversations with
     him or the children. He was granted a divorce in
     January, 1997, with sole custody of the two girls, ages
     5 and 7. He and his wife had a good marriage for 18
     years before the problems last fall. Dr. Jones has
     hired a housekeeper but he still finds the new
     responsibilities very difficult. With the additional
     pressure at work of completing the grant proposal by
     the deadline, he has been getting only small amounts of
     sleep.

Past Medical History:

General: Good health until the onset of angina pectoris two
     months ago.
Childhood Illnesses: Measles, mumps, chickenpox, scarlet
     fever.
Allergies: House dust, dog dander.
Medical: Pneumonia, February, 1990.
Accidents: Fractured femur from auto accident in 1981.
Surgery: Appendectomy, 1971.
Psychiatric: None.
Immunizations: Polio, tetanus, diphtheria, hepatitis.
Medications: Isordil 20 mg q.i.d.
                 Inderal 20 mg q.i.d.
                 Nitroglycerin 0.4 mg PRN
Transfusions: None.

Figure 9-1, cont'd Sample patient history.

HISTORY   John J. Jones   #12-12-12

Family History:

Father: Expired at age 60, acute myocardial infarction.
Mother: Alive, age 64, CVA and hypertension.
Brothers: One age 44, hypertension; second age 36, alive
     and well.
Sister: One, age 42, hypertension.
Children: Two daughters, ages 5 and 7, alive and well.

Positive for acute MI, CVA, hypertension.
Negative for adult onset diabetes mellitus, and renal,
     pulmonary or hematological disease.

Personal Social History:
     This is a 39-year-old, recently divorced, white male
     with two daughters, ages 5 and 7, whom he is raising.
     Dr. Jones has a Ph.D. from UT-Austin in biology. He
     has been at UTMB since 1980, doing research in the
     Graduate School in marine biology. He has three
     present stresses: recent divorce, job deadlines, and
     raising two daughters as a single parent. He is
     financially secure. His wife did not request a large
     financial settlement; her significant other is a very
     rich physician in private practice in California. Dr.
     Jones is Catholic and attends church each week. He has
     no time for hobbies; however, he has played golf in the
     past.

Review of Systems:

General: Patient denies heat, cold intolerance. He has a
     20 pound weight decrease and increased anxiety.
Skin: Patient denies petechiae, ecchymosis, bruising,
     rashes, lesions, mole changes, hair changes, or
     erythema.
HEENT: Patient denies cephalgia, syncope, tinnitus, visual
     changes, hearing loss, nasal discharge, epistaxis,
     bleeding gums, hoarseness, or difficulty swallowing.
     He does have dizziness and vertigo.
Neck: Patient denies masses, swelling, or painful neck.
Pulmonary: Patient denies fever, chills, coughing, sputum
     production, shortness of breath, or wheezing.
Cardiovascular: Patient has substernal chest pain,
     palpitations, and radiation of chest pain to the left
     arm. He denies syncope, or shortness of breath. He
     relates no history of heart murmur or abnormal
     electrocardiogram.
Gastrointestinal: Patient denies right upper quadrant
     abdominal pain, history of ulcer, hematemesis, melena,
     hematochezia. He does admit to nausea, diarrhea, and
     generalized abdominal cramping.

Figure 9-1, cont'd Sample patient history.

HISTORY   John J. Jones   #12-12-12

   Renal & Reproductive: Patient denies penile discharge,
        stricture, dysuria, hematuria, nocturia, or suprapubic
        pain.
   Musculoskeletal: Patient denies any muscular pain,
        weakness, coldness, erythema, or swelling.
   Neurological: Patient denies seizures, tremor, cephalgia,
        visual changes, or paresthesia. He does admit to
        suicide thoughts without specific plans.
   Lymph: Patient denies swelling or adenopathy.

Richard Rahr, PA-C

Richard Rahr, PA-C
Dictated & transcribed: 5/15/2002

Eric Greenberg M.D.

Eric Greenberg, M.D.
Attending Physician

Figure 9-1, cont'd Sample patient history.

6. *Gastrointestinal:* Dyspepsia, history of ulcer, melena, hematochezia, hematemesis, stool color, nausea, vomiting, diarrhea, constipation, changes in bowel habits, appetite, thirst, rectal bleeding, flatus, food intolerance, hemorrhoids, jaundice, ruptured spleen, colon cancer, abdominal surgery.

7. *Urinary:* Dysuria, hematuria, nocturia, frequency, hesitancy, urgency, costovertebral angle (CVA) pain, suprapubic distention.

8. *Reproductive:* Dyspareunia, discharge from genitals, venereal disease, high-risk sexual behavior, herpes, genital lesion, sexual activity.
   ➤ Men—penile abnormalities, hernia, testicular swelling or pain, vasectomy.
   ➤ Women—age of menarche, menstrual history, menstrual frequency and duration, use of pads, dysmenorrhea, menorrhagia, menopause symptoms, contraception, pregnancies, deliveries, abortions, Pap smear, abnormal Pap smear, breast examinations, breast retraction, discharges, masses, or tenderness.

9. *Neurological:* Seizures, numbness, scotoma, tremors, paresthesias, syncope, vertigo, suicide plans or tendencies, weakness of extremity, painful spine and radiation of pain, memory loss, cephalgia, visual disturbances, stroke, head injury, depression, mental disorder with treatment, anxiety, insomnia, mood changes, nightmares.

Physical Examination   The physical examination is also to be completed at the time of the visit or as soon as possible, but no later than 24 hours, after hospital admission. The physical examination is often detailed in the format given here and shown in Figure 9-2.

General   A description of the patient, this section includes age, sex, general state of health, stature,

Text continued on p. 167.

PHYSICAL EXAMINATION   John J. Jones #12-12-12

Patient Data:
      Name: John J. Jones, Ph.D.
      Record Number: 12-12-12
      Date: May 15, 2002

General: This is a 39-year-old white male who presents in
      mild acute distress with the following vital signs:
B/P 90/60   Pulse 110 (irregular)   Resp 24
Temp 36.3° C   Ht 5'11"   Wt 210 lbs

Skin: Patient has no skin rashes, lesions, erythema, or
      pigment changes.

HEENT: Normocephalic, PERRLA, normal external auditory
      canals and tympanic membranes. Good hearing at 24"
      with 512 CPS tuning fork, equal bilaterally.
      Funduscopic exam shows normal A:V ratios with clear
      disk borders. Normal nasal mucosa with midline septum.
      Normal oral and buccal mucosa with good dental hygiene
      and normal gag reflex.

Neck: Normal range of motion. No adenopathy or masses.
      Midline trachea. Good carotid pulses, equal
      bilaterally. Carotid bruit present.

Chest: Clear to auscultation and percussion (anterior and
      posterior).

Heart: Normal S_1 and S_2, with S_3 gallop. Systolic ejection
      murmurs at the left lower sternal border, grade 2/6,
      and the aortic area with radiation to carotid.

Abdomen: Normal LKKS. Normal bowel sounds. No tenderness,
      no bruit, no rebound tenderness, and no fluid levels.

Urogenital: Patient has large urethral orifice, with no
      discharge. Left testicle is larger than the right,
      both descended. No evidence of hernia. Prostate is
      smooth and non-nodular.

Rectal: Normal anal sphincter tone. No evidence of
      hemorrhoids. Stool guaiac negative.

Extremities: Good pulses. No hair changes. Full muscular
      strength. Full range of motion without joint
      crepitation. No cyanosis or rubar.

Neurological: Cranial nerves 2 through 12 intact. Oriented
      to time, place, and person. Cerebellar function
      normal. Babinski negative. No ankle clonus. Deep
      tendon reflexes are 2+ and equal bilaterally. Normal

Figure 9-2 Sample physical examination record.

PHYSICAL EXAMINATION   John J. Jones #12-12-12

muscular strength. Pin prick and sensation tests are
normal. Vibratory sensation also normal.

Lymphs: No adenopathy or edema present.

ASSESSMENT:
Problem #1   Acute myocardial infarction with previous
angina pectoris
                    Rule out aortic stenosis

PLAN:
Dx: Serial cardiac enzymes (CPK, CPK-MB, SGOT, LDH); serial
EKGs; CBC; Chest x-ray; echocardiogram; pyrophosphate
scan; thallium 201 scan. Consider angiogram, stress
test after recovery.

Rx: TPA 100 mgs over 5 hours
Heparin 5000 U every 8 hours
ASA 5 Gr daily
Atenolol 50 mg/po q daily
Demerol 50 mg every 4 hours
Bedrest - CCU
O_2 - 4 liters/minute
Liquid diet - 24 hours
Lidocaine IV 1 mg/min if PVCs controlled; raise to 2
    mg/min if needed

Patient Education:
1. Explain need to stop smoking.
2. Explain CCU care for 5-7 days and post MI followup.
3. Discuss future exercise program.
4. Explain need for stress testing and possible
   angiogram.
5. Discuss need for low cholesterol diet and weight
   loss.
6. Address ETOH intake

ASSESSMENT:
Problem #2:   **Reactive Depression**

PLAN:
Dx: Psychiatry consult.

Rx: Elavil 50 mg q.h.s.

Patient Education:
1. Inform patient it will take three weeks to get
   effect of drug.

Figure 9-2, cont'd Sample physical examination record.

PHYSICAL EXAMINATION   John J. Jones #12-12-12

ASSESSMENT:
Problem #3:   **Recent Divorce**

PLAN:
Dx: Psychiatry consult.

Rx: None

Patient Education:
        1. Explain to the patient the need for counseling for
           him and the children.

Richard Rahr, PA-C

Richard Rahr, PA-C
Dictated & transcribed: 5/15/2002

Eric Greenberg M.D.

Eric Greenberg, M.D.
Attending Physician

Figure 9-2, cont'd Sample physical examination record.

---

habitus, gait, dress, grooming, personal hygiene, sexual development, motor activity, mood, manner, affect, speech, level of consciousness, and signs of distress.

Vital Signs   The blood pressure, pulse, respirations, temperature, and weight of the patient are measured and recorded at the time of the examination.

Skin   Any lesions, color changes, erythema, dry or moist skin, rashes, ecchymosis, hair or nail changes, vascularity, edema, temperature, turgor, mobility, and thickness or thinness of skin are noted.

HEENT   Results of examination of the following aspects are noted here: hair, scalp, skull, and face; visual acuity, visual fields, eye alignment, sclera, conjunctiva, pupillary reaction to light, extraocular movements, fundus, accommodation to light, pupil size and shape, iris, eyelids, lacrimal apparatus, and eyebrows; tympanic membranes, hearing, ear discharge, auricles, canals, and Weber's and Rinne's tests; external nose, septum, turbinates, nasal mucosa, frontal and maxillary sinuses, smell, discharge, and epistaxis; lips, buccal mucosa, gums, teeth, roof of mouth, pharynx, tonsils, tongue, and salivary ducts.

Neck   Examiner records observations about stiffness, range of motion, carotid pulse, adenopathy, jugular venous distention, masses, midline position of trachea, thyroid, salivary glands, and pulsations.

Chest   Results of anterior and posterior examination for symmetry, dullness, expansion, ventilation, chest sounds, wheezing, rales, and costovertebral angle tenderness and bruit are recorded.

Breasts Palpation for nodularity, masses, tenderness, and discharge and observation for retraction, masses, drainage, nipple shape, and skin texture and color are noted.

Heart This section includes notes on heaves or lifts, thrills, the point of maximum intensity, murmurs, heart sounds, gallops, murmur radiation, displaced heart, friction rubs, venous hum, carotid artery pulse, and jugular venous distention.

Abdomen The examiner describes scars, asymmetry, bulges, peristalsis, bowel sounds, bruit, organomegaly, rebound tenderness, rigidity, hernia, tenderness, masses, ascites, liver, spleen, kidneys, femoral pulses and nodes, and suprapubic fullness or masses if applicable.

Extremities This section documents the following aspects of the arms and legs: condition of skin, color, edema, hair, size with comparison, pulses, venous patterns, lymph nodes, range of motion, muscular strength, nails, erythema or swollen joints, pain, numbness or weakness of limbs, and deformities, as well as results of palpation of joints and muscles.

Genitals For male patients, features of the penis, scrotum, testes, urethra, rectum, and prostate are recorded. Results of guaiac stool test, scars, lesions, varicocele, hydrocele, fissure, fistula, hemorrhoids, sphincter tone, and rectal masses are also noted. For female patients, results of the pelvic examination are noted: external pubic area, Skene's and Bartholin's glands, vagina, cervix, uterus, adnexae, anal sphincter, rectal fissures, fistula, hemorrhoids, rectal masses, and results of guaiac stool test.

Neurological Patient's mental status, cranial nerves, reflexes, muscle strength, and gait are noted. Results of ankle clonus, cerebellar test, Babinski's reflex, Romberg's test, and temperature and vibration test are also noted.

Assessment This section of the physical examination write-up includes a working diagnosis for each problem identified.

Plan Treatment plans for each identified problem, based on the most current information available, are listed here.

Progress Notes Progress notes should follow some systematic method of organizing the information for decision making. The SOAP method of organizing a progress note, taken from the problem-oriented medical record, is commonly used.[2]

The SOAP note has four parts, as noted here and shown in Figure 9-3:

1. *Subjective element:* The patient's expression of his or her condition, pain, complaints, reactions, and so forth.
2. *Objective element:* The physical examination findings, results of tests, laboratory findings, observations, and so forth.
3. *Assessment:* The health care professional's evaluation of the situation, which is based on both the subjective and objective elements.
4. *Plan:* Details of the course of treatment chosen.

This approach to recording progress notes provides an outline for logical progression and completeness of thought processes. Use of this system leads practitioners to disclose their reasoning and justify their actions. Progress notes should be recorded at least daily on inpatients. For an outpatient or discharged inpatient, each follow-up clinic visit would require a comprehensive progress note, as is shown in Figure 9-4.

Physician's Orders Physician's orders provide specific direction to other caregivers. Inpatient records contain a section for physician's orders, which give directions to the others on the health care team. To be effective, orders must be complete and legible and must contain few abbreviations. Only those abbreviations that are approved by the organization should be used. Orders are usually written or authenticated by the physician at the time they are given. On occasion, however, orders may be verbal, often given by telephone to approved personnel. State regulations and medical staff rules and regulations should be referenced to determine who is allowed to record or accept verbal orders. Verbal orders are to be signed by the physician at the next visit but no later

Text continued on p. 173.

JONES, John J.
UH # 12-12-12
Admitted 5/15/2002
Eric Greenberg, M.D.

PROGRESS NOTES

Date & Time	Prob. No.	Notes
5/16/2002	1	Subjective:
6 AM		This is a 39 Y/O Professor admitted with anterior myocardial infarction. The patient was given TPA with follow-up arteriogram showing good patency of the left anterior descending artery. The patient was started on lidocaine, heparin, ASA, O_2, Demerol, liquid diet, and CCU with complete bedrest.
		Patient is having chest pain with use of morphine every 3-4 hours. Patient denies SOB, edema, palpitation since admission. The patient is having a few runs of PVCs – lidocaine dosage was increased to 2 mg/min for last 12 hours with blood level pending. The patient is having nausea from medication – Phenergan 25 mg given with relief. Patient is resting without pain or nausea at 6 AM.
		Objective: B/P: 100/64 P: 96 + irregular R: 20 T: 37° C
		Chest – Clear to A & P.
		Heart – Ⓝ $S_1 – S_2$ with S_3 gallop, PMI 5ICS MCL, grade 2/6 SEM LLSB and aortic area, few PVCs
		Abd – no tenderness, no bruit, Ⓝ LKKS
		Ext – no edema
		EKG – Q wave, S-T segment elevation $V_1 – V_4$.
		Anterior M1 with few runs of salvo – 6 episodes in 8 hours.
		Enzymes – ↑ CPK – MB
		↑ SGOT
		Slight increase in LDH

S - Subjective   O - Objective   A - Assessment   P - Plan

Please sign each entry with status.
    (1) Diagnostic
    (2) Therapeutic
    (3) Patient Education

Form 5300-9/91

Figure 9-3 Sample progress note for a hospitalized patient.

JONES, John J.
UH # 12-12-12
Admitted 5/15/2002
Eric Greenberg, M.D.

PROGRESS NOTES

Date & Time	Prob. No.	Notes
5/16/2002		CXR – LVH, calcified aortic arch
continued		Arteriogram – 75% narrowing LAD coronary artery, and 70% narrowing of
		circumflex artery. Good candidate for bypass.
		PTT clotting factor – 2X control time
		Blood gases PO_2 on O_2 = 97%
		PCO_2 on O_2 = 38%
		Cholesterol = 209
		Assessment Acute myocardial infarction with previous angina pectoris
		R/O Aortic stenosis
		Plan:
		Dx: Serial enzymes, serial EKG's, follow-up stress test and echo cardiogram
		Rx: Continue heparin, O_2, bedrest, lidocaine 2 mg/ml, Demerol, CCU monitoring,
		ASA. Bedside commode at 72 hours.
		Atenolol 50 mg/po q daily. Cardiac Rehabilitation.
		Pt Ed. 1) Dietary consult with low cholesterol, low salt, and weight loss.
		2) Explain the need to relax and rest.
		3) Tell patient that his chairman said the grant will be completed and not
		to worry.
		4) Advise patient that his mother is coming to stay with children, and
		5) Brother is coming, also. Richard Rahr, PA-C
		Eric Greenberg, M.D.

S - Subjective   O - Objective   A - Assessment   P - Plan

Please sign each entry with status.
(1) Diagnostic
(2) Therapeutic
(3) Patient Education

Form 5300-9/91

Figure 9-3, cont'd Sample progress note for a hospitalized patient.

U.H. #   12-12-12
Name: John J. Jones
D.O.B.   12-01-1963
Address: 2568 Campeche Cove
           Galveston, TX 77553

OUTPATIENT CLINIC NOTES

Patient Name: ___John J. Jones_____   U.H. # __12-12-12_____

T: _36.6°_   P: _96____   R: __18____   B/P: _120/72_   WT: ____210____   HT: __5' 11"__
                                    regular

6/5/2002

Subjective:

    This is a 39-year-old white male who was discharged from John Sealy Hospital on May 29, 2002, after a two week stay for an acute myocardial infarction. The patient was admitted 5/5/2002, and spent 5 days in CCU. The additional 9 days were on the telemetry ward. He was discharged after an uneventful hospital stay. The patient is on anticoagulation with Coumadin and ASA.

    The patient is scheduled for stress test, repeat angiogram, with probable bypass surgery for regional narrowing of the left anterior descending and circumflex arteries. He will undergo thallium scan for ischemic areas of myocardium. Echocardiogram shows significant aortic stenosis that needs evaluation by the cardiovascular service.

    Dr. Jones denies chest pain, SOB, orthopnea, DOE, PND, edema, palpitation, hematuria, melena, hematemesis, hematochezia, syncope. He is on limited activity without symptoms while staying home on Rx. The patient is on

        Isordil 20 mg qid

        Atenolol 50 mg/po q daily

        ASA 5 gr q daily

        Coumadin 5 mg q daily.

    The patient is asking about driving his auto – he wants to get back to work. The patient's mother is staying with him at home with assistance from the live-in housekeeper.

    The patient has had dysuria for one day, without hematuria or nocturia.

Objective: See vital signs above.

    Chest – clear to A & P.

    Heart – normal S_1 – S_2 without gallop with grade 2/6 SEM

Form 7030-Rev. 5/87

Figure 9-4 Sample progress note for a clinic patient.

U.H. #
Name:
D.O.B.
Address:

Patient Name:____John J. Jones_____   U.H. # __12-12-12__

T:_____   P:_____   R:__18__   B/P:_____   WT:_____   HT:_____

Page 2 – 6/5/2002

LLSB and aortic area with radiation to carotid artery.

Abdomen – no tenderness, no bruit, good femoral pulse, no organomegaly.

Extremities – no edema.

CBC – within normal limits

Pro time 2X control

Urinalysis – normal

Culture & Sensitivity – normal and without growth

Chest x-ray – LVH

EKG – anterior scar without PVCs and LVH by voltage.

Assessment: S/P Acute myocardial infarction with aortic stenosis

Plan:

 Dx: Thallium scan

     Stress test

      Coronary arteriograms

     Serial EKGs

     Pro time 2X/week

 Rx: Continue on Coumadin 5 mg qid

              Isordil 20 mg qid

               Atenolol 50 mg/po q daily

              NTG 1/150 gr SL PRN

 Pt. Ed: Emphasize the need for behavioral changes of decreased stress, stop

       smoking, low cholesterol diet, and low fat diet, continue exercise program,

       and rehabilitation measures, and weight loss.   _Richard Rohr, PA-C_

Form 7030-Rev. 5/87   _Eric Greenberg, M.D._

Figure 9-4, cont'd Sample progress note for a clinic patient.

than 24 hours after being given, in most cases. Because of the legal risks of carrying out potentially hazardous treatments without proper authority to do so, many hospitals prohibit the use of oral or verbal orders. Many physicians request a PA to write such orders when necessary. Whether these orders must be countersigned by the physician depends on state laws and the medical staff rules and regulations governing each hospital.

Routine or standing orders can be used for certain diagnoses or procedures. It is important to note that routine or standing orders can be used only for services that are standard and for which little or no deviation can occur. For certain services, routine or standing orders are absolutely not appropriate, as in the case of observation services. Routine or standing orders, which are generally preprinted, are placed in the patient's record and must be signed and dated by the supervising or attending physician. Many hospitals limit the use of the standing order because it does not allow for the special needs of individual patients. Use of this type of order is very helpful, however, when it permits certain protocols to be followed in specific situations, such as a particular type of arrhythmia occurring in a coronary care unit.

Other Sections of the Record

All reports of diagnostic tests are kept in the record. They provide valuable information to the clinician. Interpretations of medical images, results of specimen testing, and recording and interpretation of electrical impulses are all examples of this type of data.

Reports of any procedures that are performed are also placed in the patient record to serve as a historical record for the person performing the procedure and to communicate information to other caregivers. If general or regional anesthesia is used, the patient record includes a report of the administration of such agents and of the patient's response. Recovery from the anesthesia is also reported, and the status of the patient during this period is noted.

The nursing section of the inpatient record comprises valuable information about the daily condition and status of the patient. Vital signs are recorded, administration of medication is documented, and nursing assessments of the patient are noted. These data can be valuable in assessing changes in the patient's condition.

Other professionals who may enter their assessments and treatments in the patient record are physical therapists, occupational therapists, dietitians, and medical technologists.

Flow Charts

Flow charts are a method of organizing data from a patient's record to help the caregiver provide the best care possible. They are frequently used in specific diseases (such as diabetes and hypertension) and in special care units. Flow charts may be kept manually, but when a computer-based patient chart record is used, the flow chart is automatically generated at each visit along with a problem list.

Discharge Summary

Used for inpatients, the discharge summary reviews the patient's entire hospitalization. An example is shown in Figure 9-5.

A discharge summary must include the admitting or provisional diagnosis and the diagnoses at the time of discharge. The principal diagnosis (the diagnosis that, after study, best explains the reason why the patient was hospitalized) should be listed first and indicated as such. All other secondary diagnoses should be listed as well. In addition, this summary includes the reason(s) for the admission, significant findings of examinations and tests, discussion of any therapies or procedures provided and the patient's response to them, and the information given to the patient at the time of discharge (including medications, physical activity, diet, and follow-up care).

PROBLEM-ORIENTED MEDICAL RECORDS

An alternative method of record keeping was developed by Lawrence Weed, M.D.[2] The format is organized around the patient's problems—hence its name. The total historical data are broken into clinical diagnoses, called problems. The first page in the patient's record is a listing of all problems—the medical, social, and psychological problems that can relate to physical findings, personal or social issues, treatments (such as radiation therapy), and organ or prosthetic implants. Figure 9-6 provides an example of a problem list, using the patient with myocardial infarction whose patient record has been illustrated in preceding figures.

DISCHARGE SUMMARY   John J. Jones   #12-12-12

Patient Data:
    Name: John J. Jones, Ph.D.
    Record Number: 12-12-12
    Admission Date: May 15, 2002
    Discharge Date: May 29, 2002

REASON FOR ADMISSION:
    Chest pain suggestive of acute myocardial infarction.

SUBJECTIVE:
    History - This is a 39-year-old white male who was
admitted after awaking at 5:30 AM with a severe substernal
pain that radiated to the left shoulder. After taking three
nitroglycerin tablets without relief, the patient came to
the emergency room at John Sealy Hospital at 6:30 AM. He
had nausea, vomiting X 1, hyperhidrosis, and shortness of
breath. He was also weak, anxious, and dizzy. The patient
had a two-month history of stable angina. He had been under
stress from a recent divorce and pressure at work because of
an approaching deadline for a research proposal he was
preparing. He was also adjusting to the role of a single
parent of two small daughters, ages 5 and 7.

OBJECTIVE:
    Physical Examination - On admission showed a 39-year-
old, well developed, white male with the following vital
signs: B/P 90/60; pulse 110; respirations 24; temperature
36.6 degrees Centigrade. The patient had an irregular pulse
with frequent PVCs. A carotid bruit, due to radiation of
grade 2/6 SEM LLSB and aortic area murmur (an AS murmur),
was heard. The patient had an S_3 gallop by auscultation.
    Laboratory Findings - EKG on admission showed an
anterior myocardial infarction with Q waves in leads V_1 and
V_4. Serial enzymes (CPK-MD, CPK, SGOT, and LDH) were all
elevated over a 7-day period. Chest x-ray showed left
ventricular hypertrophy. CBC on admission was within normal
limits. On the second day, CBC showed an elevated white
blood cell count of 15,000. Cholesterol level was 209 mgs%,
triglyerides 210, HDL 45, ratio 4.6.
    Hospital Course - The patient was admitted to the CCU
and had an uneventful five-day stay. PVCs were controlled
with lidocaine. He was transferred to 10C telemetry unit
where he stayed until discharge. The patient was
anticoagulated with heparin and ASA. This was changed to
oral Coumadin 5 mg daily before discharge. The patient was
discharged home on 5/29/2002.

Figure 9-5 Discharge summary for a hospitalized patient.

DISCHARGE SUMMARY   John J. Jones   #12-12-12

ASSESSMENT:
    Principal diagnosis - Acute anterior myocardial
infarction
       Other diagnoses -   Reactive depression
                         Aortic stenosis
                         Angina pectoris
                         Recent divorce
                         Left ventricular hypertrophy

       Procedure - 5/15/2002 - Coronary angiogram

PLAN:
    Diet - 2000 calorie, low cholesterol diet, low fat diet
          3 Gm low salt diet
    Medication -   Atenolol 50 mg/po q daily
               Isordil 20 mg q.i.d.
               ASA 5 Gr daily
               Coumadin 5 mg daily
    Physical activity - Limited activity at home. No work,
sex, or strenuous activity.
    Continue cardial rehabilitation program as an outpatient.
    Followup care - Clinic appointment for Friday, June 5,
2002.

Richard Rahr, PA-C
Richard Rahr, PA-C
Dictated & transcribed: 5/29/2002

Eric Greenberg M.D.
Eric Greenberg, M.D.
Attending Physician

Patient: John Jones, Ph.D.   Record # 12-12-12

		Active	Inactive
1.	Acute myocardial infarction with previous angina pectoris	5/15/2002	
2.	Reactive depression	10/1/2001	
3.	Recent divorce	1/8/2002	

Figure 9-6 Sample problem lists.

The record is then organized around the various problems, using the SOAP format as described previously. The chief complaint and history portion of the record are, of course, *subjective* information collected from the patient or a significant other and from old records. For each problem, the applicable parts of a traditional history (present illness, past medical history, personal/social history, family history, and review of systems) are summarized in a paragraph placed directly under the problem heading (see Figure 9-1).

The *objective* data, which include the findings on physical examination and the results of any tests, follow the list of problems. The physical examination is usually recorded in the traditional format, that is, listing the results by the parts of the body, as shown in Figure 9-2. After the initial assessment, this section includes any changes in the physical findings, as well as results of any testing or treatment (see Figures 9-3 and 9-4 for examples).

The next section in a problem-oriented record is the *assessment,* or the conclusions reached by the examiner on the basis of subjective and objective data. Assessments are separately listed for each problem. When exact diagnoses are unknown, a problem may be stated as a symptom with cause unknown. The differential diagnosis is listed in such cases to show the thinking of the caregiver.

Following each assessment is the *plan* for that problem. A plan consists of three parts: diagnosis, treatment (Rx), and patient education. *Diagnosis* in this case means the diagnostic tests needed to identify the cause or follow the case. *Treatment* can include special therapy, drugs, radiation, chemotherapy, and other modalities. *Patient education* refers to the information that the patient is given about each problem.

Organizing patient data in this way shows exactly what the medical caregiver is thinking. Each problem can easily be followed through the record. This saves valuable time for the caregiver and enables others to take over the care of the patient if necessary. Use of the problem-oriented medical record is particularly valuable in assessing a PA student's problem-solving abilities as he or she progresses through educational programs designed to develop clinicians. Use of this method by practicing professionals allows others, whether peers or the courts, to easily assess the quality of care being given to patients.

RULES FOR DOCUMENTING INPATIENT RECORDS

This section lists general guidelines that must be followed in creating a credible patient record.[1]

➤ Each page of the record should identify the patient, by name and by hospital, clinic, or private physician clinical record number.

➤ Each entry in the record should include the date and time the entry was made, as well as the signature and credential of the individual making the entry.

➤ No blank spaces should be left between entries.

➤ All entries should be written in ink or produced on a printer or typewriter.

➤ The record must not be altered in any way. Erasures, use of correction fluid, and marked-out areas are not appropriate. Such practices can cause a jury to wonder what was recorded that the caregiver did not want anyone to see.

➤ Errors should be corrected in a manner that allows the reader to see and understand the error. The following procedure is recommended:

1. A single line is drawn through the error, and the legibility of the previous entry is checked.
2. The correct information is inserted.
3. The correction is dated and initialed by the examiner.
4. If there is not enough room for the correction to be made legibly at the error, a note should be made indicating where the corrected entry can be found, and the reference is dated and initialed by the examiner. The correct information is entered in the proper chronological order for the date the error was discovered and corrected.

➤ All information should be recorded as soon as possible. Memories can fade, and important facts can be omitted.

➤ Abbreviations should be used sparingly and only used those that have been approved by the organization. The same abbreviation can have different meanings, which can be misleading.

➤ Health care givers must write legibly. It is embarrassing, and can be expensive, when caregivers cannot read their own entries in court. Because the patient record is used by so many other clinicians in providing care, it is important to the quality of care given to the patient that the record be legible.

➤ All entries must be consistent with one another. The assessment must agree with the diagnostic testing, or an explanation must be given as to why it does not.

➤ Entries should be factual accounts. Criticisms of the patient or a colleague should never occur. Records that blame or belittle others can be damning evidence in a lawsuit.

➤ All information given to the patient prior to any procedures should be recorded. This ensures and verifies that the patient was properly informed of the benefits and risks before giving consent to the procedure.

➤ Telephone contacts with the patient should be entered in the record immediately.

➤ Some method of organizing entries, such as the SOAP format, must be used to ensure that they are comprehensive and reflect the thought processes used in making decisions about the patient's care.

Following these rules results in a record that is accurate, timely, specific, objective, concise, consistent, comprehensive, logical, legible, and reflective of the thought processes of the health care providers. Not only will such a record be the best defense in a lawsuit, but it also will result in the best care for the patient.

Special Considerations for Student and Resident Entries

The only difference between entries into a patient record made by students and those made by practicing professionals concerns the obvious need for supervision of students' clinical practice while they are learning the skills and knowledge necessary to become proficient in the profession. Teaching institutions have rules for the conduct of the person assigned to supervise a student's clinical experience. These rules usually require the supervising individual's signature, in addition to the student's signature, on each entry in a patient record. This process, called countersigning, indicates that the supervisor is aware of what that student is thinking about the patient.

Further, the use of residents at teaching institutions has been addressed by Medicare in the Teaching Physician Guidelines. This document provides guidelines relative to the supervision and documentation that are required when services are provided by residents. Generally speaking, physician services furnished in teaching settings are reimbursed when the services are predominantly furnished by the physician who is not a resident, or the services are performed jointly by a teaching physician and a resident, or by a resident in the presence of a teaching physician. It is important that anyone in a teaching institution become familiar with these requirements to ensure that appropriate care is provided and documented.

DICTATING PATIENT RECORDS

Dictation can save the professional time and allows for a much more legible record. When offered this opportunity, one should be sure to take advantage of it.

Dictating information for the patient's record requires that the data be organized in the same way that it is organized before being handwritten. Other practices should be followed, however, to make dictation a worthwhile experience for both the person dictating and the person who must transcribe this information. The person dictating should:

1. Identify himself or herself with full name and title.
2. Identify the patient, using full name, medical or clinical record number, and admission date or visit date.
3. Give the date and time of dictation.
4. Indicate what information is being dictated, such as history and physical or progress note.
5. Give any special instructions about the transcription at the beginning of the dictation (such as a copy to go to a referring physician).
6. Identify each section in the record, such as "Assessment" or "Plan."
7. Speak in a normal voice, not too low or too loud.
8. Enunciate clearly and avoid mumbling.
9. Avoid talking rapidly. This can have the same effect as mumbling.

Before performing the first dictation, it is good policy for the clinician to visit the person responsible for transcribing dictation in the hospital or clinic. The clinician can ask about special instructions related to the available equipment and about the priorities that may be placed on the different types of reports submitted for transcription. In a hospital setting, where the original dictated materials are kept in the hospital record, the clinician can learn whether copies of the dictated reports are sent routinely to clinicians' offices or must be requested.

CONFIDENTIALITY OF THE PATIENT RECORD

The patient's right to privacy has traditionally imposed an ethical responsibility on the people involved in the care of that patient. Many different people may see and treat a patient during one hospitalization, and each of them needs particular information. How to protect the patient's right to privacy and yet keep all caregivers informed can be a dilemma. With the advent of the Health Insurance Portability and Accountability Act (HIPAA), the patient's right to privacy has achieved new heights. HIPAA is scheduled to be implemented in October of 2003.

The privacy rules under HIPAA include standards that protect patients' individually identifiable data. These rules apply to health plans, health care clearinghouses, and other health care providers. The information covered under this rule is broad. Protections apply to the information in many different formats, including electronic files (Internet, Intranet, private networks, and data moved from one location to another via disk, magnetic tape, or compact disk), paper records, and verbal information.

Additionally, individually identifiable data are known as protected health information (PHI). Generally speaking, PHI relates to information that identifies a patient and his or her health status.

Most health care providers, and certainly hospitals, have policies and procedures governing the release of any information about a patient. Clinicians must be aware of those policies. Generally, policies about the release of information include such items as the following:

➤ Requirement for patient consent to release any information to an outside entity, with any exceptions being outlined.

➤ Special considerations for release of information for sensitive conditions, such as alcohol, drug, or psychiatric diagnoses, and HIV-related conditions.

➤ Required data elements for a proper consent form and how long it is valid.

➤ Identification of parties who can release information to outside parties.

➤ Appropriate fees or charges for copies that may be requested.

Other issues should be addressed in separate policies. For example, individuals by title who may release information to the media could be the subject of one such policy. Another policy could indicate what information hospital employees may disclose to telephone callers regarding the condition of a patient during hospitalization. Most health care providers are in the process of reevaluating current policies and procedures in reaction to HIPAA.

All states have laws about which diseases, conditions, and events must be reported to appropriate agencies. Such incidents include births, deaths, gunshot wounds, communicable diseases, and evidence of child abuse. When reporting is required by law, confidentiality is no longer an issue. Reporting such incidents to anyone other than the responsible agency, however, would be a breach of confidentiality.

COMPUTER-BASED PATIENT RECORD (CPR) TO THE ELECTRONIC HEALTH RECORD (EHR)

The paper medical record is an impediment to effective delivery of high-quality health care. The record is difficult to access, often lacks information, and must be in a single location for a single use. Astoundingly, the paper record has changed little over the past 50 years, while expectations for use of the data contained in the record have changed significantly. These increased demands for information have forced health care systems and providers to search for alternative ways to deliver information effectively while at the same time controlling the costs incurred by doing so.

Over the past three decades, significant strides have been made in automating the record-keeping process. Technology has improved, allowing the design and implementation of electronic record-keeping systems that are easy to use.[3] You will hear many different variations of the name for an automated record-keeping system. These include *computer-based patient record (CPR), electronic patient record (EPR), computerized medical record, and electronic health record (EHR).*

The Institute of Medicine completed a study in 1991 that identified five objectives for patient record systems:

1. Support patient care and improve its quality.
2. Enhance the productivity of health care professionals and reduce the administrative costs associated with health care delivery and financing.
3. Support clinical and health services research.
4. Accommodate future developments in health care technology, policy, management, and finance.
5. Incorporate mechanisms for ensuring at all times the confidentiality of patient data.

These goals have really not changed since the initial study; however, the key definitions of the systems listed previously have evolved to fit today's health care environment.

Such systems, once they are implemented, will allow more than one user to access a record at the same time. Test results will be available as soon as the test is completed. Legibility of handwriting will no longer be a problem. The data will be quickly organized in ways that enhance the caregiver's skills, obviating the time-consuming task of creating manual flow charts. Problem lists will be updated easily. Ongoing lists of medications the patient is receiving will be easily maintained.

Movement toward an electronic health record has been a slow process. Many of the larger health care organizations struggle to integrate their older network systems with newer technology. It is often easier for the smaller providers (physician groups) to work with a practice management system and/or software in automating their record-keeping practices. There is a wide variety of technology available today that providers incorporate into clinical usage. Some of these include digital dictation systems, document imaging and scanning systems, voice recognition systems, and automated coding systems. There are also health information networks, Internet sites for exchange of information, and telemedicine applications that are widely available for use.

There are many barriers to the achievement of a computer-based patient record, including economic, technological, and behavioral issues. However, there is no question that the goal is to provide a system that incorporates the full continuum of health care data for a patient (from "cradle to grave"). The benefits, such as delivery of quality patient care and contributions to research and education, cannot be emphasized enough.

CONCLUSION

As computer-based patient records become more common, the quality of care will improve because more complete information about a patient will be easily available to everyone providing the patient's medical care. Quality health care, after all, is provided by managing information to reach the correct decision.[4,5]

CLINICAL APPLICATIONS

1. Why is it important for PAs to ensure well-documented patient records?
2. List the categories of information contained in the record of a patient's hospitalization, from admission to discharge.
3. Identify guidelines for dictating patient records.
4. Discuss typical policies for release of confidential information in patient records.
5. What are the advantages of computer-based patient records?

REFERENCES

1. Fox LA, Imbiorski W. The Record That Defends Its Friends. Chicago: Care Communications, 1989.
2. Kettenbach S. Writing S.O.A.P. Notes. Philadelphia: FA Davis, 1990.
3. Spann SJ. Should the complete medical record be computerized in family practice? An affirmative view. J Fam Pract 1990;30:457.
4. Dick RS, Steen EB (eds). The Computer-Based Patient Record: An Essential Technology for Health Care. Report by the Committee on Improving the Patient Record, Division of Health Care Services, Institute of Medicine. Washington, DC: National Academy Press, 1991.
5. Rodnick JE. Should the complete medical record be computerized in family practice? An opposing view. J Fam Pract 1990;30:460.

RESOURCES

Bates B. A Guide to Physical Examination and History Taking. St Louis: JB Lippincott, 1995. *A basic textbook that provides detailed instructions for accurately obtaining a history and performing a physical examination.*

Bazzoli F. Filling the data bucket: trends in the development of repositories and warehouses. Health Data Management 1997;5:63. *Focuses on the management of large-scale medical data by the use of repositories or warehouses, allowing better use of the data.*

Braden J. The future of HIM: an operational view. AHIMA 1998;69:44. *Discusses the restructuring and re-engineering of organizational structure that will be needed in the management of the medical record in the year 2008 in a large medical institution.*

Brandt M. Data quality: who's responsible. AHIMA 1996;67:36. *Discusses the need for high-quality medical data.*

Documentation Guidelines of Key Components for Evaluation and Management Services, 1995 and 1997.

Computer-based Patient Record, Description of Content. Prepared by the Computer-based Patient Record Institute (CPRI). Bethesda, MD: CPRI, May 1996.

Fox LA, Imbiorski W. The Record That Defends Its Friends. Chicago: Care Communications, 1989. *Booklet offering valuable information about the legal implications of entries in patient records. Short, with an easy-to-read format.*

Health Information: Management of a Strategic Resource. Philadelphia: WB Saunders, 2001. *A textbook for health information management professionals that covers the continuum of health information management from early health care delivery systems to the current state of electronic health records.*

HIPAA Regulatory Manual. Alpharetta, GA: The Medical Management Institute, 2002.

Huffman EK. Medical Record Management. Berwyn, IL: Physicians' Record Company, 1994. *Chapters 2 through 6 of this text for health information management professionals discuss the content of medical records. Chapter 15 covers legal aspects of medical records, including confidentiality issues.*

Kettenbach S. Writing S.O.A.P. Notes. Philadelphia: FA Davis, 1990. *Spells out the SOAP method of record keeping for the clinician.*

Medicare Teaching Physician Guidelines.

Pagano MP. Communicating Effectively in Medical Records: A Guide for Physicians. Newburg Park, CA: Sage Publications, 1992. *Explains how to use more effective communication techniques in the patient record.*

Ramsay A, Peterson T, Earle D. The accuracy of the computerized medical record. Top Health Rec Manage 1989;10:29. *Describes improving the medical record through the use of the computer.*

Spann SJ. Should the complete medical record be computerized in family practice? An affirmative view. J Fam Pract 1990;30:457. *Outlines the advantages of a computer-based patient record system in a family practice setting.*

Tierney LM, McPhee SJ, Papadakis MA, Schroeder SA (eds). Current Medical Diagnosis and Treatment. Norwalk, CT: Appleton and Lange, 1997. *Describes the medical information needed to write medical cases or to analyze data collected in the history and physical examination.*

Waller AA, Alcantra JD. Ownership of health information in the information age. AHIMA 1998;68:28. *Provides clear explanation of ownership rights in the various forms of health care data.*

CHAPTER 10

Interviewing and Communication Skills

Paul Lombardo and Sherry Stolberg

INTRODUCTION

Conducting an effective medical interview is essential to providing quality patient care. First impressions made during the interview are often taken by patients to be representative of the overall ability of the practitioner. Moreover, the skills demonstrated by the practicing physician assistant (PA) and the PA student during the medical interview set the tone for future interactions and significantly influence patient management decisions.

Many questions need to be answered in relation to the medical interview:

➤ Is the physical environment appropriate and one in which the patient will feel comfortable?

➤ If the interview is conducted in an inpatient setting, is the privacy of the patient as well as others in the area (e.g., roommates) protected?

➤ Is the amount of time scheduled for the interview appropriate in relation to the information available about why the patient has presented?

➤ Is the appearance of the practitioner likely to increase patient comfort during the interviewing process? For example, some elderly patients may expect the practitioner to be more conservative in dress, grooming, and approach than do younger patients.

➤ Is the patient mentally capable of giving accurate information, or should a family member, life partner, or other knowledgeable person be available to help?

➤ How might questioning need to be adjusted in order to accommodate a patient presenting with an acute or emergent problem?

➤ How might the interview be affected by the age of the patient (pediatric, adolescent, or elderly) and by the nature of the problem (sexual adjustment, otitis media, eczema)?

Finally, it is always important to remember that interviewing is a *communication skill.* Therefore, all the experience that the PA can bring to the interview is likely to improve the type and quality of the information provided by the patient. The importance of obtaining complete and accurate information is underscored when one considers how often an accurate diagnosis depends on a complete and accurate history.

In fact, communication of any sort is a two-way street. Not only will patients be influenced by the questions asked and the skill and sensitivity with which the PA attempts to elicit information, but the PA will also be influenced by the patient's responses. Successful interviews are the result of effort on the part of both the practitioner and the patient. Failed interviews usually have the same characteristic. Moreover, although communication is often thought of as a verbal skill, it is critical to remember that non-verbal communication, such as eye contact, touch, and body position, may be equally if not more important in conducting a successful medical interview.

Today, most medical providers are dealing with an increasingly diverse patient population. This fact makes it necessary for the PA to be aware of, and sensitive to, factors such as race, culture, ethnicity, religion, and sexual orientation—all of which can significantly impact a patient interview. It is easy to forget that as PAs, we come to the interview with certain biases. In order to be most effective, every PA has a responsibility to identify personal biases and ensure that they do not distort perceptions of the patient. When insensitivity to issues of human diversity interferes with the PA's ability to conduct the interview, patient care may be adversely affected. Listening well, demonstrating sensitivity to diversity issues, permitting pauses and reflection, and using silence to help give the patient time to respond are also tools that enhance effective communication. Chapter 8 provides a more detailed discussion of cross-cultural perspectives in patient care.

Empowering patients by letting them know that what they have to say is essential to their care, being willing to tell a patient "I don't know, but I'll find out," and patience in allowing trust and rapport to develop are also essential to conducting a successful interview. For PA students, in particular, it is important to remember that interviewing skills are not inborn but are the product of patience, practice, and a willingness to adopt a flexible approach based on the needs of the patient.

Because effective interviewing depends on effective communication between the physician assistant and the patient, it is important to recognize that there may be times when completion of a comprehensive interview with a patient is neither possible nor prudent. Patients with altered states of consciousness due to conditions such as trauma, metabolic imbalance, substance abuse, and severe psychiatric illness may not be able to provide comprehensive information of the type needed at the time the PA wants it. It may be necessary to delay the interview or to attempt to garner only the information essential to the immediate needs. Whenever such delay is warranted, the PA must ensure that a comprehensive interview is conducted as soon as the patient is able. Family members and past medical records can also be of help in filling in information gaps as needed for the immediate situation.

PURPOSES OF THE MEDICAL INTERVIEW

Although the tenor of the medical interview may vary with the reason for the specific patient/practitioner encounter, the interview itself serves the following purposes:

➤ To gather information relevant to the patient's problem that will assist the clinician in making an accurate diagnosis.

➤ To establish rapport between the PA and the patient.

➤ To facilitate the PA's understanding of the patient's concept of the problem.

➤ To assist in management of the patient.

➤ To provide a therapeutic outlet for patient concerns.

Gathering Information

Many diagnoses can be made on the basis of history alone. For problems that require further investigation, the selection of physical examination techniques and diagnostic studies is guided to a large extent by information gathered during the medical history.

Establishing Rapport

In today's technologically oriented health care environment, patients are increasingly asked to complete written forms or to use interactive computer formats to provide information relevant to their medical history. Although these formats may have some utility in data gathering, gaining a patient's confidence and trust is an art, and it is only during a face-to-face interview that a human relationship can be established. Through personal contact, the PA learns about the patient, and the patient learns about the individual who will be providing his or her care. Patients who have not previously been cared for by a PA may need to be educated about the profession as part of the overall effort to establish rapport. Face-to-face contact represents an ideal opportunity to educate patients about the PA's role in providing medical care and the unique relationship between PAs and physicians.

Facilitating Understanding

Understanding the way patients conceptualize their illnesses or problems is critical to the PA's ability to work with patients and effectively manage their care. The PA can play an important role in helping the patient to organize his or her thoughts about the problem at hand and may be able to correct misunderstandings and improve the patient's ability to provide the appropriate level of self-care. For example, a patient with high blood pressure may stop taking antihypertensive medication because he or she feels well, equating the illness with physical symptoms. Clearly, the patient needs to be taught that people with high blood pressure commonly have no symptoms and that the medication is prescribed to lower the blood pressure and prevent potential complications. On the other hand, patients who are concerned about a particular symptom (e.g., a patient with recurrent tension headaches who is worried about having a brain tumor) can be appropriately reassured by the PA, thus reducing the level of stress, which can be a factor precipitating some symptoms. In an age of increasing computer literacy, PAs can also help patients identify web-based sources of information. Chapter 17 provides strategies for PAs to use in guiding patients' use of the Internet.

Assisting in Patient Management

The interview can be used to direct therapy, monitor chronic problems, facilitate education about risk reduction, promote health, and provide basic patient education critical to achieving positive outcomes of therapy.

Providing a Therapeutic Outlet

The therapeutic potential of the medical interview should not be underestimated. During the interview process, the patient is offered the opportunity to discuss emotions, concerns, hopes, and fears related to the problem or illness. In this instance, the PA can help best by listening, providing reassurance and support, and introducing and exploring the possible interventions available and appropriate for the patient's needs, beliefs, and resources.

BASIC INTERVIEWING SKILLS

PA students who are just beginning to learn the skills necessary to conduct a medical interview often experience some anxiety. Concerns about not asking every single question in the universe of questions that can be asked and about missing critical information are common. It is important to remember that in many instances, the PA can contact, or even go back to, the patient if additional information needs to be gathered. Students commonly adhere tenaciously to prescribed formats for conducting the interview. Although such formats are helpful, they can be counterproductive to effective interviewing. Similar problems also confront practicing PAs, although experience in interviewing and managing patients contributes to conducting an effective interview. Experience can, of course, also color the way a particular patient presentation is approached and impede full exploration of all potential avenues of inquiry.

To minimize anxiety for PA students and to maximize productivity, it is useful to remember that some anxiety is healthy, can increase performance, and facilitates learning. Medical interviews are like the fingers on a hand: all different. Maintaining flexibility in the approach to the patient and resisting a "cookbook" approach are important. Students and practicing PAs have been inculcated with the idea that when one doesn't know or is unsure about something, one simply asks questions. This technique is as effective with respect to learning clinical interviewing skills as it is in assisting at surgery or prescribing a medication. Finally, certain techniques really can help in increasing one's interviewing effectiveness. They are described in detail in this section.

Beginning the Interview

Introductions   The PA should establish whether patients prefer the use of their surnames or first names. This is an early sign of respect for the patient. Patients should never be referred to as their diseases, for example, "the gallbladder in room 1032." Such language conveys depersonalization at a time when patients need to know that they are recognized and cared for as individuals. Some patients will not have seen a PA before, so the interviewer has the opportunity to provide during the introduction a brief explanation of the PA role and function. A statement such as, "I am a physician assistant and I will be working with Dr. Jones to help you. If you have not had contact with a PA before, I would be glad to answer any questions you may have," helps to educate patients and put them at ease.

Purpose of the Interview   The patient's cooperation and participation in the interview process can be facilitated by explaining the purpose and conduct of the interaction. For example, the PA might say, "I will be asking you questions related to your medical history and I will be doing a physical examination to evaluate your health before your operation tomorrow," or "I will be talking with you today about your complete health history, including the problem that brought you here today, your medical history, family history, and social history."

Environment of the Interview   The PA should pay particular attention to ensuring patient privacy and attempting to minimize interruptions by closing the room door, reducing outside sources of noise, and having nonemergency telephone calls held by the receptionist. Answering phones or beepers during an interview gives the message that other people or patients are more important, which may erode successful communication. If the PA must leave the room during the interview, he or she should let the patient know when the interview will continue.

Minimizing Barriers   When the PA sits behind a desk, the patient may perceive that the PA is in the "position of power." The resulting psychological distance may interfere with open communication, although the PA will also encounter patients with whom emphasizing distance and objectivity may be desirable.

Comfortable Position   Optimally, the PA and the patient should be sitting and at the same eye level. Standing while interviewing a patient is sometimes necessary but conveys the message that the PA is in a hurry. Sitting down tells the patient that the PA is devoting time to the interview and acts as an indicator of the PA's genuine interest in the patient.

Patient Attire   The patient's attire should offer adequate body coverage. This is a particularly important issue in the hospital setting because patients may be left uncovered after rounds or procedures. Both the PA and the patient are likely to be uncomfortable during the interview if they are distracted by inadequate coverage provided by the patient's body gowns or the drapes.

Reading Questions and Taking Notes Because the PA would like to establish and maintain eye contact with the patient, it is generally better to avoid reading the medical history questions and writing comprehensive notes during the interview. Reading and writing to the exclusion of maintaining eye contact may be interpreted by the patient as a lack of interest. Large clipboards and notebooks may also impede eye contact. For the PA student, practice will reinforce the memorization of medical history questions, so that reading a list of questions will not be necessary. During the comprehensive medical history, the PA can record pertinent data by pausing during the interview and saying, "I'm going to jot down a few notes about what we've talked about, and then we'll go on." For brief interviews, most practitioners write their notes at the conclusion of the encounter.

Patient's Mental Status The patient's ability to respond to questions must be evaluated early in the interview. Many factors can affect the patient's capacity to participate fully in the interview process. Altered mental status may result from medications, drugs, severe pain, or disease processes, as well as from mental health disorders. If unsure of the patient's ability to answer questions, the PA can perform a brief mental status examination before conducting the entire interview. The results will help to guide the remainder of the interaction. For example, a patient with a defect in recent memory but intact remote memory may give accurate information about childhood illnesses but may not be able to discuss the exact sequence of recent events. Case Study 10-1 illustrates this issue.

CASE STUDY 10-1

EL is a 73-year-old retired seamstress, with the chief complaint of shortness of breath. She has food stains on her clothes and appears slightly anxious.

PA: *Can you describe the shortness of breath?*
EL: I just feel breathless.
PA: *How long have you felt that way?*
EL: I just feel breathless.
PA: *Can you tell me anything else about how you feel?*

EL: I just can't breathe right.
PA: *(The PA notices that the patient is leaning forward and wears a hearing aid.) I wonder if I am speaking loud enough?*
EL: I can't hear you, dear. (The patient adjusts her hearing aid.)
PA: *Is that better? Can you hear me now?*
EL: Much better.
PA: *How long have you had trouble with your breathing?*
EL: Oh, a long time.
PA: *More than a month?*
EL: Maybe.
PA: *More than a year?*
EL: Maybe.
PA: *More than 2 years?*
EL: (The patient wrings her hands and fidgets in her chair.) I'm not sure. It's hard to keep track.
PA: *I know sometimes it's hard to keep track of time. Can I ask some questions about time? (Patient nods her head.) Can you tell me what day of the week this is?*
EL: Maybe Tuesday?
PA: *And can you tell me what year this is?*
EL: I'm not sure, . . . 1980?

Discussion: One barrier to communication was improved when the PA noticed that the patient seemed to have difficulty hearing. However, a more significant problem was then revealed. Based on the patient's verbal and nonverbal communication, the PA suspected that the patient might have a change in mental status. The patient was not oriented to time—she was mistaken in both the day of the week and the year. If the PA had not started a brief mental status examination, the patient's disorientation might have been overlooked.

Summing Up At the end of sections or at the conclusion of the interview, the PA can sum up the patient's story. This allows the patient to agree with the PA's impressions or add to or correct the information. Summing up both verifies accuracy of the information and reassures the patient that the PA understands the patient's history. At the end of the interview, the PA should inform the patient about the next step. For example, the PA may say, "Next, I would like you to put on this gown with the opening in the back, so that I can do a physical examination. I'll step out of the room while you change."

Interviewing Techniques

Formulating Questions   *Open-ended questions*[1] allow the patient to provide information in his or her own words, which tell the practitioner a great deal about the patient as well as the symptoms. Such questions help the PA better identify what the *patient* thinks is important and assist in accurate identification of the primary emotion(s) the patient is experiencing, such as anger, fear, and grief. Examples of open-ended questions include the following: "Was there any particular problem or issue that brought you here today?" "What has been troubling you?" and "How would you describe the pain?" Open-ended questions let the patient know that the PA is interested and willing to listen. They are a good medium for facilitating rapport and, as such, are particularly useful early in the interview.

Closed-ended or directed questions require a "Yes" or "No," or another very short answer. They are used to elicit more specific information, to augment the history with more detailed information, and to help focus the interview. Examples of this type of question are "Is the pain sharp or dull?" "Is there blood in your stool?" and "Does the cough wake you at night?"

Clarification and elaboration questions can be important and are considered secondary sets of questions.[2] Clarification questions ask the patient to explain or provide more detail about something that has already been stated but that the PA may not understand. An example is "Where exactly was the chest pain?" Elaboration questions are similar but ask the patient to add a new dimension of information, such as "Can you help me to better understand the other types of activity that cause your headaches to come on?"

Leading questions tell the patient the "correct answer" as perceived by the interviewer and are often judgmental. In order to maximize the accuracy of information, these questions should be *avoided.* Examples of leading questions are "Don't you think that's a little too much jogging for a man your age?" "You don't have any sexual problems, do you?" and "How much do you really drink?"

Facilitation techniques encourage the patient to go on with his or her presentation of the topic under discussion.[1] Facilitation can be both verbal and nonverbal. Examples of verbal facilitation are the use of such phrases as "please go on," repeating the patient's last words ("so you felt dizzy"), and using verbal cues such as "uh-huh." Nonverbal facilitation consists of such techniques as sitting forward and leaning toward the patient or touching the patient.

Confrontation is an attempt by the PA to bring a patient's behavior or emotional state to conscious awareness with a comment.[1] It is helpful in eliciting additional information about a primary feeling or emotion, as in "You seem worried about this chest pain." Confrontation can also help the PA reconcile perceived differences between the patient's affect and statements: "I noticed that you looked sad while we were discussing your new job. I wonder how you are feeling about that?" Many times, bringing a blocked feeling, emotion, or behavior to the surface serves to enhance communication. For example, effective communication with an angry or hostile patient may not proceed until the reason for the anger or hostility is identified and addressed. Even if the patient denies the observed feeling, emotion, or behavior, the PA has obtained valuable information. The patient may not be ready to recognize or discuss a given issue at that time. It is important for the PA to avoid using an accusatory or judgmental tone when using this technique.

Silence allows the patient to organize his or her thoughts and reflect on the interview.[1] It also gives the patient time to decide whether or not to discuss a difficult issue and may in fact be a preface to tears. Silence and tears are often difficult for the interviewer to cope with, so it is helpful to remember that silence and expressions of emotion can be therapeutic and helpful to the patient. Silence also may be influenced by culture. For example, some Native Americans may use long periods of silence effectively as a time to assess the interviewer and the situation before speaking. Chapter 8 provides additional examples of culture-based differences in communication.

Demonstrating *support* for the patient shows that the PA is sensitive to, and understands, the patient's reactions and emotions.[1] Statements such as, "I can understand that you are angry about the side effects of your medication and how being out of work for 6 months is very difficult for you," are definitive indications of your understanding and support for the patient. It is wise to *avoid* use of such statements as "I know how you feel" and "I know exactly what you're going through," because they are probably not true. In addition, such statements frequently elicit a counterstatement from the patient such as "No, you don't. What do you know about taking nitroglycerin or being out of work for six months?"

Statements of *reassurance,* which help to restore a patient's sense of confidence, hope, well-being, and dignity, are helpful in establishing trust and confidence and usually go a long way in facilitating communication between the PA and the patient.[1] They can also serve to reassure the patient that the PA remembers and is concerned about the particular illness or problem. Examples of statements of reassurance are "You've been doing very well on your diet" and "The fact that you have been drug and alcohol free for the past month is a real accomplishment." Reassurance should *not* include giving patients false hope, such as that implied by the statement, "I'm sure that everything will be okay."

Statements of *direction*[1] are used to facilitate transitions or to identify further plans. They help keep patients apprised of what the PA is going to ask and what the PA would like them to do. As a result, directive statements or questions help make patients more comfortable and increase their feeling of being full partners in the interviewing process. "I'd like you to tell me about your family history" and "Next, I'm going to do a physical examination, so I'd like you to remove your clothes and put on this gown" are examples of directive statements.

GAINING COMPETENCE

PA students and practicing PAs will quickly realize that not all the techniques described in this chapter are applicable to every patient care interaction. With the exception that most interviews start with open-ended questions, it is not appropriate to apply these techniques in a set order like the steps of a recipe. Setting the appropriate tone and flow of the interview and gathering pertinent information are important to conducting a successful medical interview. However,

the hallmark of good interviewing is flexibility in meeting the needs of the patient while eliciting the information necessary to provide quality care. As any skilled interviewer knows, the development of competence in interviewing is predicated on a good foundation of knowledge, sensitivity to patients' needs, consultation with colleagues and peers, and, most of all, practice, practice, practice!

Sample Interview

The following sample interview contains many of the interviewing techniques just discussed. Each technique is signified by the use of *italics;* the italicized line is followed by a numbered blank. If desired, the reader may write in the name (or abbreviation) of the technique being used. The techniques are confrontation (C), directed question (DQ), elaboration (EL), facilitation (FAC), open-ended question (OEQ), reassurance (RE), silence (SIL), and support (SUP). Some techniques may be used more than once. The correct answers are given at the end of the dialog.

Interview The patient is a 32-year-old white female homemaker whose vital signs are normal.

PA: *Hello, Mrs. Phillips.*
AP: Please call me Amy.
PA: *Amy, I'm Sandra Smith. I am a physician assistant in practice with Dr. Jones, and I will be talking with you about your health history and doing your physical examination today.*
AP: OK.
PA: *What brings you to the office today?*
(1_____)
AP: I have been having these terrible headaches. I'm so worried about them, I think something is terribly wrong.
PA: *Terribly wrong?*
(2_____)
AP: They are so bad. I sometimes have them all day long and sometimes I have trouble getting to sleep at night.
PA: *You seem worried about this.*
(3_____)
AP: Well, my sister died of a brain tumor 3 months ago, and she had headaches, too. [Begins to cry.]
PA: [*Offers tissues and waits.*]
(4_____)

AP: I didn't mean to cry like this. I just miss her so much and I haven't been able to cry since she passed away.

PA: *This must have been a difficult time for you.*

(5_____)

AP: Well, I've taken her two kids, plus my own two, because her husband Frank just can't cope right now. He's so broken up. I try not to let them see how I feel.

PA: *How do you feel?*

(6_____)

AP: I still think about her a lot and I miss her. We were very close. It was like her kids were my kids and vice versa. We only live a block away, and I used to see her every day. It's like there's a huge gap in my life, but I keep wondering if I'm supposed to be over it by now.

PA: *It's natural for you to still feel grief and sadness about losing your sister.*

(7_____)

In fact, it's as important for you to be able to talk about your feelings as it is for the children and other members of the family to talk about their feelings.

AP: I feel a little better already from talking to you, but what about these headaches?

PA: *Why don't you tell me more about them?*

(8_____)

AP: Well, I've had headaches for a long time, in fact, since I was a teenager, but I usually only got them once or twice a year. Pounding headaches on the right side of my head that would last a few hours, sometimes all day. My mother said she thought that they were migraines. Then, just lately, they started to get worse.

PA: *How are they worse?*

(9_____)

AP: Well, more often. Once or twice a month, and they sometimes last a whole day or even two.

PA: *When did you notice the change in the headaches?*

(10_____)

AP: About a year ago. It was about the same time that we found out about my sister's cancer.

PA: *And do the headaches feel the same now as before a year ago, except for happening more often and lasting longer?*

(11_____)

Answers   The techniques used in the dialog are as follows: (1) open-ended question; (2) facilitation; (3) confrontation; (4) silence; (5) support; (6) open-ended question; (7) reassurance; (8) open-ended question; (9) elaboration; and (10 and 11) directed questions.

Commentary   The PA would continue the interview by exploring the pattern of pain and related symptoms, including pertinent past history, family history, and social history. Open-ended questions are used intermittently but predominate early in the interview. If the PA had quickly moved to directed questions about the presenting symptom of headache, the psychological component of the patient's symptoms might have been lost. The combination of the patient's grief and her fear of cancer was contributing to her symptoms. Without that understanding, the PA would have been far less effective in evaluating and managing the problem.

NONVERBAL COMMUNICATION

Nonverbal communication is as important to a successful interview as is verbal communication. The PA should be particularly aware of, and sensitive to, the following modes of nonverbal communication.

Appearance and Grooming

It is of some interest to note that the first things that both the patient and the PA are likely to notice about each other are their respective appearance and grooming. Although styles of dress tend to differ, it is probably better for the PA to err on the side of conservatism, especially on the first interview.

There is never any excuse for poor grooming in a PA, although this aspect of nonverbal communication can easily be forgotten on a day when several patients require intensive care, especially at the end of a long day or on the day following a busy night on call. Nonetheless, the practitioner always needs to attend to grooming, even during long and busy days.

Touch

It is also important to remember that touch is a powerful (and often forgotten and unused) form of nonverbal communication. A firm handshake at the outset of an interview can contribute to setting a positive tone for open communication. More intimate contact, such as draping an arm over a patient's shoulder, is probably not appropriate (especially on the initial interview). This is usually considered to be overly intimate and may be misinterpreted. As with other aspects of the interview, however, one cannot be rigid about what is or is not appropriate nonverbal communication. The PA needs to exercise judgment in assessing what will best meet patient needs in a given situation.

Eye Contact

In most Western cultures, looking at another person directly conveys interest, and ongoing eye contact can be an important element in establishing patient rapport. It is important to remember, however, that eye contact is mediated by cultural determinants. The patient's cultural and ethnic background needs to be considered. In some cultures, looking directly into the eyes of another person is considered impolite and even a sign of disrespect. Eye contact is also mediated by psychological forces. Depressed patients often look down and away, and patients may not maintain eye contact when discussing sensitive and embarrassing issues. Therefore, in some cases (as with a depressed patient), noting lack of eye contact may be useful in establishing a diagnosis.

Comfortable Social Distance

The importance of this aspect of interviewing was previously noted. One must remember that "comfortable social distance" is also culturally mediated. To judge whether the PA and the patient are at a comfortable distance, the PA should observe whether the patient leans away or moves back while talking or listening and should adjust the distance to accommodate the patient's need.

Body Language

Body language, such as foot tapping, holding the arms tightly into the chest, and grimacing, can indicate how the interview is progressing. However, it is not wise to use body language alone to determine what a patient is feeling or experiencing because this type of expression is open to varied interpretation. For instance, a smile can indicate pleasure, embarrassment, or discomfort, depending on the situation and the patient's culture.

Speech Patterns

It is easy to become focused on the content of speech to the exclusion of its pattern, which may be equally important. Consider, for example, that rapid or "pressured" speech may indicate patient anxiety or underlying psychological problems, whereas sighing and slow speech may indicate depression.

Self-Assessment

The PA, as interviewer, is also communicating nonverbally throughout the interview. It is interesting to note that the interviewer may mirror nonverbal cues from a patient that are reflective of depression when interviewing a depressed patient or anxiety when interviewing an anxious patient. Self-assessment to identify mirrored behavior and feelings can provide important diagnostic clues.

THE IMPORTANCE OF LISTENING

Listening skills help to integrate the verbal and nonverbal communication that the PA receives from the patient. As the interviewer listens, he or she is also forming hypotheses about the patient, making determinations about what is essential and what is nonessential information, considering the differential diagnosis, assessing the additional steps required to manage the patient, and evaluating the communication itself. It is important to remember that what is heard and processed is to some extent the product of the PA's previous interaction with patients and general experience. These parameters, coupled with overall education and knowledge of medicine, allow the PA to sift through and sort a multitude of hypotheses relevant to the patient's illness or problem while attending to the patient and continuing the communication. It is the diagnostic value of the interview that is frequently given the most attention. However, the therapeutic value of listening to patients can be equally important. Frequently, patients tell the interviewer things that they do not or cannot discuss with others, not because they want a response or answer, but simply because they need a safe place in which to share highly personal information. The PA's ability to listen to patients without passing judgment is of significant value in the overall care of patients, which is an important reason for the PA to develop and hone listening skills.

USING COMMON LANGUAGE

Even when the PA and the patient speak the same language, the vocabulary and jargon of medicine can be overwhelming to the patient and may impose an unnecessary barrier to communication during the medical interview. Naturally, this barrier is compounded if the PA and the patient do not speak the same language, although the use of translators to assist the PA during the interview can help to bridge both language and cultural gaps (see Chapter 8). The PA working with patient populations for whom English is not the first language would be wise to consider learning the patients' first language or taking a specific course in medical terminology related to that language. Translator cards also are available in a number of different languages to help practitioners learn key terms necessary to elicit pertinent historical information from non–English-speaking patients.

An important role for any practitioner of medicine, but particularly for PAs, is that of translating complex medical jargon into language patients can understand. This is the reason that PA education emphasizes the need to use language that the patient can relate to when conducting an interview and during any other interaction with the patient. Doing so may involve using slang or street language. For example, when asked about sexual history, some patients may not recognize the term *syphilis*. However, simply rephrasing the question to ask whether or not they have "bad blood" (slang for syphilis) gives some patients an alternative term they recognize. Using language the patient understands also helps to prevent the miscommunication that occurs when a patient pretends to understand medical jargon so as not to seem ignorant or uneducated. Care must also be taken, however, not to "talk down" to patients who can understand more.

The interviewer must always be attuned to verbal or nonverbal patient cues that indicate confusion or a lack of comprehension. Explaining the causes, prognosis, and treatment of medical problems and illnesses to the patient is critical to providing quality care. Interpreting medical language to increase patient understanding is particularly important in the medical interview for which patient education is a goal. As a result of increased patient understanding through interpretation, patients are more likely to comply with advice on risk reduction. For example, a patient is likely to comply more fully with a diet when he or she understands what cholesterol is and why reducing an elevated cholesterol level is important. Patients are also more likely to follow a medication regimen if they are educated in advance about what the medication will do for them, what its potential side effects are, and why they may need to continue to take it even after symptoms disappear.

SPECIAL TOPICS IN INTERVIEWING

Several categories of patients and some topics present special challenges in the medical interview. This section focuses on some of them. Although this discussion is *not* intended to be a comprehensive review of the varied skills and techniques that the physician assistant may need, or of all the patient groups who will present special challenges, it *is* intended to act as a stimulus for further reading in appropriate sections of this text and related references. Chapter 31 provides additional discussion of the PA role in pediatrics.

One of the common errors made during interviewing is that of generalizing from groups to individuals, or vice versa. It can be a critical error that prevents establishing rapport with the patient. The interviewer must remember that assuming that patients will require special attention or behave in a certain way, for example, because they are a certain age, engage in a particular lifestyle, are poor, or have a certain health problem, is counterproductive to good interviewing.

Labeling the patient in such a manner may also be dangerous, to the extent that it prevents the interviewer from viewing the patient and the problem from a holistic perspective. One only needs to consider the 14-year-old girl whose life experience has given her a maturity far beyond her chronological age, the 80-year-old long-distance runner, the successful business executive who is habituated to cocaine, or the monogamous patient with acquired immune deficiency syndrome (AIDS) whose spouse is a substance abuser, to recognize the folly of generalizing from individuals to groups or vice-versa. As was previously noted, it is important for the physician assistant to remember that medical interviewing is a two-way street and that the interview itself may need to be adjusted to respond to individual patients' needs, regardless of characteristics they may share with any group.

The interviewer's disposition on a given day may also present certain problems in conducting a successful interview. Seeing a patient after 12 hours in the operating room or after a night on call may affect the PA's interviewing skills. External conditions, such as having waited 2 hours beyond the scheduled appointment time, may also affect the patient's behavior. The keys to dealing with these issues are fostering self-awareness, striving to maintain a professional approach, and practicing patience. This may not be easy, but it can be accomplished.

Interviewing Children

During the pediatric interview, a parent is often present and will be evaluating how the PA approaches and interacts with the child. It is often as necessary to put the parent at ease as it is to put the child at ease. Failure to do so may result in the transfer of parental anxiety to the child or may lead the parent to feel a need to direct the interview and provide information that might be more useful if offered by the child.

When a child is not old enough to be the historian, and questions need to be directed to the parent, the PA should try to touch the child in a nonthreatening manner, look at the child, and smile during the interview. These maneuvers help put the child at ease and establish a foundation for future interactions with both the parent and the patient. They help the parent know that the PA is concerned about both what the parent thinks and has to say *and* the child's perceptions and feelings. The interviewer must remember that during the interview, a child is also receiving impressions about how well the PA interacts with the parent, which may also influence future interactions.

Clinicians often direct questions to a parent, effectively excluding the child. This should be avoided if the child is old enough to provide cogent historical information. It is often necessary to modify questions so that they are appropriate to the child's level of comprehension and verbal ability. The PA should try to learn from the parent any special terms used at home to describe various people, objects, and activities. This will help the child understand the questions, and the PA will better understand the child's responses.

The PA should ask the child or parents what they think might be wrong and what they are really worried about. Children and parents sometimes worry about things that the PA would not necessarily consider a problem. A parent may ask, "Is my infant crying because I'm doing something wrong?" A child may wonder, "Am I sick because I've been bad?"

Children may fear people dressed in white, especially if unfamiliar instruments are being used. Street clothes may be more appropriate in the pediatric setting. Children can also be put at ease by encouragements to touch a stethoscope or reflex hammer. It may be helpful to let a child handle a new instrument first or to demonstrate its use on a parent.

Attentiveness to the appearance of the office is particularly important during the pediatric interview. The parent and child should be allowed to place themselves comfortably. For example, at certain ages, children will be much more comfortable being near or held by the parent while questions are asked. At other ages, it may be appropriate for everyone to sit at low tables or even on the floor in order to be at the appropriate eye level. Using colors and friendly pictures also helps to set children at ease. In the hospital setting, interviewing is generally done at the crib side or the bed.

Important information may be gained by observing the parents' responses while the child is speaking. Frequent interruptions and corrections by the parent may indicate the need to explore related questions in private with the child. The interviewer should remember that parental reactions that are out of proportion to the type of injury or the nature of the question may be a signal that further investigation of the problem is required. For example, in cases of child abuse or neglect, some parents may be very anxious in the face of a minor injury to the child or very calm in the face of a major injury.

Children are very aware of whether or not adults are being honest with them. The PA's failure to be truthful in response to questions asked about (or during) the interview may adversely affect a child's willingness to provide full and honest answers and is almost certain to affect the child's future interactions with both the PA and other clinicians.

Interviewing *children who are physically or mentally challenged* can be uncomfortable and anxiety provoking. It is important for a PA to recognize and acknowledge feelings of fear or despair and to develop constructive coping mechanisms. Otherwise, objectivity may be sacrificed and the interview may be compromised. Parents with a physically or mentally challenged child may also experience grief and pain. Therefore, in this situation, it is particularly important to assess the family's capacity to cope with and respond to the child's condition in an appropriate manner.

Interviewing and evaluating the child who is a *victim of abuse or neglect* is one of the most challenging responsibilities encountered in pediatrics. Anxiety and anger are not uncommon initial reactions the PA may have toward the parents or caregiver accompanying the child. During the interview with a suspected victim of abuse or neglect, it is paramount that the PA keep in mind that his or her role is to help first the patient, then the parent. Asking open-ended questions, exhibiting sensitivity, and gauging the child's capacity to answer questions at the time of the initial interview are very important. Sometimes, victims of abuse (and children, in general) try hard to act as if they are not afraid. If this is the case, it may be necessary to pose questions that use another imaginary child (or even the PA) as an example. Remarks such as, "I asked Johnny to tell me what happened when he got hurt; what do you think he said?" or "I'm thinking very hard about what you are feeling; do you know why?" can be helpful in garnering important information that the child might not offer if a more directive question were used.

It is important to know the state laws and requirements for reporting child abuse or neglect, in order to avoid some of the confusion that may occur in this potentially emotionally charged setting. The key to addressing the problem is to remember that in every state, a PA is required to report reasonable suspicions of child abuse or neglect to the appropriate agency providing child protective services. Parents should be informed that the PA is required by law to report what potential evidence has been found. This helps parents to avoid viewing the PA as being deliberately punitive or threatening and also helps to establish avenues for helping parents deal with the problem.

Interviewing Adolescents

Adolescence, with its attendant physical and behavior changes, is the developmental phase during which an individual makes the transition from childhood to adulthood (usually identified as between the ages of 12 and 21 years).[3] During this period, both dramatic and subtle changes take place in level of independence, definition of self, body image, and cognitive abilities. For example, the shift in ability from concrete to abstract thinking usually occurs during adolescence. The medical interview with a 12-year-old patient poses quite different challenges compared with the interview of a 15-year-old patient.

The initial visit with an adolescent patient may or may not include a family member. If the patient comes with a parent, it is advisable for the PA to meet with the patient and the parent individually. This helps to establish the boundaries of confidentiality early on in the patient/PA relationship. Both the adolescent patient and the parents need to understand that information given by the adolescent will not be shared without his or her permission, unless the adolescent demonstrates an imminent threat to self or others. Establishing such boundaries is not meant to diminish the parents' potential role in the patient's care. In fact, because parents are often concerned about their role in the adolescent's care, it can be helpful to let parents know that they are likely to be called on to provide important historical information as well as emotional support during patient evaluation and treatment. A final meeting with the patient and parent together provides an opportunity to give further reassurance to both and to review information and treatment plans that are not of a confidential nature.

Maintaining the boundaries of confidentiality during adolescence poses a challenge to the practitioner, particularly with regard to issues of sexuality or when the adolescent has a conflict with the parents. In addition, given the range of developmental changes that can occur from early to late adolescence, it is often necessary for the PA to adjust to the patient's changing levels of comfort with parental involvement.

When interviewing adolescent patients, the PA should try to avoid assuming a parental role. Adolescents are more likely to be open with a nonjudgmental adult figure and therefore to provide complete and accurate information. Avoiding lectures when giving information enhances the PA's relationship with the adolescent patient. Conversely, the adolescent is not searching for a peer, nor should the practitioner attempt to fill that role. The desire to be a buddy can be subtly communicated to the patient, for example, through the excessive use of slang. Trying to be a buddy may interfere with establishing and maintaining a therapeutic relationship with the patient.

The beginning of the interview with an adolescent patient is an opportunity to establish rapport. An open-ended question such as, "What issue or concern brought you here today?" may elicit a response if the adolescent is seeking help for a specific medical problem or for a school physical examination. On the other hand, if the adolescent is seeking medical attention because of developmental issues or a more sensitive matter, he or she may have more difficulty framing answers to open-ended questions. In these instances, as well as those in which the adolescent is more reserved or reluctant to speak, a directive approach may prove more effective than open-ended questions, silence, or facilitation. The PA may consider moving to a more specific discussion of school or hobbies to gain insight into issues of concern to the adolescent as well as his or her personality. Direction may take the form of embarking on the review of systems at an early stage of the interview.

Questions that provide reassurance may be particularly helpful with anxious adolescents. Examples of such questions are, "Many of my patients have questions about changes in their bodies; how about you?" and "It is often difficult to talk about physical changes during the teenage years; what have you noticed?" More talkative, less focused adolescent patients may also need to be asked more directive questions during the interview, such as, "I can see that you like to talk about school and you enjoy school. Can you tell me more about these back pains you've been having? When did they start?"

With the adolescent patient, being a good listener is crucial to establishing a positive therapeutic relationship. Demonstrating support and empathy, without condoning or enabling destructive behavior, is equally important. Independence in the adolescent

can be fostered by offering choices in scheduling appointments or selecting treatment modalities. Patients in middle to late adolescence particularly appreciate being extended the opportunity to make their own decisions. When decisions about resources and management can be made appropriately by the adolescent, the PA should extend this opportunity. In order to encourage and reinforce the patient/practitioner relationship, it is often necessary to remind the adolescent that the PA is accessible. For this reason, it is a good idea to conclude the interview or patient interaction with a statement such as, "If you want to talk more about this problem, or anything else, please remember that I'm available."

Finally, adolescence, like most other stages of human development, often contains periods of calm and periods of turbulence for both adolescents and their parents. Adolescence challenges the PA's capacity to act as advocate, educator, and resource person. Most of all, it requires being flexible enough in interviewing techniques to facilitate successful communication with patients who have different levels of cognitive development, stages of differentiation from parents, and types of problems and concerns.

Interviewing the Elderly

Modifications in the environment may be required when the PA is interviewing the elderly patient, as is discussed in more detail in Chapter 38. Elderly patients are frequently interviewed by PAs who are younger. PA students may be concerned about being taken seriously if they are younger than the patient. These concerns are often addressed, and rapport established, when elderly patients are given some time to share information regarding their life accomplishments. Recognizing and acknowledging most elderly patients' need to be independent is also a way of bridging this gap. On the other hand, addressing elderly patients by using their first names without permission or making statements such as, "I know just how you feel; my great aunt had the same problem" tends to be counterproductive.

The diminution of sensory function in some elderly patients may necessitate slowing down the pace of the interview. This adjustment is sometimes difficult for the practitioner but does make sense, especially when one considers that as people get older, they have more history to discuss. It may be helpful to take a break if it is apparent that the patient is tiring.

The PA should avoid speaking in a loud voice to elderly patients until it is established that hearing loss is a problem. Most elderly patients are capable of responding to questions if the speaker stands directly in front of them in order to be both heard and seen. It may also be helpful to speak more slowly and in a lower tone. If it is unclear whether a patient has a hearing loss, the PA should ask about the comfort level and clarity of his or her voice.

Elderly patients may not know their diagnoses, names of surgical procedures, or medications. In this event, the patient should be asked to identify family members who can help. If any family members are present, the PA should let the patient know that family members are welcome to participate in the interview, if that is the patient's wish.

Elderly patients are often fearful about the loss of sensory function and memory. The practitioner should ask about and acknowledge such fears and beliefs. The PA should recognize the symptoms of dementia and depression and be prepared to adjust the interview accordingly.

Elderly patients experience many of the same problems as younger adult patients. Therefore, the sexual, alcohol, and drug history must always be included in the medical history. In addition, it is important to ask specifically about symptoms or diseases that elderly patients often assume are "just part of getting old," such as joint pain, visual changes, and memory problems. When appropriate, the PA should inform the patient that these problems might have an organic basis and can often be treated, if not cured.

Elderly people may have beliefs and attitudes that affect the information they provide. They may regard a disease as inevitable or believe that old people are "supposed to feel lousy." "Do whatever the PA tells you to do and don't ask questions" and "The hospital is a place you go to die" are also common attitudes. It is important to identify such beliefs and attitudes and to help patients recognize the effect they may have on their overall health.

The personal and social histories of elderly patients can be of great help to the clinician in structuring an appropriate treatment plan. Discussion of topics such as a social support network and employment or occupation presents an ideal opportunity to establish rapport.

It is important to observe elderly patients carefully to get a firsthand impression of their overall physical status. Assessing their reliability as a historian early in the interview is also important. This can be accomplished through the use of a few basic screening questions (typically those used on a mental status examination to assess orientation to time, person, and place, recent and remote memory, etc.). Although it is often more time consuming, interviewing elderly patients can be rewarding for both the PA and the patient if the interviewing techniques are adapted to the needs of the elder.

Sexual History

The sexual history is an important part of the overall clinical interview and one that often causes both PA students and practitioners discomfort. Self-awareness and the ability to maintain an objective, nonjudgmental approach to the patient are critical in eliciting an accurate sexual history. Because interviewing effectiveness decreases when the practitioner is not comfortable with his or her own sexuality or is unwilling to explore personal attitudes and beliefs, PAs who have identified personal biases or weaknesses in this area need to address them.

The discussion of sexuality is an integral part of the history and can be therapeutic. It permits patients to ask questions, clear up misinformation, and be reassured that they are not alone with respect to concerns regarding sexuality. Of course, discussions of this topic also help in diagnosing such problems as sexually transmitted diseases and sexual disorders. The sexual history can also be useful as the opening to a discussion of prevention and risk management in such areas as human immunodeficiency virus (HIV) infection.

The earlier the sexual history is introduced as an integral part of the interaction with the patient, the better. Even if a patient does not choose to discuss the topic the first time it is introduced, bringing it up in the interview helps the patient know that the PA recognizes the topic as important in the context of overall health. It also helps make the patient comfortable with questions concerning sexuality during future interactions.

Many patients find it difficult to discuss problems of a sexual nature. This makes it especially important for PAs to raise the issue by asking open-ended questions that are nonjudgmental, such as "Are you sexually active?" or "Is there anything about your sexuality you would like to talk about?" Incorrect assumptions about a patient's sexual orientation or marital status may erode the rapport between the patient and the PA. Questions such as, "Are your sex partners male, female, or both?" can help to establish a nonjudgmental environment for the sexual history and promote better communication.

Patients often express concerns about the confidentiality of discussions regarding sexuality and are particularly sensitive about issues of privacy. The PA should describe the parameters of confidentiality if it seems to be an issue.

The PA should check the patient's understanding of medical terms for sexual functions. For example, a patient may not understand the term *ejaculate* but may recognize the term "come." This can be done in a nonthreatening manner by asking the patient to tell his or her understanding of the topic under discussion or by specifically asking, "Is that word familiar to you?"

It is sometimes useful to ask questions that allow the patient to select from a range of answers. For example, the phrasing in, "Some women have an orgasm every time they have sex, some women have orgasms occasionally, and some have no orgasms. How often do you have an orgasm [come] when you have sex?" tells the patient that there is no correct frequency of orgasm and helps to encourage open communication. It may also be useful to ask questions that imply that a behavior or feeling is very common, and so help facilitate discussion, for example, "Many men have experienced a time in their lives when getting or keeping an erection was difficult. Have you had that experience?"[1] Case Study 10-2 presents an example of a brief sexual history that is part of a follow-up appointment.

CASE STUDY 10-2

RT is a 48-year-old salesman who has had high blood pressure for 5 years. At his last visit, a new medication was started. His diastolic blood pressure at this visit is 4 mm higher than it was at his last visit.

PA: *Your blood pressure is a little higher than last time. How have you been feeling?*
RT: OK.
PA: *Any chest pain, shortness of breath, or headaches?*
RT: No.
PA: *Were you able to get the new medication and take it?*
RT: I got it all right, but it didn't agree with me.
PA: *Didn't agree with you?*
RT: It just didn't agree with me. (The patient looks away and blushes.)
PA: *The kinds of side effects that some people have with this medicine include tiredness and trouble sleeping, and some men have problems with erections. Did you have any of those symptoms?*
RT: Well, yeah. The last one.
PA: *Trouble with erections?*
RT: Yeah.
PA: *Some men have trouble getting erections, and some men have trouble keeping erections. Which did you notice?*
RT: Both.
PA: *Did you have those symptoms before this medicine?*
RT: No!
PA: *I can understand that you might be concerned.*
RT: You bet I am. I stopped taking that stuff after 2 weeks, and I'm not taking it again. I'd rather give up smoking and my salt shaker than go through that again.
PA: *This might be a good time to talk about smoking and salt in your diet, but I want you to know that we can try another medicine that won't affect your sexual life.*
RT: OK, let's talk.

Discussion: The PA noticed the patient's discomfort and asked questions to allow the patient to express his concerns. The patient's statement about smoking and salt suggested that he may be motivated to change some behavior at this point. The PA will use the opportunity to begin a discussion of risk factors.

The exploration of sexual problems requires the same attention to detail as exploration of any other health problem. During the interview, symptoms and circumstances related to onset, alleviating and aggravating factors, duration, and prior treatment should be investigated. It may be useful to identify the patient's understanding of the cause of the problem and his or her expectations, including whether or not the patient wants treatment. The use of drugs, alcohol, or medications, changes in relationships, external stresses, fatigue, depression, anxiety, and attempts at self-treatment (such as herbal remedies or aphrodisiacs) should also be reviewed. Misconceptions about these issues and their relationship to human sexuality should be corrected, and gaps in knowledge should be addressed.

Patients with sexual problems commonly present with other constitutional symptoms, such as headache, backache, fatigue, and depression. Often, patients will not bring up, and may not even recognize, that the underlying cause is related to sexuality. Patients with acute or chronic diseases may experience problems in sexual performance. These problems may be the result of the disease itself, such as chest pain in the post–myocardial infarction patient, or they may be a secondary psychological consequence of the disease, such as the disfiguring surgery of a mastectomy or colostomy. Sexual problems may also be the result of the treatment of disease. For example, some medications can cause erectile dysfunction. During the interview, it is very important to discuss the impact these diseases and treatments may have on the patient's sexual functioning. Brief intervention to correct misinformation may help to restore a vital part of the patient's health.

CONCLUSION

Successfully conducting the clinical interview is a challenge for both PA students and PAs with extensive practice experience. The breadth and accuracy of the information obtained are critical to the provision of quality patient care and provide the foundation for most patient management decisions. Moreover, the clinical interview sets the tone for future contacts with the patient. Therefore, interviewing is a skill every physician assistant must develop to the fullest extent possible. The time invested in developing and honing this skill not only will increase one's personal effectiveness as a physician assistant but also will make participation in the provision of health care a more rewarding experience.

CLINICAL APPLICATIONS

1. Your patient is a 14-year-old male student who has come to the office for a physical examination prior to football season. At the end of the examination, which is normal, the patient says, "I want to tell you something, but you have to promise not to tell my parents." How do you respond?

2. Assume that you are the PA in Case Study 10-1. The patient says, "I'm worried that I have Alzheimer's. What do you think?" How do you respond?

3. You are interviewing a patient who admits to using "speed balls and ice" as part of her drug history. You are not familiar with either term. How would you respond?

REFERENCES

1. Enelow AJ, Swisher SN. Interviewing and Patient Care, ed 3. New York: Oxford University Press, 1986.
2. Levinson D. A Guide to the Clinical Interview. Philadelphia: WB Saunders, 1987.
3. Oski F. Principles and Practice of Pediatrics. Philadelphia: JB Lippincott, 1990.

RESOURCES

Enelow AF, Forde DL, Brunel-Smith K. Interviewing and Patient Care, ed 4. New York: Oxford University Press, 1996. *Provides a comprehensive overview of interviewing skills, as well as chapters related to interviews with specific patient populations.*
Levinson D. A Guide to the Clinical Interview. Philadelphia: WB Saunders, 1987. *A classic text, by the author of Seasons of a Man's Life, this pragmatic and comprehensive overview of interviewing and communication skills provides the perspective of a seasoned primary care practitioner.*
Coulehan JL, Block MR. The Medical Interview, ed 4. Philadelphia: FA Davis, 2001. *This text is particularly helpful for students beginning their careers in medical interviewing.*

CHAPTER 11

Content of the Medical History

Henry Stoll and Timothy C. Evans

INTRODUCTION

History taking is the foundation of diagnosis. The material presented here is intended as a synthesis of several sources for the benefit of students who are learning the basics of medical history taking for the first time. The emphasis throughout is on the most common or most important considerations for primary care practice implicit in each symptom.

The first section is an overview of the basic parts of a complete medical history, with an emphasis on the history of the present illness (HPI). An example of a complete history, with physical findings and a problem list, follows. It is meant to tie in with the physical examination protocols and sample write-ups in Chapter 12. Subsequent sections of this chapter deal with the potential significance of various symptoms, arranged by organ system.

OVERVIEW AND COMPONENTS OF THE COMPLETE MEDICAL HISTORY

The exact content and organization of a complete medical history may vary somewhat from institution to institution. However, most complete histories have the following components:

➤ Identifying data (ID).
➤ Personal profile (PP) or social history (SH).
➤ Chief complaint (CC).
➤ History of the present illness (HPI).
➤ Past medical history (PMH).
➤ Family history (FH).
➤ Review of systems (ROS).

A brief overview of each of these components follows. For more detailed information on the content of the medical history and interviewing techniques, refer to Chapter 10 and references such as *A Guide to Physical Examination and History Taking,* by Barbara Bates.[1]

Identifying Data

Typically, identifying data are the patient's age, race, sex, and occupation. This component may also include marital status, residence, and referral source.

Personal Profile or Social History

The content of the personal profile or social history can be quite variable, depending on the individual nature and circumstances of the patient. The operating guideline for data written here should be: what *personal* information about the patient should be known to members of the health care team so that they can provide appropriate care? The data can range from religious beliefs regarding blood transfusion to socioeconomic circumstances affecting discharge planning. Typical issues addressed in a personal profile or social history include family structure (location of other family members and the patient's relations with them);

sources of strength (support systems or religious beliefs for coping with illness); interpretation of illness (patient's self-diagnosis or fears of possible diagnosis, impact of this illness on patient's lifestyle); occupation (details of occupational history as they interact with patient's stress levels, self-image, economic well-being); sources of influence (any religious, philosophical, or other beliefs that may affect health care); and communication (any difficulties staff may have in communicating with the patient).

Chief Complaint

The chief, or presenting, complaint is simply a brief statement in the patient's own words about why he or she is seeking health care. Some estimation of the duration of the problem is usually also included.

History of Present Illness

The HPI is made up of a specific set of facts. The patient may volunteer the information spontaneously, or you may have to pursue it by asking specific questions. Any complete HPI should include the following information.

Onset When did the patient become aware of the problem? Was the onset sudden or gradual?

Duration How has the reported symptom been since its onset? Has it been constant or intermittent? Has it improved, remained the same, or gotten worse? If it is an intermittent symptom, like some pains, how long does a typical episode last?

Description A general description of the problem as the patient sees it. Pain symptoms should be characterized as follows:

Location Where is the pain located?

Radiation Does it travel anywhere?

Severity How severe is it? Does it interfere with normal functions, like work or sleep?

Type of Pain Can it be described with terms such as *burning, cramplike, sharp, dull,* or *squeezing?*

Aggravating Factors What seems to make the problem worse—exercise, specific positions, drugs, foods?

Relieving Factors What seems to make the problem better—rest, position change, eating, medications?

Associated Symptoms The review of systems (ROS) questions for whatever organ system seems to be involved must be asked; for example, if the chief complaint is vomiting, ask all the gastrointestinal ROS questions. You should also inquire about other possible symptoms; for example, ask about fever if the chief complaint might be due to an infection.

Medications or Treatment for This Complaint Is the patient taking any medications now for this problem, including nonprescription medicines? Is he or she trying any nonmedical therapies for this complaint? Is the patient seeing any alternative health care providers?

Other Medications and Other Ongoing Medical Problems Briefly review all other medications and chronic medical problems, even if they are seemingly unrelated to the chief complaint.

Past Medical History (PMH) for This Complaint Has the patient ever been evaluated or treated by another health care professional for this problem? If so, document the dates, details, and results of treatment.

Family History (FH) for This Complaint Has anyone in the patient's family or close contacts had a similar illness? This may suggest either a *hereditary* problem (e.g., allergies, diabetes mellitus) or an *acquired* problem (e.g., infections, environmental exposures).

Effect on Patient's Life What effect has the problem had on the patient's life? Inability to work or sleep, emotional stress, and financial disruption can all affect diagnosis and treatment.

Past Medical History

Past medical history consists of data on all major childhood and adult illnesses and serious sequelae, including hospitalizations, operations, and serious injuries. In some formats, the PMH may also include allergies, immunizations, ongoing medications, habits (e.g., cigarette, alcohol, or drug use), and other health history data, such as dates of Pap smears, chest x-rays, and purified protein derivative (PPD) testing.

Family History

The health status of immediate family members is recorded here, along with any information on diseases that seem to run in the family, such as cancer, heart disease, and diabetes mellitus. In cases where significant inherited illnesses cross several generations, it can be useful to construct a formal family tree.

Review of Systems

The ROS is a checklist of symptoms and signs arranged by organ system. It is designed to catch any significant symptoms that the patient may have forgotten to mention or thought were irrelevant to the presenting complaint. Sometimes the ROS uncovers a symptom that is in fact unrelated to the HPI but suggests another and more serious disease. If a patient has a positive response to one question in a particular organ system, you should generally explore all the questions in that particular system. The following sections discuss the components of the ROS in greater detail.

GENERAL AND PSYCHOLOGICAL HISTORY TAKING

As the first and last sections on the ROS list, respectively, the general and psychological questions are sometimes overlooked or underexplored during medical history taking. The general questions, as their name implies, do not point to disease in any specific organ system. Sometimes a practitioner avoids asking the psychological questions because they do not seem relevant to more "physical" complaints, or because of his or her own discomfort about emotional issues. Further discussion of interviewing and communication skills can be found in Chapter 10.

General Questions

Weight Change   Important information to obtain in any history of weight change includes how many pounds have been gained or lost in what period of time, and what is the nature of the patient's appetite and food intake.

Weight gain in adults, particularly if gradual, is usually related to overeating. Less common causes include edema states and endocrine disorders (e.g., type 2 diabetes mellitus, hypothyroidism, Cushing's syndrome).

Weight loss in the absence of dieting is potentially worrisome. Weight loss with anorexia suggests cancer, psychiatric disorders (e.g., depression, anorexia nervosa), gastrointestinal irritation (e.g., alcoholic gastritis), or chronic disease of the heart (congestive heart failure), lungs (emphysema), liver (cirrhosis), or kidneys (uremia). Weight loss despite a good appetite might suggest type 1 diabetes mellitus, hyperthyroidism, or malabsorption.

Fatigue   A chief complaint of fatigue can make the practitioner feel tired before even taking the history. The differential diagnosis of fatigue is vast, and the conscientious PA will want to ensure that an organic cause is not missed. The major causes of fatigue seen in primary care practice are psychological issues such as stress, overwork, depression, and anxiety. Tiredness, or lack of energy, must be distinguished from true weakness, which may be caused by neuromuscular disorders.

Fever, Chills   *Fever* is usually suggestive of infection, but it can also be seen in some cancers (e.g., lymphoma), collagen vascular diseases (e.g., systemic lupus erythematosus), and other disorders (e.g., pulmonary emboli, drug fever, human immunodeficiency virus infection). Issues to explore with the patient with fever are duration (acute or chronic), onset (abrupt or gradual), fever pattern (constant or intermittent temperature elevation), temperature variation during the day and night, and site and method of temperature taking. Associated symptoms that would lead to a particular organ system (e.g., dysuria in urinary tract infection) or precipitating causes (e.g., travel history or insect bites) should be explored. True *chills* with uncontrollable shaking and shivering are most commonly seen with acute bacterial infection, such as pneumococcal pneumonia.

Sweating and Night Sweats   Sweating and night sweats may be seen in any illness that causes fever, but the classic associations of night sweats are with tuberculosis and lymphoma.

Psychological Questions

Any of the symptoms in the psychological section of the review of systems may require full-scale evaluation beyond what is briefly suggested here. The purpose of the ROS is to uncover potentially significant symptoms that may not be part of the patient's presenting complaints.

Memory Loss   Memory loss can be seen after destructive events in the brain, such as stroke and trauma. Delirium and dementia states also impair memory. Two common and important conditions in primary care practice that may manifest as memory loss are Alzheimer's disease and the acquired immune deficiency syndrome (AIDS) dementia complex. In dementia, recent memory usually is affected before remote memory. Memory loss can be assessed via the mental status examination.

Anxiety or Depression   *Anxiety* can be a transient, normal reaction to changes in the patient's life or environment (e.g., job loss, divorce, moving). The key issue to determine is whether anxiety is causing great emotional distress or is affecting the patient's functioning, such as through development of panic attacks or phobias.

Depression similarly can be a normal response to life events, such as bereavement, requiring little medical intervention, or it can be a disabling and even life-threatening condition. Associated symptoms that may have previously been uncovered in the HPI or elsewhere in the ROS, such as fatigue, anorexia, weight change, and insomnia, may suddenly come into focus when the question of depression is directly raised. Anhedonia, or lack of interest in things that previously brought pleasure, is a common finding in depression. Assessment of suicide risk is a necessary part of taking the history of a depressed patient.

Mood   Patients should be asked whether they are prone to prolonged (i.e., longer than 2 weeks) disturbances of mood, such as depression or irritability. A history of mood swings between depression and euphoria might suggest bipolar disorder *(old name: manic depression).*

Phobias   Fear of certain objects or situations may adversely affect the patient's work or social functioning. Asking patients whether they have certain fears, such as of flying or of speaking in public, needs to be followed by an evaluation of whether a positive response represents normal worries or actually prevents them from doing something they otherwise would normally do.

Sleep Pattern   The causes of sleep disturbance can vary from a transient stress response to serious problems. Difficulty falling asleep is common in anxiety, and early awakening is common in depression. Alcohol and drug abuse can disrupt sleep. Daytime drowsiness may be associated with sleep apnea or narcolepsy. Many psychotropic drugs also cause drowsiness.

Drug or Alcohol Abuse   If not previously covered under "Habits," an assessment of drug and alcohol use should be attempted. A nonjudgmental attitude is important in encouraging patient honesty about such practices. After quantification questions are asked (what is used, how much, and how often), attention should focus on the effects of drugs or alcohol on the patient's life or that of others, such as job loss, relationship problems, accidents, and arrests.

HEAD, EYES, EARS, NOSE, AND THROAT HISTORY TAKING

Note: **If a patient has a chief complaint of any one of the head, eyes, ears, nose, and throat (HEENT) symptoms, you must generally ask all of the HEENT ROS questions.** For example, sinusitis (nose) or refractive error (eyes) may be the cause of headaches. Allergies commonly affect the eyes

(itching, watering) as well as the nose (discharge, sneezing). Because the ears, nose, and throat are anatomically connected, infection or obstruction in one structure can lead to illness or symptoms in the others.

With certain HEENT complaints, you may also wish to ask some questions from the list of respiratory history–related questions. For example, a patient with sore throat, ear pain, or sinus congestion should also be asked about cough and sputum. A complaint of hoarseness should also lead you to ask respiratory history–related questions, such as about cough and smoking history.

Head, Headache, and Head Trauma

These topics are discussed in the section on neurological history taking (see p. 221).

Eye Symptoms

Visual Changes   Ask an open-ended question first, such as "How is your vision? Do you wear glasses or contacts?" *Gradual blurring* is usually due to refractive error as a person ages. One potential cause of blurred vision is high blood sugar—be alert to other symptoms of diabetes in this case (e.g., urinary frequency, malaise, thirst, weight loss). *Sudden visual loss* could be an emergency (retinal detachment, vitreous hemorrhage, occlusion of the central retinal artery)—evaluate or refer immediately. *Gradual visual loss* could be central (cataracts) or peripheral (open-angle glaucoma).

Scotomas   Scotomas are specks in the vision or spots where the patient cannot see. They may move around when the patient shifts gaze (suggests vitreous floaters), or they may be fixed (suggests a lesion in the retinas or visual pathways).

Diplopia   Double vision may indicate a weakness or paralysis of one or more of the extraocular muscles (EOMs).

Pain or Discharge   Sudden onset of unilateral eye pain is often due to the *foreign body/corneal abrasion* syndrome, usually with the accompanying history of something entering the eye. Infection of the eyes can be relatively benign *(conjunctivitis),* or severe and vision threatening *(herpes keratitis).* Conjunctivitis can be bacterial, viral, or allergic in origin. Clear or mucopurulent discharge can be seen in conjunctivitis and corneal infections. *Allergies* (e.g., hay fever) can cause eye itching, along with sneezing and nasal stuffiness.

Ear Symptoms

Ear Pain   The most common cause of ear pain is infection, usually otitis media (OM) or otitis externa (OE). Ask the following questions:

➤ Is the pain acute or chronic?
➤ Does the patient have PMH of ear infections?
➤ Are there associated symptoms such as fever, upper respiratory infection (URI) symptoms, and discharge? In very young children, pulling on the ears may be a symptom of OM.

Also ask about swimming ("swimmer's ear" in OE) and altitude changes (e.g., barotitis is an occupational hazard of flying).

Discharge   The most common cause is infection, either from a perforated eardrum in OM or from an OE infection, especially if due to a foreign body (FB). Ask about any discharge on the pillow in the morning. In emergency department settings, severe head trauma may result in leakage of cerebrospinal fluid (CSF) from the ears as a clear discharge.

Deafness   In addition to the regular HPI questions (onset, aggravating and relieving factors, and so forth), ask the following questions:

➤ Is the deafness unilateral or bilateral?
➤ Is it stable, progressive, or fluctuating?
➤ Is the patient occupationally or environmentally exposed to excessive noise?
➤ Is the deafness a loss of *loudness* (i.e., difficult to hear) or a loss of *speech intelligibility* (i.e., difficult to understand)? This helps differentiate conductive hearing loss (decreased loudness) from sensorineural hearing loss (decreased intelligibility).

Common Causes of Deafness   *Conductive* hearing loss commonly results from external canal obstruction (e.g., cerumen), tympanic membrane

(TM) abnormality (e.g., OM fluid or scarring), or tumor. *Sensorineural* hearing loss may be caused by congenital deafness, heredity, toxicity (e.g., aminoglycoside antibiotics, measles), aging, trauma (e.g., noise induced), or tumors.

Associated Symptoms to Ask About in Hearing Loss   The rest of the ENT ROS questions, especially those about vertigo, along with questions about the neurological ROS, the febrile/URI symptoms (e.g., symptoms of flu, labyrinthitis), and the medication history (aspirin, antibiotics, etc.) should be explored with any patient who complains of hearing loss.

Vertigo   *Vertigo* means dizziness *plus* the sensation of spinning or motion. Commonly associated symptoms include pallor, sweating, nausea, and vomiting (if severe). You must distinguish true vertigo from faintness, syncope, blurred vision, weakness, and clumsiness. To do so, first ask all the neurological ROS questions, as well as the HEENT questions. Then ask the following vertigo questions:

➤ Is the vertigo associated with medications or drugs or with anxiety or hyperventilation?
➤ Are there any URI symptoms (suggests viral labyrinthitis)?
➤ Does body position affect vertigo (transient vertigo associated with changes of position is called *benign positional vertigo*)?
➤ Does the patient tend to fall or lose balance while walking?
➤ Has there ever been loss of consciousness (LOC)?
➤ Does the patient have headache, nausea, or vomiting?
➤ Is the vertigo associated with deafness and tinnitus (Meniere's disease)?

The vestibular system consists of the semicircular canals (stuctures of the inner ear), the eighth cranial nerve, and the vestibular nuclei in the brain stem. Vertigo may result from disease in any part of this system. Vascular abnormalities, tumors, infections, trauma, and toxins can all cause vertigo.

Tinnitus   A ringing sensation in the ear or head, tinnitus is usually idiopathic. Common primary care causes are excessive noise exposure, head trauma, and ototoxic drug effects (e.g., high-dose aspirin therapy). Tinnitus may be associated with hearing loss or vertigo.

Nose Symptoms

Sinusitis   Patients may interpret a variety of symptoms as sinusitis: facial pain, headache, nasal congestion, nasal obstruction, or postnasal drip. Ask, "Do you have any sinus problems?" and then describe its symptoms—frontal facial pain, chronic nasal obstruction, postnasal drip, purulent nasal discharge, and fever. The location of pain helps in identifying the sinus involved: cheek (maxillary), nasal root and eye (ethmoid), midfrontal (frontal), or deep head (sphenoid). Achy pain is typical and may be affected by body position (e.g., upright versus recumbent or bending over).

Obstruction   For nasal obstruction, ask the following questions:

➤ Is the nasal obstruction related to the environment or season?
➤ Are there any associated symptoms (e.g., discharge, pain, sneezing)?
➤ Does the patient use medication (e.g., overuse of nasal sprays)?
➤ Is there a history of nasal polyps?
➤ Does the patient have a history of nasal trauma or deviated septum?
➤ If the patient is a child, could a foreign body be present?

Discharge   For a complaint of nasal discharge (*rhinorrhea*), ask about the amount and the color (e.g., clear and white, versus yellow or green). Are there associated symptoms (e.g., fever, pain, URI symptoms, allergies)? Sometimes nasal tightness and drying can feel to the patient like congestion or fullness, and the practitioner can mistakenly prescribe nasal drying agents. Excessive use of decongestant nasal sprays makes symptoms *worse*.

The major causes of rhinorrhea are the following:

1. Inflammation from infection, hypersensitivity (allergy), or environmental irritants (overuse of nasal sprays, termed *rhinitis medicamentosa*).

2. Parasympathetic dominance, as in pregnancy (vasomotor).

Other causes include tumor, medications (e.g., birth control pills), foreign body, and deviated septum. Association of symptoms with specific seasons or environments suggests allergies.

Epistaxis   Defined as bleeding from the nose or a nearby structure (e.g., sinus, nasopharynx), epistaxis can be either *anterior* (blood comes out the nares) or *posterior* (blood runs down the back of the pharynx). Localization is usually easy. The cause may be local or systemic (e.g., disorder of primary hemostasis). *Local* causes of epistaxis include inflammation, trauma, drying, tumor, FB, vascular abnormality, and cocaine use. *Systemic* disorders associated with nosebleeds are hypertension, vascular disease, and disorders of hemostasis (e.g., clotting disorder, leukemia, liver disease, and renal disease).

Mouth and Throat Symptoms

Teeth, Dental Care, and Dentures   The purpose of asking about the teeth is to assess the general state of the patient's dental health.

Gum Bleeding   Poor dental health (i.e., chronic gingivitis, periodontal disease) and bleeding disorders may cause gum bleeding.

Taste   Altered taste might be due to a cranial nerve problem or to liver disease (e.g., loss of desire for cigarettes in hepatitis). It is also seen as an adverse effect of some medications.

Breath   Bad breath may be due to poor dental hygiene, but it may also occur in patients with lung infection (e.g., bronchiectasis).

Hoarseness   Hoarseness can be acute or chronic. Common causes of acute hoarseness are vocal abuse (e.g., cheering) and viral laryngitis (seen with other URI symptoms). Chronic hoarseness can be associated with vocal trauma such as that caused by speaking or singing, or with cancer of the larynx, thyroid, or lung. Ask for smoking history.

Sore Throat   With sore throat, which is usually acute, the biggest distinction to be made is between a viral cause (90%) and streptococcal infection (10%). Ask about fever, URI symptoms, and dysphagia. Most patients with "strep throat" do not have associated URI symptoms. Also ask for history of culture-proven "strep throat," treatment history, and any reaction to treatment (e.g., penicillin).

Mouth Sores   Sores around the mouth suggest oral herpes. Such a finding offers an opportunity for patient education about how disease spreads (e.g., kissing, oral sex).

RESPIRATORY HISTORY TAKING

Dyspnea   Dyspnea, or shortness of breath (SOB), is the sensation of not getting adequate air in breathing. It is normal to have some degree of dyspnea in relation to heavy exercise or at high altitude. To determine whether breathing difficulty is inappropriate, you must consider the age and physical condition of the patient.

Taking a history of dyspnea involves obtaining the same sort of data required for any HPI.

Onset   When did the patient first notice SOB? Onset is important for differential diagnosis. *Sudden onset* suggests an acute process, such as asthma, pulmonary embolus, pneumonia, pulmonary edema, spontaneous pneumothorax, or hyperventilation due to anxiety. *Gradual onset* suggests a chronic process, such as chronic obstructive pulmonary disease (COPD) or congestive heart failure (CHF).

Duration   How long has the patient had SOB? Is it continuous or intermittent? If it is intermittent, how long does an episode last?

Description   *Dyspnea must always be related to activity.* The dyspnea classic for lung disease is dyspnea on exertion (DOE), unlike other forms of dyspnea (orthopnea, paroxysmal nocturnal dyspnea), which are classic for CHF. The exertion should be quantified. Typical measures include the following:
1. Number of blocks the patient can walk before onset of DOE.

2. Number of flights of stairs the patient can climb before DOE.
3. Relation of DOE to typical household tasks or self-care activities—dusting versus mopping the floor, shaving, taking a bath, or getting dressed.

This aspect of the history may be difficult to assess because patients may unconsciously slow down or modify their activities in order to avoid bringing on SOB.

Aggravating Factors   Relationship to seasons, environments, respiratory infections, drugs, exercise, dusts, pollens, emotions, occupation, and smoking should be discussed.

Relieving Factors   Ask whether anything seems to relieve the SOB, such as change of seasons, change of environment, and beginning or ceasing use of certain medications.

Effect on Patient's Life   COPD can be crippling. This question gives insight into the severity of the problem.

Associated Symptoms   Inquire about other symptoms associated with SOB. Always ask all the other respiratory ROS questions (e.g., cough, sputum), plus *smoking* and *occupational* history questions. Other important symptoms to detect include *fever* (associated with acute and chronic respiratory infections and some cancers) and *weight change* (weight loss could be associated with tuberculosis [TB] or lung cancer, weight gain with CHF). *Edema* would be an important symptom in a patient with CHF. *Wheezing* or *allergies* could point to asthma as a cause of the dyspnea.

Past Medical History   Obtain PMH for dyspnea and any lung or heart disease. Ask about birth control pills (BCPs) in a woman and about any past or present history of phlebitis (both associated with pulmonary emboli).

Family History   Ask for any FH of respiratory problems (e.g., asthma) and any current FH of infectious respiratory disease (e.g., TB or URIs).

Medications and Other Treatment   Ask whether an asthmatic patient receives any relief when asthma medications are taken. Use of diuretics or cardiac medications should be investigated for heart patients.

Wheezing
Wheezing is a high-pitched sound heard during expiration or inspiration that is caused by air movement through a narrowed or obstructed airway.

Wheezing is most commonly associated with *asthma* but may also be connected with allergies (e.g., aspirin); environmental or occupational sensitivity to inhalants; mechanical obstruction of the larynx, trachea, or a main stem bronchus (e.g., FB, tumor); emphysema; or CHF. Many acute and chronic lung diseases, not just asthma, may cause wheezing at some point.

Taking a history of wheezing involves a variation on the basic HPI questions.

Onset   When did the wheezing begin (e.g., 15 minutes ago, 2 days ago)?

Duration   Is wheezing continuous or intermittent? Is it getting better or worse, or staying the same? If intermittent (episodic), then how frequently does it occur? Are the number and frequency of episodes increasing?

Description   How severe is the wheezing? Ask the patient to describe a typical episode, including how long it lasts.

Aggravating Factors   Establish the relationship of wheezing to seasons, environments (e.g., wood-burning stoves for home heating), respiratory infections, drugs (e.g., aspirin), exercise (exercise-induced asthma), dusts, pollens, animals, and emotions. Are there any known precipitating factors?

Relieving Factors   Is wheezing relieved by use of medications, either prescribed or over the counter (OTC), by change of environment or season, or by change of position (e.g., sitting up)?

Associated Symptoms   Ask all respiratory and cardiac ROS questions. Also ask about fever, to assess for respiratory infection.

Effect on Patient's Life   Does wheezing affect the patient's ability to perform at school or on the job, for example?

Past Medical History   Obtain PMH for wheezing and atopic diseases (e.g., allergic rhinitis, asthma, and eczema).

Family History   Ask about FH of asthma and atopic diseases.

Cough
Cough is a response to irritation in the tracheobronchial tree. Examples of irritation include accumulation of mucus, inflammation, drying, cooling, and chemical inhalation.

When taking a history of cough, you want to know the same information that is required for the HPI of any complaint—onset, duration, description, aggravating and relieving factors, associated symptoms, effect, and PMH and FH (of cough or other respiratory diseases).

Regarding *associated symptoms,* you particularly want to know about *sputum, fever,* and (if the cough seems chronic in nature) *night sweats* and *weight loss. Chest pain* associated with cough may indicate pleural involvement (see "Chest Pain"). HEENT symptoms such as *ear pain, rhinorrhea,* and *sore throat* suggest URI; *sneezing* and *itchy or watery eyes* suggests allergies.

In terms of *effect,* you want to know whether the cough is interfering with work or sleep. You will also want a good *description* of the cough—how frequent, relationship to time of day or activities, if any, and severity (e.g., paroxysms of coughing versus mild throat clearing).

Of course, a *smoking history* is mandatory, especially for chronic cough (any cough lasting longer than 2 to 3 weeks). Many smokers have a chronic morning cough that produces clear or tannish sputum. You must determine whether there has been a *change* in the usual character of coughing (e.g., more frequent, more prolonged, more sputum, change in color of sputum). *A change in the character of a chronic smoker's cough may be the first sign of lung cancer.*

Sputum
It is very hard to have sputum without cough, so you will usually be taking a cough history

with this complaint. In particular, you want to know how much sputum is produced and what it looks like.

How Much? Patients have a hard time quantifying. Try asking how many teaspoons, or even cups (some smokers produce half a cup or more each morning). Smokers also tend to deny having cough or sputum unless pressed. Ask "Do you have a smoker's cough?" Another difficult situation to evaluate is the patient who swallows sputum rather than expectorating it.

What Does Sputum Look Like? Elicit appearance and character by asking the following questions:

➤ What color is the sputum? *Clear or white* sputum is usually benign, but some lung cancer sputum remains white for a long time after the onset of cough. *Yellow or green* sputum usually means respiratory infection.

➤ Is there any blood in the sputum? Blood may be bright red, rusty, or brown, depending on how fresh it is. It may appear in streaks or in large amounts.

➤ Does sputum have any foul odor or bad taste? Such characteristics are seen in lung abscess and bronchiectasis.

➤ What is the consistency? It may be thin and watery or thick and tenacious. Sputum in COPD becomes stickier and harder to bring up.

Hemoptysis Obviously, expectorating blood can be a serious problem. It is seen in TB, lung cancer, and pulmonary embolus. Fortunately, the most common cause of hemoptysis is acute bronchitis. *Warning:* make sure the blood is not coming from a nosebleed, bleeding in the mouth, or even the stomach.

Ask the usual HPI questions; be certain to include those regarding the *amount* (teaspoons, cups), *exact color* (fresh, brisk bleeding versus old blood), and *duration* (first episode versus intermittent or chronic event).

Important *associated or precipitating factors* include exertion, anticoagulant therapy, use of BCPs that may cause hypercoagulability and pulmonary infarction, and chest trauma. Always remember to ask about *weight loss* in any patient with hemoptysis or a chronic chest symptom such as cough or sputum.

Chest Pain Chest pain is not typically associated with lung disease because the lungs themselves do not have pain-sensitive nerves. However, the pleurae do; therefore, pleural involvement in a disease (e.g., inflammation, tumor) causes classic *pleuritic pain,* which is characterized as sharp, localized pain on inspiration or with coughing. This is usually easy to distinguish from chest pain of cardiac origin, which is brought on by exertion, relieved by rest, and unaffected by respiration. Pleuritic pain also occurs with chest wall trauma, such as a fractured rib.

Smoking History A smoking history is important to record because almost any respiratory symptom or disease is made worse by smoking, and because smoking is related to other diseases outside the respiratory tract (e.g., heart disease, peripheral vascular disease, peptic ulcer disease).

Try to obtain a precise quantification of the patient's smoking. Here is a suggested sequence of questions:

➤ Do you smoke?
➤ Have you ever smoked? (If the answer to question 1 or 2 is *yes,* establish what is or was smoked—cigarettes, pipes, cigars. Find out whether pipes or cigars are or were inhaled.)
➤ How long have you smoked?
➤ How much do you smoke now?
➤ Have you ever smoked more than that?
➤ Have you ever tried to quit smoking?

Smoking can be quantitated in terms of *pack years:*

Pack years = the number of packs per day (ppd) × the number of years the patient has smoked

For example:

1 ppd × 10 years' smoking = 10 pack years

2 ppd × 18 years' smoking = 36 pack years

Environmental or Occupational Inhalation
Environmental and occupational exposures to dusts, gases, fumes, and some animal byproducts can cause or aggravate a large number of chronic respiratory symptoms or diseases, as well as several acute respiratory infections. With any chronic respiratory complaint, it is most important to get a *lifetime,* detailed,

chronological occupational history. Some diseases take years to show up after exposure. For example, World War II shipyard workers with asbestos exposure are now developing lung cancer, and coal miners can eventually have anthracosilicosis. Some hypersensitivity and infectious diseases are caused by exposure to animals or organic products (e.g., farmer's lung from moldy hay, pigeon breeder's lung, and cryptococcosis). Even the travel history can be important. Coccidioidomycosis is found in the San Joaquin Valley but might be seen in a migrant laborer elsewhere.

An honest occupational history can be difficult to obtain if the patient is:

1. Seeking compensation (may exaggerate symptoms) or
2. Afraid of losing his or her job (may minimize symptoms).

Previous Chest X-Rays (CXRs)
CXRs are like electrocardiograms (ECGs): they become more valuable with age. Old films are useful for comparison when you are trying to determine whether a patient has some active disease. A small single nodule or calcification that has been radiographically stable for several years is probably benign. With growing concern over unnecessary radiation exposure, however, "routine" chest x-rays are being obtained less commonly. If a patient is asymptomatic, has a normal physical examination, and has low risk factors (e.g., no lengthy smoking history), there is little indication for a "routine" CXR as part of baseline data or for ongoing disease screening (e.g., TB or lung cancer).

TB Skin Test
Ask about this as "TB skin test" or purified protein derivative (PPD), and describe the technique.

A positive PPD skin test indicates previous exposure to *Mycobacterium tuberculosis* but does not indicate the severity or timing of previous primary tuberculosis. It also does not indicate whether the infection is still *active* (i.e., causing the patient to be ill or capable of infecting others). TB cultures or identification of the organism by other testing (e.g., deoxyribonucleic acid [DNA] probe) is needed for that diagnosis. Patients who have received bacille

Calmette-Guérin (BCG) vaccine may also have false-positive reactions to PPD.

You should be concerned about positive PPD results in *children,* persons in whom previous tests have been negative *(recent converters),* and *immunosuppressed patients* (i.e., those with cancer, alcoholism, steroid therapy, or human immunodeficiency virus [HIV] positivity).

History of Frequent Respiratory Infections, Especially Pneumonias
A history of frequent URIs is not really significant, but you might want to check into possible allergies because the symptoms can be similar (e.g., sneezing, rhinorrhea).

Recurrent pneumonia is defined as two or more separate, documented episodes with complete interim clearing, especially if the interval is less than 2 years. It suggests a weakening of the patient's normal defense mechanisms, such as by diabetes mellitus (DM), alcoholism, COPD, or cancer. Pneumonia that *persists* despite adequate antibiotic treatment is one possible presentation of lung cancer (caused by a bronchial tumor that prevents normal drainage of the infectious pus).

CARDIOVASCULAR HISTORY TAKING
Cardiac Risk Factors

Those at highest risk of coronary heart disease include persons with a past history of ischemic heart disease (myocardial infarction, coronary artery bypass graft [CABG], angioplasty, abdominal aortic aneurysm, peripheral vascular disease, symptomatic carotid artery disease), diabetes mellitus, or a constellation of risk factors that categorize them as having at least a 20% risk of myocardial infarction within 10 years. The major risk factors include age (men 45 years or older, women 55 years or older), hypertension (treated or not), cigarette smoking, family history (coronary heart disease in a first-degree male relative 55 years or younger, or in a female relative 65 years or younger), or HDL less than 40 mg/dL.

Cardiovascular Symptoms

Chest Pain In taking a history from a patient with chest pain, you must keep in mind the common societal association of chest pain with heart disease. You must be able to recognize that chest pain is the problem you are dealing with. Patients may experience and describe their symptom in a wide variety of ways. Denial mechanisms may also be at work ("It's just a little heartburn").

If you also keep in mind the four *general* anatomic sources of chest pain, you can compile a list of possible diseases to go with each. The four sources are *cardiovascular, respiratory, gastrointestinal,* and *chest wall.*

For any patient who complains of chest pain, you must take a detailed, meticulous history. Details of the history are often more important than the physical examination. Put particular emphasis on the following:
1. Description of typical episodes.
2. Aggravating and relieving factors.

Onset   You want to learn about the onset of the problem as a whole (when the patient first began having chest pains), and you want to record detailed information about the onset of typical episodes (e.g., what the patient was doing at the time, time of day, relation to meals, emotional state).

Duration   Establish the duration of typical episodes—seconds, minutes, or hours. How frequently do the episodes occur—daily, many times daily, or a few times per week? Have episodes increased lately in frequency, duration, or severity?

Description   Ask the patient to describe the sensation—sharp, dull, heavy, stabbing, like a pressure, burning. Watch for the patient's gestures—clenched fist over the sternum *(Levine's sign),* up-and-down motion over the esophagus, and so forth. A heavy or squeezing sensation is most typical of coronary artery disease (CAD). Sharp, knifelike pain is more typical of chest wall or pleuritic pain. Burning sensations are suggestive of acidic upper gastrointestinal (GI) disorders.

Location   Ask the patient to localize the pain as precisely as possible. Pointing with one finger and a vague gesture with the whole hand are both meaningful.

Radiation   There is a widespread assumption that chest pain that radiates to the left arm is classic for ischemic heart disease. This pattern is suggestive but

not the only one. Other radiation patterns are to the jaw, straight through to the back, and to the left shoulder.

Severity   Assess the severity of the pain. Remember, however, that there is *not* a good relationship between the severity of chest pain and the seriousness of its cause.

Aggravating and Relieving Factors   *This information is often the key to the diagnosis.* Chest pain brought on by exertion and relieved by rest is the classic, and still most reliable, indicator of *angina pectoris.* Aggravating factors associated with *CAD* include walking uphill, walking against a cold wind, eating a heavy meal, stressful dreaming, and emotional upset. Pain associated with coughing or deep breathing suggests a *pleuritic* or *chest wall* cause. Pain aggravated by lying down or bending over suggests a *GI* cause, like gastroesophageal reflux disease. Pain reproducible by pressing on the chest wall is diagnostic of a *chest wall disorder.* Relieving factors to ask about include rest, position change, eating, and medications.

ROS and Associated Symptoms   You must ask *all* the cardiac and respiratory ROS questions. You should ask *most* of the GI ROS questions as well, especially those that go with the upper GI tract (e.g., indigestion, dysphagia, abdominal pain). Ask the bowel movement questions if there is any possibility of a GI cause—ulcers, for example, can cause GI bleeding and melena. Then ask about the cardiac risk factors.

Medications and Treatment   Inquire about the effects of any medications the patient is taking. Prompt relief (3 to 5 minutes) of chest pain with nitroglycerin is good, but *not* absolute, proof of CAD. (Esophageal spasm can also be relieved by nitroglycerin, though it usually takes longer.) Relief with antacids might suggest reflux esophagitis as the cause of pain. Identify all medications that the patient is taking for any reason.

PMH for This Complaint   Inquire about PMH for this complaint specifically. Then broaden questioning to include any history of cardiovascular disease. Ask for details of prior workups, if known (e.g., ECGs, treadmill tests). Check for previous or ongoing respiratory, chest wall, or GI disorders.

FH for This Complaint   Inquire about any FH of heart disease. Ask whether a family member or anyone that the patient knows has recently had a heart attack. Such an event may have prompted the patient's appointment with you.

Effects on Patient's Life   Inquire not only about physical effects but also about psychological ones—fear of what a diagnosis of CAD might mean to the patient, and so on.

Orthopnea
Classic for left-sided CHF, orthopnea may also be seen in many pulmonary diseases. Some patients may experience this more as coughing or wheezing when recumbent. Quantitate the severity of orthopnea in terms of number of pillows or other measures of how erect the patient needs to be to maintain breathing comfort. Make sure that the patient props self up from necessity, not preference or habit. *Recent* onset of orthopnea is important because it should prompt a search for the precipitating event.

Paroxysmal Nocturnal Dyspnea (PND)
Similar to orthopnea, PND is even more clearly associated with CHF and pulmonary edema. Sometimes it is known as "cardiac asthma" because patients may experience more wheezing or coughing than dyspnea.

The typical scenario is of patients awakening, some time after going to sleep, very dyspneic. The patient must sit up and may go to the window for air. Associated symptoms include sweating, palpitations, and substernal tightness. A patient with pulmonary problems (e.g., bronchitis, bronchiectasis) might also awaken with coughing, but the dyspnea usually improves after sputum is expectorated.

Particular episodes of PND may be related to unusual physical activity that day, eating a large meal before bedtime, or nightmares. As with orthopnea, recent onset or increasing frequency of attacks of PND needs prompt evaluation for the precipitating cause.

Edema
A complex physical sign, edema has many possible causes. First, try to determine whether the edema is localized or generalized. *Localized* causes of edema in a limb include obstruction of the venous or lymphatic drainage (e.g., varicose veins, post mastectomy, thrombophlebitis). The three most common causes of *generalized* edema are *cardiac failure* (e.g., CHF), *liver failure* (e.g., cirrhosis), and *renal failure* (e.g., nephrotic syndrome, acute glomerulonephritis). Other causes of edema include premenstrual state, severe hypothyroidism (myxedema), and severe protein deficiency.

The following points are relevant in taking the history for a complaint of edema:

➤ Ask about edema (swelling) in general and then about particular locations (e.g., feet and ankles; tightness of rings, shoes, belt).

➤ Time of day edema occurs is revealing (worse at the end of the day and better in the morning is typical).

➤ Aggravating and relieving factors (time of day, prolonged standing, elevation of legs, tight garments or footwear).

➤ Time of month for a woman (relation to menstrual cycle).

➤ Ask for PMH of heart, kidney, or liver disease.

➤ In addition to cardiovascular ROS questions, you should ask the urinary ones (e.g., frequency, nocturia). Patients with CHF often have some degree of urinary frequency; hematuria or oliguria may be seen in renal disease.

➤ What medications and treatment is the patient using (e.g., diuretics, elevation of feet)?

Edema fluid of up to several pounds can be present in the interstitial spaces before swelling appears, so a *change in weight* alone may be significant for someone with a well-established cause of edema (e.g., CHF, chronic renal failure requiring dialysis).

Palpitations[2]
Often difficult for the patient to describe, palpitations are generally a disagreeable awareness of the heartbeat. "Skipping," "fluttering," "pounding," "racing," and other terms may be used.

There is a strong emotional component to this complaint. Many people with life-threatening arrhythmias have little or no sensation of heartbeat, and some people react strongly to any perceived palpitation.

Elicit enough information to form an accurate impression of the *frequency* and *duration* of episodes (palpitations that last minutes or longer might be significant). In addition to the other standard HPI questions, explore the following issues:*

➤ Do the palpitations occur as isolated "jumps" or "skips" *(extrasystoles/premature ventricular contractions)?*

➤ Are "attacks" of palpitation known to begin abruptly, with a very rapid heart rate (120/min or greater), with either regular or irregular rhythm *(paroxysmal atrial or ventricular tachycardia)?*

➤ Does the patient deny an association of palpitations with exercise or excitement *(atrial fibrillation, atrial flutter, fever, anemia, thyrotoxicosis, anxiety state, hypoglycemia)?*

➤ Can the patient draw an association between the palpitations and use of drugs or stimulants *(coffee, tea, tobacco, alcohol, epinephrine, ephedrine, aminophylline, atropine)?*

➤ Do the palpitations occur upon standing *(postural hypotension)?*

➤ Is the patient a middle-aged woman, and do her palpitations occur in conjunction with flushes and sweats *(menopausal syndrome)?*

➤ Do palpitations occur when the heart rate is known to be normal and the rhythm is regular *(anxiety state)?*

Murmurs   Ask whether the patient has ever been told she or he had a heart murmur. Many people have had functional systolic ("innocent") murmurs in childhood or adolescence. Pregnancy and other high-flow states can bring out murmurs, too. However, people can be born with, or can acquire, significant murmurs caused by abnormal or damaged heart valves.

---

*The bulleted material is adapted from Wilson JD, et al (eds). Harrison's Principles of Internal Medicine, ed 12. New York: McGraw-Hill, 1991. Copyright ©1991, reproduced with permission of McGraw-Hill, Inc.

Ask the following questions of the patient who knows he or she has a murmur:

➤ How long have you had your murmur? Who told you about it?

➤ Were any diagnostic tests ever done for the murmur (e.g., echocardiogram, cardiac catheterization)? Was a name or diagnosis ever given to it? Did you ever have rheumatic fever?

➤ Has the murmur ever caused you any problems in life (e.g., DOE, inability to keep up with the other kids during youth, being kept out of athletics, deferment from military service)?

➤ Do you take, or were you advised to take, prophylactic antibiotics (prevention against bacterial endocarditis), or were you advised to have surgery or follow-up tests?

Ask the rest of the cardiac ROS questions, with emphasis on cyanosis, dyspnea, and palpitations. Some patients with mitral stenosis also have cough or hemoptysis; some with aortic stenosis may have syncope; and patients with mitral valve prolapse may have palpitations.

Cyanosis   Cyanosis, which indicates insufficient oxygenation of the blood, has many causes. Cyanotic congenital heart disease and arteriovenous shunts are the most common causes in children. CHF is the most common cardiac cause of cyanosis in adults. This sign may also be seen in many pulmonary problems (e.g., emphysema, certain pneumonias, asthma).

Claudication   Claudication can be defined as angina occurring in the legs; it is brought on by exertion and relieved by rest. It usually has the same cause as angina, that is, atherosclerosis of the arteries of the legs. Claudication is usually felt as a pain or aching sensation in the calf.

Try to quantitate the claudication. In most patients, a fairly fixed, reproducible walking distance brings on the pain. Beware of one trap: the patient who can walk *any* distance "at my own pace." Be sure to ask about all the cardiac risk factors, especially *smoking*.

History of Hypertension   There are millions of hypertensive patients in the United States, but a large percentage of them are not receiving adequate treatment.

In a nonjudgmental way, ask the following questions:

➤ Have you ever been told that your blood pressure was high? When? By whom?

➤ (If yes) Were any tests done? Was a diagnosis made? Were you ever given treatment, for instance, water pills, other blood pressure pills, or a salt-restricted diet?

➤ (If yes) Are you still taking your medications? (If yes) What are they? Are you having any problems with them?

➤ (If no) Was there a reason why you stopped taking them?

Antihypertensives are associated with many potential adverse effects, such as inconvenient diuresis, effects on sexual function, and fatigue. The cost of medicine, and the difficulty patients have believing in the necessity for lifelong therapy for an asymptomatic disease are key factors also. PAs can do a great deal to increase patient compliance with hypertension treatment by taking time for education on this point.

GASTROINTESTINAL HISTORY TAKING

Appetite   Anorexia (decrease in appetite) can be a nonspecific complaint accompanying many disorders. It is most frequently the result of *nausea;* emotional causes (e.g., depression, anorexia nervosa) are also important.

Always ask for evidence of *weight change.*

Pica (unusual cravings for nonfood items, such as starch, clay, or ice) can be seen in iron deficiency anemia.

Dysphagia   Defined as difficulty in swallowing, dysphagia is a symptom of esophageal dysfunction. Common causes are pharyngitis, esophageal motor dysfunction (e.g., neuromuscular disease), mechanical obstruction (e.g., stricture, tumor), and emotional disorders (e.g., globus sensation).

Ask the following questions:

➤ Where does the food stick (localization)?

➤ What kinds of food stick (solids, soft foods, or liquids)?

➤ Is the dysphagia intermittent or progressive? (Progressive dysphagia, especially with a smoking and drinking history, suggests esophageal cancer.)

➤ Is it associated with pain (suggests esophageal spasm or inflammation)?

Food Intolerance   Intolerance of foods can be nonspecific or suggestive of several GI diseases, depending on the type of food the patient cannot tolerate. If spicy foods, coffee, and/or alcohol bothers the patient, peptic ulcer disease or gastroesophageal reflux disease (GERD) may be the cause. Fried or fatty foods suggest gallbladder disease.

Intolerance of milk and dairy products indicates lactase deficiency, which is especially common in African-Americans, Asian Americans, and Native Americans. It affects perhaps 10% to 15% of white adults.

Food intolerance can also be seen with a wide range of food allergies.

Indigestion   Indigestion is "gas," "heartburn," or a sense of fullness in the upper abdomen occurring postprandially. The medical term is *dyspepsia.* Two common causes of dyspepsia are delayed gastric emptying (e.g., obstruction at the pylorus by ulcers or tumors) and excessive upper GI gas (e.g., aerophagia).

Elicit a specific description of the patient's indigestion by exploring the following issues:

➤ Is the indigestion a belching, flatus, or both?

➤ Does it cause a burning sensation or dull discomfort?

➤ What is the relation of the indigestion to meals or specific foods?

➤ What are the patient's eating habits—eats too fast, chews properly?

➤ Is the patient under tension while eating? Are there stress factors in the patient's life at the moment?

Look for signs of anxiety, nervous tension, fatigue, depression, guilt, or fear.

Heartburn   Heartburn is a more specific and organic symptom. It represents reflux of gastric acid into the distal esophagus. Common causes of heartburn include GERD and incompetence of the lower esophageal sphincter.

The patient with heartburn will describe a substernal burning pain, frequently related to meals or specific foods or liquids. Ask for its relation to bending over or lying down, and whether it occurs at night. Often, heartburn is aggravated by spicy foods, citrus products, coffee, and alcohol. What relieves it?

Nausea Usually, but not always, nausea accompanies vomiting. Common causes of nausea include medications (cancer chemotherapy, digitalis, antibiotics, oral contraceptives); acute GI viral infections; bowel obstruction; inflammation of the appendix, gallbladder, liver, or pancreas; vertigo; pregnancy; alcohol; and psychiatric illness.

Vomiting You need a description of the vomitus. Ask about the relation of the vomiting to meals, drugs, and alcohol, and check for an association with other GI symptoms, such as abdominal pain, fever, chills, jaundice, and diarrhea. Quantity and frequency of vomiting should also be established.

The following specific aspects of vomiting should be considered:
➤ Vomiting with severe pain—occurs commonly, usually at the height of the pain (e.g., colicky abdominal pain).
➤ Vomiting with intestinal obstruction—the length of time between eating and subsequent vomiting gives some indication of the level of the obstruction.
➤ Bile vomit versus fecal vomit—fecal vomit is seen with lower intestinal obstruction.
➤ Food poisoning—suggested when several closely related patients develop vomiting at the same approximate time.
➤ Morning vomiting in alcoholism—ask for this in a suspected alcoholic, and find out whether it is relieved by alcohol.
➤ Projectile vomiting—occurs with increased intracranial pressure.

Bulimia An eating disorder characterized by episodic binge eating followed by purging behavior such as self-induced vomiting and laxative abuse, bulimia should be kept in mind in a patient with vomiting.

Hematemesis Hematemesis indicates upper GI bleeding (proximal to the ligament of Treitz or from the jejunum up). The blood may be bright red if fresh, or dark brown (like coffee grounds) if it has been in the stomach (acid denaturation) for some time.

Quantity of the bleeding is important (varices may bleed large amounts, leading to shock), as well as frequency and duration and relation to ingestion of food, alcohol, drugs (especially aspirin or nonsteroidal anti-inflammatory drugs), or vomiting (Mallory-Weiss tear). Ask about a history of bleeding disorder or anticoagulant medications.

Common causes of hematemesis include erosive gastritis (induced by alcohol or aspirin), peptic ulcer disease, esophageal varices, and reflux esophagitis. Prolonged retching and vomiting can cause a tear of the gastroesophageal junction (e.g., in bulimia or with Mallory-Weiss syndrome). You may sometimes have to distinguish hematemesis from hemoptysis, or from the swallowed blood of posterior epistaxis.

Jaundice Yellow discoloration of the skin, jaundice is caused by the accumulation of bile pigments (bilirubin). It is often first noted in the sclera.

Ask the following questions:
➤ Have you ever been jaundiced?
➤ Has anyone ever said that your skin or eyes had turned yellow?
➤ Have you ever had hepatitis or a liver disease?

Jaundice can be classified into three categories, according to how normal bilirubin pathways are interrupted: *prehepatic* (e.g., hemolytic anemia), *hepatic* (damage to liver cells themselves, as in hepatitis, alcoholism, and certain drugs), and *posthepatic* (obstruction to bile transport by gallstones or cancer of the head of the pancreas).

Other *associated symptoms* to check for include change in urine color (urine gets *dark* in hepatic causes of jaundice); change in stool color (stools get *light* in posthepatic causes); skin itching (posthepatic); and abdominal pain (might suggest gallstones or cancer of the pancreas; a dull general ache is common with any distention of the liver).

Risk factors for liver disease are as follows:

➤ Hepatitis/cirrhosis—alcohol abuse; intravenous drug abuse; consumption of impure water or food; travel to areas with poor sanitation or endemic hepatitis; known contact with a jaundiced person; sexual contact with carriers of hepatitis B; exposure to blood or blood products through transfusions or laboratory work.

➤ Toxic liver damage—especially resulting from alcohol but also from medications, industrial exposure.

➤ Gallbladder disease or recent gallbladder surgery.

➤ Family history of liver disease.

Change in Abdominal Girth Ask whether the patient has had to change clothing size. PMH of liver disease or alcohol abuse suggests cirrhosis with ascites (free serous fluid in the peritoneal cavity).

Constipation There is a wide variation in "normal" frequency of bowel movements (BMs). Symptoms of constipation include excessively dry, hard, or small stools as well as infrequent defecation. This GI disorder has many causes, both organic and functional (emotional).

Probe for an exact description of the change in the patient's normal bowel habits: Are stools smaller, thinner, harder, dryer, more difficult to expel? Is there stool remaining in the rectum? Ask about use of medications (laxatives, enemas, opiates, anticholinergics, antacids). Diet and exercise history can also be important.

Causes of constipation relate to either inadequate filling of the rectum or interference with emptying of the rectum. Constipation can be a benign, functional problem or the sign of GI malignancy. It is essential to rule out a colon or rectal carcinoma in an older person with a change in bowel habits or thinner (pencil-like) stools.

Diarrhea A wide range of "normal" BM patterns exist.

Probe for an exact description of change from the patient's normal habits, for example, frequency, character of stool (watery, blood or mucus, undigested food particles, noticeable fat content or oiliness,

particularly foul odor). Is the diarrhea acute (rapid onset, duration less than 1 week) or chronic (duration longer than 1 or 2 weeks)?

Associated symptoms and circumstances to check for include fever, chills, abdominal pain or cramps, myalgias (suggests viral enteritis), family members or friends with similar symptoms (suggests food poisoning), travel or hiking history (suggests parasites), and use of surface or well water versus city water.

Acute bloody diarrhea indicates mucosal damage; common causes are *Shigella, Amoeba,* and ulcerative colitis. Steatorrhea (excess fat in the stool) suggests pancreatic or small-bowel disease, which can lead to malabsorption syndrome with weight loss. Clay-colored stools are seen in hepatitis (due to blockage of bilirubin or bile). Ask about drugs and foods that are often related to diarrhea (e.g., antibiotics, laxatives, antacids, alcohol, dairy products).

A helpful rule is that most functional diarrhea does not awaken the patient at night; in such cases, probe for stress factors. Nocturnal diarrhea, on the other hand, suggests an organic cause.

Melena Melena is defined as the passage of black, tarry stools. Stools are very black, not just dark, and often foul smelling and sticky.

Black stools can be seen with ingestion of iron or bismuth (Pepto-Bismol).

Melena (versus hematochezia) requires time for stomach acid or intestinal bacteria to act on the blood. It usually indicates upper GI bleeding (e.g., peptic ulcer, gastritis, esophageal varices, stomach cancer, hiatal hernia).

As little as 60 mL of blood can produce melena. One GI hemorrhage can cause tarry stools for 7 to 10 days afterward.

Hematochezia Fresh blood per rectum, hematochezia usually indicates lower GI bleeding. Is this event acute or chronic? How often is blood noticed? What is the amount? To obtain a specific description, ask

➤ Is the blood on the outside of the stool or on the toilet paper (suggests hemorrhoids or an anal fissure)?

➤ Is the blood mixed in with the stool (suggests an abnormality proximal to the anus or rectum, colon cancer)?

➤ Is it accompanied by diarrhea and mucus (suggests inflammatory bowel disease, e.g., ulcerative colitis)?

Anal Discomfort and Hemorrhoids
Common symptoms of hemorrhoids are itching, mild pain with defecation, bleeding (coating the stool, on the toilet paper, or in the water in the toilet bowl), discharge of mucus from the anus, and a palpable external or internal mass. Hemorrhoids are related to excessive standing, straining at stool, pregnancy, cirrhosis, and CHF.

With rectal symptoms in patients who practice anal intercourse, you must evaluate for sexually transmitted diseases (gonorrhea, chlamydia, herpes, and syphilis). Rectal pain and fever can indicate gonorrheal or chlamydial proctitis; herpes and syphilis can cause skin ulcerations.

Abdominal Pain
There are seven questions to ask anyone with abdominal pain:

Where Is the Pain?   To localize, because the abdomen is a large area.

What Is the Pain Like?   You want to know the type of pain, for example, steady or colicky, sharp or dull.

➤ *Colicky pain* is a series of intermittent, short-lived pains that come and go, with intervals of (relative) relief in between.

➤ Spasmodic, squeezing pain suggests obstruction of a hollow organ (e.g., ureter).

➤ Steady, localized, more severe pain suggests irritation of the peritoneum.

➤ Dull, poorly localized pain suggests a visceral (abdominal organs) disorder.

When and How Did the Pain Come On?   Sudden and acute onset suggests an acute process, such as perforation or rupture.

How Long Does the Pain Last?   You want to establish whether the pain is intermittent or persistent. Intermittent pain occurs in acid-pepsin diseases and

gallbladder disease. Persistent pain may signify peritonitis or tumor.

Where Does the Pain Go?   This question seeks to determine the radiation pattern. You should learn the *patterns* of radiation that are classic for specific disorders:

➤ Gallbladder—right upper quadrant or epigastric area to top of right shoulder.

➤ Ruptured spleen—left upper quadrant to top of left shoulder.

➤ Upper GI structures (esophagus, duodenum, gallbladder, biliary tree, pancreas)—lower anterior chest (mimics angina).

➤ Pancreatitis, perforating ulcer—epigastric area to middle or upper back.

➤ Dissecting thoracic aortic aneurysm—throughout the upper chest to the back.

➤ Dissecting abdominal aortic aneurysm—down the abdomen and into the legs.

➤ Kidneys—flank pain.

➤ Ureters (renal colic, stone)—"loin to groin" (flank to genitals).

➤ Appendicitis—starts in the periumbilical region and then shifts after several hours to the right lower quadrant.

What Makes the Pain Better or Worse?

➤ Eating—pain that is better with eating suggests peptic ulcer. Pain that worsens with eating suggests pancreatitis, gallbladder disease, or small-bowel obstruction.

➤ Respiration—suggests involvement of organs lying next to the diaphragm, such as the liver, gallbladder, and spleen, or a lower lobe lung problem.

➤ Movement—pain that is worse with movement suggests peritonitis. Patients with colicky pain will writhe around during episodes.

➤ Position relief—leg flexion may ease peritonitis pain. Patients with pancreatitis may feel worse lying down but better sitting up and leaning forward.

What Else Is Going On?   You are looking for associated symptoms and PMH.

In any patient with abdominal pain, you *must* ask all of the genitourinary and gynecological/sexual history ROS questions. In any patient with upper abdominal pain, you may need to ask all of the respiratory and cardiovascular ROS questions as well.

Inquire about significant PMH of any abdominal problems or surgery, as well as any current medications or treatments. Is pain associated with fever?

GYNECOLOGICAL HISTORY TAKING
Basic Definitions
Menarche Age of onset of menstrual function, usually between 9 and 16 years in American women. Some variation exists, depending on family history, race, and nutrition. Menstruation may take 1 to 2 years to settle into a regular pattern. Menses may be anovulatory at first.

Amenorrhea Lack of menstruation. May be primary or secondary.

Dysmenorrhea Painful menstruation (primary and secondary).

Primary Amenorrhea Patient has never had a menstrual period. May be due to underdevelopment or malformation of the female reproductive organs or to endocrine dysfunction. Workup is usually initiated if a female has not had her first period by age 16.

Secondary Amenorrhea Cessation of menses after at least one presumably normal period. Most common cause is pregnancy. Other causes are lactation, menopause, malnutrition, anorexia nervosa, stress, chronic illness, and endocrine dysfunction.

Oligomenorrhea Infrequent periods. Seen normally at menarche and just before menopause.

Polymenorrhea Abnormally frequent periods (cycles shorter than 21 days).

Menorrhagia Increased amount or duration of menstrual flow (hypermenorrhea). Common causes are complications of pregnancy, tumors (e.g., leiomyomas),

and hormonal dysfunction. Bleeding may be severe enough to cause anemia.

Metrorrhagia Intermenstrual bleeding or bleeding between periods (spotting, breakthrough bleeding).

Menometrorrhagia Excessive uterine bleeding both during and between periods.

Menopause Cessation of menstruation. Declared after a woman has had no menses for 12 months. Usually occurs between mid-30s and late 50s; average age is about 51. *Premature menopause* occurs before age 35; *delayed menopause* occurs after age 58; *artificial* or *surgical menopause* occurs when ovaries are removed or made nonfunctional by medical intervention.

Abnormal Vaginal Bleeding Possible causes of abnormal vaginal bleeding include a wide range of conditions, from pregnancy and its complications to neoplasia, infections, and hormonal dysfunction.

The following questions should be asked of the patient with abnormal vaginal bleeding:
➤ When did the bleeding start?
➤ What are the duration and quantity of vaginal bleeding now, compared with previously normal periods? Ask for the specific number of tampons or pads used.
➤ Are there clots in the bleeding?
➤ Is there pain or cramping?
➤ Does the bleeding or spotting occur between periods or after intercourse?
➤ What was the date of the last menstrual period? Is pregnancy a possibility?
➤ Is there a new sexual partner?
➤ Is there any vaginal discharge or a fever (possibility of pelvic inflammatory disease [PID])?
Also inquire about perimenopausal symptoms (hot flashes, etc.).

It is useful to keep in mind the various patterns of vaginal bleeding. *Postcoital bleeding* suggests cervical disease (e.g., cervicitis, cervical cancer, or cervical polyps) or atrophic vaginitis in the older patient. *Postmenopausal bleeding* suggests endometrial cancer. *Amenorrhea* followed by heavy bleeding may indicate threatened abortion or dysfunctional uterine bleeding (DUB) related to lack of ovulation. Amenorrhea followed by spotty bleeding, plus or minus lower abdominal pain, may be caused by ectopic pregnancy.

An alternative approach to diagnosis is to remember likely causes of abnormal vaginal bleeding according to the age of the patient:

➤ Adolescence—dysfunctional bleeding (anovulatory bleeding), possible pregnancy.

➤ Younger than 40 years—accident of pregnancy (threatened abortion, ectopic pregnancy), pelvic infection (PID), contraceptive methods (BCPs, intrauterine device).

➤ Perimenopausal—functional disorder (DUB), uterine myoma (fibroids), cervical cancer.

➤ Postmenopausal—uterine cancer, cervical cancer, exogenous estrogen administration.

Dysmenorrhea
As has already been mentioned, dysmenorrhea may be primary or secondary.

Primary Dysmenorrhea   Unaccompanied by recognizable pelvic disease, primary dysmenorrhea usually begins at onset of *ovulatory* periods and tends to diminish after the first pregnancy. It is caused by high-intensity uterine contractions triggered by prostaglandins. Patients experience cramping pain in the pelvis, lower abdomen, or back that coincides with the start of menstrual bleeding and ceases when menstrual flow ends.

Secondary Dysmenorrhea   Secondary dysmenorrhea occurs in the setting of an underlying gynecological problem, such as endometriosis, PID, or intrauterine device (IUD) use. It has a later onset than primary dysmenorrhea and parallels the disease process responsible for it. Episodes may begin a few days before menstruation and may worsen or even diminish with the onset of bleeding, depending on the underlying cause.

Premenstrual Syndrome (PMS)
This disorder consists of variable symptoms experienced in the 4 to 10 days prior to menstruation, including irritability, fatigue, bloating, food cravings, mood swings, tension, depression, headaches, weight gain, and edema. Symptoms should cease with the onset of menstrual flow. The cause is still debated and is probably multifactorial.

Other Gynecological Complaints
Dyspareunia   Defined as pain with intercourse. Try to localize it. If the pain is near the outside or at the start of penetration, think of local inflammation, inadequate lubrication, or atrophic vaginitis. If the pain is felt deeper, think of pelvic disorders or pressure on a normal ovary.

Vaginismus   Involuntary spasm of the muscles surrounding the vaginal orifice, making penetration difficult or impossible. It can be physical or psychological in origin.

SEXUAL HISTORY TAKING

Taking the sexual history has two purposes: evaluating for sexually transmitted diseases (STDs) and identifying sexual dysfunction.[1]

Sexually Transmitted Disease Evaluation
Overcoming Biases and Assumptions   Do not make assumptions about sexual preference for men or women. Use gender-neutral terms such as "partner" or "person" until you have asked about sexual preference. When asking about sexual preference, avoid questions such as "Are you straight or gay?" Instead, ask "Do you have sex with men, women, or both?" Speak slowly and clearly when asking this question because some patients will be flustered by it.

Even if the patient has already spoken about a partner of one gender, you still need to ask if he or she has partners of the other gender. ("So, Jane is your steady partner. Do you ever have sex with men?") Keep in mind that some people have more than one steady partner, or have casual partners as well as one or more steady partners. Listen to the patient with empathy and acceptance. Being judgmental about someone else's sexual risk taking is counterproductive to helping him or her change it.

A patient who is in a steady relationship may have strong concerns about the partner, and a diagnosis of an STD may put severe stress on the relationship.

Avoid taking sides. You may not know the whole story, and your statements could have an unintended influence on a situation.

Specific Details Needed for STD Evaluation The following aspects of the sexual history must be elicited:

➤ Last sexual exposure (LSE).
➤ Number of partners in the past 2 months (most STDs have incubation periods of less than 2 months).
➤ Sexual practices and body sites exposed with sexual activity. When asking questions about this aspect, use exact anatomical descriptions, such as "Does he put his penis in your mouth?" Euphemisms, sexual slang, and jargon terms like "active" and "passive" may be confusing. For the most part, when evaluating STD risk, you are concerned about practices that involve penile insertion. Other sexual practices certainly have other associated risks, however (rimming, fisting).
➤ Use of protective measures, if any (condoms, spermicide).
➤ Contraceptive use and chances of pregnancy (if female).
➤ Partner's symptoms or recent health history. Patients often come to the clinic because a partner has been diagnosed with an STD—you sometimes need to ask specifically about this matter. A partner's undiagnosed symptoms can also be suggestive for the workup.
➤ PMH of any sexually transmitted diseases. Some are recurrent (e.g., herpes), and some increase the risk of acquiring other STDs (genital ulcerations increase the risk of HIV).
➤ Use of any antibiotics during the past month (may have cured or partially treated an STD).
➤ Allergies to medications.

Sexual Dysfunction
In women, problems of sexual dysfunction may be classified according to the phases of sexual response: *desire* (patient may lack desire), *arousal* (patient may fail to become aroused and to attain adequate vaginal lubrication), and *orgasm* (patient may be unable to reach orgasm much or all of the time).

In men, sexual dysfunction involves libido, erection, and ejaculation. *Libido* refers to sexual interest, which may be decreased by either psychological factors or testosterone deficiency. *Erectile dysfunction* ("impotence") is the inability to attain or maintain an erection. Its causes can be organic (e.g., medications, diabetes mellitus, arterial insufficiency), psychological, or both. *Premature ejaculation* is defined as ejaculating too soon or out of the patient's control. In *retarded ejaculation,* erections are okay, but ejaculation is difficult or is not attained. This last is a less common problem, usually seen in middle-aged or older men. Its causes are psychological, organic, or both.

GENITOURINARY HISTORY TAKING

Frequency Urinary frequency is a function of both how often voiding occurs (four to five times per day and once per night is "normal") and how much (250 to 500 mL is average) is voided.

Increased frequency or quantity may be caused by increased urine formation (as occurs with diabetes, compulsive water drinking, diuretic use), incomplete emptying (e.g., as results from chronic obstruction or benign prostatic hypertrophy [BPH]), worsened bladder irritability (cystitis, aging), or a functional problem (emotional stress).

Symptoms accompanying urinary frequency give clues as to its cause. For example, dysuria and urgency suggest infection; frequency without dysuria or polyuria suggests diabetes or urine-concentrating disorders.

Urgency For a complaint of urinary urgency, it is important to establish whether the urgency occurs with every urination. Ask about other symptoms, such as frequency, dysuria, and incontinence. Does an episode of urgency actually produce urine?

Urinary urgency suggests bladder inflammation and is most common with infection (including prostate and urethra, as well as bladder). It can also be seen with stones, tumors, and neurological disorders.

Dysuria Painful or difficult urination suggests inflammation of the lower urinary tract, usually by infection (bacterial). Other causes are stones, bladder tumors, applied chemicals, local irritation or allergies, trauma related to intercourse, and postmenopausal thinning of urethral mucosa.

Ask about fever, chills, and location of pain (e.g., suprapubic in women, urethral in men, flank pain with kidney involvement). Women can sometimes distinguish between "internal" and "external" sensations of burning. (Internal pain suggests urethritis or cystitis as the cause; external pain suggests vulvovaginitis.)

Vulvovaginitis in women can cause dysuria (e.g., by *Candida*), and not all causes are bacterial (e.g., urethral caruncle).

Keep STDs in mind during history taking, and ask the sexual history questions, too. *Chlamydia* infections of the urethra can produce a syndrome of dysuria and pyuria, yet may reveal no growth of ordinary urinary bacterial pathogens on regular cultures ("sterile pyuria"). Sexual intercourse is also associated with ordinary lower urinary tract infection in a woman, regardless of a partner's STD status (e.g., "honeymoon cystitis").

Flank Pain
Flank pain suggests a kidney problem. Flank pain associated with radiating pain to the groin and hematuria suggests a kidney stone. Fever, chills, and dysuria accompanying flank pain may be pyelonephritis.

Fever, Chills
Fever and chills are often seen in pyelonephritis or severe infections elsewhere in the body.

Nocturia
Urination at nighttime has similar causes to urinary frequency. It is commonly seen with diuretic use, in out-of-control diabetes, and in men with BPH.

Urine Color
Cloudy urine is often seen in urinary tract infection (UTI) with pyuria; sometimes it has a foul odor, too. Tea-colored urine is sometimes seen with hepatitis, along with clay-colored stools. Hematuria can be red or dark (Coca-Cola color).

Medications and foods can affect urine color: phenazopyridine (orange), hycosamine/methenam (blue/green), beets, phenolphthalein (found in OTC laxatives), and vitamins.

Hematuria
Ask whether blood is visible at the beginning of the stream, at the end of the stream, or throughout voiding. Blood only at the beginning suggests a urethral source. Blood only at the end (terminal hematuria) suggests a prostatic or bladder source. Blood throughout voiding suggests that the urine in the reservoir (bladder) is bloody, so the source is above the bladder (e.g., kidney or ureter). Be sure that the "hematuria" is not menstrual blood.

Presence or absence of pain is important. *Painful* hematuria is often seen with *cystitis* or *kidney stone.* *Painless* hematuria is often seen in *bladder cancer* (older male with smoking history), *renal cancer,* or *glomerulonephritis* (autoimmune reaction in kidneys following a streptococcal infection elsewhere; symptoms are edema, oliguria, hematuria, and hypertension).

Hematuria can also be classified as *gross* (visible to the naked eye) or *microscopic* (red blood cells visible only under the microscope).

Urinary Hesitancy and Stream Characteristics
When dealing with this issue, distinguish "shy bladder" (inability to void in the presence of another person) from difficulty in initiating stream. Ask "Do you have to wait a while for your stream to start?"

Assess continuity and force of stream in males.

Once urination has begun, 80% to 90% of the urine should pass in a continuous stream. The male patient with stream difficulties may have to strain throughout voiding to maintain flow, and the stream may slow or stop when he stops Valsalva.

Difficulty with stream usually indicates lower urinary tract obstruction (e.g., BPH in an older man) or ineffective bladder contractility. Tumors and strictures are common in men, whereas cystoceles are common in women.

Postmicturition syncope, or fainting after emptying a distended bladder, is usually seen in a male who has gotten up at night to urinate, sometimes after drinking lots of alcohol. The mechanism is vagal discharge leading to bradycardia and hypotension.

Urinary Incontinence
Ask "Do you ever lose your urine when you don't mean to, such as when you cough or sneeze, or in your sleep?"

Distinguish among the following types of incontinence:

➤ *Stress incontinence*—losing urine with coughing, sneezing, straining, or laughing.

➤ *Urge incontinence*—inability to make it to the toilet in time after becoming aware of the urge to urinate.

➤ *Overflow incontinence*—intermittent small amounts of urine lost, frequently seen in bladder outlet obstruction with bladder distention.

➤ *Total incontinence*—urine leakage or dribbling all the time.

Enuresis Involuntary urination is usually seen in childhood, although it sometimes persists into adulthood. It is often familial. An estimated 95% of children achieve total control of urination by 6 years of age. Voluntary bladder control depends on maturity of the nervous system, and enuresis may be a normal variation in the rate of maturity rather than a "disease."

As a complaint, enuresis is usually reported in a child who had achieved control but is now wetting the bed. Infection is the first consideration. Probe for stress, both emotional and physical (children will relapse temporarily if physically ill). Remember the possibility of sexual abuse.

Edema Edema with a urinary cause often is associated with gross kidney disease (e.g., acute or chronic glomerulonephritis, nephrotic syndrome, renal failure). It is also seen in heart failure and liver failure. These are causes of *systemic* edema. *Localized* edema can have other causes (e.g., venous obstruction such as varicose veins or thrombophlebitis in the legs).

Family History of Renal Disease, Hypertension, or Diabetes Hypertension either may be *caused by* kidney disease (e.g., chronic glomerulonephritis, renal artery stenosis) or may *lead to* kidney disease and failure. Diabetes mellitus can cause kidney disease and failure as a long-term complication. Some renal diseases run in families (e.g., polycystic kidneys).

Testicular Pain or Mass It is sometimes difficult for the patient to distinguish between a testicular problem and a scrotal problem when giving a history.

Testicular pain may be due to infection (epididymitis), stone, testicular torsion, or inguinal hernia. *Be sure to ask the sexual history questions.* (Gonorrhea and *Chlamydia* can both cause epididymitis in addition to urethral discharge and dysuria.) Testicular cancer usually presents as a *painless* testicular mass in a young adult male. Other causes of scrotal masses are hydrocele and varicocele.

Urethral Discharge Urethral discharge is the passage of secretions other than urine or semen. It may be associated with pain or may be noted as a staining on underwear in the absence of urinary incontinence.

Discharge is usually a complaint of men and generally implies infection of the urethra by gonococci (GC) or *Chlamydia*. Ask about associated *dysuria* as well as *amount* and *color* of the discharge. Classically, gonococcal urethritis produces thick, creamy, yellowish discharge with a great deal of dysuria; chlamydial urethritis produces scant, whitish discharge with mild or no dysuria. There are many exceptions, however, and Gram's stain and culture, or PCR identification, is required to make these diagnoses. Prostatitis can also produce a urethral discharge, especially after prostatic massage.

MUSCULOSKELETAL HISTORY TAKING

Joint Stiffness Stiffness of a joint may be due to anatomical changes in the joint or surrounding structures or to edema around the joint.

Anatomical Joint Changes Examples are degeneration of cartilage in degenerative joint disease (DJD) and adhesions from prior trauma or inflammation. Stiffness is noted after rest or immobility but should be relieved with activity in less than 30 minutes.

Edema Around the Joint This is seen in inflammatory joint diseases such as rheumatoid arthritis (RA). Edema collects in surrounding connective tissue structures and is worse after immobility (e.g., early morning stiffness). However, it is slower to dissipate with renewed activity and may persist for several hours. Any stiffness that lasts longer than 30 minutes is suggestive of inflammatory synovial disease.

Joint Swelling In taking the history for joint swelling, you should distinguish between painful and painless swelling, acute and chronic swelling, and joint (synovial thickening) and soft tissue swelling. Ask about warmth and redness.

You should also ask whether the problem is a soft swelling or a hard nodule. There are several types of hard nodules: rheumatoid nodules (over bony prominences, especially the elbow), Heberden's nodes (on the distal interphalangeal joints of the fingers, a classic sign of DJD), and tophi (gouty deposits often seen in ears and elbows).

Joint Pain The following aspects of joint pain should be explored:

Onset, Duration, and Patient Age
➤ Is the pain acute or chronic? Acute pain suggests gout or infection; chronic processes include DJD.
➤ Was the onset sudden or gradual? DJD appears gradually; RA may be sudden or gradual.
➤ How old is the patient? Suspect rheumatic fever in children; RA in young adults (20 to 45 years); septic arthritis in sexually active teens and young adults; and DJD in older adults (40 years or more).

Location of Pain
➤ Does the pain affect one joint or several? Monoarticular pain suggests gout, trauma, DJD, bursitis, or infection. Polyarticular and symmetrical involvements suggest RA. "Migratory" arthritis can be seen in rheumatic fever and gonococcal arthritis.
➤ Which joints are involved? For pain in large, weight-bearing joints (hips, knees), think of DJD. With symmetrical involvement of wrists and metacarpophalangeal (MCP) and proximal interphalangeal (PIP) joints of the hands, consider RA. Back pain in a young man suggests ankylosing spondylitis. Pain in a big toe is classic for gout.

Character of Pain
➤ Does the pain persist at rest? Aching pain accentuated by motion but persistent at rest suggests inflammatory arthritis.

➤ Is the pain severe, excruciating, and throbbing? This suggests gout or septic arthritis.
➤ Does pain radiate with associated weakness, numbness, or tingling? Such a pattern indicates nerve root involvement.

Aggravating and Relieving Factors
The following factors should aid in diagnosis:
➤ Almost all arthritis is initially worse with motion.
➤ DJD is worse after prolonged exercise or activity (e.g., aching at the end of the day, after sports, the morning after exercise).
➤ Prolonged immobility (e.g., sleep) usually results in stiffness.
➤ Aspirin and nonsteroidal anti-inflammatory drugs (NSAIDs) should be helpful in most joint pain conditions; colchicine is specifically helpful in gout.
➤ Heat should help most rheumatic pain syndromes.

Associated Symptoms
Inquire about the following symptoms:
➤ *Morning stiffness*—longer than 30 minutes suggests RA.
➤ *Swelling*—tenderness suggests inflammation, as do redness and warmth.
➤ *Limitation of motion*—shows the effect of the joint pain in limiting daily activities; may help localize the problem diagnostically.
➤ *Fever*—suggests infection, gout, or rheumatic fever.
➤ *Fatigue and malaise*—suggests RA, which is a systemic disease.
➤ *Dysuria, urethral or vaginal discharge*—GC- or other STD-related arthritis.
➤ *Recent sore throat*—"strep throat" precedes rheumatic fever; there is some suggestion of associated viral attack in RA.
➤ *Eye pain or symptoms*—several arthritides have associated eye inflammation.
➤ *Skin lesions*—psoriatic arthritis.
➤ *Recent vaccination*—rubella vaccine can be associated with polyarthralgia occurring several weeks later.
➤ *Trauma*—both recent and past; athletic and occupational factors.

Past Medical History and Family History   A PMH of acute "attacks" of joint pain suggests gout. DJD and RA tend to be persistent once they appear. Gout and ankylosing spondylitis are familial diseases. DJD, RA, and systemic lupus erythematosus (SLE) may also have some familial associations.

NEUROLOGICAL HISTORY TAKING
General Principles
Ask nondirective questions at first and then more specific questions as needed. For example, "And what happened next? And after that?" should be asked before "Did you notice ___ or ___?"

As you get to know the neurological system better, you will find it easier to ask appropriate questions. Anatomical knowledge helps you to define patterns and avoid confusion with patients who have diffusely "positive" histories.

Age of the patient is related to disease probability. For example, multiple sclerosis typically occurs in young adults, whereas strokes occur in older adults.

Onset is particularly important to define. Rapid onset for strokes differs from gradual onset for degenerative diseases.

Location and *radiation* (if any) are very important in peripheral nerve or nerve root syndromes (e.g., herniated disk).

Progression is highly important. Is the problem getting better or worse, or do symptoms wax and wane? Brain tumors get slowly and progressively worse, multiple sclerosis symptoms come and go, and stroke sequelae slowly improve.

Neurological Symptoms
Motor Symptoms   One way to approach the neurological history is to divide signs and symptoms into "positive" and "negative" (i.e., too much or too little function).

"Negative" symptoms or signs may include the following:
➤ *Weakness*—paresis (partial weakness) or plegia (total paralysis). Ascertain extent as hemi (hemisphere), para (both legs), or quad (all four limbs).
➤ *Wasting*—loss of muscle mass (atrophy or thinning).
➤ *Hypotonia*—flaccidity or hyporeflexia.

"Positive" symptoms or signs are involuntary movements, spasticity, and rigidity.

Involuntary Movements   In ascending order by size, involuntary movements include the following:
➤ *Fibrillations*—tiny twitches (visible in tongue).
➤ *Fasciculations*—muscle twitches. Can be benign or serious (e.g., amyotrophic lateral sclerosis).
➤ *Tremors*—shaking, which is usually regular and visible. Divided into *resting tremors* (Parkinson's disease) and *intention tremors* (cerebellar dysfunction). One may also see benign essential tremors (familial).
➤ *Myoclonus*—jerks. Ankle clonus has a regular, rhythmical quality.
➤ *Asterixis*—similar to myoclonus but from metabolic causes ("liver flap").
➤ *Spasms*—jumps.
➤ *Chorea, choreiform*—jerky movements that have a purposeful appearance. Seen in Huntington's chorea and rheumatic fever.
➤ *Athetosis, athetoid*—writhing movements.

Spasticity   Spasticity, or increased motor tone, is the result of exaggerated stretch reflexes (hyperreflexia). There is increased resistance to passive range of motion, but with a jerky quality ("cogwheeling" in Parkinson's disease). Ask the patient about muscle stiffness.

Rigidity   It is difficult to differentiate rigidity from spasticity, except that stiffness is present throughout the range of motion in rigidity.

Weakness   With this complaint, you must distinguish general *fatigue* from specific or generalized *muscle weakness*. Causes of weakness can be *psychogenic* (depression, anxiety) or *organic*.

Organic causes can be classified as follows:
➤ Infection (e.g., hepatitis, mononucleosis, influenza, subacute bacterial endocarditis, Guillain-Barré syndrome).
➤ Autoimmune disease (e.g., rheumatoid arthritis).
➤ Neurological disorder (e.g., Parkinson's, multiple sclerosis).

➤ Primary muscle disorder (e.g., muscular dystrophy, polymyositis).

It is helpful to elicit the following information:

➤ Acute or gradual onset. Acute onset suggests infection.

➤ Is weakness present all day, in the morning, or at the end of the day? True organic weakness gets steadily worse with exertion during the day. Psychogenic fatigue is constant or intermittent.

➤ Stress factors, such as job, family, sex, and sleep. This aspect is helpful in identifying depression.

➤ Associated symptoms. Fever, weight loss, chronic cough, and bowel changes are seen in organic disease. Double vision and difficulty chewing or speaking as the day goes on are seen in myasthenia gravis.

➤ How weakness affects the patient's daily activities, such as walking, dressing, getting things down from shelves, getting up from sitting, opening jars, and writing.

Analyze the weakness in terms of the body segment involved—distal, proximal, trunk, or face. Primary muscle diseases tend to start *proximally* (weakness in shoulders and hips), whereas neuropathies tend to start *distally* (numbness and weakness in hands and feet).

Sensory Changes   Sensory changes commonly occur in disorders of peripheral nerves and nerve roots, usually in association with other symptoms and signs of dysfunction such as weakness, pain, and loss of feeling.

A "negative" symptom would be *numbness.* Anatomical location and distribution are the keys to diagnosis. Find out whether the patient has just numbness or muscle weakness too (strokes produce both symptoms, whereas peripheral neuropathies can be sensory, motor, or both).

A "positive" symptom would be *paresthesias—* spontaneous burning, tingling sensations. *Dysesthesias* are painful, radiating sensations produced by nonpainful stimulation to the skin, such as a light touch or gentle stroking *(hyperesthesias).*

Common causes of both numbness and paresthesias are myelin sheath damage (e.g., multiple sclerosis), nerve compression or nerve root compression (e.g., tumor, herniated disk), and toxic or metabolic changes that damage nerves (e.g., diabetes mellitus).

Gait Disturbances and Incoordination   In pure form, these complaints imply cerebellar disease. You must first distinguish them from other neurological causes of muscle weakness and peripheral neuropathies (e.g., diabetic peripheral neuropathy in feet causes gait problems; basal ganglia dysfunction in Parkinson's disease leads to characteristic stooped, shuffling gait).

Evaluate cerebellar function through physical tests such as Romberg's sign, finger-to-nose test, heel-to-shin test, rapid alternating movements, and intention tremor testing.

Head Trauma   Clinically significant head trauma consists of trauma severe enough to cause the following:

➤ Produce unconsciousness or a change in the level of consciousness.

➤ Produce a localized neurological deficit or seizures.

➤ Cause hospitalization.

➤ Require consultation by a neurologist or neurosurgeon.

➤ Produce permanent neurological deficits.

If the patient has a history of head trauma, ask the following:

➤ Was there unconsciousness?

➤ Was there stupor or lethargy lasting longer than 15 minutes?

➤ Was there a localized neurological deficit (e.g., aphasia, weakness, numbness) or seizures?

➤ Was the patient hospitalized? If so, get as many details as possible.

➤ Was there a neurological consultation?

➤ Are there residual deficits? If so, have they progressed?

Serious head trauma is a significant risk for later epilepsy.

Subdural hematoma is a serious sequela of head trauma that can be missed. High-risk groups include the elderly and alcoholics. The elderly have more fragile veins; alcoholics suffer a lot of trauma; confusion in either group may be misattributed to age or the effects of alcohol, leading to a missed diagnosis.

Seizures   The international classification of seizures includes many types. The most important are:

1. Generalized seizures, which may be tonic-clonic *(old term: grand mal)* or absence *(old term: petit mal).*
2. Partial seizures. If they occur with motor symptoms *(old term: jacksonian seizures)* or sensory symptoms, there is usually no impairment of consciousness. Partial seizures that occur with complex symptoms usually involve impairment of consciousness *(old term: temporal lobe* or *psychomotor seizures).*
3. Partial seizures that become generalized.

When someone complains of loss of consciousness (LOC), first determine whether it is syncope or seizures (Table 11-1).

Hyperventilation episodes are a variation on syncope. The patient complains of anxiety, shortness of breath, perioral and finger tingling, followed by passing out.

Absence seizures, which are common in children, may last only seconds.

Partial-complex (psychomotor) seizures are characterized by repetitive actions and do not always lead to a generalized convulsion. Patients are not aware of their surroundings but they do not fall down. Such seizures may last several minutes.

Partial seizures with motor symptoms (jacksonian seizures) start locally, with involuntary movements (e.g., hand twitching), then spread, and may or may not end in generalized convulsion.

It is important to remember that not all *tonic-clonic seizures* are epilepsy. *Epilepsy* is a particular syndrome with a distinct electroencephalographic (EEG) pattern and an often unknown cause. Other causes of generalized tonic-clonic seizure include metabolic imbalances (e.g., hypoglycemia), drug or alcohol withdrawal, central nervous system (CNS) infections, focal seizures that become generalized, and high fevers in children. Age of the patient is important: idiopathic epilepsy almost never appears *after* age 30.

Partial (focal) seizures imply a pathological lesion in the brain, such as tumor, scar, or infarction.

Taking the History   Questions to ask the patient with seizures include the following:

➤ Is this the first time this ever happened to you?
➤ At what age did the seizures start? Idiopathic epilepsy begins in childhood. Tumors, trauma, strokes, and alcohol are more likely to characterize adult onset.
➤ Do you have a warning before your seizures? Common auras are unpleasant tastes or odors, visual or auditory hallucinations, repetitive motor movements, and cries or mutterings.
➤ How often do the seizures occur? They can vary from one to two times per year to many times daily.

Table 11-1   Differentiation of Syncope from Seizures

Characteristic	Syncope	Seizures
Patient position at onset	Usually standing	None in particular
Warning	Often a premonition	Sometimes an "aura"
Duration	Brief	Variable
Associated body movements	None	Shaking or moving common
Incontinence	None	May occur
Tongue biting	None	May occur
State after awakening	Alert	Often drowsy or confused ("postictal" state)
Other sequelae	Observed to be pale	May have sore muscles

➤ Can you describe what happens, step by step, as fully as you can remember it? Listen for focal symptoms that progress to generalized seizures.

➤ Do you lose consciousness?

➤ (If yes) What do other people say you did while you were unconscious? Did you fall down? Did your arms and legs shake? Did you bite your tongue? Did you lose your urine or move your bowels? Were you sore afterward? How long were you unconscious? Were you confused or sleepy when you woke up?

➤ Does anything bring on your seizures (e.g., flickering lights, sounds or music, stress, alcohol, menstrual periods)?

➤ Do you take any medication for your seizures? If so, get details.

➤ Do you take any other medications?

➤ Do you have any other symptoms? For first-time seizures, headaches, vomiting, fever, or gait disturbances might suggest CNS infection or increased intracranial pressure.

➤ Have you ever had head trauma? Meningitis? Encephalitis? A stroke? Febrile seizures in childhood? All may be associated with later epilepsy.

➤ Do you have high blood pressure? Insulin-dependent diabetes? Alcohol or drug problems? Kidney disease?

➤ Is there any family history of seizures? Some familial tendency is seen in epilepsy.

➤ How does having seizures affect your life? Epileptics often have social problems with school, jobs, and relationships and may develop emotional problems as a result.

Headaches

After the initial, spontaneous part of the history, you should be able to tell whether a patient's headaches are acute and severe, or chronic and recurrent. Acute and severe headache in a patient who has never had this type of headache before indicates serious acute illness, such as meningitis or subarachnoid hemorrhage. Ask quick, focused questions accordingly. Chronic and recurrent headaches with onset sometime in the past require the standard and detailed HPI.

Classic Headache Patterns   The most common types of headaches have classic patterns of occurrence.

Migraine headache often has an aura and may be unilateral or diffuse. Onset is early in life. There is often a family history of migraines. Throbbing pain usually characterizes a migraine headache. Photophobia and phonophobia are associated.

Muscle tension headaches have an occipital or hatband distribution. They are stress related, although it may be unconscious stress. Such headaches have a long history without significant change, despite multiple workups or medications. The pain may be dull or throbbing.

Cluster migraine occurs at night and is associated with unilateral tearing and rhinorrhea. Pain is extremely severe. Episodes occur in clusters, with long symptom-free intervals.

Brain tumor headache is distinguished by steady progression. It may be worse in the morning and is aggravated by coughing or straining. Such a headache may be confused with tension headache at first (because it is relieved by aspirin, vague in location, etc.).

Temporal arteritis causes a unilateral throbbing pain in the temple region of an older adult (older than 50 years). Vision changes are common. Patients may have fever or myalgias.

Associated Symptoms   In taking a headache history, inquire about the following symptoms:

➤ Fever—suggests infectious or inflammatory cause.

➤ Nausea, vomiting—suggest increased intracranial pressure.

➤ Blurred or decreased vision—malignant hypertension, temporal arteritis.

➤ Weakness—suggests organic intracranial process.

➤ Auras—migraine.

➤ PMH of head trauma, ear infection, sinus problems, glaucoma, hypertension—all can cause headaches.

➤ FH of headaches—common in migraines.

➤ Occupation—toxic exposures, stress factors.

➤ Stress factors—relation to muscle tension, precipitation of migraines.

ENDOCRINOLOGICAL HISTORY TAKING

The hormones secreted by the endocrine glands affect the function of other tissues and as such cause a wide variety of symptoms. Hormones may be deficient or secreted in excess. In most patients with endocrine disorders, a single hormone is abnormal. In other cases, as for example in the case of panhypopituitarism, multiple hormones may be absent.

Anterior Pituitary

The anterior pituitary secretes six hormones—growth hormone (GH), luteinizing hormone/follicle-stimulating hormone (LH/FSH), thyroid-stimulating hormone (TSH), adrenocorticotropic hormone (ACTH), and prolactin. In general, the symptoms related to these hormones are due to function or dysfunction of the associated end organ they control.

Growth Hormone   Deficiency in childhood results in growth failure and a form of dwarfism. In excess, growth hormone causes excessive proportional growth—gigantism. Excess in adulthood results in acromegaly characterized by abnormal growth of eyebrows, hands, and feet. Symptoms may also include those of diabetes mellitus, congestive heart failure, carpal tunnel syndrome, and colonic polyps or even colon cancer.

Luteinizing Hormone and Follicle-Stimulating Hormone   These hormones control ovarian cycling in women and testicular functioning in men. In adolescents, they control the onset of puberty. Symptoms related to these hormones include those associated with failure of ovarian or testicular function. In women, these involve menstrual cycling and regularity and fertility. In men, testicular failure results in decreased libido, erectile dysfunction and impaired ejaculation, and infertility.

Thyroid-Stimulating Hormone   Controlled by feedback inhibition by the thyroid hormones, TSH in turn controls thyroid hormone synthesis and secretion.

Adrenocorticotropic Hormone   This controls the synthesis and secretion of cortisol by the adrenal cortex. Excess or deficiency results in symptoms of Cushing's syndrome or adrenocortical glucocorticoid insufficiency, respectively. (See "Adrenal Cortex" later.)

Prolactin   This hormone controls lactation after parturition. Lack of prolactin results in failure of lactation. Excess prolactin may result from a pituitary prolactin-secreting tumor, many drugs (especially psychotropic drugs), hypothyroidism, nipple stimulation, and chest wall trauma. The symptoms of prolactin excess are galactorrhea (lactation at any time except following pregnancy) and amenorrhea. In men, excess prolactin causes signs of hypogonadism.

Posterior Pituitary

The posterior pituitary produces two hormones—*oxytocin* and *arginine vasopressin*. Oxytocin causes uterine muscle contraction at the time of childbirth and subsequent breast milk ejection. If oxytocin is deficient, those two important functions will fail. Arginine vasopressin (or antidiuretic hormone) causes the renal collecting duct to reabsorb water and allows production of a concentrated urine. Deficiency is called *diabetes insipidus* and results in production of a large volume of very dilute urine. An isolated state of excess arginine vasopressin results in hyponatremia, which is asymptomatic until very low sodium concentrations are reached, at which time seizures may result.

Thyroid

The thyroid hormones *thyroxine* (T_4) and *triiodothyronine* (T_3) control many metabolic functions in adulthood. In childhood, the thyroid hormones are critical for normal growth and development. When they are absent at birth, cretinism results, which is characterized by rapidly progressive failure of intellectual development. In adulthood, symptoms of hypothyroidism include fatigue, cold intolerance, weakness (especially of proximal muscles), constipation, dry skin and hair, dulled thinking, and heavy menstrual periods. Symptoms of hyperthyroidism include irritability, anxiousness, heat intolerance, tachycardia (including atrial fibrillation), easy fatigability, loose stools, and weight loss despite increased appetite.

Parathyroid

Parathyroid hormone (PTH) controls the serum calcium level and keeps it in the normal range through effects on bone and renal tubules and renal activation of *vitamin D*. Thus, the absence of PTH results in hypocalcemia, which is characterized by neuromuscular irritability, including numbness and tingling around the mouth, muscle cramps, and tetany. PTH excess results in hypercalcemia, which may be asymptomatic until the serum calcium is significantly elevated. At that point, symptoms include abdominal pain, bone pain, symptoms related to kidney stones, and eventually, if levels are very high, delirium and even coma.

Islets of Langerhans

Several hormones are produced by the several different cell types of the Islets of Langerhans in the pancreas. By far, the most important is *insulin*. Insulin deficiency causes the disease known as *diabetes mellitus*. Patients with type 1 diabetes have absolute insulin deficiency along with excess urination and thirst, weight loss, and rapid progression to a severe medical emergency condition known as *diabetic ketoacidosis*. Patients with type 2 diabetes have relative insulin deficiency but also insulin resistance. They may be asymptomatic and frequently are obese. If the blood sugar is quite elevated in these patients, they may also have polyuria and polydipsia. Additional symptoms relate to the many complications of diabetes, which include macrovascular disease (coronary heart disease and peripheral vascular disease with claudication, transient ischemic attacks [TIAs] and stroke, and impotence) and microvascular disease (neuropathy with foot numbness and pain, impotence, and gastropathy; retinopathy with decreased vision and blindness; and nephropathy with decreasing renal function and eventually renal failure).

Adrenal Cortex

The adrenal cortex makes three classes of hormones—glucocorticoids *(cortisol),* mineralocorticoids *(aldosterone),* and adrenal androgens. Of these, the most critical for sustaining life is cortisol.

Cortisol is required for normal stress response, maintenance of vascular tone, intermediary metabolism, and immune modulation. Absence (most often caused by cessation of prolonged high-dose suppressive glucocorticoid medication or by Addison's disease) results in symptoms of weakness, lethargy, hypotension, abdominal pain, anorexia, and fever, and at its worst, vascular collapse and shock.

Excess cortisol, whether endogenous or given as exogenous glucocorticoid medication, results in the symptoms of Cushing's syndrome—hypertension, glucose intolerance, centripetal obesity, muscle wasting, moon facies, abnormal fat pads between the scapulae and in the supraclavicular fossae, weakness, fatigue, hirsutism, amenorrhea, purple abdominal striae, abnormal mentation, and osteoporosis with compression fractures.

Aldosterone causes activation of a transporter in the renal collecting ducts that reabsorbs sodium in exchange for potassium. When aldosterone is deficient, symptoms of hyperkalemia, including ventricular arrhythmia, can occur. In excess, aldosterone causes one of the forms of surgically correctable hypertension due to excess sodium retention associated with hypokalemia.

Adrenal Medulla

The adrenal medulla secretes the catecholamines, epinephrine and norepinephrine. As long as the rest of the sympathetic nervous system is intact, there is no deficiency state in the adrenal medulla. When produced in excess, however, by the adrenomedullary tumor known as *pheochromocytoma,* these hormones cause hypertension that is classically episodic and is associated with headache, sweating, and palpitations.

Ovaries and Testes

The hormones of the ovary (estradiol and progesterone) and testis (testosterone) are responsible for the development of female and male secondary sexual characteristics and the maintenance of these throughout adult life. In women, these include breast development and regular menstrual cycling. In men, these include penile enlargement and male pattern musculature and hair growth. In both sexes, gonadal steroids are necessary for normal libido and fertility, and in the male for erectile function.

Metabolic Bone Disease

The three major classes of metabolic bone disease are osteoporosis, osteomalacia, and Paget's disease.

Osteoporosis—loss of bone mass due to hypogonadism, aging, or other causes—is asymptomatic until fracture occurs. The fractures are most often vertebral compression fractures that occur after menopause in women, and fractures of the hip at later ages in both men and women.

Osteomalacia (called *rickets* in childhood)—loss of the bone mineral only—has numerous causes; many of these relate to vitamin D deficiency, which causes bone pain, deformity (especially of weight-bearing bones in childhood), and fracture.

Paget's disease is an abnormality consisting of high bone turnover in discrete areas, either localized or widespread. It results in bone pain, fracture, and deafness (because of cranial nerve VIII damage in the skull foramen through which it passes and disease in the bony ossicles of the ear). Occasionally, an aggressive bone malignancy, *osteosarcoma*, arises in pagetic bone.

Lipids

The two major classes of lipids, cholesterol and triglyceride, circulate in association with apoproteins that confer specificity and therefore associated risk. Low-density lipoprotein (LDL) cholesterol is associated with increased risk of atherosclerosis, including coronary heart disease and peripheral vascular disease. Conversely, high-density lipoprotein (HDL) cholesterol is associated with a decreased risk of atherosclerosis. The symptoms of hypercholesterolemia are therefore related to atherosclerotic disease.

Triglycerides also circulate in association with apoproteins. High triglycerides have some association with atherosclerotic disease. Very high triglycerides can cause acute pancreatitis with abdominal pain, nausea, and vomiting.

DERMATOLOGICAL HISTORY TAKING

Skin lesions may be an incidental finding or may constitute the patient's chief complaint. Likewise, a skin abnormality may be a primary disease in itself or a manifestation of a systemic or underlying problem. Thus, the history should consider the skin lesion itself, including its progression, duration, and manifestations, as well as other aspects of the history and health of the patient, such as underlying diseases and non-skin symptoms, medications, travel, exposure to toxins (including topical and internal ingestions), occupation, sunlight and other radiation exposure, family history, known allergies, hobbies, pregnancy, effect of heat/cold/alcohol ingestion, and similar lesions in family, friends, or co-workers.

Cardinal symptoms of skin lesions include itching, pain, bleeding, oozing, change in color or size, swelling, redness, and warmth.

CASE STUDY 11-1

A 24-year-old woman presents to the clinic with a complaint of lower abdominal pain.

What questions need to be asked in the medical history to cover the most important possibilities in her differential diagnosis? Which organ systems on the review of systems list need to be covered?

The basic questions in a standard history of present illness will reveal nearly all of the relevant historical data in most presenting complaints. Onset, duration, description, aggravating and relieving factors, current medication, prior history and family history of this complaint, and general effect of this problem on the patient's life constitute most of the HPI. The clinician's judgment is tested in knowing which associated symptoms to ask for, in a logical and efficient manner, in order to rule in or rule out different diagnostic possibilities.

Many hospitals and medical schools have an institutional medical history and physical examination form that includes a comprehensive list of medical symptoms arranged by organ system. This "Review of Systems" list can be reproduced and carried in a convenient pocket by beginning clinicians for easy referral during patient history taking.

In this case, lower abdominal pain in a woman of reproductive age could be caused by disease of the gastrointestinal, reproductive, or urinary system. Regarding the GI system, the clinician should ask questions about bowel function (e.g., constipation, diarrhea, melena). In terms of the urinary system, questions related to cystitis, pyelonephritis, and renal stone should be asked (e.g., frequency, dysuria, hematuria). About the reproductive system, questions should be asked related to pregnancy or its complications (last menstrual period, pregnancy and menstrual history, contraceptive method, possibility of current pregnancy), endometriosis (dysmenorrhea), and pelvic inflammatory disease (e.g., sexual history, vaginal discharge, history of STDs, dyspareunia). It is almost always a good idea to ask some questions from the general, or "constitutional," list of symptoms, such as fever or weight loss.

CASE STUDY 11-2

A 43-year-old accountant presents with a 2-week history of intermittent chest pain episodes.

What history questions need to be asked to cover the most important possibilities in his differential diagnosis? Which organ systems on the review of systems list need to be covered?

Chest pain in a middle-aged adult could be caused by disease of the cardiovascular, respiratory, upper GI, or musculoskeletal system. For example, regarding the cardiovascular system, the clinician should ask all the regular questions on the cardiovascular review of systems list, plus additional cardiovascular risk factor questions such as smoking history, cholesterol, and family history of coronary artery disease. In terms of the respiratory system, the clinician should concentrate on respiratory diseases that are known to cause chest pain, such as pneumonias and pulmonary embolus. The clinician should ask questions about cough, hemoptysis, or pleuritic chest pain.

Study of the GI system reveals that certain diseases of the upper GI tract such as peptic ulcer disease or gallbladder disease can cause referred pain to the chest. The clinician should ask questions related to the pain location, its relationship to meals, description of the pain, particularly heartburn, and association with GI functions such as gas production. In terms of the musculoskeletal system, chest wall disorders can produce chest pain, so the clinician should ask questions about rib trauma, recent febrile illness (costochondritis), and point localization of pain.

CONCLUSION

Figure 11-1 shows a typical complete medical history.

CLINICAL APPLICATIONS

1. Review the available list of the most common primary care problems. Identify those problems for which a multisystem approach to the medical history would be necessary (e.g., fatigue, fever of unknown origin, headache, aches and pains). Prepare a list of specific and appropriate questions for each problem by selecting from the specific "organ system" protocols presented in this chapter. Compare your suggested history-taking lists with those of other students and practicing clinicians.

2. Talk with representatives of the various ethnic groups most commonly presenting in your clinical setting. Ask them about specific terminology that is used in their culture to describe common symptoms and ailments. Discuss the appropriate integration of these terms into your own history-taking practice.

GLOSSARY OF ABBREVIATIONS

Acronym	Definition	Acronym	Definition
ASA	Acetylsalicylic acid (aspirin)	LOC	Loss of consciousness
BM	Bowel movement	MCL	Midclavicular line
BPH	Benign prostatic hypertrophy	MCP	Metacarpophalangeal
CA	Cancer	MI	Myocardial infarction
CAD	Coronary artery disease	NSAID	Nonsteroidal anti-inflammatory
CC	Chief complaint		drug
CHF	Congestive heart failure	OC	Oral contraceptive
CNS	Central nervous system	OE	Otitis externa
COPD	Chronic obstructive pulmonary	OM	Otitis media
	disease (e.g., chronic bronchitis,	OTC	Over the counter (medication)
	emphysema)	PE	Pulmonary embolus, pulmonary
Corrected	Visual acuity score obtained with		edema, or physical examination
	patient wearing glasses or	PERRLA	Pupils equal, round, reactive to
	contact lenses		light and accommodation
CSF	Cerebrospinal fluid	PID	Pelvic inflammatory disease
CV	Cardiovascular	PIP	Proximal interphalangeal
CXR	Chest x-ray	PMH	Past medical history
DIP	Distal interphalangeal	PMI	Point of maximal impulse
DJD	Degenerative joint disease	PND	Paroxysmal nocturnal dyspnea or
DM	Diabetes mellitus		postnasal drip
DOE	Dyspnea on exertion	PP	Personal profile
DUB	Dysfunctional uterine bleeding	PPD	Purified protein derivative
ECG	Electrocardiogram		(tuberculin skin test) (PPD) or
EEG	Electroencephalogram		packs per day smoking (ppd)
ENT	Ear, nose, and throat	PUD	Peptic ulcer disease
EOMI	Extraocular movements intact	PVC	Premature ventricular contraction
FB	Foreign body	PVD	Peripheral vascular disease
FH	Family history	R	Right
GC	Gonococci	RBC	Red blood cell
GI	Gastrointestinal	ROM	Range of motion
GN	Glomerulonephritis	ROS	Review of systems
GYN	Gynecological	SH	Social history
HEENT	Head, eyes, ears, nose, and throat	SLE	Systemic lupus erythematosus
HPI	History of present illness	SOB	Shortness of breath
HTN	Hypertension	STD	Sexually transmitted disease
ICS	Intercostal space	TB	Tuberculosis
IUD	Intrauterine (birth control) device	TM	Tympanic membrane
IV	Intravenous	URI	Upper respiratory infection
L	Left	VA	Visual acuity

#	Problem	Date	Resolution (Date)
1	Hematemesis	– 6/25/02	
2	Epigastric pain	– May 2002	
	(possible peptic ulcer disease)		
3	Hypertension	– 1998	
4	Smoker x 20 years		

PATIENT NO.

PATIENT NAME

D.O.B.

PROBLEM LIST

Figure 11-1 Example of a complete medical history and physical examination notes. *(Courtesy University of Washington Affiliated Hospitals, Seattle, Washington.)*

IDENTIFYING DATA:

Age _42_ Race _W_ Marital Status _M_ Sex _M_ Occupation _Engineer_

Residence _Seattle_ Referral Source _self_

Names of parents or next of kin _Mrs. Jane Smith (wife)_

Sources of information _patient_

CHIEF COMPLAINT: _"I vomited some blood this morning"_

PRESENT PROBLEMS/ILLNESS: _This 42 y.o. WM engineer presents following an acute_ _episode of hematemesis at approx. 8:00 am on 6/25/02. Patient was in his usual state of good_ _health until approx. 1 month ago, when he began to experience episodes of epigastric pain._ _Pain is described as "gnawing," bothersome rather than severe, non-radiating, occurring 2-3_ _times per day, and lasting 1-2 hours per episode. Pain was increased by hunger or stress, and_ _decreased by food or Rolaids. Patient associates the onset of his symptoms with a stressful new_ _project at work. Pain episodes have been increasing in frequency lately, and patient was_ _awakened twice this week in the early a.m. by epigastric pain. This morning, while dressing_ _for work, he suddenly felt ill, and vomited approx. 1 cup of bright red blood. His wife drove_ _him to the ER, and he was admitted._

 Patient denies any recent appetite changes, jaundice, dysphagia, indigestion, _nausea/vomiting (other than this episode), previous hematemesis, change in abdominal girth,_ _constipation, diarrhea, melena, change in stool shape or color, anal discomfort, hemorrhoids,_ _or hernia. He denies any PMH or FH of GI problems or bleeding problems._

 Other than Rolaids, he has not taken any meds for this problem or sought medical _evaluation until the day of admission._

PATIENT NO.

PATIENT NAME

D.O.B.

HISTORY OF PRESENT ILLNESS

Figure 11-1, cont'd For legend see p. 230.

PERSONAL PROFILE/SOCIAL HISTORY

Family structure   Occupation
Sources of strength   Sources of influence
Interpretation of illness   Communication

Married with 2 children, ages 14 and 12. Other family members (mother, 1 brother)

live in town and will be helpful during this illness, if necessary. Mr. Smith sees

his family as his major source of strength, and also feels that he has a good support

system through friends and co-workers. He has been an engineer for 20 years,

and worked at his present job for the past 10 years. He thinks his current illness

is related to job stress. He has no religious or philosophical beliefs that would

conflict with any medical treatment (e.g. transfusions). He describes himself as

quiet, and someone who prefers to keep his problems to himself rather than

burden others. He appears to take a logical, matter-of-fact approach to his

current illness.

Figure 11-1, cont'd For legend see p. 230.

FAMILY HISTORY: _____

Mother _____ — alive, 62, with arthritis and psoriasis _____

Father _____ — dead, 54, car accident _____

Siblings _____ — 1 brother, alive and well _____

Spouse _____

Children _____ wife, 2 children, alive and well

Familial Diseases: _____ Denies any FH of heart disease, stroke, hypertension, diabetes, or

_____ cancer

PAST MEDICAL AND SURGICAL ILLNESS: _____

① Usual childhood illnesses.

② Broken Ⓡ arm, age 8, no sequelae.

③ Appendectomy, age 16, no sequelae.

④ Hypertension discovered, age 38.

Under care of family physician, Dr. Richard Jones.

MEDICATIONS: ____ Hydrochlorothiazide 50 mg. OD _____

Rolaids (see HPI) _____

occ. ASA for headaches _____

DRUG/TRANSFUSION REACTIONS: _____ None. No known allergies _____

SMOKING: _____ 1 pack per day x 20 yrs. _____

ALCOHOL/RECREATIONAL DRUGS: _____ 3 drinks per week. No drugs. _____

PATIENT NO.	**MEDICAL HISTORY**
PATIENT NAME	
D.O.B.	

Figure 11-1, cont'd For legend see p. 230.

REVIEW OF SYSTEMS: Check if there is no significant problem: **Circle** if there is a significant problem and record details or note "P.I." (if recorded under Present Illness) or "Past Hx" (if recorded in Past History). Items not marked are assumed to be not examined.

GENERAL
✓ Weight change   ✓ Fever-chills   ✓ Weakness
✓ Fatigue   ✓ Sweating-nightsweats

SKIN
✓ Hair-nail changes ✓ Itching   ✓ Rashes

HEAD
⟨Headache⟩   ✓ Trauma

occ. stress-related headache, relieved by aspirin

EYES
⟨Vision-glasses⟩   ✓ Blurring   ✓ Scotomata
✓ Diplopia   ✓ Pain   ✓ Discharge

Wears glasses for reading. No recent visual

changes.

EARS
✓ Pain   ✓ Discharge   ✓ Vertigo
✓ Deafness   ✓ Tinnitus

NOSE
✓ Sinusitis   ✓ Discharge   ✓ Postnasal drip
✓ Epistaxis   ✓ Obstruction

MOUTH/THROAT
✓ Sores   ✓ Teeth-dental care   ✓ Dentures
✓ Gum bleeding   ✓ Hoarseness   ✓ Taste

PULMONARY
✓ Dyspnea   ✓ Wheezing   ✓ Hemoptysis
✓ Chest pain   ⟨Cough⟩   ⟨Sputum⟩

"Smoker's cough" in a.m. with some clear

sputum production

BREASTS
✓ Masses   ✓ Pain   ✓ Discharge

CARDIOVASCULAR
✓ Palpitation   ✓ Pain   ✓ Dyspnea
✓ Orthopnea   ✓ Murmurs   ⟨Hypertension⟩
✓ Cyanosis   ✓ Edema   ✓ Claudication

see PMH

GASTROINTESTINAL
Appetite   Pain   Hematemesis ⎫
Jaundice   Hernia   Melena   ⎬ *see HPI*
Constipation   Anal discomfort   Stool shape, color ⎨
Dysphagia   Hemorrhoids   Abdominal girth ⎬
Indigestion   Nausea-vomiting-diarrhea ⎭

GENITOURINARY
✓ Dysuria   ✓ Nocturia   ✓ Hematuria
✓ Frequency   ✓ Urgency   ✓ Incontinence

SEXUAL HISTORY
✓ Syphilis   ✓ Gonorrhea   ✓ Sores-discharge
✓ Testicular pain-swelling   ✓ Impotence
✓ Sterility   Contraception   Gravida/Para/Abort

FEMALE-MENSES
Cycle/Duration/Amount/ Menopause
Dysmenorrhea   Spotting   Irregularity

ENDOCRINE
✓ Goiter   ✓ Tremor   ✓ Glycosuria/diabetes
✓ Heat-cold intolerance   ✓ Hormone therapy

ALLERGIC HISTORY
✓ Sensitivity to allergens, drugs, vaccines
✓ Eczema   ✓ Asthma ⟨Hay Fever⟩ ✓ Hives

occ. hay fever in spring

BONES, JOINTS & MUSCLES
✓ Trauma   ✓ Swelling   ✓ Pain-arthritis

BLOOD-LYMPHATIC
✓ Anemia   ✓ Bleeding tendency
✓ Transfusions   ✓ Lymph node enlargement-pain

NEUROLOGIC
✓ Syncope   ✓ Convulsions   ✓ Sensation
✓ Gait-coordination ✓ Speech   ✓ Paralysis-weakness

PSYCHOLOGIC
✓ Memory   ✓ Mood   ✓ Sleep pattern
✓ Anxiety-depression   ✓ Phobias   ✓ Drug, alcohol abuse

Figure 11-1, cont'd For legend see p. 230.

☑ **GENERAL EXAMINATION**
All items are examined.
Circle abnormal findings and describe in detail.

☐ **MODIFIED EXAMINATION**
Check areas & items examined. **Circle** abnormal findings and describe. **No mark** means not examined.

	Sitting	Supine		
BLOOD PRESSURE: RA	_96/70_	_110/88_	WEIGHT:	_165 lbs._
LA			HEIGHT:	_5' 10"_

PULSE: _96 supine – 110 sitting_

RESP. _20_   TEMP: _97.8° F._

GENERAL APPEARANCE   _Alert and oriented, somewhat pale and anxious_

HANDS/SKIN
Hair
Nails
Skin-Lesions
Texture
Color

Skin pale, cool, sl. sweaty. No rashes.

No clubbing or cyanosis. Hair clean, mod. male pattern baldness.

HEAD/EYES
Configuration
Eye position
Lids
Conjunctiva
Sclera
Cornea
Pupils (equality, light reaction)
Fundi
Visual acuity

Normocephalic. PERRLA, EOMI. Cornea and lens clear, without

opacities. Sclera white, conjunctiva pink. Fundi – red reflex present

bilat. No AV nicking, hemorrhages, exudates, or papilledema.

V.A. 20/20 corrected, bilat.

EARS
Pinna/Canal/Drum
Hearing

Canals clear, TM's intact, grey, light reflex and landmarks present.

NOSE
Septum/Mucosa

Hearing grossly intact. Nose clear – no discharge.

MOUTH/THROAT
Teeth/Gums/Mucosa
Lips/Breath
Tongue-Palate
Tonsils/Pharynx

Teeth in good repair. No gum bleeding or

lesions. Tonsils and pharynx not inflamed.

NECK/NODES
Motion
Muscle strength
Thyroid masses
Neck nodes
Inguinal/Axillary nodes

Full ROM. No adenopathy. Thyroid

smooth, not enlarged.

CHEST
Shape
Symmetry
Resonance
Breath Sounds

Percussion resonant. Clear breath sounds.

No crackles, rhonchi, wheezes, or rubs.

PATIENT NO.

PATIENT NAME

D.O.B.

PHYSICAL EXAMINATION

Figure 11-1, cont'd For legend see p. 230.

BREASTS
Masses
Tenderness
Discharge

Symmetrical. No masses.

CARDIOVASCULAR
Carotids
Neck veins
Peripheral pulses:
    radial, femoral, d. pedis
Apex impulse-,
    character/position
Cardiac sounds:
    Rate
Rhythm
S_1S_2
    A_2 P_2

PMI – 5th ICS, MCL. Regular rate
& rhythm, 96/min. S_1 and S_2
present. No murmurs or extra sounds.
Peripheral pulses intact.
Flat. No bowel sounds x 3 mins.
Marked guarding and tenderness

ABDOMEN
Shape-scars
Tenderness
Sounds
Organs:
    Liver
    Kidney
    Spleen

throughout. Rebound positive –
localizes to epigastric
area. Liver, spleen, kidneys – exam
deferred due to pain.

MUSCULOSKELETAL/ EXTREMITIES
Spine symmetry
Extremity-joints/
    muscle strength
Edema
Veins
Temperature

No obvious deformities. Extremities
symmetrical. No joint swelling or tenderness.
Strength symmetrical bilat. No edema or varicosities.
Skin sl. cool to touch.

NERVOUS SYSTEM
Mental status
Speech
Cranial nerves
Sensation   (2+=nl.)
Coordination

Reflexes:	R	L
Biceps	2+	2+
Knee	2+	2+
Ankle	2+	2+

Gait – no ataxia

Alert, oriented x 3. Speech intact and appropriate. Cranial nerves
II–XII grossly intact. Sensation, coordination, motor – all
grossly intact.

GENITALIA-RECTUM

Male	Female
Penis	Perineum
Scrotum	Vagina
Testes	Cervix-uterus
Prostate	Adnexa-ovaries

Rectum-sphincter
tone, masses, guaiac

Circumcised. No rash, lesions, or urethral discharge. Testes
symmetrical without masses. Rectal – sphincter tone intact. No
masses. Prostate smooth, not enlarged. Trace stool – guaiac (+).

Figure 11-1, cont'd For legend see p. 230.

REFERENCES

1. Bates B. A Guide to Physical Examination and History Taking, ed 6. Philadelphia: JB Lippincott, 1995.
2. Wilson JD, et al (eds). Harrison's Principles of Internal Medicine, ed 12. New York: McGraw-Hill, 1991.

RESOURCES

Bickley LS, Hoekelman RA. Bates' Guide to Physical Examination and History Taking, ed 7. Philadelphia: JB Lippincott, 1999.

Kraytman M. The Complete Patient History, ed 2. New York: McGraw-Hill, 1991 (ed 1, 1979). *In-depth approach to the systematic evaluation of symptoms. This book is the source of some of the material in this chapter.*

Walker HK, Hall WD, Hurst JW. Clinical Methods: The History, Physical, and Laboratory Examinations, ed 3. Boston: Butterworths, 1990 (ed 1, 1976). *Concise chapters on the potential significance of selected symptoms. The first edition (1976) is the source of much of the material in this chapter.*

CHAPTER 12

Performing and Recording the Physical Examination

Henry Stoll

INTRODUCTION

Physical examination of patients is a fundamental skill for all physician assistants. PA students and practicing PAs are fortunate to have access to a wide variety of excellent textbooks on the significance and proper technique of physical examination. Most textbooks, however, do not show the student or practitioner how to organize a disparate collection of physical examination maneuvers into a logical, efficient, sequential order. What is needed is a step-by-step guide, in outline form, to the most commonly performed physical examinations. Over the years, the faculty of the MEDEX Northwest Physician Assistant Program at the University of Washington has created such a set of physical examination protocols.

These protocols are organized in two columns. In the left column, the examination maneuvers are

listed in the order in which they should be performed. In the right column, important potential abnormal findings are highlighted. For reasons of space, not all possible abnormalities can be included for each maneuver.

The protocols begin with a general screening examination. This examination, which takes approximately 20 minutes to perform, is suitable for a reasonably complete comprehensive physical, such as for an annual physical checkup, insurance purposes, or hospital admission. It is followed by a series of organ-specific branching examinations, so called because they branch off the general screening examination into more detailed exploration of particular organ systems and are to be used as indicated by a patient's history or physical findings. Each of these examinations typically takes no longer than 10 to 15 minutes to perform. A complete neurological examination, taking approximately 25 minutes, finishes the set; note that even this lengthy procedure is relatively superficial in assessing mental status and aphasia.

PA students are often initially at a loss as to how to write up their physical findings once they have learned how to perform examinations. Although a case can be made that truer learning takes place when students have to struggle to create their own descriptions, they may also benefit from having good examples to imitate and from which to ultimately progress to their own prose style. Consequently, most examinations in this chapter are followed by examples of both normal and abnormal write-ups. Abbreviations are both a bane and a fact of life in medical practice. Common medical abbreviations are incorporated into the write-ups; all are defined in the glossary at the end of the chapter.

BASIC SCREENING EXAMINATION

BASIC EXAM—PROTOCOL

The left column lists the examination maneuvers in the order they are performed. The right column lists the focus, or important potential abnormal finding(s), of each maneuver.

PA student faces sitting patient.

I. Introduction
  A. States name and purpose
  B. Washes hands

II. General Appearance
  Observes patient for habitus, posture, level of comfort, signs of distress

III. Vital Signs
A. Takes or verifies temperature	Fever
B. Palpates radial pulses bilaterally	Symmetry
C. Counts radial pulse (15 seconds)	Rate, rhythm
D. Counts respirations	Rate, rhythm
E. Takes blood pressure R. arm	High BP, low BP

IV. Hands
A. Inspects palms	Erythema, moistness, tremors, thenar atrophy
B. Inspects nails	Clubbing, cyanosis
C. Inspects joints	Swelling, deformity
D. Palpates joints	Tenderness, warmth, thickening, swelling, decreased ROM

V. Upper Extremities
A. Inspects skin	Color, lesions
B. Inspects musculature	Symmetry, atrophy, involuntary movements
C. Inspects joints	Swelling, deformity
D. Palpates skin	Turgor, moistness
E. Palpates muscles	Tone, tenderness
F. Palpates joints	Tenderness, warmth, swelling
G. Tests ROM of joints (wrists, elbows)	Decreased ROM

VI. Head (scalp and face)
A. Inspection	Shape, size
B. Palpation	Deformities, lumps, tenderness

Continued

BASIC EXAM—PROTOCOL—cont'd

VII. Eyes
   A. Tests vision with pocket visual screener — Visual acuity
   B. Inspects conjunctivae and sclerae — Color, lesions
   C. Inspects and tests pupils with penlight — Size, equality, reaction
   D. Tests extraocular movements — Asymmetry, nystagmus
   E. Funduscopy (optional—do here or at XVIIIA) — Red reflex, opacities, disk, vessels, etc.

VIII. Ears
   A. Inspects auricle — Deformities, lumps, skin lesions
   B. Pulls on pinna — Tenderness
   C. Pushes on tragus — Tenderness
   D. Inspects canal with otoscope — Cerumen, discharge, foreign bodies
   E. Inspects TMs with otoscope — Color, landmarks, bulging, retraction, perforation, mobility
   F. Tests hearing (optional—do here or at XIB) — Symmetry, hearing loss

IX. Nose
   Inspects with otoscope (large speculum) — Patency, septal deviation, lesions, discharge, blood

X. Mouth and Throat—inspects with light
   A. Lips — Cyanosis, lesions
   B. Teeth — Loose, missing, caries
   C. Mucous membranes — Lesions, moisture
   D. Tongue — Color, lesions, tremor
   E. Palate — Lesions, deformities
   F. Tonsils — Presence, size, color, pus
   G. Pharynx and uvula — Lesions, color, symmetrical movement of uvula

XI. Voice and Hearing
   A. Observes voice quality — Hoarseness
   B. Tests hearing *(if not already tested)* — Symmetry, hearing loss
   PA student moves behind patient.

XII. Neck and Shoulders
   A. Observes active ROM of neck (flexion, extension, rotation) — Decreased ROM
   B. Shoulder shrug against resistance — Weakness
   C. Hands over head (biceps to ears, palms together) — Decreased ROM
   D. Palpates lymph nodes (anterior and posterior) — Size, consistency, tenderness
   E. Palpates thyroid with patient swallowing — Size, shape, consistency, nodules, tenderness

XIII. Chest
   A. Inspects—posterior view (with quiet and deep breathing) — Rate, rhythm, depth, effort
   B. Palpates spinous processes — Tenderness
   C. Percusses posterior lung fields (3 fields each lung, side to side) — Dullness, hyperresonance

BASIC EXAM—PROTOCOL—cont'd

D. Auscultates posterior lung fields (3 fields each lung, side to side, with diaphragm)	Character, duration of breath sounds, crackles, wheezes, rhonchi, rubs
E. Percusses anterior lung fields (3 fields each lung, side to side)	
F. Auscultates anterior lung fields (3 fields each lung, side to side)	

XIV. Breasts

A. Inspects—patient's hands on hips, then behind head (females only)	Masses, retractions, symmetry, skin changes

PA student instructs patient to lie down on back.

B. Inspects	
C. Palpates (4 quadrants, tail, nipples)	Consistency, tenderness, nodules, discharge
D. Palpates axillary nodes	Enlarged nodes

XV. Cardiovascular

A. Palpates each carotid *separately* (optional—do here or at D6)	Amplitude, thrills
B. Inspects precordium	PMI, pulsations
C. Palpates apex with fingertips	Location, amplitude
D. Auscultates with diaphragm	Rate, rhythm, S_1 and S_2, murmurs, gallops, rubs, bruits

    1. Apex
    2. LSB
    3. Pulmonic area (2nd L. ICS)
    4. Aortic area (2nd R. ICS)
    5. RSB
    6. Carotids *(if not already checked)*
    7. Midepigastrium
    8. Umbilicus
    9. Femorals

E. Palpates femoral pulses (optional—do here or at XVIF)	Amplitude
F. Palpates inguinal nodes (optional—do here or at XVIG)	Size, consistency, tenderness

XVI. Abdomen

A. Inspects	Scars, distention, symmetry, masses, pulsations, veins
B. Performs superficial palpation (4 quadrants)	Guarding, tenderness, masses
C. Performs deep palpation (4 quadrants)	Masses, tenderness
D. Palpates for liver edge (bimanual technique)	Size, consistency, tenderness
E. Palpates for spleen (bimanual technique)	Enlargement
F. Palpates femoral pulses *(if not already checked)*	Amplitude
G. Palpates inguinal nodes *(if not already checked)*	Size, consistency, tenderness

Continued

BASIC EXAM—PROTOCOL—cont'd

XVII. Lower Extremities
    A. Inspects skin   Color, lesions
    B. Inspects vessels   Varicosities
    C. Inspects musculature   Symmetry
    D. Inspects joints   Swelling, deformity
    E. Palpates skin   Temperature
    F. Palpates musculature   Tone, tenderness
    G. Palpates joints   Warmth, tenderness, swelling
    H. Tests ROM of joints (hip, knee, ankle)   Decreased ROM, crepitus
    I. Palpates pretibial area   Edema
    J. Palpates dorsalis pedis pulse   Amplitude, symmetry
       (if absent, checks posterior tibial pulse)
    K. Tests plantar flexion response   Present or absent
       (Babinski's reflex)
  PA student instructs patient to sit up.
XVIII. Neurological
    A. Funduscopy (*if not already checked*)   Red reflex, opacities, disks, vessels, etc.
    B. Observes forehead wrinkling   Symmetry
    C. Observes showing of teeth   Symmetry
    D. Observes tongue protrusion   Deviation from midline, tremors
    E. Tests deep tendon reflexes (DTRs)   Speed, force, amplitude, symmetry
       1. Biceps
       2. Knees
       3. Ankles
    F. Performs Romberg's test   Loss of balance
       (patient remains standing with eyes shut)
    G. Has patient extend arms with eyes shut   Drift, tremors
    H. Observes patient's gait   Ataxia
XIX. Male Genitalia
    A. Student dons gloves
    B. Inspects penis   Lesions, discharge
    C. Palpates testes   Tenderness, nodules
    D. Palpates for hernias   Bulging

  This is the end of the normal basic screening examination. Under certain circumstances, you would also add female genitalia (pelvic) examination or rectal examination with guaiac test. See other examination protocols for specific techniques and focus.

BASIC WRITE-UP—NORMAL

Vital Signs
Temp. = 98.6° F
Pulse = 80/min., reg.
Resp. = 12/min., reg.
BP = 120/80, R. arm, sitting

General Appearance
WD, WN, WM in NAD. Alert and cooperative.[a]

HEENT
Head—Normocephalic. Hair—full.[b] Scalp—clear.[c]
Eyes—VA = 20/20 OU, corrected.[d] Sclerae white, conjunctivae pink.[e] PERRL. Cornea and lens clear without opacities. Fundi—red reflex present bilat. No AV nicking, hemorrhages, exudate, or papilledema.
Ears—Auricles symmetrical without lesions or deformities, nontender to manipulation. External canals clear, no erythema. TMs intact bilat., gray, light reflex and landmarks intact.[f] Hearing grossly intact to tuning fork bilat.
Nose—Patent, no septal deviation, mucosa pink without lesions or discharge. Turbinates not swollen.
Mouth/Throat—Lips without lesions or cracking. Teeth in good repair without obvious caries. Gums pink without bleeding or recession. Mucosa pink without lesions. Tongue well papillated without lesions. Tonsils not enlarged or inflamed, without exudate. Pharynx not inflamed, uvula midline. Voice resonant without hoarseness.

Neck
Full ROM without pain. Shoulder shrug and ROM without weakness. No lymphadenopathy. Thyroid smooth, not enlarged.[g]

Chest
No chest wall deformities. No vertebral tenderness. Lungs resonant to percussion. Vesicular breath sounds throughout without crackles, rhonchi, wheezes, or rubs.

Breasts
Symmetrical without dimpling, retraction, or skin changes. No masses, tenderness, or nipple discharge. No axillary nodes.

Continued

BASIC WRITE-UP—NORMAL—cont'd

CV

PMI—5th ICS, MCL.[h] No heaves or thrills. Regular rate and rhythm, 80/min. S_1 and S_2 heard well without splits or extra sounds. No murmurs, gallops, or rubs. Neck veins nondistended, fill from above.

Pulses:

	R.	L.		
Carotid	2+	2+	No bruits	
Femoral	2+	2+	No bruits	
DP	2+	2+		(2+ = normal)

Abdomen

Flat[i] without scars. Soft, nontender,[j] no masses. Liver and spleen not enlarged. No inguinal nodes or hernias.

Extremities

Symmetrical, no deformities. Adequate muscle bulk and tone.[k] Joints—full ROM without tenderness, swelling, or stiffness. UEs—nails clear, no cyanosis or clubbing. LEs—no skin changes or varicosities. No pretibial edema.

Neuro

Cranial nerves II, III, VII, VIII, IX, X, XI, XII intact.

DTRs:

	R.	L.	
Biceps	2+	2+	
Knee	2+	2+	(2+ = normal)
Ankle	2+	2+	

Gait—Walks easily without ataxia. No tremor or drift with arms extended. Babinski—Negative.[l]

[a]Comment on mental or emotional state if patient appears anxious, confused, depressed, agitated, intoxicated, etc.
[b]Versus sparse, bald, or specific alopecia, such as tinea. Don't forget to check beard.
[c]No skin lesions, such as seborrhea or psoriasis.
[d]Vision corrected by glasses or contact lenses.
[e]Versus scleral icterus (jaundice). Conjunctivae can be pale (in anemia), injected, or inflamed.
[f]Versus perforations, scarring, redness, bulging, retractions, absence or distortion of light reflex, obscured or distorted landmarks, or visible fluid level.
[g]Versus impalpable, nodular, or diffusely enlarged.
[h]PMI is at the 5th intercostal space in the midclavicular line. The PMI shifts down and toward the axilla when the heart enlarges.
[i]Versus distended, obese, or scaphoid.
[j]Versus guarding, rigidity, or rebound tenderness.
[k]Versus atrophy, flaccidity, or spasticity.
[l]The technically correct description for this would be "plantar flexion response—downward," but most clinicians still use the terminology shown in the example.

HEAD, EYES, EARS, NOSE, AND THROAT
BRANCHING EXAMINATION

HEENT—PROTOCOL

The left column lists the examination maneuvers in the order they are performed. The right column lists the focus, or important potential abnormal finding(s), of each maneuver.

PA student faces sitting patient.

I. Introduction	
A. States name and purpose	
B. Washes hands	
II. General Appearance	
Observes patient for habitus, posture, level of comfort, signs of distress	
III. Vital Signs	
A. Takes or verifies temperature	Fever
B. Counts radial pulse (15 seconds)	
C. Counts respirations	
D. Takes blood pressure R. arm	
IV. Head—inspects and palpates	
A. Hair	Alopecia, texture, nits
B. Scalp	Redness, scaling
C. Skull	Size, contour, lumps, deformities, tenderness
D. Face	Asymmetry, involuntary movements
E. Skin	Acne, hirsutism
F. Temporomandibular joint	Pain, decreased ROM
V. Eyes	
A. Tests visual acuity	Decreased acuity
B. Evaluates visual fields	Field defects
C. Inspects	
1. Eyebrows	Hair loss, scaling
2. Eyelids and lacrimal apparatus	Redness, swelling, lesions, weakness, tearing
3. Conjunctivae and sclerae	Icterus, paleness, inflammation
4. Corneas and lenses	Opacities
D. Inspects pupils	Size, shape, equality
E. Tests pupillary reactions	Direct and consensual response
F. Tests accommodation (near reaction)	Argyll Robertson and tonic pupils
G. Extraocular movements	Asymmetry, nystagmus
H. Funduscopy	Red reflex, opacities, disk, vessels, etc.

Continued

HEENT—PROTOCOL—cont'd

VI. Ears
   A. Inspects and palpates
     1. Auricles　　　　　　　　　　　Deformities, lumps, tenderness
     2. Mastoid processes　　　　　　Tenderness
   B. Inspects with otoscope
     1. External canals　　　　　　　Cerumen, discharge, foreign bodies,
                                 swelling
     2. Tympanic membranes　　　　Color, landmarks, bulging, retraction,
                                 perforation, scarring
     3. Performs insufflation　　　　TM mobility
   C. Tests auditory acuity　　　　　Decreased hearing
   D. Performs Weber's test　　　　Lateralization
   E. Performs Rinne's test　　　　　Bone conduction versus air
                                 conduction

VII. Nose and Sinuses
   A. Inspects
     1. External nares　　　　　　　Swelling, septal deviation, perforation, discharge,
     2. Internal nares with otoscope　blood, crusting
   B. Palpates sinuses　　　　　　　Tenderness
VIII. Mouth and Pharynx
   A. Inspects
     1. Lips　　　　　　　　　　　Color, moisture, lumps, ulcers, cracking
     2. Buccal mucosa　　　　　　　Color, lesions
     3. Teeth and gums　　　　　　Inflammation, swelling, bleeding, retraction,
                                 discoloration; loose, missing, or
                                 carious teeth
     4. Palate　　　　　　　　　　Lumps, lesions
     5. Tongue　　　　　　　　　　Asymmetry, lesions
     6. Pharynx　　　　　　　　　Asymmetry, inflammation, swelling, tonsillar
                                 enlargement, exudates
   B. Tests voice quality　　　　　　Hoarseness
IX. Neck—palpates
   A. Nodes　　　　　　　　　　　Size, consistency, tenderness
   B. Trachea　　　　　　　　　　Deviation
   C. Thyroid　　　　　　　　　　Size, shape, consistency, nodules,
                                 tenderness

HEENT WRITE-UP—NORMAL

General Appearance

WD, WN, Asian F in NAD. Alert and cooperative.

Vital Signs

Temp. = 96.6° F
Pulse = 64/min., reg.
Resp. = 12/min., reg.
BP = 126/68, R. arm, sitting

Head

Normocephalic without lumps, depression, or tenderness. Hair black, full, regular texture, clean. TMJ palpated, full ROM without pain or crepitus.

Eyes

VA intact, 20/20 OU, uncorrected. Visual fields intact by confrontation testing. Eyebrows, eyelids, and lacrimal apparatus clear without redness, swelling, discharge, or lesions. Conjunctivae pink, sclerae white. Corneas clear, lens without opacities. PERRLA, EOMI. Fundi—disk, vessels, and macula well visualized. No AV nicking,[a] hemorrhages, exudates, or papilledema.

Ears

Auricles without lesions or deformities, nontender to manipulation. No mastoid tenderness. External canals patent with slight amount of soft brown cerumen present. TMs gray without scarring or perforation. Light reflex and landmarks intact and well visualized. TMs move well with insufflation. Hearing grossly intact bilat. with 512-Hz tuning fork. Weber—midline. Rinne—AC > BC bilat.

Nose

Patent bilat., mucosa pink without discharge, septum intact without deviation. Sinuses nontender.

Throat

Lips pink without lesions. Teeth intact without obvious caries. Gums pink without inflammation, bleeding, discoloration, or recession. Buccal mucosa moist without lesions. Tongue symmetrical without lesions. Pharynx nonerythematous, tonsils not enlarged, no exudate. Uvula midline, gag reflex intact. No hoarseness.

Neck

No adenopathy.[b] Trachea midline. Thyroid smooth without nodules, not enlarged.

[a]AV nicking = arteriovenous crossing point, with venous tapering underneath the arteriole (commonly seen in hypertension).
[b]No lymph nodes are palpable.

HEENT WRITE-UP—ACUTE TONSILLITIS AND SEROUS OTITIS MEDIA

General Appearance
WD, WN, Asian F in NAD, but appears to have pain with swallowing. Alert and cooperative.

Vital Signs
Temp. = 100.8° F
Pulse = 88/min., reg.
Resp. = 16/min., reg.
BP = 126/68, R. arm, sitting

Head
Normocephalic without lumps, depressions, or tenderness. Hair black, full, regular texture, clean. TMJ palpated, full ROM without pain or crepitus.

Eyes
VA intact, 20/20 OU, uncorrected. Visual fields intact by confrontation testing. Eyebrows, eyelids, and lacrimal apparatus clear without redness, swelling, discharge, or lesions. Conjunctivae pink, sclerae white. Corneas clear, lens without opacities. PERRLA, EOMI. Fundi—disk, vessels, and macula well visualized. No AV nicking, hemorrhages, exudates, or papilledema.

Ears
Auricles without lesions or deformities, nontender to manipulation. No mastoid tenderness. External canals patent with slight amount of soft brown cerumen present. TMs gray, somewhat injected, and retracted, but without gross redness or bulging. Clear fluid level seen on L. No scarring or perforation. TMs nonmobile with insufflation. Hearing grossly intact but slightly decreased on L. with 512-Hz tuning fork. Weber—lateralizes to L. Rinne—BC > AC on L., AC > BC on R.

Nose
Patent bilat., mucosa pink without discharge, septum intact without deviation. Sinuses nontender.

Throat
Lips pink without lesions. Teeth intact without obvious caries. Gums pink without inflammation, bleeding, discoloration, or recession. Buccal mucosa moist without lesions. Tongue symmetrical without lesions. Pharynx moderately erythematous, tonsils 2+ enlarged, with moderate amount of yellowish exudate. Uvula midline, gag reflex intact. No hoarseness.

Neck
2-3 cm. anterior cervical nodes present bilat., mildly tender. Trachea midline. Thyroid smooth without nodules, not enlarged.

RESPIRATORY BRANCHING EXAMINATION

RESPIRATORY EXAM–PROTOCOL

The left column lists the examination maneuvers in the order they are performed. The right column lists the focus, or important potential abnormal findings, of each maneuver.

PA student faces sitting patient.

Maneuver	Focus
I. Introduction	
A. States name and purpose	
B. Washes hands	
C. Puts on face mask and/or offers face mask to patient if TB is suspected	
II. General Appearance	
A. Observes patient for habitus, posture, level of comfort, signs of distress	Anxiety, lip pursing, noisy breathing, nasal flaring
B. Inspects nails for clubbing, cyanosis	
C. Inspects lips for cyanosis	
III. Vital Signs	
A. Takes or verifies temperature	Fever
B. Counts radial pulse	Rapid pulse
C. Counts respiratory rate	Rate, rhythm, depth
D. Takes blood pressure R. arm	
PA student moves behind patient.	
IV. Posterior Inspection	
A. Inspects for AP diameter	Barrel chest
B. Checks alignment of vertebral column	Scoliosis
C. Observes quiet respiration	Symmetry and extent of movement
D. Observes deep respiration	Symmetry and extent of movement
V. Posterior Palpation	
A. Checks symmetry during deep respiration with both hands on lower rib cage	Symmetry
B. Palpates for tactile fremitus, apices to bases, side to side	Increased, decreased
C. Palpates for tactile fremitus, posterolaterally	Increased, decreased
VI. Posterior Percussion	
A. Percusses lung fields, apices to bases, side to side	Dullness, hyperresonance
B. Percusses lung fields, posterolaterally	Dullness, hyperresonance
VII. Posterior Auscultation	
A. Instructs patient to take deep breaths through the mouth	

Continued

RESPIRATORY EXAM—PROTOCOL—cont'd

B. Instructs patient to stop if dizzy	
C. Auscultates lung fields, apices to bases, side to side, througout inspiration and expiration	Character and duration of breath sounds; crackles, rhonchi, wheezes, rubs; distant or absent breath sounds
D. Auscultates lung fields, posterolaterally	Character and duration of breath sounds; crackles, rhonchi, wheezes, rubs; distant or absent breath sounds

PA student moves in front of patient.

VIII. Anterior Inspection	
A. Chest is adequately exposed	Use of accessory muscles, rib retractions
B. Observes quiet respiration	Use of accessory muscles, rib retractions
IX. Anterior Palpation	
A. Checks position of trachea	Deviation
B. Palpates for tactile fremitus, apices to bases, side to side	Increased, decreased
C. Palpates for tactile fremitus, anterolaterally	Increased, decreased
X. Anterior Percussion	
A. Percusses lung fields, apices to bases, side to side	Dullness, hyperresonance
B. Percusses lung fields, anterolaterally	Dullness, hyperresonance
XI. Anterior Auscultation	
A. Instructs patient to take deep breaths through the mouth	
B. Instructs patient to stop if dizzy	
C. Auscultates lung fields, apices to bases, side to side, throughout inspiration and expiration	Character and duration of breath sounds; crackles, rhonchi, wheezes, rubs; distant or absent breath sounds
D. Auscultates lung fields, anterolaterally	Character and duration of breath sounds; crackles, rhonchi, wheezes, rubs; distant or absent breath sounds
XII. Special Maneuvers	
A. Auscultates for post-tussive crackles bilat.	Persistent crackles
B. Auscultates for whispered pectoriloquy bilat.	Consolidation
C. Auscultates for egophony (E-to-A change) bilat.	Pleural effusion, consolidation

RESPIRATORY WRITE-UP—NORMAL

General Appearance
WD, WN, WF in NAD, sitting comfortably.

Vital Signs
Temp. = 98.4° F
Pulse = 68/min., reg.
Resp. = 12/min., reg.
BP = 110/64, R. arm, sitting

Inspection
Even, symmetrical respirations with no labored breathing or use of accessory muscles. No abnormalities of chest configuration or AP diameter. No clubbing or cyanosis.

Palpation
Trachea in midline. No splinting. Chest expansion even, symmetrical. Tactile fremitus intact, equal bilat.

Percussion
Percussion note resonant throughout.

Auscultation
Vesicular breath sounds throughout, inspiration > expiration. No crackles, rhonchi, wheezes, or rubs. Post-tussive crackles, whispered pectoriloquy, egophony—all negative.

RESPIRATORY WRITE-UP—PNEUMONIA AND LEFT LOWER LOBE CONSOLIDATION

General Appearance
WD, WN, WF appearing moderately ill.

Vital Signs
Temp. = 103.2° F
Pulse = 112/min., reg.
Resp. = 24/min., reg.
BP = 124/76, R. arm, sitting

Inspection
Moderately increased, regular breathing, with some extra use of accessory muscles seen. No abnormalities of chest configuration or AP diameter. No clubbing or cyanosis.

Palpation
Trachea midline. No splinting. Chest expansion even, symmetrical. Tactile fremitus *increased* over LLL posteriorly, otherwise of regular and equal intensity elsewhere.

Percussion
Percussion note *decreased* over LLL posteriorly, otherwise resonant and symmetrical throughout rest of lung fields.

Auscultation
Bronchial breath sounds and numerous *crackles* heard in LLL posteriorly; crackles do not clear with cough. Whispered pectoriloquy and egophony *positive* in LLL posteriorly. Other lung fields clear, with vesicular breath sounds and no crackles, rhonchi, wheezes, or rubs.

CARDIOVASCULAR BRANCHING EXAMINATION

CV EXAM—PROTOCOL

The left column lists the examination maneuvers in the order they are performed. The right column lists the focus, or important potential abnormal finding(s), of each maneuver.

PA student faces sitting patient.

I. Introduction
  A. States name and purpose
  B. Washes hands

II. General Appearance
  A. Observes patient for habitus, posture,   Anxiety, pallor, sweating, cyanosis
     level of comfort, signs of distress
  B. Observes lips and nails   Cyanosis, clubbing

III. Vital Signs
  A. Takes or verifies temperature   Fever
  B. Palpates radial pulse bilat.   Symmetry
  C. Counts radial pulse   Rate, rhythm, contour
  D. Counts respirations   Rate, rhythm, depth, effort
  E. Takes BP bilat.   High or low BP, asymmetry
  F. Takes postural BP and pulses   Postural hypotension

PA student moves behind patient and opens gown.

IV. Posterior Palpation and Auscultation
  A. Palpates presacral area   Edema
  B. Percusses lungs posteriorly, mid to bases,   Dullness, hyperresonance
     side to side
  C. Auscultates lungs posteriorly, mid to bases,   Crackles
     side to side, with diaphragm

PA student instructs patient to lie on back and expose chest.

V. Anterior Inspection, Palpation, and Auscultation
  A. Inspects precordium   PMI, pulsations
  B. Palpates
     1. Apex with fingers   PMI
     2. Left sternal border with ball of hand   Thrills, pulsations
     3. Pulmonic area with ball of hand
     4. Aortic area with ball of hand
  C. Auscultates with diaphragm   Murmurs, gallops, rubs
     1. Apex
     2. Left sternal border (LSB) in small steps
     3. Pulmonic area (L. 2nd ICS)
     4. Aortic area (R. 2nd ICS)
     5. Right sternal border (RSB)
     6. Epigastrium
  D. Auscultates with bell
     1. Apex S_3 and S_4, murmurs
     2. LSB in small steps
     3. Carotids while patient holds breath   Bruits, aortic murmur

Continued

CV EXAM—PROTOCOL—cont'd

PA student instructs patient to lie in left lateral decubitus position.

VI. Auscultates apex with bell   Mitral murmurs, S_3 and S_4

PA student instructs patient to sit up, lean forward, exhale, and hold breath.

VII. Auscultates LSB and apex with diaphragm   Aortic murmurs

PA student instructs patient to lie down, and head of bed is elevated to 30 degrees.

VIII. Pulses, Abdomen, Lower Extremities

A. Inspects neck veins (identifies internal jugular)	Distention
B. Strips neck veins	Direction of filling
C. Palpates liver edge, measures if enlarged	Hepatomegaly in CHF
D. Observes neck veins while palpating RUQ of abdomen (hepatojugular reflux)	CHF
E. Palpates aorta and auscultates *(bed lowered—optional)*	Width, pulsations
F. Auscultates over renal arteries	Bruits
G. Palpates femorals and auscultates	Symmetry, bruits
H. Inspects lower extremities	Skin color changes, hair loss, varicosities, ulcers, nail changes
I. Palpates calves	Warmth, tenderness, cords
J. Palpates pretibial region	Edema
K. Palpates dorsalis pedis and posterior tibial pulses bilaterally	Amplitude, symmetry

CV WRITE-UP—NORMAL

General Appearance

WD, WN, BF in NAD, resting comfortably in bed. No cyanosis or clubbing.

Vital Signs

Temp. = 98.2° F

Pulse = 80/min., reg., sitting; 82/min., standing

Resp. = 12/min., reg.

BP = 136/86, R. arm, sitting; 134/86, standing

Lungs (Posterior Exam)

Resonant to percussion, no dullness. Vesicular breath sounds, no crackles at bases bilat.

Heart

Inspection and Palpation—PMI 5th ICS, MCL. No heaves or thrills. Neck veins nondistended, fill from above (or: no NVD)

Auscultation—S_1 and S_2 audible throughout, with physiologic splitting of S_2. No murmurs, rubs, gallops, or extra sounds heard with patient supine, leaning forward, or in LLD position.

Continued

CV WRITE-UP—NORMAL—cont'd

Pulses

	R.	L.		
Carotid	2+	2+	No bruits	
Radial	2+	2+		
Femoral	2+	2+	No bruits	(2+ = normal)
DP	2+	2+		
PT	2+	2+		

Abdomen
Liver edge not palpable. No hepatojugular reflux.[a]

Lower Extremities
Skin warm, hair present on toes. No rubor, cyanosis, ulcers, or other skin changes. No calf tenderness or warmth. No pretibial or sacral edema.

[a]Hepatojugular reflux (HJR). Note that it is *reflux* (i.e., backflow), not *reflex*.

CV WRITE-UP—CARDIOMEGALY AND CHF SECONDARY TO AORTIC STENOSIS

General Appearance
WD, WN, elderly WF in NAD, sitting up somewhat uncomfortably in bed with moderately rapid breathing. Slightly cyanotic, no clubbing.

Vital Signs
Temp. = 98.2° F
Pulse = 104/min., reg., sitting; 108/min., standing
Resp. = 28/min., reg.
BP = 168/86, R. arm, sitting; 164/88, standing

Lungs (Posterior Exam)
Resonant to percussion, no dullness. Vesicular breath sounds throughout. Fine inspiratory crackles present at bases bilat., do not clear with cough.

Heart
Inspection and Palpation—PMI 5th ICS, AAL, with forceful impulse seen and felt. No heaves or thrills. Neck veins distended at 45 degrees, fill from below.
Auscultation—S_1 and S_2 audible throughout. S_3 gallop[a] present, heard best at apex. Grade IV/VI harsh, systolic murmur present, heard best at R. 2nd ICS, with radiation to the carotids bilat.[b]

CV WRITE-UP—CARDIOMEGALY AND CHF SECONDARY TO AORTIC STENOSIS—cont'd

Pulses

	R.	L.		
Carotid	2+	2+	No bruits[b]	
Radial	2+	2+		
Femoral	2+	2+	No bruits	(2+ = normal)
DP	2+	2+		
PT	2+	2+		

Abdomen

Liver edge palpable 6 cm below costal margin, span 14 cm by percussion. Hepatojugular reflux is positive.

Lower Extremities

Skin cool, hair present on toes. Slightly cyanotic in fingers and toes. No rubor, ulcers, or other skin changes. 3+ pitting edema present bilat. No sacral edema.

[a]An S_3 sound is commonly heard in CHF. Any S_3 or S_4 sound can be called a gallop if it is heard at a heart rate greater than 100/min. Otherwise, it is just called an S_3 or S_4 sound.
[b]A harsh, systolic sound heard in the carotids could be a bruit or a transmitted aortic stenosis murmur. If it is heard bilaterally, that would be more consistent with a transmitted murmur.

GASTROINTESTINAL BRANCHING EXAMINATION

GI EXAM—PROTOCOL

The left column lists the examination maneuvers in the order they are performed. The right column lists the focus, or important potential abnormal finding(s), of each maneuver.

PA student faces sitting patient.
- I. Introduction
    - A. States name and purpose
    - B. Washes hands
- II. General Appearance
    - A. Observes patient for habitus, posture, level of comfort, signs of distress
    - B. Checks sclerae for icterus   Jaundice

Continued

GI EXAM—PROTOCOL—cont'd

III. Vital Signs
    A. Takes or verifies temperature   Fever
    B. Palpates radial pulses bilat.   Symmetry
    C. Counts radial pulse   Rate, rhythm
    D. Counts respirations   Rate, rhythm
    E. Takes blood pressure   High BP, low BP
    F. Takes postural BP and pulses   Postural hypotension
  PA student instructs patient to lie supine with abdomen completely exposed from below breasts to pubis.
IV. Inspection
    A. Inspects abdomen from several angles: Contour, scars, striae, dilated veins, bulges,
       head of bed, laterally, from feet   asymmetry, masses, pulsations, peristalsis
    B. Inspects from side and at feet during
       normal and deep breathing
PA student moves to right side of patient.
  V. Auscultation
    A. Warms stethoscope
    B. Auscultates with diaphragm   Bowel sounds, bruits
       1. Periumbilical area
       2. Right upper quadrant (RUQ)
       3. Left upper quadrant (LUQ)
       4. Left lower quadrant (LLQ)
       5. Right lower quadrant (RLQ)
VI. Percussion
    A. Percusses lightly in 4 quadrants   Tympany, dullness
    B. Percusses liver borders, marks borders,   Enlargement
       measures liver span
    C. Percusses for spleen in lowest intercostal   Enlargement
       space of L. anterior axillary line, with
       normal and deep inspiration
  PA student instructs patient to place hands at sides and to flex the knees. PA student explains exam and instructs patient to identify any tender areas.
VII. Palpation
    A. Lightly palpates with flats of fingers   Tenderness, rigidity, masses
       (starting systematic sequence in area
       other than patient's source of pain)
       1. LLQ[a]
       2. Suprapubic
       3. RLQ
       4. RUQ
       5. Epigastrium
       6. LUQ
       7. Umbilicus   Hernia
    B. Deeply palpates with flats of fingers   Masses
       (starting systematic sequence in area
       other than patient's source of pain)

GI EXAM—PROTOCOL—cont'd

       1. LLQ[a]
       2. Suprapubic
       3. RLQ
       4. RUQ
       5. Epigastrium
       6. LUQ
       7. Supraumbilical area   Aortic enlargement
     C. Palpates for liver edge starting at RLQ   Enlargement, hardness, blunt edge, irregular
       (bimanual technique)   contour
     D. Palpates for spleen, starting at LLQ   Enlargement
       (bimanual technique)
PA student instructs patient to move onto right side.
     E. Palpates for spleen (bimanual technique)   Enlargement
PA student instructs patient to sit up.
     F. Performs blunt percussion of costovertebral   Tenderness
       angles (CVA) bilat.
 VIII. Rectal or Rectovaginal Examination
     A. For male patient, performs rectal   Tenderness, mass, sphincter tone, GI bleeding
       examination (see p. 263)
     B. For female patient, performs pelvic   Tenderness, adnexal or uterine mass, bleeding
       examination (see p. 259)
PA student instructs patient to return to supine position.
  IX. Special Tests
     A. For peritoneal irritation
       1. Checks for rebound tenderness while   Peritoneal inflammation
         observing patient's face for reaction
       2. Checks for referred rebound tenderness   Peritoneal inflammation
         while observing patient's face for
         reaction
       3. Questions patient appropriately
         for any pain upon release of
         examining hand
     B. For appendicitis
       1. Performs obturator test (R. leg only)   Appendicitis
       2. Performs psoas test (R. leg only)—   Appendicitis
         either flexes hip or rolls patient on
         L. side
     C. For acute cholecystitis Hooks liver and has Tenderness
       patient take a deep breath
       (Murphy's sign)
     D. For ascites
       1. Palpates flanks for fullness   Ascites
       2. Checks for fluid wave using patient's   Ascites
         hand for damper
       3. Checks for shifting dullness   Ascites

[a]Palpation may start elsewhere than LLQ but should then proceed systematically.

GI WRITE-UP–NORMAL

General Appearance
WD, WN, WM in NAD. Alert and cooperative.

Vital Signs
Temp. = 98.6° F
Pulse = 80/min., reg., sitting and standing
Resp. = 12/min., reg.
BP = 120/80, sitting; 118/80, standing

Inspection
Flat, nonobese. No scars or lesions. Sclerae nonicteric.

Auscultation
BS normoactive. No bruits.

Palpation
Soft, without guarding. No pain to superficial or deep palpation in all quadrants. Liver and spleen not palpable with deep inspiration. Liver span 9 cm by percussion. No masses. No CVA tenderness.

Rectal
Sphincter tone intact. No masses or tenderness. Prostate smooth, nontender, not enlarged. Trace brown stool; guaiac negative.

Special Tests
No rebound tenderness. Obturator and psoas tests negative. No flank fullness, fluid wave, or shifting dullness.

GI WRITE-UP–PERFORATED ULCER

General Appearance
WD, WN, WM, lying on a stretcher, reluctant to move because of pain.[a] Pale, anxious, and sweating. Alert and oriented.

Vital Signs
Temp. = 97.8° F
Pulse = 96/min., lying; 110/min., standing
Resp. = 24/min., shallow
BP = 110/88, lying; 96/70, standing

Inspection
Mildly obese, not distended. Old, well-healed, 8-cm horizontal surgical scar in RLQ.[b] Sclerae nonicteric.

GI WRITE-UP–PERFORATED ULCER–cont'd

Auscultation
  BS absent during 3 minutes of listening.[c] No bruits.

Palpation
  Marked guarding and tenderness throughout with light palpation; some rigidity in upper abdomen. Palpation of liver and spleen deferred due to pain. No apparent masses. No CVA tenderness.

Rectal
  Sphincter tone intact. No masses or tenderness. Prostate smooth, nontender, not enlarged. Trace black stool; strongly guaiac positive.

Special Tests
  Rebound tenderness present, localizes to epigastric area. Obturator and psoas tests negative. No flank fullness. Fluid wave and shifting dullness palpations deferred due to pain. Murphy's sign negative.

[a]Pain with movement and consequent reluctance to move are typical of peritonitis (versus colicky pain, which makes patients quite restless).
[b]This would be consistent with a prior appendectomy.
[c]Hypoactive bowel sounds are common in peritonitis.

GYNECOLOGICAL (PELVIC) BRANCHING EXAMINATION

PELVIC EXAM–PROTOCOL

The left column lists the examination maneuvers in the order they are performed. The right column lists the focus, or important potential abnormal finding(s), of each maneuver.
  PA student faces patient, who is sitting, undressed below the waist but with drape.
  I. Introduction
    A. States name and purpose
    B. Washes hands
  PA student instructs patient to assume a lithotomy position. PA student drapes patient appropriately, prepares light source, puts on gloves, and seats self comfortably.
  II. Inspection and Palpation
    A. Inspects external genitalia
      1. Pubic hair   Lice, nits
      2. Labia minora   Excoriations, rash, lesions, swelling

Continued

PELVIC EXAM–PROTOCOL–cont'd

3. Urethra	Caruncle, prolapse
4. Clitoris	Enlargement
B. Spreads labia with right hand, then inspects and palpates Bartholin's and Skene's glands	Swelling, tenderness, discharge
C. Milks urethra (optional)	Discharge
D. Retracts clitoral hood (optional)	
E. Separates labia with middle and index fingers and asks patient to bear down	Cystocele, rectocele

III. Speculum Examination
   A. Lubricates closed speculum with warm water
   B. Inserts right index finger into vagina and locates cervix (optional)
   C. Holding speculum in left hand, depresses pubococcygeus muscle with right index finger; instructs patient to relax this muscle
   D. Inserts obliquely turned speculum at 45-degree angle, avoiding anterior structures
   E. Rotates speculum gently to horizontal position and inserts to full length
   F. Opens speculum blades slowly, identifies cervix, and secures blades open

IV. Cervical and Vaginal Examination

A. Inspects cervix; removes excess mucus with swab if necessary	Color, lesions, bleeding, discharge

   B. Obtains Pap smear
      1. Inserts cytobrush into os, turns through one 360-degree turn, rolls onto slide
      2. Using wooden spatula, scrapes through at least one 360-degree turn, applies on slide
      3. Fixes specimens immediately
   C. Obtains other cultures from cervix or vagina (optional)

D. Reinspects cervix	Bleeding

   E. Holding blades of speculum open, loosens locking mechanism, then allows blades to close slightly

F. Rotates speculum gently and inspects vaginal walls	Inflammation, discharge, lesions

   G. Gently withdraws speculum, continuing to inspect the vagina as speculum is withdrawn

PA student stands.

V. Bimanual Examination
   A. Lubricates gloved index and middle fingers and introduces them into posterior fornix

PELVIC EXAM—PROTOCOL—cont'd

B. Identifies and palpates cervix	Consistency, mobility, tenderness
C. Using vaginal fingers as reference points, palpates body of uterus with abdominal hand using dipping motion, from umbilicus in midline	Size, shape, consistency, mobility, tenderness, masses
D. Places vaginal fingers into right vaginal fornix, using same bimanual technique, and palpates right adnexa	Ovarian size, adnexal masses, tenderness
E. Places vaginal fingers into left vaginal fornix, using same bimanual technique, and palpates left adnexa	Ovarian size, adnexal masses, tenderness

VI. Rectovaginal Examination
  A. PA student changes gloves
  B. Slips middle finger into rectum and index finger into vagina while asking patient to bear down
  C. Palpates rectovaginal septum
  D. Using rectovaginal fingers as a reference point, repeats the bimanual examination — Masses, retroverted uterus
  E. Withdraws fingers, tests stool for guaiac blood (optional)

PA student assists patient to the sitting position and offers tissues for cleaning.

PELVIC EXAM—ELEMENTS OF NORMAL WRITE-UP

Elements that should be part of any write-up of a gynecological examination are as follows:

Ext—BUS
  For external inspection, comment on pubic hair distribution, skin lesions, redness, or inflammation. BUS—comment on any swelling, redness, tenderness, or discharge from any of these structures.

Vagina
  Note the mucosal color, the presence or absence of rugae, normal or abnormal discharge, lesions, and muscular support.

Cervix
  Note color, whether nulliparous or multiparous, any discharge coming from the os, lacerations, lesions, ectopy, or friability. Note the presence of an IUD string, if applicable.

Continued

PELVIC EXAM—ELEMENTS OF NORMAL WRITE-UP—cont'd

Uterus

Normal findings are often abbreviated to "NSSC," meaning normal size, shape, and consistency. Also comment on position, mobility, and tenderness.

Adnexa

If the ovaries are not palpable, say so. If they are palpable, describe their size. Note the presence of any masses or tenderness.

Rectovaginal

If there are no new findings, you can write "RV confirms." Comment on sphincter tone, rectal masses, and stool, including guaiac testing.

GYN WRITE-UP—NORMAL

General Appearance

WD, WN, young adult WF in NAD.

Vital Signs

Temp. = 98.6° F
Pulse = 80/min., reg.
Resp. = 16/min., reg.
BP = 116/64

Ext—BUS

Sexually mature pubic hair pattern, no redness or lesions. No urethral discharge.

Vagina

No redness or discharge. Mucosa rugated.

Cervix

Nulliparous. No discharge, lesions, or ectopy.

Uterus

Retroflexed. NSSC. No cervical motion tenderness.

Adnexa

Left ovary palpable—1 × 2 × 2 cm. Right ovary not palpable. No adnexal masses or tenderness.

Rectovaginal

Confirms above. Sphincter tone intact, no masses. Trace stool; guaiac negative.

GYN WRITE-UP—PELVIC INFLAMMATORY DISEASE

General Appearance
WD, WN, adolescent WF, appearing somewhat uncomfortable.

Vital Signs
Temp. = 100.6° F
Pulse = 88/min., reg.
Resp. = 16/min., reg.
BP = 104/72

Ext—BUS
Sexually mature pubic hair pattern, no redness or lesions. No urethral discharge.

Vagina
Rugated, mucosa not inflamed. Moderate amount of yellowish discharge present.

Cervix
Nulliparous. Thick yellow discharge visible from os. No cervical lesions or ectopy seen.

Uterus
Small, anteflexed. Tender to manipulation.[a]

Adnexa
Markedly tender to palpation, L. greater than R. No masses felt. Ovaries not palpated.

Rectovaginal
Confirms. Sphincter tone intact, no masses. Trace stool; brown, guaiac negative.

[a]Some examiners write as "positive CMT" (cervical motion tenderness).

MALE GENITOURINARY AND RECTAL BRANCHING EXAMINATION

MALE GU/RECTAL EXAM—PROTOCOL

The left column lists the examination maneuvers in the order they are performed. The right column lists the focus, or important potential abnormal finding(s), of each maneuver.
  I. Introduction
     A. States name and purpose
     B. Washes hands
     C. Dons gloves
 II. General Appearance
     A. Observes patient for habitus, posture, level
        of comfort, signs of distress

Continued

MALE GU/RECTAL EXAM—PROTOCOL—cont'd

PA student sits facing patient, who is standing and disrobed below the waist.

III. External Genitalia
A. Inspects pubic hair	Amount, distribution, lice, nits
B. Inspects penis	
1. Skin	Warts, chancres, vesicles, nodules, ulcers
2. Foreskin	Phimosis, paraphimosis
3. Glans	Balanitis
4. Urethra	Discharge
C. Palpates penis	Induration
D. Inspects scrotum	Lumps, swelling, ulcers, redness
E. Palpates each testis and epididymis	Size, shape, consistency, tenderness, mass
F. Palpates spermatic cord	Varicocele, nodules
G. Inspects inguinal and femoral areas	Bulges
H. Palpates inguinal areas	Lymphadenopathy
I. Palpates for hernias bilat.	Bulge on straining

PA student instructs patient either to bend over examination table and spread buttocks with hands or to lie on left side with knees drawn up.

IV. Rectal Examination
A. Inspects perianal area	Hemorrhoids, ulcers, inflammation, warts and excoriations, fistula, fissure, discharge
B. Explains procedure to patient	
C. Inserts gloved, lubricated finger while patient bears down	
D. Evaluates sphincter	Tone, tenderness, induration
E. Evaluates prostate	Size, shape, consistency, nodules, tenderness
F. Evaluates rectal wall with rotary motion	Induration, nodules, irregularities
G. Removes finger, wipes off excess lubricant from patient, and offers tissue	
H. Examines stool from glove and does guaiac testing	Melena

MALE GU/RECTAL WRITE-UP—NORMAL

General Appearance
WD, WN, young adult BM in NAD.

External Genitalia
Well-developed male escutcheon without lice or nits.
Penis—No skin lesions. Uncircumcised, foreskin retracts easily, Urethra midline, without discharge.
Scrotum/testes—No scrotal swelling, lesions, or redness. Testes descended, symmetrical, no nodules or tenderness. No scrotal masses or hernias. No inguinal adenopathy.

Rectal
Perianal area without redness or lesions. Sphincter tone intact. Prostate smooth, not enlarged, without tenderness or nodules. No palpable rectal masses. Stool soft and guaiac negative.

MALE GU/RECTAL WRITE-UP—GENITAL HERPES

General Appearance
WD, WN, young adult WM in NAD.

External Genitalia
Well-developed male escutcheon without lice or nits.
Penis—15-20 small vesicles on erythematous bases, grouped in clusters along shaft and glans, tender to touch. Circumcised. Urethra midline, without discharge.
Scrotum/testes—No scrotal swelling, lesions, or redness. Testes descended, symmetrical, no nodules or tenderness. No scrotal masses or hernias. Tender, 3-cm inguinal node palpable on L., negative on R.

Rectal
Perianal area without redness or lesions. Sphincter tone intact. Prostate smooth, not enlarged, without tenderness or nodules. No palpable rectal masses. Stool soft and guaiac negative.

MUSCULOSKELETAL BRANCHING EXAMINATION

KNEE EXAM—PROTOCOL

The left column lists the examination maneuvers in the order they are performed. The right column lists the focus, or important potential abnormal finding(s), of each maneuver. *Note:* All maneuvers must be performed on *both* knees.
PA student faces sitting patient.
I. Introduction
  A. States name and purpose
  B. Washes hands
II. General Appearance
  Observes patient for habitus, posture, level of comfort, signs of distress
PA student instructs patient to lie supine with both knees exposed.
III. Inspection
  A. Observes general thigh and leg configuration, valgus and varus deformities
  B. Inspects knee joints for alignment, obvious effusion

Continued

KNEE EXAM—PROTOCOL—cont'd

IV. Palpation
  A. Palpates bony landmarks
    1. Patella   Pain, crepitus
    2. Tibial tubercle   Pain, swelling
    3. Adductor tubercle
    4. Joint line, medially and laterally   Pain, bony ridges
    5. Head of fibula
  B. Palpates for effusion   Effusion
    1. Milking suprapatellar pouch and
       patellar fossa
    2. Ballottement of patella while
       compressing suprapatellar pouch
  C. Palpates quadriceps group contraction   Strength, tone
  D. Measures quadriceps circumference
      (at least 5 in. above patella)   Atrophy
  E. Evaluates ROM   Decreased ROM
    1. Tests active flexion and extension
       of knees
    2. Tests passive flexion and extension
       of knees
V. Joint Stability Tests   Pain, laxity
  A. Tests stability of medial collateral ligament
    1. Straight
    2. At 20-30 degrees of flexion
  B. Tests stability of lateral collateral ligament   Pain, laxity
    1. Straight
    2. At 20-30 degrees of flexion
  C. Performs patellar apprehension test
    1. Attempts to dislocate patella   Pain, laxity
      a. With knee extended
      b. With knee flexed at 20-30 degrees
    2. Observes patient's face during test   Apprehension
  D. Performs drawer test (patient's knee flexed   Pain, laxity
    at 90 degrees) to evaluate
    1. Anterior cruciates
    2. Posterior cruciates
VI. Meniscus Tests
  A. Palpates joint lines   Tenderness
  B. Performs McMurray's test (attempts to trap   Palpable or audible "click"
    menisci through rotation and straightening
    maneuvers)
PA student instructs patient to resume sitting.
VII. Muscle Group Power Tests (patient sitting)
  A. Quadriceps (resists in slight flexion)   Strength, atrophy
  B. Hamstrings (resists flexion at 90 degrees)   Strength, atrophy

KNEE WRITE-UP—NORMAL

General Appearance

WD, WN, adult WF in NAD, sitting comfortably.

R. and L. Knees

Inspection—No obvious effusions or bony abnormalities. Patellas nondisplaced. Active and passive ROM intact bilat. Quads are well developed, and both thighs measure 48 cm at 5 in. above the patella.[a]

Palpation—No effusion by milking and ballottement techniques. Joint lines and bony landmarks nontender bilat. Patellar apprehension test is negative bilat.

Ligament testing—Medial collaterals and lateral collaterals without laxity to stress testing, both straight and in mild flexion. Drawer tests negative bilat. McMurray's negative bilat. Quads and hamstrings strength 4+/4+ against resistance.

[a]Or 5 in. proximally from the superior edge of the patella, to be more precise.

KNEE WRITE-UP—MEDIAL COLLATERAL LIGAMENT TEAR

General Appearance

WD, WN, adult WM, unable to bear weight on R. leg.

R. Knee

Inspection—Moderate swelling over medial joint space. Patella nondisplaced. 2+ tenderness with either active or passive ROM, though ROM is intact. Quads are well developed and thigh measures 48 cm at 5 in. above the patella.

Palpation—No effusion by milking and ballottement techniques. 2+ tenderness along medial joint line; lateral joint line and other bony landmarks nontender. Patellar apprehension test is negative.

Ligament testing—Moderate laxity and greatly increased tenderness in medial joint space with valgus stress testing. Drawer test negative. McMurray's negative. Quads and hamstrings strength 4+/4+ against resistance.

L. Knee

Inspection—No obvious effusion or bony abnormalities. Patella nondisplaced. Active and passive ROM intact. Quads are well developed and thigh measures 48 cm at 5 in. above the patella.

Palpation—No effusion by milking and ballottement techniques. Joint lines and bony landmarks nontender. Patellar apprehension test is negative.

Ligament testing—Medial collateral and lateral collateral ligaments without laxity to stress testing, both straight and in mild flexion. Drawer test negative. McMurray's negative. Quads and hamstrings strength 4+/4+ against resistance.

SPINE EXAM–PROTOCOL

The left column lists the examination maneuvers in the order they are performed. The right column lists the focus, or important potential abnormal finding(s), of each maneuver.

PA student faces sitting patient.

I. Introduction
  A. States name and purpose
  B. Washes hands

II. General Appearance
   Observes patient for habitus, posture, level of comfort, signs of distress

III. Vital Signs
   A. Takes or verifies temperature
   B. Counts radial pulse (15 seconds)
   C. Counts respirations
   D. Takes blood pressure R. arm

PA student stands behind standing patient.

IV. Inspection and Palpation
   A. Observes posterior spine
     1. Shoulder height   Inequality
     2. Scapular prominence   Asymmetry
     3. Pelvic levelness   Pelvic tilt
   B. Palpation
     1. Palpates paraspinous muscles   Spasm
     2. Palpates vertebral bodies   Tenderness, prominence
   C. Observes laterally   Abnormal curvatures
     1. Cervical lordosis
     2. Thoracic kyphosis
     3. Lumbar lordosis
   D. Observes anteriorly   Asymmetry
     1. Rib prominence
     2. Waistline symmetry

V. Range of Motion
   A. Evaluates cervical ROM   Decreased ROM
     1. Flexion (viewed from side)
     2. Extension (viewed from side)
     3. Rotation (viewed from front)
     4. Lateral bending (viewed from front)
   B. Evaluates thoracolumbar ROM   Pain, decreased ROM
     1. Rotation (while hips are stabilized and
        viewed from front)
     2. Lateral bending (viewed from front)
     3. Flexion (viewed from side and rear)
       a. Inspects scapular and flank areas   Scoliosis
       b. Inspects for reversal of lumbar lordosis
       c. Observes for 1 or 2 phase recovery
          when patient returns to erect position
     4. Extension (viewed from side)

SPINE EXAM—PROTOCOL—cont'd

VI. Gait
    A. Instructs patient to walk across room   Limp, ataxia
    B. Instructs and observes toe walking (S1)   Weakness
    C. Instructs and observes heel walking (L5)   Weakness
  PA student instructs patient to sit.
VII. Neurological Assessment
    A. Inspects calf circumference   Atrophy
    B. Elicits knee reflexes (L4)   Asymmetry
    C. Elicits ankle reflexes (S1)   Asymmetry
    D. Strokes dermatomes innervating both feet   Hypesthesia
      1. L4 (medial leg)
      2. L5 (lateral leg and dorsum of foot)
      3. S1 (lateral foot and sole)
    E. Tests strength of extensor hallucis longus   Weakness
      bilat. (L5)
    F. Performs sitting straight leg raising (SLR),   Radicular pain
      bilat.
  PA student instructs patient to lie supine.
VIII. Supine SLR Tests
    Performs SLR on sciatic nerve bilat., including   Radicular pain
      passive dorsiflexion of the foot

Under some circumstances, further examinations would be indicated in a patient with back pain. Prostate pathology can cause back pain, so a rectal exam would be indicated in a male patient older than age 50. Abdominal aortic aneurysm can be a cause of back pain, so abdominal palpation would be indicated in patients with suggestive symptoms.

SPINE WRITE-UP—NORMAL

General Appearance
  WD, WN, BM in NAD, sitting comfortably.

Vital Signs
  Temp. = 97.8° F
  Pulse = 68/min., reg.
  Resp. = 12/min., reg.
  BP = 132/76, R. arm, sitting

Inspection
  Cervical lordosis, thoracic kyphosis, and lumbar lordosis intact without accentuation or flattening. No scoliosis or abnormal curvature noted. Shoulders and pelvis level.

Palpation
  No paravertebral muscle tenderness or spasm. Vertebral bodies symmetrical and nontender.

Continued

SPINE WRITE-UP–NORMAL–cont'd

ROM

Full cervical ROM without pain. Full forward spinal flexion to within 2 in. of the floor with smooth recovery. Backward extension and rotation side to side intact without pain. Patient able to touch fibular heads bilat. on lateral bending.

Gait

Symmetrical without limp. Heel and toe walking intact.

Neuro

No calf muscle atrophy.
Reflexes–Patellar 2+ bilat.; Achilles 2+ bilat. Sensation intact to light touch over L4, L5, and S1 dermatomes.
Dorsiflexion of great toe intact without weakness bilat.
SLR–No pain elicited sitting, supine, or prone.

SPINE WRITE-UP–ACUTELY HERNIATED DISC AT L5-S1

General Appearance

WD, WN, BM in moderate discomfort, sitting uncomfortably in a chair.

Vital Signs

Temp. = 97.8° F
Pulse = 68/min., reg.
Resp. = 12/min., reg.
BP = 132/76, R. arm, sitting

Inspection

Cervical lordosis, thoracic kyphosis, and lumbar lordosis intact without accentuation or flattening. No scoliosis or abnormal curvature noted. Shoulders and pelvis level.

Palpation

Moderate paravertebral muscle tenderness in lumbosacral area without spasm.[a] Vertebral bodies symmetrical and slighly tender in LS area.

SPINE WRITE-UP—ACUTELY HERNIATED DISC AT L5-S1—cont'd

ROM
Full cervical ROM without pain. Forward spinal flexion markedly limited by pain. Backward extension also limited by pain. Rotation side to side is intact with slight pain at extremes of movement. Patient able to touch fibular heads bilat. on lateral bending with some effort.

Gait
Walks stiffly with slight limp on R. side. Heel walking intact. Toe walking produces pain in the right lower back.

Neuro
No calf muscle atrophy.
Reflexes—Patellar 2+ bilat.; Achilles 2+ on L., 0+ on R. Sensation intact to light touch over L4, L5, and S1 dermatomes on L.; some diminished sensation along R. lateral foot.
Dorsiflexion of great toe intact without weakness bilat.
SLR—Produces pain radiating down the R. leg when either leg is raised; pain is increased by dorsiflexing the R. foot.

aParavertebral muscle spasm is common in acute musculoskeletal strain; it would not usually be seen in herniated disk.

SHOULDER EXAM—PROTOCOL

I. Introduction
   A. States name and purpose
   B. Washes hands
II. General Appearance
   Observes patient for habitus, posture,
   level of comfort, signs of distress
III. Vital Signs
   A. Takes or verifies temperature
   B. Palpates radial pulse bilat.   Checks pulses distally in trauma
   C. Counts radial pulse (15 seconds)
   D. Counts respirations
   E. Takes blood pressure R. arm
  Patient sitting with both shoulders adequately exposed.
IV. Inspection: Compare Both Shoulders
   A. Anteriorly   Swelling, deformities, scars, muscle atrophy,
     1. Clavicle   discolorations, etc.
     2. Acromioclavicular (AC) joint
     3. General contour of both shoulders
   B. Posteriorly
     1. Scapula   High scapula, winging of scapula
     2. Neck (cervical spine)   Kyphosis, scoliosis
     3. Upper back (thoracic spine/trapezius)   Kyphosis, scoliosis, symmetry

Continued

SHOULDER EXAM–PROTOCOL–cont'd

V. Palpation: Compare Both Shoulders
  A. Anteriorly
    1. Sternoclavicular joint   Pain, deformity, swelling, crepitance
    2. Clavicle
    3. Coracoid
    4. AC joint (flex and extend shoulder
       to locate)
    5. Acromion
    6. Rotator cuff and biceps tendon–long head
       a. Below anterior lateral border of   Location of subacromial bursae, supraspinous
          acromion   pain, swelling
       b. Biceps tendon–long head   Pain, swelling, deformity
          (ext/int rotates arm and palpates
          tendon in the bicipital groove)
  B. Posteriorly
    1. Spinous process of C-spine   Pain, deformity, spasm, trigger points
    2. Trapezius (superior aspect)
VI. Range of Motion
  A. C-spine   Decreased ROM, pain
    1. Flexion
    2. Extension
    3. Rotation (bilat.)
    4. Lateral flexion (bilat.)
  B. Shoulder bilat.
    1. Active
       a. Abduction (raise arms overhead,   Decreased ROM, pain
          palms touching)
       b. Extension
       c. Flexion
       d. Abduction/external rotation (hands
          behind head, touch opposite scapula)
       e. Adduction/internal rotation
          (hands behind back, touch
          opposite scapula)
    2. Passive (checked when active ROM
       is impaired)
       a. Flexion
       b. Extension
       c. Abduction
       d. Adduction
       e. Internal rotation (arm at side, elbow
          flexed at 90 degrees)
       f. External rotation (arm at side, elbow
          flexed at 90 degrees)

SHOULDER EXAM—PROTOCOL—cont'd

VII. Neurological Exam
   A. Muscle strength (bilat.)   Weakness
     1. Shoulder
       a. Flexion (C5-C6)
       b. Extension (C5-C8)
       c. Abduction (C5-C6)
       d. Adduction (C5-T1)
       e. Internal rotation (C5-T1)
       f. External rotation (C5-C6)
     2. Elbow
       a. Flexion (C5-C6)
       b. Extension (C7)
     3. Wrist
       a. Flexion (C7)
       b. Extension (C6)
   B. Sensory: sharp/dull, comparing bilat.   Decreased sensation
     1. Deltoid region, axillary nerve (C5)
     2. Thumb, dorsal aspect (C6)   Radial nerve
     3. Middle finger, palmar aspect (C7)   Median nerve
     4. Little finger, palmar aspect (C8)   Ulnar nerve
     5. Arm, medial aspect (T1)
   C. DTRs (bilat.)
     1. Biceps (C5)
     2. Brachioradialis (C6)
     3. Triceps (C7)
VIII. Special Tests
   A. Compression test (for C-spine origin)   Pain in C-spine, or referred down extremity along
     1. Patient sitting   a dermatome
     2. Presses down upon top of patient's
       head
   B. Acromioclavicular (AC) stress test: passively Pain due to AC joint or degenerative arthritis
     adduct patient's arm across body
   C. Impingement signs (imply rotator cuff
     pathology)
     1. Passively bring arm through frontal   Anterior pain due to rotator cuff degeneration,
       flexion into maximal elevation directly   tendonitis, or tear
       overhead
     2. With elbow flexed, passively abduct arm Pain felt in shoulder
       to 90 degrees, internally rotate arm as it
       is slowly brought across the chest
     3. Painful arc test   Pain between 60 and 120 degrees suggests
       Patient actively abducts arm to   rotator cuff tendonitis; past 100 to 120 degrees
       120 degrees   implies AC joint disorders

Continued

SHOULDER EXAM—PROTOCOL—cont'd

D. Tests for rotator cuff tears
  1. Drop arm test
    a. Passively abducts arm to 90 degrees
    b. Actively lowers arm slowly
  2. With both arms abducted, push down bilaterally while patient resists
E. Tests for biceps tendinitis
  1. Elbow flexed, arm at side, patient supinates forearm against resistance
  2. Speed's test: arm supinated and elbow extended, patient flexes shoulder and arm forward against resistance
F. Apprehension test
  1. Abduct to 90 degrees at shoulder with elbow flexed
  2. Externally rotate arm while pressing proximal humerus down and forward

Incomplete tears; unable to lower arm slowly and smoothly, or arm drops to side quickly with complete tear
Shoulder with tear will be weaker

Pain in bicipital groove

Pain in biceps tendon

Shoulder instability
Apprehension on patient's face

Note: The shoulder is a classic area for referred pain. Problems with the C-spine, the heart (e.g., MI), or irritation to the diaphragm (e.g., gallbladder disease) can all cause referred shoulder pain. If the shoulder exam is negative, then a complete examination of the chest, abdomen, and cervical spine needs to be performed in a patient complaining of shoulder pain.

SHOULDER WRITE-UP—NORMAL

General Appearance
WD, WN, WM in NAD.

Vital Signs
Temp. = 98.6° F
Pulse = 80/min., reg.
Resp. = 16/min., reg.
BP = 120/80, R. arm, sitting

Neck
No deformities of C-spine noted. No tenderness of spinous processes or trapezius. Full ROM without pain. Compression test neg.

Shoulders
No muscle atrophy, redness, warmth, or deformities noted. Sternoclavicular (SC) joints, clavicles, and acromioclavicular (AC) joints intact and nontender. Rotator cuff and biceps tendon nontender bilat. Active full ROM of both shoulders. DTRs 2 + biceps, brachioradialis, and triceps. Sensation intact to pinprick (C5-T1). Muscle strength of shoulder, elbow, and wrist 5/5 bilat. AC stress test, impingement signs, and Speed's test are neg. Shoulders are stable.

SHOULDER WRITE-UP–ROTATOR CUFF TEAR

General Appearance
WD, WN, WF in moderate discomfort.

Vital Signs
Temp. = 98.2° F
Pulse = 84/min., reg.
Resp. = 12/min., reg.
BP = 136/84, L. arm, sitting

Neck
No deformities of C-spine noted. No tenderness of spinous processes or trapezius. Full ROM without pain. Compression test neg.

Shoulders
No muscle atrophy, redness, warmth, or deformities noted. SC joints, clavicles, and AC joints intact and nontender on L. Patient unable to abduct R. shoulder secondary to pain, full ROM on L. Passive ROM intact bilat. Drop arm test positive on R. DTRs 2 + bilat. for UEs. Sensation intact for UEs bilat. Muscle strength equal bilat. for elbows and wrists. AC stress test, impingement signs, and Speed's test negative bilat.

NEUROLOGICAL EXAMINATION

Equipment

The following equipment is needed to conduct a neurological examination:
➤ Materials for olfactory testing.
➤ Snellen card.
➤ Oto-ophthalmoscope.
➤ Cotton.
➤ Disposable object for sharp/dull testing.
➤ Tuning fork.
➤ Tongue blade.
➤ Reflex hammer.
➤ Objects for identification (key, coins, etc.).

NEURO EXAM–PROTOCOL

The left column lists the examination maneuvers in the order they are performed. The right column lists the focus, or important potential abnormal finding(s), of each maneuver.
PA student faces sitting patient.
I. Introduction
  A. States name and purpose
  B. Washes hands
II. General Appearance
  Observes patient for habitus, posture, level of comfort, signs of distress
III. Vital Signs
  A. Takes or verifies temperature   Fever
  B. Counts radial pulse (15 seconds)
  C. Counts respirations
  D. Takes blood pressure R. arm

Continued

NEURO EXAM–PROTOCOL–cont'd

IV. Mental Status
    A. Observes level of consciousness, mood, etc.   Altered or abnormal consciousness
    B. Asks patient to state   Orientation
        1. Name
        2. Address
        3. Today's full date
        4. Present location
    C. Tests recent memory with recall of
        three objects (must wait at least 2 min.
        before recalling)
    D. Tests receptive ability with performance of   Receptive aphasia
        complex command
    E. Tests expressive ability with naming of   Expressive aphasia
        common objects
    F. Tests simple arithmetic ability or ability to
        spell backward
V. Cranial Nerves
    A. Olfactory (CN I)   Anosmia
        1. Tests bilat. with patient's eyes closed
    B. Optic (CN II)
        1. Tests visual acuity   Decreased acuity
        2. Tests visual fields in each eye separately   Field defects
        3. Funduscopic exam   Red reflex, optic atrophy, papilledema
    C. Oculomotor, trochlear, and abducens
        (CN III, IV, and VI)
        1. Checks pupil size   Size, shape, equality
        2. Tests pupil response directly and
            consensually
        3. Tests accommodation   Argyll Robertson and tonic pupils
        4. Tests extraocular movements,   Asymmetry, ptosis
            including nystagmus
    D. Trigeminal (CN V)
        1. Tests sensation in three areas   Sensory loss
            a. Light touch
            b. Pinprick
        2. Tests corneal reflex   Absence of blinking
        3. Tests chewing muscles   Weak contraction
    E. Facial (CN VII)
        1. Tests facial muscles
            a. Brow wrinkling   Weakness, asymmetry
            b. Showing of teeth   Weakness, asymmetry
        2. Tests eyelid muscles against resistance   Weakness, asymmetry
    F. Auditory (CN VIII)
        1. Tests gross hearing bilat.   Decreased hearing
        2. Tests lateralization
        3. Tests bone versus air conduction bilat.

NEURO EXAM–PROTOCOL–cont'd

G. Glossopharyngeal and vagus (CN IX and X)
  1. Observes swallowing — Paralysis
  2. Observes palate during phonation — Asymmetry
  3. Elicits gag reflex bilat. — Asymmetry
H. Spinal accessory (CN XI)
  1. Tests against resistance
    a. Shoulder shrug — Weakness
    b. Head rotation — Weakness
I. Hypoglossal (CN XII)
  1. Observes protruded tongue — Fasciculations, asymmetry, atrophy, deviation
  2. Tests tongue movement bilat. — Weakness

VI. Cerebellar
  A. Performs Romberg's test (must do with patient's eyes open, then closed; feet together, arms at sides) — Loss of balance
  B. Observes gait
    1. Normal walking — Ataxia
    2. Tandem walking — Ataxia
  C. Tests RAMs of upper extremities bilat. — Incoordination
  D. Tests finger-to-nose, eyes open and closed bilat. — Incoordination
  E. Tests toe tapping bilat. — Incoordination
  F. Tests heel-to-shin bilat. — Incoordination

VII. Motor System
  A. Inspects and palpates muscle masses — Atrophy, involuntary movements
    1. Upper extremities
    2. Lower extremities
  B. Checks passive ROM of flexor and extensor muscle groups at major joints — Flaccidity, spasticity, rigidity
    1. Hands
    2. Wrists
    3. Elbows
    4. Shoulders
    5. Feet
    6. Knees
  C. Tests muscle groups at major joints against resistance — Weakness, paralysis
    1. Hands (grip strength)
    2. Fingers and thumb
    3. Wrists
    4. Elbows
    5. Shoulders (arms extended)
    6. Feet
    7. Knees
    8. Hips (flexion, abduction, and adduction)

Continued

NEURO EXAM–PROTOCOL–cont'd

VIII. Sensory System
    A. Tests for light touch over
        1. Shoulders (C4)
        2. Inner forearms (T1)
        3. Outer forearms (C6)
        4. Thumbs (C6)
        5. Little fingers (C8)
        6. Medial calves (L4)
        7. Lateral calves (L5)
        8. Little toes (S1)
    B. Compares side to side on all areas in VIIIA
        1. Shoulders (C4)
        2. Inner forearms (T1)
        3. Outer forearms (C6)
        4. Thumbs (C6)
        5. Little fingers (C8)
        6. Medial calves (L4)
        7. Lateral calves (L5)
        8. Little toes (S1)
    C. Compares proximal to distal at least once on upper extremities and lower extremities
    D. Tests for sharp/dull over
        1. Shoulders (C4)
        2. Inner forearms (T1)
        3. Outer forearms (C6)
        4. Thumbs (C6)
        5. Little fingers (C8)
        6. Medial calves (L4)
        7. Lateral calves (L5)
        8. Little toes (S1)
    E. Compares side to side on all areas in VIIID
    F. Compares proximal to distal at least once on upper extremities and lower extremities
    G. Tests vibratory sense, comparing side to side
        1. Upper extremities (any DIP joint)
        2. Lower extremities (IP joint big toe)
    H. Tests position sense
        1. Finger (PIP joint)
        2. Toes (IP joint)
    I. Tests point localization
    J. Tests extinction
    K. Tests stereognosis (identifying objects in the hand)
    L. Tests graphesthesia (identifying numbers "written" on the palm)

Right column annotations:

- Anesthesia, hypesthesia, hyperesthesia
- Analgesia, hypalgesia, hyperalgesia
- Sensory loss (G)
- Sensory loss (H)
- Sensory loss (I)
- Sensory loss (J)
- Sensory loss (K)
- Sensory loss (L)

NEURO EXAM—PROTOCOL—cont'd

IX. Reflexes
    A. Tests DTRs   Hyperactive reflexes, decrease or
        1. Biceps   absence of reflexes
        2. Triceps
        3. Brachioradialis
        4. Patellar
        5. Achilles
    B. Tests superficial reflexes   Absence of reflexes
        1. Upper abdomen
        2. Lower abdomen
    C. Tests for Babinski's reflex   Upper motor neuron lesion
        (plantar response) (patient must be supine)
X. Special Tests: Meningeal Signs
    A. Tests for Kernig's sign   Pain, resistance
        (knee extension with hip flexed)
    B. Tests for Brudzinski's sign   Pain, resistance, hip and knee flexion
        (flexes neck with patient supine)

NEURO WRITE-UP—NORMAL

General Appearance
    WN, WD, middle-aged WM in NAD.

Vital Signs
    Temp. = 98.2° F
    Pulse = 72/min., reg.
    Resp. = 12/min., reg.
    BP = 136/86, R. arm, sitting

Mental Status
    Alert, oriented × 3. Short-term memory, receptive and expressive abilities, serial 7s—all intact.

Cranial Nerves
    I-XII intact.

Cerebellar
    Romberg's negative. Gait—walks well without assistance, no ataxia. RAMs, finger-to-nose, and heel-to-shin—all intact.

Motor
    Full ROM of all extremities without rigidity or spasticity. Strength equal, appropriate for age in UEs and LEs. No atrophy, fasciculations, or involuntary movements.

Continued

NEURO WRITE-UP–NORMAL–cont'd

Sensory
Intact to light touch, sharp/dull, vibratory, proprioception, point localization, extinction, stereognosis, and graphesthesia testing.

DTRs[a]

(2+ = normal)

Meningeal Signs
Kernig's and Brudzinski's both negative.

[a]The downward-pointing arrows on the feet indicate a negative Babinski's reflex; a positive Babinski's would be indicated by drawing the arrows going up. An alternative way to chart reflexes would be to create a table similar to that used in charting pulses. (See following write-up.)

NEURO WRITE-UP–LEFT-SIDED CVA

General Appearance
WN, WD, elderly WM lying comfortably in bed, in NAD.

Vital Signs
Temp. = 98.6° F
Pulse = 84/min., reg.
Resp. = 16/min., reg.
BP = 108/102, R. arm, sitting

Mental Status
Alert, oriented to place and person, but not time. Patient has moderate difficulties with speech. Patient is able to name objects, but struggles for the proper words and pronunciation. Patient can follow simple orders. Short-term memory is impaired (i.e., cannot remember three previously named objects when asked about them later).

Cranial Nerves
I–Intact.
II–VA 20/40 bilat., with glasses. Visual fields grossly intact by confrontation method, but patient has some difficulty with the instructions. Funduscopy–widespread vessel narrowing seen. AV nicking seen at 4:00 and 8:00 in L. eye, and 6:00 in R. eye. No hemorrhages, exudates, or papilledema seen.

NEURO WRITE-UP—LEFT-SIDED CVA—cont'd

III, IV, VI—PERRLA, EOMI. No ptosis.

V—Facial sensation intact to light touch and pinprick. Corneal reflex intact bilat. Jaw strength intact.

VII—Some drooping and weakness of R. lower face. R. upper facial muscles slightly weaker than L., but almost symmetrical. R. eyelid can be forced open more easily than L.

VIII—Hearing grossly intact bilat. Weber's—midline. Rinne's—AC greater than BC bilat.

IX, X—Swallowing and gag reflex intact. Uvula elevates in midline.

XI—Moderate R.-sided weakness to shoulder shrug and turning head against resistance.

XII—Tongue movement intact bilat.

Cerebellar

Romberg's and gait not tested (patient unable to stand without assistance). RAMs, finger-to-nose, and heel-to-shin—all intact on L. side, but unable to perform on R. side due to weakness.

Motor

Full ROM of L. arm and leg without rigidity or spasticity. Strength equal, appropriate for age on L. side. R. side—moderate-to-severe weakness of R. arm and leg (worse in leg), with some increase in general muscle tone. No atrophy, fasciculations, or involuntary movements bilat.

Sensory

Intact to light touch, sharp/dull, vibratory, proprioception, point localization, stereognosis, and graphesthesia testing on L. side. Some perception of sharp/dull on R. arm and leg (though decreased in comparison with L.), but otherwise has fairly complete sensory loss on R. side.

DTRs

	R.	L.	
Brachioradialis	3+	2+	
Triceps	3+	2+	
Biceps	3+	2+	(2+ = normal)
Abdominal	0	2+	
Patellar	3+	2+	
Achilles	3+	2+	
Babinski	positive	negative	

Meningeal Signs

Kernig's and Brudzinski's both negative.

CASE STUDY 12-1

The patient is a 72-year-old woman with a 20-year history of type 2 diabetes who is seen in your clinic on an irregular basis. She presents for a minor acute problem. You do not have time to do a full physical examination, but you would like to use this brief visit as an opportunity to check for common complications of diabetes that have not been monitored for some time in this patient. What sections of the physical examination would you try to cover in the short time available?

Knowledge of appropriate physical examination maneuvers to be performed depends on the clinician's knowledge of the long-term complications of diabetes, as well as any specific patient complaints. A brief, focused physical examination should proceed according to the discussion in the following paragraph.

Although cardiac complications of diabetes are common and important, these are often not easily assessed by physical examination. Therefore, only a brief heart examination would be warranted. Blood pressure evaluation and auscultation for bruits over the carotid and femoral arteries are important. Common, serious, but often asymptomatic complications of diabetes can develop in the eyes and feet. Therefore, even a brief examination should include funduscopy and careful examination of the feet for ulcers and skin infection. Impaired vibratory sense is an early sign of diabetic neuropathy and can be assessed easily as part of the foot examination. Checking skin folds for signs of fungal infection is another relatively brief but important assessment.

GLOSSARY OF ABBREVIATIONS

Acronym and Definition		Acronym and Definition	
AAL	Anterior axillary line	LS	Lumbosacral
AC	Air conduction	LSB	Left sternal border
AP	Anteroposterior	LUQ	Left upper quadrant
AV	Arteriovenous	MCL	Midclavicular line
BC	Bone conduction	NAD	No acute distress
BCP	Birth control pill	NSSC	Normal size, shape, and consistency
BF	Black female	NVD	Neck vein distention
bilat.	Bilateral or bilaterally	Oriented × 3	Oriented to time, place, and person
BM	Bowel movement or black male		
BP	Blood pressure	OU	Both eyes
BS	Bowel sounds	PERRLA	Pupils equal, round, reactive to light and accommodation
BT	Bowel tones		
BUS	Bartholin's glands, urethra, Skene's glands	PIP	Proximal interphalangeal
		PMI	Point of maximal impulse
CHF	Congestive heart failure	pt	patient
CMT	Cervical motion tenderness	R	Right
CV	Cardiovascular	RA	Rheumatoid arthritis
CVA	Costovertebral angle or cerebrovascular accident	RAMs	Rapid alternating movements
		reg.	Regular or regularly
DIP	Distal interphalangeal	RESP	Respiration
DP	Dorsalis pedis pulse	RLQ	Right lower quadrant
DTR	Deep tendon reflex	ROM	Range of motion
EOMI	Extraocular movements intact	RSB	Right sternal border
ER	Emergency room	RUQ	Right upper quadrant
GI	Gastrointestinal	RV	Rectovaginal
GYN	Gynecological	SLR	Straight leg raising
HJR	Hepatojugular reflux	T	Thoracic
ICS	Intercostal space	TM	Tympanic membrane
IUD	Intrauterine (birth control) device	TMJ	Temporomandibular joint
L	Left	UE	Upper extremities (arms)
LE	Lower extremities (legs)	VA	Visual acuity
LLD	Left lateral decubitus	WD	Well developed
LLL	Left lower lobe	WF	White female
LLQ	Left lower quadrant	WM	White male
LMP	Last menstrual period	WN	Well nourished

CASE STUDY 12-2

A 28-year-old woman presents with a 3-month history of episodic joint pain, mostly in her wrists and fingers. She is a graduate student and notes fatigue and early morning stiffness. She has a part-time job as a clerk typist.

Your differential diagnosis includes conditions such as rheumatoid arthritis and carpal tunnel syndrome. What physical examination maneuvers do you need to include?

Elements of the musculoskeletal and neurological physical examinations would be appropriate. Vital signs should be checked for temperature elevation. A brief but comprehensive musculoskeletal survey should be carried out, examining all extremity joints for signs of inflammation (e.g., heat, redness, swelling, pain, and decreased range of motion). Particular attention should be given to the joints of the wrist and hand. Specific neurological tests related to carpal tunnel syndrome, such as Tinel's and Phalen's signs, should be performed (see physical examination reference texts such as Bates or DeGowin [listed in Reference Section] for details on these procedures).

CONCLUSION

Figure 11-1, which can be found on p. 230-236 provides a complete medical history and physical examination for a hypothetical patient.

CLINICAL APPLICATIONS

1. Review the physical examination procedures discussed in this chapter, and describe how you might modify them for use with patients in a variety of settings (e.g., bedridden patient, patient in a less than private examining area, unconscious patient, frightened pediatric patient).

2. Review the available list of the "most common" primary care problems. Identify those problems for which a "multisystems" approach to the physical examination would be necessary. Prepare a list of specific and appropriate physical examination procedures for each problem by selecting from the specific "organ system" protocols presented in this chapter. Compare your suggested physical examination plan with those of other students and practicing clinicians.

RESOURCES

Binkley LS, Hoekelman RA. Bates' Guide to Physical Examination and History Taking, ed 7. Philadelphia: JB Lippincott, 1999. *Probably the most popular textbook for teaching physical examination skills in PA programs.*

DeGowin RL, Brown DD. DeGowin's Diagnostic Examination, ed 7. New York: McGraw-Hill, 2000. *A classic reference, most suitable for graduate PAs.*

Hoppenfeld S, Hutton R. Physical Examination of the Spine and Extremities. New York: Prentice-Hall, 1976. *A superb reference for the musculoskeletal examination.*

Seidel HM, Ball JW, Dains JE, Benedict GW. Mosby's Guide to Physical Examination, ed 4. St. Louis: Mosby, 1999. *A competitor to Bates and a good alternative for teaching physical examination skills.*

CHAPTER 13

Utilizing Diagnostic Studies

David B. Buck[†] and Geraldine A. Buck

INTRODUCTION

Diagnostic studies are an important adjunct to clinical findings in patient care, and the physician assistant will experience both affirmation and frustration with the technological evaluation of patients. The rewards of affirmation accompany the confirmation of diagnoses and clinical suspicions with diagnostic studies. Sentiments of frustration summarize the complexity of keeping abreast of new technology and methodologies, mastering a cost-effective approach to the use of diagnostic tests, and dealing with the inadequacies and limitations of diagnostic studies. The objective of this chapter is to provide a basic understanding of key concepts necessary to minimize the frustrations

related to the use of diagnostic studies. The chapter discusses factors influencing the use of diagnostic studies, an overview of tests commonly used in primary care, practical applications for the collection and handling of specimens, and, finally, an approach to the interpretation of diagnostic studies.

RATIONALE AND CHOICE OF STUDIES

The United States spends more money per capita on health care expenditures than any other country in the world—14% of the gross domestic product in 2001.[1] Burgeoning health care costs are attributable in part to the use of expensive technologies that have proliferated over the past two decades, and to ineffective utilization of diagnostic studies based on anecdotal experience, patient preferences, financial

[†]Deceased

incentives, and individual practice prerogatives.[2] Beginning in the 1980s, guidelines for cost containment began to emerge to promote the effective use of limited health care resources.[3-5] Today, clinical practice guidelines based on cost effectiveness analysis[6] continue to be developed through the application of evidence-based medicine principles, which allow health care providers to choose a course of diagnostic investigation based on scientific evidence.[7]

Several clinical guidelines have been designed for the use of diagnostic tests. The most universally accepted reasons for testing are to:

➤ Confirm suspected diagnosis(es).
➤ Monitor the progression/regression of disease process(es).
➤ Aggregate prognostic indicators.
➤ Monitor therapeutic response and/or levels.
➤ Measure fitness.[8]

For example, a positive urine pregnancy test in a sexually active female patient who missed her last expected menstrual cycle confirms the probable diagnosis of pregnancy. The use of serial pulmonary function studies, particularly the spirograph or flow-volume loop, displays the role of monitoring the progression of diseases, such as chronic obstructive pulmonary disease (COPD), and the regression of acute exacerbations of asthma. When diagnostic studies are used to accumulate prognostic information, a conglomerate of studies is typically needed. A patient diagnosed with a neoplastic disease, for example, may require a bone marrow aspiration and biopsy, liver and spleen scans, bone scan, and multiple biochemical tests to synthesize the prognosis. Examples of using diagnostic tests to monitor therapeutic response include serial serum glucose testing in the patient with diabetes mellitus and the measurement of actual levels of therapeutic agents such as phenytoin and digoxin. Documenting fitness status for sports or employment requires variable types of testing according to the activity for which an individual is being tested. Fitness testing may require a resting or exercise electrocardiogram (ECG), antibody titers documenting immunity to communicable diseases, or toxicology tests for identification of illicit drugs.

Woolf and Kamerow best summarize the rationale for the use of diagnostics; it applies to PAs as well as physicians:

> "The 'thorough' physician, rather than being someone who orders all possible tests, should be the physician who considers all effects, benefits, and risks to ensure that testing is beneficial to those who receive it... 'Competent' physicians should be expected to seek reliable evidence of improved clinical outcome, rather than relying on assumptions that testing is beneficial."[9]

Statland and Winkel[10] define "appropriate practices" for the use of tests as "such practices that maximize use of laboratory resources while a defined strategy proposed to solve the problem is implemented." Hence, the PA must define the problem and devise an approach to it. This approach requires the selection of studies based on clinical information and evidence gathered through the history and physical examination, review of prior medical records, and the application of one's knowledge base to the epidemiology and prevalence of the suspected disease or diagnosis. Additional consideration must be given, prior to requesting diagnostic studies, to potential risks to the patient, financial expense for both the patient and the health care system, and most important, what impact the test may have on the management of the case.

Underutilization and *overutilization* are terms applied to deviations from "appropriate practices." *Underutilization* consi   ering too few tests or not requesting that r   made available when they are needed.[10] Und   on of diagnostic studies, according to Statland and Winkel, "prevents the stated strategy from being implemented"[10] and tends to be the focus of medical legal disputes. In this regard, underutilization has the potential to negatively affect cost containment efforts as well as patient care. Conversely, *overutilization,* described as ordering too many tests or ordering tests too frequently, results in excessive costs.[10] The PA must be conscious of the tremendous expense to the health care system of inappropriate utilization of diagnostic studies—both underutilization and overutilization—and must strive to select necessary and appropriate diagnostic tests.

Primary care provi   t be cognizant of the multitude of indica   traindications, and procedures for each system of the body and all disease processes. Beyond an awareness of available tests, the PA needs an approach to test selection, sequencing, and frequency. Test *selection* depends primarily on the diagnosis being entertained, the yield of a test's methodology in contrast to its potential complications for a given patient, and the possible impact of the test result on the management plan. The *sequencing* of diagnostic studies is related to the results of preliminary tests, to the clinical status of the patient, and with a hospitalized patient, to the anticipated length of stay and the guidelines of the utilization review team. *Frequency* of testing is determined by disease progression or resolution and the need for monitoring of therapy.

Test selection, sequencing, and frequency can best be demonstrated by the case of a patient suspected of having coronary artery disease (CAD). Appropriate selection of diagnostic studies in this case is based on the epidemiology and prevalence of CAD, the patient's risk factors, such as hypertension, obesity, and smoking, and the clinical manifestations assessed through the history and physical examination. Provided that the clinical evidence warrants diagnostic evaluation, tests such as an ECG and lipid profile would be selected first. Depending on the results of these tests and the patient's condition, additional studies of higher specificity may or may not be indicated. An exercise ECG, 24-hour Holter monitoring, a multi-gated angiogram, an echocardiogram, or a cardiac catheterization may be necessary to identify the pathological process precipitating the symptoms in this patient. The clinical diagnosis, patient status, and therapeutic modalities employed dictate the frequency of testing as a reflection of the quality of care. Additional factors in the frequency of testing are clinical practice guidelines and the health care organizational structure.

OVERVIEW OF COMMON LABORATORY STUDIES

Procedures in the clinical laboratory can be described as qualitative, semiquantitative, or quantitative. *Qualitative tests* identify the presence or absence of a measurable substance, and results are generally reported as either "positive" or "negative." Examples of qualitative tests are serological identification tests for antibodies to viral illnesses such as infectious mononucleosis and rubella. *Semiquantitative tests* provide an estimation of the concentration of the test substance, in addition to identifying the presence of the analyte. Examples of semiquantitative tests include the components of urine dipsticks, which not only identify the presence of hemoglobin, protein, and glucose but also provide a fairly accurate estimation of the concentration of these constituents within the test specimen. *Quantitative tests* are those that furnish a precise numerical value. Chemical analyses of serum for levels of electrolytes, glucose, blood urea nitrogen, and creatinine are examples of quantitative tests, all of which are reported in numerical values for comparison of the patient's test results with a reference interval.

Diagnostic testing procedures may be performed for a variety of reasons, ranging from targeted screening to diagnosis-specific testing. Screening tests are used to detect a specific disease in persons suspected of having a particular disease or condition[11]; they are most effective when used to identify high-risk individuals early in the course of a disease, prior to the onset of symptoms. Diseases for which targeted screening positively affects patient outcomes are breast and cervical cancers, congenital hypothyroidism, and phenylketonuria.[5] Screening for hyperlipidemia can identify asymptomatic individuals with elevated lipid levels within high-risk populations such as diabetics, men, and postmenopausal women. The PA may recommend lifestyle modifications or treatments to reduce the risk of atherosclerotic plaque formation, coronary artery disease, and cerebrovascular accident for the patient with high lipid levels.

By and large, only a limited number of clinical laboratory tests are capable of confirming a specific diagnosis. Most laboratory tests are used to detect common abnormalities that fit into patterns associated with specific diseases. These test results must be evaluated in light of the entire clinical picture because the same laboratory test results are abnormal in several disease states. The PA must evaluate the results of a battery of tests in combination with the historical and physical findings to arrive at a specific diagnosis. For example, the white blood cell (WBC) count, performed as part of the complete blood count (CBC), might reveal leukocytosis (elevated WBC count), which can be representative of infection, inflammatory responses, leukemia, or normal physiological states. To differentiate the cause and interpret the clinical significance of the elevation in WBC count, the clinician must evaluate the patient with the abnormal test result. The following case illustrates this point.

CASE STUDY 13-1

A 19-year-old female patient without a history of chronic disease presents complaining of fever for the past week. The onset of the fever, ranging from 100.2° F to 101.0° F orally, was abrupt, and the pattern is remittent. There is minimal resolution of the fever with acetaminophen, 650 mg every 4 to 6 hours. The patient admits to experiencing easy fatigue, lassitude, anorexia, and "body aches" for the past week as well.

The physical examination reveals an ill-appearing young woman with an oral temperature of 101.4° F. Mild pallor of the mucous membranes and splenomegaly are the only remarkable findings. A CBC is ordered, which reveals an elevated WBC count.

The differential diagnosis for the triad of fever, splenomegaly, and leukocytosis in this patient is extensive. The major areas of concern to the PA include infectious causes such as hepatitis B virus (HBV), Epstein-Barr virus, infective endocarditis, and Lyme disease. Immunological abnormalities such as rheumatoid arthritis, systemic lupus erythematosus (SLE), drug fever, and hemolytic anemias must also be considered. Lymphoma, leukemia, and solid tumors are neoplastic diseases of grave concern to the astute clinician faced with such a clinical presentation.

The interpretation of the leukocytosis in light of the history and physical findings depends on several factors—the actual degree of leukocytosis (the exact WBC count) and a search for essential clinical information through an extensive history and physical examination and additional diagnostic studies. The degree of increase in the WBC count is often helpful, although never exclusionary, in determining the cause. A mild elevation of the WBC count may indicate an inflammatory response, whereas an extremely elevated WBC count occurs in leukemia and severe infectious processes. The additional information gained through in-depth history and physical examination and the progression of the clinical course determine the studies required to make the diagnosis. Tests for infectious causes include cultures, serological antigen and antibody tests, and tests specific to target organs, such as echocardiography for endocarditis. The immunological diseases require testing for specific abnormal antigens and antibodies. Finally, the neoplastic diseases typically necessitate the utilization of multiple invasive tests, such as bone marrow biopsy and aspiration, as well as noninvasive studies, computed tomography (CT) scans or magnetic resonance imaging (MRI), and serial blood testing for blood cell counts, tumor markers, and potential metastatic effects of the malignant disease.

Examples of diagnosis-specific tests include antigen identification tests, which identify individual protein markers that are often unique to the antigen. Rapid antigen tests used to diagnose pneumococcal meningitis detect either capsular antigens or the *Streptococcus pneumoniae* C-polysaccharide of the cell wall, allowing for timely and specific diagnosis and treatment.

Clinical laboratories are divided into the following specialty areas: hematology, clinical chemistry, microbiology, urinalysis, blood bank, and histology/cytology. Although an in-depth discussion of the clinical laboratory tests available in each of these departments of the laboratory is beyond the scope of this chapter, the most common diagnostic studies for each specialty are summarized in Table 13-1 and are briefly described in the following pages.

Hematology

Complete Blood Count   In hematology, one of the oldest and most common test procedures is the complete blood count (CBC), which typically includes the white blood cell (WBC) count, red blood cell (RBC) count, measurement of hemoglobin, hematocrit, red blood cell indices, platelet count, and white blood cell differential count. Reference intervals for each type of count or measurement vary slightly, depending on the laboratory and methods used, but generally, men

Table 13-1 Common Laboratory Studies

Name of Test	Specimen Type	Collection Instructions	Turnaround Time	Special Instructions or Notes
HEMATOLOGY				
CBC	Venous/capillary blood	Purple-top tube/EDTA	10-30 min	Differential count may or may not be included
WBC differential count	Venous/capillary blood	EDTA tube or blood smear	15-30 min	May be manual or automated
RBC morphology	Venous/capillary blood	EDTA tube or blood smear	15-30 min	Request specifically
Reticulocyte count	Venous/capillary blood	Purple-top tube/EDTA	30-45 min	Requires special stain
Erythrocyte sedimentation rate	Venous blood	Purple-top tube/EDTA	75-90 min	Specimen ≤2 hr old
IMMUNOHEMATOLOGY (BLOOD BANKING)				
Blood typing	Venous/cord blood	Red-top tube only	10-15 min	Patient identification and specimen labeling are vital and essential for all immuno-hematology procedures
Crossmatching	Venous/cord blood	Red-top tube only	30-60 min	
Indirect Coombs' test	Venous blood	Red-top tube only	30-60 min	
Direct Coombs' test	Venous/cord blood	Red-top tube only	15-30 min	
COAGULATION TESTS				
Platelet count	Venous/capillary blood	Purple-top tube/EDTA	10-15 min	Platelet estimate from peripheral smear
PT	Venous blood	Blue-top tube/sodium citrate	15-20 min	Refrigerate plasma if >1 hr to testing
APTT	Venous blood	Blue-top tube/sodium citrate	15-20 min	Refrigerate plasma if >1 hr to testing
Fibrinogen	Venous blood	Blue-top tube/sodium citrate	15-20 min	Refrigerate plasma if >1 hr to testing
FSP	Venous blood	Special manufacturer's tube	15-30 min	Obtain special tube from laboratory
URINALYSIS				
Macroscopic urinalysis	Freshly voided urine	Midstream clean catch	5-10 min	Refrigerate if >30 min to testing
Microscopic urinalysis	Freshly voided urine	Midstream clean catch	15-30 min	Refrigerate if >30 min to testing
Urine pregnancy testing	Freshly voided urine	Midstream clean catch	30-60 min	Filter urine if + for blood
CHEMISTRY				
Glucose	Venous/capillary blood	Gray-top/capillary tube	15-30 min	Gray tube to inhibit glycolysis
Glycosylated hemoglobin A_{1c}	Venous blood	Purple-top tube	1-7 days	Index of long-term glucose control
Electrolytes (Na, K, Cl, CO_2)	Venous/capillary blood	Red/speckled-top tube	30-60 min	Do not draw blood from arm with IV line
Creatinine and BUN	Venous/capillary blood	Red/speckled-top tube	30-60 min	

Liver function tests (LFT)	Venous/capillary blood	Red/speckled-top tube	30-60 min	Includes total bilirubin, direct bilirubin, AP, LDH, total protein, albumin, ALT (SGPT), GGT
Amylase/lipase	Venous blood	Red/speckled-top tube	30-60 min	Lipase more specific than amylase
Cardiac enzymes	Venous blood	Red/speckled-top tube	30-60 min / 1-2 days	Includes CPK, LDH, AST (SGOT); CPK isoenzymes performed on abnormals
Cholesterol/lipid profile	Venous blood	Red/speckled-top tube	2-3 days	12-hr/overnight fast preferred
Biochemical profile (SMA)	Venous blood	Red/speckled-top tube	45-60 min	Variable types and numbers of tests
Thyroid studies (TFT)	Venous blood	Red/speckled-top tube	2-3 days	Specify tests necessary: TSH, T_4, T_3 RIA
Drug screen	Urine/venous blood	Fresh urine/red-top tube	2 hr to 7 days	Consent form may be necessary
Alcohol level	Venous blood	Gray-top tube	30-60 min	Consent form may be necessary; do not use alcohol/betadine
Therapeutic drug levels	Venous blood	Red/speckled-top tube	2 hr to 7 days	Specify drug; digoxin, phenytoin, ASA
Hormone/vitamin tests	Urine/venous blood	Contact laboratory for specific requirements for patient preparation and specimen collection	2 hr to 7 days	Specify drug; digoxin, phenytoin, ASA

MICROBIOLOGY

Culture and sensitivity tests				
Pharyngeal/nasopharyngeal	Swab of pharynx/nasopharynx	Transport swab	24-48 hr	No sensitivity for GABHS; for gonococcus, see below
Sputum	Deep cough expectoration	Sterile container with lid	48-72 hr	Collect aerobic and anaerobic samples; incubate
Blood	Venous blood	Liquid culture media	7 days	Refrigerate specimen until plated
Urine	Fresh midstream urine	Sterile container with lid	24-72 hr	Salmonella/Shigella—special transport media
Stool	Fresh stool	Sterile container with lid	48-72 hr	
Vaginal/urethral/rectal for gonococcus	Discharge	Martin-Lewis agar with CO_2	48 hr	Plate specimen for transport on warm agar
Wound/exudate	Discharge	Transport swab/anaerobic tube	48-72 hr	Requirements vary with suspected pathogen
Cerebrospinal fluid	Cerebrospinal fluid	Sterile tube	48-72 hr	Must incubate specimen immediately
Joint fluid	Joint fluid	Sterile tube	48-72 hr	Note suspected pathogen
Mycobacterium cultures	Sputum, urine, joint fluid, CSF, skin, tissue biopsy	Sterile tube/container with lid	4-6 wk	Use acid-fast bacilli smears to follow organism load

Chlamydial and viral cultures require special collection and transport media; contact laboratory for requirements and transport media, but they require special media and long growth periods, up to several weeks.

Continued

Table 13-1   Common Laboratory Studies—cont'd

Name of Test	Specimen Type	Collection Instructions	Turnaround Time	Special Instructions or Notes
STAINING				
Gram's staining	Any specimen for culture and sensitivity testing	As listed above for specific specimen	15-30 min	Identifies shape, configuration, and staining reaction (+/−) for bacteria with cell walls
Wright's staining	Capillary/venous blood	Thick and thin blood smears	1-7 days	Various forms of malarial parasites in RBCs
Acid-fast bacilli (AFB) staining	Any specimen for Mycobacterium culture	As listed above for specific specimen	1-3 hr	AFB organism load noted via sequential smears
India ink stain	Cerebrospinal fluid	Sterile tube	15-30 min	Positive with cryptococcal meningitis
Ova and parasite studies	Stool, sputum, tissue biopsy	Sterile container identified	1-7 days	Forms and types of parasites
Cellophane tape test	Perianal	Specimen tape on glass microscope slide	15 min to days	Pinworm eggs/worms identified
Wet preparation or mount	Vaginal/urethral discharge	Sterile tube with saline	15 min	Trichomonads, yeasts, clue cells visualized
SEROLOGICAL AND ANTIGENIC TESTS				
RPR/VDRL	Venous/cord blood	Red/speckled-top tube	1-7 days	Biological false-positives occur
FTA-ABS/MHA-TP	Venous/cord blood	Red/speckled-top tube	1-7 days	Confirmatory tests for positive RPR/VDRL
TORCH test	Venous/cord blood	Red/speckled-top tube	1-7 days	Toxoplasmosis, rubella, CMV, herpes
HIV testing	Venous/cord blood	Red/speckled-top tube	1-7 days	ELISA test + confirmed with Western blot; p 24 antigen utilized for infant HIV testing
Hepatitis testing	Venous blood	Red/speckled-top tube	1-7 days	Request antigen and antibodies specific to type of hepatitis suspected (A, B, C)
Mono spot test	Venous blood	Red/speckled-top tube	15-30 min	Includes varying rheuma-tological, oncological, and endocrinological tests (ANA, RA, CEA, alpha-fetoprotein, anti-insulin/thyroid)
Immune system tests	Venous blood, tissue biopsy	Red-top tube, container	Variable by test	
Rapid strep test	Pharyngeal swab	Sterile cotton swab	15-30 min	Negative result requires throat culture
Cryptococcal antigen Skin tests	Cerebrospinal fluid Specific antigen of sus-pected disease injected intradermally to invoke local immune response	Sterile tube	15-30 min	Use for variety of bacteriological, viral, tuberculous, fungal, parasitic diseases

have higher RBC, hemoglobin, and hematocrit values than women. WBC and platelet counts are typically similar in healthy men and women. Most CBCs are performed by automated cell-counting instruments, which count the numbers of WBCs, RBCs, and platelets; photometrically measure the hemoglobin concentration; measure the mean corpuscular volume; and mathematically calculate the hematocrit, mean corpuscular hemoglobin value, and mean corpuscular hemoglobin concentration on the basis of direct measurements obtained from the specimen sample. The types and percentages of white blood cells reported in the differential count are determined enzymatically for each specimen through an automated counter. The specimen is collected in a purple-top blood collection tube with ethylenediaminetetraacetic acid (EDTA) anticoagulant. The CBC specimen remains stable at room temperature for several hours; however, it is preferable to analyze the specimen as soon after collection as possible, to allow for accurate identification of the cellular components on the peripheral smear. After 4 to 6 hours, the cellular elements may become distorted and the WBCs may disintegrate, causing a falsely decreased WBC count.

Abnormalities of *white blood cell count* and red blood cell count are common. Leukocytosis (an elevated WBC count) is often caused by bacterial infections but can also be seen in a wide variety of other conditions such as leukemia, allergic reactions, inflammatory processes, drug reactions, and viral or other infectious diseases.[12] The differential count of WBCs is helpful in suggesting the underlying cause of the leukocytosis. Classically, an increase in polymorphonuclear WBCs occurs with bacterial infections, whereas an increase in lymphocytes is associated with viral diseases. Eosinophilia is associated with allergic reactions and invasive parasitic infections. Any of the white blood cell lines may be involved when leukemia is the cause of the leukocytosis. Leukopenia has its own varied list of causes, which include overwhelming sepsis, viral illnesses, cancer chemotherapeutics, and aplastic anemia.

Red blood cell counts are commonly low with any cause of anemia or acute blood loss. *RBC indices,* used in the classification of anemia, are calculated on the basis of the RBC count, hemoglobin, and

hematocrit values. The mean corpuscular volume (MCV), calculated or measured directly by the cell-counting instrument, is defined as the average volume (size) of the erythrocytes. The mean corpuscular hemoglobin (MCH) value is the average weight of hemoglobin per erythrocyte, and the mean corpuscular hemoglobin concentration (MCHC) is the average hemoglobin concentration per erythrocyte.[13] The RBC indices, although not diagnostic, may suggest the underlying cause of the anemia. Anemia may be classified on the basis of the MCV as normocytic (89 ± 9 fL), microcytic (<80 fL), or macrocytic (>100 fL), depending on the average size of the RBCs. Evaluation of the MCH and MCHC enables further classification of anemia as normochromic or hypochromic. Thus, anemias are described as normocytic/normochromic, microcytic/hypochromic, or macrocytic/normochromic, depending on the MCV and MCH/MCHC determinations.

Sickle cell anemia is an example of a normocytic/normochromic anemia, in which the MCV, MCH, and MCHC values are within their reference intervals, but the RBC count and hemoglobin concentration are low. Iron deficiency anemia is a classic example of a microcytic/hypochromic anemia, with MCV values typically in the range of 70 fL. The MCH and MCHC are often also depressed as a result of the low numbers of RBCs and low hemoglobin values. Increases in the MCV suggest the megaloblastic causes of anemia, namely vitamin B_{12} and folate deficiencies and pernicious anemia.

The CBC provides a screening mechanism for the various anemias. The number of RBCs, the amount of hemoglobin, and the volume of packed RBCs (the hematocrit), in conjunction with the RBC indices of the MCV, MCH, and MCHC, allow the PA to categorize the anemia in a manner that allows for the workup of the specific anemia suspected. The following case depicts the usefulness of the CBC as an initial test to differentiate the types of anemia. The reader is reminded that RBC, hemoglobin, hematocrit, and RBC index abnormalities may warrant the use of additional tests, such as microscopic evaluation of a stained peripheral blood smear for RBC morphology and the reticulocyte count, as well as serum vitamin B_{12}, serum folate, serum iron, and total iron-binding capacity (TIBC) measurements, to evaluate the common treatable causes of anemia.

CASE STUDY 13-2

A 67-year-old white female patient, with a past medical history (PMH) of gastric polyposis, presents complaining of increasing weakness for 6 months accompanied by intermittent episodes of vertigo and palpitations for 4 months. She admits to a 15-lb weight loss over the past 3 months. She denies fever; night sweats; anorexia; changes in skin, hair, or nails; polydipsia; polyphagia; polyuria; melena; hematochezia; hematemesis; and easy bruising or bleeding. There is no PMH or family history of anemia, leukemia, hyperthyroidism, diabetes mellitus, or cancer. She admits to smoking cigarettes, 1 pack per day, for 50 years and drinking 2 glasses of red wine per week for most of her adult life. She takes no over-the-counter, prescriptive, or illicit medications. On physical examination, the patient appears older than her stated age of 67 years; she is thin and pale but in no acute distress. Vital signs include the following: blood pressure, 140/80, sitting; pulse, 104/min; respirations, 20/min; and temperature, 99.8° F, oral. Her skin is pale with rapid turgor and pallor of the nail beds. The palpebral conjunctivae are pale pink and moist. Sclerae are icteric. The thyroid is smooth, symmetrical, nontender, and without masses or goiter. Jugular venous pressure is 4 cm at 45 degrees. The cervical, axillary, and inguinal lymph nodes are nonpalpable. The lungs are resonant to percussion with scattered bibasilar wet crackles. The cardiac examination reveals a bounding point of maximal impulse (PMI) displaced 3 cm lateral to the left midclavicular line and a regular rhythm at 104/min with a grade I/VI systolic ejection murmur along the left sternal border. The abdomen is soft and nontender with a liver span of 11 cm in the right midclavicular line. The spleen is nonpalpable; no masses are encountered. Rectal examination is heme negative. Pelvic findings are unremarkable for vulvar lesions, masses, or tenderness of the uterus or adnexa. The cervix is closed, pink, and parous without lesions. The neurological examination reveals diminished vibratory and position sensations in a stocking-glove distribution. Muscle strength is 4/5 in the upper extremities and 3/5 in the feet and lower legs. Patellar reflexes are 1/4 bilaterally. The Romberg test is positive and the gait is ataxic. The initial laboratory results of a CBC with manual WBC differential and RBC morphology and reticulocyte count are shown at the end of this case study (normal intervals shown in parentheses).

In addition to the history and physical findings, the initial diagnostic studies for this patient reveal multiple clues to the type of anemia (macrocytic/normochromic anemia with depressed erythropoiesis), and they direct clinical attention to the categories of diagnostic studies necessary to make a diagnosis while using the laboratory in a cost-effective manner. To complete the evaluation of this patient, serum B_{12} and folate measurements, bone marrow analysis, and possibly a Schilling test and serological testing for antibodies to intrinsic factor and/or parietal cells may be necessary to confirm the working diagnosis of pernicious anemia.

WBC	3.9×10^3/cu mm ($5 - 10 \times 10^3$/cu mm)
RBC	2.2×10^6/cu mm ($3 - 5 \times 10^6$/cu mm)
Hemoglobin	7.0 g/100 mL (14 ± 2 g/100 mL)
Hematocrit	20% (42 ± 3%)
MCV	114 fL (89 ± 9 fL)
MCHC	33% (32%-36%)
Platelet count	132,000/cu mm (150,000-400,000/cu mm)
Differential count of WBCs	84% segmented neutrophils with hypersegmented neutrophils seen; 3% band cells; 10% lymphocytes; and 3% monocytes.
Morphology	Platelets appear decreased, with several misshapen thrombocytes; there is generalized macrocytosis, with macro-ovalocytes and slight poikilocytosis.
Reticulocyte count	0.3% (0.5%-1.5%)

The *reticulocyte count* is useful in measuring the bone marrow's ability to respond to anemia and circulatory blood loss. Reticulocytes are immature erythrocytes containing nuclear remnants, most of which are found in the bone marrow. Under normal circumstances, only about 1% of peripherally circulating erythrocytes consist of reticulocytes.[12] When erythropoiesis is stimulated, higher numbers of reticulocytes are found in the circulating blood if the bone marrow is functioning normally. When treatment for anemia is initiated, rising reticulocyte counts suggest a favorable response to treatment, whereas a low or unchanging reticulocyte count suggests depletion of the erythroid elements of the bone marrow, which may be irreversible.[13] Specimens for reticulocyte counts are collected in purple-top blood collection tubes containing EDTA (anticoagulant).

A more recent addition to hematology testing is the quantification of T-cell lymphocyte subsets by phenotyping of the cell-surface receptors via flow cytometry. Assessing the numbers of CD4 and CD8 lymphocytes is useful in monitoring the status of transplant and human immunodeficiency virus (HIV) patients.[12]

Tests for Coagulation and Hemostasis The analysis of coagulation factors and hemostasis is routinely performed within the hematology laboratory. Prothrombin time (PT), activated partial thromboplastin time (APTT or PTT), fibrinogen, fibrin split products (FSPs), and factor assays are the common tests of coagulation. The *PT* is used to evaluate the extrinsic pathway of coagulation and to monitor warfarin therapy, which inactivates this division of the coagulation pathway. The *APTT* is used to evaluate the intrinsic pathway and to monitor heparin therapy, which disrupts the intrinsic pathway. Patient results for the PT and the APTT are compared with laboratory controls to evaluate the functioning of each subdivision of the coagulation pathway, or to monitor anticoagulation therapy for effectiveness. *Fibrinogen levels* are often measured because fibrinogen is rapidly depleted with active bleeding. Coagulation studies are performed on freshly collected specimens anticoagulated with sodium citrate, in blood collection tubes with a light blue top. The presence of *fibrin split products* can help in the diagnosis of disseminated intravascular coagulation (DIC), an often fatal, late complication of

several life-threatening conditions. FSP specimens require the use of a special tube available in the hematology laboratory and prompt analysis to yield clinically useful information.

Factor assays measure specific coagulation factor activity in vitro. The antihemophilic factor (VIII) is one such coagulation factor with clinical importance. By factor assay methods, the laboratory is able to measure the percentage of factor VIII activity, a value that the clinician can then use to diagnose hemophilia or to titrate the amounts of cryoprecipitate needed to normalize hemostasis and prevent uncontrolled bleeding. Deficiencies of other coagulation factors exist and can be identified by similar methods.

Thrombocytopenia generally is associated with hematological diseases, such as leukemia, lymphoma, and hypersplenism, and can be found secondary to cytotoxic effects of drugs and other chemotherapeutic agents, or it may be idiopathic. Increased platelet counts are encountered in chronic inflammatory states such as rheumatoid arthritis, after splenectomy, and secondary to hemorrhage.[12]

Clinical Chemistry

The clinical chemistry laboratory is responsible for analysis of the chemical constituents of blood, body fluids, tissues, and secretions. The most common tests are measurements of serum electrolytes, serum glucose, blood urea nitrogen, creatinine, biochemical profiles, and arterial blood gases. Red-top or red-speckled-top specimen tubes are used for these tests, with the exception of arterial blood gas (ABG) measurements, for which a heparinized syringe is needed. The routine chemistry specimen is permitted to clot prior to centrifugation; once centrifuged, the serum is extracted from the specimen tube and analyzed.

Serum electrolyte analysis includes the measurement of serum sodium, potassium, chloride, and carbon dioxide levels. These electrolytes are monitored to evaluate acid-base balance and hydrational status as well as to identify electrolyte imbalances from other causes. Electrolyte determinations are important to the assessment and successful treatment of sustained vomiting, in which electrolyte depletion may occur as a result of the fluid loss. Patients prescribed potassium-wasting diuretics may experience severe potassium loss and become predisposed to cardiac dysrhythmia. Patients with end-stage renal failure may have potassium retention because of the inability to excrete the electrolyte, a state that also carries the risk of cardiac dysrhythmia. Many other conditions also cause disequilibrium of electrolytes, making electrolyte testing one of the most commonly requested clinical chemistry procedures.

The *serum glucose measurement* is used to evaluate and monitor carbohydrate metabolism and glucose regulation. Glucose tests may be performed randomly as a screening for abnormal glucose regulation, after a 12-hour fast, or 2 hours after eating (2-hour postprandial). Each of these determinations has its own reference interval, related to the expected response of the body to the different levels of glucose present at various times of the day. Individuals with a deficiency or absence of insulin production tend to have elevated levels of serum glucose and may have detectable levels of glucose in their urine. The most common cause of this hyperglycemic state is diabetes mellitus, but several other causes, such as steroid administration, must be considered. If glucose is the only test to be performed on the blood sample, or a delay in the analysis is anticipated, it is preferable that a gray-top blood collection tube be used, which contains sodium fluoride to inhibit cellular utilization of glucose. The addition of sodium fluoride stabilizes the specimen so that it will more accurately reflect the true serum glucose level.

Blood urea nitrogen (BUN) and *creatinine tests* are performed on serum specimens to evaluate the filtering capabilities of the kidneys. Creatinine, the end product of creatine metabolism, is excreted at fairly constant rates from skeletal muscle in the absence of muscle-wasting disease. Urea, the end product of protein metabolism, is also excreted at a fairly constant rate. Under normal conditions, the urea-to-creatinine ratio is approximately 10:1.[12] Measuring the BUN and creatinine levels allows a functional evaluation of the kidneys to be made. Loss of renal filtering capacity results in retention of these byproducts within the bloodstream, with elevation of either BUN or creatinine or both. The BUN-to-creatinine ratio may be helpful in determining whether the underlying cause is prerenal, infrarenal, or postrenal.

The *biochemical profile* is a panel of clinical chemistry tests used as a screening mechanism for several major organ systems—hepatic, renal, and endocrine. Tests typically included in this profile are total protein, albumin, total bilirubin, lactate dehydrogenase (LDH), aspartate aminotransferase (AST), alanine aminotransferase (ALT), and alkaline phosphatase (AP) measurements for liver function; BUN and creatinine measurements, as described previously, coupled with uric acid and phosphorus measurements to evaluate kidney function; and calcium and glucose measurements for endocrine function. In addition to evaluating the liver and kidneys, the biochemical profile may be used to detect abnormalities typical of other diseases. Diseases of bone may demonstrate abnormalities in calcium, phosphorus, alkaline phosphatase, and total protein levels. Gallbladder disease may manifest as elevated alkaline phosphatase with normal levels or slight elevations of AST, ALT, and total bilirubin. Elevations of LDH and AST in the presence of otherwise "normal" enzyme levels may suggest a cardiac cause for these abnormalities. Additional tests are often required to fully evaluate abnormalities identified on this screening profile. Moreover, in the outpatient setting and current health care policy climate of cost containment, the use of broad-based screening panels such as the biochemical profile is being limited. Third party payment for diagnostic studies is made only for those tests deemed appropriate and necessary by documented findings in the patient's history and physical examination.

Arterial blood gas evaluations are an important tool for monitoring the diffusion capacity of the lungs and the resorptive abilities of the kidneys. The maintenance of acid-base balance is heavily influenced by the regulation of oxygen and carbon dioxide exchange in the lungs and by the excretion and retention of electrolytes at the kidneys. Measuring the arterial blood gases yields information concerning these functions. Arterial blood is collected in an airtight, heparinized syringe, and the dissolved gaseous constituents within the specimen are measured. Because of the volatile nature of gases, the specimen must be placed on ice and transported to the laboratory for immediate analysis. A specimen more than 10 to 15 minutes old will have undergone significant deterioration; the test results from such a specimen will be of limited clinical utility because of the rapid degradation of the gases. The specimen is analyzed for the arterial pH, the partial pressure of arterial carbon dioxide ($paCO_2$), the partial pressure of arterial oxygen (paO_2), the bicarbonate (HCO_3) level, the base excess, and the oxygen saturation percentage. ABG evaluations are ordered when the oxygenation, acid-base, or electrolyte status of the patient is in question. Patients may require ABG analysis if they have shortness of breath, renal insufficiency, or cardiac dysrhythmia; are on artificial ventilation; or have postoperative status.

Microbiology

The microbiology laboratory is responsible for the identification of pathogenic bacteria, viruses, fungi, parasites, and other disease-causing organisms. Recent advances in molecular diagnostic studies, such as the development of DNA probes, polymerase chain reaction (PCR), and immunofluorescence assay (IFA) techniques, allow for the detection of pathogenic microorganisms directly from clinical specimens[12]; however, the standard tests of routine cultures and antimicrobial sensitivity remain the most commonly used studies in the microbiology laboratory. Specimens may be collected from any source, but they are generally limited to throat, sputum, blood, cerebrospinal fluid (CSF), urine, stool, genitalia, tissue, and wound drainage. On the basis of knowledge of the normal and common pathogenic organisms present in these body systems, the microbiologist is able to select the appropriate growth media to culture and identify most disease-causing microorganisms. Once isolated from culture and positively identified by biochemical tests, the microorganism is exposed to selected antimicrobial drugs to determine the mean inhibitory concentration of the drug necessary to eradicate it. If the organism is "susceptible" to treatment by the antimicrobial agent, that agent may be selected as therapy for the patient's infection. The reader is directed to standard texts of clinical microbiology for more information about normal flora of the body systems and sensitivity testing.

In addition to routine culture and sensitivity testing, *Gram's stain* is a rapid and valuable microbiological identification method. All clinicians should be familiar with and adept at performing Gram's stain because most clinically significant bacteria are stained by this method. By evaluating Gram's stain and noting the morphology of any microorganisms present, one may initiate empirical antibiotic therapy that is effective against the class of microorganism identified on the stained smear. *Rapid antigen tests* may also provide valuable information regarding the cause of infection, allowing for early initiation of therapy.

Fungal cultures may be performed on most types of specimens submitted for routine culture. If fungal infection is suspected as the cause of a patient's illness, fungal cultures should be specifically requested. Four to six weeks may be required for the adequate growth and identification of a fungus by culture techniques. Potassium hydroxide (KOH) wet mounts of hair, nail, and skin scrapings may be microscopically examined for identification of fungal elements when dermatophytoses are suspected.

Viral cultures are used to detect and isolate viruses such as herpes and enterovirus. With newer centrifugation-enhanced techniques, many viruses can be detected in 1 to 2 days as opposed to the usual 7 to 14 days. HIV testing is typically performed by enzyme-linked immunosorbent assay (ELISA), and a positive test is confirmed with Western blot assay. A rapid HIV antibody detection test that uses a synthetic peptide enzyme assay allows patient feedback in a single visit, and may encourage seropositive patients to return for confirmatory test results and to adopt risk-reducing behaviors sooner.[14] Gene sequencing assays to detect mutations of HIV are used in an attempt to battle antiviral drug resistance.

Tuberculosis cultures are performed by the microbiology laboratory. Sputum and other specimens, such as cerebrospinal and synovial fluids, may be submitted for acid-fast bacilli (AFB) or fluorochrome staining and *Mycobacterium* culture. Acid-fast and fluorochrome staining are specialized techniques employed to identify species of *Mycobacterium* that do not readily stain with standard Gram's stain. *Mycobacterium* species appear as red rods, or "acid-fast bacilli," against a dark blue-black background when stained by carbolfuchsin (AFB). *Mycobacterium* culture requires 4 to 6 weeks for successful growth of the organisms[12] because they have strict growth requirements and are extremely slow-growing, even on specialized culture media.

The microbiology laboratory is also responsible for identification of disease-causing *parasites* of the blood, muscles, and gastrointestinal tract. *Plasmodium* species, the causative agents of malaria, are identifiable on "thick and thin" blood smears collected from infected patients. Gastrointestinal (GI) parasites, such as *Giardia lamblia,* may be identified by examining a smear of prepared stool for the presence of active trophozoite or encysted forms of parasites. *Trichinella spiralis,* the causative agent of trichinosis, is identified by finding the cyst in a muscle biopsy specimen. Many other parasites may also be identified by the microbiology laboratory. Although relatively uncommon among residents of highly industrialized nations, parasitic infection may be found in severely immunocompromised persons, among residents of or emigrants from developing countries, and in people who travel outside the United States, Canada, and Europe.

Serological markers of disease are often detected by a subdivision of the microbiology lab, the serology department. Serology tests are performed to identify the presence of antibodies to specific antigens. The presence of antibodies in a patient's serum suggests exposure to the corresponding antigen. Serially measuring the level of antibody present enables one to observe a rise in the titer of the antibody in a patient who has been recently exposed to the antigen. Specimens are collected during the acute phase of illness and 2 to 3 weeks later, during the so-called "convalescent phase," and they are serologically tested against the suspected antigens, which are chosen on the basis of clinical information. The diagnosis is confirmed when a rise in antibody titer is observed in the convalescent specimen. Additionally, serological tests may confirm a diagnosis when specific antibodies are identified that would not normally be present without exposure to the causative antigen-carrying organism. For example, the ELISA test for HIV, when positive, suggests HIV infection because the test would be negative if the patient had never been exposed to the HIV. Confirmation of positive ELISA tests is performed by identifying antigenic markers via Western blot analysis methods as a means of ruling out causes of false-positive ELISA tests.

Blood Bank (Immunohematology)

The blood bank is responsible for the collection and storage of blood and blood products used in transfusion therapies. The standard tests performed by the blood bank include blood group and Rh typing, crossmatching for transfusion, and identifying unusual antigens or antibodies.

The major *blood types* are type A, in which the A antigen is present on the red cell membranes; type B, in which the B antigen is present; type O, in which neither antigen is present; and type AB, in which both antigens are present. The *Rh factor* is also determined. Approximately 85% of the population have detectable Rh antigen on their red blood cell membranes and are designated Rh positive. The remaining 15% have no detectable Rh factor and are designated Rh negative.

Blood bank specimens are routinely tested for the presence of unusual serum antibodies by the *antibody screening* procedure. A patient's serum is tested against known antigens and is observed for agglutination reactions, which confirm the presence of clinically significant antibodies with the potential to cause a fatal transfusion reaction. When the antibody screening result is positive, a more complete antibody identification panel is performed to identify the antibody and determine its clinical significance.

The *crossmatch* is performed to determine the suitability of specific transfusion products for a patient. The compatibility of blood products for transfusion is determined by mixing the patient's serum with a portion of the red blood cells from a unit of blood and subjecting the mixture to varying temperatures with and without reaction-enhancing additives. Test tubes in which no agglutination reactions occur are considered compatible; this means that no antigen-antibody reactions have been identified, suggesting that the blood product does not contain antigens corresponding to antibodies in the patient's circulation. Compatible units are reasonably safe for transfusion. Incompatible units of blood are those in which agglutination reactions occur, either macroscopically or microscopically, during any phase of the crossmatch procedure, and these units are not recommended for transfusion. If blood products containing an antigen are given to a patient with a corresponding antibody, a potentially fatal transfusion reaction can occur.

It is noteworthy to mention that before being administered, human blood or blood products intended for transfusion are tested for the presence of HIV, HBV, and hepatitis C virus (HCV), as well as the syphilis bacterium. Units found to have any of these contaminants are discarded.

Urinalysis

Urinalysis is an inexpensive yet important and often overlooked laboratory test that provides clinically relevant information about the kidneys and urinary system. Urinalysis is composed of two parts—the biochemical analysis and the microscopic examination.

Biochemical analysis is performed with the urine dipstick, a strip of biochemical reagent pads that undergo color reactions when reacted with urine. Characteristics measured by the dipstick include pH, specific gravity (SG), and the presence or absence of protein, glucose, ketone, blood, nitrite, leukocyte esterase, bilirubin, and urobilinogen. Normal urine has a pH between 5.0 and 7.0. Acidic urine (pH <5.0) is seen with ketosis or a diet high in meats; alkaline urine (pH >7.0) may be the result of the presence of urea-splitting bacteria or a vegetarian diet. The specific gravity of urine, normally between 1.005 and 1.030, reflects the function of the tubules in their concentrating and diluting abilities. Repeatedly low specific gravity readings are often seen in acute renal failure. Urinary protein, usually negative by dipstick testing at normal excretion levels, may be present with fever, strenuous exercise, and intrinsic renal disease. Glucose is usually not present in the urine unless the renal threshold for glucose (180 mg/dL) has been exceeded, as is typical in uncontrolled diabetes mellitus. Blood, either intact or as hemolyzed cells, is not found in the urine of healthy individuals but is seen in disease states ranging from infections, tumors, and stones to autoimmune diseases such as SLE. Nitrites, a byproduct of bacterial action, are detected when large numbers of bacteria are present, as in a urinary tract infection. Leukocyte esterase is

detected when significant numbers of white blood cells are present; the WBCs represent inflammatory processes not limited to infections. Urinary bilirubin and urobilinogen are usually absent unless hepatobiliary disease prevents excretion of these substances via the usual routes, or unless an acute hemolytic process overwhelms the hepatobiliary system.

If any abnormalities are found on biochemical analysis of the urine, *microscopic evaluation* of urine may be performed on centrifuged or uncentrifuged specimens. The urinary sediment is examined for the presence of organized and unorganized elements, including the numbers of red and white blood cells, epithelial cells, and casts per high-powered microscopic field; the quantity of bacteria or crystals present is also noted. Red blood cells are associated with renal calculi, urinary tract infections, and carcinoma of the urinary system, whereas RBC casts are typically associated with acute glomerulonephritis. WBCs and WBC casts are indicative of inflammatory processes, including urinary tract infections, with WBC casts highly suggestive of pyelonephritis. Many other conditions, such as chronic renal failure, congestive heart failure, diabetes mellitus, and autoimmune diseases, commonly cause casts to be present in the urinary sediment; their presence is typically a poor prognostic sign of renal function.

Histology/Cytology

The histology/cytology laboratory is responsible for the preparation, staining, and evaluation of cell and tissue specimens under the direction of a pathologist. Tissue biopsy specimens, body fluids, and surgical and postmortem specimens may be stained by histocytological methods and microscopically examined for the numbers and types of cells present, as well as for the presence of dysplastic or malignant cells. Tumor staging is established by histological examination of tissue and lymph node specimens.

The Papanicolaou (Pap) smear is used in the screening and diagnosis of precancerous and cancerous lesions of the uterine cervix, for hormonal assessment, and to aid in the diagnosis of inflammatory diseases of the female genital tract.[13] Pap smear specimens are obtained by vaginal speculum examination or by colposcopy. Cells from the endocervix, cervix, and posterior fornix are collected for routine Pap smear, whereas cells from the vaginal wall are collected for hormonal assessment.[13] The results of the Pap smear may be affected by careless specimen collection or thick cell preparation, the use of lubricating jelly, or recent douching. Conditions such as the use of medications (e.g., tetracycline), heavy menstrual bleeding, and infection can also adversely affect the reading of the Pap smear, and the test should not be performed when these conditions exist.[13] As with all diagnostic studies, the test result is only as good as the specimen submitted for analysis. Careful technique in the collection, preservation, and labeling of the specimen is essential to a quality reading and effective screening.

DIAGNOSTIC PROCEDURES

The most commonly used diagnostic procedures are summarized in Table 13-2 and are described briefly in the following pages.

Diagnostic Radiology

The visualization of internal structures by radiographic techniques is invaluable in the diagnosis and treatment of a multitude of disorders and illnesses. The use of diagnostic radiographic studies continues to grow as newer and safer techniques are developed. Some of the more common techniques include plain radiographs (x-rays), tomography, computed tomography, magnetic resonance imaging, ultrasonography, and nuclear medicine scans. All these techniques, with the exceptions of MRI and ultrasonography, carry the risk of radiation exposure each time a patient undergoes a procedure. The value of the information gained by such procedures must be carefully weighed against the risks to the patient before any study is requested. Only when the value of the information is sufficient to outweigh the risks to the patient should radiographic studies be ordered.

Plain radiographs or plain films are by far the most common diagnostic radiographic studies available and used. Radiographs allow visualization of bone, air-filled and fluid-filled structures, and to some extent the soft tissues. X-rays, having a shorter wavelength than visible light, are used to penetrate opaque structures in order to visualize the internal composition.[15] Depending on the density of the structure being radiographed, areas of shadow and lightness will appear on the radiographic film. Areas of the film that represent dense structures, such as bone, will appear whiter than surrounding areas; this quality is *radiopacity* or *radiodensity*. Areas of the film that represent fluid-filled or air-filled structures, such as the intestines and lungs, will appear more gray or black, depending on their relative densities; the gray to black appearance is called *radiolucency*.

Plain radiographs are employed for studies of the chest and extremities; for flat plates of the abdomen or the kidneys, ureters, and bladder (KUB); and for barium swallows and enemas. In each of these films, the contrasting radiopacity of bone or the contrast medium helps to delineate the radiolucency of air-filled and fluid-filled structures, so that evaluations of positioning, size, or continuity may be made. Plain radiographs are routinely necessary to confirm or rule out the presence of bony fracture or dislocation.

Tomographs are specialized x-rays of soft tissue structures that are poorly visualized by plain radiographic techniques. Mammographies are tomographs of breast tissue that help to identify the presence of cystic or solid breast masses with malignant potential. Other tomographic studies have been largely replaced by computed tomography (CT) scans.

In *computed tomography,* a thin beam of x-rays is passed through the patient and sensed by electronic detectors that convert the conventional tomographic x-rays into electronic pulsations. The electronically converted information is automatically fed into a computer, which calculates the average absorption of the x-ray beam and generates a precise, cross-sectional slice (picture) of the structure on the basis of thousands of computed picture elements, all appearing in varying shades of gray. The image is viewed on the computer screen, and the computer generates a permanent photographic record of the images. The x-ray dose per slice is comparable to the exposure from conventional radiographic studies.[15] Contrast material is routinely used for CT scanning, as a means of enhancing the visibility of selected structures that are in close proximity to other structures of similar density. For example, the GI tract may be better

Table 13-2   Common Diagnostic Procedures

Name of Test	Examples	Indications	Duration	Special Instructions and Contraindications
RADIOLOGICAL STUDIES				
Radiographs without contrast	CXR, KUB, bone films	Screening and diagnosis	15-30 min	Cooperative, nonpregnant patient
Radiographs with contrast	IVP, barium, upper or lower GI	Screening and diagnosis	1-2 hr	Cooperative, nonpregnant patient; allergy to contrast medium
Mammography		Screen for breast cancer	30-45 min	No powder/deodorant use day of test
Nuclear medicine studies	Lung, liver/spleen, bone, gallbladder, thyroid scans	Screening and diagnosis	1-4 hr to 24-48 hr	Cooperative, nonpregnant patient; no breast-feeding for 2-4 days after the study
Computed tomography with or without contrast	Head, chest, abdominal CT	Image bone, internal organ(s) structure and characteristics	1-3 hr	Cooperative, nonpregnant patient
Angiography	Arteriography, venography	Screening and diagnosis	1-2 hr	Cooperative, nonpregnant patient; allergy to contrast medium
Magnetic resonance imaging	Brain stem, spine, joints	Define anatomy of structures	1-2 hr	Cooperative patient without metal joints, prosthetic heart valves, vascular clips
Ultrasonography	Abdominal/pelvic organs	Image soft tissues of body cystic vs. solid masses	45-90 min	Cooperative, nonobese patient
PULMONARY FUNCTION TESTS				
Spirometry	Pre- and post-bronchodilator	Screen for obstuctive/restrictive disease patterns	15-20 min	Cooperative patient
Lung volumes	Total, reserve, inspiratory, etc.	Measure lung capacities	30-40 min	Cooperative patient
Flow-volume loop		Obstructive lung diseases	15-20 min	Cooperative patient
Arterial blood gases	pH, PaO_2, $PaCO_2$, HCO_3	Arterial O_2, CO_2, acid-base	30-60 min	Cap specimen, put on ice to transport
CARDIOVASCULAR TESTS				
Electrocardiogram	Resting, exercise, Holter	Detect ischemia, infarction, dysrhythmias, hypertrophy	15 min-24 hr	Cooperative patient
Thallium scan		Detect ischemic myocardium	2-3 hr	Exercise test and IV ^{201}Tl before scan

Continued

Table 13-2 Common Diagnostic Procedures—cont'd

Name of Test	Examples	Indications	Duration	Special Instructions and Contraindications
CARDIOVASCULAR TESTS—cont'd				
MUGA scan	With/without exercise test	Ejection fraction, wall motion	1-3 hr	
Echocardiogram	M-mode, real-time, transesophageal	Valvular function, wall motion/thickness, pericardial effusion	45-60 min	Cooperative, nonobese patient
Doppler flow studies	Arterial/venous	Detect obstruction of vessel(s)	30-60 min	No smoking 20-30 min before test
NEUROLOGICAL STUDIES				
Electroencephalography	Awake/sleeping With/without photic stimulation	Detect epilepsy, brain death	1-7 hr	Sedative/hypnotic, anticonvulsant drugs interfere with results
Electromyography	Extremital	Neuromuscular damage	1-2 hr	Cooperative patient
Myelography	Lumbar, cervical	Spinal tumor, ruptured disk	1-2 hr	MRI, CT scans have replaced most myelography
FIBEROPTIC ENDOSCOPIC STUDIES				
Bronchoscopy		Biopsy, culture, foreign body removal	30-60 min	Local anesthetic required, sedative/tranquilizer 1 hr before
GI endoscopy	Gastroscopy, colonoscopy, endoscopic retrograde cholangiopan-creatography	Visualize GI tract, biopsy	15-45 min	Local anesthetic, IV benzodiazepam
Laparoscopy		Visualize ovaries/tubes, liver	30-60 min	Local or general anesthesia
Cystoscopy		Visualize urinary tract, prostate	45-60 min	Local or general anesthesia
Arthroscopy	Knee, shoulder, wrist	Visualize joint for biopsy, repairs	45-60 min	General anesthesia
CYTOLOGICAL STUDIES				
Papanicolaou smear	Cervical/vaginal	Cancers, hormonal response	5-10 min	Cell fixative required
Tissue biopsy	Any bodily tissue or fluid	Screen for cancer, culture, transplant rejection	Varies by test	Preservative may be needed
Chromosomal studies	WBCs, skin, amniotic fluid	Genetic/oncological diseases	2-3 wk	Chemotherapy interferes with results

visualized when the study is enhanced with orally ingested contrast material, helping to differentiate the intestinal tract from other abdominal organs. Blood vessels can be distinguished from ducts when intravenous contrast material is used. In some instances, such as suspected gallbladder obstruction, CT scanning may be performed both before and after ingestion of contrast material to determine whether bile duct obstruction is present.

Computed tomography scans should be reserved for the study of special problems and should not be used for screening procedures for which other, less expensive or safer procedures may adequately diagnose a problem. One exception to this general rule is the case of head trauma, in which CT scanning is the recommended study of choice.[15] CT scans are useful for evaluating thoracic and mediastinal structures, intra-abdominal organs and masses, the brain and its blood supply, and lymphatics and blood vessels throughout the body.

Ultrasonography is the use of sound waves to produce a visual image of internal structures. Sound waves are transmitted readily through fluids but are deflected by bone, air, and barium.[15] In ultrasound scanning, a transducer applied to the skin through a layer of jelly emits sound waves and detects the echoes of the sound waves as they are deflected off the internal structures encountered in their path. These echoed wave deflections are converted into electrical energy to produce a cross-sectional image on a monitor. The monitor is capable of generating a permanent photographic record of these images. Unlike plain radiographs and CT scans, ultrasonography does not carry the risks of ionizing radiation, so it is a useful technology for visualizing the female reproductive organs. Pelvic ultrasound scanning assesses intrauterine pregnancy, ectopic pregnancy, and fetal growth and development. Ultrasonography is also useful in ascertaining whether a mass is cystic or solid, as well as in determining the size, positioning, and continuity of intra-abdominal structures such as the pancreas and abdominal aorta. *Echocardiography* is ultrasound scanning of the heart that permits visualization of cardiac valve function, blood flow across the cardiac valve opening, myocardial contraction, and determination of the left ventricular ejection fraction. Echocardiography is indicated for evaluation of heart murmurs, congenital anomalies, contraction abnormalities, and some cases of congestive heart failure.

Magnetic resonance imaging (MRI) is a technique that employs a strong magnetic field and radiofrequencies in short pulses, causing the body to emit its own radiofrequency. The body's signal is relayed to a computer, which generates an image from the information.[16] MRI provides excellent visualization of soft tissues, ligaments, tendons, nerves, joints, and bone; all have different MRI characteristics without the interference of fatty tissues, which is often encountered on CT scanning, and without the use of ionized radiation. MRI is exceptionally well suited for visualization of intervertebral disks and the joints and surrounding tissues. MRI is relatively expensive, especially compared with plain radiography. Contraindications to MRI include any implanted prosthetic device, such as a large artificial joint, a cardiac pacemaker, or a prosthetic cardiac valve, which may be adversely affected by the magnetic field.

Nuclear medicine scans are conducted by introducing selective radioisotopes into the body and scanning for their uptake into body tissues and fluids. Examples of nuclear medicine studies include radioactive iodine uptake of the thyroid, brain scans, liver scans, kidney scans, bone scans, and ventilation-perfusion (V/Q) scans of the lungs. Nuclear medicine studies are based on the theory that certain radioisotopes have an affinity for specific body tissues. When administered, the selective isotope accumulates in the target organ. Measuring the amount of radioactive uptake allows an image to be generated on the basis of the distribution of the isotope within the target organ. Areas of homogeneous uptake, of excessive uptake (hot spots), and of poor uptake (cold spots) can be identified, which may localize areas of hyperfunctioning or hypofunctioning. Nuclear medicine scans also identify areas of circulatory obstruction, as when the V/Q scan of the lungs is used to identify pulmonary vessel obstruction by pulmonary emboli. Nuclear medicine scans are used to search for metastatic tumors. Most tumors stand out as "cold spots," except in the case of bone tumors, which have increased radioactive uptake.[13] In most procedures, nuclear medicine scans expose the patient to less ionizing radiation than is emitted by plain radiographs.[13]

Electrocardiograms

Electrocardiography (ECG) is the study of the electrical conduction system of the heart. By applying surface electrodes to the patient's skin, one can obtain tracings of the electrical activity of the heart for examination. The electrodes are divided into three reference systems: limb leads—leads I, II, and III; augmented leads—leads aVR, aVL, and aVF; and precordial leads—V_1 through V_6. Correct placement of the 12 leads is critical for accurate ECG tracings to be obtained. Cardiac dysrhythmia, atrial and ventricular hypertrophy, myocardial ischemia and infarction, and axis deviation are but a few of the abnormalities found on ECG. Single-lead electrocardiographs, known as Holter monitors, may be worn around the clock by patients in whom infrequent dysrhythmias are suspected. By using a Holter monitor to record heartbeats over extended periods, the physician assistant may identify underlying disease not found on routine ECG. Postoperative cardiac patients also wear Holter monitors during the 3 to 5 days immediately after surgery for constant monitoring of the cardiac rhythm to allow for rapid and early detection of deteriorating cardiac status. Patients requiring antiarrhythmic medications also may wear Holter monitors to enable evaluation of the efficacy of treatment.

Electrocardiography is performed as part of the exercise stress test, in which the patient is maximally exercised while continuous ECG tracings record the myocardial response to the demands of exercise; this provides identification of the presence or absence of coronary artery disease. Some indications for ECG include a complaint of chest pain, shortness of breath, or other symptom suggestive of cardiopulmonary disease; preoperative screening; and the evaluation of hypertensive and diabetic patients who are at increased risk for cardiac disease.

Fiberoptic Endoscopic Examinations

Fiberoptic endoscopic devices consist of flexible tubing that contains a series of lighted mirror lenses and optic fibers. These instruments transmit light around corners, twists, and bends, allowing direct visualization of body systems not easily visualized by other means. These fiberoptic scopes can be inserted into orifices, cavities, and hollow organs for diagnostic and therapeutic purposes.[13] Visualization, biopsy, sclerotherapy, dissection, and foreign body retrieval may be accomplished by fiberoptic endoscopic technique.

Fiberoptic scopes have been developed for use in the mediastinum, bronchi, gastrointestinal tract, female reproductive tract, urinary tract, and joints.[13] Many surgical procedures are now carried out with the use of fiberoptic scopes. For example, tubal ligation, cholecystectomy, and appendectomy may be performed by laparoscopic techniques. Arthroscopy permits visualization of many joints and makes surgical repair of the joints possible without major disruption of the surrounding ligamentous and muscular tissues. All fiberoptic examinations require the use of local or general anesthesia for patient comfort.

Pulmonary Function Studies

Pulmonary function studies are designed to detect the presence and extent of lung dysfunction when obstructive or restrictive disease is suspected. Restrictive lung diseases are characterized by loss of the normal elasticity of the lungs and chest wall, which results in patient inability to inspire the normal volume of air. Examples of causes of restrictive lung diseases include asbestosis, tumor, and kyphoscoliosis. Obstructive lung diseases are characterized by impedance to air flow during expiration, with prolongation of the expiratory phase of respiration. Examples of obstructive lung disease include chronic bronchitis, emphysema, and asthma. Indications for pulmonary function studies include evaluation of a patient with dyspnea, detection of cardiac or pulmonary disease, periodic examination of patients with high-risk occupations, and assessment of tolerance to anesthesia with intubation during a surgical procedure.[13]

Common pulmonary function studies include *spirometry, flow-volume loops,* and *diffusion studies. Spirometry* is used to gather quantitative information about the effectiveness of the forces involved in moving the chest wall and lungs. In spirometry, measurements are made of the forced vital capacity (FVC) and forced expiratory volumes (FEV$_1$ and FEV$_3$). The FVC is the measure of the maximum volume of air that can be rapidly exhaled upon maximum deep inspiration; FEV_1 and FEV_3 are the volumes of air exhaled within 1 second and 3 seconds, respectively. Vital capacity (VC) is the measure of the largest volume of air that can be exhaled from the lungs upon maximum inspiration. Residual volume (RV) is the volume of air remaining in the lungs after maximum expiration. Total lung capacity (TLC) measures the volume of air within the lungs on maximal inspiration. By comparing patient results with predicted normalized values based on age, gender, weight, and height, one can determine whether restrictive or obstructive disease is present.

Flow-volume loop procedures measure the same parameters as spirometry, with the addition of a maximal forced inspiration at the end of the forced expiratory maneuver. With flow-volume loops, it is possible to determine the peak inspiratory flow rate (PIFR), peak expiratory flow rate (PEFR), and forced expiratory flow rates (FEFRs). Flow-volume loops are useful in the diagnosis of small airways disease.[13]

Diffusion studies, which measure the numbers of functioning capillaries in contact with functioning alveoli, are used in the diagnosis of pulmonary vascular disease.[13] Many other types of specialized pulmonary function studies are available. Textbooks of pulmonary medicine should be consulted by readers wishing to learn additional details.

SPECIMEN COLLECTION

The type of specimen submitted for laboratory analysis is dictated by the information being sought. In all cases, clinical specimens must be collected, handled, and processed with adherence to universal precautions as outlined by the Centers for Disease Control and Prevention (CDC). The reader is referred to CDC publications for the specifics of universal precautions, which can be accessed through the CDC web site at: www.cdc.gov/ncidod/hip/blood/UNIVERSAL.HTM.

Generally, each specimen must be collected in a clean specimen container appropriate to the test being requested. All specimens for culture and sensitivity must be collected in the appropriate sterile container, preferably prior to the initiation of antibiotic therapy. Many tests have special specimen collection requirements, and the advice of the laboratory should be sought prior to collecting the specimen. As common sense suggests, all specimens need to be delivered to the laboratory as soon as possible after collection. The sooner a specimen arrives in the laboratory, the sooner testing begins and the sooner results are made available. Generally speaking, the longer a specimen waits before testing is completed, the less likely that the quality of results obtained from the specimen will be good.

Body Fluids

Whole blood is collected in blood collection tubes or syringes that contain the appropriate anticoagulant to inhibit coagulation. Routine hematology tests require a purple-top blood collection tube containing EDTA, a chelating anticoagulant. EDTA preserves the morphology of the cellular elements of blood, making it a satisfactory anticoagulant for hematological studies. Green-top blood collection tubes contain heparin, which stabilizes the red blood cell membranes. These tubes are used for specialized hematology studies, such as red cell fragility tests and several specialized chemistry tests. Light-blue-top blood collection tubes contain sodium citrate and are used for coagulation studies.

Clotted blood is obtained in red-top and red-speckled–top blood collection tubes, which contain a silicon coating and a serum separator, respectively. The blood collected into these tubes is allowed to clot for 15 to 30 minutes prior to centrifugation. Once centrifuged, the serum is separated from the clotted red blood cell mass. Serum specimens are required for routine chemistry, serology, and blood bank tests.

Blood for culture and sensitivity must be collected by aseptic technique into a sterile syringe. Once the blood has been drawn into the syringe, the syringe is withdrawn from the patient's vein, and the needle is replaced with a new, sterile, large-bore needle. The culture bottles are inoculated directly from the syringe, each with 5 mL of blood. Alternatively, blood may be collected by aseptic technique into yellow-top blood collection tubes that contain transport growth media. Two yellow-top tubes are needed for each blood culture requested. The inoculated blood culture bottles or yellow-top tubes must be delivered promptly to the microbiology laboratory. See Table 13-3 for a summary of blood collection tubes.

Table 13-3	Blood Collection Tubes	
Color of Container Top	**Additive/Anticoagulant**	**Uses**
Red	Silicon coating, no anticoagulant	Serum studies
Red speckled	Serum separator, no anticoagulant	Serum studies
Purple	EDTA anticoagulant	Hematology studies, special chemistry
Light blue	Sodium citrate anticoagulant	Coagulation studies
Green	Heparin anticoagulant	Special hematology and special chemistry
Gray	Sodium fluoride additive	Glucose, ethanol
Yellow	Liquid growth media	Blood culture

Many other types of blood collection tubes are available for an array of special tests. The PA is advised to consult the laboratory before collecting any blood test specimen that may require specialized collection procedures.

Urine is collected in a clean specimen container for routine urinalysis, either by having the patient void into the container or by pouring the urine from a bedpan or catheter collection bag into the specimen container. Urine for culture and sensitivity must be collected by aseptic technique. The patient is instructed to cleanse the genital area around the urethral meatus and then to collect the midstream portion of the urine. The first morning specimen is always preferred for any urine test. Urine specimens are collected for 24 hours for a variety of chemical analyses. For most 24-hour urine specimens, some type of preservative is added to the specimen container. The laboratory should be consulted for specific preservative requirements. All urine specimens must be refrigerated until delivered to the laboratory, to prevent bacterial overgrowth. As with any specimen, prompt delivery to the laboratory is essential for maintaining the quality of the specimen.

Cerebrospinal fluid is collected by standard lumbar puncture, under sterile conditions, into sterile specimen containers provided in lumbar puncture kits. The CSF must be transported to the laboratory within 5 to 10 minutes of collection for immediate analysis. A CSF specimen should never be allowed to sit at the patient's bedside. Likewise, it should not be refrigerated prior to microbiological culture and

staining for microorganisms because many of the causative organisms of meningitis are fastidious and fragile in suboptimal conditions outside the body. Protein, glucose, cell counts, and other enzymatic or serological tests of CSF are not adversely affected by refrigeration.

Semen is collected by the patient into a sterile specimen container. The patient must be advised to deliver the semen specimen to the laboratory within 20 minutes of collection to allow for accurate evaluation of motility, viscosity, and viability of the sperm. The specimen should be kept as close to body temperature as possible during transport and is never refrigerated.

Stool specimens are collected into wide-mouth containers appropriate to the volume of stool required for testing. Specimens for ova and parasites and for stool culture are collected into standard-sized, sterile specimen containers. These specimens are best delivered to the laboratory within an hour of collection and should not be refrigerated unless lengthy delay is anticipated. Stool specimens collected for 24 hours for fecal fat evaluation are put in wide-mouth, clean, gallon-sized metal containers with tight-fitting lids; refrigeration is recommended.

Synovial, thoracentesis, and *paracentesis fluids* are collected by sterile technique in sterile containers of appropriate size. If synovial fluid is submitted to the laboratory in the aspirating syringe, the needle must be removed and the syringe capped prior to transport of the specimen to prevent accidental percutaneous injury. These specimens may be refrigerated unless culture for anaerobic organisms is requested.

Surgical and Postmortem Specimens

Surgical specimens are collected during an operation by the surgical team under sterile conditions. Each specimen is placed in a sterile container and is delivered to the laboratory by the circulating nurse or another surgical team member immediately upon completion of the surgical procedure. At times, biopsy specimens are collected and are taken to the laboratory during operation for immediate examination by the pathologist. The surgical procedure is completed once the pathologist confirms the tissue diagnosis.

Postmortem specimens are collected by the pathologist or the pathology assistant during a postmortem examination. Blood, body fluids, tissue, and body secretions may be submitted for examination.

Body Secretions

Sputum is collected from the patient, who is instructed to deeply and forcefully cough to expectorate the lung secretions into the sterile specimen container. The patient should avoid contaminating the sputum with secretions from the oropharynx. Patients who have tracheotomies or are on artificial ventilation may be suctioned for collection of sputum specimens.

Exudates are collected from sites as close as possible to the suspected source of infection. When a swab is used to obtain exudative material, it is important that the swab remain moist to prevent desiccation of the bacterial organisms. Swabs may be used to collect exudate from the skin, pharynx, urethra, cervix, rectum, or wound. Routine exudate specimens may be refrigerated; however, when anaerobic or gonococcal infection is suspected, refrigeration should be avoided.

Gonococcal specimens should be collected on a sterile swab and immediately inoculated onto room temperature, specialized growth plates such as those containing Thayer-Martin or Martin-Lewis agar. The swab is gently rolled in a Z pattern over the surface of the agar to inoculate the plate. The agar plate is then placed in an airtight plastic bag containing a carbon dioxide pellet. Once the bag is securely closed, the pellet is crushed, releasing CO_2 into the bag. The specimen is then delivered promptly to the microbiology laboratory for incubation at 37°C.

The following case history demonstrates the proper use of clinical laboratory and diagnostic procedures for diagnosis and management.

■ CASE STUDY 13-3

A 28-year-old white male surgical technician, without significant PMH, presents complaining of nausea and vomiting for 2 days, accompanied by anorexia, fever, myalgias, and fatigue. He has also noted that his urine has been darker than normal for the past week. He denies weight loss, photophobia, cough, coryza, and change in stool color or bowel habit. He denies a PMH and family history of hepatitis, cholecystitis, peptic ulcer disease, renal calculi, and pyelonephritis. He admits to smoking one pack of cigarettes per day for 12 years, drinking a six-pack of beer every weekend, and engaging in protected oral and vaginal intercourse with two female partners two to three times per week. He denies intravenous drug use, homosexual activity, and recent percutaneous needle-stick injury at work. He also denies hepatitis B vaccination.

On physical examination, the patient appears his stated age, well developed, well nourished, diaphoretic, flushed, alert and oriented to person, place, time, and purpose, and in no apparent respiratory distress. Vital signs: blood pressure, 130/76 in both arms, and pulse, 104/min and regular, while seated; blood pressure, 126/78 in the right arm, and pulse, 104/min standing; respirations, 20/min, shallow and unlabored; weight, 80 kg; height, 170 cm. Conjunctivae moist, slightly icteric bilaterally. Buccal mucosa is pink and moist, without jaundice. Cervical lymph nodes are palpable, approximately 1 cm in size, mobile, smooth, and slightly tender throughout. Lungs are resonant to percussion and have vesicular breath sounds bilaterally at the bases on auscultation. Heart examination reveals a bounding PMI, not sustained, 1 cm in diameter in the left midclavicular line in the 5th intercostal space, with an apical rate of 104/min and a regularly, regular rhythm.

No lift, heave, pulsation, murmur, rub, or gallop is noted. Abdominal examination reveals a flat, nondistended, symmetrical abdominal wall with slightly hyperactive bowel sounds in all quadrants. The liver span measures 12 cm in the right mid-clavicular line by percussion. Tenderness is elicited over the liver during percussion. The abdomen is soft, with right upper quadrant guarding and tenderness to palpation. The liver edge is smooth and tender, palpable 3 cm below the right costal margin without masses or nodules. The spleen and kidneys are nonpalpable. No masses are palpated in other quadrants. No rebound tenderness is noted. Rectal examination reveals a smooth rectal wall and a symmetrical, nonenlarged prostate. No masses or tenderness are noted. Stool test for occult blood is negative. Initial laboratory results are as follows (normal indices shown in parentheses):

Aspartate transaminase (AST)	428 IU/L (0-36 IU/L)
Alanine transaminase (ALT)	353 IU/L (4-24 IU/L)
Total bilirubin	5.4 mg/dL (0.5-1.5 mg/dL)
Alkaline phosphatase (AP)	90 IU/L (20-90 IU/L)
Total protein (6.5–8.0 g/dL)	6.8 g/dL
Albumin (3.5-5.5 g/dL)	4.8 g/dL
PT	11 sec (11 sec)
WBC	4.8×10^3/cu mm ($5\text{-}10.0 \times 10^3$/cu mm)
Polymorphonuclear neutrophils (PMNs)	48%
Lymphocytes	35%
Monocytes	6%
Eosinophils	2%
Atypical lymphocytes	9%

Serological tests for hepatitis B surface antigen (HBsAg) and hepatitis B envelope antigen (HBeAg) are positive; those for anti-HBsAb and anti-HBeAb are negative.

This patient has presented with fairly typical signs and symptoms of viral hepatitis, which are confirmed by laboratory identification of hepatitis antigen markers. Additionally, the functional impairment of the liver is assessed by liver function studies. The patient should undergo repeat studies during the recovery period to evaluate his immune response. Hepatitis antibodies should appear as the hepatitis B antigens are cleared from the circulation. Until the immune system begins producing antibodies, the serum protein level will remain in the normal range; upon antibody production, there will be a slight increase in the total protein level, with a normal albumin fraction indicating an increase in the globulin portion of the proteins. The prothrombin time, another protein produced by the liver, should remain in the normal range throughout the acute illness. An increasing PT is a sign of chronic hepatic injury and hepatocellular dysfunction. The levels of liver enzymes—ALT and AST—as well as the byproduct of hemoglobin metabolism—bilirubin—should decrease to the normal range over several weeks as evidence of decreasing hepatocellular damage and patient recovery. Serial evaluation of liver function tests is indicated to assess the recovery of normal hepatic function.

INTERPRETATION OF DIAGNOSTIC STUDIES

The valid use of diagnostic studies requires an approach to their interpretation. To understand the value of a diagnostic result, the PA must apply a few basic principles of statistics and probability in relation to the clinical findings for a given patient. The first concept is that of normal value ranges. Normal values represent 95%, or ±2 standard deviations (SD), of a normal population, without regard to the prevalence of a disease. This means that 5% (or the 2.5% at each end of the spectrum of results—the third standard deviation) of the normal population will have an "abnormal" test result (Figure 13-1).

A further caveat regarding "normal" values and the interpretation of diagnostic studies relates to the increasing probability that the more tests that are performed on an individual patient, the greater will be the number of "abnormal" results. Recall that for one test, 5% of the normal population will fall outside the "normal" range of ±2 standard deviations. Thus, the probability of an abnormal result in the absence of disease for one test is 5%. For 20 tests, as in a biochemical profile, the probability of having at least one abnormal test result is 64%. In clinical terms, this

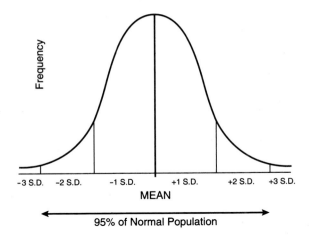

Figure 13-1 Normal range distribution graph.

means that when 20 tests are performed for one patient, the chance that all 20 test results will be "normal" is only 36%! According to Fernandes,[17] "In published studies, these abnormal test results that do not reflect disease have been calculated to be as high as a third of (all) biochemical screening." In evidence-based medicine, this is the rationale for limiting broad-based screening profiles and recommending that only specific studies be used based on the findings in the patient's history and physical examination.

To apply this concept to the interpretation of test results, the PA must use caution and review the clinical data obtained from the history, physical examination, and prior medical records where applicable. Often the presence of a single abnormal test result is truly without clinical significance and does not represent disease in a given patient. When this is the case, and all other parameters of the clinical evaluation are unremarkably normal, the "abnormal" test is typically repeated once and then periodically followed up as clinically warranted. It is important to note that an "abnormal" result in the range of ±3 standard deviations is not usually in the extreme of abnormal; rather, it tends to be just outside the normal range.

To demonstrate this point, consider a patient who has one abnormal result on the biochemical profile—a lactate dehydrogenase (LDH) value that falls outside the normal range (±2 SD). Recall that the enzyme LDH is found in a variety of places, such as the heart, lungs, liver, kidneys, and muscle. In the absence of clinical symptoms or signs and without any other abnormal results, such as an elevation in AST or alkaline phosphatase, it is highly unlikely that the "abnormal" LDH value represents clinical disease.

The limitations of diagnostic testing are summarized in terms of the sensitivity and specificity and positive predictive value for a given test. *Sensitivity* is "the incidence of true positive results obtained when the tests apply to a group known to have the disease."[17] *Specificity* is the "incidence of true negative results when the test is applied to a group known to be free of the disease."[17] In essence, a test result may fall into one of four categories—true-positive, false-positive, true-negative, or false-negative (Table 13-4). True-positive results represent a positive test result in persons with a disease; the sensitivity of a given study is the number of true-positive test results. False-positive results are abnormal results in persons without disease. True-negative results are those results within the normal range or negative in persons without disease. The specificity of a given test is the rate of true-negative results. Finally, false-negative results fall within the normal range or are negative in persons with disease.

Table 13-4 Categories of Test Results

	True	**False**
Positive	Positive result when disease is present = sensitivity	Positive result when no disease is present
Negative	Negative result when no disease is present = specificity	Negative result when disease is present

The clinical effects of false-positive results include inappropriate diagnoses and, frequently, extensive diagnostic workups. Occult blood testing of stool is notorious for false-positive results. Patients should be instructed to avoid red meat in their diet and to discontinue iron supplementation for several days prior to stool testing in an effort to decrease the number of false-positive results. The false-positive occult blood test result may, however, lead to evaluation via barium enema or colonoscopy.

False-negative results, in which case the diagnostic studies have failed to detect the given disease, may lead to a missed diagnosis if the diagnostic testing results are weighed more heavily than the history and physical findings. Accepting the two types of limitations that false-negative results place on interpretation of the clinical picture is essential to accurate and timely patient management. For example, rheumatological diseases such as the arthritides are commonly present for several years before any diagnostic studies yield positive results because the abnormal substances causing disease are present in quantities too minute for detection by the studies. The clinical diagnosis is therefore based on the clinical findings and the expertise of the clinician. When the abnormal substances eventually become detectable by diagnostic studies, the positive results confirm the clinical diagnosis.

Another limitation that false-negative results place on diagnostic studies is caused by interference factors. Echocardiographic and radiographic studies are known to yield false-negative results in patients who are morbidly obese; thus, the diagnostic studies are of limited value and have the potential to miss significant findings. For example, a morbidly obese male is admitted to the hospital for a fever of unknown origin (FUO). The patient is evaluated for endocarditis by a routine echocardiogram at the urging of the infectious disease fellow because of clinical evidence of microembolism. The echocardiogram is negative, and the workup for the FUO continues for several days as the patient succumbs to the disease. On autopsy, an enormous fungal vegetation is found in the aortic root. Excessive focus on the falsely negative echocardiogram combined with too little acknowledgment of the clinical findings and progressive deterioration of the patient's clinical status led to an early death for this patient.

To increase the utility of interpretation of diagnostics, the clinician needs to consider the positive predictive value of a diagnostic test in conjunction with the prevalence of the disease being sought. *Positive predictive value* is the probability that a positive result will be correct. The positive predictive value increases when the disease prevalence is high and the sensitivity and specificity of a given test are held constant. (*Prevalence* is the number of persons per 100,000 who have the disease; *incidence,* with which prevalence is often confused, is the number of new cases of the disease per year.[17]) The following classic examples of positive predictive value and disease prevalence illustrate their importance to the interpretation of diagnostic studies.

If a disease is found in a population of 10,000 at a rate of 10%, and the sensitivity and specificity of the study are each 90%, then the positive predictive value of the study is 50%. This number is derived from the number of true-positive test results (a positive result in a person known to have the disease) divided by the number of total positive results (true-positives plus false-positives). If the disease prevalence is only 0.1% in a population of 10,000, however, with the sensitivity and specificity again held constant at 90% each, the positive predictive value of the study will be 0.9%.[5] See Table 13-5.

The clinical significance of positive predictive values lies in the impact that a positive test result has on the patient's physical and psychological well-being, the expense of additional diagnostic studies, and clinical management. When there is disease prevalence of 10%, half of the patients with a positive result will be falsely labeled as having a disease. If the same study is applied to a population with 0.1% disease prevalence, then the number of persons incorrectly labeled by a positive test result will be 999 of 1008, or 99%. Conversely, the number of true-positive results found is 9 of 1008, or 0.9%. In clinical terms, the positive result in a member of a population with 0.1% disease prevalence is more likely to represent health rather than disease.

Table 13-5   Relation of Positive Predictive Values of a Test With Disease Prevalence

	Disease Prevalence of 10%		Disease Prevalence of 0.1%	
	Positive (+) Result	**Negative (−) Result**	**Positive (+) Result**	**Negative (−) Result**
Disease present	900 (true +)	100 (false −)	9 (true +)	1 (false −)
Disease absent	900 (false +)	8100 (true −)	999 (false +)	8991 (true −)
Totals	1800	8200	1008	8992
Positive predictive value*		900/1800 = 50%		9/1008 = 0.9%

*Positive predictive value $= \dfrac{\text{No. true + results}}{\text{Total no. + results}}$.

CONCLUSION

The utilization of diagnostic studies is essential to the practice of medicine. Study selection and interpretation require knowledge of available tests, astute clinical reasoning skills, and the ability to interpret the results within the limitations of the tests. Factors such as cost containment, the effects of study results on patient management, and the risk-benefit ratio of performing diagnostic studies are imperative considerations for the thorough clinician in the practice of evidence-based medicine.

As in all areas of medicine, advances and newer technologies in diagnostic studies continue to accrue rapidly. For clinicians, both the neophytes and the seasoned, technological advances offer an opportunity to provide high-quality patient care, with the challenge to balance the effects of testing on the patient and on society at large. Responsible, educated utilization of diagnostic studies is the goal for competent health care providers of the 21st century.

CLINICAL APPLICATIONS

1. Discuss the periodic diagnostic evaluation of a patient with a known diagnosis of diabetes mellitus. Consider costs and effects on management in your deliberations.
2. Outline the workup for each category of anemia:
   ANEMIA WITH NORMAL MCV
   ANEMIA WITH MCV <80
   ANEMIA WITH MCV >110
3. What is a cost-effective approach to the diagnostic evaluation of tender versus nontender hepatomegaly? Review common causes of each clinical problem prior to outlining the diagnostic approach.

REFERENCES

1. Heffler S, Smith S, et al. Health spending projections for 2001-2011: the latest outlook. Health Affairs 2002;21:207.
2. Epstein AM, McNeil BJ. Variations in ambulatory test use: what do they mean? Medical Clinics of North America 1987;71:705.
3. American College of Emergency Physicians. Guidelines for Cost-Containment on Emergency Medicine. Dallas: American College of Emergency Physicians, 1983.
4. Sox H (ed). Common Diagnostic Tests: Use and Interpretation. Philadelphia: American College of Physicians, 1987.
5. Woolf SH. Practice guidelines: a new reality in medicine. II: Methods of developing guidelines. Archives of Internal Medicine 1992;152:946.
6. Mushlin AI, Ruchlin HS, Callahan MA. Cost effectiveness of diagnostic tests. The Lancet 2001;358:1353.
7. Sackett DL, Straus SE, et al. Evidence-Based Medicine: How to Practice and Teach EBM, ed 2. Edinburgh: Churchill Livingstone, 2000.
8. Knottnerus JA, van Weel C, Muris WM. Evaluation of diagnostic procedures. British Medical Journal 2002; 324:477.
9. Woolf SH, Kamerow DB. Testing for uncommon conditions: the heroic search for positive test results. Archives of Internal Medicine 1990;150:2451.

10. Statland BE, Winkel P. Utilization review and management of laboratory testing in the ambulatory setting. Medical Clinics of North America 1987;71:719.

11. Labus JB, Lauber AA. Patient Education and Preventive Medicine. Philadelphia: WB Saunders, 2001.

12. Henry JB (ed). Clinical Diagnosis and Management by Laboratory Methods, ed 20. Philadelphia: WB Saunders, 2001.

13. Fischbach FT. A Manual of Laboratory and Diagnostic Tests, ed 6. Philadelphia: Lippincott, Williams and Wilkins, 2000.

14. Irwin K, Olivo N, et al. Performance characteristics of a rapid HIV antibody assay in a hospital with a high prevalence of HIV infection. Annals of Internal Medicine 1996;125:471.

15. Squire LF, Novelline RA. Squire's Fundamentals of Radiology, ed 5. Cambridge, MA: Harvard University Press, 1997.

16. Newhouse JH, Wiener JI. Understanding MRI. Boston: Little, Brown, 1991.

17. Fernandes JJ. Realistic expectations of laboratory testing. Journal of the American Osteopathic Association 1991;91:1223.

RESOURCES

Henry JB (ed). Clinical Diagnosis and Management by Laboratory Methods, ed 20. Philadelphia: WB Saunders, 2001. *This classic textbook of clinical laboratory medicine includes basic principles of laboratory science and the methodologies of testing for all areas of the clinical laboratory. Clinical interpretations of abnormal test results are discussed.*

Fischbach FT. A Manual of Laboratory and Diagnostic Tests, ed 6. Philadelphia: Lippincott, Williams and Wilkins, 2000. *The clinically oriented text is organized by subdivisions of the clinical laboratory. A discussion of each diagnostic study includes a brief explanation of the test in terms of basic physiology and pathophysiology. The indications, procedure, and normal values are given for each test.*

Squire LF, Novelline RA. Squire's Fundamentals of Radiology, ed 5. Cambridge, MA: Harvard University Press, 1997. *A classic introduction to radiology for medical education. The text introduces the basic principles of radiology and offers easily understood explanations of radiographic concepts. Photographs and case histories enhance the text.*

Wallach JB. Interpretation of Diagnostic Tests, ed 7. Philadelphia: Lippincott, Williams and Wilkins, 2000. *This text outlines the diagnostic study findings for individual diseases organized in an organ system approach.*

www.cdc.gov *The web site of the Centers for Disease Control and Prevention (CDC) provides access to news and documents, including guidelines for universal precautions.*

C H A P T E R   1 4

Clinical Procedures

Edward M. Sullivan

INTRODUCTION

The ability to perform clinical procedures is a necessary skill for practicing physician assistants (PAs) and PA students alike. Procedures often provide valuable information that may aid in the diagnosis and treatment of a patient's disease. No matter how routine and uncomplicated a clinical procedure may seem to a health care provider, it must always be regarded as a unique and personal experience for the patient.

Preparing the patient for the procedure both mentally and physically remains a challenge to all health care providers. Preparation skills must be developed and applied often. The PA must have a complete understanding of the procedure to be performed, a command of the anatomy, an attention to detail, and an awareness of the goal that is to be accomplished by each procedure.

A majority of all clinical procedures are painful in some way to the patient. Many times, the patient's ability to cope with a procedure lies in the sure hands of the clinician. A positive, gentle manner combined with a thoroughness in the explanation will instill confidence in the patient, as well as in the other health care providers assisting with the procedure. A patient who has a complete understanding of what is to be accomplished is much more likely to cooperate with specific requests and is better prepared to handle any difficulties that may be encountered. Finally, no matter how many times a PA or PA student may have performed a clinical procedure, he or she must keep in mind that it may be the first time for the patient, and that the better prepared the patient is, the more satisfying the outcome will be.

Mr. W, a 19-year-old male, was crossing the street outside the emergency department when he was struck by a car. He was transported to the emergency department, where the PA evaluated his injuries. In addition to multiple lacerations and contusions, internal bleeding was suspected. The patient was conscious. An intravenous line was started, heart monitoring was initiated, a urethral catheter was inserted, and blood was drawn for a complete blood count and other baseline studies. A computed tomography (CT) scan of the abdomen was negative. Based on the appearance of the injuries and the history and physical examination findings, x-rays were taken of both legs and ankles. A 4-cm laceration on the left lateral forearm was sutured, and multiple other superficial lacerations were irrigated and closed with Steri-Strips (Life-Assist, Inc., Rancho Cordova, California).

The PA talked to Mr. W about each step and asked if Mr. W would like to have someone called to come to the hospital. Mr. W's father arrived at the emergency department within 30 minutes. The PA explained the nature of Mr. W's injuries and the plan to admit him to the hospital for repair of a compound fracture of the left tibia.

WOUNDS AND THEIR TREATMENT

Any consideration of an invasive clinical procedure must begin with an understanding of wounds and their healing process. This chapter provides only a brief overview of wounds because a detailed explanation of the biochemistry is beyond the scope of this discussion. The resource list at the end of the chapter provides sources for more comprehensive study and an in-depth discussion of specific types of wounds.

Definitions

A *wound* can be defined as any break in the normal anatomical relationship of tissues. Wounds can be classified as *internal* (those inside the skin) and *external* (those involving the skin). This chapter concentrates on external wounds because of their relationship to the performance of clinical procedures.

Wounds caused by any clinical or surgical procedure are classified, according to degree of contamination and risk for infection, as clean, clean-contaminated, contaminated, or dirty, as follows:

➤ *Clean:* A clean wound is typically a surgical incision made under sterile conditions. For the most part, wounds caused by clinical procedures are performed under sterile conditions and therefore can be considered clean.

➤ *Clean-contaminated:* A wound that begins as a clean wound but has experienced a potential source of contamination is clean-contaminated. One example is the opening of the colon during a bowel anastomosis. In this case, special precautions should be initiated to prevent spillage.

➤ *Contaminated:* A contaminated wound may have begun as a clean wound or may have been made under nonsterile conditions and has a greater incidence of infection. Some examples are a knife or glass laceration, the bowel opened during an operation with spillage of the contents into the surrounding sterile tissue, and the opening of an abscess, whether accidentally or by design, without containment of the enclosed infected material.

➤ *Dirty:* A dirty wound is one that begins in any form other than those previously described.

Wound Healing

Wounds heal by forming scars. The process of forming scars is traditionally divided into three main phases:
1. Inflammatory or exudative phase.
2. Fibroplastic or proliferative phase.
3. Maturation phase.

Inflammatory or Exudative Phase   Wound healing begins immediately after an injury has occurred to otherwise normal tissue. The inflammatory phase, which usually lasts 2 to 4 days, serves to cleanse the wound of dead tissue and foreign objects by a sequence of physiological and biochemical events, beginning with an immediate vasoconstriction to minimize blood loss. This vasoconstriction is brief, lasting approximately 10 minutes, and is followed by a histamine-induced vasodilatation and a migrating of leukocytes into the wound. Serum enters the wound from gaps between endothelial cells, aiding the activation of platelets, kinin, complement, and prostaglandin components of the clotting cascade. Lymphatics are blocked by dilating venules. Polymorphonuclear neutrophils (PMNs) and mononuclear leukocytes (MONOs) are then deposited into the wound to begin the cleaning process.

Hemostatic Factors   The hemostatic factors of wound healing are all activated within the first 1 to 2 minutes after an injury. One of the first is the *activation of platelets,* which adhere to one another and to the edges of the wound, forming a plug that attempts to cover the wound. This plug or clot soon retracts and stops the loss of blood. The kinins are a group of polypeptides that influence smooth muscle contraction, which induces hypotension. Additionally, they increase the permeability of small blood capillaries, serving to increase the amount of blood flow, which in turn increases the amounts of other hemostatic factors previously mentioned.

Another hemostatic factor is *complement.* Its main job is to produce bacteriolysis and hemolysis by accumulating fluid within a cell, causing it to eventually rupture. *Prostaglandin* acts to increase vasomotor tone, capillary permeability, smooth muscle tone, and the aggregation of platelets. *Fibronectin* aids in the migration of neutrophils, monocytes, fibroblasts, and endothelial cells into the wound and also promotes the ability of these cells to adhere to one another, creating a framework of fibrin fibers. Fibronectin is found in abundance within the first 48 hours, gradually decreasing as protein synthesis begins to produce the collagen fibers that will eventually be the scar. The wound appears red and swollen and is painful and warm to the touch at this stage.

Fibroplastic or Proliferative Phase   The second phase of wound healing can begin only when the wound is covered by epithelium. This phase begins on or about the third day after an injury and continues for approximately 24 days. An injured patient must have a normal amount of circulating calcium (Ca), platelets, and tissue factor in order for the second

phase to begin. If these three substances are present as blood is exposed to air, prothrombin will be converted to thrombin. Thrombin acts as a catalyst in the conversion of fibrinogen to fibrin fibers, which stabilize the clot.

Fibroblasts are normally located in the perivascular tissue, and once they get into the wound, they produce several substances essential to wound repair, ending with the formation of collagen fibers. *Collagen* is the principal structural protein found in tendons, ligaments, and fasciae. Arranged in bundles, it strengthens and supports these tissues. Collagen levels rise continuously for approximately 3 weeks and have a negative feedback mechanism related to the number of fibroblasts found in the wound. As collagen increases, the number of fibroblasts decreases, eventually causing a decrease in the production of collagen. The rapid gain in tensile strength during this phase is directly related to the remodeling of collagen from a randomly arranged fiber mesh to a more organized formation of fibers that respond to the local stress found at the wound site.

At this stage, although less swollen, inflamed, and painful, the wound may look its worst. The scar may appear beefy red and may feel hard and raised. This is normal and should be expected. If the wound remains painful and inflamed at this stage of the healing process, however, some foreign material may have been retained, and re-exploration may be warranted.

Maturation Phase   During this third phase of wound healing, metabolic activity remains high, but there is no increase in collagen production. This phase is sometimes referred to as the "remodeling phase" because of the rearrangement of the collagen fibers from their initial haphazard appearance after production to one of more organization. This pattern is determined by the anatomical location of the wound and the amount of stress placed on the skin and the scar at that location.

This phase usually begins at 3 weeks and can be active for a year or longer, depending on the health status of the person. The appearance of the scar becomes less conspicuous. It begins to flatten out and gradually begins to resemble normal skin tissue. The scar becomes more supple and more permanent as the cross-links of collagen are reorganized.

Factors That Affect Wound Healing

The health of an individual can greatly affect the time involved in the healing of a wound. Proper wound closure is paramount to the successful healing of an injury, but many other factors influence this process. The surgical technique, the type of injury, the degree of contamination, and the health status and biochemical makeup of the patient all play important roles in the final outcome of an injury. Suturing and other techniques of wound closure are discussed later in the chapter, but first, some consideration of the biochemical factors and the health status of an individual with a wound is warranted. Some of the factors that directly relate to the healing process are as follows:

➤ *Oxygen:* Fibroblasts are very closely related to the partial pressure of oxygen (Po_2) in the circulating blood. A Po_2 of less than 30 mm Hg severely retards the healing process by lowering the production of collagen in the cytoplasm of the fibroblast. Disease processes such as small vessel atherosclerosis, chronic infection, and diabetes mellitus can be greatly affected by the oxygen delivery system.

➤ *Hematocrit:* There must be an adequate supply of hemoglobin in the blood to carry oxygen to the tissues.

➤ *Steroids (anti-inflammatory):* Steroids slow the inflammatory phase of the healing process by inhibiting macrophages and fibrogenesis. Anabolic steroids and vitamin A, on the other hand, can reverse the effects of anti-inflammatory drugs by restoring the monocytic inflammation process of the wound.

➤ *Vitamin C:* Vitamin C is important to the maturation process of fibroblasts.

➤ *Vitamin E:* In large doses, vitamin E can decrease the tensile strength of a wound by lowering the accumulation of collagen.

➤ *Zinc:* Epithelial and fibroplastic proliferation is slowed in patients exhibiting a low serum zinc level.

➤ *Anti-inflammatory agents:* Aspirin and ibuprofen decrease collagen synthesis in a dose-related fashion.

➤ *Age:* Both tensile strength and wound closure rates decrease as a person ages.

➤ *Mechanical stress:* Wounds involving the skin over joints, where the stresses are greatly increased by normal usage, take longer to heal. The delay is due to the constant stretching and tearing of the collagen mesh, which results in re-initiation of the entire wound-healing process.

➤ *Nutrition:* Poor nutrition results in absence of the essential building blocks of protein for collagen production, prolonging the inflammatory phase and inhibiting fibroplasia. Glucose supplies energy for leukocytes to function. Fats are necessary for synthesis of new cells.

➤ *Hydration:* A well-hydrated wound, not a wet wound, epithelializes faster than a dry wound. Keeping a wound covered by a dressing enhances the humidity of the wound and speeds the healing process.

➤ *Environmental temperature:* Wound-healing time is shortened by environmental temperatures greater than 30° C. Wound-healing time can increase by as much as 20% in temperatures of 12° C or less, owing to vasoconstriction and lowering of the capillary blood supply.

➤ *Denervation:* Denervated skin is less susceptible to local temperatures and more prone to ulceration. Paralytics develop massive, rapidly destructive ulcers that can be five times worse than in the patient with an intact nervous system.

➤ *Infection:* The ability of local tissue defenses to cleanse the wound is greatly diminished by a larger number of pathogenic organisms. Infection prolongs the inflammatory phase of the healing process.

➤ *Idiopathic manipulation:* Overhandling and rough handling of tissue by health care providers along with tight sutures can result in tissue ischemia and poor healing.

➤ *Chemotherapy:* Anticancer drugs decrease the fibroblast proliferation.

➤ *Radiation therapy:* Acute radiation injury is manifested by stasis and occlusion of small vessels, resulting in the formation of ulcers at the point of ischemia.

➤ *Diabetes mellitus:* Defective leukocyte function and microvascular occlusion may occur secondary to hyperglycemia in diabetes mellitus. High glucose levels interfere with the ability of cells to transport ascorbic acid, resulting in a decrease in the production of collagen.

Tensile Strength All the factors just described can affect the tensile strength of a wound during the healing process. *Tensile strength* is defined as the greatest force a substance can bear without tearing apart. The tensile strength of a wound is directly related to time, and is very low for approximately the first 3 weeks following an injury and a primary closure. Extreme care must be taken to protect the newly formed scar from re-injury at this time. The strength of the wound increases rapidly during the early stages of the maturation phase as the collagen fibers are rearranged and simplified according to the mechanical stresses applied to the scar. Although the wound needs 6 to 7 additional months of maturing before the final cosmetic result should be evaluated, the scar no longer gains strength after the maturation phase.

Wound Anesthesia

Injection of a local anesthetic for painless clinical and minor surgical procedures is an important tool that is readily available and easy to use. The ability to remove the pain whenever a clinical procedure is warranted not only provides a sense of relief for the patient but gives the practitioner the option to perform the procedure at his or her own pace. This option minimizes the cost and time commitment and usually results in a more favorable outcome for both the patient and the clinician. Local anesthetic agents have redefined the "office procedure," making it a significant alternative to hospitalization. Suturing of minor lacerations and the performance of office-based clinical procedures are the hallmark of PA practice. Therefore, a good understanding of these agents and their properties is an important aspect of PA education. The practicing PA should have the knowledge and ability to perform clinical procedures wherever and whenever possible, thus enabling the physician to concentrate on the more seriously ill patients.

Anesthesia is used in a number of different ways. The most common is *local,* whereby just the area around the wound is anesthetized. A *hematoma block* is local anesthetic injected directly into a hematoma. This is primarily used in fractures where there is some internal bleeding around the fracture site. The anesthetic is allowed to filter throughout the surrounding tissue and fracture site. Once an adequate amount of anesthesia has been achieved, the fracture can be set. A *field block* is the injection of an anesthetic around a given surgical operative site. A *nerve block* targets a specific nerve at a distant site from the area of the proposed surgery. A *digital block* is used to numb an entire finger or toe. This is especially useful when a laceration of a finger or toe is massive and a local infiltration would result in increased swelling and a more difficult closure. The clinician injects anesthetic at the base of the finger or toe, usually a minimum of two injection sites, one on each side of the digit. Lastly, a *regional block* is used to anesthetize a large specific area; for instance, an epidural block (regional) allows the parturient patient to remain awake during the delivery of her child. A digital block may be referred to as a regional block in some instances. Regional blocks may affect the motor activity of the affected area.

The properties of the ideal local anesthetic are few and simple. It must be easy to administer and have a rapid onset. Its effect must last as long as needed for a given procedure, and it must dissolve completely, with no adverse effects or toxic effects either locally or systemically. Local anesthetics work by blocking depolarization of a nerve impulse. Of the numerous anesthetic agents available on the market today, lidocaine is probably the most widely used for local anesthesia. It is manufactured in a variety of solutions, but the two most commonly used for local anesthesia are 1% and 2%. One percent lidocaine works very well in blocking pain stimuli while leaving the sensations of touch and pressure relatively intact. Two percent lidocaine usually blocks all stimuli from a wound area.

Two other agents, procaine hydrochloride (Novocain) and bupivacaine hydrochloride (Marcaine), are well known and warrant some discussion. Novocain has a rapid onset, usually about 4 to 7 minutes, and lasts approximately 1 hour. Lidocaine has an equally rapid onset but may last approximately 3 hours. Marcaine takes longer to reach its anesthetic level but lasts up to 10 hours.

Choosing the right anesthetic for the wound takes a significant amount of skill that is developed with years of wound evaluation and experience. The clinician must also be aware of the possible complications involved in the use of these agents. Some general rules to avoid any complications are of value, and the safety of the patient should always be of primary concern, as with the use of any medication.

1. Use the least amount of local anesthetic to gain the maximum amount of anesthesia for a given wound.
2. Almost all the local anesthetic agents on the market today give the patient a sensation of burning on injection. Therefore, when injecting, go slow and wait for some of the anesthetic effects of the agent to begin working before continuing.
3. Always aspirate when attempting to inject an agent into the body. If there is a blood return, remove the needle and apply local pressure to ensure hemostasis.
4. Be aware of the signs of an allergic reaction, such as wheezing, hives, and hypotension. Always be prepared to support the airway with ventilations if necessary. Although a true allergic reaction to lidocaine is rare, extra precautions should be taken if the patient reports any history of this type of allergy.

The last area for potential complications concerns those local anesthetics that contain a vasoconstrictive agent. Epinephrine, in concentrations of 1:100,000 or 1:200,000, is most commonly used to prolong the effects of the local anesthetic. Because of its vasoconstrictive action, it may also be used to control or decrease bleeding. It is this use for which the potential for complications arises. The local anesthetics that contain epinephrine should *never* be used in areas of the body that have terminal vasculature, such as the ears, tip of the nose, fingers, penis, and toes. The vasoconstricting action can lead to tissue death and gangrene in such areas. There is also a higher potential for wound infection because prolonged vasoconstriction delays the highly effective cleansing agents from entering the wound. Adherence to meticulous

hemostasis is also important under these conditions to control the potential for increased bleeding once the effects of epinephrine wear off.

The anesthetics mentioned in this discussion are easy to use and readily available. The resource list at the end of this chapter provides in-depth studies of these agents.

Sutures

Numerous types and sizes of suture materials are available. A significant number of different sutures may be used to adequately repair any given wound. What type of suture should be used for what type of wound? What type of suture should be used on the face, and can that same suture be used on the leg, arm, or abdomen? Because of the confusion involving these issues, a brief explanation of sutures and their properties is warranted. The following discussion provides some general principles to help in the selection of a dependable suture for a specific area of the body and a specific type of wound.

Suture Types   Sutures can be divided into two categories—absorbable and nonabsorbable. Absorbable sutures may be either *natural* (e.g., plain catgut, chromic catgut) or *synthetic* (e.g., Vicryl, Dexon). Nonabsorbable sutures may be either *multifilament* (e.g., silk, cotton) or *monofilament* (e.g., nylon, propylene, stainless steel wire).

When evaluating a wound for primary closure, the clinician must keep in mind the ideal qualities of a suture and must choose the most appropriate suture for each particular wound. The ideal suture:

➤ Maintains adequate tensile strength until its purpose is served.
➤ Causes minimal tissue reaction.
➤ Avoids serving as a nidus for infection.
➤ Is nonallergenic and noncarcinogenic.
➤ Is easy to handle and tie.
➤ Holds knots well.
➤ Is inexpensive.
➤ Is easily sterilized.

Absorbable sutures should be used when the suture needs to function for a short time and cannot be recovered when its use is completed, as for the inner layer of a bowel anastomosis. The suture serves only to approximate the mucosa and to assist in temporary hemostasis until the body's hemostatic mechanism can secure permanent hemostasis and wound closure. The suture used most often for this type of anastomosis is catgut. Absorbable catgut sutures, which are obtained from the small intestine of cattle or sheep, excite an inflammatory response within the wound that eventually leads to their absorption. Plain catgut sutures lose approximately 50% of their initial tensile strength in just 7 days. Chromic tanning of plain catgut (chromic catgut), on the other hand, prolongs the absorptive time and the life of this suture to about 3 weeks. The synthetic absorbable sutures (Vicryl, Dexon) do not excite as extensive an inflammatory response. Their chief advantage is their uniform loss of tensile strength. Research has shown that these sutures lose their strength at a steady rate for about 21 days, at which time they have none.

Silk, throughout the years, has been the most commonly used nonabsorbable suture. It is easily obtained at a lower cost than the monofilaments and is comfortable to work with. Additionally, it holds knots securely. The major disadvantages of using silk include the following:

1. The tissue reaction it stimulates, which although less than that produced by catgut sutures, is more than that of the synthetic monofilaments.
2. Its construction as a multifilament.

A multifilament suture is made of many filaments or fibers intertwined, producing numerous interstices (spaces between the fibers) that when contaminated with bacteria serve as a continuous nidus for infection. The interstices are small enough to deter body host defenses but large enough for bacteria to multiply. Cotton suture has the same advantages and disadvantages as silk; however, cotton is slightly weaker than silk initially but maintains its tensile strength in the tissue for a longer period.

Monofilament sutures (nylon, propylene, stainless steel wire) share the advantages of prolonged high tensile strength, low tissue reaction, and lack of interstices. Their chief disadvantages are difficulties for the clinician in handling and tying knots. More throws (seven or eight) are required in a single knot in order to maintain its security. The monofilaments are also more expensive and are less readily available than silk and cotton.

Suture Sizes Suture sizes are expressed, in order of decreasing size, as follows: 2, 1, 0, 00 (2-0), 000 (3-0), 0000 (4-0), 00000 (5-0), and so forth. The larger sizes (2, 1) are used for heavy work (i.e., bone, retention sutures of the abdomen), whereas the smallest sutures (12-0 and smaller) are used exclusively in microvascular surgery.

Choice of Suture The question still remains: what type of suture should be used? Because of the numerous types and sizes of suture available to the clinician, the choice of suture for each specific purpose reverts to personal preference and wound closure experience. Because many possible different sutures can be used to close a wound, Table 14-1 is supplied as a general guide for the novice in choosing the type of suture according to the anatomical location of the wound. Multifilament sutures (silk) should not be used on the skin. The skin contains an overabundance of bacteria, and the interstices of the multifilament greatly increase the incidence of wound infection.

Retention Sutures A special type of suture that needs to be mentioned is the *retention suture,* which is placed as noted in Figure 14-1. Observe that the retention suture encompasses all of the abdominal wall layers. After placement, the retention sutures are tied over a skin bridge—usually a plastic, red rubber catheter—to prevent the suture from cutting into the skin and causing areas of skin necrosis. This type of suture is used to decrease the tension on a healing fascial wound in order to prevent dehiscence. A heavy (2, 1), nonabsorbable, monofilament suture is chosen and then is removed after an adequate period of healing, usually 3 to 4 weeks. Obviously, most wounds heal without retention sutures, and the judgment of the clinician dictates closure of the wound with this type of procedure. Patients at high risk of wound dehiscence are those with poor nutrition, cancer, diabetes, obesity, massive trauma, or long-term systemic steroid ingestion, and those in whom contamination occurs during surgery with a high likelihood of wound infection. In these patients, retention sutures are most often considered.

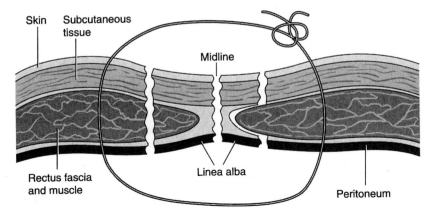

Figure 14-1 A retention suture must contain all layers of the abdominal wall from the peritoneum to the skin.

Table 14-1	Suture Size and Type According to Wound Location	
Location of Wound	**Suture Size**	**Suture Type**
Skin		
Face	5-0, 6-0	Nylon
Hands	4-0, 5-0	Nylon
Scalp	3-0, 4-0	Nylon
Extremities, abdomen	3-0, 4-0	Nylon
Subcutaneous tissue	3-0, 4-0	Vicryl, Dexon
Fascia	0	Prolene
	2-0	Stainless steel wire
	0	Surgilon
Peritoneum*	2-0, 3-0	Vicryl, Dexon
Bowel anastomosis		
Inner layer	3-0, 4-0	Catgut
Outer layer	3-0, 4-0	Silk, propylene

*The peritoneum is usually included with fascial suture but may be closed separately.

Suture Needles Two basic types of needles are used with suture material in surgery—tapered and cutting (Figure 14-2). A *tapered needle* has a sharp point and a round body. Tapered needles are much less traumatic than cutting needles. *Cutting needles* are beveled and have sharp, knifelike edges. A general rule is that cutting needles are used for skin suturing and tapered needles are used for most other tissues.

Sutures come prepackaged with a label telling the size, type, and length of the suture and the type

and size of the suture needle. Labels are usually color-coded according to the type of suture material contained.

Skin sutures should be removed when they have fulfilled their purpose. The longer sutures remain, the more inflammatory the response they elicit, which ultimately results in a larger, more noticeable scar. The clinician must weigh the odds of creating an unsightly scar against the chance of a wound dehiscence if the sutures are removed prematurely.

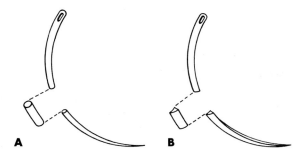

Figure 14-2 **A,** Tapered needle. **B,** Cutting needle.

The following is a guideline for when to remove sutures according to location:

Face	3-4 days
Scalp	5-7 days
Trunk	6-8 days
Extremities	7-14 days; longer for areas under maximal tension

Wound Closure

Wounds, however they are created, require proper and timely attention to facilitate the best possible outcome. As the clinician approaches a wound, whether it is a result of an accident or a specifically designed surgical incision, a few general principles can aid in deciding how best to close it. The history plays an important role in determining the cause of the wound and, moreover, the possibility of contamination. The history also reveals valuable information about the health status of the patient, which may influence the final decision on how the wound should be treated. Surgical wounds are almost always closed primarily because of the controlled atmosphere in which they are created. Acute, accidental wounds need much more evaluation prior to treatment. Often the decision focuses on the size and shape of a wound and the degree of contamination suspected.

Historically, there are three methods of treating wounds, and timing is the most critical aspect to consider when choosing among them.

Primary Closure The immediate suturing, stapling, or taping of a wound yields the best possible outcome (Figure 14-3). The two factors to consider in deciding whether a wound can be closed primarily are

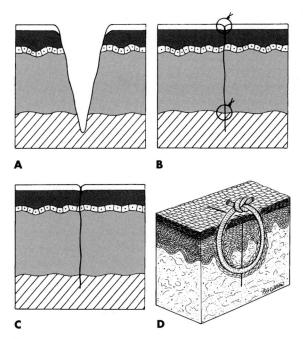

Figure 14-3 Primary wound closure. Closing a wound primarily—within the first 8 hours—will yield the least possible scarring. **A,** Simple laceration. **B** and **D,** Correct placement of a simple interrupted stitch. **C,** The best possible result of a laceration closed primarily. *(**A** and **C** from Westaby S. Wound Care. St Louis: CV Mosby, 1986; **D** from Schultz BC, McKinney P. Office Practice of Skin Surgery. Philadelphia: WB Saunders, 1985.)*

the amount of tissue loss and the degree of contamination. Clean, surgical wounds fall into this category, as well as lacerations from sharp objects, such as a glass, knife, or sharp piece of metal, in which there is almost no tissue loss and contamination is minimal. Generally, an accidental wound is not closed primarily if it is more than 8 hours old.

Delayed Primary Closure The wound is left open, usually because of a great amount of bacterial contamination. Through a process that is not fully understood, the wound develops a resistance to infection over the next 4 to 5 days (Figure 14-4). This development occurs only if the wound is cleansed of all foreign material and is loosely packed with a sterile dressing. The wound is then closed by approximation of the two sides using as little suture as possible.

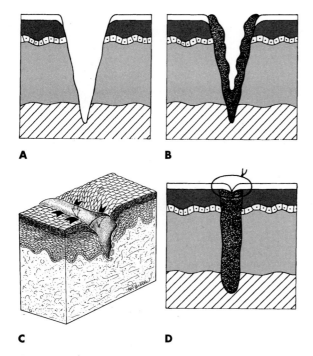

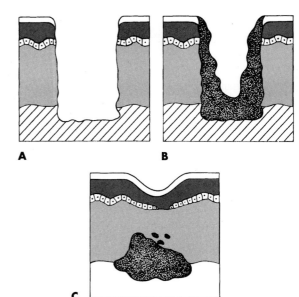

Figure 14-4 Delayed primary closure results in a larger and more noticeable scar. **A,** Simple laceration. **B** and **D,** The laceration is allowed to granulate. **C,** Correct placement of a simple interrupted stitch on the fourth or fifth day with the absence of any sign of infection. *(A, B, and D from Westaby S. Wound Care. St Louis: CV Mosby, 1986; C from Schultz BC, McKinney P. Office Practice of Skin Surgery. Philadelphia: WB Saunders, 1985.)*

Figure 14-5 Allowing a wound to heal secondarily is usually done if there is a large amount of tissue loss or an overabundance of bacterial contamination. **A,** Wound with a large amount of tissue loss. **B,** The wound is allowed to granulate completely until **(C)** epithelialization covers the entire area, which may take weeks or months. *(From Westaby S. Wound Care. St Louis: CV Mosby, 1986.)*

Healing by Secondary Intention A wound treated by secondary intention typically involves a large amount of tissue loss or heavy contamination by bacteria. In this case, the wound closes by the process of epithelialization and contraction rather than any type of suturing (Figure. 14-5). The wound is carefully observed throughout the healing process, which may take weeks or months. All wounds heal in this manner if they can remain free of bacteria and no fistula or sinus tract develops. The cosmetic result of this type of closure is extremely poor, however, and may require numerous trips to a plastic surgeon.

Wound Suture

The principles of wound suturing are few and simple. Ideally, when the clinician is evaluating a wound for primary closure, he or she wants to produce the best possible result with the least amount of pain by using the most appropriate material with the least financial cost to the patient. A person's skin is his or her showcase to the world, and wounds and scars create physical changes that often affect self-image. The psychological aftermath of scars can be deeper than the wound itself. Every health care provider must be aware of how an injury has affected the patient. Additionally, the clinician must be ready to address these needs by referring the patient to a plastic surgeon or a psychologist, as well as by perfecting suturing technique.

Two things make scars visible—color and shadows. The clinician has very little control over the color of the patient's skin, but the smaller the scar, the less likely it is that a color change will occur. Shadows, however, are created by a centralized light source catching a subject at an angle. Even the very smallest elevation or indentation of a scar makes it visible (Figure 14-6). This problem is expertly

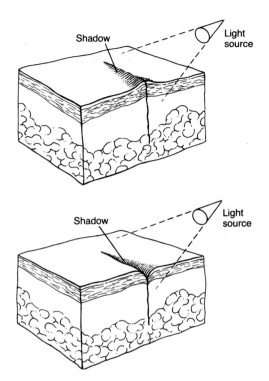

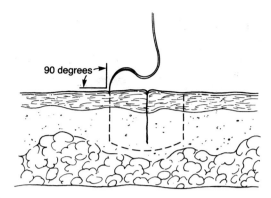

Figure 14-7 The suture needle should enter the skin at a 90-degree angle to the surface.

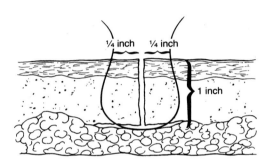

Figure 14-8 The depth of the stitch should be greater than the width. This principle will help evert the wound edges. In this example, the suture enters and leaves ¼ inch from the wound, for a total depth of ½ inch; the depth is 1 inch.

Figure 14-6 A single centralized lighting source creates a visible shadow. The least amount of scar elevation or indentation can cause a shadow.

addressed by good portrait photographers in their use of multiple lighting sources to obliterate all possible shadows. The only way for the clinician to address this concern is to make the scar as flat as possible because a flat scar leaves no shadow.

First Principle   The first principle of wound repair is to close the wound in layers, making sure that each layer of skin, from the deep fascia to the epidermis, butts up against its counterpart on the other side. Perfect epithelium-to-epithelium matching and a technique called "everting of the skin edges" give the best possible result (Figure 14-7). The key is to remove tension from the outer wound edges by placing absorbable sutures inside deep lacerations and matching them layer to layer. This arrangement will support the skin and removes any underlying abnormal pull on the skin. Correctly placed layered stitches can result in a closure that may not even need skin sutures.

The skin edges can be everted by making sure that
1.   The depth of the stitch is greater than the width.
2.   The stitch reaches the bottom of the wound.
Adherence to this principle automatically everts the skin edges (Figure 14-8). As the suture needle is placed in the skin, it should follow a direction that is oblique, back, and away from the wound edge. This creates the desired bottleneck effect of the stitch in the wound (Figure 14-9). In a wound that has been closed with this technique, the tissue will fall back into place when the sutures are removed, and the scar will eventually flatten.

Second Principle   The second principle of wound repair is to match any landmarks that are readily identifiable. Before the first stitch is placed, the wound

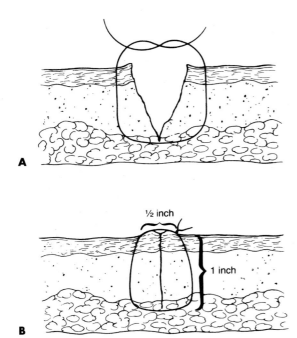

Figure 14-9 Gathering more tissue within the stitch at the base of the wound (**A**) will create the desired bottleneck effect (**B**) and aid in everting the wound edges.

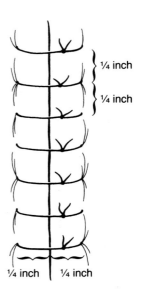

Figure 14-10 The "quarter-inch rule." Consistency in the spacing between sutures ($\frac{1}{4}$ inch) and the distance of the suture from the wound edge ($\frac{1}{4}$ inch) greatly enhances healing of the wound.

should be inspected for the location and identification of landmarks (e.g., creases or wrinkles, birthmarks, old age spots, tan lines, hairlines, the vermilion of the lip, eyebrows, eyelids, tattoos). The first stitch should be placed in the landmark or as close to it as possible to match it precisely. Stair-step effects in linear lines, especially on the face, are visible, and extreme caution should be taken to avoid this result.

Third Principle

The third principle is the need for proper placement of the sutures. In 95% of the lacerations seen in the emergency department, one side of the wound is longer than the other. Care must be taken in attempting to correct this imbalance. Taking more tissue between stitches on one side than on the other will create what is known as a dog-ear. To avoid a dog-ear effect, it is essential to place the sutures at the same distance along each side of the wound. In the absence of landmarks, measuring may be necessary. A good rule to follow is to measure $\frac{1}{4}$-inch down one side of the laceration from the apex, to

place the stitch in the skin about $\frac{1}{4}$-inch from the wound edge (Figure 14-10), and then to repeat the procedure on the other side. This method gives the most accurate closure possible.

Wound Tension

Wound tension is another aspect of suturing that must always be considered. The amount of tissue captured within a suture loop, no matter how little, creates a potential for ischemia by the overzealous use of force when the knot is tightened. The reduced capillary blood flow within the suture loop can result in a dangerous necrosis, provoking a prolonged inflammatory response and eventually a breakdown in healing. Wound dehiscence is common when care is not taken to reduce the tension within each suture placed in the wound. The wound edges should be brought together so they merely touch, and no other tension should be exerted. In most wounds, edema created by the inflammatory response increases the amount of tension in the suture loop. This could be disastrous if the suture line is already

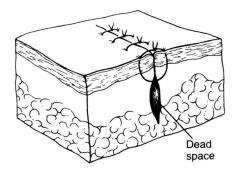

Figure 14-11 Dead space occurs when the stitch fails to reach the base of the wound. The shallowness of the stitch leaves an open area that is an ideal nidus for bacterial growth, leading to infection. Absorbable synthetic sutures are ideal for placement in the base of the wound to eliminate any dead space.

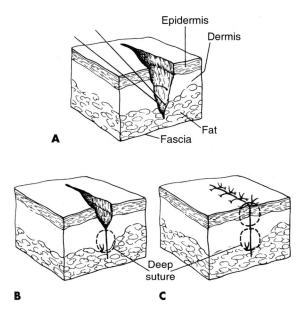

Figure 14-12 A-C, Proper placement of a deep, internal absorbable suture. Absorbable synthetic sutures are ideal for placement in the base of the wound to eliminate any dead space **(B).** The wound is then closed primarily **(C).**

compromised by an overzealous tightening of the sutures. Approximating the edges so that dead space is eliminated and tension is minimal should be the goal in each wound closure.

Dead Space   Dead space occurs when a suture placed in the skin does not encompass the entire wound (Figure 14-11). A hematoma will develop in the dead space. Hematoma is historically a great culture medium for bacteria. This happens in deep wounds in which the skin suture has not reached the full depth of the wound. In this case, deep sutures using absorbable suture material should be used (Figure 14-12). Caution should be taken to avoid the overuse of deep absorbable sutures. These sutures act as foreign objects, and the inflammatory response around them may result in prolonged healing or wound dehiscence. Additionally, deep sutures should not be used in overly contaminated wounds. In the presence of an abundance of bacteria, any additional material, whether in the form of a hematoma or a suture, will delay the healing process. A few well-spaced, deep sutures can remove the dead space and lessen the tension on the outermost layers of the wound, resulting in a minimal "good" scar that will need no revision.

Poor Technique   What causes "bad" scars? Understanding how poor technique may cause bad scarring

gives the clinician insight as to what to avoid when attempting to close a wound. Speed is one of the most notorious culprits in the poor results of a wound. The clinician must never sacrifice a good cosmetic result for speed.

Rolling of one of the wound edges is also a result of poor technique (Figure 14-13). One edge of epithelium is rolled under the other. The raw wound edge lying on top of the normal epithelial skin surface will not heal, and when the sutures are removed, that portion of the wound will open, resulting in a much bigger scar. If the skin edges do not butt up together, the capillaries ooze, resulting in a hematoma pocket. This raises the incidence of infection by 50%. It is better to evert the skin edges drastically so the raw surfaces of the wound are exposed. In this case, the wound will produce granulation tissue over the raw area, and when the stitches are removed, the ridge will flatten and the scar will shrink, resulting in a fairly good scar.

Occasionally, although very diligent and adhering to these principles, the clinician will find the remains of a dog-ear at the end of a procedure. Plastic surgeons use a procedure to remove the excess tissue, called a "dog-ear maneuver" (Figure 14-14), as follows:

1. Undermine the area involving the dog-ear, using blunt dissection (Figure 14-15), between the dermal layer and the fascial layer of the skin.
2. Cut a straight line away from the apex of the dog-ear, at an angle of 45 to 55 degrees, just the length of the dog-ear.
3. Measure the resulting triangular piece of excess skin on that side.

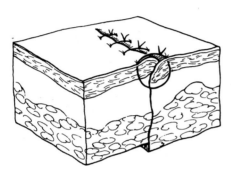

Figure 14-13 Poor technique can result in rolling of one wound edge over the other. Care must be taken to ensure that equal amounts of tissue on either side of the wound are enclosed within the stitch. The scar resulting from wound edge rolling is readily avoidable if care is taken to match the internal levels of tissue.

4. Re-drape the excess skin to determine just how much of the dog-ear should be removed.
5. Cut and remove the excess tissue, and close the new wound primarily.

The clinician and the patient are at the mercy of the wound and resulting scar. Although scars are always present after a wound, there are a number of ways to deal with them. It is possible to hide scars, disguise them, or improve them. All of these procedures require additional surgery, however, which in some cases is not possible. The basic, overriding principle should be to make the scar right the first time.

Occasionally, a wound may need débridement prior to primary closure. *Débridement* is the careful removal of dead or damaged tissue in addition to any unwarranted foreign material from the wound. This procedure should be considered when wounds, such as crush injuries, create jagged edges that have obliterated any previously existing landmarks. The goal of the clinician at this point is to create a more manageable wound that will produce a better cosmetic result and minimize the opportunity for any bacterial growth.

The basic technique of instrument-assisted wound closure is shown in Figures 14-16 and 14-17. The key here is to be certain that the first knot laid down on the wound is a square knot. A minimum of six throws, or three knots (two throws equaling one knot), should be used with each suture placed in the wound.

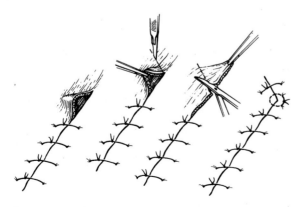

Figure 14-14 Procedure for eliminating a dog-ear. See text for explanation.

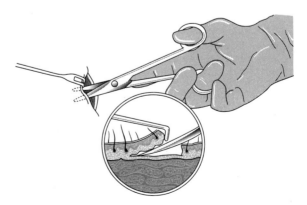

Figure 14-15 Undermining the skin at different levels releases tension on the entire wound and can give a better result.

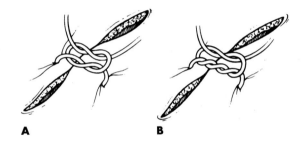

A **B**

Figure 14-16 **A**, Square knot. **B**, Surgeon's knot.

These principles are crucial to all wound closures. They can be improved and altered as a student becomes more sophisticated in suturing. When wounds are large or have a great amount of tissue loss, however, even the most respected plastic surgeons return to these basics for initial wound closure with difficult wounds.

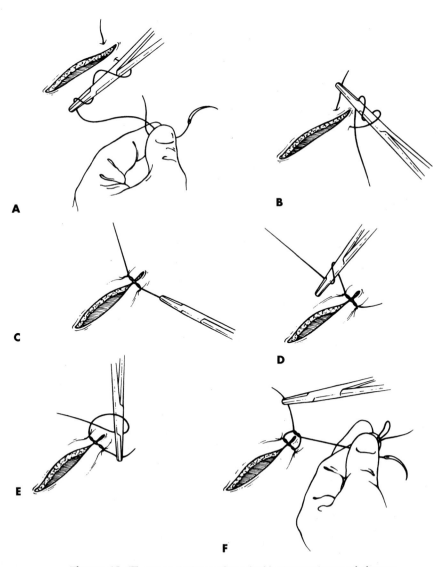

A **B**

C **D**

E **F**

Figure 14-17 The technique of surgical instrument wound closure.

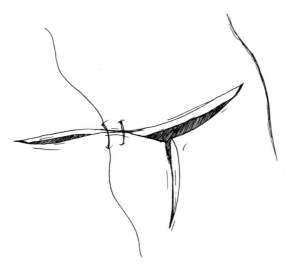

Figure 14-18 The first loop of a square knot is made and tightened until the desired tension is in place.

Special Considerations and Problems in Wound Closure

Nylon suture is difficult to handle because the thread is very stiff and has a tendency to slip. It is useful to use a locking technique to achieve proper tension on the wound edges (Figures 14-18 to 14-20).

A commonly encountered problem is a triangular flap with a sharp point (Figures 14-21 to 14-24).

The following technique can be used with minimal compromise of the blood supply. Occasionally, the margins of a wound will be ragged and contused. The wound can be converted into a nicely incised surgical wound by excision of a 2- to 3-mm wound margin. This can be most easily accomplished by using a No. 15 surgical blade on a scalpel to cut into the dermis along a predetermined line that is safe to excise. Cut along the line created by the scalpel with a pair of surgical cutting scissors, excising the margins of the wound in a perpendicular fashion. Do not excise tissue on the scalp or the eyebrows. This will create a prominent hairless scar.

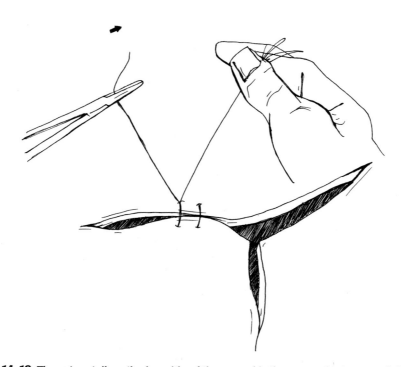

Figure 14-19 The suture tail on the low side of the wound is then moved into a parallel position with the second tail on the up side of the wound, keeping both tails taut as they are placed in this proximity.

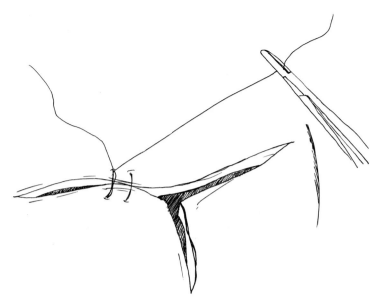

Figure 14-20 When the "lock" is secured by tension on the opposite stitch end, it will be possible to release the suture originally on the low side of the wound without slippage. The second throw of the square knot should be placed from behind the lock. Any other position will allow the tension on the lock to be released. Additionally, placing the lock on the low side of the wound may correct minor differences in skin height. Locking the suture in this fashion, on the low side, will raise the low side and depress the high side.

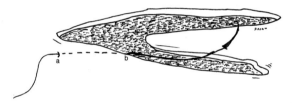

Figure 14-21 For closure of a triangular flap wound with a sharp point, pass the needle through the skin at point *a* and exit through the dermis at point *b*, which is inside the wound.

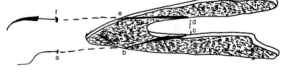

Figure 14-23 After following the steps in Figures 14-21 and 14-22, reenter the dermis at point *e* and pass the needle out through the skin at point *f*, approximately the same distance from the wound edge as point *a*. Tie the suture in a normal fashion.

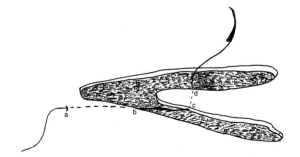

Figure 14-22 After following the procedure shown in Figure 14-21, pass the needle transversely through the dermis at the tip of the wound flap from point *c* to point *d*, being careful to maintain the same depth of the suture on both sides of the wound.

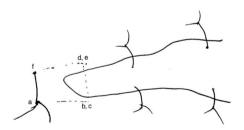

Figure 14-24 After the steps shown in Figures 14-21 to 14-23 are completed, the entire wound is sutured closed.

The elderly and those who have been long-term steroid users create a special situation that does not occur in the general population. Their skin is very thin and fragile, and it is common to see large avulsed flaps of this type of skin from relatively minor trauma. It is very difficult to close these flaps normally because the sutures will tear through the skin, which is like tissue paper. Steri-Strips and tincture of benzoin work very well. Paint the flap and surrounding skin with benzoin and allow it to dry, being careful not to get any benzoin in the wound itself. Then place the Steri-Strips on the wound, drawing the wound edges close together, and allow them to remain in position for about 3 weeks.

Some wounds should not be closed primarily. *Grinder injuries* are notorious for getting infected, despite the amount of brushing and irrigating of the wound that is done. Lacerations of the lower leg caused by objects thrown by a *lawn mower* nearly always get infected. *Human bites* are heavily contaminated with bacteria. *Dog bites* usually involve crush injury and bacterial contamination. A dog's tooth is a blunt instrument, and the biting mechanism is such that the bite does not create a sharp incision. The first effect is to crush the tissue and then puncture it. Because of the angle of closure of the dog's jaw, a bottle-shaped defect in the tissue is created and there is usually a tearing of the tissue as the bite is completed. Calcareous plaques from the dog's teeth may be deposited deep in the wound and act as foreign bodies. *Wounds more than 12 hours old* are frequently heavily contaminated with bacteria and should not be closed primarily. The "golden period" for all wounds to be closed primarily is within the first 6 hours of injury.

There are two ways to deal with these types of wounds. The first is to let the wound heal by secondary intention. This is satisfactory if the wound is small. Most grinder injuries, injuries caused by objects thrown by lawn mowers, and many dog bites fall into this category. The second option is to perform a delayed primary closure, as described previously in this chapter. These types of wounds should be anesthetized, irrigated and cleansed profusely, and then dressed. The dressing should be changed every day, and antibiotic treatment should be initiated. After 5 days, the wound should be re-anesthetized and sutured as a primary closure. Never put absorbable sutures in a wound at high risk for infection because they will act like foreign bodies and decrease the resistance of the wound to infection.

The preceding guidelines can be adjusted for facial injuries because the face, with its rich vascular supply, has a high resistance to infection. The major concern here is getting the best cosmetic result. For this reason, most dog bites and wounds more than 12 hours old on the face are closed primarily. Always use antibiotic coverage in these cases.

Dermabond

The newest wound closure material is put out by Ethicon (Cornelia, Georgia) and is a topical skin adhesive called DERMABOND; it can be thought of as a super glue for the skin. It is very easy to use and will leave an airtight hard coating over the wound when applied correctly. "DERMABOND is intended for topical application only to hold closed easily approximated skin edges from surgical incisions, including punctures from minimally invasive surgery, and simple, thoroughly cleansed, trauma-induced lacerations. It can be used in conjunction with, but not in place of, subcuticular sutures."

"DERMABOND should not be used on any wound with evidence of active infection or gangrene, or on wounds of decubitus etiology. It should not be used on any mucosal surfaces or across mucocutaneous junctions (e.g., oral cavity, lips), or on skin that may be regularly exposed to body fluids or with dense natural hair (e.g., scalp). It should not be used on patients with a known hypersensitivity to cyanoacrylate or formaldehyde, and great care must be taken if it is used near the eye. Other areas to avoid with this material are high–skin tension areas such as knuckles, elbows, and knees, unless the joint will be temporarily immobilized during the healing period."

This super glue for the skin is fast drying and can adhere to just about any surface, including stainless steel. There is no need for a dressing when DERMABOND is used. (See Figure 14-25, *A* to *D*.)

PROCEDURE FOR WOUND CLOSURE WITH DERMABOND ADHESIVE

The procedure will require two persons to perform properly.
1. Make sure the wound is clean, dry, and hemostatic.
2. Using two pairs of Adson forceps with teeth, each person should grasp the skin approximately 2 mm from the corners of the wound and retract away from each other, pulling the skin edges as close together as possible.
3. Apply the DERMABOND liquid over the approximated wound edges, covering the wound completely.
4. Remove excess liquid from any area wider than 5 mm around the wound before it has a chance to dry.
5. Maintain tension until the liquid has dried and become adherent to the skin.
6. Remove the forceps.
7. The DERMABOND will peel away naturally in 7 to 10 days, after the wound has healed.

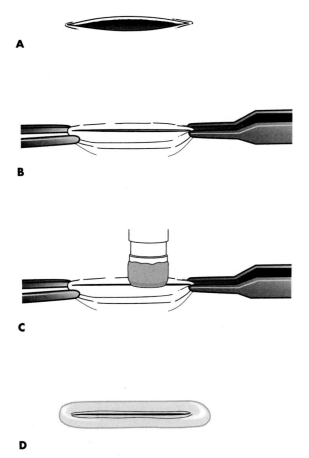

Figure 14-25 DERMABOND wound closure technique. **A,** Clean open wound. **B,** Wound edge approximated by retraction with Adson forceps. **C,** DERMABOND is applied to the closed wound surface. **D,** The wound is closed and DERMABOND is in place.

Dressings

A basic wound dressing consists of four parts. The first part is a nonadherent base that allows the wound to breathe while maintaining a high level of humidity over the wound. The second part is an absorbent gauze sponge that allows the wound to drain and does not obstruct the gaseous exchange that aids in wound healing. An obstructive sponge may result in the drying of the exudate, creating a new wound each time the dressing is changed. The third part is a gauze wrapping that allows free movement of gases through the dressing and holds the first two parts in place. The last part is some sort of adhesive to hold the entire dressing in place.

There are several new semipermeable, occlusive, nonadherent dressings on the market. Some are more expensive than others, and the decision as to which dressing to use for a specific wound remains with the clinician's experience and knowledge of the patient. For example, the farm worker may need much more in the way of wound protection, resulting in a bulkier dressing, than the office worker.

Petrolatum-based antibacterial ointments (e.g., bacitracin, polymyxin B sulfate, silver sulfadiazine, neomycin sulfate) may be applied to the surface of the closed wound often. This aids in maintaining a moist environment over the wound. High humidity between the wound and the dressing causes rapid epidermal healing and helps prevent drying of the wound surface, thereby avoiding a "scab," which prolongs the healing process by creating a gas-impermeable state. Repeated removal and re-creation of the "scab" also slows the healing process by creating a new wound each time the scab is removed, thereby re-initiating the inflammatory phase of healing and resulting in a bigger and less cosmetic scar.

The dressing also maintains the heat of the wound by providing a thermal insulator between the wound and the environment. The heat of the wound must remain as close to body core temperature as possible. Phagocytic and mitotic activity decrease greatly in temperatures below 30° C. Removing the dressing from a wound that has a high humidity can drop the temperature of the wound to as low as 12° C, and the resulting recovery to full mitotic activity can take up to 3 hours. Every attempt should be taken to shorten the time involved in changing a dressing and to maintain the temperature of the wound at or above a 30° C environment.

A dressing must also be impermeable to air-borne microorganisms. Wounds that are infected despite the available phagocytic processes do not heal. In *strike-through,* an overabundance of exudate produced by the wound results in soaking of the dressing through to the outer layer. This provides a wet pathway from the surface of the dressing to the wound for any airborne microorganisms. Strike-through can take as little as 6 hours, and the resulting infection can drastically prolong the healing process.

The optimum dressing for any wound has the following characteristics:

➤ Is sterile.
➤ Is big enough to cover the wound.
➤ Must have enough absorptive qualities for dry and heavy wound exudates.
➤ Must be comfortable and have good handling capabilities, both wet and dry.
➤ Must maintain a good shelf-life (must remain sterile in storage).
➤ Must be easily disposable.

In summary, the objectives of a dressing are simple and, when they are met, the healing process can be shortened by days. These objectives are:

➤ To maintain a high humidity between the wound and the dressing.
➤ To remove excess exudate and toxic compounds.
➤ To allow gaseous exchange.
➤ To provide thermal insulation to the wound surface.
➤ To be impermeable to bacteria.

➤ To be free from particles and toxic wound contaminants.
➤ To allow removal without causing trauma during dressing change.

COMMONLY PERFORMED CLINICAL PROCEDURES

This section describes some of the clinical procedures most commonly conducted in the delivery of health care. As the clinician becomes more confident and sophisticated in the ability to perform these tasks, he or she may refine or streamline individual procedures and develop preferences. Each description is simply one proven way to complete a given procedure and obtain the desired results.

Injections

Injections are used to deliver a variety of substances, including drugs, vaccinations, and skin test antigens, through the skin by means of a needle. The types of injections most commonly used are intramuscular, subcutaneous, and intradermal.

Intramuscular Injections

Indications Intramuscular injections are used for drugs that are not easily absorbed orally, when an intermediate rate of onset and duration of action are preferred, and when parenteral delivery is necessary.

Contraindications Intramuscular injections should not be given at any site where a dermatitis or cellulitis exists.

Equipment The following equipment should be assembled:

➤ Alcohol wipes.
➤ Syringe of appropriate size dependent on the volume to be injected.
➤ Needle. Selection of needle depends on the depth of insertion and the viscosity of the drug. In general, adults require a 19- to 22-gauge, 1½-inch needle. An obese patient may require a longer needle.
➤ Substance(s) to be injected.
➤ Sterile gauze sponge.
➤ Self-adhesive bandage.

PROCEDURE FOR INTRAMUSCULAR INJECTION

1. Fully expose and palpate the anatomical landmarks. The muscle being injected should be at rest and should be non–weight bearing.
2. Prepare the skin with an alcohol wipe, starting at the injection site and extending outward in a circular motion, using the bull's-eye method, for about 5 cm.
3. Fill the syringe with the desired amount of fluid to be injected.
   a. Wipe the rubber stopper of the vial of medication with an alcohol wipe.
   b. Pull the plunger of the syringe back to the mark signifying the amount of medication to be withdrawn from the vial, filling the syringe with air.
   c. Insert the needle through the center of the rubber stopper of the vial.
   d. Invert the vial.
   e. Inject air into the vial.
   f. Withdraw the desired amount of medication into the syringe, making it as free of air bubbles as possible.
4. Pull the subcutaneous tissue slightly to one side.
5. Rapidly plunge the needle perpendicular (a 90-degree angle) into the surface of the skin.
6. Insert the needle to a depth of ½ to 1 inch.
7. Aspirate to ensure that the needle is not in a blood vessel. If blood returns, do not inject at this site, but withdraw the needle and apply pressure to encourage hemostasis. Repeat steps 5 and 6.
8. Inject the medication slowly.
9. Withdraw the needle.
10. Massage the area briefly with a gauze sponge.
11. Apply a self-adhesive bandage, if necessary.

Injection Sites

DELTOID MUSCLE   Use the main body of the deltoid muscle, which lies lateral and a few centimeters below the acromion. Large volumes (greater than 2 mL) and irritating solutions should not be given at this site.

GLUTEAL MUSCLE   The gluteal muscle is the most common and preferred site of injection in adults and in children older than 2 years. A large volume of solution can be injected into the muscle, and the skin over the area is thin and easily pierced. The site for injection into the gluteal muscle should always be in the upper outer quadrant of the buttock, in order to avoid injury to the sciatic nerve and superior gluteal muscles.

VASTUS LATERALIS MUSCLE (LATERAL THIGH)   The vastus lateralis is the preferred injection site in infants. Although it may be used in adults, it is painful because of the fascia lata. The injection should be given into the bulk of the muscle.

POSSIBLE COMPLICATIONS   The following complications may occur with intramuscular injections:

➤ Injection into blood vessels may cause a toxic reaction, injury to the vessel, or a hematoma.
➤ Injection into a deep nerve may cause pain, paresthesias, and possible permanent damage to the nerve.
➤ The needle may break off and become embedded in the muscle.
➤ Sterile and septic abscesses at the injection site may occur if equipment is not sterile, the injection site is not properly cleansed, or a site is overused.

FOLLOW-UP   No special follow-up is required.

Subcutaneous Injections

Indications   Subcutaneous injections are to be used for drugs that require slow absorption and long duration of action.

Contraindications Subcutaneous injections should not be given at any site where a severe dermatitis or cellulitis exists.

Equipment The following equipment should be assembled:
➤ Alcohol wipes.
➤ Syringe of appropriate size, depending on the volume to be injected.
➤ Needle: 25- to 27-gauge, 3/4 to 1 inch.
➤ Substance(s) to be injected.
➤ Sterile gauze sponge.
➤ Self-adhesive bandage.

Possible Complications Local reactions can occur with repeated injections over the same site.

Follow-up No specific follow-up is required.

PROCEDURE FOR SUBCUTANEOUS INJECTION

1. Fully expose the area.
2. Prepare the skin with an alcohol wipe, starting at the injection site and extending outward in a circular motion, using the bull's-eye method, for about 5 cm.
3. Fill the syringe with the desired amount of medication to be injected, usually 2 to 3 mL.
4. Pinch up the subcutaneous tissue into a roll between the thumb and the forefinger.
5. Insert the needle with one quick motion at a 45-degree angle to the skin at the midpoint of the roll.
6. Advance the needle about three fourths of its length.
7. Release the roll of skin.
8. Aspirate to ensure that the needle is not in a blood vessel. If blood returns, do not inject at this site; withdraw the needle and repeat steps 4 through 7.
9. Inject the medication slowly.
10. Withdraw the needle.
11. Apply pressure with a gauze sponge over the site.
12. Apply a self-adhesive bandage, if necessary.

Intradermal Injections

Indications Intradermal injections are used to test for hypersensitivity to extrinsic allergens and for infection by tuberculosis, nontuberculous mycobacteria, and certain fungal infections.

Contraindications Intradermal injection should not be given at any site where dermatitis or infection exists. Patients with a previous positive tuberculin skin reaction should not be retested.

Equipment The following equipment should be assembled:
➤ Alcohol wipes.
➤ Tuberculin syringe.
➤ Needle: 27-gauge, ½ inch.
➤ Substance(s) to be injected.
➤ Sterile gauze sponge.

Injection Sites The ventral forearm is the most common site used. The back may be used for extensive allergen testing.

Possible Complications Severe local skin reactions may develop in hypersensitive patients.

Follow-up Patients should be instructed about when to return to have the skin reaction read, usually in 48 to 72 hours. If the skin reaction is positive, the diameter of the cutaneous induration should be measured and recorded.

Venipuncture

Venipuncture is one of the most frequently performed clinical procedures. It is a skill that can be learned and perfected through frequent practice to minimize patient discomfort. Venipuncture is used to obtain blood samples for analysis; to administer fluids, medications, blood, and blood products; and to treat polycythemia.

Phlebotomy

Indications Phlebotomy is used to obtain blood samples for laboratory analysis and to remove blood in the treatment of polycythemia.

PROCEDURE FOR INTRADERMAL INJECTION

1. Prepare the skin with an alcohol wipe. Let the skin dry.
2. Fill the syringe with the desired amount of solution, usually 0.1 to 0.2 mL.
3. Hold the skin taut between the thumb and the index finger.
4. Hold the needle bevel up and angle it about 10 to 15 degrees (almost parallel) to the skin.
5. Insert the needle into the dermis for about two thirds of its length.
6. Inject the solution. A wheal should form immediately.
7. Withdraw the needle. Discard the gauze in an appropriate container.
8. Record the following information on the patient's chart: type of test, date and time done, and exact location of each test injection mode.

Contraindications   Phlebotomy should not be performed if there is evidence of phlebitis, cellulitis, lymphangitis, scarring, recent venipuncture, or venous obstruction at the proposed site of venipuncture. Phlebotomy should not be performed in the same arm in which an intravenous line is positioned.

Equipment   The following equipment should be assembled:
➤ Tourniquet.
➤ Alcohol pads.
➤ Disposable latex gloves.
➤ Vacutainer needle holder or syringe (5, 10, or 20 mL).
➤ Vacutainer needle or a 20-gauge needle for the syringe. If a large amount of blood is to be drawn, it is best to use an 18-gauge needle. Needles smaller than 22-gauge should be avoided because the blood sample tends to hemolyze in the small bore. A butterfly needle may be needed for small veins.
➤ Properly labeled specimen Vacutainer tubes.
➤ Sterile gauze pads.
➤ Self-adhesive bandage.

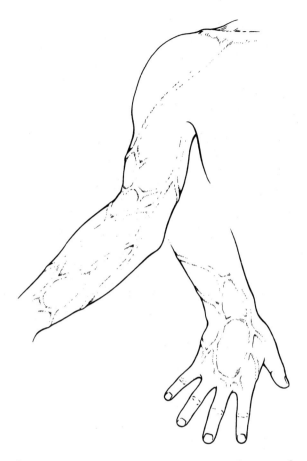

Figure 14-26 Arm and hand anatomy most commonly used for venipuncture.

Site Selection   The arm is the best site for phlebotomy, especially in the antecubital fossa (Figure 14-26). The superficial veins of the arm are more easily observable and accessible, distinct, and palpable. Vein selection is determined by size, elasticity, and distance below the skin. In general, the most easily palpable vein, even though it may not be the most visible, should be selected for phlebotomy. To aid in selection of a vein, the clinician can:
➤ Apply the tourniquet first to observe for a suitable vein.
➤ Have the patient open and close his or her fist to help pump blood from muscles into the superficial veins.

➤ Lower the extremity to a dependent position.

➤ Apply warm soaks to the area.

➤ Gently tap repeatedly over the vein with the tips of the fingers.

When a suitable vein cannot be found in the forearm, one of the superficial veins on the dorsal surface of the hand may have to be used.

These veins are small and collapse easily and so should not be used to draw large amounts of blood.

Patient Preparation The procedure should be explained to the patient to help reduce anxiety and elicit cooperation. The patient should be positioned comfortably with the arm resting on an even, solid surface.

Peripheral Intravenous Catheterization

Indications Peripheral intravenous (IV) catheterization is used to administer fluids, medications, blood, and blood products. In most cases, catheter placement

---

PROCEDURE FOR PHLEBOTOMY

1. Apply the tourniquet above the antecubital fossa so that it may be removed quickly with one hand. Do not apply the tourniquet too tightly, to avoid causing patient discomfort and blood stasis. The tourniquet should be removed if cyanosis is observed in the arm. Generally, it should not remain on for longer than 1 minute.
2. Select the vein site. Palpate and trace the path of the vein with the index finger, or use one of the methods previously described.
3. Cleanse the skin with the alcohol pads and allow the area to dry.
4. Put on gloves.
5. Grasp the patient's arm firmly with the nondominant hand and stabilize the vein, using the thumb to anchor the vein by drawing the skin taut.
6. Insert the needle, bevel up, under the skin at an angle of 15 to 30 degrees with a quick motion. A sensation of resistance will be felt, followed by ease of penetration as the vein is entered.
7. Transfer the blood as required by equipment chosen.
   a. If using a syringe, withdraw the desired amount of blood into the syringe.
   b. If using a Vacutainer system, hold the Vacutainer needle and unit steady with the hand used to do the venipuncture. Push the vacuum tube forward onto the needle, and look for the inflow of blood into the Vacutainer. Allow the tube to fill until the blood flow ceases. Remove the tube from the holder. If multiple tubes are needed, insert the next tube into the holder and repeat the procedure. The shutoff valve automatically covers the butt end of the needle, stopping blood flow until the next tube is inserted.
   c. If using a butterfly catheter, remove the cap at end of the tubing and attach a syringe. Withdraw the required amount of blood into the syringe.
8. Release the tourniquet.
9. Place a sterile gauze pad just above the venipuncture site.
10. Remove the needle quickly and smoothly, and slide the gauze down to the site with a moderate amount of pressure. Maintain pressure until bleeding has ceased.
11. Apply a self-adhesive bandage.
12. If a syringe was used, fill the appropriate tubes by puncturing the rubber stopper of the tube with the needle and allowing vacuum to fill the tubes.
13. If using tubes containing an additive, mix them immediately by gently inverting them 10 to 12 times each.
14. Make sure all tubes are properly labeled.
15. Used needles should not be recapped but should be disposed of directly into an appropriate needle disposal container, which should be readily available.

into the vein is preferred over needle placement because a catheter lasts longer and is better tolerated by the patient. The catheter-over-needle unit (Angiocath) is the most common type used. A butterfly intravenous line may be preferred for patients requiring brief venous access and immediate removal of the line.

Contraindications Catheters should never be placed where there is cellulitis, phlebitis, lymphedema, or pitting edema of the extremity. Previous mastectomy or other axillary surgery by which ipsilateral venous drainage may have been impaired is another contraindication. Hyperosmolar fluids and agents known to cause chemical phlebitis should not be administered through peripheral veins. Arteriovenous shunts should never be used for placement of routine intravenous lines.

Equipment The following equipment should be assembled:
➤ Tourniquet.
➤ Povidone-iodine (Betadine) antiseptic skin preparation sponges.
➤ Tape to secure the intravenous line. Prepare two 4-inch lengths of ½-inch-wide tape.
➤ Catheter-over-needle (Angiocath) unit or butterfly needle of appropriate diameter for the rate and type of fluid to be infused (see "Catheter Selection").
➤ Bottle or bag of IV fluid or blood products with proper tubing.
➤ Disposable latex gloves.
➤ Transparent sterile dressing, antiseptic or antibiotic ointment, and labels.

Catheter Selection Considerations in selecting the correct catheter include the size and condition of the vein and the viscosity of the fluid to be infused. The following guideline can be used:

14-16 gauge	Trauma or major surgery
16-18 gauge	Blood and blood products, administration of viscous medications
20-22 gauge	Most patient applications
24 gauge	Pediatric patients and neonates

Site Selection The veins most suitable for intravenous therapy are found at the dorsum of the hand, the volar aspect of the proximal ulnar forearm, and the radial aspect of the forearm just proximal to the wrist. In general, the following principles should be followed:
➤ Use distal veins first.
➤ Use patient's nondominant arm when possible.
➤ Avoid veins at areas of flexion, such as the antecubital fossa.
➤ Select a vein that will not interfere with the patient's daily living activities.
➤ An ideal vein has not been used previously and is relatively straight.

Patient Preparation Explain the procedure fully to the patient to minimize anxiety and elicit cooperation. The patient should be in a comfortable position with the extremity to be used resting on a solid surface.

Possible Complications Hematoma formation, extravasation, phlebitis, cellulitis, bacteremia, and sepsis may occur. Daily inspection of the site and aseptic technique are essential to minimize the chances of complications. Intravenous sites should be changed every 3 to 4 days to reduce the probability of phlebitis, or they should changed at the first signs of phlebitis or infection.

Arterial Blood Gas Sampling
Radial Artery Puncture
Indications Arterial blood gas (ABG) levels, used in a variety of clinical problems, may be determined using samples of arterial blood. ABG sampling has become an important and commonly used procedure. The most common site is the radial artery; alternative sites are the brachial and femoral arteries.

Contraindications Poor collateral circulation in the hand, as determined by the Allen test, or no palpable pulse in the radial artery is an absolute contraindication. The Allen test should always be done before a radial arterial puncture (see procedure for the Allen test in box). Arterial puncture should not be done over areas of cellulitis or local infection. It is relatively contraindicated in patients with bleeding disorders

---

PROCEDURE FOR PERIPHERAL INTRAVENOUS CATHETERIZATION

1. Assemble and prepare the intravenous fluid and tubing. Run the fluid through the tubing to flush all air from the system, and recap the end of the tubing.
2. Apply a tourniquet 4 to 6 inches above the proposed site in a way that allows quick removal. The tourniquet should be tight enough to stop venous flow, but not arterial flow.
3. Select the vein to be used. The techniques used for phlebotomy can be used to help palpate and visualize a suitable vein for catheterization.
4. Palpate the course of the vein. Make sure it is long enough to accept the catheter to be used.
5. Put on gloves.
6. Cleanse the skin around the insertion site with the antiseptic sponges.
7. Inspect the catheter-over-needle unit to ensure that the beveled tip of the metal needle is well beyond the tip of the catheter and that the catheter slides easily.
8. Anchor the vein by gently applying pressure and pulling distally with the thumb of the nondominant hand.
9. Insert the needle, bevel up, through the skin at an angle of 15 to 30 degrees, either on top or to the side of the vein. Insert the needle and the catheter into the vein. A "pop" will be felt, and blood will flow back into the hub of the needle.
10. Advance the needle and the catheter until both have entered the lumen of the vein.
11. Gently and gradually advance the catheter into the vein while withdrawing the needle. Palpate the catheter through the skin as it is advanced inside the vein. Applying gentle pressure just proximal to the end of the catheter prevents blood from leaking back through or around the catheter.
12. Make sure the entire length of the catheter is inside the lumen of the vein.
13. Release the tourniquet and remove the needle.
14. Attach the intravenous tubing, and check for leakage along the entire system.
15. Secure the catheter in place with tape, and apply an antiseptic or antibiotic ointment to the puncture site. Apply the transparent sterile dressing. Loop and tape the IV tubing onto the forearm to prevent accidental dislodgment of the IV catheter.
16. Label the insertion site with the catheter gauge, date and time of insertion, and initials of the person performing the procedure.

---

and patients on anticoagulant and thrombolytic therapy. When essential to management, arterial puncture should be done into the radial artery, with careful monitoring and prolonged postpuncture compression.

Equipment The following equipment should be assembled:
- Glass syringe, 3 to 5 mL.
- Plastic syringe, 3 to 5 mL, containing 1% lidocaine without epinephrine.
- Two needles, 25-gauge, ½ -inch.
- Heparin, 10,000 U/mL solution, 1 mL.
- Povidone-iodine (Betadine) skin preparation sponges.
- Rubber stopper.
- Rolled towel.
- Crushed ice.
- Sterile gauze sponges.
- Sterile gloves.

Preparation of the Syringe To heparinize one 5-mL glass syringe and 25-gauge needle, withdraw 0.5 mL heparin into the syringe. Hold the syringe with the needle up, pull the plunger to the end of the syringe, and expel all the heparin through the needle. This procedure leaves an adequate amount of heparin in the syringe and needle. Too much heparin left in the syringe gives an artificially low pH.

Patient Preparation   Explain the procedure to the patient to facilitate patient cooperation and reduce anxiety. Tell the patient to expect some discomfort and pain. It is important that the patient keep as still as possible.

Possible Complications   Thrombus, embolus, or hematoma may occur at the puncture site, causing vascular obstruction. Transient spasm may also occur. Ischemia or gangrene of the hand or fingers can also occur. The patient should be instructed to notify the physician or PA if the hand becomes numb, painful, cold, or blue. A consultation with a vascular surgeon should be arranged immediately if arterial flow is compromised in any way.

Brachial Artery Puncture   The use of the brachial artery should be reserved for situations in which the radial artery cannot be used. Potential complications from the brachial artery are more common, and the procedure is often more painful. The contraindications, equipment, syringe preparation, and patient preparation are the same as for radial arm puncture.

Possible Complications   The possible complications of brachial artery puncture are essentially the same as for radial artery puncture. Any signs of arterial compromise seen in the forearm, hand, or fingers should prompt an immediate consultation with a vascular surgeon.

PROCEDURE FOR RADIAL ARTERY PUNCTURE

1. Palpate the radial artery, and perform the Allen test to assess the adequacy of the ulnar artery collateral flow to the hand (Figure 14-27).
   a. Occlude both the radial and ulnar arteries while the patient makes a tight fist and elevates the arm.
   b. Allow the hand to blanch, and lower the arm to waist level.
   c. Have the patient open the hand. Release the pressure over the ulnar artery while maintaining pressure over the radial artery.
   d. Normal skin color should return to the ulnar side of the palm within 6 seconds, with color returning to the whole palm quickly. Failure of the hand to regain color within 6 seconds signifies inadequate ulnar collateral circulation, and radial artery puncture is contraindicated.
2. Extend the patient's supinated wrist to about 30 degrees by placing a rolled towel under the wrist.
3. Palpate the artery to determine where the pulsation is most prominent.
4. Cleanse the skin over the puncture site with the antiseptic sponges.
5. Put on gloves.
6. Anesthetize the skin over the puncture site with the 1% lidocaine. Care should be taken not to inject into the circulation.
7. Relocate the point of maximal impulse with the nondominant hand. Facing the patient, hold the syringe with the dominant hand like a pencil, bevel up.
8. Gently insert the needle through the skin at an angle of 45 to 60 degrees (Figure 14-28). Advance the needle toward the point of maximal impulse until arterial blood returns into the syringe. The needle and syringe may be advanced until the periosteum of the radius is encountered. If blood returns, allow the syringe to fill itself.
9. If no blood is obtained, slowly withdraw the needle and syringe and continue to observe for blood return. If this is still unsuccessful, withdraw the needle to a position just under the skin and repeat the attempt, redirecting the needle toward the point of maximal impulse.
10. Collect the desired amount of blood and remove the needle quickly. Immediately apply direct pressure with a gauze sponge over the puncture site for 10 minutes.
11. Expel all air bubbles from the syringe. Gently roll the syringe between the fingers to mix the blood with the anticoagulant, embed the needle in a rubber stopper, and place the syringe on ice. Make sure the syringe is properly labeled and transported to the laboratory immediately.

PROCEDURE FOR BRACHIAL ARTERY PUNCTURE

1. Fully extend the patient's arm, with the forearm supinated.
2. Palpate the brachial artery at the medial side of the antecubital fossa.
3. Prepare the skin with antiseptic sponges.
4. Anesthetize the area with the 1% lidocaine, taking care not to inject into the circulation.
5. Locate the point of maximal pulsation, face the patient, and hold the syringe with the dominant hand like a pencil, bevel up.
6. Insert the needle through the skin at an angle of 60 to 90 degrees, and advance the needle slowly toward the point of maximal pulsation. Watch for return of arterial blood into the syringe. If no blood is obtained, withdraw the needle to just under the skin and attempt again.
7. Once the amount of blood needed is collected, withdraw the needle. Immediately apply direct pressure with a gauze sponge over the puncture site for 10 minutes.
8. Expel all air bubbles from the syringe. Gently roll the syringe to mix, embed the needle in a rubber stopper, and place the syringe on ice. Make sure the syringe is properly labeled and transported to the laboratory immediately.

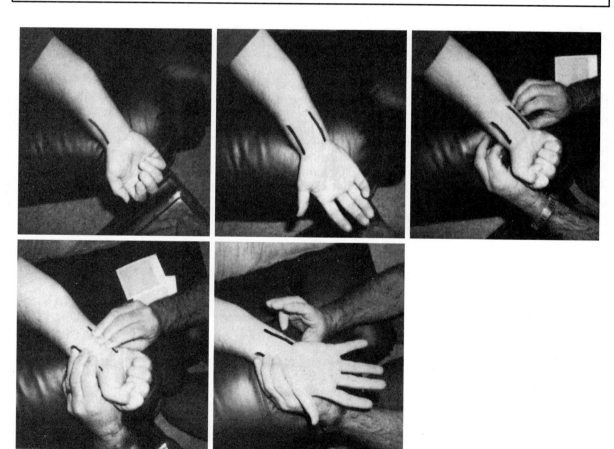

Figure 14-27 Allen test. See text for explanation. *(Photographs by Christopher Sullivan.)*

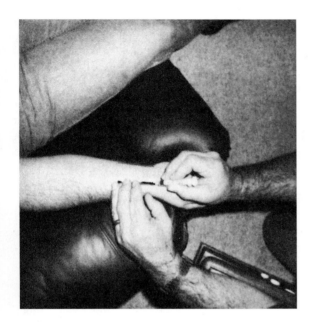

Figure 14-28 Technique for obtaining an arterial blood gas sample from the radial artery. The needle should enter the skin, bevel up, at an angle of 45 to 50 degrees. *(Photograph by Christopher Sullivan.)*

Femoral Artery Puncture Although many believe that femoral artery puncture is the easiest to obtain, it should still be used only when radial arterial blood cannot be obtained. The close proximity of the femoral vein makes inadvertent venous sampling common. There is also a risk of embolization to the distal extremity. Postpuncture bleeding that is undetected can occur. The technique used for femoral artery puncture is similar to that for radial and brachial artery puncture, except for anatomical considerations. The differences in procedure are as follows:
➤ The patient should be in a supine position with the hip extended and slightly externally rotated. The femoral artery can be palpated just distal to the inguinal ligament in the groin.
➤ The needle should be inserted perpendicular to the skin surface.

Possible Complications The possible complications in femoral artery puncture are essentially the same as for radial artery puncture. Any signs of vascular com-

promise seen in the leg, foot, or toes should prompt an immediate consultation with a vascular surgeon.

Lumbar Puncture

Lumbar puncture (LP) is an important diagnostic procedure that provides cerebrospinal fluid (CSF) from the lumbar subarachnoid space. It is used diagnostically in both emergency and nonemergency situations and is used therapeutically to give medication intrathecally.

Indications Lumbar puncture is indicated for the following situations:
➤ Suspected meningitis.
➤ Follow-up of meningitis therapy.
➤ Suspected subarachnoid hemorrhage.
➤ Aid to diagnosis of miscellaneous neurological diseases or complaints.
➤ Diagnosis and staging of neoplastic disease.
➤ Intrathecal administration of antimicrobial or antineoplastic agents.
➤ Administration of spinal anesthesia.
➤ Reduction of CSF pressure.

Contraindications Lumbar puncture is contraindicated by the presence of:
➤ Unexplained increased intracranial pressure (papilledema).
➤ Suspected intracranial mass lesion.
➤ Suspected spinal cord mass lesion.
➤ Local skin infection over the lumbar area.
➤ Bleeding coagulopathy or anticoagulation therapy (relative contraindication).

Equipment Prepackaged lumbar puncture kits are available that contain all the equipment needed to perform the procedure. The kits should include the following essential items:
➤ Spinal needles, 22- and 20-gauge, with stylet.
➤ 25-gauge, ½-inch needle.
➤ 22-gauge, 1½-inch needle.
➤ 5-mL syringe.
➤ 1% lidocaine with epinephrine.
➤ Three-way stopcock and manometer.
➤ Sterile collection tubes (minimum of three).
➤ Sterile towel and barrier.
➤ Sterile gauze sponges.

➤ Mask, goggles, and sterile gloves.
➤ Povidone-iodine solution and materials for skin cleansing.
➤ Self-adhesive bandage.

Patient Preparation   Informed written consent is usually required, unless the procedure is an emergency and the patient is confused or lethargic. The procedure should be explained fully to the patient before it is begun to reduce anxiety and elicit cooperation.

Patient Positioning   Patient positioning is the most important step in performing a successful lumbar puncture. In most cases, the lateral decubitus position should be used. In patients with scoliosis, marked obesity, or ankylosing spondylitis, the sitting position may be more beneficial.

To achieve the lateral decubitus position:
1. Place the patient on the side in the fetal position.
2. Put a pillow under the patient's head to keep the spinal axis parallel to the bed.
3. The patient's spine should lie along the edge of the bed, with the bed raised until the spine is at mid-chest level for the seated clinician.

To achieve the sitting position:
1. Have the patient sit on the edge of the bed facing away from the clinician.
2. Have the patient bend over a bedside table with the arms resting on the table and the head, knees, and hips flexed.
3. Raise the bed until the lower lumbar spine is at mid-chest level for the seated clinician.

Site Selection   The site used most commonly for needle entry is the L3-L4 interspace, although the L4-L5 interspace may be used. The fourth lumbar vertebra is at the level of the iliac crest.

To facilitate locating the landmarks after the skin has been cleansed, mark the skin with a ballpoint pen or an impression from a fingernail. The location of needle entry should be the exact midpoint of the interspace between the spinous processes.

Possible Complications   Several complications of lumbar puncture may occur, such as cerebral herniation, bloody CSF, and headache.

Cerebral Herniation   A mass lesion, cerebral abscess, or increased intracranial pressure could result in cerebellar herniation through the foramen magnum upon removal of CSF. When these conditions are suspected, lumbar puncture should be deferred until a more definitive evaluation can be undertaken.

Bloody Cerebrospinal Fluid   Bloody CSF may occur from a traumatic tap or a subarachnoid hemorrhage. A traumatic tap occurs when the spinal needle passes through the subarachnoid space into the ventral epidural plexus. Features that may signify a traumatic tap rather than a previous intracranial bleed are:
➤ Normal cerebrospinal pressure.
➤ Decline in amount of blood after several tubes have been obtained.
➤ Decline in the red blood cell count in successive tubes.
➤ Absence of xanthochromia.
➤ Subsequent lumbar puncture at higher interspace, showing clear CSF.

Headache   This usually occurs as a result of persistent CSF leakage through the dura, or removal of large amounts of CSF. Using the smallest spinal needle possible and prescribing bedrest for several hours after the procedure usually can minimize the risk of headache. Analgesics, bed rest, and oral hydration usually relieve the symptoms.

Follow-up   The patient should be instructed to remain prone for 1 to 3 hours after lumbar puncture to minimize the risk of postpuncture headache. If headache develops, bedrest, oral analgesics, and adequate hydration are indicated. The patient should be instructed to contact a physician if the headache persists.

If a therapeutic agent was injected, the patient should be placed in the Trendelenburg position for 30 to 60 minutes after the procedure.

PROCEDURE FOR LUMBAR PUNCTURE

1. Put on the mask, goggles, and sterile gloves and prepare all equipment. Assemble the manometer and stopcock, and have the specimen tubes ready for use.
2. Draw up the 1% lidocaine into the 5-mL syringe with the 25-gauge, ½-inch needle.
3. Cleanse and prepare the skin with the iodine solution, starting at the needle site and working outward until a wide sterile field has been prepared. Drape the back.
4. Locate the needle site and administer the 1% lidocaine. First raise a skin wheal, and then infiltrate into the deeper tissues between the spinous processes. Aspirate for blood return before injecting the lidocaine.
5. Hold the spinal needle between the index and middle fingers with one thumb over the stylet and the other thumb stabilizing the needle. Avoid touching the tip and shaft of the needle.
6. Introduce the needle perpendicular to the skin, and advance the needle at an angle of 30 to 45 degrees, directing the needle toward the umbilicus. The bevel of the needle should be up if the patient is in the lateral decubitus position or to the side if the patient is in the sitting position.
7. As the needle is slowly advanced, a distinct "pop" is felt as the needle penetrates through the ligamentum flavum and the arachnoid membrane. If no pop is felt, the stylet should be removed after frequent small advancements to look for CSF return. Advancement too far through the subarachnoid space will result in piercing of the ventral epidural venous plexus, with a subsequent traumatic tap.
8. If bony resistance is encountered, withdraw the needle to the subcutaneous tissue, redirect the needle more caudally, and try again.
9. Once CSF begins to flow, discard the first few drops of fluid. Do not aspirate because a nerve root might become trapped against the needle and incur injury.
10. Measure the opening pressure.
    a. Have the patient carefully straighten the legs to decrease intra-abdominal pressure.
    b. Attach the three-way stopcock to the manometer, remove the stylet, and attach the stopcock and manometer to the hub of the needle. The lever of the stopcock should be toward the patient.
    c. Rotate the lever back toward the clinician. The CSF will fill the manometer, and the opening pressure can be measured. Normal pressure is 65 to 195 mm H_2O. If the pressure is elevated, check the patient's position to make sure it is not causing jugular or abdominal compression. CSF pressure should decrease with inspiration and increase with expiration.
11. Fill the specimen tubes. Drain the CSF from the manometer into the first tube. Remove the manometer and collect the remaining samples. Replace the stylet in the needle shaft halfway to block the flow between samples.
12. The first tube should be labeled for Gram's staining and bacterial culture, the second for glucose and protein tests, and the third for a cell count and differential. If further information is needed, more samples should be obtained.
13. If therapeutic injection is necessary, inject the solution slowly over 30 seconds after removing at least an equivalent volume of CSF.
14. Replace the manometer and measure the closing pressure.
15. Replace the stylet and remove the needle.
16. Remove residual iodine from the skin, and cover the puncture site with a self-adhesive bandage.

Urethral Catheterization

Indications   The insertion of a Foley catheter through the urethra to the bladder for urinary drainage is a very common bedside procedure indicated for both diagnostic and therapeutic reasons.

Contraindications   Urethral trauma and inability to pass the catheter through the urethra into the urinary bladder are contraindications to the procedure.

Equipment   Disposable Foley catheter trays are generally available for use. The essential items are:
➤ Foley catheter of proper size. Most adults tolerate a 16F or 18F rubber catheter with a 5-mL balloon. (The larger the F number, the larger the diameter.)
➤ Drainage bag and connecting tube.
➤ Sterile specimen cup.
➤ Sterile syringe containing 5 mL of sterile water.
➤ Sterile lubricating jelly.
➤ Antiseptic cleansing solution and cotton swabs.
➤ Emesis basin or small tray to catch urine.
➤ Sterile towels to drape the area.
➤ Sterile gloves, mask, and goggles.

Patient Preparation   The necessity for catheterization and the procedure itself should be explained to the patient. The female patient should be supine with both legs raised (lithotomy position). The male patient should be supine with legs flat.

Possible Complications   Infections such as cystitis, pyelonephritis, and bacteremia from long-term indwelling catheters can occur. Traumatic catheterization may cause hematuria, as can creation of a false urethral passage.

Follow-up   Routine Foley catheter care is important. Keep the urethral meatus area clean, and keep the bag below the level of the bladder to prevent gravity drainage of contaminated urine from the tube into the bladder. Removing the catheter as soon as possible will reduce the risk of infection. Make sure to deflate the balloon before removing the catheter.

Nasogastric Intubation

The insertion of a nasogastric (NG) tube is common in both hospital and emergency department settings. It is an uncomfortable procedure for most patients.

Indications   Nasogastric tubes are inserted to facilitate gastric lavage, both therapeutic and diagnostic, as well as for gastric decompression.

PROCEDURE FOR URINARY CATHETERIZATION IN FEMALES

1. Put on the mask, goggles, and sterile gloves, and drape the genital area with sterile towels.
2. Use the antiseptic packet to moisten the cotton swabs. Cleanse the outside of the labia and the urethral meatus with the swabs. Stroke from anterior to posterior in a downward stroke, using a new cotton swab each time.
3. Lubricate the tip of the catheter with the sterile lubricating jelly. Insert the catheter into the urethral meatus until urine returns, and then advance the catheter another 4 to 5 cm.
4. Collect a urine specimen in the sterile cup, and let the rest of the urine drain into the basin.
5. If the bladder is markedly distended, it should be drained gradually; generally, no more than 1000 mL of urine should be drained at a time.
6. Inflate the balloon with the sterile water. Pull on the catheter gently to ensure that the balloon is in place.
7. Connect the catheter to the drainage bag. Tape the distal catheter to the inner aspect of the patient's thigh.

PROCEDURE FOR URINARY CATHETERIZATION IN MALES

1. Put on the mask, goggles, and sterile gloves, and drape the genital area with the sterile towels.
2. Use the antiseptic solution to moisten the cotton swabs. Grasp the shaft of the penis, hold it erect, and retract the prepuce if the patient is uncircumcised. Cleanse the glans from the meatus to the corona of the glans with downward strokes, using a new cotton swab each stroke.
3. Lubricate the end of the catheter tip with the sterile lubricating jelly. Holding the penis at a 90-degree angle to the body, advance the catheter into the meatus, through the urethra, and into the bladder until urine returns.
4. If the bladder is markedly distended, it should be drained gradually; generally no more than 1000 mL of urine should be drained at a time.
5. Inflate the balloon with the sterile water. Pull on the catheter gently to ensure that the balloon is in place.
6. Connect the catheter to the drainage bag. Tape the distal catheter to the inner aspect of the patient's thigh.

Contraindications In semiconscious or fully unconscious patients, nasogastric tube insertion should not be attempted without inserting an endotracheal tube first to prevent aspiration. Massive facial trauma or basilar skull fracture contraindicates nasogastric intubation. When there is evidence of head or neck injury, obstruction of the nose, throat, or esophagus should be ruled out first. Esophageal burn, such as from the ingestion of corrosive acids or alkali, and esophageal atresia or stricture also contraindicates insertion of a nasogastric tube.

Equipment The following equipment should be assembled:
➤ Nasogastric tube of proper diameter. Two types of NG tubes are in common use—the single-lumen tubes (Levin) and the double-lumen sump (Salem's sump) tubes. The single-lumen tubes are best for decompression, and the double-lumen sump tube is best for continuous lavage or irrigation of the stomach. Both may be used for either purpose. Most adults require a 16F to 18F tube. The limiting factor is the size of the nostril or any deviation of the nasal septa.
➤ Suction syringe, 30 mL.
➤ Suction tube and suction device (wall or portable suction).
➤ Sterile lubricating jelly.

➤ Glass of water and a straw.
➤ Emesis basin.
➤ Disposable latex gloves, goggles, and gown.
➤ One 4-inch-long piece of ½-inch tape and benzoin.

Patient Preparation The procedure should be explained to the patient, especially the fact that introduction of the tube will produce gagging. The patient should be in a comfortable sitting position and leaning on a backrest. If the patient is unconscious, position supine with the head slightly elevated. It is important that the patient maintain cervical flexion, to enable the entrance to the trachea to be closed when the patient swallows and to allow the tube to enter only the esophagus.

Possible Complications Accidental placement of the tube into the tracheal airway, aspiration pneumonia, sinusitis, gastric erosion with hemorrhage, and nasal mucosa erosion or necrosis may occur with nasogastric intubation.

Follow-up The tube should be checked to ensure proper functioning and should be removed as soon as possible. If the tube is left in for an extended period, the nostril should be monitored periodically for signs of necrosis.

PROCEDURE FOR NASOGASTRIC INTUBATION

1. Put on the gloves, goggles, and gown.
2. Determine the tube length needed by measuring from the patient's ear to the umbilicus, and mark the length on the tube.
3. Lubricate the distal end of the tube with the jelly.
4. With the patient's neck flexed, insert the tube into one of the nostrils, along the nasal floor, and toward the posterior pharynx. When the tip of the tube reaches the back of the throat, resistance is met and the patient may gag.
5. Have the patient drink small sips of water through a straw, and every time the patient swallows, advance the tube. If the tube slips into the trachea, violent coughing and gagging will occur. Withdraw the tube if this occurs, and repeat the attempt. The most important step is timing the advancement of the tube with swallowing.
6. Advance the tube into the stomach. Entry into the stomach can be determined when the measured mark on the tube reaches the opening of the patient's nasal passage.
7. Check for the tube's placement in the stomach by aspirating for stomach contents. Inject air down the tube while listening over the epigastrium for the sound of air bubbling into the stomach. If no sound is heard, reposition the tube and inject more air. Obtain a chest radiograph to confirm correct tube placement.
8. Secure the tube to the nose with tape and benzoin. The tube should not exert pressure or traction on the nostril when the patient moves.

CLINICAL APPLICATIONS

1. List the factors that affect wound healing.
2. List the causes of "bad" scars that can result from poor suturing technique.
3. List the equipment needed for each of the following clinical procedures:
   - ➤ Phlebotomy.
   - ➤ Peripheral intravenous catheterization.
   - ➤ Arterial blood gas sampling.
   - ➤ Lumbar puncture.
   - ➤ Urethral catheterization.
   - ➤ Nasogastric intubation.
4. If you were entering a rotation or new job situation in which you would be performing the procedures listed in item 3, how would you develop a reminder system for the equipment needed and the steps of each procedure?

RESOURCES

Chestnut MS. Office and Bedside Procedures. London: Prentice-Hall, 1992.

Cosgriff JH. An Atlas of Diagnostic and Therapeutic Procedures for Emergency Personnel. Philadelphia: JB Lippincott, 1978.

Edgerton MT. The Art of Surgical Technique. Baltimore: Williams & Wilkins, 1988.

Klippel AP, Anderson CB (eds). Manual of Emergency and Outpatient Techniques. Boston: Little, Brown, 1979.

LaRocca JC. Pocket Guide to Intravenous Therapy, 3rd ed. St. Louis: Mosby, 1997.

Mayhew HE, Rodgers LE. Basic Procedures in Family Practice: An Illustrated Manual. New York: Wiley, 1984.

McGregor IA. Fundamental Techniques of Plastic Surgery and Their Surgical Applications. New York: Churchill Livingstone, 1989. *This book describes the proper use of surgical tools and their handling, from simple repairs of uncomplicated skin lacerations to more complicated plastic surgery techniques.*

Nealon TF Jr. Fundamental Skills in Surgery. Philadelphia: WB Saunders, 1979. *This is an excellent book for the beginning student in surgery. It covers the basics of surgical tools, gowning, gloving, and operating room conduct to the proper use of surgical drains, local anesthesia, sutures, and patient monitoring equipment.*

Rohrich RJ. The Biology of Wound Healing/Techniques of Wound Closure/Abnormal Scars/Envenomation. Selected Readings in Plastic Surgery, Vol. 5 No. 1. Dallas: Baylor University Medical Center, 1988.

Schultz BC, McKinney P. Office Practice of Skin Surgery. Philadelphia: WB Saunders, 1985. *This book covers basic outpatient skin surgery techniques and instruments. It describes skin preparation, anesthesia, scar formation, and basic wound closure.*

Shila R. Manual for IV Therapy Procedures, 2nd ed. Oradell, NJ: Medical Economics Books, 1985.

Swanson NA. Atlas of Cutaneous Surgery. Boston: Little, Brown, 1987. *This book describes the basic techniques in skin closure. It covers instruments that are normally used for cutaneous surgery, describes their proper uses, and provides some basic instruction in biopsies, incisions, excisions, and wound closures with a variety of techniques.*

Trott A. Wounds and Lacerations. St Louis: Mosby, 1991. *This book covers emergency department treatment of wounds and lacerations. There is an excellent introduction to wound anesthesia, wound cleansing, and irrigation, as well as to the principles and techniques of basic laceration repair, complicated lacerations, problems and solutions, stapling, and dressing and bandaging techniques.*

Van Way CW III, Buerk CA. Surgical Skills in Patient Care. St Louis: Mosby, 1978.

Westaby S. Wound Care. St. Louis: Mosby, 1986. *This book provides a practical understanding of wounds and their definitive care, from the smallest cellular response to injury to the care of nonhealing wounds involving large areas of cutaneous destruction. It also provides a basic understanding of wound closure and drainage, sutures, and dressings and describes some methods to treat common wounds involving specific areas of the body.*

CHAPTER 15

Pharmacology: The Use of Medications

John R. White, Jr.

INTRODUCTION

The prescribing of sophisticated drugs, until recently the exclusive purview of physicians, is unquestionably one of the most important and powerful tools in modern medical practice. The statutory authority to prescribe is increasingly being extended to physician assistants (PAs), nurse practitioners, and pharmacists.[1] The responsible, safe, and effective use of this privilege is an essential element of practice and a serious responsibility for PAs as professionals.

To the student or new graduate physician assistant, the thought of choosing from a bewildering array of drugs, using them effectively and safely, dealing with a competitive industry, and, in general, managing this new responsibility is intimidating indeed. This chapter describes the legal basis of prescribing, outlines general principles for choosing drugs, discusses some specific suggestions on communicating with the pharmacist and the patient, and touches on some of the ethical and practical implications of prescribing. With solid grounding in these basic principles, the fledgling prescriber can approach therapeutic decisions appropriately and with relative confidence. It is the purpose of this chapter to serve as an introduction to the thought processes and communication skills essential for conscientious prescribing. Physician assistant training program curricula contain significantly more detail. This chapter should serve as a basis for further discussion. Information on specific drugs, such as indications, side effects, and dosage, is available in several excellent resource works, some of which are described at the end of the chapter.

LEGAL BACKGROUND

The authority to prescribe medications in the United States is determined by state law. In 1973, North Carolina enacted legislation allowing physician assistants to prescribe from a limited formulary developed by the State Board of Medical Examiners.[2] Several other states followed suit, and in 1978, the Washington State Supreme Court upheld this authority when it was challenged by a suit from the State Nursing Association.[3] The legal principle on which this decision was based is that of "agency," that is, that the PA is an "agent" of the physician, and that orders from the PA are equivalent to those from the physician.[4]

Research on physician assistant prescribing has revealed three important patterns that have strengthened the case for expanded authority. First, prescribing habits of PAs are very similar to those of physicians in terms of appropriateness and safety. Second, very few PAs have been disciplined for misuse or abuse of the privilege. Finally, states that allow physicians to delegate prescribing have a higher percentage of PAs practicing in rural areas.[5]

As of 2002, only two states do not allow for some form of prescriptive authority for physician assistants (Figure 15-1). There is wide variation among state laws as to the specific requirements of and restrictions

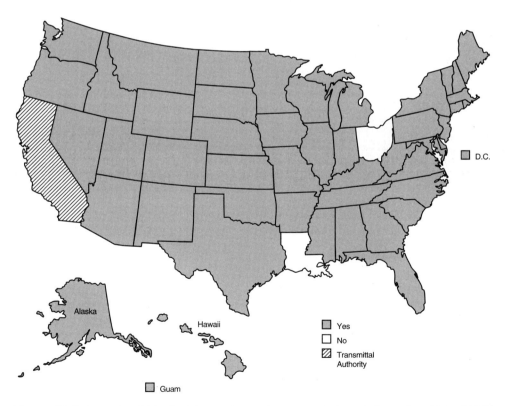

Figure 15-1 States in which physician assistants have prescriptive privileges (as of May 2002). Information supplied by the American Academy of Physician Assistants.

on PA prescribing. Some states use a "formulary" approach, by which the Board of Medical Examiners has a list of specific drugs from which PAs may prescribe. Other states take a more general delegatory approach and allow the physician/PA team to develop its own prescribing protocols. It is the responsibility of all prescribers to know and comply with the laws of the state in which they practice.[6]

DRUG CLASSIFICATION AND REGULATION

Approval and regulation of therapeutic agents is the domain of the U.S. Food and Drug Administration (FDA). The FDA classifies drugs either as over the counter, that is, available without a prescription, or legend, meaning that they bear the legend statement, "Caution: Federal law prohibits dispensing without a prescription." These determinations are based on drug safety, the conditions for which it is indicated, and in some cases, the strength or dosage form. The FDA determines the conditions or indications for which a drug may be advertised, labeled, or otherwise marketed. This determination does not, however, limit the manner in which a physician (or other prescriber) may use an approved drug. Accepted medical practice, in other words, often includes use of drugs that is not reflected in package labeling that shows FDA-approved uses. For example, many angiotensin-converting enzyme inhibitors such as enalapril or lisinopril are used in the management of diabetic proteinuria, although only captopril is FDA-approved for this use. Unfortunately, non-FDA-approved uses of drugs are not published in the commonly used *Physicians' Desk Reference (PDR)*, but they are included in some references, such as *Drug Information for Health Professionals: United States Pharmacopeial Convention* (see Resources).

The FDA also categorizes drugs according to their safety in pregnancy or potential for harm to the fetus. Owing to the ethical problem in performing controlled studies on pregnant women, the human data for most drugs are incomplete, and these ratings are largely based on animal studies. The difficult decision to prescribe any drug for a pregnant woman must be made on an individual basis with a clear understanding of the risk-benefit ratio (Table 15-1).

Drugs that have the potential for abuse or addiction are further regulated by the U.S. Drug Enforcement Agency (DEA). These include opiate

Table 15-1	Key to FDA Use-in-Pregnancy Ratings*
Category	**Interpretation**
A	Controlled studies show no risk. Adequate, well-controlled studies in pregnant women have failed to demonstrate risk to the fetus.
B	No evidence of risk in humans. Either animal findings show risk but human findings do not, or if no adequate human studies have been done, animal findings are negative.
C	Risk cannot be ruled out. Human studies are lacking, and animal studies are either positive for fetal risk or lacking as well. However, potential benefits may justify the potential risk.
D	Positive evidence of risk. Investigational or postmarketing data show risk to the fetus. Nevertheless, potential benefits may outweigh the potential risk.
X	Contraindicated in pregnancy. Studies in animals or humans, or investigational or postmarketing reports, have shown fetal risk that clearly outweighs any possible benefit to the patient.

From Gara N. Physician Assistants: Presenting and Dispensing Summary. Alexandria, VA: American Association of Physician Assistants, 1992.
*The Food and Drug Administration's Pregnancy Categories are based on the degree to which available information has ruled out risk to the fetus, balanced against the drug's potential benefits to the patient. Ratings range from "A," for drugs that have been tested for teratogenicity under controlled conditions without showing evidence of damage to the fetus, to "D" and "X," for drugs that are definitely teratogenic. The "D" rating is generally reserved for drugs with no safer alternatives. The "X" rating means there is absolutely no reason to risk using the drug in pregnancy.

and synthetic narcotics, sedatives, stimulants, and hallucinogens, which are collectively referred to as "controlled substances." Controlled substances are classified into one of five categories or schedules according to their potential for abuse or addiction (Table 15-2), and for this reason are sometimes referred to as "schedule" drugs. Providers who are legally authorized to prescribe controlled substances—including PAs in many states—must comply with DEA rules and sometimes with additional state regulations regarding prescription format, refills, and record keeping.

GENERAL PRINCIPLES OF DRUG THERAPY

The decision to implement drug therapy and the choice of appropriate drugs are complex undertakings. Careful consideration of host factors, suspected or known causes of disease, and the properties and actions of available drugs is always required. In addition, the clinician should remember that drugs are not always the best solution to a clinical problem. Often, a nonpharmacological therapeutic plan is the best choice for the patient. The following case will be used in the discussion that follows, to illustrate the process

of deciding to use drug therapy and choosing from available agents.

CASE STUDY 15-1

Mr. C, a 48-year-old man with a past history of asthma, presents to the clinic with a 3-day history of upper respiratory infection (URI) symptoms—an increasingly productive cough, burning substernal chest pain, mild shortness of breath, and a low-grade fever. Careful history and physical examination and a normal chest x-ray lead to a diagnosis of acute asthmatic bronchitis.

THE RISK-BENEFIT RATIO

Given that virtually all drugs carry some degree of risk, whether to the patient, society, or the biosphere, all decisions to prescribe drugs should be predicated on evidence that the potential benefit will outweigh this risk. Often, the expectations of patients can make this point a challenge to the provider—it takes less time to write a prescription than to persuade the patient that a medication is not necessary! By the same token, once the decision has been made to use drug therapy, the choice of drugs often rests on consideration of the

Table 15-2   Key to Controlled Substances Categories*

Category	Interpretation
C I	High potential for abuse. No accepted medical use.
C II	High potential for abuse. Use may lead to severe physical or psychological dependence. Prescriptions must be written in ink or typewritten and must be signed by the practitioner. Verbal prescriptions must be confirmed in writing within 72 hours and may be given only in a genuine emergency. No renewals are permitted.
C III	Some potential for abuse. Use may lead to low to moderate physical dependence or high psychological dependence. Prescriptions may be oral or written. Up to five renewals are permitted within 6 months.
C IV	Low potential for abuse. Use may lead to limited physical or psychological dependence. Prescriptions may be oral or written. Up to five renewals are permitted within 6 months.
C V	Subject to state and local regulation. Abuse potential is low. A prescription may not be required.

Modified from Gara N. Physician Assistants: Presenting and Dispensing Summary. Alexandria, VA: American Association of Physician Assistants, 1992.
*Products listed with the symbols shown here are subject to the Controlled Substances Act of 1970. These drugs are categorized according to their potential for abuse. The greater the potential, the more severe are the limitations on their prescription.

risk-benefit ratio. In this respect, the guiding principle, as always, is, "First, do no harm."

DRUG ALLERGIES

Hypersensitivity reactions, or drug allergies, are allergic reactions to chemicals that occur after previous sensitization to that compound or to other compounds with structural similarities. The clinical effect of hypersensitivity reactions can range from mildly bothersome to life threatening and even fatal. Comprehensive medication histories should be taken on all patients because a missed allergy can be fatal, and because patients frequently erroneously label adverse effects of medications as allergies. A complete history includes medications to which the patient is "allergic," along with the specific untoward effects the medications had in that particular patient. This type of history will provide the practitioner with a great deal more information than a simple list of drugs under the rubric of allergy. For example, many patients will state an allergy to codeine—nausea—which is not usually a true allergy but is a simple adverse effect of opiate narcotics.

The clinician should understand that an allergic response to a compound increases the likelihood of an allergic response to compounds with "similar" molecular structures. For example, a patient who has an allergic response to penicillin is also more likely to be allergic to antibiotics in the cephalosporin category than is a patient with no allergic history. Because of chemical similarities between sulfonamides and sulfonylureas, patients who are allergic to sulfonamide antibiotics may also be allergic to sulfonylurea hypoglycemic agents. Cross-reactivity exists among several categories of medications.

Allergic responses may be divided into four discrete categories by immunological mechanism.[7] Type I reactions are mediated by immunoglobulin (Ig) E antibodies. During this type of reaction, several mediators, including histamine, leukotrienes, and prostaglandins, are released, causing vasodilation, edema, and a general inflammatory response. This type of allergic response can affect the gastrointestinal tract (food allergy), the respiratory system (rhinitis and bronchoconstriction), the vasculature (shock), and the skin (urticaria and atopic dermatitis).

Penicillin-induced anaphylactic shock, which can be fatal, is an example of a type I reaction. Type II, or cytolytic, reactions are mediated by IgM and IgG antibodies and the subsequent activation of the complement system. Cells in the circulatory system are most frequently affected by type II reactions. Methyldopa-induced hemolytic anemia and quinidine-induced thrombocytopenia are examples of type II reactions. Arthus reactions, serum sickness, or type III reactions are mediated primarily by IgG and the deposition of antigen-antibody complexes in vascular endothelium. Certain anticonvulsants, iodides, and other drugs have been linked to type III reactions. Delayed hypersensitivity, or type IV, reactions are mediated by macrophages and sensitized T lymphocytes. Contact dermatitis caused by poison ivy is an example of a type IV reaction.

CASE STUDY 15-2

Although acute bronchitis in an otherwise healthy patient is often a self-limiting condition that will resolve with fluids, rest, and symptomatic therapy, Mr. C's asthma puts him at increased risk for complications. Antibiotic therapy is not unreasonable. His dyspnea and wheezing also suggest the need for a bronchodilator. In response to further questioning, Mr. C admits that he has been taking theophylline tablets for his asthma. He is supposed to take 200 mg twice a day, but he says he often forgets. He knows of no drug allergies.

LIMITING THE ARMAMENTARIUM

A very helpful practical suggestion for the neophyte prescriber faced with the bewildering array of available products is this: strive to know well a few drugs in each therapeutic class. With careful choices based on proven efficacy and safety, the beginner will gradually become comfortable with them and will rarely find it necessary to diverge from the chosen list. Until PAs reach this level of comfort, it is well worth their time to look up a drug each time they prescribe it.

The usual offending organisms in acute bronchitis include *Streptococcus pneumoniae, Haemophilus influenzae,* and *Moraxella catarrhalis,* as well as viruses. Classes of antibiotics covering this spectrum (excluding viruses) that are appropriate to use in this situation are extended-spectrum penicillins (e.g., ampicillin), second-generation cephalosporins (e.g., cefaclor), sulfonamides (e.g., trimethoprim, sulfamethoxazole), macrolides (e.g., erythromycin), and some tetracyclines (e.g., doxycycline) and quinolones. Effective bronchodilation is often achieved either with xanthines such as theophylline or with any of several beta-agonist sympathomimetics (e.g., albuterol).

ROUTES OF ADMINISTRATION

The next decision to be addressed is how to get the drug into the patient. With the current marketing of new "delivery systems" (designed for patient convenience and compliance), this is an increasingly complex choice because we must consider available dosage forms and routes of administration.

Dosage form is the physical form in which the drug is administered. Tablets, capsules, solutions, suspensions, gases, and ointments are all examples of dosage forms. The physical properties of a given dosage form can have a significant effect on how rapidly and completely the drug is delivered to the target tissue. For example, drugs taken orally must be in solution if they are to be absorbed into the circulation. Drugs that are already in solution or suspension are obviously absorbed faster than tablets or capsules, which must first dissolve.

The traditional routes of administration are oral (taken by mouth and absorbed by the gastrointestinal tract), topical (applied directly to the skin or mucous membranes), and parenteral (any route that bypasses the gastrointestinal absorption system). Parenteral injection choices are the direct intravenous route, intramuscular and subcutaneous routes, and intra-arterial and intrathecal (into the spinal column) routes for special applications. Other parenteral routes are inhalational (via the lungs), sublingual (absorbed by the oral mucosa), transdermal (placed on the skin for absorption into the circulation), and rectal.

The above-mentioned antibiotic classes and the xanthines are all available in a variety of oral and parenteral dosage forms. Sympathomimetics are most often inhaled using a metered-dose inhaler or nebulizer, although oral and parenteral preparations of some are available.

PHARMACOKINETICS AND PHARMACODYNAMICS

The study of how drugs are absorbed, distributed, metabolized, and excreted is known as pharmacokinetics. The study of how drugs produce an effect on the body is pharmacodynamics. Although a detailed discussion of these fields is beyond the scope of this chapter, it is critical that the prescriber understand some basic principles and consider their implications for therapy and patient education.

The first principle to consider is that of bioavailability—the fraction of the drug taken that actually reaches the systemic circulation. Bioavailability of an orally administered drug is influenced by two major factors: absorption of the drug by the gastric mucosa and metabolism of the drug as it passes through the liver from the portal system (the first-pass effect). These in turn are influenced by the properties of the drug itself, as well as by host factors such as other gastric contents, gastric motility, and the state of liver enzymes.

Although ampicillin itself is not very well absorbed, an alternative—amoxicillin—is well absorbed. As is often the case, variations in bioavailability of the other antibiotics are compensated for by the dosage schedule. Xanthines are variably absorbed and, as will become apparent, must be dosed very carefully. Inhaled sympathomimetics are rapidly absorbed directly from the lungs to the systemic circulation. Proper use of the inhaler, however, is essential to ensure delivery of the desired dose to the lungs.

The distribution of a drug to various body tissues is primarily influenced by its relative solubility in water and by the degree to which it becomes bound to plasma proteins. The important thing to remember is that it is the free (unbound) drug that is dissolved in the plasma that is available to produce an effect. Drugs that are hydrophobic, such as barbiturates, are largely distributed to fat and muscle tissue, whereas some drugs, such as warfarin, have a very high affinity for plasma proteins. In both cases, a small fraction of the originally absorbed drug is left freely dissolved and therefore able to produce an effect. Competition for protein-binding sites is one of the major mechanisms of drug-drug interactions.

None of the drugs being considered for Mr. C is protein bound to a clinically significant extent.

The third major pharmacokinetic variable is the rate of excretion from the body, or clearance. The major routes of drug excretion are the kidney, liver (through the bile), gastrointestinal tract, and lungs. Small amounts of drugs may also be excreted in saliva, sweat, and breast milk. (This may be significant for a nursing infant.) The most important concepts of clearance for the prescriber are those of half-life and steady state. Simplistically speaking, the half-life of a drug is the time it takes for 50% of a dose of that drug to be cleared by the body. A steady state is achieved when the rate of administration of a drug is equal to the rate of clearance, thereby keeping the plasma concentration constant. Although drug half-lives are often given or estimated, we must use these with caution because many host factors, such as age, disease states, and drug interactions, influence the actual clearance. In some cases in which relatively toxic drugs are being used (e.g., theophylline), serum concentrations can be measured to assure that the drug concentration is within the therapeutic range. Additionally, patient-specific pharmacokinetic parameters (i.e., clearance, half-life, and volume of distribution) may be calculated with pharmacokinetic equations using drug concentration data and patient characteristics. Most often, these calculations are done on request by a clinical pharmacist and can be of great assistance in the assessment of compliance, efficacy, toxicity, and future dosing regimens.

For antibiotic therapy of bronchitis, the route of excretion is not a major issue. For a urinary tract infection, however, it may be, because the drug would have to concentrate unchanged in the urine. In addition, the desired effect of most antibiotics does not depend on a constant plasma concentration, but rather on adequate peak levels. On the other hand, steady state is very important when one is considering the xanthine bronchodilators. Theophylline has a "narrow therapeutic window," which means that the therapeutic plasma concentration is very close to the toxic plasma concentration.

Pharmacodynamics is a complex field, and this chapter is too limited to explore it. The reader should remember, at least, that no drug has just one effect, and that there virtually always are desired (or therapeutic) effects and undesired (or toxic) effects associated with a drug. Perhaps the most important knowledge a prescriber must have is what the potential toxic effects of a prescribed drug are, how to monitor for them, and what action to take should they appear. Patient education plays a major role in this respect, as is explored later.

Antibacterial drugs generally act either by causing the death of the organism (bactericidal activity) or by simply inhibiting its reproduction (bacteriostatic activity). If the host immune system is impaired for any reason, or if the condition is resistant to immune mechanisms (as is bacterial endocarditis), then bactericidal effect may be necessary to prevent a relapse. Amoxicillin and cefaclor are both bactericidal, whereas erythromycin seems to be either bactericidal or bacteriostatic, depending on the dose. Sulfonamides are bacteriostatic. Other than an allergic reaction, the only significant toxic effect among the three agents being considered in this case is the well-known gastrointestinal upset associated with erythromycin. The two classes of bronchodilators both work by increasing the supply of cyclic adenosine monophosphate (cAMP) in smooth muscle cells, but they do so by different mechanisms. Mr. C is taking his theophylline inconsistently, so his level is probably subtherapeutic. In this case, an argument can be made for reinforcing his compliance with the theophylline and adding a sympathomimetic. To minimize cardiac side effects, a beta$_2$-selective agent such as albuterol is preferred.

DRUG INTERACTIONS

Another vastly complex area is how drugs interact with one another in vivo. Most interactions occur by one of three major mechanisms:

1. Pharmacokinetic interference with absorption, distribution, metabolism, or excretion.

2. Pharmacodynamic mechanisms such as additive or competitive receptor binding.
3. Combined toxicity.

Most prescribers become familiar with a few well-known and common drug interactions over time; therefore, they must consult reference books and trust that their patients' pharmacists will detect potential interactions among the drugs they supply.

CASE STUDY 15-5

It is well known that macrolide antibiotics (excluding azithromycin) can inhibit the metabolism of theophylline, thereby increasing theophylline effect. Because theophylline has a narrow therapeutic window, administration of macrolides may, in fact, cause theophylline toxicity. In this case, the most appropriate choice of antibiotic is either amoxicillin, a second-generation cephalosporin, or a sulfonamide. The only other interaction to consider is the potential combined toxicity of theophylline and a sympathomimetic, which in this case will probably not be clinically significant.

COST EFFECTIVENESS

With all other therapeutic considerations being equal, the choice of a specific agent may be a question of relative cost. With the current public focus on rising health care costs and the advent of managed health care systems, relative cost of prescribed drugs is an increasingly important and complex issue.

One major factor that influences drug costs is whether a drug is produced under patent or is available in a generic form. The pharmaceutical company that develops a new drug is allowed an exclusive patent on it for 14 years. When the patent has expired, other companies are free to produce and market the drug under its generic, or chemical, name, while the original company maintains the proprietary name and often sells the agent at a higher price. In most cases, the generic preparations are therapeutically equivalent to the brand name product. Many insurance companies and professional organizations are developing policies on generic prescribing, and in some systems, a pharmacy and therapeutics committee or a formulary committee may have input on these decisions. In addition, public third party payers such as Medicare

and Medicaid have very specific restrictions on what drugs they will pay for. It is our bias that with a few notable exceptions, generic preparations, when available, should be used.

Another factor related to cost is variability in price among retail outlets. Especially with medications taken on a long-term basis, patients can realize a significant savings by doing some comparison shopping. This is not only a direct benefit for them, but it may affect compliance as well. On the other hand, it is safer for a patient who is taking multiple medications to purchase them all at one pharmacy.

Amoxicillin is chosen because it is inexpensive, is well tolerated, has no significant drug interactions in this case, and is often effective in uncomplicated bronchitis. Compliance with theophylline therapy should also be reviewed with the patient. Lastly, he will be placed on an albuterol inhaler. The next step is to decide what communication is necessary to accomplish this goal.

COMMUNICATION WITH THE PHARMACIST

A pharmacist is a professional member of the health care team who is trained and authorized by law to stock and dispense medications on the order of an authorized prescriber. A pharmacist completes 5 to 8 years of education and is very knowledgeable about the actions and side effects of drugs. Pharmacists can be a valuable resource to the prescriber by assisting in choosing medications, dosing medications, reviewing regimens for drug interactions, and counseling patients regarding their medication.

THE PRESCRIPTION

Once the PA has evaluated a patient, arrived at a diagnosis, and determined that drug therapy is indicated, he or she must communicate the order to the pharmacist. This is done with the prescription. A prescription for noncontrolled substances may be written on a preprinted form or any blank paper. A prescription may also be transmitted over the telephone by speaking directly to a licensed pharmacist or pharmacy intern. Although it is common practice for this duty to be delegated to the prescriber's office personnel, this practice may lead to communication errors and should probably be avoided. Schedule II controlled substances may not be prescribed over the telephone, and some states require specially numbered, duplicate forms. The prescription for any controlled substance must contain a valid DEA number.

However the order is transmitted, it must contain certain legal elements. Incomplete or sloppily written prescriptions are the source of many dangerous medication errors, much patient confusion leading to poor compliance, and hours of wasted time for the pharmacist. The following list describes all of the elements of a complete prescription, with suggestions for accuracy in each:

➤ The date the prescription was written.

➤ Prescriber identification: Name, professional degree, office address and telephone number, and DEA number if required.

➤ Patient identification: Name, address, age, sex, and weight.

➤ Superscription: Rx, an abbreviation of a Latin phrase meaning "take thou."

➤ Inscription: The name of the drug and the strength. This should be the strength of each dosage unit, not the total dose to be taken by the patient. Abbreviations for drug names should be used only if the prescriber is certain that they will be clearly understood by the pharmacist.

➤ Subscription: Instructions to the pharmacist regarding the dosage form and the number of dosage units to dispense. Instructions should be specific about the dosage form (i.e., tablets, capsules, suspension), and a quantity must be specified if it is a liquid or semisolid (e.g., 120-mL suspension or 30-g tube). For controlled substances, quantities should be written in words as well as numbers to guard against alteration, such as "Dispense: thirty (30) tablets."

➤ Signa: Instructions to the patient. These should be as simple, complete, and specific as possible and should include how much to take, when to take it, and why it is being taken. "As directed" and "usual directions" should be avoided; such instructions are confusing and dangerous and are even illegal in some states.

➤ Refill information: The number of times (or time period) that the patient may renew the prescrip-

tion without authorization from the prescriber. Prescriptions for schedule II controlled substances may not be refilled, and schedule III to V controlled substances have a 5-refill or 6-month limit.

➤ Container information: Unless the prescriber specifies otherwise, medications will be dispensed in childproof containers, which may create problems for elderly or arthritic patients.

➤ Generic substitution: In most cases, the pharmacist may substitute a generic preparation for a prescribed brand, unless the prescriber specifies "dispense as written" on the order. Most preprinted forms contain two spaces for the prescriber's signature, with the space on the left labeled "substitution permitted" and the other labeled "dispense as written."

➤ Warnings: The prescription should specify what if any warning labels should be attached to the medication vial. "May cause drowsiness" and "Do not take with alcohol" are examples.

➤ Prescriber's signature.

The use of abbreviations and symbols in prescription writing is unavoidable. The prescriber should, however, make every effort to ensure that such abbreviations are clear and standard to avoid confusion. Table 15-3 lists standard prescription abbreviations. A common technique is the use of lower case roman numerals for numbers (e.g., "iii tabs p.o. tid" to specify three tablets by mouth three times daily). Above all, the prescription should be legibly and clearly written.

> **CASE STUDY 15-6**

The decision is made to treat Mr. C with 250 mg of amoxicillin by mouth three times daily for 10 days. In addition, he is to be given an albuterol inhaler to use four times daily. Figure 15-2 shows complete prescriptions, legibly written, for this treatment.

INPATIENT ORDERS

Inpatient orders differ only slightly from the preceding description. Because they are usually written in the patient's chart on a preprinted, duplicate order form that is stamped with the patient's identifying

Table 15-3   Standard Abbreviations Used in Prescriptions

Abbreviation	Meaning	Abbreviation	Meaning
DOSE		**FREQUENCY**	
dr	Teaspoonful	hs	At bedtime
g, gm	Gram	pc	At meals
gr	Grain	prn	As needed
gtt	Drops	q	Every
mcg, µg	Microgram	qd	Every day
mg	Milligram	qid	Four times a day
ROUTE		qod	Every other day
ad	Right ear	stat	At once, immediately
as	Left ear	tid	Three times a day
au	Each ear	ut dict	As directed
od	Right eye	**MISCELLANEOUS**	
os	Left eye	aa	Of each
ou	Each eye	cap	Capsule
po	By mouth	c	With
supp	Suppository	n.r.	No refill
vag	Vaginally	qs ad	Add a sufficient amount to make
FREQUENCY			
ac	Before meals	rep	Repeat, refill
ad lib	Freely at pleasure	ss	One half
bid	Twice a day	sig	Directions for use
h	Hour	tab	Tablet

Modified from Katzung BG. Basic and Clinical Pharmacology, ed 4. Norwalk, CT: Appleton & Lange, 1989.

data, the prescriber does not have to supply this information. In addition, medications are generally continued until the provider writes a discontinue order or the patient is discharged, or unless an expiration policy exists for that medication. Therefore, the elements of the hospital order are the same as the "body" of the outpatient prescription—inscription, subscription, and signa.

DISPENSING

Some states have specific laws allowing physician assistants to dispense medications under certain circumstances.[7] The purpose of these rules is generally to serve the patient's best interest when the services of a pharmacist are not available or in emergency situations. In some cases, they also allow for the dispensing of office samples. In most states, the laws specify that the PA must comply with labeling regulations when dispensing.

CASE STUDY 15-7

Mr. C is finally ready to receive his prescription. What information should the PA discuss with him before he leaves?

PATIENT EDUCATION

It is tempting, in a busy office setting, for the clinician to simply hand the patient the prescription and send him or her to the pharmacy. It is critical to the success and safety of the treatment, however, that the provider give careful instructions about what to do with the prescribed drug. Even though most pharmacists repeat the instructions when dispensing the drug, good patient education by the provider influences the outcome of

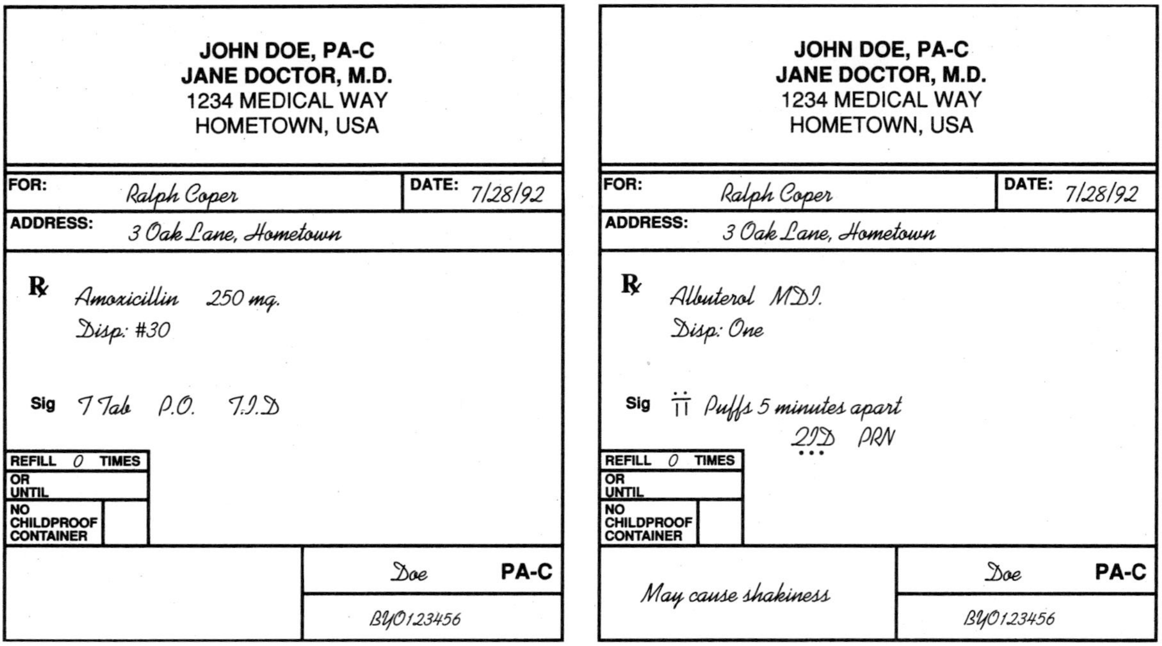

JOHN DOE, PA-C
JANE DOCTOR, M.D.
1234 MEDICAL WAY
HOMETOWN, USA

FOR: Ralph Coper DATE: 7/28/92
ADDRESS: 3 Oak Lane, Hometown

℞ Amoxicillin 250 mg.
Disp: #30

Sig 1 Tab P.O. T.I.D

REFILL 0 TIMES
OR UNTIL
NO CHILDPROOF CONTAINER

Doe PA-C
BY0123456

JOHN DOE, PA-C
JANE DOCTOR, M.D.
1234 MEDICAL WAY
HOMETOWN, USA

FOR: Ralph Coper DATE: 7/28/92
ADDRESS: 3 Oak Lane, Hometown

℞ Albuterol MDI.
Disp: One

Sig ii Puffs 5 minutes apart
QID PRN

REFILL 0 TIMES
OR UNTIL
NO CHILDPROOF CONTAINER

May cause shakiness

Doe PA-C
BY0123456

A **B**

Figure 15-2 Sample prescriptions for **(A)** amoxicillin and **(B)** albuterol. (Prescription format from Katzung BG. Basic and Clinical Pharmacology. Norwalk, CT: Appleton & Lange, 1989.)

treatment to a great extent. The principal areas to reinforce with the patient include the following:

- ➤ The reason for the treatment.
- ➤ The expected outcome and how and when to take the medication.
- ➤ What side effects to be alert for.
- ➤ What to do if side effects should appear.
- ➤ Any precautions to take.

Every patient has the right to a full explanation of his or her condition, the rationale and risks of drug therapy, and what other options, if any, exist. With this explanation and the guidance of the provider, the patient becomes a fully consenting participant in his or her care rather than simply a consumer of service. As part of this process, a discussion of what toxic effects are commonly encountered is essential. Because the required listing of reported side effects in drug package inserts is often intimidating, it is the provider's role to explain the important side effects in perspective and to give specific instructions about what to do if they should appear.

The provider should confirm that the patient will be able to obtain the medicine and comply with instructions. Often, the involvement of a spouse or other caregiver is valuable at this point to enhance compliance. Very specific suggestions about when to take the medication and how to remember to do so are helpful, for example, "Keep it in the kitchen and take it when you start to fix each meal," and "Keep it by your toothbrush so you'll remember to take it at bedtime." In addition, care should be taken not to assume that the patient knows even something that may seem obvious. Therefore, instructions such as "Be sure to take the foil off the suppository before you insert it" are often not unreasonable. In addition, the duration of therapy should be explained, and the patient encouraged to take the medication until it is gone.

With long-term drug therapy, it is important to review instructions at each visit and to reinforce and monitor compliance. Repeated instruction on the proper use of inhalers, for example, can greatly enhance the success of this therapy.

The PA gives Mr. C his prescription for amoxicillin. He confirms that he is able to pay for it and will go straight to the pharmacy next door. He is told to take one tablet three times a day with water. The PA explains that some antibiotics are better absorbed on an empty stomach and suggests that Mr. C take the amoxicillin when he starts to prepare each meal. The PA also gives him an albuterol inhaler from office samples, along with thorough instructions and a demonstration of its proper use. Finally, the PA recommends that Mr. C take his theophylline as prescribed and return in 3 days for a blood theophylline level.

Mrs. C, who is present for the conversation, states that she will help him remember to take the medicine. Mr. C is told to be alert for any side effects of the amoxicillin, especially skin rash, palpitations, or diarrhea, and to stop the medicine and call the clinic immediately if any should appear. The PA also alerts Mr. C to the fact that the combination of bronchodilators may make him feel a little "shaky" and dry in the mouth.

As with many elements of PA practice, a final critical consideration in prescribing is that of documentation. The patient's office chart should contain complete treatment information, including dosages, precautions, and follow-up. All medications approved for refill should also be noted in the chart. Attention to detail in this respect is a matter of good medical practice and can only help PAs and their patients overall.

THE PHARMACEUTICAL INDUSTRY

The production and sale of therapeutic drugs in the United States represents a huge industry worth many billions of dollars. Even a small market share of a single drug can mean millions in profit to a company. It is no wonder that drug manufacturers have large marketing departments dedicated to encouraging the prescribing of their products. The individual prescriber encounters such encouragement through advertisements in professional journals and through contact with company representatives, or "detailers." These representatives make routine calls to providers' offices and often have displays at professional

meetings. Although pharmaceutical industry support of educational meetings and materials is a valuable contribution, prescribers must exercise care to avoid any potential conflict of interest. Professional organizations, including the American College of Physicians and the American Academy of Physician Assistants, are in the process of developing guidelines for interaction with this industry.[8]

Industry representatives often give free samples of their products to prescribers. Many providers consider accepting these samples useful to patients who could not otherwise pay for medications. Often, however, such samples are of more expensive, brand name products, so starting patients on these can be more costly in the long run. In addition, the PA must consider the time spent in detail visits. Although these can be good sources of information about new products and community trends, the PA may be able to use this time more productively by seeing more patients.

In the final analysis, the new prescriber would do well to consider two suggestions about dealing with the pharmaceutical industry. The first is to examine all product claims with as critical an eye as he or she would any piece of medical literature. The second is that it may not be the best policy to be among the first to use a new drug. Conversely, one should probably not stubbornly refuse to change an old habit in the face of convincing evidence that there is something better. Keeping these caveats in mind, PAs can achieve a mutually beneficial relationship with the pharmaceutical industry.

ETHICAL AND PRACTICAL CONSIDERATIONS OF PRESCRIBING

As has been mentioned, the prescribing of potentially dangerous drugs is a tremendous responsibility. Although it is often referred to as prescriptive authority, the ability to do so is best considered a privilege and treated with care. Perhaps extra considerations for physician assistants reflect the dependent nature of the practice and the necessity of close coordination with the supervising physician. A consistent approach to the following issues among the health care team can prevent misunderstandings.

It is not uncommon for a friend or family member, who knows of a PA's skills and training, to ask informally for information or medical advice. Although this occurrence is often a boost to the ego, it is fraught with danger and should be carefully planned for. The difficulty involved in maintaining professional objectivity when dealing with family members or friends is well known. One must also consider that the legal authority (in most states) to treat patients extends only to those who have an established relationship with the supervising physician. Finally, it may be helpful to consider the potential consequences, both legal and emotional, of a complication or bad outcome.

By the same token, a PA might be tempted to treat himself or herself by taking from office samples rather than making the effort to see another health care provider. To that temptation, one can simply answer by quoting Voltaire: "He who is his own physician has a fool for a doctor." In many states, prescribers are legally prevented from prescribing controlled substances for themselves.

A prescriber faces another difficult situation when he or she knows or suspects that a patient is seeking to obtain drugs for other than therapeutic use. The PA can only be alert to this possibility and should not be too quick to label someone as a drug-seeker simply because his or her pain is not convincing. Perhaps taking a philosophical approach can be helpful: That drug-seeking behavior is itself the problem for which intervention is indicated. On the other hand, the PA does not want to become known as an "easy mark." Reasonable caution includes protecting prescription pads from theft, protecting prescriptions from alteration, and being alert to common ploys, such as lost prescriptions, uncommon allergies, and inconsistent stories. In addition, local knowledge of the resources available for referral and help with problems of substance abuse and addiction can be useful.

CONCLUSION

The authority to prescribe medications is a privilege extended to physician assistants in many states. When exercising this authority, it is incumbent on the practitioner to understand the rules and regulations regarding the prescribing of medications. The choice of medication used in each situation must be tailored to the individual patient and the disease being treated.

Considerations should include the risk-benefit ratio, drug allergies, the most appropriate route of administration, pharmacokinetics and pharmacodynamics, possible drug interactions, and cost. Pharmacists are a readily available source of information and should be used. Prescriptions should be accompanied by patient education in order to ensure compliance. When used in an appropriate fashion, pharmacological therapy can be one of the most effective tools clinicians have at their disposal.

CLINICAL APPLICATIONS

1. Interview pharmacists from a large health care system (e.g., managed care organization, academic health center, hospital system) that uses a closed formulary for its providers. Discuss how drugs are chosen for, or excluded from, the formulary. Who makes the decisions? What are the criteria? Is there a research component to the decision making (evidence based)? What is the role of pharmaceutical companies in influencing these decisions?

2. Interview practicing pharmacists to whom you may refer patients. Find out what type of relationship they ideally would like to have with a physician assistant. Describe typical patterns of communication between pharmacists (or PharmDs) and prescribers in your community, and recommend strategies for providing optimal patient care through maximizing this communication.

REFERENCES

1. Gara N. Regulation of physician assistant prescribing. J Am Acad Physician Assist 1990;3:71.
2. NC Gen Stat § 90 (1973).
3. Washington State Nurses Association v Board of Medical Examiners, 93 Wash 2d 117, 605 P2d 1269 (1980).
4. Creighton H. Law for the nurse supervisor: physician's assistant medication orders. Superv Nurse 1981;12:46.
5. Willis JB. Prescriptive practice patterns of physician assistants. J Am Acad Physician Assist 1990;3:39.
6. Gara N. Physician Assistants: Prescribing and Dispensing Summary. Alexandria, VA: American Academy of Physician Assistants, 1992.
7. Hardman JG, Limbard LE (eds). Goodman and Gillman's: The Pharmacologic Basis of Therapeutics, ed 9. New York: McGraw Hill, 1996;67–68.

8. Caton L, et al. Roundtable: exploring the ethical relationship between pharmaceutical companies and physician assistants. J Am Acad Physician Assist 1992;5:209.

RESOURCES

Hardman JG, Limbard LE (eds). Goodman and Gillman's: The Pharmacologic Basis of Therapeutics, ed 10. New York: McGraw-Hill, 2000;67–68. *The "gold standard" reference in the field of pharmacology, containing detailed information by drug class.*

Knobin J, Anderson PO (eds). Handbook of Clinical Drug Data, ed 10. Hamilton, IL: Drug Intelligence Publications, 2002. *This is a comprehensive pocket-sized handbook of drug information that is well referenced, nonbiased, and arranged by drug class. It contains many useful sections on such topics as common adverse drug effects and drug interactions.*

Handbook of Nonprescription Drugs, ed 12. Washington DC: American Pharmaceutical Association, 2000. *This nonbiased, comprehensive review is a full-sized text that contains information about all over-the-counter drugs.*

Herfindal ET, Hart LL, Gourley D (eds). Clinical Pharmacy and Therapeutics, ed 7. Baltimore, London: Williams & Wilkins, 2000. *This is a therapeutics text that discusses the clinical use of drugs by disease state. The text is accompanied by a companion book of patient cases demonstrating the pharmacological management of all major and some rare diseases.*

Mosby's 2001 GenRx: The Complete Reference for Generic and Brand Drugs. St Louis: Mosby, 2001. *This is a compendium of medications arranged by generic name, which includes information needed by prescribers found in other commonly used references such as the Physicians' Desk Reference (PDR), information about drug costs, and generic equivalency information. The text is available on CD/ROM.*

Drug Information for Health Professionals: United States Pharmacopeial Convention. Rockville, MD: United States Pharmacopeia, 2000. *This is the official pharmacopeia for the United States, published by the American Society of Health Care Systems Pharmacists, which includes both FDA-approved and nonapproved uses of medications not found in other compendia such as the PDR.*

CHAPTER 16

Health Promotion, Disease Prevention, and Patient Education

William R. Duryea

Rationale for Preventive Interventions	**Physical Examination**
Patient Education and Counseling	**Screening Tests and Procedures**
• **Case Study 16-1**	**Immunizations**
	Conclusion

RATIONALE FOR PREVENTIVE INTERVENTIONS

Most physician assistants (PAs) are trained in primary care and have the capability as primary care clinicians to provide a broad range of health promotion and disease prevention (HPDP) services. Such services involve, in large measure, patient education and counseling about lifestyle issues and high-risk behaviors that are known to have negative consequences on patients' health and well-being. In their role as mid-level providers, PAs are in a key position to initiate HPDP programs in their practices and can ensure that such programs are carried through for all patients according to a systematic plan of action.

PA education programs around the country currently provide experiences by which students can learn the elements of health promotion and disease prevention. Unfortunately, although preventive medicine has become one of the important components in virtually every primary care physician assistant's didactic experience, the academic experience does not always carry over to clinical practice. There are as many reasons for that as there are practice settings, but certainly one factor that often mitigates against providing routine preventive medical services is cost, in both time and money.

One could convincingly argue that practices employing PAs should be able to increase the time spent with each patient in order to include preventive interventions. However, is the added task of providing preventive services worth the effort? Some clinicians may answer, "No, because patients don't listen anyway." Obviously, such a position is self-defeating and avoids determining the real or potential value of providing the service.

Frame[1] has evaluated preventive interventions directed at atherosclerotic and infectious diseases, cancer, and metabolic and behavioral conditions. He considers such interventions useful if they meet the following criteria:

➤ The disease or condition must have a significant effect on the quality or quantity of life.

➤ Acceptable methods of treatment must be available.

➤ The disease or condition must have an asymptomatic period during which detection and treatment significantly reduce morbidity or mortality.

➤ Treatment in the asymptomatic phase must yield a therapeutic result superior to that obtained by delaying treatment until symptoms appear.

➤ Tests that are acceptable to patients must be available at reasonable cost to detect the condition during the asymptomatic period.

➤ The incidence of the condition must be sufficient to justify the cost of screening.

The U.S. Preventive Services Task Force[2] (USP-STF) has assessed the effectiveness of more than 150 interventions, giving specific recommendations for counseling, screening (including history, physical examination, laboratory tests/diagnostic procedures), and immunizations for patients at various levels of risk for their age groups. The USPSTF continues to update its recommendations regarding these interventions.[3,4] Other groups that have issued recommendations on this subject include the Canadian Task Force on the Periodic Health Examination,[5-9] the American Cancer Society,[10] the American Heart Association,[11] and the American College of Physicians.[12] Duryea[13] has addressed the use of primary care PAs in the provision of services for adult health maintenance.

The purpose of this discussion is to provide a framework for preventive services that PA students should learn, and that physician assistants may find practical to initiate or expand upon in their clinical practice settings. In this regard, the preventive services described constitute a selective group of interventions that may be readily incorporated into any primary care practice and offered to those considered to be low-risk patients. Because this group of interventions is geared to low-risk patients, practitioners may want to augment them with others recommended for patients with known risk factors.[2,3] For example, no attention is given here to issues surrounding developmental disorders, speech problems, and behavioral and learning disorders in pediatric patients. Once identified, patients with such disorders would constitute higher risk groups, for whom specific interventions outside the scope of this discussion would be appropriate.

The preventive medicine measures that are addressed in this chapter should be provided at four levels: patient education and counseling, physical examination, laboratory screening tests and procedures, and immunizations. To be effective, these preventive services should become an integral part of routine health care, appropriately scheduled according to patient sex and life stage as well as generally accepted guidelines.[1-12] To ensure that HPDP services are being provided and that issues are being addressed according to the practice's plan, a schedule should be inserted in each patient's chart with a tickler file as a reminder. It is suggested that the preventive medicine file be a separate unit of the overall file for each patient, so that:

1. The schedule of HPDP interventions is easily identified.
2. There is continuity in logging of information.
3. The patient's HPDP status is readily accessible. (A sample flow sheet for scheduling HPDP services is given in Figure 16-1.)

Preventive services are likely to be accepted by clinicians if they are relatively easy to perform, have good patient acceptance, and have demonstrated effectiveness as preventive tools. If a preventive intervention does not result in an improved outcome, such as identification of cancer at an early-enough stage to possibly effect a cure, there is no reason to perform it.

The comprehensive review by USPSTF[2-4] of current scientific evidence on the clinical effectiveness of interventions for the prevention of a large number of target conditions forms the basis for the recommendations described here. Aside from immunizations and screening tests, the most effective preventive services that PAs can provide are those that address the health practices of patients, with the intention of changing their personal health attitudes and behaviors long before clinical disease develops. In this respect, health-promoting behaviors should be emphasized in the practice's patient education program. The section that follows addresses patient education, emphasizing important issues that PAs should discuss with patients during a routine health visit.

Pt. Name____ Id #____	D A T E	A G E	...18	21	24	27	30	33	36	39	40	41	42	43	44	45	46	47	48	49	50	51	52	53	54	55	+...
PROCEDURE/TEST																											
1. BREAST EXAM										★	★	★	★	★	★	★	★	★	★	★	★	★	★	★	★	★
2. MAMMOGRAPHY																					★	★	★	★	★	★	★
3. OCCULT BLOOD TESTING						★				★		★		★		★		★			★	★	★	★	★	★	★
4. DIGITAL RECTAL EXAM						★				★		★		★		★		★			★	★	★	★	★	★	★
5. SIGMOIDOSCOPY																					★		★		★		★
6. PAP SMEAR			★	★	★	★	★	★	★	★	★		★		★		★		★		★	★	★	★	★	★	★
7. CHOLESTEROL										★		★		★		★		★			★	★	★	★	★	★	★

Figure 16-1 Sample flow sheet for screening tests and procedures. A similar sheet can be developed for scheduling pediatric health promotion and disease prevention interventions (e.g., immunizations, parent/patient education).

PATIENT EDUCATION AND COUNSELING

An important requirement of effective patient education and counseling is that primary care PAs have an excellent understanding of their patients' personal health behaviors, particularly those that increase their risks for preventable diseases. The development of this understanding goes beyond knowledge of the patient's history of smoking cigarettes, drinking alcohol, and having casual sex with multiple partners. An insight into the attitude of the patient toward such issues is equally important and will bear on the PA's approach to education and counseling. (An example is provided in Case Study 16-1.) An effective educator practices what he or she preaches and should be prepared to be challenged by patients regarding the relative value of particular interventions. An obese patient probably spent many years getting to that condition, and the habits of overeating and lack of exercise are usually well ingrained and resistant to change. Good education must be persistent, tempered by understanding of the patient's ability to handle the program, and carried through with continual encouragement and reassurance.

CASE STUDY 16-1

Mark, a 15-year-old high school student, has been smoking about ½ pack of cigarettes a day for 3 years. He has been advised about the health risks of smoking but has made no attempt to quit. Mark describes smoking as "Just something that I do with friends—it relaxes me." He denies alcohol, marijuana, and other drug use.

Mark has come to the office for his first hepatitis B immunization. While discussing the vaccine, the PA asks about Mark's sexual activity. Mark says that he started dating Michele about 3 months ago, but they are not having intercourse. The PA asks about Michele's smoking habits, and Mark says, "She doesn't smoke at all. She doesn't really like me to smoke, so I don't smoke around her."

The PA sees an opportunity to encourage Mark to quit smoking and asks if Michele has made any other comments about smoking, such as the smell of his clothes. Mark admits that she has made comments about his "cigarette breath." The PA asks if Mark has thought about quitting, and Mark agrees that this would be a good time to try. The PA discusses various alternatives for smoking cessation, and Mark sets a quit date.

Discussion

Health risks of smoking are less likely to provide compelling motivation for smoking cessation in adolescent patients than issues related to appearance and peer group activities. On the other hand, parents may be motivated to quit smoking by being given information about the impact of secondhand smoke on their children.

An important objective is to encourage a shift of responsibility for health-promoting behavior from the physician assistant to the patient. Patients must be prepared to "buy into" the program of preventive services offered by the practice and must begin to accept responsibility for their own health. This may be difficult at first because of the traditional nature of the clinician/patient relationship. Very simply, patients come into the office with a problem, expecting the clinician to take charge of the treatment plan and to make them well. This passive patient role applies to the provision of preventive services also. Therefore, for the HPDP program to succeed, it is important that patients be invested with a stake in the plan; it must be made clear to them that a favorable outcome depends on their patience, understanding, and active participation. This is not to discharge the PA's responsibility for being actively in charge of the HPDP program and for promoting it throughout the practice and in the community.

Community health education is an important emerging responsibility for PAs. Many are going outside their immediate practice environments, taking the HPDP message to area schools, youth groups, and community service organizations. Their practices may sponsor health fairs, local marathons and fun runs, golf tournaments, and other recreational activities. Community involvement also has a political dimension, and PAs are becoming more proactive in addressing community health problems (e.g., public safety, accident prevention, pollution) and in seeking favorable legislation for the development of healthful and safe community environments.

Direct one-on-one discussions with patients are paramount in many HPDP interventions because direct exchanges personalize the issues and allow the clinician to assess a patient's understanding, attitude, and likelihood of compliance with the program. However, other methods have proved effective in promoting a practice's HPDP program. The education and counseling of patients on HPDP issues can be, and probably ought to be, a "multimedia" event. The waiting room is an often-underused patient education area that can be regarded as an opportunity for laying out literature, hanging posters, and using other visual aids to draw attention to HPDP subjects. Patient examination rooms also afford opportunities for "advertising" wellness issues and can be equipped with audiotape players, video monitors, and computer-aided instruction to provide more comprehensive coverage of patient-specific issues (e.g., getting a teenager's attention about the dangers of unprotected sex with multiple partners).

Whatever the methods used, PAs should strive to make patient education an integral part of every patient's routine health visit. The approach varies according to time available for the visit, behaviors to be addressed, and anticipated problem areas that may have to be discussed with the patient in greater depth. In any case, the overall strategy should allow for education and counseling in three general areas: risk reduction, wellness promotion, and anticipation of potential problems. Priorities given to the specific matters to be addressed in each of these general areas are determined by a patient's age, sex, and risk categories. For infant and pediatric patients, most counseling will involve the parents and should cover issues of diet and exercise, injury prevention, dental health, and the child's environment (e.g., effects of passive smoking). Teenage and adult patients should also be counseled about diet and exercise, injury prevention, and dental health; and issues of substance use or abuse and sexual practices should be added to their education and counseling plan. Specific subjects recommended for a comprehensive primary care program of patient education and counseling are listed in Table 16-1. As was mentioned previously, to ensure that education and counseling for all patients are covered over time, a

Table 16-1 Patient Education and Counseling Program*

BIRTH TO 18 MONTHS (PARENTAL COUNSELING)

Diet	Breast-feeding, nutrient intake (especially iron-rich foods)
Injury prevention	Child safety seats; smoke detectors; hot water heater temperature; stairway gates, window guards, pool fence; storage of drugs and toxic chemicals; syrup of ipecac and poison control telephone number
Dental health	Baby bottle tooth decay
Environment	Effects of passive smoking

AGES 2 THROUGH 6 (PATIENT AND PARENTAL COUNSELING)

Diet and exercise	Sweets and between-meal snacks; iron-enriched foods; sodium; caloric balance; selection of an exercise program
Injury prevention	As for birth to 18 months; also bicycle safety helmets, firearms, matches
Dental health	Regular tooth brushing and dental visits
Environment	Effects of passive smoking

AGES 7 THROUGH 12 (PATIENT AND PARENTAL COUNSELING)

Diet and exercise	Fat (especially saturated fat); cholesterol; sodium; sweets; between-meal snacks; caloric balance; selection of an exercise program
Injury prevention	As for ages 2-6
Dental health	As for ages 2-6
Environment	As for ages 2-6

AGES 13 THROUGH 64

Diet and exercise	As for ages 7-12; also iron and calcium for females (add complex carbohydrates and fiber for older patients)
Substance use	Tobacco and alcohol (cessation/primary prevention); driving and other dangerous activities while under the influence; treatment of abuse
Sexual practices	Sexually transmitted diseases (partner selection, condoms, oral and anal sexual practices); unintended pregnancy and contraceptive options
Injury prevention	Safety belts and bicycle and motorcycle helmets; firearms; smoke detectors; violent behavior (especially males)
Dental health	As for ages 2-6; also flossing
Environment	Effects of passive smoking

AGES 65 AND OVER

Diet and exercise	As for ages 13-64
Substance use	As for ages 13-64; also tobacco cessation; limiting alcohol consumption
Injury prevention	As for ages 13-64; also prevention of falls; hot water heater temperature; inquire about vision and hearing problems, functional status, symptoms of transient ischemic attacks
Dental health	As for ages 13-64
Primary prevention	Benefits of glaucoma testing

*Based on U.S. Preventive Services Task Force recommendations.[2,3] (The value of patient education regarding breast, oral cavity, skin, and testicular self-examinations for early detection screening remains to be demonstrated.)

checklist reminder system should be used in the routine chart record for all patients in the practice (see Figure 16-1). By such means, a deliberate, scheduled approach to preventive medicine can be maintained, regularly reviewed, and updated throughout the patient's relationship with the practice.

PHYSICAL EXAMINATION

All new patients, whether they are at low or high risk for preventable disease, require a full head-to-toe physical examination on their first routine health visit. After that initial visit, authorities agree that the provision of preventive services requires a more focused and selective approach in terms of which segments of the physical examination are to be done and when.[1-12] Current evidence questions the efficacy of regular (i.e., annual) head-to-toe comprehensive physical examinations to screen for preventable diseases in terms of time spent and cost to the patient. This does not dismiss the PA's responsibility to take a pertinent history and to perform a complete physical examination when the patient presents with any new medical or surgical problem. The intervention involved in such a case is outside the protocol for the practice's HPDP program for that patient.

Greater selectivity in the provision of a range of preventive services is an important finding in the reports of the USPSTF and others.[1-12] This implies greater selectivity in performing segments of the physical examination as well, with the degree of selectivity corresponding to the patient's level of risk for preventable disease. Moreover, the selection of segments of the physical examination to be performed regularly in the program of HPDP services must be based on their documented effectiveness as screening tools for early detection of disorders and diseases widely acknowledged to be preventable or correctable (e.g., obesity, hyperlipidemia, hypertension, atherosclerosis, vision and hearing deficits, breast cancer, colorectal and prostate cancer). In this respect, the periodic screening examination for low-risk patients should contain scheduled elements, some at fixed intervals and others at discretionary intervals, that focus on patient weight, blood pressure, vision and hearing, breast examination, and digital rectal examination (see Box).

SCREENING TESTS AND PROCEDURES

The USPSTF defines screening tests as "those preventive services in which a special test or standardized examination procedure is used to identify patients requiring special intervention."[2] An array of screening regimens is becoming available to clinicians without clear evidence of their effectiveness in terms of:

1. How accurately they can detect conditions earlier than they are detected without screening.
2. Whether accurate early detection significantly improves outcome.

Authorities[1-12] indicate that certain preventable conditions carry significant morbidity and mortality in this country, and that effective screening tests can improve outcome. Among these conditions are hyperlipidemia and atherosclerosis, colorectal cancer, cervical cancer, and breast cancer. In this context, it seems prudent to include in the primary care regimen of preventive services for low-risk patients the tests listed in the Box.

ELEMENTS OF PERIODIC SCREENING EXAMINATION FOR THE LOW-RISK PATIENT

Weight	At least once yearly (height and weight for infants up to 18 months of age at more frequent intervals, left to clinical discretion).
Blood pressure	Measured routinely every time patient seeks care.
Vision and hearing	For children aged 2-6 years and the elderly, with intervals left to clinical discretion.
Breast examination	Annually beginning at age 40; mammography every 1-2 years for women over 40 years of age, and every year after age 50.
Digital rectal examination	Periodic, with interval left to clinical discretion.

SCREENING TESTS FOR THE LOW-RISK PATIENT	
Mammography	Every 1-2 years for women over age 40, and every year after age 50.
Occult blood testing	Periodic, with interval left to clinical discretion.
Papanicolaou testing (Pap smear)	Recommended for all sexually active women, beginning with onset of sexual activity or at age 18, then every 1-3 years (according to clinical judgment) until at least age 65 (longer if previous results were abnormal).
Serum cholesterol measurement	Annually for men ages 35 and older, and for women ages 45 and older.
Sigmoidoscopy	Periodic, with interval left to clinical discretion.

IMMUNIZATIONS

There is proven benefit to including immunizations among the primary preventive services offered to asymptomatic persons. It is clear that certain infectious diseases are almost completely preventable if childhood immunizations are given according to schedule. These include immunizations against tetanus, diphtheria, pertussis, *Haemophilus influenzae* type b infection, poliomyelitis, measles, mumps, and rubella. The evidence is less clear regarding the efficacy of vaccines available for normal adults. Although measles and tetanus vaccines are about 95% effective, pneumococcal vaccine and annual influenza vaccines may be only about 70% effective. Despite their somewhat lower rate of effectiveness, the latter two vaccines afford acceptable levels of prophylaxis and are recommended by the Immunization Practices Advisory Committee (ACIP).[14-16] Guidelines for the immunization of normal infants and children have been issued by the ACIP[14,17,18] and the American Academy of Pediatrics.[19,20] A summary schedule of immunizations for normal infants, children, and adults is given in Table 16-2.

CONCLUSION

As programs for preventive services continue to evolve, physician assistants will be assuming more responsibility for delivering them. Therefore, it is incumbent upon PAs to understand the full range of services that should be provided in the areas of patient education and counseling, screening tests, and immunizations. It is also important that such services be integrated into routine health visits, with schedules of delivery and appropriate follow-up action when required. As delivery of preventive services becomes more routine, patients will become more accustomed to dealing with HPDP issues. With continual reinforcement of those issues by PAs, patients will better understand the importance of behaviors and attitudes that promote wellness.

CLINICAL APPLICATIONS

1. What should be included in preventive medicine measures for the following patients? Each patient is healthy and without specific risk factors for disease. Include patient education and counseling, physical examination, laboratory screening tests, and immunizations.
   a. 5-year-old girl (include parental counseling).
   b. 15-year-old male adolescent.
   c. 30-year-old woman.
   d. 40-year-old man.
   e. 50-year-old woman.
   f. 65-year-old man.
2. What techniques and materials could be used to improve the patient education environment in a typical waiting room and examination room?
3. Describe some opportunities in your community for becoming more active in community health education. How would you go about making contacts and developing a community health education project?

Table 16-2   Summary Schedule of immunizations[13-20]

Age	Vaccine/Toxoic	Administration
Birth	Hepatitis B vaccine (HBV)	One 0.5-mL dose intramuscularly (IM)*
2 months	Diphtheria-tetanus-acellular pertussis (DTaP)	One 0.5-mL dose IM
	Inactivated poliovirus vaccine (IPV)†	One 0.5-mL dose given subcutaneously (SC)
	Haemophilus influenzae type b conjugate vaccine (Hib)‡	One 0.5-mL dose IM
	Pneumococcal conjugate vaccine (PCV)	One 0.5-mL dose IM
4 months	DTaP #2, IPV #2, Hib #2, PCV #2	As above
1-4 months	HBV #2	As above
6 months	DTaP #3, Hib #3, PCV #3	As above
6-18 months	HBV #3, IPV #3	As above
12-15 months	Hib #4, PCV #4	As above
	Measles-mumps-rubella (MMR)	One 0.5-mL dose SC
12-18 months	Varicella-zoster vaccine (VZV)	One 0.5-mL dose SC
15-18 months	DTaP #4	As above
4-6 years	DTaP #5, IPV #4, MMR #2	As above
11-14 years	Tetanus-diphtheria (Td)	One 0.5-mL dose IM (repeat every 10 years throughout life)
2-18 years	Hepatitis A vaccine (HAV)§	Two 0.5-mL doses (2nd dose after 6 months)
50 years	Influenza vaccine‖	One 0.5-mL dose IM (repeat yearly, with current vaccine)
65 years	Pneumococcal polysaccharide vaccine	One 0.5-mL dose IM

*Recombivax HB® or Engerix-B® given at a dose of 0.5 mL IM for infants of mothers negative for hepatitis B surface antigen (HBsAG). Children of HbsAg-positive mothers should complete the 3-dose series within 2 months after birth.
†Two IPV products are licensed in the U.S.: Ipol® and Poliovax®. Both contain the same three antigenic types of poliovirus.
‡Three Hib conjugate vaccines are available for use. If PRP-OMP (PedvaxHIB® or Comvax® [Merck]) is administered at 2 and 4 months of age, a dose at 6 months is not required. Do not use DTaP/Hib combination products for primary immunization in infants at 2, 4, or 6 months. A booster dose of Hib conjugate vaccine is recommended at 12-15 months.
§HAV is recommended for all children in this age range living in states or communities where hepatitis A infection rates are twice the national average. Consult local public health authorities for current information.
‖Influenza vaccination is now recommended as a component of pre-adolescent assessment. The vaccine can be given as early as 6 months of age. Children who receive their first dose of influenza vaccine when they are 8 years of age should be given a second dose no sooner than a month later. Dosage is 0.25 mL for ages 6 to 35 months, and 0.5 mL for age 3 years.

REFERENCES

1. Frame PS. A critical review of adult health maintenance (pts. 1-4). J Fam Pract 1986;22:341-346, 417-422, 511-520; 23:29-39.
2. U.S. Preventive Services Task Force. Guide to Clinical Preventive Services: An Assessment of the Effectiveness of 169 Interventions. Baltimore: Williams and Wilkins, 1989.
3. U.S. Preventive Services Task Force. Guide to Clinical Preventive Services, ed 2. Baltimore: Williams and Wilkins, 1996.
4. U.S. Preventive Services Task Force (USPSTF). Screening Adults for Lipid Disorders. Am J Prev Med 2001;20:73.
5. Canadian Task Force on the Periodic Health Examination. The periodic health examination. Can Med Assoc J 1979;121:1193.
6. Canadian Task Force on the Periodic Health Examination. The periodic health examination: 1984 update. Can Med Assoc J 1984;130:1278.
7. Canadian Task Force on the Periodic Health Examination. The periodic health examination: 1986 update. Can Med Assoc J 1986;134:721.
8. Canadian Task Force on the Periodic Health Examination. The periodic health examination: 1988 update. Can Med Assoc J 1988;138:617.

9. Canadian Task Force on the Periodic Health Examination. The periodic health examination: 1989 update. Can Med Assoc J 1989;141:209.

10. American Cancer Society. Report on the cancer-related health check-up. CA 1980;30:194.

11. American Heart Association. Cardiovascular and risk factor evaluation of healthy American adults: a statement for physicians by an ad hoc committee appointed by the steering committee. Circulation 1987;75:1340A.

12. American College of Physicians. Periodic health examination: a guide for designing individualized preventive health care in the asymptomatic patient. Ann Intern Med 1981;95:729.

13. Duryea WR. Adult health maintenance: a guide for primary care PAs. J Am Acad Physician Assist 1990;3:607.

14. Immunization Practices Advisory Committee. Update on adult immunization: recommendations of the Immunization Practices Advisory Committee (ACIP). MMWR 1991;40:1.

15. Advisory Committee on Immunization Practices (ACIP). Summary of Adolescent/Adult Immunization Recommendations. www.cdc.gov/nip/recs/adult-schedule.pdf (accessed 2/21/02).

16. Advisory Committee on Immunization Practices (ACIP) and American Academy of Family Physicians. General Recommendations on Immunization. MMWR 2002;51:1.

17. 2000 Red Book: Report of the Committee on Infectious Diseases, ed 25. Elk Grove, IL: American Academy of Pediatrics, 2000.

18. Hemophilus b conjugate vaccines for prevention of *Hemophilus influenzae* type b disease among infants and children two months of age and older: recommendations of the Immunization Practices Advisory Committee (ACIP). MMWR 1991;40:1.

19. American Academy of Pediatrics. Committee on Infectious Diseases. Recommended Childhood Immunization Schedule—United States, 2002. Pediatrics 2002;109:162.

20. Hepatitis B virus: a comprehensive strategy for eliminating transmission in the United States through universal childhood vaccination. Recommendations of the Immunization Practices Advisory Committee (ACIP). MMWR 1991;40:1.

RESOURCES

American Health Foundation. Preventive Medicine. New York: Academic Press. *A bimonthly international journal devoted to practice and theory. The official journal of the American Society of Preventive Oncology. An excellent source for the latest in cancer detection and prevention research.*

Campos-Outcalt D (ed). Twenty Common Problems in Preventive Health Care. New York: McGraw-Hill, 2000 (510 pp). *Contributors employ recommendations from the U.S. Preventive Services Task Force (USPSTF) and the Centers for Disease Control and Prevention (CDC) to present 20 of the most common clinical preventive medicine issues facing today's health care providers. Preventive health care is covered in depth for three age groups: infants and children, adolescents and young adults, and adults. An excellent resource for clinicians and PA educators.*

Ferri FF(ed). Clinical Advisor. Philadelphia: Mosby, 2001 (1375 pp). *Clinical preventive services focusing on the periodic health examination; childhood, adolescent, and adult immunizations; and chemoprophylaxis are given excellent coverage in Section 5.*

Noble J (ed). Textbook of Primary Care Medicine, ed 3. Philadelphia: Mosby, 2001 (2048 pp). *The benefits of the periodic health examination versus the annual physical examination are compared in the section on "Core Issues and Special Groups in Primary Care." The elements of preventive care, the components of the periodic health examination, and special issues in the elderly are presented (Chapter 4), as well as information on immunizations and travel (Chapter 5) and health screening and prevention in adolescents and young adults (Chapter 7).*

Rakel RE, Bope ET (eds). 2002 Conn's Current Therapy. Philadelphia: WB Saunders, 2002 (1314 pp). *Current immunization practices (up to December 2001) and issues to be addressed with patients planning to travel to foreign countries are well covered in Section 2 (pp 141-155). Such issues as pretravel advice; preparation of an individualized medical kit; malaria prevention; required and recommended immunizations; prophylaxis and treatment of traveler's diarrhea; and post-travel care are thoroughly presented.*

Wallace, RB (ed). Maxcy-Rosenou-Last: Preventive Medicine and Public Health, ed 14. Norwalk, CT: Appleton and Lange, 1998 (1275 pp). *Encyclopedic coverage of communicable diseases and their control; environmental health issues; behavioral factors affecting health; noncommunicable and chronic disabling conditions; public health methodology; and health care planning, organization, and evaluation. A valuable resource for all students of preventive medicine, epidemiology, and public health.*

CHAPTER 17

Utilizing Consultants and Community Resources

Albert Simon and Ernest L. Stump

INTRODUCTION

The process of seeking consultation and community referral is an integral part of every practitioner's practice pattern. Since the beginning of medical practice, health care providers have sought counsel about difficult patients. As the complexity of medical practice increases, it is logical that one would seek expert advice about the treatment and management of conditions out of the realm of one's expertise or resources.

Physician assistants (PAs), as dependent practitioners, consult with other health care practitioners as a routine portion of their daily practice. This is especially true for the consultation that goes on between PAs and their supervising physicians. Every PA uses some form of consultation with the physician-super-

visor. There is a great deal of latitude as to the form that process of consultation takes. For some PAs, the supervising physician is on site and acts as a consultant for review of elements of every case. Other PAs practice in locations remote from their supervisors and tend not to consult as frequently. Most PAs also use individuals other than their supervisory physicians for consultation. The primary reason for consultants is the need for expert opinions when decisions are made regarding patient care.[1] In addition, consultants expand the knowledge base for a PA in areas related to the PA's practice.

Providers today are confronted with the changes that result from the growth of managed care. PAs have to understand the rules concerning referrals that govern many interactions for specialty consultation. These include the lack of ability of the patient to self-refer, criteria that may exist for the use of special testing referral (e.g., use of magnetic resonance imaging in cases of low back pain), and constraints of cost. While these types of rules have added complexity to the provider/patient interaction, they have also added new responsibility. As a patient's primary care provider, the PA must have the ability to appropriately use the system as an advocate on the patient's behalf.

Technology has also entered the referral arena. Telemedicine is increasingly used as a method of providing access to specialty consultation services. This technology also provides access to services that were previously unavailable in certain remote areas or in areas that could not support certain services because of a small population base. It is important for the PA to understand the basics of using this new technology as a resource for modern practice.

When a referral or consultation is needed, the PA must be cognizant of the resources available in the community. These include human resources, in the form of other health care providers, as well as helping organizations. This chapter discusses methods of consultation and the appropriate use of community resources through patient referral.

USING CONSULTANTS

For patients to make their way to specialty services, they must have a means of moving along the medical hierarchy. This pathway has been dubbed the "referral chain."[2] Patients may enter the referral chain from a number of starting points and may be referred by a general practitioner to a specialist, by a specialist to a specialist, or by a specialist to a general practitioner. Each of the providers along the chain may be used as a consultant. The goal of the referral chain (and thus the use of consultants) is to guide patients to the appropriate level of medical care.

Primary care practitioners often initiate the entry of the patient into the realm of specialists. Indeed, in countries with national health care systems, primary care providers are looked upon as the gatekeepers to more expensive specialist care.[3] The following two cases illustrate the types of situations in which consultations typically occur.

CASE STUDY 17-1

A 42-year-old female presents with a history of headache and slurred speech. These symptoms have been progressive over the past month or two. On examination, the PA finds cranial nerve deficits and refers the patient for immediate computed tomography (CT) scan. The examination reveals a cerebral tumor. The patient is referred for immediate neurosurgical consultation.

CASE STUDY 17-2

A 63-year-old woman with advanced degenerative joint disease has been under the care of a general practitioner for several years for management of the arthritis. She now needs specialty referral to an orthopedist for hip replacement.

Both of these cases depict patients moving from primary care situations to the use of specialists or subspecialists. Referral in the other direction, from specialist to primary care provider, is also appropriate, as is shown in the following case.

CASE STUDY 17-3

Mr. W is a 65-year-old white man with a number of medical problems. During each 6-month period, Mr. W sees a cardiologist, a pulmonologist, and a neurologist. Each of the specialists involved in this case has prescribed at least one medication. On the last visit, the neurologist refers the patient to a family practitioner.

Mr. W's situation is not uncommon. This patient is involved with multiple specialists, each providing quality medical care but focused from a specialty perspective. In these cases, consultation with family practitioners or general internists is entirely appropriate. The inclusion of primary care providers serves to help coordinate the patient's overall treatment. It is easy for a patient (usually an older patient) receiving care from multiple specialists to be "lost in the shuffle," with no one to coordinate care from the broader perspective.

Another aspect of the consultation that should not be neglected is its role in the process of medical education.[4] In days past, consultations between specialists and primary care providers would occur at the bedside. Currently, this exchange more often occurs via letter. Even without personal contact between the health care providers, an opportunity for teaching still exists in the consultation process. The detailed information about the patient possessed by the primary care provider can teach the consultant. The consultant obviously has detailed expertise to pass on to the primary care provider relative to specific disease processes. For this education to be substantive, communication must be effective. With the appropriate use of consultation, the patient, the referring provider, and the consultant all may benefit.

Consultants are used in any situation in which special skills are needed. Referral to a consultant may be to a specialist, a subspecialist, or a primary care provider, as the situation dictates. The referral chain can be considered effective if the patient reaches the appropriate health care provider within a time that is not detrimental to his or her medical condition.

Choosing a Consultant

After the decision to make a referral has been made, the PA must choose the consultant. What attributes are desirable in a consultant? First, a consultant must be *qualified*. This usually means being board certified in the area of practice. Board certification certainly speaks to competence on one level. The "fit" of the consultant in the referral chain may extend beyond board certification. A visit to the consultant's practice allows the PA the chance to talk at length with the consultant. The visit also serves to showcase the consultant's facilities, making the PA aware of the range of services he or she may provide. The PA may then develop a sense of the consultant's approach to patient care and his or her perspectives and priorities as they pertain to practice. With the advent of managed care, the provider may be limited in the consultants who may be used, unless the patient wishes to go "out of the system" and pay out of pocket for the service. A consultant should also be *available*. This availability should extend to both the provider and the patient. The consultant should be available for inquiries via telephone and for "bedside consults" in the hospital. The patient should also benefit from the consultant's availability by not having to wait unduly for an appointment with a referral. It may also be

important to know what forms of insurance are accepted by the consultant.

Making the Referral

For the consultant to adequately perform his or her job, appropriate information must be transmitted. In a patient referral, it is customary to send a typed letter that contains a synopsis of the history of present illness, past medical history, pertinent physical findings, and current medications, including the current form of treatment and the results. Most important, the reason for requesting the consultation must be included. This last statement may seem self-evident, but a review of the literature reveals that such may not be the case. In a study of 500 nonurgent referrals to the Manchester Royal Eye Hospital by general practitioners and ophthalmic opticians, many of the baseline data were found to be lacking. In only 27.5% of cases was an adequate medical history provided, and in only 13% was any drug information provided. Fully 43.7% of patients' referral records to this specialty eye hospital from general practices contained no evidence that an ocular examination had been performed.[5] Other studies have reviewed referral letters from general practitioners and found that a high percentage (59.4%) were barely adequate or were poor.[6] The following is information needed for any patient referral:

➤ Introductory sentence (identifies patient).
➤ Synopsis of history of present illness.
➤ Pertinent past medical history and review of systems.
➤ Social or personal history as it relates to the case.
➤ Physical examination findings.
➤ Statement of why the consultation is being initiated.
➤ Follow-up instructions the patient has received.

In the outpatient setting, referral information is dictated in a short letter (usually one or two pages) and mailed directly to the consultant. Occasionally, this letter is sealed and given to the patient to carry by hand. The office staff at the referring practice usually phones to make the appointment with the consultant's office for the patient. The contact from the referring office staff should ensure that the patient has an appointment within a reasonable time. A sample referral letter is shown in Figure 17-1.

Deborah R. Jones, M.D.
Family Practice
Suite C Benlo Place
Altoona, PA 16601

June 1, 2002

David Smith, M.D.
Neurology
501 Howard Avenue
Altoona, PA 16601

Dear Dr. Smith:

Please allow me to introduce Mr. James Walker. Mr. Walker is a 37-year-old white male who has been a patient in our practice for the last five years. Mr. Walker presented to my office earlier this week with a complaint of photopsia in his right eye. The photopsia has occurred two times during the past month. Each time the photopsia occurs, it lasts approximately fifteen minutes. The patient states that at the conclusion of the photopsia, he feels somewhat washed out. On the last occasion, Mr. Walker reported a mild headache located over the left frontal area. The photopsia is not associated with any other symptoms; particularly, I note a lack of nausea, vomiting, or other sensations of aura, such as unusual smells. Mr. Walker denies any history of vertigo, dizziness, or paresthesia. He denies any ataxia or problems with coordination. A similar episode occurred approximately one-and-a-half years ago, at which time he sought attention from his optometrist. The optometrist examined Mr. Walker's fundus and advised him to return should this particular problem occur again. He had no further episodes until this month. He presented to our practice at this time because of the increased frequency of the episodes.

He is in generally good health, with the following ongoing medical problems: Mild hypertension that has been well controlled by Lisinipril, 10 mg q d at HS. He is mildly obese and struggles to maintain his weight at a reasonable level; I have recommended that he lose approximately 20 pounds. Finally, we have found on one occasion that his serum cholesterol was elevated to 232. I have recommended a level one diet. His cholesterol will be rechecked within six months. There is no history of migraine headache or other neurological maladies in his past or family history. Mr. Walker is a chairman of a medium-sized corporation here in Altoona and indicated that he feels that he is under quite a bit of stress in his job. He does admit to difficulty sleeping, particularly in falling asleep, and sometimes has early morning awakening. He also indicates that he suffers from bruxism.

Physical examination reveals a mildly obese, well-developed, well-nourished white male in no acute distress. Skin is warm and dry. **HEENT**—benign bilaterally, no evidence of embolic phenomenon or hypertensive retinopathy. The thyroid is not enlarged. **Thorax and lungs**—clear to auscultation and percussion. **Cardiovascular system**—heart rate at 86 with regular rate. II/VI systolic ejection murmur located at Erb's point without radiation. No clicks or heaves are present. Pulses are all equal at 2/4; no bruits are heard at the carotid, aortic, or renal areas. **Abdomen**—soft without tenderness or organomegaly. **Musculoskeletal**—full range of motion without deformity; strength is 5/5 and equal at all. **Neurological**—cranial nerves 1 through 12 are intact. Motor—gait and station are intact. Romberg is negative. Coordination and rapid alternating movements are performed well. Sensory—intact to touch and sharp/dull through all major dermatomes. Stereognosis and graphesthesia are intact bilaterally. Reflexes— +2/4 and equal bilaterally, no clonus noted. Mental status—affect is appropriate, recent and remote memory are intact.

My thought at this point is that these phenomena represent the onset of ocular migraines; perhaps the stress is playing a role. I am interested in getting your opinion relative to the photopsia. Could this represent early multiple sclerosis or other neurological processes? Please evaluate Mr. Walker and relay your impression to me. I have instructed Mr. Walker to make an appointment to see me 2 weeks after your examination and diagnostic workup are complete. I am also sending Mr. Walker for ophthalmological referral to rule out primary retinal disease.

Thank you for seeing this patient in consultation.

Sincerely,

John Williams, PA-C

Figure 17-1 Sample referral letter.

In the institutional setting, a standardized form is usually provided for requesting consultations. This form can be obtained from the unit manager or ward secretary. Once the form is completed, ward staff members generally process the request and notify the consultant. One may elect to designate the consultation as *emergent,* in which case the consultant is called immediately; as *urgent,* whereby the consultant is notified within a couple of hours; or as *routine,* by which the patient is generally seen in the next day or two. A word concerning emergent consultations may be appropriate here. An emergent consultation implies the need for immediate intervention necessary to prevent the patient's condition from deteriorating. This type of consultation is generally expensive for the patient and stressful for the consultant. Many practitioners have witnessed the abuse of this designation. People are called in from home to see a patient and perform diagnostic studies, only to realize that by the time the studies are finalized, the requesting practitioner is no longer available to act on the information generated.

In cases that are very complicated or emergent, the provider usually elects to call the consultant and discuss the case personally. This allows the provider to establish a clear sense of the case with the consultant and to be informed about additional initial management or laboratory studies needed before the consultant sees the patient.

Many providers forget that one of the most frequent referrals is to the radiologist. Yet often a patient is sent for an upper gastrointestinal (GI) or other radiological procedure without the radiologist's being notified of the history and physical findings. Each consultant needs adequate information on which to base recommendations. Some consultants do not have the advantage of seeing the patient, and few have the background knowledge of the case that the referring practitioner has. The responsibility of the referring provider is to transmit as much of the essence of the case to the consultant as possible in a succinct form. Consultants should also be obliged to inform the referring health care provider of their findings, recommendations, and treatments. This is usually accomplished by a follow-up letter sent to the referring provider shortly after the consultation has been completed. Failure of the consultant to engage in this practice is a common source of dissatisfaction for the referring provider.[7]

Referral Rates

In today's climate of practice comparisons and nonanalytical data, a provider may wonder how many patients should be referred. Is the PA referring too many or too few patients? The literature provides little clear guidance on these points. Referral rates vary by practitioner, by location, and by specialty. It does seem clear that consultations are requested for a variety of personal, medical, and friendship reasons.[8]

Although managed care is affecting referral rates, it is not clear exactly what impact it is having or whether it is appropriate. Gomez and colleagues[9] studied residents' behavior in connection with a managed care curriculum presented during their residency experience. A lower rate of referrals was one outcome of this experience. The investigators indicated that the lower rates of referral might have been due to the intimidation of scrutiny of these behaviors by colleagues. The authors go on to warn against undercare that may result from this trend. At present, it seems prudent to recommend that a referral be made when the circumstances dictate. These parameters include the personal characteristics of the practice. Scientifically, no clues currently exist as to whether practitioners in general practice refer too few or too many patients.[10]

Patient Considerations

The referral situation holds the potential for great benefit for the patient, but also for the patient to become alienated from the primary care provider. Should the referral to a consultant be made without a proper explanation, the patient may feel "dumped off" or perhaps lost in the "doctor shuffle."

A good way to avoid disgruntled feelings is to rely on good basic patient interaction techniques. The patient who is involved in the decision making and consideration of treatment options is apt to be more accepting of the notion of the referral. The idea and reasons for the referral should be introduced to the patient. The provider should point out that the consultant will indicate preferences for treatment, but that through the process of negotiation, the patient will have a role in approving which treatment option is chosen. The primary care provider may then reassure the patient that he or she will be available to help discuss any treatment options, should the patient desire.

The primary care provider must be sure to follow up with a referred patient, inquiring about how the patient perceived the consultant. The provider should try to evaluate the level of the patient's satisfaction with the consultant visit. Patient dissatisfaction can rank high as a reason for treatment failure. In these situations, basic skills become quite important. In a study of patients needing a second opinion, a group of dissatisfied patients indicated that the physician had not spent enough time with them, even though 90% of this group indicated that the physician had asked appropriate questions and 60% believed that their questions were answered adequately.[11]

The provider should also review the consultant's recommendations with the patient and put them into a workable perspective relative to the practice orientation. Again, it is important for the patient to be an active participant in deciding on a treatment plan. If the patient is not invested in the process, he or she cannot relate to following medication regimens or making behavioral changes critical to the management of the illness.

CASE STUDY 17-4

Ms. Q is a 32-year-old woman who presents complaining of a frontal headache. She just moved into the area and joined a managed care plan to provide her health care. She is somewhat put out when the PA sees her because she had wanted to consult a specialist for her headache, as she had done under her old health care plan. She does not understand why she has to see the PA before she goes to the neurologist.

Managed Care and Referrals

Over the past several years, the percentage of patients covered under a managed care system has been steadily increasing. The amount of penetration of managed care into a particular population varies geographically. It is reasonable to conclude that all PAs

will work with some percentage of their patients in a managed care system. For many practitioners, the differences in providing care to patients in a managed care system can be confusing. Providers in a managed care system are required to be able to prescribe from a formulary and to adhere to rules governing referrals. Indeed, some question how well the present system of medical education prepares practitioners to function within such a system.[8,12]

When referrals are made to consultants in this type of system, there is usually a protocol to follow. Patients are often unable to self-refer to specialists (with the exception of obstetrics and gynecological services, which often do not require a referral from the primary care provider). Under managed care, referral to a specialist physician requires that patients first see their primary care provider, who then determines the need for the referral and the appropriate venue. This approach increases the rates of referral from primary care physicians for patients in certain demographic groups.[13] Recent research also shows that patients under managed care tend to use the emergency room less frequently. The study suggested that patients who had a primary care physician also used the emergency room less frequently, even if they were not under managed care.[14]

How should PAs respond to the issue of referral under a managed care system? PAs will need to learn to work within its rules to facilitate care for patients. At the very least, physician assistant educational programs should devise a curriculum to acquaint PA students with the skills they will need to function in the managed care environment. Practicing physician assistants must learn the rules of managed care as they encounter them in their daily practice. Under no circumstance should any rule of referral be used as a reason not to connect patients with the care that they require. In this new system, the PA's role as an advocate for the patient is more important than ever.

With the lack of self-referral capability, patients often feel powerless. This may lead to anger on the part of the patient, as is illustrated in Case Study 17-4, or the feeling that needed medical care is being withheld to save money. PAs must continue to be partners with their patients. Using the steps discussed here will allow one to create a successful referral process that will satisfy the patient's needs, form the basis for a facilitative process between the generalist and the specialist, and provide satisfaction to all parties involved.

First, engage all of the parties involved. Try to meet with the specialty consultant health care providers. Discuss approaches to various common referral issues. This type of encounter is an opportunity to discuss the ways that primary care and specialty care providers can work together to provide top-quality, seamless patient care. Educate patients on how the system works, why referrals are made, and the capabilities (and limitations) of primary care versus specialty care.

Next, anticipate ahead of time the need for referral and build that possibility into the discussion with the patient about his or her disease. Keep communication open between the referring health care provider, the patient, and the specialist. Make sure everyone knows what is happening and why. Finally, assess the situation to determine whether the treatment or process can be improved. It is critical to get feedback from all of the parties involved to make this assessment. These steps can allow quality monitoring of the referral process and are based on suggestions made by Rosenthal and associates.[15]

The goal when establishing a referral base within a managed health care system is to provide top-quality patient care in a rational, cost-effective manner. By partnering with the specialty providers and the patient, one can promote both quality health care and satisfied consumers.

Nontraditional Consultants

The United States has experienced a dramatic increase in the number of immigrants arriving over the past two decades. Before 1980, most immigrants coming to the United States were from European nations. Since that time, the demographics have shifted and now the vast majority of immigrants are from non-European nations. Along with their values and culture, patients from other countries bring experiences in health care systems very different from traditional Western medicine. In attempts to provide culturally competent patient care to this diverse population, consultations with traditional healers from

these various cultures are increasingly common. Originally dismissed as nonscientific, Curanderos, Shamans, Santiguadoras, and other traditional healers are now increasingly acknowledged as powerful allies to Western medicine. Although they may be accessing care within the U.S. health care system, many people hold deep-seated beliefs in methods of treatment rooted in their culture and values; this is discussed in greater detail in Chapter 8. The recommendations below provide strategies for working with patients who use traditional healers.

Negotiate the treatment plan with the patient and discuss how you are willing to work with the traditional healer for the patient's benefit. Encourage the patient to continue on the necessary course of Western therapy and keep you informed about additional treatments employed by the traditional healers. Use the LEARN model to assist in reducing cultural barriers and increasing patient compliance in your culturally diverse patients[16]:

L   Listen with understanding to the patient's perception of the problem.

E   Explain your perceptions and strategy for treatment.

A   Acknowledge and discuss differences in perceptions.

R   Recommend treatment with respect to the patient's cultural perceptions.

N   Negotiate agreement, keeping in mind the patient's conceptual framework of disease.

Employing traditional healers in the treatment plan for these patients can often assist in the patient's recovery. During the patient interview, it is helpful to inquire what the patient believes is causing the illness. This line of questioning may reveal that the patient believes an evil spirit or other entity is at the root of the problem. When patients hold these beliefs, it may be helpful to consult with traditional healers.

In many areas of the United States, traditional healers may be located by contacting local religious leaders in the community. Often, these individuals can help to provide insight about the culture and values of your patient, and they will usually be aware of what traditional healers are available in the area. Other contacts that may be helpful include ethnic organizations and alternative therapy units of larger hospitals.

If your practice has a large culturally diverse population, it may be wise to establish relationships with local nontraditional healers to facilitate future referrals. Most traditional healers are willing to work with Western practitioners to assist in the patient's recovery.

CASE STUDY 17-5

Mr. W is an 86-year-old Hispanic male who is unable to drive because of vision problems secondary to his diabetes. He and his wife live on a small ranch just outside of town. Mrs. W does drive, but her vision is also failing and she is uncomfortable driving farther than about 10 miles from their home. She is unable to drive at night. Mr. W is in need of a specialty consultation that is available only in a large community about 160 miles away (3 ½ hours by automobile). The Ws do not want to make the drive, but the PA needs to have the consultant see the patient.

Using Telemedicine Consultation

Case Study 17-5 illustrates a situation in which access to expert consultation without causing the patient to travel would be quite desirable. Using available telemedicine technology to provide consultative services is becoming more and more common in medical practice in the United States. Telemedicine technology has evolved to the point that it is reasonably priced, reliable, and practical.

Providers generally prefer to work with a system that provides video and audio quality that allows a conversation and examination to take place much as if the consultant were in the room with the patient. This level of interaction is referred to as real-time video capability. The signal sent under this system has only a slight delay that is not very noticeable. Real-time video is the standard of practice for consultations in which the patient will participate, either to give the history, have a physical examination performed, or both. Other methods are available to send data (i.e., x-rays, electrocardiogram [ECG], or other static images) that do not require real-time interaction.

To provide real-time interaction for a telemedicine consultation, it is likely that the data will be sent over telephone cables (i.e., ISDN, ATM, or T1) or via satellite. No matter which of the two types of transmission is used, the basic equipment and principles of consultation will be much the same for the provider. The basic setup of equipment usually includes the following:

1. A television screen on which to view the people on the other end (in this case, the consultant).
2. A second television, which serves as a monitor, to show how the PA's end looks to the consultant.
3. A box that looks like a big videocassette recorder (VCR) (this is the codec, the device that sends and receives the information).
4. A microphone and a camera.

Telemedicine units have the capability of plugging in many diagnostic instruments. This allows the use of the oto-ophthalmoscope and the stethoscope to send video and audio elements of the physical examination. Actually, any instrument with a standard connection (RS 232) will play through the units, allowing any type of scope to be attached and the accompanying video and audio data to be sent. This provides the ability to conduct a rather thorough physical examination and history. Other images may be viewed by the use of a document camera, which displays x-rays and ECGs with adequate detail for interpretation.

Many rural and frontier communities have found that the addition of telemedicine capabilities has allowed services to be provided on a local level. The consultation service is usually provided by a large academic medical center or referral hospital. The equipment can be used for consultations of a nonemergent nature or to receive emergent aid from experts.

Conducting the telemedicine referral requires several different skills. The telemedicine consultation is conducted live with the consultant viewing the patient from a remote location. For most patients, this type of interaction with a health care provider will be unique. Thus it is imperative to obtain the patient's permission to conduct the consultation using this technology. Once the patient agrees, education about how it will be different from other consultations should be delivered. It is ideal to be able to give the patient a tour of the facilities and demonstrate the equipment prior to the consultation. A conversation with the consultant prior to the presentation will also help to establish what type of information the consultant is interested in obtaining, so that the proper equipment is ready. Of course, it will be necessary for the referring health care provider to actually conduct the examination at the direction of the consultant.

Other issues need to be considered in conducting a telemedicine consultation. Most centers have a permission form for patients to sign to indicate that they agreed to the consultation using technology instead of the traditional method. It is important to remember that the legal responsibility for care of the patient rests (in most states) with the referring health care provider who is in physical contact with the patient. Some facilities record the consultation for future reference (most telemedicine systems have a VCR interface that allows for recordings to be made). Should this be the case, the patient's permission should be obtained, and the recording treated as privileged material along with the rest of the patient's record.

If the consultation crosses state lines (referring provider and patient in one state and consultant in another), an issue arises concerning the licensing requirements for the consultant. Performing a consultation on a patient from state A by a consultant in state B may be considered practicing medicine in state A. Thus it is important to ensure that those participating in the consult have met all legal requirements.

A final consideration for the consultation is the acceptance by third party payers of this type of consult. In many areas of the United States, telemedicine consultation is not considered reimbursable. It is advisable to obtain a determination prior to the consultation so that the patient is not placed in an awkward position if payment is denied after the service has been performed.

Although still an evolving technology, telemedicine consultation is becoming more widely available, providing access to specialty services in areas where they were previously unavailable. These services may save the patient travel time and money. Like any medical service, telemedicine consultation must be integrated into the practice setting. Patients should be educated about the benefits of this type of consultation. PAs should learn the skills needed to participate

in telemedicine services because they likely will be refined and offered in a greater number of geographic locations.

Internet Consultations

With the advent of the Internet, many patients go "on-line" to gather information about their health, any diseases they may have, or symptoms they are experiencing. Most patients will be interested in finding information from various web sites; others will actually seek a diagnosis and perhaps treatment. Guidelines for the PA who is attempting to help patients obtain useful information on-line follow:

1. Ask patients what questions they have about their illness.
2. Refer patients with Internet access to reputable web sites that you know provide quality information.
3. Ask patients about what information they obtained from the Internet and what sites they frequent for health issues.
4. Indicate your willingness to help the patient evaluate health information received from the Internet.
5. Discuss potential pitfalls with obtaining "on-line" diagnoses and treatments.
6. Ask patients to send you links to helpful sites for use with other patients.

By following these guidelines, you will help patients get the most out of the resources available on the Internet.

USING COMMUNITY RESOURCES
The Case of the S Family

Before the discussion of community resources begins, let us consider the following case. It will help the reader understand how a PA becomes involved in referrals to community resources.

CASE STUDY 17-6

The S family has been coming to a general practice for years. The previous PA worked with them for several years. Mr. S is 48 years old, and Mrs. S is 46. They have five children: Mary (17), John (15), Sean (11), David (9), and Beth (1). Mrs. S is a diabetic and has been treated for depression in the past. Mr. S has struggled for years with control of his hypertension. The new PA notes from the chart that Mr. and Mrs. S have both had drug and alcohol problems in the past. Mr. S is in the office today for his regular appointment.

After introducing herself and explaining her transition into the practice, the new PA mentions the fact that Mr. S's blood pressure is 170/100. Mr. S indicates that he sometimes forgets to take his medication because he has many other things on his mind these days. When the PA asks for details, Mr. S describes his current situation.

Mr. S has worked in the local automobile plant for years. That plant is now closing, and in the next 6 months, he will be out of a job. Mrs. S has never worked outside the home, choosing to stay home with the children. Mrs. S has become depressed again and has called the local mental health center for services. Her name has been added to its waiting list. Mr. S has tried desperately to pull his wife out of this depression but has been unsuccessful. He states that she has alluded to thoughts of suicide. A great deal of the responsibility for the care of the children has now fallen to Mr. S. He seems able to manage fairly well with Beth and David. David presents difficulty sometimes because his borderline mental retardation makes it difficult for him to understand his mother's disinterest. John and Sean, according to Mr. S, are doing okay at home. However, he states that he has had calls from the school informing him that John has been getting into fights and that Sean refuses to socialize, appearing withdrawn. The most recent family upset has come with Mary's announcement that she is pregnant. Mrs. S blames Mr. S for letting this happen because he should have taken more responsibility for the family when she became depressed. Mrs. S claims he is a poor father, and she has proposed divorce.

Mr. S remarks that it feels good to tell someone about all of this. He then asks whether there is any further help the PA can suggest.

At first glance, this scenario may seem overwhelming to approach. The practitioner at any level of experience who has a sound knowledge of community resources could, however, use a systematic approach to assist this patient. In fact, it would be considered a clear opportunity for community involvement integrated with a realistic treatment and prevention plan for the patient. The reader should remember this scenario while reading the section on community resources. At the conclusion of the chapter, a discussion of one approach to Mr. S's problems is presented.

Community resources vary widely, and there are often crossover relationships and duplicate services within a single community. A particular community service agency, such as a family service agency, may have services for families, individuals, and groups. A mental health center in the same community may also have services for families, individuals, and groups. These agencies may use one another's services and refer patients back and forth, depending on the nature of a client's needs, the agency's ability to serve that client at that particular time, and the desires of the client or the family. In addition, a client may need to use more than one service within a community. Because many community resources provide multiple services, choosing to which agency a patient should be referred is sometimes difficult. The novice soon discovers what the experienced user of community resources knows, namely, that no matter how many services a community resource provides, there are often waiting lists, or it may be difficult to find the appropriate resource for a particular patient.

These situations may overwhelm the PA. It would seem easier to simply ignore this part of the differential diagnosis and eliminate it completely from the treatment plan. Experienced practitioners are aware, however, that community resource referral is an essential part of the differential diagnosis and treatment plan, for several reasons, including the following. First, there are simply times when no physical reason can be found for a patient's complaint. Patients may believe that they must have a physical complaint in order to see the practitioner. This admission ticket is their way past the receptionists and office nurse to the patient room, where they look to the practitioner to discover their real needs and reasons for the office visit. Second, many medical diagnoses and treatment plans require the community resource referral for completeness. Consider the following case.

CASE STUDY 17-7

A patient comes to the office for her regular prenatal check. She is 25 weeks pregnant. The PA notices that she is wearing heavier makeup than usual and seems to avoid eye contact. When the PA inquires about her behavior, the patient begins to cry and says that her boyfriend hit her after consuming a lot of alcohol. She explains that her boyfriend feels pressured to provide for the baby and to get married. He is young, she says, and had different plans for his future.

To simply treat this situation as a routine prenatal visit would be an act of negligence on the part of any clinician. Recognizing that this patient needs a different kind of treatment plan fulfills the patient's needs as well as the clinician's obligation to treat and heal. There are many potential referral sources for this particular scenario, such as:

➤ A family service agency to assist with the relationship difficulties, that is, to enable the patient's boyfriend to deal with his feelings about the pregnancy, to provide counseling for abusive behavior, and to assist the patient in making decisions about the relationship.

➤ A legal services or attorney referral to advise the patient on legal action she can take to protect herself from further incidents of abuse.

➤ Possible drug and alcohol assistance services for the patient's boyfriend.

The clinician in this scenario must act as the catalyst and facilitator by identifying services for the patient. The patient must ultimately determine what assistance she will or will not accept. It is the responsibility of the clinician to be knowledgeable about the assistance available, to facilitate referral by discussing the idea with the patient and significant others, and to make the initial referral to the appropriate community service agency.

An Overview of Typical Community Services

As has been discussed previously, there is overlap of services among community service agencies. As a result, any attempt to discuss community resources can be a difficult task. Various approaches have been used to illustrate the community network of services. Many focus on an outline of services for children, school

guidance services, mental health services, services for the elderly, home care services, and self-help and mutual help groups. For the purposes of this chapter, five specific *areas* have been identified as problem categories for the family—personal/social, financial/employment, addiction, legal, and health. Examples of each category, along with the possible community service responses available for each identified family problem, are listed in Table 17-1 and discussed in this chapter. The brief explanation of each community service listed serves as a helpful reference for the reader. The lists of services shown in Table 17-1, however, are not to be viewed as all-inclusive; in fact, they fall far short of that. They are also not to be viewed as representative of any particular agency's services.

Physician assistants must recognize that it is necessary to become knowledgeable about the network of community services available in their particular practice areas. They must also be aware of individual agency resources; many communities now have a human service directory that can be of invaluable assistance in helping the practitioner discover these resources. Finally, PAs must be aware of community services that are not available. Ultimately, it is the PA's responsibility to integrate all three of these areas of knowledge into the treatment plans for their patients.

Assistance With Personal and Social Problems

Table 17-2 shows which of the community resources discussed here are generally available for personal and social problems.

Family service agencies are probably the most generic of all community service providers. Counseling for individuals and families is often the core of services offered by this type of agency. Counseling can address personal, legal, educational, financial, and other difficulties. With such a broad base, additional supportive programs are chosen according to the agency's perception of community needs. Many family service agencies use a sliding fee scale for payment, which makes them ideal for people with limited incomes.

Mental health services and centers provide evaluation, diagnostic, and treatment services for people of all ages who are experiencing emotional or mental health difficulties. These centers use professionals from many disciplines. Psychiatrists, psychologists,

Table 17-1   Categories of Family Problems and Possible Community Resources
Available to Assist With Them

Problem Area	Examples	Community Resources Available to Help
Personal/social	Marital counseling	Family service agencies
	Mental retardation/emotional problems	Mental health centers
	Child or adult physical or sexual abuse	Family planning centers
	Spouse abuse	Private psychiatrists, psychologists, and social workers
	Sexual assault	
	Adolescent pregnancy	Child welfare agencies
	Child or adult education	Mental retardation centers and services
	Child care and companionship	
	Adult or elder care	Senior citizen centers
	Individual and family counseling	Big Brothers and Big Sisters
	Psychological testing	Private and public day care centers and homes
	High school equivalent education or career counseling	Employee assisted day care centers
	Early childhood development	Personal care boarding and nursing homes
	Post-traumatic stress disorder	
	Acquired immune deficiency syndrome (AIDS)	Adult day care centers
		School special services for exceptional children
	Bereavement	
	Eating disorders	Adult education centers
	Anxiety	Centers for special learning
	Depression	Head Start programs
	Job stress	Religious communities
Financial/employment	Unemployment	Departments of public welfare
	Housing	Emergency financial services
	Transportation	Budget and credit counseling
	Budgeting	Offices of employment security
	Cash assistance	Domestic relations resources
	Discrimination	Housing authorities and resource groups
		American Rescue Workers
		Salvation Army
		Goodwill Industries and Skills Training & Employment Programs
		Equal Employment Opportunity Commission and human relations commissions
Addiction	Drugs	Alcoholics Anonymous
	Alcohol	Alanon and Alateen
		Narcotics Anonymous
		Drug and medical clinics
		Inpatient rehabilitation facilities
		Relapse programs

Table 17-1 Categories of Family Problems and Possible Community Resources Available to Assist With Them—cont'd

Problem Area	Examples	Community Resources Available to Help
Legal	Incarceration DUI convictions Legal services Juvenile delinquency	Adult probation and parole offices, including DUI programs Juvenile probation offices Legal aid services Victim/witness programs
Health	Aging Handicapped (physically or educationally disabled) Hospitalization Home health needs Immunizations and state health laws Nutrition Cancer	Food banks Support groups Hospital social services Associations for blind and visually handicapped Associations and services for learning disabled Community nursing services Easter Seals Society Vocational rehabilitation March of Dimes State health centers

social workers, and nurses are usually an integral part of the treatment approach. A sliding fee scale is usually applied. Crisis intervention services are usually available on a 24-hour basis.

Family planning centers offer educational, screening, and testing services for women regarding pregnancy and gynecological problems. A sliding fee scale is usually applied.

Psychiatrists, psychologists, and social workers in private practice are valuable to the community. Their services range from individual psychotherapy to marital and family counseling to psychological testing. Many people in need of help find the private practice service area a more comfortable environment. Provision of service is based on ability to pay.

Child welfare agencies provide protective, adoptive, foster care, and institutional services for children (18 years of age and younger) in the community. These agencies are mandated service providers for situations of physical, emotional, and sexual abuse and exploitation of children. In recent years, abuse and exploitation assistance has become the core of these agencies' community work. Many child welfare agencies have direct

working relationships with governmental juvenile parole and probation departments.

Mental retardation services and centers are sometimes directly tied to mental health services in a community and sometimes are private services. They offer vocational assistance, advocacy, and supervision to mentally retarded community members. Services are also provided to anyone caring for a mentally retarded family member in the home.

Senior citizen centers are the central providers of services to the elderly in a community. Their services range from in-home care, adult day care, services, transportation, and employment to volunteer programs. Protective services for the abused or exploited elder family member are also available.

In *Big Brothers* and *Big Sisters* programs, same-sex companionship is provided to children from single-parent families. Emphasis is placed on assisting a child in his or her development through contact with a positive role model.

Private and public day care centers furnish child care to parents interested in entering or remaining in the workforce. Educational programming and development

Table 17-2 Community Resources Available for Specific Personal and Social Problems and Needs*

Community Resource	Adolescent Pregnancy	Adult and Elder Care	Adult Physical and Sexual Abuse	Anxiety	Child Physical and Sexual Abuse	Child Care and Companionship	Child and Adult Education	Depression
Family service agencies	X		X	X			X	X
Mental health centers			X	X	X		X	X
Family planning centers	X						X	
Private practice psychologists and social workers			X	X	X			X
Child welfare agencies					X		X	
Mental retardation centers and services		X	X				X	
Senior citizen centers		X	X				X	
Big Brothers and Big Sisters						X		
Private and public care centers and homes		X				X		
Employee-assisted day care						X		
Professional care boarding and nursing homes		X						
Adult day care								
School special services for exceptional children	X					X		
Adult education centers						•		
Centers for special caring								
Head Start programs								
Religious communities						X	X	

*An X indicates that assistance is available from the resource for the problem.

for children are emphasized in many of these centers. A range of fees is available for low-income families. Some employers provide day care services to employees. These services, called employee-assisted day care, are typically located near or on the site of the business. This service is considered an employee benefit and is provided at a competitive fee for employees only.

Personal care boarding and nursing homes offer care to people who are no longer able to maintain themselves in their own homes. Assistance in activities of daily living is available for elders in this type of facility. Nursing homes provide a range of nursing and medical care needs to the elderly person in poor health.

In *adult day care* arrangements, elderly individuals unable to take responsibility for themselves are supervised and monitored while their primary caregivers are at work or otherwise unable to care for them.

Special services for exceptional children are often provided through the local school district. Mentally retarded, socially or emotionally disturbed, learning disabled, physically handicapped, speech handicapped, and mentally gifted students are eligible for such services.

In community *adult education centers,* interested adults can obtain a high school graduate equivalency certificate or receive special training. Career

Table 17-2 Community Resources Available for Specific Personal and Social Problems and Needs*—cont'd

Job Stress	Marital Counseling	Mental Retardation/ Emotional Problems	Spouse Abuse	Sexual Assault	Individual and Family Counseling	Psychological Testing	High School Equivalency and Career Counseling	Early Childhood Development
X	X		X	X	X	X		
	X	X			X	X		
X	X				X	X		
		X			X	X		
		X			X	X		
		X			X	X		
		X				X		
							X	
			X			X		X
								X
	X				X			

counseling services are also available for individuals seeking employment after being unemployed, unable to work for an extended time, or wishing to change their current employment status.

Centers for special learning provide assistance to children with developmental difficulties. *Head Start programs* prepare low-income children and children with special needs for entering kindergarten.

An often-overlooked community resource is the *religious community* (e.g., church, synagogue, temple). Many have religious leaders who are trained in both pastoral and personal counseling. Some religious denominations also have special programs for youths and adults. A patient may prefer assistance of this nature for personal or social problems.

Financial and Employment Assistance Table 17-3 shows which services from the community resources discussed here are generally available for financial and employment problems.

The *department of public welfare* is a state agency providing cash assistance, assistance for medical care, and similar services to low-income or needy people.

Many community service resources, such as family service agencies and agencies affiliated with

Table 17-3   Community Resources Available for Specific Financial or Employment Problems*

Community Resource	Unemployment	Housing	Transportaion	Budgeting	Cash Assistance	Discrimination
Departments of public welfare	X	X	X	X	X	X
Emergency financial services					X	
Budget and credit counseling	X			X		
Offices of employment security	X					
Domestic relations resources					X	
Housing authorities and resource groups		X				
American Rescue Workers		X				
Salvation Army		X		X		
Goodwill Industries and Skills Training & Employment Programs	X					
Equal Employment Opportunity Commission and human relations commissions	X	X				X

* An X indicates that assistance is available from the resource for the problem.

particular religious denominations, provide one-time *emergency financial assistance* to persons in need.

Budget and credit counseling are available both publicly and privately to people needing help with money management.

State or local *offices of employment security* (unemployment offices) assist people with job placement, job testing, and other employment services, in addition to processing unemployment insurance claims.

People who need financial support for children from the legally responsible parent who is unwilling or reluctant to meet his or her financial care responsibilities are assisted in obtaining such support by *domestic relations resources.*

Housing authorities and *resource groups* help low-income and moderate-income people of all ages obtain housing.

American Rescue Workers and the *Salvation Army* offer emergency shelter on a temporary basis for people in need.

Both *Goodwill Industries Skills Training* and *Employment Programs* provide employment and training for mentally retarded and mental health consumers. The *Equal Employment Opportunity Commission (EEOC)* and *human relations commissions* investigate complaints of potential discrimination in the areas of sex, ethnic or religious origin, housing, and employment.

Assistance for Addiction Problems

Table 17-4 shows which services from the community resources discussed here are generally available for addiction problems.

Alcoholics Anonymous is a self-help group comprising recovering alcoholics who help one another maintain their sobriety and help others attain it. *Alanon* and *Alateen* are related self-help groups that assist adults or teens in coping with alcohol dependence in a family member or friend.

Another self-help group, *Narcotics Anonymous,* is composed of individuals who are recovering from dependency on drugs. Addicted individuals learn to cope with life without using drugs.

Drug and alcohol clinics provide outpatient services to individuals dealing with drug and alcohol problems. Group therapy and counseling are usually offered. Referral to inpatient treatment facilities after evaluation of individual needs is also an integral part of services provided by drug and alcohol clinics. An *inpatient rehabilitation facility* offers a battery of treatment services for addicted persons judged to require intensive treatment.

Relapse programs offer services on an outpatient basis. Group sessions are intended to assist individuals who have abstained from drugs and alcohol but have had a recent relapse of use.

Legal Assistance

Table 17-5 shows the services available for legal problems from the community resources discussed here.

Adult probation and parole departments are responsible for the supervision of all adult parolees and probationers from the prison and court systems. Family members of these individuals may need to communicate through these departments special needs or difficulties they are experiencing.

Juvenile probation departments are responsible for the supervision of juvenile offenders who have been either put on probation or institutionalized. Such departments assist parents in dealing with a juvenile on probation. They also monitor special programs involving juvenile offenders. Reintegration into the community after institutionalization and community service opportunities are examples of these programs.

Legal Aid services help eligible people who cannot afford to hire a private attorney deal with civil legal matters such as divorce, child custody, landlord and tenant matters, and bankruptcy.

Through *victim/witness* programs, victims of or witnesses to crimes obtain compensation or referral to community social service agencies for counseling or other appropriate services.

Assistance With Health Care and Related Problems

Table 17-6 shows resources available for specific health problems and needs.

Food banks give food to individuals and families on a limited basis in times of emergency and crisis when other services such as food stamps are not available or eligibility for them has not yet been determined.

A vast array of *support groups* are available to individuals, particularly in the health field. Groups for health-related concerns and diseases such as cancer, diabetes, Parkinson's and Alzheimer's diseases, and epilepsy have been formed in many communities. Other support groups offer help to single parents dealing with a delinquent teenager or to victims of sexual assault or other crimes.

Table 17-4 Community Resources Available for Specific Addition Problems and Needs*

Community Resource	Drugs	Alcohol
Alcoholics Anonymous		X
Alanon		X
Alateen		X
Narcotics Anonymous	X	
Drug and alcohol clinics	X	X
Inpatient rehabilitation facilities	X	X
Relapse programs	X	X

*An X indicates that assistance is available from the resource for the problem.

Table 17-5   Community Resources Available for Specific Legal Problems and Needs*

Community Resource	Incarceration	DuI	Legal Aid Services	Juvenile Delinquency
Adult probation and parole, including DUI programs	X	X		
Juvenile probation offices	X	X		X
Legal aid services			X	
Victim/witness programs			X	

*An X indicates that assistance is available from the resource for the problem.

Table 17-6   Community Resources Available for Specific Health Problems and Needs*

Community Resource	Aging	Handicapped (Physically or Educationally Disabled)	Hospitali-zation	Home Health Needs	Immuni-zations and State Health Laws	Nutrition	Cancer
Food banks	X	X				X	
Support groups	X	X	X	X			X
Hospital social services		X	X	X		X	X
Associations for blind and visually handicapped		X	X				
Community nursing services	X	X	X	X	X	X	X
Easter Seals Society		X	X	X			
Vocational rehabilitation		X	X				
March of Dimes		X		X			
State health centers	X				X	X	
Associations and services for learning disabled		X					
American Cancer Society							X

*An X indicates that assistance is available from the resource for the problem.

Hospital social services and *case management services* help patients and their families cope with the stress accompanying hospitalization. Follow-up referrals to community service agencies and medical facilities are also provided.

Associations for the blind and visually handicapped offer preventive programs and educational services to minimize the incidence of loss of vision. They also assist impaired individuals by furnishing special equipment, transportation, and counseling.

A *community nursing services* agency supplies nursing care, physical therapy, nutritional education, prenatal services, hospice home services, and counseling to patients in their own homes.

The *Easter Seals Society* offers an extremely broad range of assessment and treatment services to people of all ages and varying economic status in the community. Its services include speech and language, orthopedics, hearing evaluations, equipment rentals, summer camps, psychological testing, and day care.

The primary focus of the *March of Dimes* is prevention of birth defects through educational programming. Prenatal patients, for example, may be referred for education services.

Vocational rehabilitation agencies formulate programs to increase the employability of people with learning, physical, mental, or addictive problems.

State health centers provide immunizations and health guidance to individuals. Community health education is also a priority.

Associations for learning disabilities assist children and adults with developmental disabilities to gain referral and information for services, legal rights, tutoring, and advocacy.

The American Cancer Society offers information, support services, and advocacy for people and families living with cancer.

Conclusion: Help for the S Family

In Case Study 17-6, Mr. S has already given the PA one clue as to his needs. He needs someone with whom to discuss his situation and to sort out and develop alternatives to his circumstances. Although this counseling component is well within the realm and abilities of the PA, it must be carefully weighed with the time such an undertaking would require and how that would fit with a busy practice. Even if the time is available, a community referral for this patient and his family should address the need for family and marital counseling. The S family appears to be a prime candidate for referral to a family service agency, where a multiservice approach could be taken. The PA could continue to see Mr. S for support and coordination of the community resources, either as part of his regular medical appointments or as separate appointments. The PA might also consider meeting with the S family to discuss the need for referral to a family service agency. This would lend support to Mr. S's efforts to help his family and could almost be seen as a prescription for this dysfunctional family. The PA, acting as community resource coordinator, could also help by contacting the local mental health center to facilitate assistance for Mrs. S. Other community resources for this family would include mental retardation services for David, to help him understand what is happening at home, and a contact with the school system to discuss John's and Sean's behavior. All of this, of course, would be done with the S family's permission.

CLINICAL APPLICATIONS

1. You are the family practice PA caring for Mr. W in Case Study 17-3. What is your role, and how can you help to coordinate Mr. W's health care?

2. You are the PA seeing Ms. Q in Case Study 17-4. How will you describe your function to Ms. Q and explain why she cannot self-refer to a neurologist?

3. Based on your history and physical examination findings, you believe that Ms. Q needs a neurological consultation. Her managed care plan refuses this referral. How will you handle this situation?

4. You are the PA caring for Mr. S in Case Study 17-6. How will you present the array of community resources available to your patient and his family? What will you say that will educate Mr. S about the usefulness of these resources, while making sure that he knows that you want to continue as his PA?

REFERENCES

1. Braham RL, Ron A, Ruchlin HS, et al. Diagnostic test restraint and the specialty consultation: original articles. J Gen Intern Med 1990;5:95.
2. Jones RB, Larizgoita I, Casado I, Barric T. Clinical audit: how effective is the referral chain for diabetic retinopathy? Diabet Med 1989;6:262.
3. Wilkin D, Metcalfe DH, Marinker M. The meaning of information on GP referral rates to hospitals. Community Med 1989;11:65.
4. Langley GR, Tritchler DL, Llewellyn-Thomas HA, Till JE. Use of written cases to study factors associated with regional variations in referral rates. J Clin Epidemiol 1991;44:391.
5. Jones NP, Lloyd IC, Kwartz J. General practitioner referrals to an eye hospital: a standard referral form. J R Soc Med 1990;83:770.
6. Westerman RF, Hull FM, Bezemer PD, Gort G. A study of communication between general practitioners and specialists: original papers. Br J Gen Pract 1990;40:445.
7. Eaglstein WH, Laszlo KS. Patient referrals to a dermatologist: the referring physician's perspective. Arch Dermatol 1996;132:292.
8. Bienia R, Heuser G, Bienia B. Consultation patterns in an urban hospital setting. Va Med 1989;116:371.
9. Gomez AG, Grimm CT, Yee EF, Skootsky SA. Preparing residents for managed care practice using an experienced-based curriculum. Acad Med 1997;72:959.
10. Roland MO, Green CA, Roberts SOB. Should general practitioners refer more patients to hospitals? J R Soc Med 1991;84:403.
11. Sutherland LR, Verhoef M. Patients who seek a second opinion: are they different from the typical referral? J Clin Gastroenterol 1989;11:308.
12. Roberts KB, Starr S, Dewitt TG. The University of Massachusetts Medical Center office-based continuity experience: are we preparing pediatrics residents for primary care practice? Pediatrics 1997;100:E2.
13. Franks P, Clancy CM. Referrals of adult patients from primary care: demographic disparities and their relationship to HMO insurance. J Fam Pract 1997;45:47.
14. Gill JM, Diamond JJ. Effect of primary care referral on emergency department use: evaluation of a statewide Medicaid program. Fam Med 1996;28:178.
15. Rosenthal TC, Riemenschneider TA, Feather J. Preserving the patient referral process in the managed care environment. Am J Med 1996;100:338.
16. Berlin EA, Fowkes WC. Teaching framework for cross-cultural care: Application in the family. West J Med 1983;139:934.

RESOURCES

Braham RL, et al. Diagnostic test restraint and the specialty consultation: original articles. J Gen Intern Med 1990;5:95. *A well-written article that examines the effects of consultants on the diagnosis and management of patients admitted to a university teaching hospital. The article describes the differences in patient outcomes and hospital stays when consultants were and were not used.*

Wilkin D, et al. The meaning of information on GP referral rates to hospitals. Community Med 1989;11:65. *Describes variations in referral to specialty services by general practitioners in the United Kingdom. Wide variations in referral rates were discovered, but no indications of the appropriateness of the referral could be drawn by observation of the referral rates alone. Suggestions were made concerning the use of referral rate data in the development of quality assurance and other health policy considerations.*

Westerman RF, et al. A study of communication between general practitioners and specialists: original papers. Br J Gen Pract 1990;40:445. *Analyzes referral letters from general practitioners to specialists in medicine, dermatology, neurology, and gastroenterology. A panel of general practitioners and specialists reviewed the letters and the replies from specialists.*

CHAPTER 18

Using the Medical Literature: Lifelong Learning Skills

Robert W. Jarski

INTRODUCTION

Early 20th century medical training primarily involved apprenticeships. Medical information was conveyed between individual practitioners informally by word-of-mouth and more formally through textbooks that were considered "authoritative." The validity of available medical information was established by "experts," who discussed various topics around conference tables. The scientific basis of disease had not yet entered mainstream medical practice—a concept that seems unimaginable today. However, the scientific era of medicine became widespread with the publication in 1910 of the Flexner Report, which recommended that medical practice should be based on science and that medical curricula should include basic science coursework such as anatomy, physiology, and microbiology.[1] Modern medical practice has replaced the expert's word with evidence-based information and, when possible, scientific verifiability.

Physician assistants (PAs) are educated in their chosen profession to be, first and foremost, excellent clinicians who apply scientific principles to the art of medical practice. The role of the PA focuses on the use of evidence-based scientific information while skilled and humane patient care is provided. In order to use scientific information effectively, PAs need to stay up-to-date and clinically competent in a complex medical information environment. To practice in this environment, PAs use a multifaceted system of information not only in their reading and use of the Internet, but also in gathering and generating a patient's clinical information.

Clinical information can be broadly classified as either subjective or objective. The three drawings in Figure 18-1 demonstrate some of the characteristics of objective information. Because the information contained in the drawings is directly observable, in the clinical sense, it is "objective." The lines in Figure 18-1, *A,* appear unequal in length, the lines in Figure 18-1, *B,* appear nonparallel, and each number in Figure 18-1, *C,* appears to be in *one* location in relation to the box. Most observers would initially agree with these conclusions. Nevertheless, the horizontal lines are actually equal in length, the vertical lines are parallel, and each number can be interpreted as residing in more than one location in relation to the box. The initial conclusions drawn about these pictures were based on imperfect information. The nature of an imperfect information environment shows that PAs should constantly validate findings, even though they are "objective." This would appear to be a simple task. The task is actually not simple, and "facts" that are able to withstand genuine tests of truthfulness and validity occur rarely.

Yet clinicians use volumes of information they believe to be fact and often accept others' unverified observations as fact. Clinical experience alone is not sufficient for maintaining competence. The founder of the Alderson-Broaddus College PA Program, Dr. Hu C. Myers, said in 1973: "Clinical experience is doing the same thing over, and over, and over—wrong."

Throughout their professional careers, astute PAs who are lifelong learners reexamine their observations, thinking, and information, primarily through literature, the Internet, and other medical information sources. To be successful lifelong learners, PAs must be knowledgeable about how medical information—which is the foundation of clinical practice—is

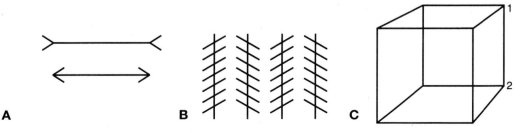

Figure 18-1 Examples of objective information. See text for discussion.

generated and presented for clinicians' use. In a nutshell, PAs must be informed consumers of medical information.

HOW DEPENDABLE ARE MEDICAL INFORMATION SOURCES?

Even though PAs rely on medical information sources, not all information to which they are exposed is accurate. Among the various medical information sources, peer-reviewed journals in either hard copy or electronic form are considered the most dependable and most highly quality controlled. Most readers, however, are surprised to learn that as many as two thirds of studies appearing in the *best* U.S. medical journals have been marked by flaws that invalidated their conclusions. Fortunately, the review process that was initiated approximately 2 decades ago and is still used today can potentially reduce the number of flawed articles to approximately 26%.[2] The reader must therefore be alert for flawed information, which may appear in one of every four articles. In addition, several studies have found that numerous published articles that had been fully retracted in print because of honest errors were later cited repeatedly in medical journals. For example, one investigation found that 82 retracted articles had been later cited in the literature 733 times.[3]

Even well-controlled experimental studies and randomized clinical trials using placebos that are free of any known methodological problems are sometimes difficult to interpret. For example, in experimental studies, subjects who take a placebo regularly have better outcomes than subjects who comply erratically.[4] Many other reported therapeutic effects are currently unexplained by conventional medical science.

Methods of generating and presenting medical knowledge are complex and obviously imperfect. Relying on others for interpreting new information is not sufficient; PAs must cautiously evaluate medical information for themselves, taking into account their own patient population, biases toward treatment methods, and practice style, which is shaped by past experiences and personal attitudes and philosophies of health care.

GOALS AND OBJECTIVES

The goal of this chapter is to describe practical methods for using medical information sources, especially the medical literature. Specifically, the reader will learn the following:

1. How to classify and effectively deal with the magnitude of medical information available from a variety of sources.
2. How to locate and select medical information for remaining competent and current in practice.
3. How to screen new information to help detect faulty reports and identify those that are dependable and clinically useful.
4. How to interpret and apply statistical information using a "rule of thumb" approach.

PRACTICING IN THE INFORMATION AGE

PAs practice in the postindustrial information age in which the volume of scientific knowledge is increasing exponentially. To remain current and thereby competent in practice, PAs must learn new information throughout their professional lifetime. In the evidence-based medical environment, PAs must also interpret and critically evaluate published research. After graduating from their academic programs, PAs typically learn about new medical developments through journals and other periodicals, conferences, textbooks, and various audiovisual and electronic sources (such as the Internet, educational television, audiotape, CD, and DVD.).

The task of maintaining current knowledge in any medical discipline may initially seem impossible. Each year, from medical journals alone, approximately 350,000 new biomedical articles are indexed by the National Library of Medicine.[5] It is neither necessary nor desirable, however, for PAs to assimilate all new medical information published in journals. A PA can remain current by reading in a specific way only a few carefully selected journals. A recommended system is presented later in this chapter.

THE VARIETY OF MEDICAL INFORMATION SOURCES

In the broadest sense, PAs learn new information both informally and formally. Informal sources, such as word-of-mouth transmission of knowledge, are often useful and readily available (sometimes to excess), but few or no quality control safeguards help ensure the accuracy and reliability of that information. Formal information sources include textbooks, professional conferences, various audiovisual and electronic media, and journals. In addition, dissertations and theses can be invaluable to PA readers. Each information source provides a slightly different type of content, and each has advantages and disadvantages.

Textbooks

Textbooks generally summarize and recapitulate information that has been previously published elsewhere. Most textbooks do not present original research data (information new to the store of recorded knowledge). Textbooks have the advantages of being practical and portable, and they require no expensive, bulky, or special equipment to use. In addition, the reader can write personally meaningful notes on the pages, and information listed in a book's index is readily accessible.

Textbooks provide ample information for orientation purposes. Sometimes, however, they lack sufficient depth and detail about specialty topics. At some point, most PAs outgrow the information level of the textbooks in their specialty. A second limitation is that some textbooks lack scientific scrutiny. They are not always systematically reviewed for scientific validity and technical accuracy, as are the best medical journals. There is, however, some degree of review for textbooks compiled and evaluated by conscientious editors who have subject area expertise.

Because of publication lag times, most textbooks do not contain current information about new medical developments. Following their discovery, it takes approximately 2 to 5 years for new data to appear in most textbooks. This is because of printing and editing complexities, and because debatable and unsettled issues are generally omitted. For some very dynamic health care developments, for example, recent developments in study of the human immunodeficiency virus (HIV) and the acquired immunodeficiency syndrome (AIDS), cardiovascular disease prevention, and health care policy, this amount of lag time is unacceptable. Textbooks are probably clinicians'

most used medical information resource, but at some point, PAs find it necessary to consult more timely and in-depth sources.

Professional Conferences

Information presented at professional conferences tends to be timely, and it may undergo some quality control for accuracy and reliability. Abstracts of presentation content are typically screened by a panel of reviewers, and if the presentation includes a question and answer period, an astute audience may provide some content review. Presentation of scientific information at conferences sometimes precedes its publication in journals, although not all presentations are published. A presentation's content can be original research or a review of a clinical topic. The important distinctions between original research and clinical review articles are discussed later in this chapter.

Audiovisual and Electronic Media

Modern technology, including the Internet, has made sophisticated audiovisuals accessible to nearly all health care providers regardless of practice setting. Audiotapes are relatively inexpensive and can be used while one is commuting or vacationing. Modem-accessible computerized medical news networks have made information on recent developments quickly available to practitioners. More costly media, such as videotapes, videodisks, and computerized presentations, can be accessed through most hospital libraries. Many of these media are furnished to institutions by subscription and can be as timely as journals. Some computerized media are user-interactive to suit the needs of individual learning and personality styles, and the content can be selected to match particular practice needs. High-resolution graphics, motion, and sound can communicate complex clinical information in new and creative ways.

The disadvantages of audiovisual media include cost and the need for specialized equipment. These media are not as accessible and conveniently transported as are textbooks or printed journals. None fits easily into a coat pocket. Although it is possible to referee these media, the review process used for many of these information sources is not as systematic as it is for quality journals.

Doctoral Dissertations and Master's Theses

Although most clinicians fail to think of them, dissertations and theses may be invaluable information resources. A thesis is the report on a research project that is conducted as a requirement of some master's degree programs. A dissertation is the report of a research project that is conducted as part of an academic doctoral degree, such as the PhD, EdD, DPH, or DSc. A dissertation is evaluated and determined by a panel of scholars to be a significant contribution to the store of knowledge. Some master's level PA programs and scholarly allopathic (MD) and osteopathic (DO) training programs require a major paper or thesis; in some programs, a dissertation is completed as part of the PhD degree in conjunction with a medical degree.

The structure of a dissertation or thesis is similar to that of a research article, except that each of the five major sections (introduction, literature review, methods, results, and discussion) accounts for an entire chapter. A dissertation or thesis is a book, rather than an article, about a study. Many articles published in medical and health journals are derived from dissertation and thesis research.

Dissertations and theses are useful when the PA needs the following:

1. A comprehensive review about a topic area.
2. In-depth detail about a particular study (e.g., individual questionnaire items used in a survey).

The literature review in dissertations is usually comprehensive if not exhaustive, and it may encompass peripherally related topics. A dissertation can therefore be a quick and excellent source of a literature review.

Nearly all dissertations written in North America are catalogued and abstracted in the bound index *Dissertation Abstracts International,* which is available in most libraries and on the Internet as DISS. Hard copies of dissertations may be purchased through University Microfilms International, 300 Zeeb Road, Ann Arbor, MI 48106. The cost is approximately $20 to $50. A copy of a dissertation or thesis is also available from the library of the college or university at which the work was completed.

Clinicians may not always need the specific information presented in a dissertation's methods and results sections, but the more general information contained in the introductory chapter and discussion and the comprehensive literature review may be particularly useful. A dissertation or thesis written on one's topic of interest can be a time saver and a gold mine of information.

Journals

A journal is "an unbound periodical usually containing multiple articles on different subjects by different authors that is published under the general editorial supervision of an identified editor or group of editors."[6]

The best modern medical journals use a systematic process of quality control in an attempt to help ensure the accuracy and scientific worth of published information. Most are published weekly or monthly to provide current information. Even so, there is, on the average, a lag time of approximately 6 to 10 months between an article's submission to the journal and its appearance in print. The period between data collection and publication is even longer. Some journals, however, maintain a special "fast track" that is reserved for the occasional item of medical news that is of major importance; publication time may be only days or weeks for such urgent information.

The major medical journals are available in most hospital libraries and in some community libraries; a few are provided free of charge to members of certain professional groups, including PAs. Because of their quality control, timeliness, and availability, peer-reviewed journals may be considered one of the PA's most important and practical information resources. For these reasons, the remainder of this chapter emphasizes scientific information presented in journals.

THE PEER REVIEW PROCESS

In the modern peer review process that is used by the best medical journals, a submitted article is systematically evaluated by a panel of experts for scientific worth and accuracy prior to publication. The peer review process is generally synonymous with the term "refereeing." Although the particulars of the procedure may vary somewhat, a manuscript submitted by an author to a journal is referred to approximately three content experts identified by the journal's editorial staff; if the article involves the statistical analysis of data, a methodological expert may be one of the reviewers.[7]

Peer reviewers may serve on the journal's editorial board, may be selected from a pool of experts maintained by the journal, or may be guest reviewers. They advise acceptance, revision, or rejection of articles, and their advice is relayed to the journal's editor or a designee. For purposes of correspondence and negotiation, the journal editorial staff acts as a "middle-person" between the article's author(s) and the peer reviewers. An article's final disposition is generally left to the journal's editorial staff.

Although some flaws go undetected by this process, peer-reviewed journals are considered more reliable information sources than are textbooks and periodicals that print unrefereed manuscripts. For more information about how the review process affects the quality of journal articles, refer to Relman[6] and to a special issue of *JAMA*[8] that is dedicated entirely to the topic of medical journal peer review.

TYPES OF MEDICAL ARTICLES

Medical journals present a variety of article types whose quality, style, and structure vary considerably. To evaluate journal articles and appropriately decide which articles to read, a PA must differentiate among the various types: *full-length* versus *short,* and *clinical review* versus *research.* Research articles are further classified according to two major types: *basic* and *applied.*

Short articles can be divided into several categories: media reviews, case reports, poetry, humor, letters to the editor and other types of commentaries, and editorials. A lengthy editorial with the scholarly use of references may be considered a full-length article. *Full-length articles* can be subdivided into research and clinical review.

Research Articles

Research is the organization or discovery of information or facts that help revise theories, help interpret known phenomena, or result in the practical application of information or facts. A research article presents this information in a fairly consistent format that includes four sections:

1. Introduction, which contains an orientation to the problem, a brief literature review, and the study objective or purpose statement.
2. Methods, which describe the patients or subject sample studied, instrumentation, procedures, and any statistical tests used.
3. Results.
4. Discussion.

These four sections are almost always labeled with the corresponding headings. A research article typically addresses a specific topic (i.e., the study objective) in a very detailed way by presenting data.

Research articles can be further categorized as applied or basic research. *Applied research* (sometimes referred to as clinical research) has direct application or relevance to patients, known diseases, or familiar problems. *Basic research* addresses theoretical models, experimental methods, or hypothetical problems. The practical application of the information learned through basic research might not be currently known; the information is used to further knowledge and not necessarily to help us manage today's patients directly. The information presented in numerous basic research articles, however, is later applied to actual clinical problems and real patients. Basic research is often conducted at the cellular or biochemical level and through animal studies. These studies are sometimes misunderstood by uninformed lay commentators who fail to connect basic research with meritorious scientific developments. Although many basic research studies may seem remote from immediate, practical applications, innumerable medical breakthroughs are attributed to basic research.

What about "library research"? The colloquial definition of *research* differs from the definition used in referring to the medical literature. In medicine, it is more accurate to call library research a literature review. *Literature reviews* present and comment on information found in both research and clinical review articles.

Clinical Review Articles

Clinical review articles differ from research articles in their purpose, appearance, structure, and content. Clinical review articles are typically literature reviews and analyses that critically examine a clinical topic, problem, or disease. They do not present *new* data, but rather are collections and reviews of information that have already been reported. Depending on what is to be emphasized, clinical review articles assume a variety of styles; they also do not adhere to a consistent format and do not include a methods or results section.

As secondary sources of information, textbooks resemble clinical review articles; they are not original reports on new findings but rather collections of previously reported information put into an easily usable form that is suitable as an overview and for teaching. Clinical review articles typically address broader subject areas than research articles. An example of a clinical review article title is "The Risks and Benefits of Exercise During Pregnancy," and an example of a research article title is "The Effects of Maternal Exercise on Fetal Responses to Sound During the Second Trimester."

Differentiating Research and Clinical Review Articles

Understanding the differences between research articles and clinical review articles enables clinicians to communicate more effectively when writing or talking with others about published medical information. To test whether the reader has comprehended the distinctions made in the preceding section, he or she is encouraged to complete the nine-item "quiz" in the text box that follows. Each numbered item lists a characteristic primarily of a clinical review article (C) or a research article (R). The reader should write either C or R on the line after the phrase and then compare choices made with the answers in the footnote.

In regard to items 8 and 9, some may believe that clinical review articles, rather than research articles, are easier for clinicians to read and for authors to write. This is probably the case because PA education involves extensive use of clinical review information but limited experience in interpreting original research. Once the research format is learned, however, reading a research article may actually be easy because the format is straightforward, consistent, and predictable. As a rule, research

---

CLINICAL REVIEW VS. RESEARCH ARTICLE*

1. Very narrow in scope._____
2. Good for an overall review about a topic. _____
3. Good for learning the very latest information about your clinical specialty._____
4. The structure of the article varies considerably. _____
5. Analyzes experimental studies already published._____
6. Contains original numerical or descriptive information._____
7. The structure is fairly consistent and predictable._____
8. Easier to read._____
9. Easier for the author to write._____

*Answers: 1. R; 2. C; 3. R; 4. C; 5. C; 6. R; 7. R; 8. R; 9. R.

---

articles are also shorter. For these reasons, research articles may actually be less difficult to read than would be expected.

THE ANATOMY OF MEDICAL ARTICLES

Clinical review articles are generally easy to understand and apply because PAs are conversant with this type of content through their formal education and clinical practice. Clinical review articles usually follow a format that is analogous to the patient presentation, and they use familiar information and terminology. A research article, on the other hand, presents some new terms, statistical tests, and a less familiar (yet simpler) format. Enhancing one's practice by becoming an informed consumer of current research information is easier than most clinicians realize. Once readers understand the anatomy of such articles, they can readily glean information from them. Most clinicians who have not been oriented to research do not feel proficient in reading and interpreting research articles. One approach recommends that readers become familiar with the anatomical landmarks of each type of article.

Anatomy of a Research Article

The anatomy of a research article is presented first because it is consistent and simple. The more variable format of clinical review articles is discussed later.

Whether an article reports basic or applied research, the overall scheme is: broad–narrow–broad. That is, an article starts with general information (usually including a brief literature review) that orients the reader to the topic. Information then becomes focused on the specific, narrow question that is addressed in the study; this is the study objective or purpose statement. The specifics of the methodology and results are likewise narrow and are focused on the particular study. Then, the information that has been learned is broadened and generalized. The author explains how study information can be used or applied by others.

Virtually all research articles appearing in medical journals have the same anatomical features. The overall scheme resembles two funnels placed end-to-end (Figure 18-2). The specific anatomical features are discussed below.

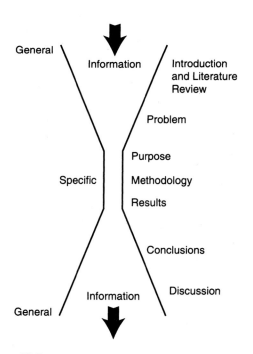

Figure 18-2 The "dual funnel" model.

Introduction   The introduction is an orientation to the study's purpose. It begins with a description of the circumstances that led to the specific project or investigation. The orientation consists of the following:

1. Background (which often entails a literature review).
2. Statement of the problem that stimulated the project's beginning.
3. Specific objective, purpose, question, or hypothesis to be addressed.

   When an article contains new or unfamiliar terms, these are defined in the introduction. The purpose statement is the article's nucleus, and it usually appears at the end of the introduction.

Literature Review   As a summary of the pertinent published information relative to the article's topic, the literature review should help orient the reader and should demonstrate that the author is familiar with known information pertaining to the topic—the "wheel is not being recreated." It often provides the rationale or basis for the present study. For example, if the purpose is to help resolve a medical controversy about treatment, the literature review describes the previously published contending reports. Spoken quotations from authoritative sources may be incorporated, even if the information has not yet been published. A short literature review may be (and usually is) incorporated into the introduction and furnishes a meaningful examination of the topic area. The literature sources found in dissertations and theses are extensive. In journal articles, however, the literature review is brief and focused.

Methods   The methods section describes what was actually done when the study was carried out. This section should be sufficiently clear and detailed so that the study may be duplicated by others. The methods section describes these points:

1. Subjects.
2. Instrumentation used (including questionnaires).
3. Procedures carried out.
4. Statistical analysis for evaluating and summarizing the data.

Results   The factual observations and numerical data obtained in the study are presented in the results section. Generally it is short; presents the data as tables, figures, photographs, and so forth; and is free of commentary. Commentary is reserved for the discussion section that follows. Results appearing in tables are supported by text that guides the reader through the most important points.

Discussion   Because the discussion section explains the meaning of the results, it complements the introduction and the literature review. Conclusions may appear anywhere in the discussion section or may be presented separately. The conclusions represent what was learned in this study and should not generalize or extrapolate beyond the data. The remainder of the discussion section *is* the place where the author expands on the study's findings, comments, and speculates. The discussion usually includes recommendations for future investigators and addresses the limitations of the study. The implications for clinical practice and the author's recommendations to health care providers are added in the discussion. In short, the discussion makes the results meaningful and usable to readers who are not as familiar with the topic area as the author.

References   The references cited in this article are listed at the end. Recommended readings may also be listed separately.

Abstract   Nearly all U.S. medical journals begin with an abstract, which is designed to give the reader a brief overview of the article's content. The abstract is a synopsis of the main purpose, the methods, and the most important results and conclusions. An abstract may also present a very brief background of the study and definitions of unfamiliar terms; when included, these usually appear before the purpose statement.

Publishers impose strict word limitations on abstracts. Because they are very brief, they do *not* present all essential content. An abstract is useful for superficially scanning an article but does not replace an actual reading. The abstract alone provides insufficient information for correctly understanding the content. For example, an abstract might not contain a study's secondary purpose(s), detailed methods, all

significant results, nor all of the conclusions. Most importantly, a reader might not agree with the abstract's cursory content after reading the full-length article. Except for purposes of "triage"—choosing which articles to read in their entirety—abstracts have very limited usefulness. (See the following section, "Reading the Selected Journals.")

The various sections of a research article are almost always arranged in the sequence described. Just as an efficient, symptom-directed physical examination is aided by knowledge of a patient's anatomy, the efficient reading of an article is based on familiarity with typical anatomical landmarks.

Qualitative Research Articles

A research subspecialty, qualitative research, has the following characteristics:

➤ Data are collected in the natural setting rather than in the laboratory.
➤ It is descriptive rather than numerical, using words, photographs, videotaped recordings, and so forth, as findings and results.
➤ It is concerned with processes rather than experimental outcomes.
➤ It generates hypotheses rather than tests them.[8]

Qualitative research is used daily in clinical practice and is very familiar to PAs, although it is not always recognized by name. The medical history is an example. Open-ended questions are used to obtain descriptive, verbal data directly from patients. During the medical interview, reactions and communication cues help guide the investigative process. Physical examination and laboratory and imaging data are then used to test hypotheses generated by the interview (i.e., differential diagnosis).

As expected, the anatomy of qualitative research articles varies somewhat from the more commonly encountered quantitative research articles described earlier. In qualitative research articles, the purpose statement is broader and the methods do not include the statistical treatment of data. The other components, however, are basically similar.

Anatomy of a Clinical Review Article

Unlike research articles, clinical review articles vary considerably in their objective and scope.

Their structure therefore varies as well. Clinical review articles have most or all of the following components:

1. Introduction.
2. Patient presentation/history.
3. Physical examination.
4. Laboratory and imaging findings.
5. Diagnosis.
6. Treatment/management.
7. Prevention and patient education.
8. Follow-up.
9. Discussion.
10. Conclusions.
11. Abstract.[9]

A discussion typically brings together and analyzes the earlier components. As with the research format, the discussion may be extensive and helps readers understand and apply the article's content by commenting upon, clarifying, and analyzing the information previously presented.

Being able to recognize the components of a clinical review article enables the reader to quickly find the sections of greatest interest. The components, however, are less predictable than are those of a research article. Both clinical review articles and research articles are invaluable for helping the PA to stay current in practice.

HOW TO STAY CURRENT

Medical literature is typically used for browsing, searching, and keeping up,[6] and it represents one of the legs of the three-legged stool of evidence-based medical practice. Evidence-based medicine is a system of medical decision making that incorporates the clinical capabilities of the health care provider, pathophysiological knowledge, and patient preferences, with research information published in the literature. Steps involve the following:

1. Precisely defining the patient problem.
2. Searching and critically evaluating the relevant literature.
3. Deciding how to use the information for disease management (this is generally done by a team of providers).[10]

Refer to Chapter 19 for a detailed explanation of evidence-based medicine.

Browsing

Although browsing through the literature may be enjoyable and useful for stimulating new ideas, it is inefficient. Busy clinicians are rarely able to browse through a medical library's holdings and successfully locate the fund of information needed for modern practice.

Searching

Searching uses various databases to locate articles on specific topics. This method of locating literature is especially useful for the PA who urgently needs current and precise clinical information. For example, the PA with a patient in whom a diagnosis of lupus cerebritis is suspected may need information that he or she had learned while a student but has since forgotten. Because recent advances have been made in diagnosing and treating this autoimmune disorder, textbook information would be unsatisfactory. A search for information about this or other health-related topics could effectively use the various computerized literature databases, such as MEDLINE, a computerized form of *Index Medicus*. Certain utility packages such as GratefulMed and PubMed provide user-friendly access to the parent database, MEDLINE. Computerized databases produce reference lists, abstracts, and in some cases full articles, in response to selected words that appear in an article's title, abstract, and key word list.

In addition to MEDLINE, other computerized databases to health care–related information have been compiled: CINAHL (or the Cumulative Index to Nursing and Allied Health Literature), PsycFIRST and PsycINFO (for psychological topics), ERIC (for educational topics), and SportDiscus (for topics related to medical aspects of sport and exercise). More than 1000 other computerized indexes are available. MEDLINE is the most widely used database for medical topics; because it is a tax-subsidized service of the National Library of Medicine, searches cost less than half as much as those provided by most other computerized databases. Most hospital libraries provide their staff members with access to MEDLINE and other health care–related databases.

Database programs used for locating medical information are user-friendly and easy to learn in a few minutes. Because they can be accessed directly by the user, literature databases are helpful for those who need to quickly locate a large number of article citations about most any topic. It may be helpful for the clinician to consult a terminology index, such as *Medical Subject Headings Supplement to Index Medicus* or an on-line thesaurus, to identity appropriate key words.

Computerized literature searches are highly recommended because of their thoroughness, efficiency, and timeliness. Many journal citations may be located electronically within a few days to 1 month of publication. In addition to topic searches, author searches can be used to locate articles. Searches may be limited to the English language, to particular blocks of time by year, or to human subjects (excluding lower animal studies).

Because they are easy and often enjoyable to do, many clinicians perform their own searches. However, many hospital libraries provide this service conducted by librarians. It often involves completing a form that a librarian uses to conduct the search. However, many clinicians have been frustrated by searches that seemingly yield a low proportion of useful articles or, on the other hand, an unwieldy large number. When a librarian conducts a search on the basis of sketchy information provided on such a form, sometimes an inappropriate topic is searched because greater detail was needed. For example, searching the topic of "stress" could lead to the discovery of article listings on stress fractures, stress testing, stress incontinence, and psychological stress. With limited details and no feedback from the clinician, it is difficult for the librarian to clarify which key word(s) will locate the type of citations the clinician had in mind. Librarians take special courses and continuing education to learn and keep up with the vast and rapidly evolving database systems. There is no substitute for consulting and personally interacting with librarians to make one's ideas and needs clear. It takes only about 10 to 30 minutes, which in most cases is a good time investment. When a serious or comprehensive literature search is indicated, a librarian's specialized skills are invaluable.

Keeping Up

Most PAs use journals for learning up-to-date medical information so they can remain competent throughout their professional lifetime. MEDLINE lists more than 3000[5] medical periodicals of varying quality and usefulness. To keep up in practice, it is not only impossible but unnecessary for PAs to read most medical journals. Nearly all medical developments that are essential for practice are reported by a few of the best journals. This does not mean that other journals do not publish information of importance to PAs, but relevant follow-up studies and commentaries about vital medical developments tend to appear in a few top-rated journals. By reading as few as three or as many as five well-selected journals, the average clinician will have encountered within approximately 1 year nearly all the new information that is important for practice.[6]

The PA should select one or two general medical journals, one or two journals on his or her specialty, and at least one PA journal. General medical journals report on the "news" of medicine; examples are *JAMA, New England Journal of Medicine, British Medical Journal,* and *The Lancet.* Radio and television news media often have privileged access to news-oriented journals 1 or 2 days in advance of publication. Clinicians should therefore be prepared for patients who have learned about new medical developments before they appear in print.

There is a broad range of quality among specialty journals. They should be selected according to the types of problems seen most frequently in one's practice (e.g., *American Journal of Cardiology* for PAs practicing in cardiology) or to coincide with one's practice philosophy (e.g., *American Journal of Health Promotion*).

The most-read PA journals are *Clinician Reviews, Physician Assistant,* and *Journal of the American Academy of Physician Assistants.* In addition, state societies publish periodicals that provide news and information of importance to PAs practicing within each state or district. All PAs should follow the medical, legal, and professional issues directly affecting their unique professional role by regularly reading selected PA periodicals.

READING THE SELECTED JOURNALS

Once three to five journals have been selected, each issue should be read in a way that helps ensure comprehension of important information in the least amount of time. All abstracts should be scanned for identification of articles that are interesting or potentially useful and relevant to one's practice; if an article does not qualify, it may be skipped. With this approach, some issues are read completely, and others not at all.

This plan for keeping up works effectively when the PA analyzes and evaluates the content of articles. This is possible when *full articles* are read, not just the abstracts. The usefulness of abstracts is limited to "triage" on a journal's articles, as was explained earlier.

Alternative methods for keeping up have also been successful. To help identify articles relevant to their practice, some PAs use the various medical article summaries or indexes that are published periodically, such as *Current Contents,* which is distributed monthly by the Institute for Scientific Information, 3501 Market Street, Philadelphia, PA 19104. Whatever method is selected, it should meet the following criteria:

1. Suit the PA's own learning style.
2. Involve the reading of entire articles.
3. Be used regularly.

Only by using a systematic approach can busy clinicians keep up with new developments and effectively deal with the magnitude of available new medical information.

STARTING A REPRINT FILE

The purpose of starting a reprint file is to organize selected, unbound literature so that it can be readily accessed when needed for reviewing, referencing, and sharing with patients and colleagues. Reprints can be made from journals, books, or pamphlets. Although this is a personal undertaking aimed at meeting an individual's professional needs, a plan using the principles discussed in the following paragraphs may save time.

Although computerized systems are becoming increasingly useful, use of hard copy files often facilitates access to, and distribution of, materials for patients and colleagues. After initially reading an article that will be included in one's reprint file, the PA should obtain a copy and write at the top of the first page the major points that made him or her want to keep the article. Making notes in the margins and marking important paragraphs are also ways to save time later and to make reprints personally useful.

When indexing articles, one should decide on the categories that meet particular practice needs. These may be found as headings in the annual index issue of most general medical journals. If a category contains too many articles (approximately 15 to 30), it should be subdivided. For example, cardiology may be divided into diagnosis, treatment, and prevention. Diagnosis may be further subdivided into invasive and noninvasive procedures. If an article fits more than one category, a page that cross-references the article should be added to the other category, or a second copy of the article should be filed there. A specialized need, such as the collection of one particular author's work, can also constitute a category. A file drawer should be reserved exclusively for storing the reprint file.

The benefits of a well-organized reprint file include having convenient access to information, a personally meaningful collection of information that can be used for formal and informal presentations at a moment's notice, and information that can be exchanged with others. In this regard, the PA should mark each reprint with his or her name as well as the information needed to cite it as a reference (full title of the article, the journal or book, and the chapter author(s), publisher, date, and inclusive page numbers). Copyright laws should be respected when published material is photocopied, but most legislation permits the making of single copies for personal use.

Computerized programs for storing and retrieving articles are becoming increasingly practical and useful for rapidly accessing information and producing electronic and hard copies.

SCREENING TESTS FOR EVALUATING THE MEDICAL LITERATURE

Screening tests can help PAs in assessing the medical information they use. Some of the characteristics should send up a "red flag" in the reader's mind when they are encountered. These screening tests are based on the information presented in this chapter, and they are intended to help the reader pull together the most important ideas. (See also the later section, "Statistically Related Screening Tests for Medical Articles.")

Limitations Versus Flaws   Every study has limitations. The perfect study has not yet been published. Even in the best of studies, sampling always carries the risk of not representing the total population. Strictly controlled laboratory studies have the limitation of not reflecting the actual clinical situation. Most if not all studies have methodological limitations that affect the results.

A limitation must not be confused with a flaw. A flaw invalidates a study's conclusions, but a limitation merely defines the applicability of the conclusions. An example of a flawed study is one in which an instrument was not calibrated before experimental measurements were taken (such as a sphygmomanometer that unknowingly varied in one direction by 12 mmHg). In this case, the results are simply not accurate. An example of a limitation, on the other hand, can be seen in a drug study on men between the ages of 35 and 50 years. It cannot be known from the study whether the drug has the same effect on younger or older men or on women. The study's conclusions are limited to men within the age range that was investigated. It would be inappropriate to discredit the entire study because of this limitation.

Just as every study has limitations, almost every study contains useful information. The reader must evaluate the particulars in each article and decide what information is suitable for his or her own practice. In the article itself, the authors *should* point out the study's limitations; to do so is considered honest and professionally responsible. The reader should beware of studies that do not admit to any limitation. He or she should not totally dismiss a study because it has limitations, but should look for the limitations and consider them when applying the article's information to actual practice situations.

"Proof"   A single study does not "prove" anything. When an important finding is reported, the results should be able to be duplicated elsewhere by other investigators. All medical studies have limitations, and clinicians should almost never change their practice based on the findings of a single study. A single article that warrants a change in practice is rare, and PAs should wait until the results are verified through follow-up studies.

The concept of *proof* is reserved almost entirely for pure theoretical sciences, such as certain subdisciplines of mathematics. Proof does not apply to most, if any, medical studies. Rather, studies provide *evidence* that supports or refutes what is currently thought to be true; it is likely that today's "truth" will be replaced by tomorrow's new findings.

The statistical technique of *meta-analysis* has been developed to combine study results.[11] It is used to estimate treatment effects reported in similar studies conducted by different investigators. Individual scientific studies are like pebbles that accumulate until they form a "mountain" of medical knowledge. In reference to medical studies, there are more single pebbles than mountains. If each of the more than 350,000 articles published each year "proved" something, there would be no unanswered question.

Secondary References   Secondary information may be unreliable. Of 150 citations from three of the most prestigious surgical journals, 38% were found to contain major quotation errors.[12] Whenever possible, authors should use original information sources, and readers should beware of articles that cite mostly secondary information.

Outdated References   Because scientific information is constantly evolving, an article's references should be as recent as possible. Occasionally, a classic study or historical reference point may be legitimately cited. In addition, some old citations may appropriately reflect a past period of research or scientific dialog on a topic that has not received recent attention. Articles that cite clearly outdated references are suspicious.

Missing Data   All studies must account for any "lost" subjects or missing data. Readers should look for the number of subjects that were initially sampled and the reasons why any of their data were not included in the final results.

Reputation An article's worth should be evaluated on its own merit. There is a tendency for professionals to try to shortcut proper evaluation by assuming that an article contains reliable information because of the good reputation of the author or an institution. Although this principle occasionally works, it is frequently erroneous. In some institutions, "publish or perish" pressure may cause quality to give way to quantity. (See the earlier section in this chapter, "How Dependable Are Medical Information Sources?")

On the other hand, a publication may be suspect if it is from an institution that has a product to sell or that advocates a particular dogma in view of overwhelming evidence to the contrary. Although the best journals attempt to control quality through the refereeing process, there is no substitute for each reader being an informed and critical consumer of medical information. Evaluating each work on its own merit is an essential skill as important as interpreting laboratory tests or physical examination findings. Although the reputation of the source may be a general guide to an article's quality, each article must be individually evaluated.

Words That May Indicate Quality Certain words may provide clues that reflect the quality of the medical information provided. Responsible reports contain words that accurately represent findings, but pretentious reports that attempt to overstate or sensationalize medical information tend to use extreme words (Table 18-1). Words such as "may," "probably,"

Table 18-1 Words That May Indicate the Quality of Medical Literature

Likely to Indicate Credibility	Suspicious
Shows	Always
Supports	Never
Suggests	Proves
Provides evidence	Disproves
Helps validate	Indisputable
Adds credence	Definitely
Probably	Unquestionably
May	
Might	

and "sometimes" do not make sensational news headlines, but such descriptions accurately portray medical information that is, out of necessity, based on probability statements, variability among patients, and incomplete knowledge. Often, media reporters cover developments ranging from astronomy to breast implants, and they cannot possibly provide information that is sufficiently reliable for clinical practice. PAs must read complete reports and evaluate their possible relevance to clinical practice.

Volunteers Most studies depend on volunteer subjects because of ethical considerations. Humans and their tissues and body fluids cannot be involved in studies without informed consent. A study should account for possible differences between those who volunteer and those who do not. For example, subjects who volunteer for a study on exercise may have lifestyles, attitudes, health habits, and a body composition very different from those who refuse to participate because exercise was part of the study protocol. Such differences must be considered in the interpretation of findings.

Generalizability Readers should be alert for studies that attempt to apply findings to inappropriate groups that substantially differ from the subjects in the study sample. Differences in age, co-morbidities, health status, sex, socioeconomic and cultural backgrounds, and other possible intervening variables may limit the application of study results to other populations.

Intervening Variables When an article indicates that the Japanese are healthier than Americans because they eat more fish, consider that they also eat more rice and soybean products, exercise more, use different water supplies, and have different lifestyle habits. Studies should control for the various other factors that could be responsible for an observed effect.

The Hawthorne Effect An experimental variable called the Hawthorne effect was originally described in a study that attempted to investigate how varying light levels affected workers' productivity. The results showed that subjects consistently improved their performance independent of the lighting conditions. Improvement was attributed to subjects' perception that they were "special" because they were asked to participate in an experimental study.

Subjects in a study tend to behave in ways they think are expected of them by the research staff. One way to help control for behavioral differences is to use a placebo in a double-blind fashion, so that neither the subjects nor the experimenters know who is receiving actual treatment and who is receiving a treatment analog. In this way, both experimental and control subjects are treated alike, and the Hawthorne effect is less likely to be introduced as a source of experimental error.

Is the Subject Sample Appropriate for the Study Question?
The subjects of a study should be capable of showing the desired effect. For example, a treatment intended to improve myocardial contractility in post–myocardial infarction patients should be tested on a sample of these patients rather than on individuals free of cardiovascular illnesses. Testing a group of healthy subjects may not show a comparable treatment effect.

Survey Studies

Surveys are useful for describing a group's characteristics for documentation of baseline information, norms, and reference points for future research. On the surface, survey research may appear simple. However, like any other type of research, it must be carefully planned and conducted with the use of appropriate information procurement techniques to help assure validity and reliability of the results.[13,14] Because of the relevance of survey research to the PA profession, screening tests for its evaluation are described here.

Was a Survey Indicated?
Because of the numerous limitations of survey research, it should be clear to the reader why the survey method of investigation was selected over more reliable methods. For example, a description of a population's health status in relation to blood pressure is obtained more reliably by a review of clinic records than it is by a search for the same information through patient surveys.

Was a Standard Instrument Used?
Previously published instruments with established reliability and validity are preferred to unique instruments that do not allow comparisons with other studies. New instruments should be used only when previously developed instruments are not available or are unsuitable for the question(s) being investigated.

General Versus Specific Information
The design of a study should be suited to the study question(s). If the desired information is general in nature, queries should be open ended.[14] Pointed or quantified questions are appropriate only after relevant issues have been identified by qualitative research methods.

Low Return Rates
Because some subjects do not respond to surveys, sampling bias is a serious consideration in any type of survey research. Short of a response rate of 95% or greater (to be compatible with an error rate of $P \leq 0.05$), there is no specific "good" level. One must always consider what the study results would have shown if nonrespondents' results had been included. When possible, nonresponding subjects should be checked for possible biases and the reasons for their nonresponse, and this information should be reported. If a biased sample was selected, even a 100% return rate would not represent the population from which the sample was obtained. If attrition among subjects was random rather than systematic, there is some assurance that the data from respondents represent the population that is being studied. Sampling methods and survey designs that are well thought out help increase return rates.[13-15] Readers should be alert for all sources of biases, especially if potentially embarrassing or otherwise emotionally sensitive information was sought. Subject confidentiality or anonymity should have been ensured in all cases, and articles should describe the methods used.

Investigator or Subject Bias
To help increase the generalizability of study results, sampling should normally be independent of economic, political,

religious, educational, and other biases. Readers must be alert for these and other problems that may limit the study.

Narrow Interpretation of Data   In good survey studies, relationships among questions are explored and comparisons are made between groups within the study (internal validity) and those with previously published reports (external validity). Survey data that are analyzed one variable at a time, isolated from the effects of other variables, seldom further a reader's knowledge or understanding.

STATISTICAL TERMS AND TESTS

Statistics is simply a way to present and compare large amounts of information as meaningful and usable summaries. No reader would want to actually see a study's hundreds or thousands of data entries. The raw data do not create a useful or meaningful picture of the results. An average with its standard deviation, however, is a valuable representation that is readily understood at a glance.

For some clinicians, the term *statistics* conjures up notions of complex mathematical formulas, peculiar applications of logic, and sometimes fear and nausea. Probably some of this reaction is the result of previous attempts to clarify general concepts through the overuse of specific formulas involving unfamiliar symbols and terms. Even after completing a bona fide statistics course, many clinicians have complained that they are unable to apply their knowledge to medical problems. As with electrocardiogram interpretation, statistics is quickly forgotten if it is not purposefully applied and practiced.

When clinicians without special statistical training attempt to read medical literature or attend or give journal club presentations, they often feel limited by their incomplete understanding of the clinical implications of statistical terms and tests. Most clinicians understandably do not have in-depth knowledge about statistics, yet they rely heavily on medical information that is based on statistical concepts. It is therefore necessary for the PA to recognize and understand the *fundamental* terms and tests that appear repeatedly in medical articles.

Knowledge of statistical concepts adds a new level of understanding and enjoyment to the reading of medical literature and helps reduce the frustration that results when unfamiliar or confusing information is encountered. Some authors believe that it is virtually impossible for the PA to read medical literature without having some understanding of research methodology.[8] The Accreditation Review Commission on the Education of the Physician Assistant, Inc. (ARC-PA) has included interpretation of medical literature as a curricular standard for all PA educational programs.

The goal of this section is to introduce the reader to minimal statistical knowledge and the most commonly encountered terms and tests used in medical literature. This goal is accomplished primarily by the use of principles rather than numerical formulas, in an attempt to maximize understanding while minimizing apprehension.

Although some clinicians may find a more detailed mathematical approach more suited to their particular learning style and knowledge level, the approach used here is primarily conceptual, not mathematical. It attempts to keep technical terminology and formulas to a minimum. Readers may find it useful to consult a statistician, an informed colleague, or a recommended statistical reference[8,11,13,15,16] for specific mathematical information.

A "RULE OF THUMB" APPROACH TO MEDICAL STATISTICS

Familiarity with only a few basic terms and tests helps in establishing a foundation on which can be built an understanding of the statistics used most commonly in the medical literature. The model in Table 18-2 classifies the world of statistics into two types of data and two types of tests.

Types of Data

In the simplest sense, there are two types of data—categorical and numerical. (Although it is not essential at this point, the reader may recall that categorical data come in two forms, nominal and ordinal, and numerical data also come in two forms, interval and ratio.) An example of categorical data is "smoker, nonsmoker." Note that these are exclusive categories—someone belongs to either one group or the

Table 18-2   Simple Classification of Common Statistical Data and Tests

Type of Test	Type of Data	
	Categorical	**Numerical**
Relationship	Rho*	Pearson's *r**
	Odds ratio	Regression analysis
	Relative risk	
	Kendall's tau	
Difference	Chi-square*	*t*-test*
	Fisher's exact test	ANOVA
	Median test	ANCOVA
	Sign test	MANOVA
	Mann-Whitney U	
	Kruskal-Wallis ANOVA	

*Prototype test.

other. It makes no sense to associate these categories with numerical values.

An example of numerical data used to *quantify* smoking history is pack years. When data are numerical, they can be analyzed for frequency of occurrence along a continuum and according to whether or not the frequencies describe a normal bell-shaped curve. Numerical data can therefore be used in establishing reference values, quantitative levels at which pathology occurs, and so on. Blood glucose level is a familiar reference value. If the average blood glucose level is 94 mg/dL with a normal range of 72 to 116 mg/dL,

the range includes 95% of the population. Expressed as a 95% confidence interval, 95% of patients have blood glucose values between 72 and 116, and 5% have values that are above or below these.

Unlike categorical data, numerical data do not fall into mutually exclusive groups. In a sense, categorical data are "looser" or less precise than numerical data; they require the use of specific tests for their analysis (nonparametric tests); numerical data typically require the use of parametric tests (see Table 18-2).

Types of Tests

For analysis of the two types of data, there are basically two types of tests—those that evaluate relationships and those that detect differences. *Tests of relationship* show how variables might be related or associated with one another, such as diuretic dosage with blood pressure, and serum cholesterol level with coronary artery occlusion. Tests of relationship are usually exploratory tests that help determine whether there is a "co-relationship" or correlation. Regression, or applying the "line of best fit," also refers to tests of relationship. Correlation is probably the most commonly used statistical test found in the medical literature, and all readers should be very familiar with the concept. Correlation may be further demonstrated diagrammatically (Figure 18-3).

Tests of difference help determine the degree of contrast between sets of numbers. Figures 18-4, *A,* and 18-4, *B,* are examples of how this distinction appears when two numerical averages are compared. If an antihypertensive drug is being compared with a

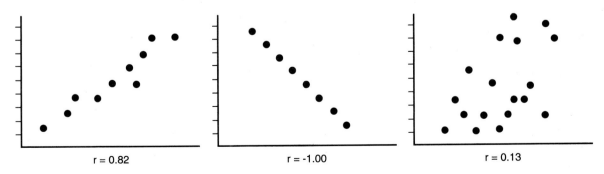

r = 0.82   r = -1.00   r = 0.13

Figure 18-3 Correlation. A correlation (or *r* value) close to 1.0 or −1.0 indicates a high degree of association between the variables tested; *r* values close to 0 suggest little or no association.

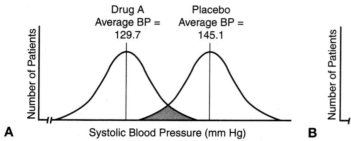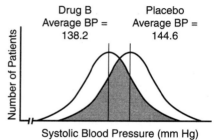

Figure 18-4 In **A**, there is a significant difference between the average blood pressure of patients receiving the drug and the average of patients receiving placebo. In **B**, there is a small difference between the averages, and it is neither statistically nor clinically significant. In both **A** and **B**, the *shaded areas* represent the blood pressure values that do not differentiate patients receiving the drug from those receiving placebo.

placebo, the clinician wants to know whether the average blood pressure of patients receiving the drug is really different (or statistically different, i.e., beyond random chance alone) from the average blood pressure of patients receiving the placebo.

Differentiating between categorical and numerical data is essential because these two types of data are analyzed with the use of different kinds of tests. Categorical data are analyzed by means of a group of tests known as "nonparametric" tests, and numerical data are analyzed with appropriate "parametric" tests. Further definitions of parametric and nonparametric are not necessary at this point.

A "RULE OF THUMB" GUIDE TO STATISTICAL TESTS

In-depth understanding of all statistical tests is neither necessary nor possible for most busy clinicians. The following prototype tests are recommended as a basis for understanding medical statistics.

Prototype Tests of Relationship

Pearson's *r* (also known as the product-moment correlation coefficient, or simply "correlation") is the recommended prototype for learning about tests of relationship using numerical data. The rho (or Spearman-Brown correlation) is the prototype for tests of relationship using categorical data (see Table 18-2).

Prototype Tests of Difference

The *t*-test (or Student's *t*-test) is the recommended prototype for tests of difference according to

numerical data. The *t*-test compares two averages. There are several versions of the *t*-test, including one for independent (unmatched) data and one for dependent (matched) pairs of data. For example, dependent data result from having a premeasure and a postmeasure on each subject in a sample; each subject's postmeasure depends to some degree on his or her premeasure. An example of unmatched data is comparison of the average weight of a group of men with the average weight of a group of women. Matching is not possible because the groups are independent—the results of one group do not affect or depend on the results of the other.

Whether the groups are dependent or independent, once the concept of the *t*-test is understood, the reader has a solid base of statistical knowledge on which to build and apply sophisticated adaptations of the *t*-test, such as analysis of variance and analysis of covariance. The chi-square (specifically, the chi-square test of independence) is the prototype for tests of difference using categorical data (see Table 18-2).

USING THE PROTOTYPE TESTS FOR UNDERSTANDING UNFAMILIAR ONES

Over time, the reader will encounter numerous statistical tests in the medical literature. With the advent of computers, even more tests with increased sophistication are being developed. Nearly all, however, can be conceptualized as one of the four prototype tests: Pearson's *r*, rho, *t*-test or chi-square. That is, when readers encounter new or unfamiliar tests and consult appropriate texts for guidance and details, they will find that most of the unfamiliar tests resemble one of the familiar prototypes.

The statistical tools used in epidemiologic studies further increase the number of terms encountered. Many epidemiological terms and tests, however, are identical or similar to those already presented. Appropriate texts should be consulted for more detailed applications to epidemiology.[11]

A GUIDE TO COMMON STATISTICAL TERMS

Some of the terms most commonly encountered in medical statistics are presented in the text box on the following pages. A complete description of statistical terminology is beyond the scope of this chapter; appropriate references should be consulted when necessary.[8,11,13,15,16] Understanding of these commonly encountered terms, along with the prototype tests described previously, should provide a solid foundation for reading articles that deal with medical statistics.

STATISTICAL APPLICATIONS

After working through the preceding "minicurriculum," the average clinician without an extensive statistics background may ask whether this statistical knowledge base is sufficient for getting through a professional lifetime of reading and properly interpreting medical literature. Most will find that these concepts will sufficiently familiarize them with the information needed to grasp the statistical data generally encountered in their professional reading. In addition, PAs will be prepared to communicate effectively with statisticians, colleagues, and others when they participate in journal clubs or professional meetings, or when they seek research project consultation.

Practicing the use of these statistical concepts is necessary for ease of understanding. Such practice arises from thoughtful reading of the medical literature, including the methods section of research articles. Too many well-meaning clinicians study statistics and are later discouraged when they seem unable to apply what they have learned. Learning to apply statistics is comparable to learning to read x-rays; most agree that new clinicians cannot "really" read x-rays until after they have studied approximately 1000 films. Only then do significant anatomical landmarks and shadows become apparent—what was initially "invisible" later seems obvious.

The good news is that PAs do not need to practice using the statistical concepts on 1000 journal articles before they can gain new insights; most find that they have increased their proficiency after working through only about 10 research articles involving statistics. Each time, the reader should ask: "Are the data being analyzed categorical *or* numerical?" and "Is the goal to identify a relationship *or* a difference among the variables?" What initially seemed incomprehensible becomes "second nature," just as performing a physical examination does, once it has been learned. Once learned, the rewards are many.

STATISTICS-RELATED SCREENING TESTS FOR MEDICAL ARTICLES

The following screening tests help readers in assessing statistics-related information found in the medical literature. These tests are based on the information presented in the medical statistics section of this chapter. They can be used for evaluating articles in conjunction with the general medical literature screening tests described earlier.

Claiming "Significance" Without Stating the Acceptable *P* Value (or Alpha Level)   A study should report the *P* value that will be considered statistically significant. An alpha level is sometimes confused with the *P* value; the *alpha level* is the level of significance that is selected *before* a study begins. In medical studies, the alpha level (or *P* value that will be accepted as significant) is almost always 0.05. Readers should be suspicious of studies that use values greater than 0.05. Incidentally, rounding off *P* >0.050 to 0.05 is not valid; for example, 0.051 is *not* considered significant.

No Statistical Test Indicated   A study that reports "statistical significance" without indicating the statistical test that was used warrants extreme suspicion. If no significance was detected by the test used, a *P* value does not necessarily need to be reported; "NS" or "not significant" is acceptable and sufficient in these cases. In all cases, however, the statistical test must be indicated.

One-Tailed Tests   One-tailed tests consider only one side of a data distribution. This has the effect of ignoring unfavorable results in some studies. Among almost any group of patients given a treatment, some improve and some do not. Most researchers agree that both favorable and unfavorable results should be considered when clinical results are evaluated; this is accomplished in two-tailed tests. When a one-tailed test is used, the acceptable significance or P value is halved. For example, a one-tailed P value of 0.045 appears significant because it is less than 0.05, but the two-tailed P value is actually 0.09, which is not significant.

One-tailed tests may be acceptable under some conditions, when it is certain that one side of a data distribution is not important or is nonexistent. These conditions are rare in medicine, however, and even in these instances, it is not wrong to use the more conservative two-tailed result. Readers should be suspicious when a study indicates that a one-tailed test was used.

COMMON STATISTICAL TERMS

General Terms

Bias	A tendency toward a particular, nonrandom pattern of observation; a prejudice
Confidence interval	The values between which a specified percentage of the population being described lies. A 95% CI 135 to 145 for sodium means that 95% of patients have values between 135 and 145 mEq/L, and 5% have values outside this range
Convenience sample	A sample that is used because of easy access; a convenience sample may be biased, and it may not accurately represent the population from which the sample was taken
Data	Plural of datum
Datum	A single observation or phenomenon
n	The number of subjects, observations, measurements, etc.
Normal distribution	A gaussian or symmetrical, bell-shaped curve
P	The probability of a chance occurrence; in medicine, the acceptable P value used for routine hypothesis testing is usually 0.05, that is, 5% or less of the observations occur randomly, and 95% occur not because of chance (such as individual patient variation) but because of treatment; also known as statistical significance
Population	The group that a study attempts to describe or represent; this is usually done by studying a sample from the population and inferring that the results of the sample reflect the population
Random sample	A sample in which all elements of a population have an equal chance of being selected
Reliability	The extent to which a test provides the same value repeatedly; precision; reproducibility
Sample	The part of a population selected to represent the entire population
Sensitivity	The degree to which a test is likely to detect a true-positive result; low sensitivity produces false-negative results, and very high sensitivity may produce false-positive results
Specificity	The degree to which a test accurately detects the variable in question; low specificity produces false-positive results

Insufficient Information Reported   In addition to indicating the statistical test used and what data were tested or compared, additional information is required for proper evaluation of statistical results. The following minimum information should also be reported: a *t*-test should include the *n* values, the averages, and their corresponding standard deviations (or standard errors), as well as the *P* value (see text box entitled "Common Statistical Terms"). F tests (e.g., analysis of variance, analysis of covariance, multivariate analysis of variance) should report the *n* values, the averages and their standard deviations, and whether or not significant differences were detected. If a significant difference was found, a follow-up or post hoc test (which detects the values that were significantly different) must be reported along with the corresponding *P* value(s). In all cases, whenever a mean is reported, a corresponding standard deviation (or

---

COMMON STATISTICAL TERMS—cont'd

Systematic error	An error repeated according to a nonrandom pattern
Tails	The extreme ends of a distribution curve
Validity	The extent to which a test measures what it says it measures; accuracy

Descriptive Statistics
These numerical summaries help the reader understand at a glance the nature of a data set.

Measures of Central Tendency

Mean	The sum divided by the *n*; the statistic referred to as the "average"
Median	The number that divides a group in half so that 50% are above the number and 50% are below
Mode	The number or value occurring most frequently

Measures of Variability

Range	The extreme values of a group between which all values lie
Standard deviation	A number representing the amount of variability on either side of a mean; ±2 standard deviations captures 95% of the values in a normal curve; the most common measure of variability
Standard error	Also called standard error of the mean; a measure of variability that accounts for errors in sampling by relating the mean obtained from the study sample to a hypothetical mean representing the population from which the sample was derived

Terms Used Especially in Epidemiology

Incidence	The number of new cases of a disease during a particular interval of time (usually per year)
Odds ratio	The odds of having a risk factor if a condition (e.g., disease) is present divided by the odds of having the risk factor if the condition is not present; for example, an odds ratio of 2 represents twice the risk
Prevalence	Estimated risk of having a particular disease at a particular time considering all cases, both old and new
Relative risk	The probability of developing an outcome (e.g., a disease) when a risk factor is present (e.g., smoke) divided by the probability of developing the outcome when the risk factor is not present; similar to the odds ratio in case-control studies

standard error) should accompany the mean value; many medical editors have made this a journal requirement.

Tests like the chi-square should report the categorical groups that were tested, the *n* values (or counts) for each group, and the *P* value. If any of the counts is lower than 5 in any cell of a 2-by-2 chi-square design (that is, where two rows and two columns are compared), a Fisher's exact test should be used rather than the chi-square.[11]

Tests of correlation should indicate the specific test used, the variables compared, the *n* value, and the correlation coefficient. Because tests of correlation are usually exploratory in nature and because most readers attribute erroneous value to statements of "significance," when in fact the correlation coefficient is close to zero, many authorities suggest *not* reporting *P* values. To report them, however, is not erroneous, and they may be useful for interpretation of correlation results when the *n* is low and the correlation coefficient is close to 1.0 or −1.0.

Using Numerical (Parametric) Tests on Categorical (Nonparametric) Data
Studies must use appropriate statistical tests according to the type of data being analyzed, as was described earlier. The parametric tests that are capable of detecting smaller effects than nonparametric tests are generally reserved for numerical data with a sufficiently high *n*, distributed in a normal symmetrical curve. Nonparametric tests should be used for categorical data; special tests are indicated for certain classes of small numbers whose distribution might be skewed or otherwise not normal.

Assuming Causality from Correlations
Correlation shows that factors are *associated,* which is very different from a cause-and-effect relationship. Even though there is a high correlation between subjects' body height and frequency of basketball dribbling, this does not mean that dribbling caused them to grow or that growing caused them to dribble. Height and dribbling are only associated, not causally related. Correlational studies are usually exploratory. If a relationship is found, more refined follow-up experimental studies can help in determining cause-and-effect relationships.

Seemingly High Correlation Coefficients
In general, *r* values greater than 0.85 reflect a close association between two variables and are considered predictive; 0.65 to 0.85 is moderate; 0.35 to 0.65 is low; and less than 0.35 reflects only a slight relationship.[15] However, to gain a perspective that is useful for evaluating clinical studies, *r* should be squared. This results in the Pearson's coefficient of reliability that reflects the variability that two measures have in common. For example, if diastolic blood pressure predicted systolic blood pressure where $r = 0.70$, $r^2 = 0.49$ or 49%. This means that only 49% of the variation in systolic blood pressure was accounted for by the variation in diastolic blood pressure, and more than half (51%) of the variation could *not* be accounted for. Furthermore, even when a correlation is perfect (i.e., 1.0 or −1.0), this does not reflect causality (see preceding discussion). Studies using correlation must be interpreted with this limitation in mind.

Very Small *n*
Small subject numbers are suspicious for several reasons. With a small *n,* sampling errors and biases are likely, and variability reduces the chance that a significant *P* value will be detected when it really exists. In addition, normal distributions cannot be inferred when the *n* is small. Because a normal distribution is required for most parametric tests, a small *n* generally invalidates the results.

For nonparametric tests, special calculations help one to deal with small numbers. For example, with a small *n,* the Fisher's exact test should be used instead of the chi-square. (See previous section, "Insufficient Information Reported.")

Very Large *n*
Most readers are impressed with studies that report a very large number of subjects. Although a large *n* reduces the problems cited previously in regard to very small numbers, a study using a very large *n* may show statistical significance when the clinical effect is low or even nonexistent.

Marks[17] describes a study in which two antihypertensive drugs were compared. The mean systolic blood pressure of subjects taking drug A was lower than that of the other subjects, who were taking drug B. The calculated *P* value was 0.001, which is considered statistically significant. The mean systolic blood pressure of subjects taking drug A was 140.2 mm Hg; that of those taking drug B was 140.3 mm Hg. This *statistically* significant finding may be attributed to the study's very large *n*—involving hundreds of patients. The *clinical* significance of 140.2 mm Hg versus 140.3 mm Hg, however, is nonexistent. A very, very large *n* may detect very, very small between-group differences. Statistical significance is a function of several factors, the most important of which are the variability among results (expressed as standard deviation) and the sample size *(n)*.

Power analysis is a method of estimating the minimum sample size required for a study.[11,13] Studies using sample sizes that far exceed such estimates may boast minute differences that are not clinically significant, as is shown in the previous example. Because *P* values can sometimes be lowered by increasing the *n* in cases in which there is a negligible clinical effect, readers are cautioned to carefully evaluate studies that involve very large subject numbers.

Randomization Appropriate randomization in procuring subjects can help reduce selection biases. Many studies fail, however, to indicate the method of randomization used. In human research, truly random samples are rare and difficult to come by, especially when there are relatively small subject numbers. Studies that report "randomization" without describing the method used to actually achieve it may have used a convenience sample with inherent selection biases.

CONCLUSION

As lifelong learners, PAs use the medical literature as their primary information source to stay current and competent in practice, and for applying the principles of evidence-based medicine. Although peer-review mechanisms can help ensure some degree of content accuracy, PA readers should assess medical information for themselves, taking into account the many human and technical factors that affect the discovery and reporting of medical information. Readers must evaluate medical information as a jury would evaluate complex subjective and objective evidence of varying reliability, importance, and relevance.

Appropriate screening tests are likely to identify factors that may limit the dependability of medical information; adequate scrutiny of journal articles involves reading them entirely. For those articles involving numerical information, understanding of some basic statistical concepts increases comprehension, reading enjoyment, and lifelong learning.

CLINICAL APPLICATIONS

1. Why should PAs develop skills to critically evaluate and use the medical literature instead of relying only on their experience in clinical practice?
2. What are the advantages and disadvantages of textbooks as a source of medical information?
3. What is the average time lag between an article's submission to a journal and its appearance in print?
4. You are treating a patient for hypertension with dietary recommendations and an antihypertensive medication. She asks you about a television show that mentioned nutritional supplements as a treatment for hypertension. You are unfamiliar with this modality and decide to search the medical literature for information. What key words would you include in your search? Describe the criteria you would use to evaluate the validity of the literature.
5. Identify the categories of articles for a reprint file that would be useful for you. Where would you keep a reprint file, and how would you review and update the articles it contains?

REFERENCES

1. Ludmerer KM. Time to Heal: American Medical Education from the Turn of the Century to the Era of Managed Care. New York: Oxford University Press, 1999.
2. Sheehan TJ. The medical literature. Arch Intern Med 1980;140:472.
3. Pfeifer MP, Snodgrass MS. The continued use of retracted, invalid scientific literature. JAMA 1990;263:1420.
4. Palumbo PJ. Statistics and the practicing physician. Mayo Clin Proc 1988;63:835.
5. National Library of Medicine. Journals Indexed in MEDLINE, 2001. Bethesda, MD: National Library of Medicine, 2001.
6. Relman AS. Journals. In: Warren KS (ed). Coping with the Biomedical Literature. New York: Praeger Publishers, 1981.

7. The American Medical Association. Editorial peer review in biomedical publication: the first international congress. JAMA 1990;263:1317.

8. Neutens JJ, Rubinson L. Research Techniques for the Health Sciences. Boston: Allyn and Bacon, 2001.

9. DeDonato RE. How to write and publish a clinical article. Physician Assist 1989;13:112.

10. Evidence-Based Medicine Working Group. Evidence-based medicine: a new approach to teaching the practice of medicine. JAMA 1992;268:2420.

11. Riegelman RK. Studying a Study and Testing a Test. Philadelphia: Lippincott, Williams and Wilkins, 2000.

12. Evans JT, Nadjari HI, Burchell SA. Quotational and reference accuracy in surgical journals. JAMA 1990; 263:1353.

13. Gall MD, Gall JP, Borg WR. Educational Research. Boston: Allyn and Bacon, 2002.

14. Rea LM, Parker RA. Designing and Conducting Survey Research. San Francisco: Jossey-Bass Publishers, 1997.

15. Currier DP. Elements of Research in Physical Therapy. Baltimore: Williams & Wilkins, 1990.

16. Blessing JD. Problem-Based Learning for the Physician Assistant. Philadelphia: FA Davis, 2001.

17. Marks RG. Designing a Research Project. Belmont, CA: Lifetime Learning Publications, 1982.

RESOURCES

Blessing JD. Problem-Based Learning for the Physician Assistant. Philadelphia: FA Davis, 2001. *This is a well-written text by and for PAs who wish to understand the medical literature or who are planning a research study. It contains numerous diagrams and figures that easily guide the reader through some difficult to understand concepts.*

Gall MD, Gall JP, Borg WR. Educational Research. Boston: Allyn and Bacon, 2002. *Although this is a text for educational researchers, it is one of the most user-friendly yet comprehensive works available for explaining the range of scientific methodology. Examples come from education, and they can be easily translated into medical cases.*

Currier DP. Elements of Research in Physical Therapy. Baltimore: Williams and Wilkins, 1990. *A recommended reference text on the topics of clinical research, methodology, and biostatistics. Concise and clearly written; excellent clinical examples are used throughout.*

Riegelman RK. Studying a Study and Testing a Test. Philadelphia: Lippincott, Williams and Wilkins, 1999. *An effective physician-authored text that has become a classic work among health care providers for interpreting epidemiological data. Accompanied by a CD-ROM.*

Neutens JJ, Rubinson L. Research Techniques for the Health Sciences. Boston: Allyn and Bacon, 2001. *One of the most practical texts for explaining the breadth of health sciences research. It is enjoyed by clinicians across the health care disciplines.*

CHAPTER 19

Evidence-Based Medicine

Anita Duhl Glicken

INTRODUCTION

The dawning of the information age has had a major impact on society, giving rise to a cultural and technological revolution that has dramatically changed the delivery of health care. Rapid availability of information from across the world has transformed medical decision making. Although practitioners are still likely to seek consultations and to compare the results of treatments with their colleagues down the hall, they are now also able to seek the opinions of international groups of experts. As physician assistants (PAs) seek out the best treatments and outcomes for their patients, they may come to rely increasingly on the wealth of emerging literature that critically evaluates new treatments and ongoing standards of care. This paradigm of evidence-based medicine (EBM) is

the application of the best available evidence to the decision-making process of patient care.

HISTORY OF EBM

The formal evolution of EBM can be traced back to the early 1970s, a period of strong debate about the shortcomings of medicine. Archie Cochrane, an early critic of the medical profession for its repeated failure to conduct timely systematic reviews of accumulating clinical evidence, lived to see the first organized responses to his critique in the late 1980s. In 1988, Ian Chalmers and colleagues published a database of neonatal randomized controlled trials, followed in 1989 by the release of their important book, *Effective Care in Pregnancy and Childbirth*.[1] At the conclusion of this book, Chalmers, Enkin, and Keirse reported

413

their own perspectives on the treatments they reviewed, based on conclusions formed in the preceding articles. The authors concluded that, although some strategies and forms of care were very useful, others were of questionable value. Moreover, some interventions commonly thought to be useful were in fact of little benefit or were even harmful to patients. In 1992, a similar publication, *Effective Care of the Newborn Infant,* provided a compilation and review of all existing neonatal randomized clinical trials (RCTs).[2]

Several developments in medicine during the late 1970s and early 1980s helped to stimulate this early effort. The need and demand for health care increased owing to the following:

1. An aging population.
2. New technology and knowledge.
3. Increased expectations on the part of professionals and their patients.

However, the growth of available resources for health care had not risen at the same rate as the increase in demand. As a result, there had been increasing pressure on health care organizations and professionals to demonstrate that procedures and practices were both clinically sound and cost effective. Evidence-based medicine became an important thread in the fabric of the health care industry, ensuring that available resources are allocated effectively and that the services provided are of high quality.

In 1991, the National Health Service (NHS) launched an evaluative culture through the establishment of a Research and Development Program. In 1992, this program developed two important centers for evidence collation, in which certain forms of evidence are synthesized to produce systematic reviews and meta-analyses. The United Kingdom (UK) Cochrane Center at Oxford and the NHS Center for Reviews and Dissemination were both funded as part of the Research and Development Program. The Cochrane Center undertakes the meta-analysis of randomized controlled trials. The Collaboration represents a global community whose role is to collaborate with others in building and maintaining a core database of systematic up-to-date reviews of randomized controlled trials of health care, and to arrange for these reviews to be readily accessible through various electronic media. Many of the reviews focus on specific questions of importance to the NHS, principally in areas of effectiveness and cost effectiveness of health care interventions and management and organization of health care services.

Evidence-based medicine was further developed in 1992 with the publication of an article entitled "Evidence-Based Medicine: A New Approach to Teaching the Practice of Medicine" in *the Journal of the American Medical Association.*[3] This paper, published by the newly formed, evidence-based medicine working group, was the precursor to many subsequent articles that described the process and practice of EBM. By 1998, more than 850 articles had been published. Now specific search engines are dedicated to finding articles with the use of an EBM methodology; there are more than 150 EBM-related web sites, including centers for evidence-based medicine, child health, dentistry, emergency medicine, mental health, nursing pathology, and pharmacotherapy. In 1998, EBM became the focus of major curriculum reform for medical schools because both the Liaison Committee for Medical Education and the Medical Schools Objectives Project identified it as a priority. One of the first-known EBM curricula in PA education was launched at the University of Colorado in 1995, and many PA programs now teach EBM or are currently integrating it into their curriculum.

WHAT IS EBM?

Evidence-based medicine is the application of the best available evidence to patient care. Most practitioners recognize that the ideas underlying EBM are not new; clinicians have always consulted literature. However, for decades, the gap between research and practice has grown larger, leading to expensive, ineffective, or harmful decisions. The term "evidence-based medicine" was coined at McMaster Medical School in Canada in the 1980s to label a specific clinical learning strategy, which had been under development there for longer than a decade.[3]

FOUR CORE SKILLS OF EBM

Typically, evidence-based practice is recognized as having four core skills:

1. Formulating a clear, researchable question for a clinical problem.

2. Searching the literature for relevant clinical articles.
3. Evaluating (critically appraising) the evidence for its validity and usefulness.
4. Implementing useful findings in clinical practice.

This new paradigm of evidence-based practice is designed to enhance clinical judgment, not to replace it. Although the practitioners of the past relied heavily on expert opinion and testimonial evidence, the clinicians of today have an opportunity to explore a high grade of evidence in rigorous research, thereby generating a new standard for medical practice.

This chapter provides an overview of the four core skills, followed by a step-by-step approach to critical appraisal of medical research.

Core Skill 1: Formulating a Question

As an exercise, think about the patients seen in clinic last week. Take 5 minutes to brainstorm on your questions about these patients. Typically, it does not take long to generate a long list of questions from clinical practice. Alternatively, consider the following case scenario:

CASE STUDY 19-1

Mary P, a 75-year-old white female, presents to the office with complaints of fatigue and cough, which she has had for 2 weeks. She was last seen 3 months ago for a follow-up visit for stable hypertension.

Many questions might be generated from this case. Consider the following two lists of questions:

List 1

1. What are the causes of pneumonia?
2. What physical examination findings would be expected from acute bronchitis?
3. What information would help differentiate acute bronchitis from bacterial pneumonia?
4. What treatments are available for acute bronchitis?

List 2

1. In patients presenting with fatigue and cough, with possible pneumonia, does a chest x-ray or oxygen saturation level more accurately confirm the diagnosis?

2. In patients with acute bronchitis, does the use of a bronchodilator in aerosol form relieve symptoms of cough and wheezing as compared with placebo?
3. In patients with acute bronchitis, do α agonists reduce the duration of cough compared with placebo or erythromycin?
4. In patients with acute bronchitis, do antibiotics prevent nonsuppurative complications of a hemolygic streptococcal pharyngitis?

Notice that List 1 of questions is typical of beginning PA students. Students might ask general questions about the disorder—acute bronchitis—attempting to find what can be called "background" knowledge.[4] Well-built clinical questions about background knowledge usually have two components—a question **root** (who, what, when, where, why, and how) and a verb (causes) AND an aspect of the health condition at hand (disorder, syndrome, finding, concern). "What are the causes of pneumonia," from the previous list, is an example of a background question.

The second list of questions is typical of those asked by practitioners with more experience. They are specific questions about how to best care for this patient with bronchitis, seeking what can be termed "foreground" knowledge. Well-built questions about "foreground" knowledge usually have three or four components. These include the following:

➤ The patient or problem.
➤ The intervention of interest.
➤ The comparison intervention, when relevant (such as for questions about therapy or diagnostic tests).
➤ The clinical outcomes of interest.

Review the questions you created at the beginning of this section to determine whether they were background or foreground questions. If they were background questions, how might you change them to make them foreground questions? The distinction between types of questions is an important one because answers to different types of questions are often found in different places. Textbooks often answer background questions, whereas foreground questions are typically answered in medical journals and places where information can be updated routinely as new data emerge.

Core Skill 2: Searching the Literature

Evidence-based medicine clinicians face two major challenges in accessing medical knowledge:

1. Finding the most relevant and reliable information to address a clinical problem at hand.
2. Keeping abreast of important new developments in the expansive mass of published research.

Both of these rely on skills of searching the Internet for literature. Mastering appropriate and efficient searching techniques is the second step in becoming an evidence-based medicine practitioner.

The goal of a search strategy is to retrieve the most reliable information in as short an amount of time as possible. Priority is given to sites that are most likely to yield valid information and to cover large amounts of research on a topic. Therefore, we first search for reliable sources of integrative literature. If these time saving resources do not provide the information we seek, we next search MEDLINE, which is the "gold standard" but is a more time-consuming database. MEDLINE is a service of the U.S. National Library of Medicine (NLM) and is an acronym for their online Medical Literature Analysis and Retrieval System. This comprehensive database has catalogued over 10 million journal articles since 1966. Most of the information a clinician needs can be found in this database. The challenge, however, is to understand how the information is catalogued so that it can be accessed efficiently. If we are still unsuccessful in finding what we need, then specific medical information searches are performed. Finally, if we have still not found the required information, we may dredge the Internet by putting any related search term into one of the many general search engines, remembering to be cautious with respect to the quality of data. Many excellent EBM textbooks[5] or your local medical librarian can familiarize you with the mechanics of navigating your search if you are unfamiliar with the particular search engines and databases available to you. Most search engines use some form of "MeSH terms"—medical subject headings or keywords. Some of these are not intuitively obvious, others are menu driven, allowing you to select from a range of topics and modifiers for your search.

Sources of Integrative Literature   As has been previously noted, in EBM we frame the clinical question, identify and retrieve all relevant information, appraise it, and integrate it so that we can apply it to our patients. This often takes a great deal of time, more than is allowed in a brief office visit. A number of sites present information in which this sequence of steps has already been done. Integrative literature provides summary findings or recommendations in the form of overviews, meta-analysis, and/or practice guidelines of consensus statements.

Just because the literature has been integrated does not guarantee it is valid. As responsible readers, we need to be certain that each step has been rigorously performed. Critical appraisal takes time, but groups that assemble many reviews or guidelines often use a uniform methodology that is available as a supporting document. Reading once the group's supporting article enables us to assess their entire body of work. If we are satisfied that their method of assembling literature is rigorous, we can use the review with confidence. We typically assume that the review or guideline is evidence-based and that its host site is likely to be an efficient and reliable location for use in the future.

Some examples of sites you may find useful in your search for valid integrative literature include the following:

➤ Cochrane Collaboration (Cochrane Database of Systematic Reviews—CDSR) is a rapidly growing collection of updated systematic reviews. These reviews are generated by an international group of individuals and institutions dedicated to summarizing all randomized controlled trials relevant to health care. Their process of compiling reviews is rigorous, focusing on a particular clinical question. All available trials are critically appraised. Studies that meet specific quality criteria are summarized quantitatively, using meta-analysis. Summary findings are also presented qualitatively.

➤ The Database of Abstracts of Reviews of Effectiveness (D.A.R.E.) is a comprehensive collection of reviews from around the world (including those from the Cochrane Collaboration). Reviewers at the National Health Service Center critically appraise each article. Following quality reviews, detailed structured abstracts describing the methodology, results, and conclusions are produced. Comments on the overall quality of reviews and their implications for health care are also included. Of particular note is that this vast database is indexed not only by keywords, but also by the official Medical Subject Headings, or MeSH terms of the MEDLINE database, which can improve the specificity of our search.

➤ NIH: Health Services Technology Assessment Text. The National Library of Medicine provides documents useful in health care decision making. This site has many guidelines and references for clinicians sponsored by the Agency for Health Care Policy and Research. This site also contains the complete U.S. Preventive Health Series Task Force Guidelines from 1996, as well as consensus documents and research sponsored by the National Institute of Health.

➤ National Guidelines Clearinghouse. This site provides a broad spectrum of clinical practice guidelines from more than 100 institutions and organizations. The U.S. Department of Health and Human Services Agency for Health and Policy Research (AHCPR) sponsors this site in partnership with the American Medical Association (AMA) and the American Association of Health Plans (AAHP). Structured abstracts facilitate critical appraisal. The site allows you to display comparable guidelines on a table that enables you to compare issues of relevance, rigor, and generalizability. The site also links to the full text of the guidelines.

The sites described here may provide the data you need to answer your specific clinical question; however, often the information required is so new that it is not yet available in these sources. Additional sources are available to help you obtain the most recent information. These sources will also help you stay up-to-date with emerging trends and new data as an EBM practitioner. Many major journals have web sites. Most provide free access to the abstracts; some also provide free access to full text and figures. They can often be found with the use of a search engine like MEDLINE and the name of the journal. If the journal has an electronic site, it will also typically be found at an ejournal. Sites are updated before or on the day of publication. Information may be available here before the articles are indexed in MEDLINE. Most good electronic journal sites have their own search engines, for example, *Annals of Internal Medicine, British Medical Journal, Journal of the American Medical Association, Lancet,* and *New England Journal of Medicine.*

Reviewing summaries of key articles excerpted from journals is another way to view current research findings. Reading prereviewed summaries from publications that have scanned many journals for quality articles can be a very efficient use of time when one is looking for the latest research on common clinical issues. There are many such publications available to PAs. The three publications discussed in the following paragraph pay particular attention to the rigor and validity of the articles reviewed.

Published bimonthly, the *American College of Physicians Journal Club (ACPJC)* abstracts key articles from a number of "core" internal medicine journals (e.g., *American Journal of Medicine, Annals of Internal Medicine, Archives of Internal Medicine, BMJ, JAMA, Lancet, New England Journal of Medicine, Journal of Internal Medicine*). Articles are selected according to their perceived importance and rigor, judged by specific criteria from the *User's Guide to the Medical Literature.* A content expert reviews each article. A commentary follows each summary, describing any significant methodological problems and providing a context of previous literature as well as recommendations for clinical applications of the study findings. A select group is available for free; the entire list is available with payment or through a library.

The journal *Evidence-Based Medicine* is generated by means of identical procedures, is published bimonthly, and also requires a subscription fee but may be available at no charge through your local medical library. *EBM* has a broader focus than does *ACPJC,* reviewing more than 100 journals that focus on family practice, surgery, psychiatry, pediatrics, obstetrics, and gynecology. *EBM* also publishes about 50% of the abstracts reviewed in *ACPJC.*

Best Evidence is an electronic presentation of all issues of *ACPJC* (1991-present) and *Evidence-Based Medicine* (1995-present). *Best Evidence* also includes editorials from *ACPJC* and notes from *Evidence-Based Medicine*.

Core Skill 3: Critical Appraisal of the Literature

The following sections of this chapter build upon the principles discussed in Chapter 18, Using the Medical Literature. Before continuing, it is suggested that the reader review the distinction between research articles and clinical review articles. The critical appraisal skills outlined here refer only to medical research articles, not clinical review articles.

Published medical research can be broadly classified as either studies or integrative literature. Studies are considered descriptive if they "describe" individual variables (e.g., the prevalence of characteristics of a particular disease) or analytical if they "analyze" the association between two or more variables (e.g., intervention and mortality). A majority of the studies that we evaluate are of the analytical type. Analytical studies are divided into four basic study designs: experimental, cohort, case-control, and cross-sectional. Detailed descriptions of the various study types are found in any research methods textbook.

Integrative literature "integrates" information derived from individual studies within a particular framework to provide a summary finding or recommendation. Examples of integrative literature are overviews, meta-analyses, practice guidelines, decisional analyses, and cost-effectiveness analyses. Meta-analysis is a statistical method of combining data from independent studies.

The Evidence-Based Medicine Working Group has published its approach to systematic evaluation of the diversity of published medical research, in a series of journal articles entitled "User's Guide to Medical Literature." These guides contain a series of questions that are individually tailored to multiple types of studies (e.g., therapy, diagnosis, harm, prevention), as well as integrative literature (e.g., overview, decision analysis, practice guidelines, and cost effectiveness studies). The method discussed in this chapter incorporates the general framework of these publications, which considers a study's validity, results, and application to patient care. This discussion differs in two respects:

1. Instead of a different set of questions for each type of study, a single set of questions is used for studies of risk, diagnostic tests, intervention, and prognosis.
2. This discussion places the study within a context of other relevant knowledge (i.e., other literature, biological plausibility) to help assess whether the result is believable.

Core Skill 4: Implementing Useful Findings

The skills outlined previously will help the PA to analyze the research literature and to determine the believability of a study. An additional skill set is required to apply the findings of research studies to individual patients. The steps outlined below will contribute to this core skill.

STEPS IN CRITICAL APPRAISAL
Overview

The following sections focus primarily on the evaluation of analytical studies because analytical studies provide much of the emerging information needed for practice. This model is adapted from a discussion by Daniel Friedland in his book entitled *Evidence-Based Medicine: A Framework for Clinical Practice,*[6] in which he described the following five steps for systematic analysis of a study:

Step 1.   Do I want to evaluate the study?
Step 2.   What is the study outline/method?
Step 3.   Is the study finding believable?
Step 4.   What is the clinically relevant finding?
Step 5.   Will the study help me in caring for my patient?

Each step will be addressed individually. Steps 1 to 3 relate directly to Core Skill 3: Critical Appraisal of the Evidence. Steps 4 and 5 pertain to Core Skill 4: Implementing Useful Findings.

The format in Table 19-1, Matrix for Critical Appraisal, is provided to assist you to organize an evaluation of a research study. It is suggested that you follow the Matrix through each step of the discussion that follows.

Table 19-1   Matrix for Critical Appraisal*

CITATIONS
Step 1. Do I Want to Evaluate the Study? (INR)
Is the study Interesting,
Novel,
Relevant?
Step 2. What Is the Study Outline/Method?
Research Question
Subjects/Target Population   Temporal and Geographic Characteristics.
                                                               Intended Follow-up.
                                                               Sampling.

Predictor Variable Defined
Outcome Variable Defined
Findings
Step 3. Is the Study Finding Believable?
Do the subjects and variables accurately   Subjects:
   represent the research question?   Predictor Variable:
                                                               Outcome variable:
                                                               ? Chance.
Are findings attributable to other factors?   ? Bias.
   (Chance, Bias, Confounders)   Bias in Selecting Study Subjects.
                                                               Biases in Following Up on the Study Subjects.
                                                               Biases in Executing or Measuring the Predictor Variable.
                                                               Biases in Measuring the Outcome Variable.
                                                               Biases in Analyzing the Data.
                                                               ?Confounders.
Are the findings believable within the context   ? Consistency with Other Literature.
   of other knowledge?   ? Biological Plausibility.
                                                               ? Analogy.
Step 4. What is the Clinically Relevant Finding? (Likelihood ratios [LRs] for diagnostic tests; disease-specific
mortality [DSM]; patient-specific mortality [PSM] and/or life expectancy [LE] for prognosis; absolute risk reduc-
tion [ARR]; number needed to treat [NNT]; discounting for therapy)
Weighing Costs and Benefits
Step 5. Will the Study Help Me in Caring for My Patient?
Are the Subjects Adequately Described and Applicable to My Patient?
Is the Predictor Variable Adequately Described and Applicable to My Patient?
Will the Finding Result in an Overall Net Benefit for My Patient?

*For a Matrix for Critical Appraisal that can be used as a worksheet, see Appendix 3, p. 1006.

Step 1. Do I Want to Evaluate the Study?

You must have a motivation to evaluate a study. By developing a habit of browsing the literature, you will soon recognize the factors that interest you. Typically, clinicians are looking for information that extends previous knowledge about the topic. You will want to evaluate studies that are relevant for your practice and then determine whether study questions are phrased in a clinically meaningful way and whether outcomes are stated with respect to short-term impact on patients or long-term morbidity and mortality. Much of this information can be found in the article's abstract, which will help you identify whether or not you want to evaluate the study further.

Step 2. What Is the Study Outline/Method?

The outline of the study consists of the research question, the study method, and the findings (Figure 19-1). The **research question** represents knowledge we are seeking and considers the association between a given predictor and an outcome in a given population. A predictor is something that precedes, affects, or tests for the outcome. Therefore, predictors might be a risk, an intervention, a prognostic factor, or a diagnostic test. The outcome is whatever is being affected by the predictor or is being diagnosed. For example, consider the following question.

CASE STUDY 19-2

We are familiar with the drug fluoxetine, a selective serotonin reuptake inhibitor (SSRI), for treating depression. In a patient with type 2 diabetes, what is the efficacy of fluoxetine in improving glycemic control, as evidenced by decreased fasting blood glucose levels, decreased HbA1c levels,

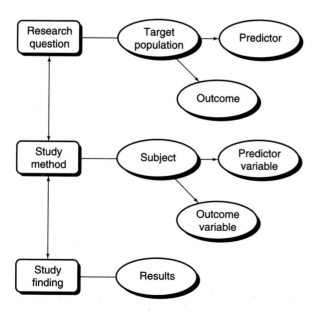

Figure 19-1 Outline of a research study.

and weight loss? In this example, fluoxetine would be the predictor. Glycemic control (as evidenced by decreased fasting blood glucose levels), decreased HbA1c levels, and weight loss would be the outcomes in a target population of patients with type 2 diabetes.

When outlining the study method, one should consider the type of study design, the subjects, and the variables. As was mentioned earlier, analytical studies analyze the association between a predictor and outcome variables. Analytical studies are classified as one of four study designs—experimental, cohort, case-control, and cross-sectional.

The double-blind, randomized, controlled trial is considered the model experimental design. Subjects are randomly assigned to either an intervention or a control group. "Double-blinding" means that neither the researcher nor the patients are aware of which group they are in. Single-masking implies that only the patient is unaware of which therapy is being received.

In the cohort study, the researcher collects data about patients over a period of time and associations are made between the predictor and outcome variables. In case-control studies, associations are made between the predictor and outcome variables by the selection of groups on the basis of whether an outcome is present or absent. The researcher then looks within each group to identify whether the given predictor variable has occurred.

In cross-sectional studies, a group of study subjects are evaluated at a single point in time, and associations are then made between predictor and outcome variables. Additional information on these study designs is available in Blessing's *A Physician Assistant's Guide to Research and the Medical Literature*.[7] Friedland has identified three questions to help differentiate between these analytical study designs[6] (Figure 19-2).

Because it is typically not feasible to study all of the subjects in a population, a group is chosen that is representative of the problem through a selection process. Subjects are described according to key factors, which frequently identify inclusion or exclusion criteria. These include temporal characteristics, such

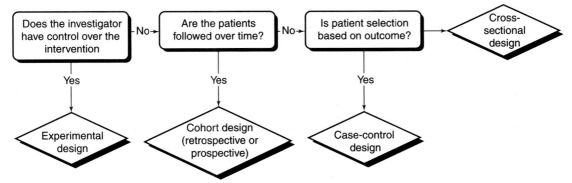

Figure 19-2 Differentiating study designs.

as the dates of the recruitment period or the length of follow-up. Other information may include geographical characteristics, which detail where the study took place or whether it was a multicenter trial. One of the most important pieces of information related to subjects is the sampling strategy used to select the representative population. For example, were the subjects a random sample, or were they enrolled consecutively? Some mention of attrition tells us how many subjects dropped out of the study before completion.

The variables tell us how the predictor and outcome were defined and measured or implemented. For example, consider the following question:

> ### CASE STUDY 19-3
>
> Do women between the ages of 15 and 30 who receive medroxyprogesterone acetate injections (Depo-Provera) have decreased bone mineral density (BMD) compared with women using no hormonal contraception? If you were evaluating this study, you would note in your outline how the variables define the predictor and the outcome. The predictor variable would be how the authors defined and measured the use of Depo-Provera. Similarly, the outcome variable—decreased BMD—can be expressed as a percentage of bone loss (determined by dual x-ray absorptiometry).

A study finding is the final piece of the outline. This is the association between the predictor and the outcome variables in the subjects who were studied. The level of statistical significance is typically presented, along with the magnitude of the outcome (typically presented as a P value or a confidence interval). Outlining the study in your mind and/or using the matrix in Table 19-1 will help you decide whether the study you found is likely to yield the information you are seeking. In addition, you will use the outline to organize your thinking as you proceed with a critical appraisal of the study.

Step 3. Is the Study Finding Believable?

The first question to be considered when the validity of any study is explored is whether the subjects and variables accurately reflect the research question. For example, we have already determined that the target population is defined by a set of inclusion and exclusion criteria. We need to be sure that the subjects in the study actually meet these criteria.

> ### CASE STUDY 19-4
>
> A randomized clinical trial of a new acne medicine for adolescents was conducted by randomly assigning 100 adolescents with severe acne to the new medicine and 100 with severe acne to a placebo. Ninety percent of the adolescents randomly assigned to the new medication experienced "very satisfying" results with a decrease in the number of facial lesions. The placebo group had no apparent improvement. How would it affect the study if it was later determined that as many as 50% of the adolescents in the treatment group had only moderate or intermittent skin problems, or that 24% of the population were older than

25 years of age? In either of these cases, the study would not answer the intended question and instead would be testing a different association.

Because the variables of the study also must accurately represent the predictor and the outcome, we must consider how they are measured. If the variables are inaccurate, the association between them will not be meaningful, no matter how rigorously the study attempts to limit other confounding variables. If the patients and variables accurately represent the research question, we go on to explore whether the association between the predictor and outcome is valid and believable, given what we know about existing knowledge on this topic.

To determine if the association between the predictor and the outcome variable is valid, we assess whether the predictor was responsible for the finding, or whether the finding is attributable to other factors. Two things help in determining whether the finding can be explained by other factors—study design and study source.

First, we consider whether the study design is descriptive or analytical. If there is no comparison or control group, the study can only describe an occurrence in a given population and cannot analyze associations between outcomes.

CASE STUDY 19-5

For example, consider a study of children with otitis media and antibiotic therapy. If the study does not include a control group and describes only the population of children taking antibiotics, we cannot conclude anything about the association between the antibiotics and resolution of the otitis media. If, however, the study does include a comparison group, the study is analytical and can determine whether the antibiotics might have cured the otitis media. With a comparison group, we can determine whether the outcome is due to the predictor variable, rather than reflects the natural resolution of the illness.

The strength of an analytical study design is also based on its susceptibility to chance, bias, and other confounding factors. The experimental study design

is typically considered the strongest design and the least susceptible to bias, followed by the cohort study, the case-control study, and the cross-sectional study design. Another factor that affects study design validity is whether the study is prospective or retrospective. Prospective studies are stronger because they outline a predictor variable, follow the subjects forward in time, and then record an observable outcome. In this case, we can be more certain that the predictor variable preceded the outcome variable. Retrospective studies look backward at the predictor and the outcome, which makes it less clear that the finding is attributable to the predictor variable; the outcome could have caused the predictor.

The source of the study is another important piece of information. This includes the study's sponsorship, the author's reputation, and the credibility of the journal. Pharmaceutical companies are likely to fund original research on new drugs; however, they may also be less likely to publish research that sheds unfavorable light on their products. Clearly, if the journal and the author have a known reputation, one feels more comfortable with the appraisal process that has gone on before publication.

Three major factors also affect the credibility of the findings: chance, bias, and confounding factors (Figure 19-3).

The researcher considers the effect of chance when presenting the power of the study, the *P* value, and the confidence interval. The power of a study dictates the

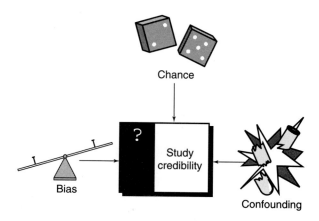

Figure 19-3 Chance, bias, and confounding factors.

probability that a specific magnitude of association will be found between the predictor and outcome variables, if such an association exists. This is calculated before a study takes place and takes into consideration the number of subjects, the estimated magnitude of effect, and the precision of the measures that are being used. A power of .8 (80% probability) is typically used and is considered satisfactory in detecting a specific effect of size that has been determined before the study. A review of common statistical terms and tests is included in Chapter 18.

The P value is the probability that the association between the predictor and the outcome variables could have occurred strictly by chance, when in reality there was no association between predictor and outcome. If the P value is less than .05 (less than a 5% chance of finding an association when no association exists), the finding is considered statistically significant and unlikely to be due to chance alone.

Just as the power statistic informs the design of a study, the width of the confidence interval helps us determine whether more precise variables or a greater number of subjects might have allowed the researcher to find a particular association. The confidence interval (CI) represents the range of values that are statistically compatible with the estimate of the study result. When 95% confidence intervals are used, we can determine whether or not the reported data are statistically significant with a P value less than or equal to .05.

For example, a study that reports symptom reduction of 10% (95% CI, 7%-20%) implies that the data are statistically compatible with an effect as small as 7% or as large as 20% at a significance level of .05. Typically, the CI is expressed as a span for an odds ratio to the patient. (Remember that the odds ratio represents the proportion of subjects with the event divided by the proportion of subjects without the event.) For odds ratios, 1 represents the point at which the odds of disease are the same whether or not the risk factor is present. Therefore, an odds ratio of 1 is actually the same as the null hypothesis, which states that the risk of having the disease is the same whether the risk factor is present or absent. If a 95% CI around the observed odds ratio does not extend beyond 1, it can be concluded that the odds ratio is

statistically significant with a P value less than or equal to .05. The same strategy applies to relative risks. Consider the following study:

CASE STUDY 19-6

Imagine a study in which the odds ratio of skin cancer and sun exposure was 8(6, 10). The 8 indicates the odds ratio for the sample; that means that the odds of having skin cancer are increased 8-fold for those with sun exposure. An odds ratio of 1 would mean that the odds are the same of having skin cancer if you had sun exposure as they are if you had none. The confidence interval on this odds ratio tells us with 95% confidence that the odds ratio in the larger population is between 6 and 10. The lower confidence limit is 6 (much greater than 1), and this allows us to be quite sure that a substantial odds ratio is present not only in our sample, but in the larger population from which our sample was obtained. Consider an odds ratio for the same problem with an odds ratio of 8(−2, 9). In this case, the observed odds ratio is greater than 1; however, the lower limit of our 95% confidence interval extends below 1, indicating that we should be uncertain about whether sun exposure actually increases the risk of skin cancer.

Bias in a study is often a matter of judgment. Unlike the confidence interval, there is no statistic that indicates that bias is present in the study. Bias can be defined as "any process that tends to produce results or conclusions that differ systematically from the truth".[8] There are exhaustive lists of potentially biasing factors available in most research textbooks. The reader should review Chapter 18 for screening tests used in evaluating the medical literature. You can identify some of the most significant sources of bias by using your study outline and reviewing the study method and study findings. In this way, you can explore the issue of bias with respect to the selection and follow-up of study subjects, the execution and measurement of the predictor variable, and the measurement of the outcome variable and analysis of the data.

For example, in studying a new diagnostic procedure, the investigator must convince us that an appropriate spectrum of patients are represented in the data.

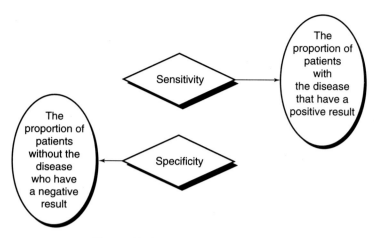

Figure 19-4 Sensitivity and specificity.

If the diseased patients all have more advanced illness than the nondiseased patients, we are more likely to find a false-negative test result in the diseased population. The nondiseased subjects are similarly less likely to have a false-positive result. This type of sampling would overestimate the sensitivity and specificity of the test in a population with a broader spectrum of the disease (Figure 19-4).

When the study population for experimental randomized controlled trials is critically appraised, it is important that both study and control groups are equally likely to have the identified outcome. For example, in a study of a new treatment for preventing high blood pressure, if the patients in the comparison group are all overweight, the comparison group is more likely to have the outcome than the study group patients. That might lead us to believe that the intervention was more successful than it actually was. Alternatively, in a case-control study, the presence of the predictor variable should not influence the process of group selection.

Additional bias may occur during follow-up of study subjects. Consider what happens to the data analysis when the patients drop out or are lost to follow-up. Consider a study designed to test the efficacy of a new, noninvasive treatment for carpal tunnel syndrome in a population of factory workers who do repetitive tasks. How would the findings be affected if this population typically leave the work-place to seek other opportunities when affected by this problem?

Bias can also be present in the predictor variable. Consider the effect on the magnitude of the finding if some people did not really receive the intervention as planned, or received an additional therapy or different therapy. For example, in a study evaluating the effects of a new medication on depression, what would happen if some of the patients also enrolled in an outside exercise program? We would have a difficult time determining which intervention actually caused an effect.

Bias also could occur in measurement of the predictor variable. This is a particular concern in case-control studies in which the subjects and controls are selected based on the outcome variable. Retrospective interview data from these subjects may be compromised by the subject's memory of the exposure, or the data may be inaccurate owing to the researcher's inability to accurately and completely locate data in charts or medical records.

Investigator bias might also occur if the researcher is not blind to the outcomes. For example, if the researcher's hypothesis is that the outcome variable is attributable to a particular predictor variable, for example, lung cancer is attributable to exposure to electromagnetic waves, the investigator may be unconsciously more persistent in eliciting a history of exposure from patients with lung cancer.

Measurement of the outcome variable is also subject to bias from both the subject and the investigator. If blinding is not present and subjects are aware that they have received an intervention, they may change their behavior or fail to report negative findings. For example, if patients receive a new homeopathic treatment for headaches, they might also modify their diet or exercise routine or fail to report some minor headaches that were not as severe as those that they were experiencing before the intervention.

Most clinicians assume that reputable journals have individuals in the peer review process who evaluate whether an appropriate statistical test was used in analyzing the relationship between the predictor and outcome variables. However, one particular issue that does not relate to the test itself, but rather to the process of analysis in randomized controlled trials, warrants further mention. Many studies fail to indicate whether an intent-to-treat analysis was used. Intent-to-treat means that groups are analyzed according to their original assignments, in spite of the fact that some members of the control group may have, for whatever reason, ended up receiving the intervention, and members of the treatment group did not. Intent-to-treat analysis is important for preserving the random allocation assigned to the study subjects. For example, consider what would happen if patients in the treatment group got well before the intervention and therefore did not receive it. If they were then analyzed as part of the control group, it would bias the results of both groups in that the control group would be healthier than the treatment group at the outset of the intervention. This would introduce bias in the results in favor of the control group.

Bias can occur during the design, implementation, or analysis phase of a study, through intrinsic errors in the process such as those outlined earlier. Confounded results emerge from an extrinsic cause. A confounder causes a skewed result in the outcome variable and is related to the predictor variable. For example, referring back to Case Study 19-1, what if an author conducts a study of the use of fluoxetine for weight loss in type 2 diabetes, and some members of the population under study are also diagnosed with co-morbid depression?

The author can limit the effect of confounders on the study population by excluding subjects with the particular confounder from the study population. Alternatively, subjects and controls in the study can be matched based on the confounder. If these strategies are not implemented at the front end of the study, researchers can also attempt to control for confounders in the data analysis process, either through stratification of the data or by using multivariate analysis. In a critical appraisal, the important determinant related to confounders is whether the author of the study has attempted to control for these.

As a clinician, you will consider all of these issues as you evaluate a study's validity. However, you should also ask how the study's findings relate to other knowledge you may already have or may find in the literature. If the finding is not believable within the context of other knowledge, you may be reluctant to integrate this new information into your practice. Any time we read a new study finding, we consider what we knew before. We consider this information in light of what was known and reevaluate or review what we now believe about the issue (Figure 19-5).[6]

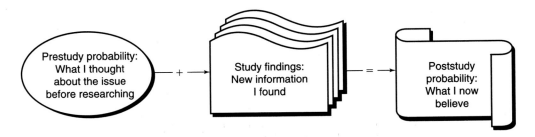

Figure 19-5 Clinical decision making.

Several factors are weighed as we qualitatively assess this issue. We may look to the information's consistency with other literature. Is there literature that would support the present finding? For example, we are exploring the use of fluoxetine for weight loss in type 2 diabetes in Case Study 19-1; does other literature report this outcome from fluoxetine use in other populations? We also would consider the biological plausibility of our findings. Does the pathophysiology that we already know make sense in terms of the study? Are there analogous situations wherein this intervention has been shown to be an effective treatment? These factors influence our judgment about the validity of new study findings.

In conjunction with our consideration of the potential impact of chance (*P* value, confidence intervals), bias (systematic, intrinsic factors), and confounding factors (extrinsic factors), we can make a reasonable judgment about whether the outcomes reported are truly associated with the predictor variable. If we determine that this is the case, we proceed to consider whether this information will help us in providing care for the patient.

Step 4. What Is the Clinically Relevant Finding?

An understanding of a limited number of key concepts and statistical calculations will help a clinician recognize the clinically relevant finding. Most statistical calculations are presented in a journal article;

however, it is important for clinicians to understand what the statistics mean for the patient and how to interpret these findings in the context of clinical practice. Figure 19-6 presents a selection of these calculations, and Chapter 18 discusses statistics as well. Because a majority of the clinical studies we will use involve interventions in patient care, we will review these in greater detail.

As clinicians, we select what treatments to use with our patients. This selection is often based on a qualitative evaluation in which we weigh the risks and benefits of a particular therapy for the patient. We can also assess quantitatively the relative value of an intervention. Studies of intervention may report the benefit of a given therapy as a relative risk reduction (RRR). This may not represent the true impact on our patient population. A better way of expressing the benefit of an intervention may be the absolute risk reduction (ARR) and the number needed to treat (NNT).

> **CASE STUDY 19-7**
>
> For example, two studies of cardiac arrest were undertaken with different populations. Both studies used the same therapy and received the same follow-up for 4 years. Study A's intervention group had a 5% cardiac event rate, with a control group event rate of 10%. Study B's treatment group had a 10% cardiac event rate, with a control group rate of 20%. In both cases, the therapy reduced the relative risk of cardiac arrest by 50%.

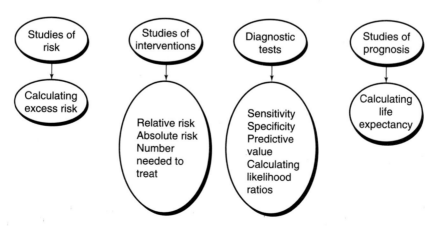

Figure 19-6 Statistical calculations.

$$RRR = \frac{\begin{array}{c}\text{Incidence of outcome control group} -\\ \text{Incidence of outcome study group}\end{array}}{\text{Incidence of outcome control group}}$$

In Study A, the RRR = {10 – 5}/10 = 50%; in Study B, the RRR = {20 – 10}/20 = 50%. It would seem that the therapy had the same impact on both study populations. The absolute risk reduction (ARR) would indicate, however, that the impact on the populations is actually very different.

$$\begin{array}{c}\text{ARR} = \text{Incidence of outcome in control group} -\\ \text{Incidence of outcome in study group}\end{array}$$

For Study A, the ARR over 10 years equals 10 – 5 = 5%; in Study B the ARR = 20 – 10 = 10%. This means that for every 100 patients treated during a 10-year period, five cardiac arrests were prevented in Study A and ten cardiac arrests were prevented in Study B. The number needed to treat (NNT) follows from this. This represents the number of patients we need to treat in order to prevent one outcome event. This is the inverse of the ARR if the ARR is in the form of a fraction or is 100 divided by the ARR, if the ARR is displayed as a percentage.

In Study A, the NNT = 100/5 = 20, and for Study B, the NNT = 100/10 = 10. Therefore, in Study A, 20 patients were treated to prevent one cardiac arrest, whereas in Study B, 10 patients were treated to prevent one cardiac event. The impact of the intervention is obviously greater in Study B. The NNTs for these studies were calculated over a 4-year period. Therefore, for Study A, the NNT of 20 over 4 years is equivalent to treating 80 patients to prevent one cardiac arrest per year (NNT = 20/4 = 80 per year). This is why it is important to make sure that studies you compare follow patients for comparable lengths of time. Generally, the less time patients are followed, the less opportunity there is for an effect to be seen. This would result in a smaller ARR and a larger NNT.

We perform the same steps if the intervention is harmful. We calculate the absolute risk increase (ARI). The inverse of the ARI is the number needed to harm (NNH). This would tell us the number of patients we would need to treat to observe a single adverse event. For clinicians, it is particularly important to remember that your patient may be sicker or healthier than the one in the study you are reading. In that case, you would adjust the NNT for your particular patient. The amount of the adjustment would depend on your assessment of your patient's anticipated risk relative to the study population. For example, if the NNT for a study is 15 and you estimate that your patient's risk of outcome without intervention would be three times that of the study group, the NNT for your patient is 15/3 = 5.

New models incorporate ethical decision making, weigh costs and benefits, and can be completed at the patient's bedside. These models incorporate the probabilities of various outcomes of a treatment and the outcome probabilities of no treatment in addition to a consideration of patient preferences for treatment. Although these models are quite complex, it is important to recognize that the patient's perspective is a critical piece in clinical decision making that should not be overlooked.

Another way of saying this is to consider a process known as discounting. In discounting, we consider that future life may be "discounted" over present life. In other words, a patient might value his or her present life over a future life. This implies that a patient may not want to take a risk today for the promise of a health benefit in the future. Informing patients of up-front risks is essential toward reaching a mutual decision regarding treatments and outcomes.

Step 5. Will the Study Help Me in Caring for My Patient?

The final question clinicians must ask in evaluating studies is whether the information reported would assist them in caring for a particular patient. First, we refer to the information we reviewed in Step 2, Outline of the Study. We explore the target population and determine if it was adequately described, so that we can compare our patient to the study group. Similarly, we determine whether the predictor variable and/or intervention was adequately described and comparable to treatments under consideration for your patient. We may also want to consider whether local resources are available to implement the intervention or test. Finally, we consider whether the finding will provide the patient with an overall net benefit.

If we have determined in Step 3 that the findings were valid and that the study subjects and predictor variables relate to our patient, then we can determine that the clinically relevant result will provide useful information for our clinical decision making.

CONCLUSION

The guidelines in this chapter will help busy PAs and PA students separate the "wheat from the chaff" and focus attention on those published articles that have direct clinical application to patients. Clinicians must continue to exercise caution, however, as they embrace new medical literature for the "truths" it contains. Even the best-quality literature may be filled with discrepancies with respect to an individual patient's situation. For example, what if the literature describes a daily treatment for a condition that your patient can only access weekly, or the literature describes efficacy in a population older or younger than your patient?

Clearly, clinical judgment remains the predominant factor in determining patient care. So why bother with peer-reviewed research when making clinical decisions, particularly when so many clinicians remain appropriately uneasy about this element of the medical process? The more we know in medicine, the more questions we seem to be asking, including what to do with the new information we have gained. Probably one of the strongest arguments for mastering EBM skills is that we are challenged to continually attempt to find better solutions for our patients. Discrepant literature will continue to be an important force in medicine, promoting additional research and dialogue on the efficacy of practice and the quality of care.

CLINICAL APPLICATIONS

1. Identify a researchable question, and use the Matrix for Critical Appraisal, Table 19-1, to work through a study related to the question.

2. Differentiate between experimental, cohort, case-control and cross-sectional studies. What are the advantages and disadvantages of each? Find an example of each type of study in the medical literature.

3. List six possible causes of bias in a study.

REFERENCES

1. Chalmers I, Enkins M, Keirse M. Effective Care in Pregnancy and Childbirth. New York: Oxford University Press, 1989.
2. Sinclair JC, Bracken MB. Effective Care of the Newborn Infant. New York: Oxford University Press, 1992.
3. Evidence-Based Medicine Working Group. JAMA 1992; 268:2420 (Nov 4).
4. Sackett DL, Straus SE, Richardson WS, Rosenberg W, Haynes RB. Evidence-Based Medicine: How to Practice and Teach EBM. 2nd ed. Edinburgh: Churchill Livingstone, 2000.
5. Greenhalgh T. How to Read a Paper: The Basics of Evidence Based Medicine. London: BMJ Publishing Group, 1997.
6. Friedland D, Go AS, Davoren JB, Shlipak MG, Ben SW, Subak LL, Mednelson T. Evidence-Based Medicine: A Framework for Clinical Practice. Connecticut: Appleton & Lange, 1998.
7. Blessing JD. A Physician Assistant's Guide to Research and the Medical Literature. Philadelphia: FA Davis, 2001.
8. Sackett DL. Bias in analytic research. J Chron Dis 1979;32:51.

RESOURCES

DePoy E, Gitlin LN. Introduction to Research: Understanding and Applying Multiple Strategies. 2nd ed. St. Louis: Mosby, 1998. *This research textbook is designed for students in allied health professions and human services. Compared with most research texts, it is readable and interesting. The authors address both qualitative and quantitative methods.*

Greenhalgh T. How to Read a Paper: The Basics of Evidence Based Medicine. London: BMJ Publishing Group, 1997. *A good beginning text for students and practitioners, this book discusses searching the literature, assessing methodological quality, appraising different types of papers, and implementing findings.*

Riegelman R. Studying a Study, Testing a Test. Baltimore: Williams and Wilkins, 2000. *A text for students and practitioners on evaluating the validity and value of the medical literature; the accompanying CD-ROM contains self-assessment questions and may be used for CME credits. The book has many clinical examples and provides a step-by-step, active-participation approach to a clinical review of the medical literature.*

Sackett DL, et al. Evidence-Based Medicine: How to Practice and Teach EBM. Edinburgh: Churchill Livingstone, 2000. *A short and concise book that demystifies EBM. The authors include study cards for summarizing points, and a CD-ROM provides additional case examples.*

CHAPTER 20

Dealing With Stress and Burnout

Ruth Ballweg

INTRODUCTION

As part of physician assistant (PA) training, most of us receive extensive information about stress. We learn that almost all change creates stress, and most of us optimistically believe that stress can be "managed." Typical classroom presentations generally include the concepts of "good" and "bad" stress, the Holmes-Reye Stress Scale as a teaching and evaluation tool for patients, and recommended treatment plans (exercise, decreased caffeine intake, improved nutrition, and even short-term psychotherapy) for patients with stress. This chapter does not attempt to duplicate that information. Rather, the chapter seeks to identify and discuss the specifics of stress and burnout as they apply to physician assistants, recommends strategies for prevention, and suggests a range of treatment interventions.

THE DECISION TO BECOME A PHYSICIAN ASSISTANT

Ironically, whether we choose to look at it this way or not, PAs all become personal experts on stress as part of our medical education. The consideration of any medical career creates stress. The prospect of long hours, personal sacrifice, a commitment to care of patients sometimes at the expense of family, and the recognition of the intensity of a medical career have demanded serious consideration. Many PAs at some point considered becoming physicians. This consideration was at least understandable to our teachers, mentors, family, and friends. Becoming a nurse also made some sense ("You'll always have a job"). The relatively new career of physician assistant commonly was neither understood nor supported. Fortunately, the admissions process for most physician assistant programs has favored the selection of risk-taking and pioneering individuals who see the PA profession as a unique opportunity. Candidates are often referred to practicing PAs who are willing to provide firsthand knowledge of and experiences within the PA profession.

Nevertheless, the first stress for successful candidates to PA programs has been the job of answering the question, "You're going to become a what!?" Even the most understanding friend may still ask, "When will you be a doctor?" The most supportive parent may still not understand why being a PA is a separate and different career with its own satisfactions and rewards.

THE EXPERIENCE OF STRESS IN TRAINING

Next come the adventure—and the stress—of PA training. Asked about the difference between PA and physician training programs, many of the founders of PA education are quick to point out that both physician assistant and nurse practitioner (NP) programs, although designed to train new types of primary care providers, were also intended to be a proving ground for new concepts in medical education. Problem-based learning, the use of simulated patients and videotaping to teach patient interviewing skills, and new types of clinical training experiences were used early on in PA and NP programs, prior to their more recent appearance in medical schools. Objectives and competency-based learning also were used to make PA training extremely efficient. As a result, the curriculum of most PA programs is intended to present an incredible amount of information in a very short time. PA program directors often say, "It's not that the material is so hard, but that it comes in truckloads."

In addition to simple acquisition of information, the relatively short duration of PA training—compared with that of physicians—demands that the PA student develop a professional identity in an extremely responsible role very quickly. This rapid role transition actually accounts for much of the stress PA students experience. Students entering the PA profession as a first career choice generally have a successful college career as a foundation for their

PA training but may have had little exposure to patient care. Thus, the stress for these students is often that of developing a way of relating to patients as well as seeing themselves as decision makers on the health care team. People who enter PA programs as second career students—former registered nurses (RNs), licensed practical nurses (LPNs), military corpsmen, paramedics, surgical/respiratory/radiology/laboratory technicians, and other allied health personnel—may have had identities as members of the health care team but generally find that they have to relinquish their former identities in order to assume their new role of physician assistant.

Recognizing these concerns, PA program admissions committees often seek and choose applicants who are flexible, trainable, proactive, and proficient in multiple tasks. Students less adaptable to the extremely rapid didactic and clinical experiences required of them in PA training may become alienated from classmates who are enthusiastically moving ahead on an exciting career path.

Another unique aspect of PA training that often creates some short-term stress but may actually decrease long-term stress is the necessity of dealing with gender issues as part of training. The PA profession has been proud of its track record of training men and women side by side. Included in this training has been extensive small-group work to teach interviewing and physical examination skills. Course work is also required to include primary care topics dealing with sexuality, parenting, death and dying, cross-cultural issues, and family dynamics. In studying these topics, students are forced to confront their own opinions and biases as they apply to interactions not only with their colleagues but also with their future patients.

One solution for stress in the didactic year is to focus on planning for the future in the clinical year. This diversionary tactic is probably most appealing for students with prior clinical experience, who feel that they are "just putting in time" in the classroom until they can "really perform" in the clinical setting. In contrast, students with more extensive academic experience and less clinical identity may approach the clinical year with increasing anxiety. Regardless of each group's anticipatory viewpoint, the clinical year brings certain predictable stresses:

➤ No matter how well the program has prepared the site and used it in the past, some members of the physician, nursing, and administrative staff, in at least some sites, still will not know what a PA is or does.

➤ Medical students assigned the same clinical placements will often not know what a PA is and may at first perceive the PA student as a threat. This will seem very strange to the PA student, who feels too frightened or incompetent to understand how he or she could possibly be a threat to anyone.

➤ The process of relocating from site to site is disorienting. The health care system may, for the first time, appear extremely fragmented to the PA student, who may not have realized that medicine is practiced so many different ways in so many different settings.

➤ The demand for documentation (charting) as to both detail and timeliness is much greater than the student had expected.

➤ Other health care workers question PA students very aggressively about their career choice. What seem like "attacks" are often discovered to be the questions of individuals who are considering PA training for themselves.

➤ When required to make complex decisions about patient care, the student realizes how judgmental he or she has been about other health care providers in the past.

Throughout the process of didactic and clinical training, the impetus is toward greater recognition of how much there is to know. Other providers may make disparaging comments about the limited knowledge base of the new PA, with little recognition of past experience or of the serious decisions he or she may have been required to make in previous employment settings.

STRESS IN CHOOSING THE FIRST JOB

As the student approaches graduation, the job decision becomes the next developmental obsession. Students who enter PA training with a well-defined idea of their employment choices may suddenly see other variables, often as a direct result of their clinical training experiences. Opportunities to pay back student loans in exchange for service to specific populations (rural or inner city underserved) may significantly influence a student's employment choice.

Program faculty members describe new episodes of stress for recent graduates, who face an extremely wide range of employment choices, many of which offer salaries and "perks" that have rarely been paid to practicing PAs in the past. In contrast to the employment scene in the mid-1980s, when the number of new PA jobs roughly equaled the number of new PAs entering the job market, the current market offers multiple positions for each graduate. Each graduate is now faced with the task of avoiding those jobs that are inappropriate, as well as seriously considering those offers that provide the best short-term and long-term opportunities.

The choice of the first PA job also shapes each PA's ultimate view of his or her new profession. Much of the initial stress for new PAs in their first jobs is directly related to the acceptance of PAs in the specific employment setting. This is a particular concern if other members of the health care team are not informed about PAs. It is very difficult to adjust to a new role and employment setting while also being called upon to educate administrators, nursing and medical staff members, credentials committees, and billing clerks about PA issues. This stress can be significantly reduced by negotiation of an orientation process as part of an employment contract, seeking the assistance of PA program administrators in providing technical assistance to new PA employment sites, or enlisting the assistance and support of other PAs practicing in the institution or community. Some PA graduates believe that one criterion of the "perfect PA job" is current or recent employment of a PA at the site who has enthusiastically and proactively pioneered the PA role.

Other graduates deliberately seek sites where there has not been a previous PA role model. They see the opportunity to be the "first PA" as one of great potential, stressful though it may initially be.

EDUCATING CONSUMERS

New graduates are often unprepared for the number of patients and health care professionals asking, "What is a physician assistant?" It is important that

PA programs train their students and graduates not only to expect these questions but also to regard them as opportunities. Unfortunately, some PAs stressfully view each such encounter as further proof that PAs are still not accepted and that the profession, state and national PA organizations, and PA programs are not doing their job of public education. In fact, health care consumers are frequently confused by the wide diversity of careers represented in any clinic and should be encouraged to ask about the training and credentials of those providing their care.

RELATIONSHIPS WITH PRECEPTORS

The dependent nature of PA practice makes the relationship between PA and preceptor a potential source of both satisfaction and stress. Here again, the messages given to new PAs by PA training programs about the relationships between PAs and preceptors set the stage for collaboration or dysfunction. Like all other relationships, the preceptor/PA collaboration requires work. The preceptor needs to be well informed about the background and current clinical expertise of the PA. This may appropriately require frequent observation and supervision early in the employment period. In fact, little or no supervision from a preceptor at the start of a PA job—especially for a new graduate—should be seen as a "red flag."

Appropriate supervision from the precepting physician is one of the greatest stress relievers for a PA. Similarly, the physician may have chosen to be a PA preceptor because of the opportunity that the relationship provides for sharing the challenges and frustrations of medical practice.

The fact that there is a formal backup for knowledge, decision making, and consultation makes the PA profession particularly attractive for many potential PA candidates. PAs, however, need to learn to use this collaborative relationship for teaching and support. Each new job requires a renegotiation of this communication. An important stress reduction tool is to plan on regular case review and journal assignments in addition to whatever chart review is required by state law. Insistence on a theme of "lifelong learning" early in an employment setting fosters communication and decreases stress. The intense and emotional demands of medical practice are most easily shared with those who are there at the same time seeing the same patients. The opportunity to review individual cases and specific encounters often allows the preceptor and the PA to leave these cases at work and to make the transition to personal and family time more efficiently.

RELATIONSHIPS WITH ADMINISTRATORS

With health care increasingly being provided by large systems, the relationships of PAs, which formerly were primarily with physicians, now include health care administrators. Although the physician may provide clinical supervision and oversight, the administrator may develop and negotiate jobs, supervise and evaluate personnel, and manage patient scheduling and follow-up. Thus although PAs were required in the past to speak the "language of medicine," they now must also be able to speak the "corporate language of business." A lack of understanding of concepts such as productivity, quality improvement, supervisory relationships, capitation, per member per month costs, and risk sharing will put the PA at a disadvantage.

In addition, the communication styles of administrators may vary vastly from those that PAs are accustomed to with physician preceptors. Notes on charts and hallside consultations may be replaced with memos requiring written responses. Written evaluations of clinical performance may involve complicated spreadsheets and graphs. Electronic communication skills will most likely be required for all providers.

Although some PAs and PA students may initially feel that the best coping mechanism is to avoid the transition to administrative relationships, probably a better strategy would be to quickly acquire the skills to interact effectively with health care administrators in these new and evolving relationships.

STRESS ON THE JOB

Once on the job, PAs report a variety of stresses. Holmes and Fasser,[1] using the Health Professions Stress Inventory to survey 2334 PAs, found that PA stress levels were relatively low. The highest stresses were reported in the following areas:

➤ Caring for the emotional needs of patients.
➤ Dealing with difficult patients.

➤ Feeling that opportunities for advancement on the job were poor.

➤ Feeling ultimately responsible for patient outcomes.

➤ Keeping up with new developments in order to maintain professional competence.

➤ Trying to meet society's expectations for high-quality medical care.

These stresses may be categorized into three types: patient care issues, formal professional issues, and role ambiguity issues.

Patient Care Issues

Caring for the emotional needs of patients, dealing with difficult patients, and feeling ultimately responsible for patient outcomes are patient care issues shared by the PA with other health care professionals. Because they are shared concerns, the solution to these stresses is also best shared by colleagues. Family members and friends can be supportive of health care professionals, but because of confidentiality and a lack of specific shared experiences, it is difficult and sometimes even inappropriate for them to "debrief" their health care professional family member or friend about specific patient care stresses. Some employment settings provide support groups for their health care providers. In addition to formal support networks, social events with co-workers also effectively reduce stress. Although many PAs use other PAs for support in patient care issues, it is valuable to see all members of the health care team as part of a support network because different viewpoints may bring different insights to a situation or incident.

One of the best published resources on stress in the helping professions is Christina Maslach's *Burnout—The Cost of Caring*.[2] In reviewing patient care stresses, Maslach believes that a large part of the problem is that health care professionals, as students and as practitioners, are often so busy acquiring facts and proficiency in procedures that they do not learn the relatively simple interpersonal skills that will carry them through difficult situations and reduce stress on the job.

Surprisingly, interpersonal skills are often not recognized as a major necessity for providers. They are considered secondary to other professional skills—extras rather than essentials, the "icing on the cake" rather than the cake itself. This viewpoint is sadly in error for it trivializes an essential aspect of the relationship between provider and recipient. It fails to recognize that both of them are human beings whose personal attitudes and feelings can affect not only the delivery of care, but also how and even whether it is accepted.[2]

Recognizing that health care professionals may have been taught to deal with specific crisis situations, Maslach is concerned that it is in fact the daily encounters, producing incremental stress, for which daily "garden variety" interpersonal skills should be gained. Maslach lists three of these skills as examples:

1. **How to Start, Stop, and Keep Things Going:** Just like true love, the course of helping relationships does not always run smoothly. Getting things started on the right foot often depends on how you greet the other person, whether there is any initial social talk to reduce tension and "break the ice." Similarly, bringing things to a successful halt depends on whether you interrupt the person (and how you do so), how you announce that time is up, whether you evaluate the progress that has been made, how you say good-bye, and so on.

2. **How to Deal With Different People:** The infinite variety of human beings is what makes working with people so interesting, exciting, and challenging. It is also what makes it so difficult at times. The approach that a practitioner uses with one client may not work with someone else because of differences in sex, age, cultural backgrounds, personality, values, attitudes, and so forth. Although practitioners often long for a single strategy that will work well with everybody, the truth is they need to have several different strategies in their hip pocket, ready to be used when appropriate.

3. **How to Talk About Unpopular Topics:** All too often in helping relationships what needs to be said is what one person does not want to say and the other does not want to hear. Practitioners dread these difficult moments, and it is here, more than anywhere else, that they express a

need for additional interpersonal skills. The topics that are most difficult to handle are how to ask tough questions, how to discuss sensitive issues, and how to deliver bad news. Special skills training for these problems would go a long way toward alleviating the emotional exhaustion of burnout.[2]

Formal Professional Issues

Formal professional issues are potential stressors for physician assistants. Although significant progress has been made in many areas of the country, medical practice acts in some states are still harshly restrictive of PA practice. Reimbursement policies also vary dramatically from state to state and region to region. Institutions that have not previously employed PAs may need help in adapting their credentialing processes for the effective utilization of physician assistants. Relatively new graduates may have a poor appreciation of the rapid progress that has been made by the PA profession in removing barriers to practice. As a result, new PAs may feel helpless and hopeless. One of the best solutions is political involvement. State PA academies are always seeking the energies of PAs willing to serve on a wide range of committees, all ultimately dealing with the expansion of PA practice. Although some PAs have initially believed that they did not have either the time or the skills for such involvement, almost all PAs who have become engaged in these activities have found that the sense of "making a difference" is a strong deterrent to stress and burnout.

One stress that may be somewhat more pressing for PAs than for other providers is keeping up with new developments in order to maintain one's professional competence. Initially trained in a primary care model with broad skills, physician assistants are first certified by an examination that tests primary care knowledge. The re-certification examination may be less applicable to the practicing PA's knowledge base, although it may be a barrier to employment.

Although it is difficult for most health care professionals to keep up with continuing developments in the medical field, PAs are among the few health care professionals who must undergo periodic re-certification by examination at 6-year intervals. In addition,

the profession is the only one in which re-certification is tied directly to state registration and the right to work.[1]

Role Ambiguity Issues

Aside from the specifics of regulation, certification, and credentialing, the ambiguity of the PA profession is both the good news and the bad news. Many PAs have chosen the profession because of its limitless aspects. Other PAs are distressed by the fact that the PA career lacks precise definition with clearly delineated standards of practice, consistent legislation, and reimbursement standards throughout the country.

Trying to meet society's expectations for high-quality medical care in a time of rapid change in the health care system is both exciting and terrifying. Because it is a relatively new career, new opportunities for PAs are constantly being developed, often by creative and innovative members of the profession. Here, expectations are the critical factors. It is to be hoped that:

➤ PA program applicants have researched the profession as part of their entry process into training.
➤ PA programs have given the students exposure to practicing PAs serving as role models and providing realistic insights into both the frustrations and satisfactions of their jobs.
➤ PA students in their clinical rotations have sought to achieve an understanding of the emotional context of their jobs as part of their training.
➤ Practicing PAs regard questions from consumers about physician assistants as opportunities to educate them not only about PAs but also about the variety of health care professions that exist today.

BURNOUT

We are all concerned when stress turns to burnout. Originally thought of as a syndrome characterized by emotional depletion and exhaustion, burnout is now better understood as a state and process that begin as a response to work-related stressors.[3] Holmes and Fasser[1] describe the process as moving through tedium ("the experience of physical, emotional, and mental exhaustion precipitated by stress and characterized by feelings of strain, emotional and physical depletion, and negative attitudes toward self, environment, and life") into burnout. "The cumulative effects of sustained tedium in the work environment produce tension, irritability, and fatigue, which end in a defensive reaction of detachment, apathy, cynicism, or rigidity, referred to as burnout."[1]

Personal Characteristics

Some individuals seem more prone to burnout than others. According to Maslach,[2] "burnout is more likely if the person is younger, less mature, and less self-confident; is impulsive and impatient; has no family commitments but needs other people who can provide approval and affection; has goals and expectations that are not in tune with reality." Armstrong and colleagues[4] list four types of individuals most susceptible to burnout: "Those who assume too much responsibility and feel driven to achieve goals; those who view their jobs as the major reason for living and fail to develop outside activities; those who place a heavy emphasis on completing the task regardless of the cost; and those who are truly overworked."

Identifying Burnout

One of the biggest problems with burnout is that we are least able to identify it in ourselves until it is a critical problem. Thus, we must rely on our friends, family members, and colleagues to be our "early warning systems." Similarly, we must provide this same assistance to other friends in health care. Colon[3] suggests that clinicians should always "maintain a high index of suspicion. . . for symptoms of burnout." Complications can include depression, substance abuse, and even suicide. Appropriate and supportive referrals for assessment and treatment are particularly important.

Maslach[2] also believes that employers should be on the alert for burnout.

The organization should institute standard reviews, or pre-burnout "checkups" at periodic intervals (1 month after starting the job, then every 3 months or so). When such reviews are a ritualized and regular procedure for all staff, then no one person has to accept the burden of alerting you to the fact that you are beginning to get singed around the edges.

Assessment and Treatment

In assessing individual situations of burnout, three questions are important[2]:
➤ What is the individual's role?
➤ What roles do other people play?
➤ What role does the institution play?
Answers to these three questions will give some direction to a treatment plan.

On an individual level, Maslach describes the physical and psychological dysfunction accompanying burnout. "Exhaustion, illness, depression, irritability, increased use of alcohol and drugs—these are some of the personal costs."[2] Personal strategies might include a redefinition of work style and the search for a better balance between professional and private life.

In terms of patients and co-workers, interpersonal symptoms are changes in relationships with clients, such as callous and insensitive behavior. Colon[3] describes the "clues" of burnout in physician assistants:

> A classic example is when the clinician jokes about patients' illnesses, calls patients by symptoms, and becomes less trusting and less sympathetic toward them. Another sign is overall loss of concern and feeling for patients. Occasionally, however, the opposite is true: a burned out clinician becomes too involved with patients, or overidentifies with them—and commits a considerably greater number of hours than required for their care.

Strategies for interpersonal aspects of burnout most often include the assistance of others in the same or similar situation to offer perspectives and solutions. In some situations, the best treatment plan might also call for the assistance of a therapist experienced in the concerns of health care providers.

Burnout at the institutional level may be the result of unrealistic workloads, barriers to practice, inefficient staffing patterns, and poor management. Maslach[2] describes the effects of burnout at the institutional level as being "reflected in high rates of absenteeism, turnover, and complaints about staff performance." Strategies for a dysfunctional employment setting include "redesigning jobs, changing organizational policies, devising explicit structures and contracts, establishing flexible leaves and support services, and improving the training programs for staff."[2]

One of the most important aspects of burnout treatment (and prevention) is increasing an individual's sense of personal power, because it is "powerlessness" that makes one feel most trapped. Maslach discusses "ways in which the individual exerts some active control in a situation rather than just passively acquiescing to it. The person changes the work routine, redefines goals, utilizes downshifts, takes breaks, seeks out positive feedback, engages in decompression activities and so forth. All of these activities involve *choice* and *initiative*—the hallmarks of freedom and autonomy."[2] Believing that individual health care providers (PAs in this case) generally have more power than they realize, Maslach further notes that "by wiggling around in the job and finding out what can change and what cannot, the practitioner can counteract the helplessness and 'the hell with it all' attitude associated with burnout."[2]

The other well-known strategy for treating burnout is working toward the goal of re-establishing some balance in one's life. At the simplest level, this includes eating balanced meals and establishing realistic sleep and exercise patterns. Further activities include developing interests outside work and cultivating friendships and relationships away from the health care environment. Placing greater emphasis on family and leisure time has been effective for some individuals. Others have chosen to seek additional education or training as a way of expanding their horizons. Many health care providers see therapists as needed for help in balancing their lives.

CASE STUDY 20-1

Dennis is a 34-year-old paramedic enrolled in the first year of a physician assistant program. It is now halfway through the didactic year of training. His classmates are concerned that he has become increasingly "negative" toward the program in which he is enrolled. This seems particularly unusual to them because he had been working toward getting into this specific program for longer than 5 years prior to admission—expanding his clinical experience, enrolling in basic science coursework to fulfill the prerequisite requirements for program admission, and volunteering in community programs serving the homeless.

When his faculty advisor meets with him Dennis says he feels that much of the coursework is either "too soft and a waste of time" or "not appropriate to what PAs need to know." He feels that he is "not getting what he has paid for" from the program. The faculty advisor, who was also a former paramedic, suggests that he meet with some practicing PAs from similar backgrounds to find out their opinions on these issues. He provides him with three contacts, and they plan to meet again in a week.

The student meets with two of the graduates who are available that week. One works in a general internal medicine outpatient clinic, and the other is employed in a rural private practice. They both describe similar concerns during didactic training and independently share with him that, in retrospect, they feel that their frustration during didactic training was actually more related to their own role transition. One PA says that during his didactic training, he did not really understand the very broad roles that PAs are expected to play within the health care system. Therefore, he kept trying to "manage" his learning by focusing it down to specific areas (what he *thought* PAs "needed" to know). This strategy had worked during his paramedic career but turned out to be ineffective for a PA student. This PA suggests that the student look at the "bigger" picture and try to be less resistant and more flexible in his approach to the curriculum.

The second PA specifically wants to talk about the "softer stuff" in the curriculum. She says that she initially thought the behavioral science content of the program was totally unnecessary, until she got into her clinical year. In the first week of her first rotation (general internal medicine), she was "blown away" to find out how many of her patients had some behavioral science component to their illness. Not only that, but they also expected her to be comfortable talking about these issues. Even more surprising was the fact that she had gained competency in these skills during the didactic year, despite her resistance to these issues. Now she says it would almost be fun to take the behavioral science course again, if only she had the opportunity.

The student returns to meet with his advisor. He reports on his contact with the graduates, and they discuss the findings. Although Dennis says he still has concerns about what he is learning, he seems much less hostile and anxious. He says that he plans to try to be more flexible about his approach to the curriculum and his own learning. He also has made plans to keep in contact with both the graduates he has met. One of them has offered her clinic to him as a potential training site. He says that he really feels good about this. The student and his advisor schedule a follow-up appointment at the end of the quarter, or sooner if needed.

CASE STUDY 20-2

Jo is a senior student who has only three more clinical clerkships prior to her graduation. She has been a strong student throughout both the didactic and clinical years but suddenly seems to be behind in submitting her written assignments, including chart notes, patient care logs, and a research paper on "the perfect PA job." Her faculty advisor contacts her and arranges to visit Jo in her clinic, a VA outpatient site.

In meeting with Jo at the start of the day, the faculty advisor asks her how things are going and gets the following response: "I can't seem to get caught up. I can't sleep. I just can't do this!" She also says that she has a hard time fitting in regular meals, has totally abandoned her daily exercise routine, and has been just too busy to even interact with her fellow classmates on e-mail. Further conversation reveals that Jo is also engaged in negotiations with four potential employers, all in sites where she has previously been assigned for clinical rotations. She is receiving almost daily calls from all of these sites and feels that she has to make a decision immediately. At the same time, she notices that she is having trouble making decisions about even the most simple patient care issues.

The faculty advisor suggests that she needs to prioritize her concerns. If she spends too much time on future employment negotiations, she may not successfully complete the program. If she is ill—from not eating, not sleeping, and abandoning her social contacts—she will probably not be able to fulfill her job responsibilities in a new employment setting. In addition, she may be at risk for board examination failure if she continues to be distracted from her learning during the remaining 3 months of training. The student says, "Of course—why do you think I'm not sleeping!?"

They discuss a variety of strategies, including even a timeout from the program. Finally, they agree on the following actions:

➤ Complete any outstanding assignments as the highest priority, beginning with the copies of chart notes and patient care logs.
➤ Eat breakfast and lunch on a more regular schedule, attempt to re-institute an exercise routine, and decrease caffeine consumption.
➤ Delay job negotiations at least until the completion of this rotation.
➤ Re-establish contact with at least two fellow students.
➤ Plan for weekly follow-up with faculty advisor.
➤ Consider referral for supportive therapy if not improved.

CONCLUSION

Given the complexity and intensity of the health care system within which we all work, it is normal to expect that we will all be regularly subjected to significant amounts of stress. It is also important to acknowledge that we generally have anticipated this stress as part of our career choice. We may not, however, have always gauged accurately the emotional costs of pioneering what still is a relatively new career. We also may not always have recognized the importance that good interpersonal skills, strong support systems, and well-chosen jobs play in job satisfaction.

Unfortunately, it is not unreasonable to predict that everyone in health care will experience some form of burnout during his or her professional life. As Colon[3] points out, "Stress is a particularly urgent problem for PAs. Their unique position in health care delivery can intensify other stressors of medical practice.

Consequently, PAs must be especially on guard against burnout—in themselves, in other PAs, in supervising physicians, and in support staff."

Although PAs are generally very satisfied with their career and actively promote it to individuals choosing health care careers, we must be realistic in recognizing the sources of stress as well as satisfaction. It is only by recognizing those stresses and satisfactions that we are best able to evaluate our current professional and personal lives and make the ongoing choices that will sustain our health as individuals.

CLINICAL APPLICATIONS

1. Begin a personal "stress" log to document your progress in the program. On a daily or weekly basis, list all of those issues and concerns that you believe are contributing to your stress. Divide your list into two categories: (1) Things you can do something about and (2) things you cannot do anything about. Develop a strategy for attacking and resolving the items on the first list.

2. Interview at least one preceptor to whom you are assigned in your clinical year. Ask about his or her perception of common stresses in professional practice and abilities to resolve these stresses. Discuss what involvement he or she has with colleagues for mutual support.

REFERENCES

1. Holmes SE, Fasser CE. Occasional stress among physician assistants. J Am Acad Physician Assist 1993;6:172.
2. Maslach C. Burnout—The Cost of Caring. Englewood Cliffs, NJ: Prentice-Hall, 1982.
3. Colon EA. Burnout. Physician Assist 1986;10:18.
4. Armstrong M, King M, Meller B. Avoiding orientation burnout: a practical guide designed to help inservice instructors. Nurs Manage 1982;13:27.

RESOURCES

Alexander DA, Klein S. Caring for others can seriously damage your health. Hosp Med 2001;62:264.

Badger JM. Understanding secondary traumatic stress. Am J Nurs 2001;101:26 (quiz 32–3).

Carius M. Avoiding "training toxicity"—staying human during residency. Ann Emerg Med 2001;38:596.

Cherniss C. Beyond Burnout: How Teachers, Nurses, Therapists and Lawyers Recover from Stress and Disillusionment. New York: Routledge, 1995.

DiGiacomo M, Adamson B. Coping with stress in the workplace: Implications for new health professionals. J Allied Health 2001;30:106.

Figlery CR (ed). Compassion Fatigue: Coping with Secondary Traumatic Stress Disorders in Those Who Treat the Traumatized. Philadelphia: Brunner/Mazel, 1995.

Holland JW. A Doctor's Dilemma: Stress and the Role of the Career. New York: New York University Press, 1995.

Leatz CA, Stolar MW. Career Success/Personal Stress: How to Stay Healthy in a High Stress Environment. New York: McGraw-Hill, 1992.

Meier DE, Back AL, Morrison RS. The inner life of physicians and care of the seriously ill. JAMA 2001;286:3007.

CHAPTER 21

Employment: Building Your Career

Donald M. Pedersen

INTRODUCTION

To find an employment situation that is both professionally satisfying and financially rewarding is a primary concern of senior physician assistant (PA) students nearing the end of an intense curriculum. Will the rewards be there? Will the hard work and sacrifice pay off? In this chapter, various concepts are explored to help the new graduate maximize the opportunity for success in obtaining that first PA job.

NATIONAL STATISTICS

Physician assistants work in all 50 states, plus Washington, D.C., Guam, and Puerto Rico; around the world with the military; in multiple charitable and humanitarian aid efforts; and in various major corporations. Currently, there are nearly 60,000 clinically practicing PAs in the United States. PAs practice in virtually all health care settings and in every medical and surgical specialty.[1] Just under 30% of all PAs practice in rural areas (with a population of less than 50,000 people), and just over one half of all PAs are in primary care, with 34.5% in family or general practice. A full 21% of PAs practice in surgical specialties. Nearly three quarters of PAs practice in outpatient settings, and more than 88% are still engaged in clinical practice. The most comprehensive demographic study of the profession, compiled annually by the American Academy of Physician Assistants, is entitled *General Census Data on Physician Assistants.*[2]

Physician assistant was one of the 20 "Hot Professions" profiled in the November 11, 1991, issue of *U.S. News and World Report.*[3] The physician assistant profession was again profiled by *U.S. News and World Report* in 1997 as the number one hot career track for the health professions.[4] In 2002, the U.S. Bureau of Labor Statistics ranked PAs number 12 of the 15 fastest-growing occupations from 2000 to 2010.

THE SEARCH
Constituent Chapters of the American Academy of Physician Assistants (AAPA)

Each state has a constituent chapter of the AAPA, and most, if not all, chapters publish a state chapter newsletter or a web site. A job listing section is a common feature of these venues. A local listing of job possibilities in the state of one's choice could be invaluable. Membership in the state chapter may be required for one to receive this benefit, but the cost of student membership is typically quite low ($5 to $10 on average). It would be wise to ask whether the newsletter in question carries a job listing and whether copies of previous issues could be received as a membership benefit.

State AAPA chapters often sponsor continuing medical education (CME) courses as their major moneymaking events. Attendance at these events can also provide leads on unadvertised jobs, such as potential jobs that have not yet come to the formal

marketing stage but are being contemplated by physicians or health care organizations. As in many occupations, most job information for PAs is passed by word of mouth in a rather informal arrangement; knowing the right people and being in the right place at the right time can make all the difference. If the constituent chapter has a mechanism for recording a PA student's name and job requirements, take advantage of the opportunity.

Programs as a Resource

If there is a physician assistant training program in the PA student's preferred state for employment, this program is an important potential source of information on available jobs. Often, the state constituent chapter and the PA program work closely in delivering the services described previously. In addition to these activities, however, PA programs offer a wealth of information with regard to the practice climate for PAs, as well as which specific practices use and train physician assistants.

Key State PAs

In every state, certain key PAs, by their nature, have consistently remained involved in the profession as constituent chapter leaders, as advocates for the profession in legislative battles, as mentors for students, as public educators, and as participants in many other uncompensated and typically unrecognized activities over countless years. Identifying and contacting these individuals can yield valuable information. A request through a local CME program, a local PA program, or a state constituent chapter usually reveals the names of the key players. Their knowledge of local politics and their institutional memory can serve PA students well in the job search.

Professional Journals

Professional journals are another source of job information. Often, the classified ads are the sections reviewed first, not only by those seeking a first job and those interested in a change of work environment, but also by providers in stable, long-term positions who like to keep abreast of the trends in the marketplace, particularly salary trends. The profession currently has four major peer-reviewed journals: *Journal of the American Academy of Physician Assistants, Physician Assistant, Clinician Reviews,* and *Advance for Physician Assistants.*

Journal of the American Academy of Physician Assistants
This journal is published monthly by Medical Economics and is the official journal of the AAPA. A subscription is a member benefit that costs nonmembers $50 annually. The journal is dedicated to the education and advancement of the PA profession. The goal of the journal is to improve health care by publishing current information and research on clinical care, education, health policy, and professional issues. Job opportunities are included and typically all pertinent details are given, including information on how to directly contact a potential employer.

Physician Assistant
This journal is published monthly by Lippincott, Williams & Wilkins. Founded in 1976, it is the oldest of the PA journals and is available free to members of the AAPA. For nonmembers, the subscription rate is $58. *Physician Assistant* publishes a broad range of peer-reviewed clinical articles to support PAs in their pursuit of clinical excellence and to provide a forum in which PAs can consider their role in health care delivery. Job opportunities, listed in the classified advertisements, are arranged according to specialty.

Clinician Reviews
This journal, aimed at both PAs and nurse practitioners (NPs), is published monthly by Jobson Publishing. It is designed to keep these providers informed of the latest advances in health care and their application to clinical practice. Articles and features cover major areas of medicine and surgery. Summaries of significant articles in the leading medical literature are included, along with reports from medical meetings. Jobs are listed in the "Marketplace Express," which provides complete information on positions available nationally and internationally.

Advance for Physician Assistants
This PA journal is published monthly by Merion Publications and provides clinical and news information to physician assistants. Its mission is to provide practical, readable, up-to-the-minute clinical articles, practice and professional news, health coverage, and profiles from today's physician assistants. Jobs are listed by region in the "Career Opportunities" section of the journal.

Other Publications
Numerous other publications that can aid in the job search are available. AAPA members receive *AAPA News,* which is published twice monthly and contains a "PA Career" section that profiles current job opportunities across the nation. Additionally, this publication runs occasional articles on issues related to the job search. *NEWSLine for Physician Assistants* is intended to serve as a news and information source. This periodical includes a comprehensive "Employment Opportunities" section and can be quite helpful to the new graduate. *Clinician News,* which has been added as a resource from the publishers of *Clinician Reviews,* also provides job information and is published six times per year. *PA Today* has been published for several years and contains job information arranged by state. *PA Careers* is also available to help you in your search.

Job Placement Services
Many job placement firms are now directing their efforts toward the placement of PAs. For the most part, fees for the services of these agencies are paid by the hiring party. PA program faculty members usually advise caution in dealing with agencies and in particular recommend very careful reading of any contract to determine the responsibilities of those who sign. Information about these firms can be found in the advertising sections of professional journals. In communicating with an agent, or "headhunter," the student should ask for names of PAs who have been placed by the agency. He or she also should ask specific questions to determine the firm's familiarity with PA practice in the geographic areas where the student wishes to work.

Other Services
Other useful information may be obtained from the sources listed in the box on p. 442.

PA EMPLOYMENT RESOURCES

FAST FAX: The AAPA has a FAST FAX service that has a directory of documents on many topics of interest to the new graduate. The service can be reached by calling 1 (800) 286-2272.

Yearly Census Data: The AAPA provides yearly information on PAs, including practice demographics, individual salary profiles, and customized reports.

Internet Sites: The reader is referred to the Internet for further help with the job search. Following are some specific web sites that may offer assistance:

- www.aapa.org
- www.apap.org
- www.nurse.net/jobs/pa.html
- www.flintweb.com/employment.html
- www.careersonline.com.au/show/hosp/hosp.html
- www.hotjobs.com
- www.medconnect.com/newjobs/newspeclty.htm
- www.travcorps.com
- www.medical-admart.com
- www.provserv.com/pa-np.html
- www.AJB.dni.us/index.html
- www.healthcareers.com
- www.healthstaf.com/mainset_careeropps.htm
- www.occ.com
- www.careermosaic.com
- www.joblocator.com

THE RÉSUMÉ

One can think of a résumé as an advertisement about oneself, the primary purpose of which is to garner an interview with the physician or organization with which one desires to work. The résumé is neither an autobiography nor a 10-page description of everything one has ever done or been involved in. Conversely, it is not a brief outline of work experience or a simple compilation of job descriptions. Any graduate PA possesses the basic credentials to practice in the field. The PA must avoid the situation in which he or she eliminates job prospects by distributing a résumé that detracts from relevant skills and qualifications. Some common pitfalls in résumé preparation, as described by Tom Jackson of the Catalyst Group,[5] are the following:

- ➤ A sloppy and hastily written look.
- ➤ Vague and confusing content.
- ➤ Failure to stress skills and accomplishments.
- ➤ An excess of irrelevant information that obscures important points.
- ➤ A writing style that is unclear and hard to follow.
- ➤ Lack of visual appeal.[5]

Developing the Personal Biography

Education should be described at the beginning of the personal biography, which is the first step in developing the résumé. Of interest to potential employers is the college experience, including degrees obtained. Some states require a minimum of a bachelor's degree for PA practice. PA education should be recorded, along with the program certification date. Many new graduates choose to list the specific rotations or preceptorships that they have completed. The National Commission on Certification of Physician Assistants (NCCPA) certification warrants documentation because most states require initial national certification. The date of one's certification or the date one plans to sit for the national examination should be listed. Graduate courses or degrees as well as postgraduate training should also be detailed. Because most PA students come from the ranks of a variety of allied health disciplines, it is important to include training obtained before entrance into the PA program. For example, a graduate who is interested in an orthopedic PA position and has previously been an x-ray technician, or a graduate who desires to work as a PA in an emergency room setting and has been a paramedic, will stand out from other applicants by virtue of previously acquired skills and credentials.

Membership in professional and other organizations and the extent of involvement not only can demonstrate commitment to the profession but also can provide insight into civic, social, political, and cultural orientation. The graduate may need to use discretion in this type of disclosure, first assessing a potential employer's posture relative to the organizational affiliations.

Skills developed through formal and informal processes can be an invaluable selling point. Consider the employer who not only is involved in patient care but also is actively engaged in conducting research. An applicant who, through schoolwork or previous employment, has been involved in research design or technical writing may have an advantage over other applicants. One strength of the PA profession lies in the heterogeneous backgrounds of its students and the diversity they eventually bring to the PA workforce. Because the applicant pool for any given job is composed of individuals with a common credential, a candidate may be favored because of additional skills and whether these skills, along with PA training, can be used to address the potential employer's personnel needs.

Awards and recognition can enhance the biography and the résumé and help the reviewer gain further insight into the applicant's employability.

Hobbies and interests are generally of interest to those who review résumés. Information regarding the nonprofessional aspect of a graduate's life can facilitate a better understanding of how he or she might fit into the position and integrate with the clinic or hospital staff. The number of years involved and the degree of competence attained in a given area of interest would be informative, as would details on how the extracurricular activity might have some application to the professional role.

Work history, the final descriptive section of the personal biography, consists of a chronological listing of positions held. It begins with the most recent and works backward no farther than 10 years. Gaps in employment that cannot be accounted for by time spent in school or other training should be explained. Unpaid work or other experiences that have relevance to the position being applied for should also be catalogued. Each description should list the duties performed and relate briefly what was accomplished in the position. Names of supervisors and the address and telephone number of each employing organization should be included. Previous work experiences of value to a potential employer should also be described.

References are individuals who will honestly and candidly convey information regarding the applicant and his or her performance in many spheres, including personality traits, habits, work performance, emotional stability, and integrity. The applicant must choose references wisely and must have complete confidence in what they might disclose to a potential employer. It is common practice for employers to check with the officials of an applicant's PA education program regarding academic and behavioral performance. Anyone who has burned bridges during PA training is well advised to reevaluate his or her stature with the alma mater.

Compiling a personal biography is an introspective process. Transforming the personal biography into a functional résumé is the next step. The graduate should keep in mind that the main function of the résumé is to obtain an interview with the prospective employer. Anything that does not contribute to getting the interview should be eliminated.[5] Things such as the names and ages of children, lengthy descriptions of leisure activities that have nothing to do with job targets, and lists of personal friends and references tend to clutter the résumé and detract from the essential information being communicated.

Organizing the Résumé

The organization of the résumé can take one of three forms: the chronological, the functional, or a combination of the two.

The chronological résumé, as the name implies, is a listing of current and former jobs in reverse chronological order. This is probably the most widely used format and has several advantages—ease of preparation, familiarity to professional interviewers, and emphasis on a steady employment record. The drawbacks are that it can reveal employment gaps, it may emphasize areas that the applicant may want to minimize, and skill areas might be difficult to discern.

The functional résumé is organized to highlight the qualifications of the applicant, with little emphasis on specific dates. The advantages are that it stresses selected skill areas, it can help camouflage a spotty employment record, it allows for the emphasis of professional growth, and positions not related to current career goals can be played down. One disadvantage is that employers might be suspicious of it and will want to see supplemental documentation of work history.[5]

The combination résumé is similar in format to the functional résumé, but company names and dates of employment appear in a separate section. This format allows an applicant to stress the preferred and most relevant skill areas and at the same time satisfies the employer's desire to know specific names and dates. It offers an opportunity to emphasize the applicant's most relevant skills and abilities, allows gaps in employment to be played down, and can be varied to emphasize chronology and de-emphasize functional descriptions, or vice versa.[5] By its nature, the combination format can take longer to read, and an employer can lose interest unless it is very succinctly written.

In some cases, a well-composed letter can be used as an alternative to the résumé, particularly by one who has little work history related to the position sought, or by an applicant who is making a career change. Because most new PA graduates are indeed making a career change, a well-formulated letter as an alternative may be appropriate. However, a potential employer may also ask for a résumé, which is usual and customary. In this case, the most appropriate type would be a functional or combination résumé because it would be desirable to emphasize skills acquired in the past, as well as the newly acquired PA training. A cover letter to the potential employer is essential regardless of the presence of a résumé.

Résumé Layout

Some specific tips on the layout of your résumé follow:

➤ Lines should be single-spaced and the total length should be a page or two. Long résumés have a smaller chance of being read carefully.

➤ An attractive amount of white space should be retained; top, bottom, and side margins should be at least 1 inch; paragraphs should be separated by double spacing.

➤ Paragraphs should be kept short (i.e., no more than eight to ten lines).

➤ Long ideas should be broken into short sentences or phrases.

➤ Each new category of information (e.g., education, work experience) should be emphasized in such a way that readers can find specific information quickly.

➤ Unnecessary and obvious captions such as "Name" and "Address" should be avoided.[5]

Other Resources

For information beyond these basics, the reader is referred to the multitude of reference texts on this subject, many of which include examples of various résumé formats. These can be reviewed at local libraries or purchased at bookstores.

SELLING ONESELF

Having completed training, prepared a résumé, and researched the local or national job market, the graduate must next approach job situations that seem the most promising. Because the résumé is standardized, a cover letter directed to the appropriate individual, specifically detailing interest in the desired position, can allow the graduate to make a personal pitch based on his or her analysis of the employer's needs. It can also demonstrate knowledge of the practice or, in some cases, persuade the individuals involved that they could indeed benefit by including the applicant in their practice. The cover letter should be no longer than one page in length and should always conclude with a request for an interview. If referred to the practice by a person influential in the field, the applicant should mention this fact, taking care not to overdo it. The purpose of the letter is to get a foot in the door, especially if a formal job opening has not been announced but the position represents the ideal career move.

The Interview

Nearly all employers use the interview to help in selection and evaluation of future employees. It is virtually impossible to land a job without being interviewed.[5] Often, it is not necessarily the most qualified person who gets the job. The first choice of employers may be the person who makes the best first impression and is the most skilled at finding a job. The interview is an opportunity for both parties to become better acquainted and to determine whether their expectations surrounding the position in question are mutually compatible. Is the position right for the applicant, and is he or she right for the position?

The structured interview follows a format similar to the structure of a chronological résumé. Work experience, education and training, outside activities and interests, and other achievements are discussed in turn. While gaining a better understanding of these areas of concern, the interviewer will also discover information about the applicant's personality, as well as social, communication, analytical, and decision-making skills. Research demonstrates that interviewers actually talk about 65% of the time during the interview, and interviewees talk 35% of the time.[5] Most interviewers would agree that they appreciate the interviewee who talks and asks questions—it makes their job easier.

The unstructured interview follows no particular order, and questions are often asked spontaneously. Physicians are likely to conduct an unstructured interview. However, the applicant should count on a more structured interview if a clinic business or personnel manager is involved. It is important to find out who makes the hiring decisions. If these decisions are made by individuals other than those with whom the applicant would be working, he or she should arrange to meet with the supervising physician and other providers in the clinic to determine whether they would be compatible.

There is no substitute for being prepared. In general, interviewers make their decisions on the basis of appearance, perceived or demonstrated motivation, communication skills, academic standing, and personality. Not surprisingly, command of speech is often used as a way to measure intelligence and competence.[5] It has been noted that interviewers are more influenced by unfavorable information than by the reverse. Thus, lack of preparation, overconfidence, cockiness, put-ons, falseness, superficiality, and late arrival can severely affect one's chance of success. Employers are looking for applicants with ambition, poise, sincerity, trustworthiness, articulateness, analytical ability, and initiative who also look neat and clean and do not display an extreme style of dress.[5] In the health care field, it is an advantage to live the healthy lifestyle one preaches to one's patients, and such a lifestyle may well provide an edge in the job market. In the interview, the applicant should relax and be genuine. He or she should use the techniques learned in stress management class to channel nervous energy and use it for a positive effect. A firm handshake and direct eye contact are a good start in the process of selling oneself.

PA Program Productivity Records

Many PA programs require that students keep a log of the patients they see during the clinical year of training for the purpose of documenting the volume and variety of patient contact. The graduate can use these log records advantageously in the application and negotiation process. A new PA can gain a realistic idea of earning potential by translating the volume and variety figures from the patient logs into actual practice charges. This allows for more effective negotiation of the contract by providing a basis of real and relevant numbers, as opposed to speculation or reliance on national data. As a caveat, the literature suggests that PAs can see 70% to 90% of the patients in a family practice setting, and they can do so at a 90% productivity rate compared with the supervising physician.

Additional Certificates and Credentials

Special recognition in surgery obtained through the NCCPA could be of particular importance to an orthopedic surgeon with whom a PA might like to work. Likewise, the Advanced Cardiac Life Support certificate acquired as part of training would be of interest to individuals who are staffing a hospital emergency room, or who practice at a remote site 50 miles from nowhere in which the applicant would like to work. Additionally, training and experience acquired before PA certification is attained can bolster one's negotiating position. Certain practice settings might lend themselves better to a PA who was a nurse or a paramedic first.

CONTINUED EMPLOYABILITY

It is imperative that PA graduates become familiar with the laws that govern PA practice in the state in which they first find employment. In some states, a temporary licensure or registration is granted that allows PA practice for new graduates until national board scores are released. Other states do not allow PAs to practice until after they have attained certification. This situation may have an impact on the decision to make a home in one state versus another.

FINANCIAL COMPENSATION

Compensation for services rendered can take many forms. Unfortunately, the category that preoccupies the minds of most new graduates is salary. Although this is understandable, given the time and ever-increasing cost of PA education, salary is only one of the many benefits to consider when one is evaluating a job offer.

Based on demonstrated competence and the quality of care provided throughout two decades of practice, the demand for PA services fueled an increase in salaries for PAs during the late 1980s and early 1990s. During this time, there was a twofold rise in PA salaries.[6] Presently, according to AAPA national census data (based on the 2001 census of AAPA members and nonmembers), the median total annual income from the primary employer for respondents who work at least 32 hours per week for their primary employer and who are not active duty military or self-employed was $67,743, with a mean salary of $71,046. Comparable figures for respondents who graduated in or after 2000 (new graduates) were $58,578 and $59,839, respectively.[7,8]

According to Cannon,[9] to negotiate effectively, a PA must know the following:

1. What PAs in his or her specialty and practice setting earn around the country.
2. What PAs in his or her specialty and practice setting are making in the particular locale.
3. What other health care providers are making per hour in the particular locale.
4. The local standard charges for medical services the PA will be providing.

Knowing these facts will help PAs to define a reasonable salary structure and make a case for their asking price. New graduates should consider a confirmed salary, especially if productivity is in question, a specialty practice setting is desired, or a significant amount of on-the-job training is anticipated. They should, however, leave the door open to renegotiate for a salary plus a percentage or a salary plus a bonus after they feel comfortable in the practice setting. It is important to gain a full understanding of the expectations of the employer, including hours per week, time spent on call, and additional benefits, before making a decision on the appropriate salary level. Likewise, a PA should not accept a job offer until the financial compensation and benefits package have been fully negotiated.

BENEFITS

The personal benefits accrued through employment can be as important as the most sought-after salary. Some benefits might be considered luxury items, whereas others are critical to a PA's professional well-being.

Continuing Medical Education

CME is a fact of life in the PA profession. Maintaining current national certification by NCCPA requires 100 hours of CME for each 2-year period. State laws vary on this requirement, and the potential employer must understand the importance of CME not only from a regulatory standpoint but also from a quality of care perspective. Keeping current is a professional responsibility, one that the PA shares with the employer. Thus, sharing the cost is a reasonable approach; the applicant should start high and negotiate down if necessary. A physician employer or interviewer may be receptive to the idea of CME benefits, but an applicant who is negotiating with a nonclinician may need to state the case for this important benefit, which requires both time and money. Ten paid days per year is a good place to start, but fewer than five would not be realistic. A specified amount of money set aside each year for travel, fees, and accommodations is the general arrangement. A national conference in a major, distant city can easily cost $2000 to $3000 for 1 week of CME and may garner 20 to 30 Category 1 CME credits. A negotiated amount of $2500 to $5000 annually would be a reasonable employer share of CME costs.

Vacation

Life in the patient care "trenches" can be physically demanding and mentally taxing. Provider burnout is often mentioned in the professional literature. To a new graduate entering a profession he or she may have long sought after, the idea of vacation time may not be of much importance. A word of caution: time spent away from the practice is critical, not only for the personal satisfaction that avocational activities bring, but also for the renewal and revival that are brought back to the practice. In a large corporate practice setting, a PA may be locked into a standard package of benefits, including vacation time. If there is room to negotiate, it would be helpful for the PA to know what is standard practice in the community.

Sick Leave

Sick leave is an important consideration in any employment situation. A defined amount of time and how the time can be used should be spelled out to avoid confusion. For example, can it be used when a family member is sick and needs tending to, or only for periods of personal illness or injury? The question of carrying sick time forward and accumulating a number of weeks or months should be clarified, as well as whether unused sick leave can be converted into vacation time according to some standardized formula.

Maternity or Family Leave

Nearly half of all practicing PAs are women. Although maternity leave is not entirely a women's issue, contracted maternity benefits of some sort are an important consideration for all female PAs of childbearing age. Questions to be answered include the length of time off, whether a salary will continue, whether other benefits such as health insurance will continue, what continued responsibilities the PA might have during time off, whether an alternative job structure such as part-time work is an option, and whether a leave of absence is a possibility. Policies may already be in place, and some employers are more receptive than others to the idea of family leave for both male and female providers. Specific answers to these questions are varied and often conditional. In Canada, maternity leaves average 4 to 5 months; in Sweden, employees are given 18 months of paid parental leave. One author recommends 2 months as the minimum amount, adding that less than 6 weeks is physically and emotionally difficult.[9] Another consideration is whether sick leave benefits can or must be used for maternity leave.

Health, Life, and Disability Insurance

The need for health insurance is obvious and critically important. Our current national rate of uninsured people underscores the need to provide for self and family. Through their training, PAs have probably been touched by the calamity the lack of health insurance can bring to individuals and families. In past years, the physician-employer may have offered his or her services or the services of the clinic in the event of an employee's personal or family illness. Although well intentioned, this approach could leave the PA sorely lacking if a catastrophic illness or injury were to occur. A health insurance policy with benefits clearly spelled out is mandatory for the health and well-being of both PAs and their families.

Disability insurance and life insurance are somewhat more negotiable and might be considered icing on the cake if acquired as benefits of employment. An interesting twist on this issue is the idea of a life insurance policy taken out on the supervising physician with the PA as the beneficiary. Because PAs are interdependent providers, the death of a supervising physician can lead at best to a lapse of employment for the PA, or at worst to a complete job switch, perhaps necessitating a change in geographic location.

Retirement Benefits

An area that is often neglected in negotiations for a clinical position is the issue of eventual retirement. The capital to live comfortably in one's retirement years must come from somewhere, so a plan needs to be in place. The options are limitless and ever-changing, and as such are clearly beyond the scope of this text. The applicant should inquire about plans already available for other providers in the practice. Most financial consultants would advise beginning some plan immediately, no matter how small. A PA involved in a nonprofit arrangement can qualify for many supplemental annuity benefit plans. Some of these plans are self-pay, and some plans are a combined effort between the employee and the employer. These plans and other financial vehicles can allow employees to shelter money before it is taxed, thus lowering taxable income while accumulating a substantial nest egg for use at a later date when a lower tax bracket would apply. The applicant should consult a financial advisor or take advantage of the consultants used by the practice to maximize savings potential and to outline the best possible tax strategy.

Professional Fees

Membership and plans for involvement in professional societies are included in many employment arrangements. Annual dues for the AAPA provide many benefits, not the least of which is the availability of technical assistance and effective political involvement from an extremely motivated and knowledgeable staff. AAPA membership also includes newsletters, magazine subscriptions, and reduced registration rates at the national PA conference. Each state also has a constituent chapter of the national organization, with dues ranging from $50 to $100. Becoming active on a local and national level can ensure that PAs will continue to enjoy a positive professional atmosphere.

There are also local licensure or registration fees to pay. The fee to apply initially is higher than the annual or biennial fee required to maintain current regulatory credentials. It is important to know what these fees entail and to negotiate for their payment by the practice. To maintain national certification from the NCCPA, a fee and documentation of the required amount of CME (85 credits) must be submitted every 2 years. The initial NCCPA certifying examination costs more than $400, and the re-certification examination, which is required every 6 years to maintain national certification, is more than $200. Making a potential employer aware of these ongoing professional financial requirements may work to the applicant's advantage. Often, this category of benefit is lumped in with a CME fund. If this is the case, the substantial membership and certification fees may limit the PA's ability to attend desired CME activities.

Malpractice Insurance

No PA job applicant should conclude negotiations without settling on the extent of malpractice coverage that is prudent for that particular practice setting. Most commonly, PA insurance is added as a rider to the policy carried by the supervising physician. Individual policies are available through a number of insurance carriers and may indeed prove to be a better choice, particularly if the PA has multiple practice sites and multiple employers. Geographic location and practice specialty dictate the cost of coverage. Having the supervising physician check on the cost of adding a PA to the policy is appropriate. Information on individual coverage is available through the AAPA.

CONTRACTS

A written contract that spells out all the preceding topics is essential to avoid future frustration or disenchantment with the employer. The contract could be reviewed on an annual basis as part of a performance evaluation. A written contract provides a basis for ongoing negotiations. Verbal promises can be forgotten or distorted, but a document that is mutually agreed upon and signed protects both parties.

OWNERSHIP, PARTNERSHIP, AND OTHER PRACTICE OPTIONS

Nationwide, PAs are developing a wide range of practice situations. Outright PA ownership of practices through purchase, hiring physicians to satisfy the need for supervision, establishing corporations to own practices, and creating partnership arrangements are but a few of the ways in which PAs are exercising the entrepreneurial spirit. A review of the existing state laws governing PA and physician practice is of paramount importance in considering the legal and ethical implications of such arrangements because some states have statutes or rules that prohibit many of these practice options. Knowledge of the statutes and rules pertaining to PA practice is prudent, as is legal consultation.

Dependent practice is the cornerstone of the PA profession, and any practice arrangement that erodes the relationship between the PA and the supervising physician is unacceptable. This is not to say that independent action and problem solving are not integral parts of PA practice regardless of the setting. PA practice must take place within a framework of responsible supervision. If this basic tenet can exist within a nontraditional practice arrangement, such an arrangement should by all means be explored by the PA and potential partners, employees, or employers.

RURAL PRACTICE SUPPORT BENEFITS

By its nature, rural practice presents additional challenges to the PA in terms of lifestyle and support mechanisms. Housing and locum tenens capabilities are particularly important in this setting. A request for paid housing would not be out of the question in a geographically remote region where available housing is scarce. The ability to get away from the practice for vacation and CME is critical. (All the vacation and CME benefits in the world are useless if coverage for the practice cannot be found.) The interested applicant should explore the existence of locum tenens services on a state or national level and make clear that time away from the practice needs to be assured.

CASE STUDY 21-1

A senior PA, with 20 years of experience in the same clinical site, is seeking a new job rather than remain with his clinic, which has been purchased by a large for-profit health care system. As part of his transition, he consults a career counselor for advice on how to approach the job search. Because he had felt that the counselor would simply help him "design" his job search, he is somewhat startled to hear the counselor's recommendations.

First, the counselor advises him to "deal with his feelings about his decision." The counselor suggests that this type of change is similar to a grieving process and that this type of change should be approached as a process that will take some time to complete. In the meantime, the PA must be prepared to answer questions in job interviews about why he has made this choice. The trick will be to present the decision in a positive light rather than to display anger and negativity about the previous employment setting. The counselor points out that employers are not enthusiastic about hiring employees with "baggage," regardless of the amount of clinical experience.

The counselor then advises the PA to "practice" with some mock job interviews. Again, the PA is puzzled: "I've been doing this forever. Why should I have to do a dress rehearsal?" The counselor explains that the job market is different today from what it was 20 years ago and that the PA may need to meet with a range of interviewers—administrators as well as the physician-preceptor. Therefore, greater attention is needed in preparing for both the interview "style," as well as its "content."

Finally, the counselor asks the PA to prepare a list of "negotiating points" or "highest priorities" to assist him in clarifying his search. The counselor points out that what experienced providers are seeking in a job is generally very different from those job attributes sought by new graduates. The counselor advises the PA to be clear about his preferences during the employment interview.

In summary, the counselor advises the PA to prepare for job interviews by having answers to any questions that might be asked about PA practice, having answers about optimum relationships with other providers (physicians and NPs), and clearly communicating strengths and priorities in addition to past clinical experience.

CASE STUDY 21-2

A new PA accepts her first job as a "contract" worker with an emergency department in a medium-sized hospital. She is proud because her hourly salary, when calculated for a full year, is about 20% higher than what is being paid to her classmates.

She is excited to receive her first paycheck and quickly deposits it in the bank without really looking at the attached pay stub. She does the same with the second check. Upon receiving the third check, she notices that the amount "earned" is identical to the amount "paid." She goes to her supervisor, who refers her to the payroll office of the hospital. In meeting with a staff person there, she is surprised to find that her salary does not include benefits and that as a "contract worker," she is required to pay her taxes (quarterly) as well as provide her own benefits (CME, health insurance, disability insurance). Fortunately, she is covered under the hospital's malpractice insurance. In addition, she will not receive any vacation or sick leave; instead, she simply will not be paid for this time off.

After her shock, she decides to consult a personal accountant and to reevaluate her job situation.

CONCLUSION

At present, there is much discussion and debate relative to the appropriate mix and number of health care practitioners needed in the future. What the future holds for PAs in the existing managed care marketplace is not entirely clear. Over the past 5 years, there has been a proliferation of both PA and nurse practitioner programs, with unprecedented numbers of graduates in both disciplines being produced. In the face of a pending physician oversupply during the next decade, the PA graduate of today faces greater challenges in finding initial employment. An in-depth discussion on this topic can be found in a recent issue of *Journal of the American Academy of Physician Assistants*.[10] Additionally, the Association of Physician Assistant Programs (APAP) commissioned a blue ribbon panel to explore the issues surrounding PA program expansion. The report of the panel provides an excellent synopsis of the issues regarding workforce supply and demand. The complete report can be found in "Perspective on Physician Assistant Education."[11] PA graduates not only will need to sell themselves in the future but will need to sell their profession to the corporate powers that play an ever-increasing role in the way health care is delivered today. A keen knowledge of the history of the profession, the significance of the educational process, the credential mechanism for programs and individuals, and the data relative to PA practice, including cost effectiveness and productivity, will be crucial to the graduates of the future.

CLINICAL APPLICATIONS

1. List and describe all of the potential information sources on available jobs (e.g., newspaper ads, state academy job listings) that should be collected before one applies for and selects a job. Discuss how you might screen these jobs to choose which jobs to apply for. What are your highest priority issues (e.g., hours worked, benefits, preceptor availability) in choosing your first job?

2. Do you think it is important to ask an employer to pay professional dues in the American Academy of Physician Assistants or your state PA chapter? In other professional organizations? Why or why not?

3. Compare your previous experiences with job interviews (pre-PA) with those of other colleagues. Were common questions asked? What was the interview environment? What was the expectation for "appropriate dress" for the interview? How might PA job interviews be different from other job interview situations?

4. Seek out and interview PA graduates who have recently begun practice or changed jobs. Ask their advice about the job interview situations they encountered. What recommendations do they have for you?

REFERENCES

1. Physician Assistant: A Quarter Century of Quality Care. Alexandria, Va: American Academy of Physician Assistants, 1992.
2. General Census Data on Physician Assistants. Alexandria, Va: American Academy of Physician Assistants, 2001.
3. Hot tracks in 20 professions. U.S. News World Report 1991;111:97.
4. 20 hot job tracks. U.S. News World Report 1997;123:96.
5. The Catalyst Group. Marketing Yourself: The Catalyst Guide to Successful Résumés and Interviews, 6th ed. New York: Bantam Books, 1986.
6. Willis J. Explaining the salary discrepancy between male and female PAs. J Am Acad Physician Assist 1992;5:280.
7. General Census Data on Physician Assistants 2001. Alexandria, Va: American Academy of Physician Assistants, 2001.
8. General Census Data on Physician Assistants 1991. Alexandria, Va: American Academy of Physician Assistants, 1991.
9. Cannon CS. Professional issues for PA mothers. J Am Acad Physician Assist 1992;5:261.
10. Cawley JF, Jones PE, Hooker RS. Are there (a) too many, (b) too few, or (c) just enough PAs? J Am Acad Physician Assist 1997;10:80.
11. Carter RD, Cowley JF, Hooker RS, et al: Perspective on physician assistant education. Physician Assist Progr Exp 1998;9:20.

RESOURCES

Susan Ireland. The Complete Idiot's Guide to the Perfect Résumé. New York: MacMillan General Reference Publications, 1996. *Rated as one of the top publications on this subject, this book helps the reader to focus on the appropriate information to be included in a professional résumé. The guide includes templates for building résumés, tips for job hunters, and suggestions for feeling confident during the job search.*

From Program to Practice: A Guide to Beginning Your New Career. Alexandria, Va: American Academy of Physician Assistants, 1997. *This comprehensive guide provides details and recommendations on every aspect of the transition from student to graduate. This publication is usually provided to senior PA students through their program.*

Donaldson MC, Donaldson M, Frohnmeyer D. Negotiating for Dummies. Foster City, Calif: IDG Books, 1996. *General information about the negotiation process that can be applied to job negotiations. This book also includes valuable information for use in negotiating with patients, health care administrators, and other health care providers.*

Tysinger JW. Resumes and Personal Statements for Health Professionals. Tucson, Ariz: Galen Press Limited, 1994. *Providing guidance on strategies to describe accomplishments and emphasize strengths, this publication also includes examples of actual résumés and personal statements.*

Marino K. Résumés for the Health Care Professional. New York: John Wiley & Son, 1993. *Sample cover letters, thank-you letters, and résumés are provided by the author. The author also includes interview tips and identifies the 25 tough questions most often asked by interviewers, answers to these questions, and key questions the interviewee should ask in return.*

CHAPTER 22

Financing and Reimbursement

Michael Powe

INTRODUCTION

For most Americans, managed care continues to be the dominant force responsible for the way in which their health care is delivered. Recently, however, it has become an increasingly difficult task to define managed care. Conceptually, managed care sought to bring greater continuity and cost-effective access to health care. Practically speaking, managed care, in part, was characterized by the ability of managed care organizations (MCOs) and other payers to control access and direct patients to specific health care practitioners and hospitals. This task was accomplished through the use of gatekeepers, pre-certification techniques, and other methods that led to reduced access to care or, in some cases, denial of services based on the managed care organization's determination that the services provided did not meet its definition of medical necessity. We have begun to see a shift back toward increased consumer choice and flexibility, sometimes referred to as *consumer-driven health care,* that eliminates many of the restrictions and barriers put in place by MCOs. The problem is that as MCOs relax some of their restrictive rules and consumers gain more control over their

health care, we are experiencing a resurgence of the very issues that brought about managed care in the first place—double-digit increases in health insurance premiums.

Managed care organizations and insurance companies, along with the primary purchasers of health care services—employers and federal and state government agencies—are again facing the complex challenge of attempting to balance the competing goals of containing health care costs while at the same time maintaining or increasing appropriate access to care. Ongoing changes and the often complex coverage rules and regulations can be confusing to patients and health care practitioners alike. Those practitioners who fail to understand the underlying philosophies driving this country's health care delivery system run the risk of being at a competitive disadvantage in the health care marketplace.

Concerns about access to care, appropriate utilization of services, and cost remain at the forefront of our health care system. Rising costs and the realization that resources are not unlimited have magnified the debate as to who should control decisions regarding access to and availability of services and

452

who should be responsible for paying for those services. Payment or reimbursement for professional services affects delivery of and access to health care services. It is essential for the consumer to understand both the official and unofficial rules about how public and private payers view coverage of medical and surgical services delivered by physician assistants (PAs).

PROFESSIONAL SERVICES

Physician assistants deliver physician-quality medical and surgical services that would otherwise be provided by a physician. Numerous objective reports and studies have verified that within the PA's scope of practice, the quality of care is the same as that provided by physicians. In addition, patient satisfaction with services provided by PAs is nearly equal to that associated with physician services as part of the physician/PA team concept of delivering health care.

When dealing with public and private payers, it is useful to avoid the term "physician assistant services" because this can be construed to refer to a separate set of services not already included in the patient's benefit package.

GOVERNMENT-RUN PROGRAMS

There are two government-run health programs for the general public—Medicare and Medicaid.*

Medicare

Medicare, which provides coverage to more than 39 million people, is available for the aged (over 65 years), the disabled who have received cash benefits under Social Security for at least 24 months, and those with permanent kidney failure (e.g., end-stage renal disease). The Medicare program is administered

---

*Although the federal government sponsors the Federal Employee Health Benefits Program (FEHBP) and the Civilian Health and Medical Program of the Uniformed Services (CHAMPUS), now known as TRICARE, these programs operate much like private insurance programs. These two programs are open only to government/military employees and retirees, and their spouses and dependents.

by the federal government and is funded through a combination of Medicare premiums or taxes, general fund revenues, and patient deductibles and co-payments.

Medicare insurance is divided into two parts—A and B. Medicare Part A pays for hospital facility costs, health care personnel who do not provide physician-type professional services, some inpatient care in a skilled nursing facility (SNF), home health care, and hospice care. Medicare Part B pays for professional services delivered by physicians and physician assistants, durable medical equipment, and other medical services and supplies not covered by Part A.

Medicare Part A   Generally, Part A does not recognize individuals but rather pays institutions such as hospitals on an all-inclusive rate basis. Hospitals, for example, are paid by Part A for inpatient care based on a patient-specific diagnosis-related group (DRG). This lump-sum DRG payment is intended to cover certain employee costs, overhead costs of the institution, and supply costs during the patient's stay in the hospital. This prospectively determined DRG payment is meant to cover all facility-related costs associated with the patient's care for the particular admission. If the hospital can deliver the necessary treatment to the patient for less than the DRG payment amount, the hospital keeps the difference. If the hospital's costs for delivering care are higher than the DRG payment, the hospital loses money. Currently, there are some 523 DRGs, as determined by the Centers for Medicare and Medicaid Services, the government agency that administers the Medicare and Medicaid programs.

Administratively, payments to hospitals are made by *intermediaries,* who are under contract to the federal government to administer the Part A program in their service areas. Intermediaries are typically insurance companies, such as Blue Cross.

Medicare Part B   Medicare Part B pays for professional services provided in hospitals, nursing homes, private offices, or a patient's home. Part B also covers services provided "incident to" the physician's care. As with Part A, Medicare contracts with private insurance companies, such as Blue Shield, to administer the Part B program on behalf of the federal government. The administrators of the Part B program are called *carriers*.

Most Medicare beneficiaries receive services on what is commonly referred to as a *fee-for-service* basis. Under such an option, if a patient walks into a physician's office with a broken arm, the physician takes an x-ray, reads the x-ray, sets and casts the fracture, and bills Medicare for the services provided. The value of the service is determined according to the Resource-Based Relative Value Scale (RBRVS).

Fee-for-service gives the beneficiary maximum flexibility in selecting the physician or other practitioner of choice. However, the patient's out-of-pocket expenses can be highest under the fee-for-service arrangement.

Medicare beneficiaries must satisfy an annual deductible before Medicare pays for any services they receive. (Some Medicare health maintenance organizations [HMOs] and managed care plans may waive the deductible payment.) Once the deductible ($100 for office-based services and $812 for a hospital admission, as of 2002) has been met, Medicare covers 80% of the fee schedule amount, and the patient is responsible for the remaining 20%. Medicare's fee schedule amount is generally less than the medical practice's usual charge for the service or the amount the practice charges private payers. This is best shown by a list of the typical fees assessed for the patient who became dizzy and fell off a ladder, as described in Case Study 22-1.

CASE STUDY 22-1

Patient: John Jackson, Provincetown, Massachusetts

Practitioner: Samuel Smith, MD, Provincetown, Massachusetts

Medical problem: Patient was on a ladder changing a light bulb. Patient became dizzy, fell, and is suspected to have a broken arm.

Services Provided	Charge	Fee Schedule
Office visit	$55	$40
X-ray	$65	$55
Casting	$50	$45
Total	$170	$140

Although the fees the physician normally charges amounted to $170, Medicare's approved fee schedule allowed the physician to charge only $140. The actual Medicare payment to the practice would be $112 ($140 × 80%), with the patient being responsible for the 20% (or $28) difference, assuming that the patient has paid his $100 deductible and the physician participates with Medicare.

Physician Assistants   PAs are covered by law under Medicare's fee-for-service plan. PAs may be covered under Medicare's managed care plans, also known as Medicare+Choice or Medicare HMOs, at the discretion of the managed care entity that runs the plan. Table 22-1 details Medicare's coverage policy. If a PA provides a physician service that would be covered by Part B of Medicare if provided by a physician, the PA's service is covered in all settings.

For some time, PAs have been covered for services delivered in hospitals, nursing facilities, and rural health professional shortage areas, and for first-assisting at surgery. Rates of reimbursement have ranged from 65% to 85%. However, services provided by PAs in nonrural health professional shortage area offices and clinics were covered only when billed under the "incident to" billing method, which required the constant on-site presence of the physician. In 1997, the Balanced Budget Act extended coverage to all practice settings at one uniform rate.[1] As of January 1, 1998, Medicare pays the PA's employer for medical and surgical services provided by the PA at 85% of the physician's fee schedule. This includes the office or clinic setting even when the physician is not physically present, if allowed by state law.

The PA's employer bills for the services delivered by the PA, and payment is made to the employer. The employer is required to accept assignment for services

Table 22-1   Medicare Policy for Physician Assistants

Setting	Supervision	Reimbursement Rate	Services
Office or clinic when physician is not on-site	State law	85% of physician's fee schedule	All services PA is legally authorized to provide that would have been covered if provided personally by a physician
Office or clinic when physician is on-site	Physician must be in the suite of offices	100% of physician's fee schedule*	Same as above
Home visit or house call	State law	85% of physician's fee schedule	Same as above
Skilled nursing facility and nursing facility	State law	85% of physician's fee schedule	Same as above
Office or home visit if rural health professional shortage area	State law	85% of physician's fee schedule	Same as above
Hospital	State law	85% of physician's fee schedule	Same as above
First-assisting at surgery in all settings	State law	85% of physician's first-assist fee schedule†	Same as above
Federal rural health clinic	State law	Cost-based reimbursement	Same as above
HMO‡	State law	Reimbursement is on capitation basis	All services contracted for as part of an HMO contract

*Using carrier guidelines for "incident to" services.
†85% × 16% = 13.6% of primary surgeon's fee.
‡Some Medicare HMO risk contracts may exclude nonphysician providers.

provided by the PA. In all cases, the PA must be supervised by a physician; however, the degree of supervision is determined by state law. Typically, when billing is submitted under the PA's name and Medicare provider number at 85%, general supervision is required. General supervision simply requires that the physician and the PA have access to electronic (e.g., telephone) communication. The PA's employer can be a physician, physician group, hospital, nursing home, group practice, professional medical corporation, limited liability partnership, or limited liability company. As of 2002, the Medicare program expanded the abil-

ity of PAs to have an ownership interest in a practice. Rules that became effective in April of 2002 allow PAs to own an approved Medicare corporation that is eligible to bill the program.

"Incident to" Services   Medicare has a long-standing policy of covering medical services provided by PAs in physicians' offices and clinics under what is called the "incident to" provision, at 100% of the physician's fee schedule. Even with the expansion of PA coverage at the 85% reimbursement rate in all settings through the Balanced Budget Act of 1997, "incident to" remains an appropriate billing mechanism for PAs as long as Medicare's more restrictive billing requirements are followed.

If medical services provided by PAs are to be billed under the "incident to" provision, the following criteria must be met:

➤ The service must be one that is typically performed in the physician's office.

➤ The service must be within the PA's scope of practice and in accordance with state law.

➤ The physician must be in the suite of offices (providing direct supervision) when the PA renders the service.

➤ The physician must personally treat the patient during the patient's first visit to the practice; any established patient who presents with a new medical condition must also be treated by the physician. PAs may provide the follow-up care.[2]

➤ The physician is responsible for the overall care of the patient and should perform services at a frequency that reflects his or her active involvement and participation in the ongoing management of the patient's treatment.

Direct supervision does not require that the supervising physician be in the same room with the PA, but he or she must be in the office suite and immediately available to provide assistance and direction throughout the time the PA is providing the service, if necessary.

Medicare HMOs

In addition to the fee-for-service program, Medicare allows its beneficiaries the option of receiving care from certain health maintenance organizations. Not all HMOs are approved to participate in Medicare's HMO option. In general, these plans must cover all hospital fees (Part A) and professional services (Part B) that are covered under the Medicare fee-for-service plan. Often, the benefits offered by Medicare HMOs are more generous than those offered in the fee-for-service plan.

Medicare-approved HMOs are paid a predetermined monthly amount of money for each Medicare enrollee. Salaries and benefits of PAs are considered allowable costs, and services provided by a PA are covered.

A recent development is that Medicare allows beneficiaries to receive care from health plans under the Medicare Choice program, also known as Medicare Part C. Medicare Choice plans are HMOs and other types of managed care plans that are paid a predetermined, capitated monthly fee to cover beneficiaries; they typically also offer enhanced benefits (such as routine physicals, pharmaceuticals, and/or coverage for eyeglasses). Health plans operating under the Medicare Choice designation have the option of determining whether PAs are covered providers. As of 2002, approximately 10% of all Medicare beneficiaries were enrolled in a Medicare Choice plan.

Certified Rural Health Clinics

In the mid-1960s, the maldistribution of physicians had reached a crisis. The supply of physicians had become insufficient to meet the demands of smaller, isolated rural communities. Although PAs were well accepted by residents in these rural communities, Medicare and Medicaid coverage for their services was not available in most cases.

In 1977, Congress passed the Rural Health Clinic Services Act (Public Law 95-210) in an effort to increase the availability of primary health care services to rural areas of the country. Federal certification as a rural health clinic (RHC) allows the clinic to be reimbursed by means of a cost-based methodology, as opposed to the fee-for-service payment system. Medical care provided by a PA in a certified RHC is covered at the same basic rate as that provided by a physician, as long as the PA is practicing in accordance with state law and state regulatory requirements. Physicians who provide care in designated underserved areas receive a 10% bonus payment. At the present time, that bonus payment is available only to physicians.

Each rural health clinic has a per patient reimbursement rate (generally based on the clinic's overall costs and the number of patients treated on a yearly basis) that the clinic receives for each patient encounter. There is a maximum per patient encounter amount that will be paid.

To be eligible for federal RHC status, the clinic must be located in a nonurbanized area that is designated by the federal government as either a health professional shortage area (HPSA) or a medically underserved area. In addition, the clinic must have a PA, a nurse practitioner, or a certified nurse midwife on-site and available to patients at least 50% of the time the clinic is open.

Medicaid

Medicaid, authorized by Title XIX of the Social Security Act, is a program jointly funded by federal and state governments that provides medical assistance for low-income individuals, families with dependent children, the aged, and the disabled. Although the federal government sets basic guidelines, establishes a basic set of core benefits, and pays 50% to 80% of the cost of Medicaid (depending on the state's per capita income), individual states actually administer the program. The Medicaid program, which began on January 1, 1966, covers more than 36 million people.

In their Medicaid programs, states may cover medical and surgical services provided by PAs. The decision as to whether to cover PAs rests solely with the state, except with respect to federally certified rural health clinics. If a clinic is designated by the federal government as a certified RHC, the state's Medicaid program must cover PA-provided services in the clinic.

As Medicaid costs rose in the late 1980s and early 1990s, states began to experiment with more cost-effective methods of providing care to beneficiaries; fee-for-service programs were shifted to managed care delivery systems. To make many of these changes, states were required to get permission from the federal government in the form of 1915 and 1115 waivers, which provided states with exemptions from the traditional guidelines of the Medicaid program.

One of the popular concepts that states have used to lower costs, and ideally to improve the quality of care, is to assign Medicaid beneficiaries to a specific health care provider, known as a primary care provider (PCP). The rationale is that beneficiaries will have better continuity of care and will be more likely to access the health care system at the appropriate time and place if one specific provider is responsible for directing their overall care. The PCP is able to refer the beneficiary to specialist and hospital inpatient care services as required. The federal government allows PAs to serve as PCPs, and some states allow PAs to assume that role.

Provisions of the Balanced Budget Act (BBA) of 1997 allow states greater flexibility in using managed care methods within their Medicaid programs without having to get formal approval (through the waiver process) from the federal government. The BBA of 1997 also contained language beneficial to PAs by giving states the authority to name PAs as primary care case managers (PCCMs) under the Medicaid program. A PCCM is typically paid a small monthly fee to act as a gatekeeper or coordinator of care for beneficiaries. States may cover PAs at the physician's rate of reimbursement or on a discounted fee basis. Coverage may apply in all practice settings and for all medical services, or there may be limitations. Table 22-2 shows the most current information on how states cover PAs under their Medicaid plans.

The Balanced Budget Act of 1997 provided nearly $24 billion in funding over the next 5 years for a new children's health care initiative. The State Child Health Insurance Program (SCHIP), established as Title XXI of the Social Security Act, represents the single largest expansion of health care coverage by the federal government since Medicare more than 30 years ago. SCHIP entitles states to receive block grants to initiate or expand coverage for low-income children. This program has the potential of reducing the number of uninsured children in this country by 40%. At the discretion of the state, PAs may be covered providers under SCHIP.

PRIVATE INSURANCE

Private health insurance companies can be problematic regarding coverage of medical services provided by PAs, but not because the insurers fail to cover PA-provided medical services. Most

Table 22-2   Coverage for Physician Assistants in State Medicaid Programs

State	PA Covered Provider	Reimbursement Rate (% Physician Fee)	Physician Supervision Requirements*	Services Covered
Alabama	Yes	100%	Physician on-site	All medical services cited in PA law, except assisting at surgery
Alaska	Yes	100%	Physician on-site except in RHCs and FQHCs	
Arizona†	Yes	100%		
Arkansas	Yes	100%	Physician on-site 50%	All medical services cited in PA law
California	Yes	100%	Same as PA law	All medical primary care, including home care
Colorado	Yes	100%	Physician on-site*	All medical services cited in PA law
Connecticut	Yes	100%	Physician present except in freestanding clinic	All except nonsupervised inpatient services; only "incident to" in physician office
Delaware	Yes	100%		All medical services cited in PA law
District of Columbia	No			
Florida	Yes	80%	Same as PA law	All medical services cited in PA law
Georgia	Yes	90%	Physician present except in RHCs and FQHCs	All medical services cited in PA law
Hawaii	Yes	100%	Same as PA law	All medical services except assisting at surgery
Idaho	Yes	85%	Same as PA law	All medical services cited in PA law
Illinois	Yes	100%	Same as PA law	Services within physician's scope of practice
Indiana	Yes	100%	Same as PA law*	All medical services cited in PA law
Iowa	Yes	100%	Same as PA law	All medical services cited in PA law

Table 22-2 Coverage for Physician Assistants in State Medicaid Programs—cont'd

State	PA Covered Provider	Reimbursement Rate (% Physician Fee)	Physician Supervision Requirements*	Services Covered
Kansas	Yes	75%	Same as PA law	Office visits and H&Ps; home visits; nursing home visits, H&Ps, and recerts; subsequent hospital visits
Kentucky	No—fee for service Yes—managed care (proposed)	100%	Physician face-to-face contact	
Louisiana	No			
Maine	Yes	100%	Same as PA law	All medical services cited in PA law; limits on settings in which services are covered (e.g., no birthing centers)
Maryland	Yes	100%	Physician on-site*	All medical services cited in PA law
Massachusetts	Yes			Routine well-care services to beneficiaries under age 21; and obstetric care
Michigan	Yes	100%	Same as PA law	All medical services cited in PA law
Minnesota	Yes	90%	Same as PA law	All delegated tasks
Mississippi	No			
Missouri	No			
Montana	Yes	80%	Same as PA law	All medical services cited in PA law
Nebraska	Yes	100%	Same as PA law	All medical services cited in PA law
Nevada	Yes	PA rate‡	Same as PA law	All medical services cited in PA law
New Hampshire	Yes	100%	Same as PA law	All medical services cited in PA law
New Jersey	No			
New Mexico	Yes	100%	Same as PA law	All medical services except assisting surgery
New York	Yes	100%	Same as PA law	All medical services cited in PA law

Continued

Table 22-2   Coverage for Physician Assistants in State Medicaid Programs—cont'd

State	PA Covered Provider	Reimbursement Rate (% Physician Fee)	Physician Supervision Requirements*	Services Covered
North Carolina	Yes	100%	Same as PA law	Only "incident to" services
North Dakota	Yes	75%	Same as PA law	All medical services cited in PA law
Ohio	Yes	85%-100%	Same as PA law	All medical services
Oklahoma	Yes—fee for service	75% for output fee for service		10.4% for first-assisting (fee for service)
	Yes—managed care	EPSDT, laboratory, x-rays at 100%		Primary care provider status in rural areas
Oregon	Yes	100%	Same as PA law	All medical services cited in PA law
Pennsylvania	Yes	100%	Same as PA law	All medical services cited in PA law except assisting at surgery
Rhode Island	Yes			
South Carolina	Yes	100%	Physician on-site	All medical services cited in PA law
South Dakota	Yes	90%	Same as PA law	All medical services cited in PA law
Tennessee	Yes	100%	Same as PA law	All medical services cited in PA law
Texas	Yes	100%	Same as PA law	All medical services cited in PA law
Utah	Yes	100%	Same as PA law	All medical services cited in PA law
Vermont	Yes	90%	Same as PA law	All medical services cited in PA law
Virginia	No			
Washington	Yes	100%	Same as PA law	All medical services cited in PA law
West Virginia	Yes	100%	Same as PA law	All medical services cited in PA law
Wisconsin	Yes	90%	Same as PA law	All medical services cited in PA law
Wyoming	Yes	100%	Same as PA law	All medical services cited in PA law

EPSDT, early periodic screening, diagnosis, and treatment; FQHC, federal qualified health clinic; H&P, history and physical examination; RHC, rural health clinic.
*In the case of federally certified rural health clinics, the state Medicaid program cannot establish supervisory requirements more stringent than those found in the state PA law. Consequently, the "physician on-site" requirement does not apply to Medicaid reimbursement in RHCs unless it is a requirement of the Medical Practice Act.
†Arizona Health Care Cost Containment System (AHCCS).
‡Reimbursement based on PA-assigned relative value unit.

insurance companies do cover services provided by PAs. The problem is that there are more than 1000 insurance companies, HMOs, and preferred provider organizations (PPOs) operating in the United States, and they often differ in both how services delivered by PAs are covered and how claim forms should be submitted. Even within the same insurance company, PA coverage policies can change based on the particular plan type, the specific type of service being provided, and the part of the country in which the service is delivered. Although many private payers do not separately credential or issue provider numbers to PAs, they do usually cover at the physician rate services provided by the PA.

As of 2002, 11 states had some type of reimbursement mandate in place requiring payment by third party payers.

Many businesses have opted to no longer purchase medical coverage for their employees from MCOs and insurance companies; instead, many are self-insuring (paying out of their company funds the full cost of providing insurance/paying claims) and are using insurance companies only for claims processing and other administrative tasks, also known as administrative services. These self-insured companies are free to design their own benefit plans and to decide which practitioners are eligible to deliver care. Employee health plans for businesses that are self-insured are exempt from state reimbursement mandates.

Because of the potential variation, it is virtually impossible to present a complete picture of specific private insurance plan coverage policies, as has been done with respect to Medicare and Medicaid. Instead, this section attempts to outline basic concepts that can help in the determination of whether medical services provided by PAs are covered by the specific plan in question.

Covered Versus Direct Payment

As the Director of Health Systems and Reimbursement Policy for the AAPA, I occasionally receive calls from PAs who have contacted a particular insurance company and were told that PAs are not reimbursed. Upon closer examination, the medical services provided by the PA were covered, but the insurance company did not pay directly to the PA. Instead, payment for the PA's services was made to the employing physician. The following case study may better explain the dilemma.

CASE STUDY 22-2

A PA once called the AAPA to say that she was told by a major insurance company that it would not reimburse for a service provided by a PA. The insurance company was immediately contacted by AAPA staff, and the following question was asked: "Are physician medical services covered when performed by PAs in the physician's office under the supervision of the physician when billed under the physician's name and provider number?" The answer was that yes, of course, those services would be covered. The lesson to be learned is that how you ask the question will often determine the kind of answer you get.

Instead of asking whether PAs can bill for services or whether the insurer will pay to the PA, it may be more useful to ask whether services performed at the direction and with the supervision of a physician are covered by a particular plan. It is important to keep in mind that PAs are acting as legal agents of the supervising physician. Generally, the services performed by a physician assistant are deemed to have been delegated by the supervising physician.

The American Medical Association (AMA) issued a policy statement in 1978 recommending this approach to physicians. The policy states:

The AMA has recommended that reimbursement for services of a physician assistant be made directly to the employing physician. In instances where the PA is providing services in a physician's office and in conjunction with the physician, the cost of such services would appropriately be a part of the physician's charge, as is now the case with other personnel he [or she] employs. When the PA provides physician services to a patient under the direction of, but in a location physically remote from, the employing physician, AMA has recommended that the physician bill for such services on the basis of the usual, customary, and reasonable charges concept insofar as this may be established by custom and experience for the physician assistant.

GLOSSARY

A

Administrative Services Only (ASO)   Self-insured businesses often contract with an insurance company for clerical and claims processing only. The insurance company provides only administrative services to the self-insured companies. Policy language and coverage terms are determined by the self-insured business, not the insurance company. Thus, even though the claim form may carry the name of an insurance company, the patient is not covered by a policy issued by that company.

Assignment   When doctors and other suppliers of services covered by Medicare Part B accept assignment, they agree to accept Medicare's approved charge as payment in full and will not bill the patient for the difference between the Medicare-approved charge and the practice's actual charge.

C

Capitation   A method of paying for health care services whereby a practitioner or hospital is paid a fixed amount per patient to provide covered medical care for a specified period of time. Typically paid on a per month basis, the amount of payment does not change even if the actual cost of treating the patient exceeds the predetermined, fixed amount. Payment adjustments may be made at the end of a specified period of time.

Case Management   The process by which all health-related aspects of a patient's care are managed by a designated health professional. Case managers provide coordination for designated components of health care, such as appropriate referral to consultants, specialists, hospitals, and ancillary providers and services. Case management is intended to ensure continuity of services and proper accessibility so that fragmented health care systems or the improper utilization of facilities and resources can be overcome. It also attempts to match the appropriate intensity of services with the patient's needs.

Co-payment (Co-pay)   An amount of money that the insured pays directly to a provider (practitioner or facility) for medical services. For example, many health plans have an 80%/20% provision in their policies. After the deductible, the insurer pays 80% of medical costs while the insured pays 20% up to a certain dollar amount. This 20% is known as the co-payment.

Cost-Based Reimbursement   A method of reimbursing medical services based on the global facility costs incurred in treating the patient (as opposed to a pre-established fee for each individual medical service). Certified Rural Health Clinics (RHCs) are reimbursed on a cost-based method. That is, the actual cost of the facility (rent or mortgage), utilities, medical provider(s) and clerical staff salaries, equipment, and so forth, is divided by the number of patients treated in the clinic within a year to yield the per patient reimbursement amount to which the clinic is entitled. There is a ceiling on the per patient amount that RHCs can be reimbursed under this system. The cap tends to increase each year based on a medical inflation formula determined by the Centers for Medicare and Medicaid Services (CMS).

CPT Codes   Current Procedure Terminology codes represent a system developed by the American Medical Association (AMA) to describe medical procedures performed by physicians. The 5-digit CPT codes, which are also used by physician assistants because PAs provide physician services, are updated annually. Beginning in 1993, the AMA and the Health Care Financing Administration (now CMS) embarked upon a formal effort to open up the CPT coding system to certain other nonphysician practitioners whose services in the past had not been adequately described by the CPT system.

GLOSSARY—cont'd

Credentialing   The process of reviewing a practitioner's qualifications (i.e., education, training, experience, or demonstrated ability) for the purpose of determining whether he or she meets the criteria for clinical privileging.

D

Diagnosis-Related Group (DRG)   A classification system of approximately 523 disease categories used by Medicare and other insurers to determine payment rates for services provided to patients in hospitals.

Discharge Planning   Cost-control technique that determines the appropriate time for patients to be released from the hospital and organizes posthospital care.

E

Evaluation and Management Services (E&M Services)   Often described as cognitive or medical decision-making services, these are patient evaluation and management functions performed during patient office visits, outpatient and hospital visits, or consultations. E&M services consist largely of taking the patient's history, examining the patient, and participating in medical decision making. Under Medicare's Resource-Based Relative Value Scale (which went into effect January 1, 1992), CMS has attempted to upgrade the value (and fee schedules) of E&M services while holding down the fees paid for surgical and more technical types of services.

Explanation of Benefits (EOB)   An explanation, prepared by the third party payer or administrator, of the covered and reimbursed medical benefits; or an explanation for the denial of such benefits.

F

Fee-for-Service   A system of payment for health care services whereby a fee is rendered for each service delivered (sometimes known as indemnity insurance).

Under a fee-for-service system, costs increase not only if the fee for the service increases, but also if more "units" or services are provided. This traditional method contrasts with that frequently used in the prepaid sector, whereby services are covered by a fixed payment made in advance independent of the number or volume of services rendered.

G

Gatekeeping   The process by which a primary care provider (or other trained individual) is the first point of contact for a patient who is seeking care. The gatekeeper evaluates the patient's medical needs and coordinates all diagnostic testing and referrals required for appropriate medical care. If the patient is to receive referrals to specialists and hospitals, the care must be preauthorized by the gatekeeper unless there is an emergency. Gatekeeping functions are closely related to those of a case manager.

Global Payment   The bundling of procedures (and payment) that are provided to a patient as opposed to paying separately for each procedure.

H

Health Maintenance Organization (HMO)   A type of prepaid health insurance in which a patient pays a monthly membership fee. In exchange, the HMO provides all the patient's medical care. If a patient joins an HMO, he or she agrees to obtain all health care from the HMO and its affiliated providers, except in emergencies.

I

Indemnity Insurance   Traditional health insurance that pays for provided services on a service-by-service basis. The physician normally charges a fixed fee; if the patient's insurance does not cover the entire fee, the patient typically must pay the difference. Also commonly referred to as a fee-for-service plan.

Continued

GLOSSARY—cont'd

Independent Practice Association (IPA) Sometimes referred to as an HMO without walls. Practitioners in the IPA agree to treat HMO patients in their own private offices. IPA doctors bill the HMO, not the patient, for medical services. Rates are generally discounted.

M

Managed Care Refers to a health plan that attempts to control costs by closely monitoring and managing patient treatment decisions, limiting referrals to outside providers, and generally requiring preauthorization for hospital care and surgical procedures. Health Maintenance Organizations or Preferred Provider Organizations are often considered to be prototype managed care providers. However, a traditional fee-for-service plan could be considered a managed care entity if it has set procedures for utilization review, or requirements such as hospital pre-certification.

P

Preexisting Condition A physical or mental condition that exists prior to the purchase of a health insurance policy or the enrollment of an individual or family into a health care plan. Limits on preexisting conditions may take the form of higher premiums, exclusion of payment for certain medical treatment(s) for a set period of time, or total exclusion of coverage. A preexisting condition should not affect enrollment into most HMOs.

Preferred Provider Organization (PPO) A discounted fee-for-service health plan in which health care practitioners agree to charge the payer a discounted fee for treating patients. Beneficiaries are given a list of these "preferred providers" by the payer and are encouraged to use them. Typically, use of a practitioner not on the "preferred" list results in greater out-of-pocket expenditures or decreased benefits for the patient.

Prior Authorization The evaluation of a patient's medical need and the approval for medical care before the procedure is performed; monitoring and controlling a patient's access to medical care.

Q

Quality Assurance (QA) Activities and programs intended to assure the quality of care in a defined medical setting. QA programs typically include peer or utilization review procedures to remedy any identified deficiencies in quality. A successful quality assurance program should also have a mechanism for assessing its relative effectiveness.

R

Rural Health Clinic (RHC) Also known as a certified Rural Health Clinic. The Rural Health Clinic Services Act (Public Law 95-210) was passed in 1977 in an attempt to increase the availability of primary care health services in rural areas. The RHC Act provides Medicare and Medicaid payments for covered services furnished in an RHC by physician assistants (PAs), nurse practitioners (NPs), and certified nurse midwives (CNMs). The RHC Act requires that a PA, NP, or CNM staff the RHC at least 50% of the time the clinic is open. Federal RHC regulations also require that the clinic be under the general (not full-time) direction of a physician and that a physician be physically on-site at the clinic at least once every 2 weeks. State laws, which may be more restrictive than federal RHC regulations regarding provisions such as supervision, must be followed.

T

Third Party Administrator (TPA) An entity that provides only administrative services for businesses that self-insure their employee health plan. Services typically include utilization review, administration of claims payment, and benefit design. TPAs are not financially at risk for actually paying claims.

GLOSSARY—cont'd

Third Party Payer   An organization that acts as a fiscal intermediary between the medical practitioner and the consumer of health care. Examples include insurance carriers and the government (through the Medicare and Medicaid programs).

U

Utilization Management   A systematic method for reviewing and controlling a patient's use of medical services and a provider's utilization of medical resources. This process usually involves data collection, utilization review, and/or authorization (especially for services such as specialist referrals and hospitalizations). Typically, managed care organ-

izations establish procedures for reviewing the medical care of subscribers to ensure that care is provided in the most appropriate setting and is delivered by the most appropriate provider.

W

Workers' Compensation   A state-administered program (sometimes known as industrial insurance) that covers payment for work-related injuries. Under this system, the employer assumes the cost of employee medical treatment and/or lost wages due to job-related injury or disease. The state may act as the "insurance entity," or this function may be handled by private insurers.

CONCLUSION

For more than 35 years, PAs have proved their ability to deliver quality medical and surgical care. As this country continues to redefine its health care system and search for ways to keep health care costs under control, even more payers and health care-related organizations will realize the important role that PAs play in the health care system. One must not forget, however, that health care is a business. In addition to delivering physician-quality medical care, PAs must be cognizant of their economic and noneconomic value to the system. Understanding the financing and payment mechanisms of the health care system is an important step in that direction.

CLINICAL APPLICATIONS

1. Describe the concept of "consumer-driven health care."
2. Differentiate between Medicare Part A and Medicare Part B.

3. Define "incident to" services, and list the criteria that must be met for reimbursement for services provided by PAs under this policy.
4. Describe Medicare Choice plans.
5. Define the method by which payment is made to certified rural health clinics.
6. Discuss the responsibility of PAs to understand the financing of health care and to advocate on behalf of reimbursement for medical and surgical services delivered by PAs.

REFERENCES

1. Medicare Carriers Manual, Part 3: Claims Process, Section 2050, May 1997.
2. Medicare Program Memorandum, Transmittal No. AB-98-15, April 1998.

RESOURCES

Medicare Carriers Manual, Part 3: Claims Process, Section 2050, May 1997. *This manual contains the Health Care Financing Administration's interpretation and implementation instructions regarding laws passed by Congress that affect the Medicare program.*

Medicare Program Memorandum, Transmittal No. AB-98-15, April 1998. *This memorandum summarizes changes in Medicare coverage and payment policy that affect physician assistants, as required by the Balanced Budget Act of 1997.*

Medicare Program Memorandum, Transmittal No. 1744, March 12, 2002. *This memorandum summarizes the Balanced Budget Act of 1997 and incorporates the expansion of Medicare coverage that allows PAs to be employed by Ambulatory Surgical Centers and to have an ownership interest in an approved corporate entity that is eligible to bill the Medicare program.*

CHAPTER 23

Health Insurance and Managed Care

Ruth Ballweg and Keren H. Wick

Health Insurance Coverage and Noncoverage	**Managed Care Competencies**
Trends in Health Insurance Coverage	**Continuing Medical Education**
Managed Health Care	**Emerging Managed Care Issues for PAs**
History of Managed Care	**Conclusion**
The Concepts of Managed Care	**• Case Study 23-1**

HEALTH INSURANCE COVERAGE AND NONCOVERAGE

Health insurance coverage—who has it and who doesn't—is one of America's top public policy dilemmas. Depending on the state and the point in time, an average of 16% of Americans (more than 43 million people) do not have health insurance coverage. In the past, the uninsured were most often the poorest and the most disadvantaged. Now however, many of these individuals have access to health care through Medicare, Medicaid, and even some state plans. Figure 23-1 provides an overview of the uninsured population.

Increasingly, the uninsured group is composed of working low-income families, recent college graduates, contract workers, and part-time employees. As a result, the political clout of the uninsured has changed significantly. Almost everyone has a close friend or family member who is in this predicament. With this increased awareness of the problem, policymakers, legislators, and other decision makers are faced with rising pressure to solve the problem of a lack of health coverage and access to care.

An increasing percentage of those who are insured receive this benefit from government-funded programs—although we may not think of them that way (Figure 23-2). Governmental programs include Medicare, Medicaid, the CHAMPUS program for retired military personnel, as well as a variety of insurance plans for federal, state, and local governmental workers. In many states, more than half of the insured are covered under governmental plans. New Children's Health Insurance Plan funding will increase these numbers even further.

In a historical context, we have moved toward governmental funding in a relatively short time, beginning in the 1960s with the creation of Medicare and Medicaid. Over time, coverage has been gradually extended—beginning with citizens at either end of the life span, and moving toward increased coverage for those in the middle (governmental workers and retirees)—creating the possibility that all citizens will

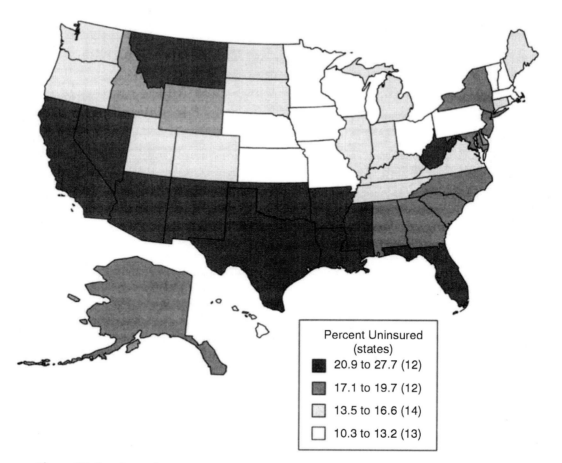

Figure 23-1 Uninsured Americans by state. *Reprinted by permission. Calculations by A. Shields based on Current Population Survey data presented in: Fronstin P. Sources of Health Insurance and Characteristics of the Uninsured: Analysis of the March 1999 Current Population Survey. EBRI Issue Brief No. 217. Washington, DC: Employee Benefit Research Institute, 2000.*

ultimately have access to some type of health care coverage. Despite nationwide resistance to the idea of socialized medicine, interest is growing in the more palatable idea of universal coverage, which could be a blend of some public-private partnership that would encounter less opposition from current third-party payers. Many health policy experts feel that this can be achieved only when health insurance is "decoupled" from an individual's employment setting, as it is in many European countries, and provided as a separate benefit to everyone.

In the meantime, physician assistants and all other health care providers must factor in the patient's insurance coverage—or noncoverage—as they determine optimum *and available* treatment options. Knowledge of the types of coverage and an understanding of insurance concepts and terminology allow providers to practice more efficiently and to maximize care for each individual patient.

TRENDS IN HEALTH INSURANCE COVERAGE

Since its inception, U.S. health insurance has expanded from initial catastrophic coverage for acute hospitalizations, surgery, and traumatic events to broad coverage that typically includes outpatient and inpatient services, pharmaceuticals, rehabilitation, and even mental health

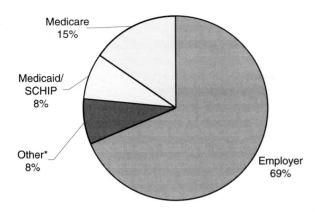

Figure 23-2 Primary source of health coverage among the insured population, 2000. *Reprinted by permission. Chart from: Underinsured in America: Is Health Coverage Adequate? Fact Sheet 4060. Menlo Park, CA: The Henry J. Kaiser Family Foundation, 2002.*

and dental benefits. As these benefits have expanded, interest in controlling costs has increased.

The most dramatic cost-control trend has been the movement away from traditional fee-for-service, which essentially has no cost controls, to more structured plans that control access to providers and services through the use of primary care gatekeepers. Although fee-for-service coverage is still available—at relatively high costs—most of America's insured receive their care through health plans that manage their care delivery through some sort of controlled network of physicians and hospitals. The relatively new point-of-service (POS) plans are a hybrid of fee-for-service and preferred provider (PPO) plans; they allow the consumer to obtain care through extended networks but at a higher cost. Figure 23-3 illustrates the rapid move away from fee-for-service care to

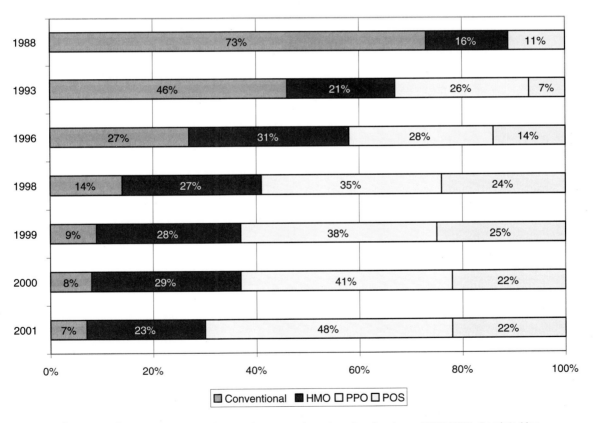

Figure 23-3 Health plan enrollments for covered workers by plan type, 1988-2001. *Reprinted by permission. Employer Health Benefits: 2001 Annual Survey. Menlo Park, CA: The Henry J. Kaiser Family Foundation, 2001.*

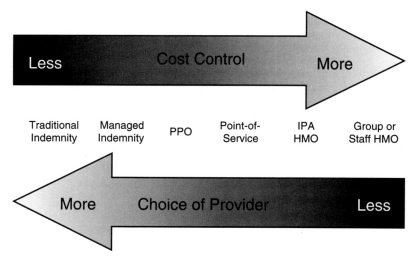

Figure 23-4 The spectrum of health care plans. *Reprinted with permission. Dowling WL. The Future of Managed Care. Presented at the 28th Annual Advances in Family Practice and Primary Care Course. Seattle, WA: University of Washington, September 14, 2000.*

PPOs, formal health maintenance organizations (HMOs), and the new POS plans.

Generally speaking, the lower the cost of coverage (to both the employer and the consumer), the greater will be the attempt to manage health care utilization (Figure 23-4). With increasing costs of health care, the emerging trend is to pass these costs back to individual consumers through higher premiums, changing or decreased benefits, and larger co-pays. It will be interesting to see if these increased consumer costs finally force the issue of universal coverage to the forefront of public debate.

MANAGED HEALTH CARE

For the purposes of this chapter, the term *managed care* will be used in its broadest sense—to include all attempts at cost control in health care. Therefore, the discussion will not be limited to formal staff-model HMOs, but will include PPO and POS plans as well.

Over the past 15 years, enrollment in managed care plans has increased dramatically at the expense of the traditional fee-for-service model. In 2001, only 7% of employees were covered under a traditional plan. In the managed care population, a shift had occurred

away from HMOs toward PPO and POS plans.[1] In 2001, 57% of Medicaid enrollees received coverage under a managed system.[1] With the move of Medicare and Medicaid patients into managed delivery systems and with the application of managed care concepts to service delivery in all types of health care settings, PAs should assume that they will be involved in some sort of managed care during their careers. This places a responsibility on PA training programs and PA professional organizations to prepare students as well as practicing PAs to meet the demands of a managed care practice. The growth in the market penetration of managed care creates for the PA an obligation—and opportunity—to "obtain a broader education."[2]

HISTORY OF MANAGED CARE

Managed care is a relatively new concept. The first formal health maintenance organization was created by Henry Kaiser in 1938 as a strategy for providing available and efficient health care for workers on the dam construction on the Colorado River (Boulder/Hoover Dam) and the Columbia River (Grand Coulee Dam). The Kaiser Health Plan was quickly expanded to provide care for Kaiser's shipyard workers during World War II.

Closely following the Kaiser development was the Group Health Cooperative, a consumer-run system that grew out of the union movement in Seattle. Both of these not-for-profit systems were quick to hire PAs. The Group Health Cooperative served as a training site for trainees in the first class of the MEDEX Northwest Physician Assistant Program in 1969 and hired 3 new graduates. The Kaiser system's Research Center in Portland, Oregon, assigned a prominent researcher—Jane Record—to monitor the development and performance of these new professionals. Dr. Record produced many studies, all supporting the utilization of PAs in managed care settings.

Although managed care systems in their various iterations have commonly employed PAs, national employment surveys have probably underreported the involvement of PAs in managed care. In retrospect, it appears that PAs have indicated that they were working in managed care only if they were employed by the traditional staff-model HMO. In fact, much of managed care is provided through other systems, including fee-for-service settings that incorporate capitated managed care contracts as a portion of their market share.

Some of the most significant confusion about managed care seems to be the differentiation between for-profit (e.g., Columbia/HCA) and not-for-profit (e.g., Kaiser or Group Health) managed care organizations (MCOs). As a result, a passionate backlash against the for-profit managed care organizations, which transfer cost-savings or profits to highly paid executives and stockholders, is often misdirected toward not-for-profit entities, which redirect any cost-savings back into patient care. Obviously, the economic incentives and the decision making in these two settings are dramatically different. Unfortunately, health care providers making employment choices may not identify or understand these major differences as they make their career decisions. In recent years, the not-for-profit sector accounted for only one third of the HMO market.[1]

Although it is easy to think of managed care as an all-or-nothing proposition, in fact the transition to managed care is a gradual process that has been described as occurring in stages. Thus, regions of the country in which managed care is well established are in later stages of managed care development or evolution, and other regions would be in earlier stages.[3]

In stage 1 of managed care, less than 10% of the population is enrolled in MCOs. As managed care emerges (stage 2), enrollment will have increased to 10% to 15% (including managed Medicare and managed Medicaid). Health care systems develop regional hospital networks, upgrade clinical information systems, defer capital investments in expanded facilities, and encourage primary care–based medical groups. The strategy here is to build primary care and consolidate tertiary care into efficient systems.

Stage 3 of managed care sees an increase in enrollment to 15% to 25%. During this phase, systems are actively merging and expanding and beginning to capitate primary care groups and networks. Clinical pathways and guidelines are developed, and employers who contract for health care begin to use provider performance data as a factor in their choice of health plan. Stage 3 brings what is sometimes seen as a dramatic restructuring of staff and management as a strategy for cost reduction.

With enrollments of 25% to 40%, stage 4 brings with it regional networks to begin clinical consolidation and the removal of providers with low clinical and cost performance. Although capitation began with primary care providers, in stage 4 it moves to hospitals and specialists. Population-based protocols are put in place for managing many clinical diagnoses and decreasing hospitalizations.

Managed care at stage 5 has been characterized as "post-reform." In this phase, there is regionalization of high-tech services to maximize resources and skills. Buildings will have been reconfigured for team and group practice, and complete computerization of clinical information systems will have been accomplished.

This scenario may seem overwhelming, but it is taking place, in all phases, in various regions of the country. The agenda of federal policymakers to move Medicaid and Medicare patients into managed care contracts is introducing managed care even to states such as Alaska and Idaho, where it has seemed unthinkable.

THE CONCEPTS OF MANAGED CARE

Managed care employers often make the assumption that providers entering their systems are well versed in managed care concepts, but in fact this is seldom the case. Table 23-1 lists the major managed care concepts that should be understood by PAs.

All of the health professions are being forced to play "catch-up" in terms of how they educate both their students and their graduate practitioners on the evolving health care systems. PA programs are increasingly including managed care topics in their curricula. In some programs, this may involve a health policy or a health care finance course; in others, managed care topics may be integrated into didactic and clinical courses. Table 23-2 summarizes managed care principles that can provide a core knowledge base for PAs learning about managed care.

MANAGED CARE COMPETENCIES

Ideally, educators and human resource planners should define competencies that managed care will require of its clinicians, and then formulate how to develop the relevant skills in PA students and providers. As is the case when learning any complex system that assumes a fundamental shift in focus, an overview of the central concepts and the various ways in which they are applied must precede a more detailed topical focus.[6,8,9] This gives learners a perspective on the entire landscape, complete with a map and a compass, before they plunge into the managed care jungle. It is essential that clinicians, including PAs, have a basic conceptualization of MCO structures, economics, and legal issues to be able to protect their patients and themselves in practice.[8,10] Even a PA who is not required to be involved in the administrative details of the supervising doctor's practice will benefit from this knowledge. The PA may be his or her own only advocate for appropriate inclusion in a contract that the supervising physician signs with an MCO. Failure to ensure a defined role for the PA can make the whole practice less efficient.[11] Table 23-3 lists several topics, in outline form, that should feature in one way or another in a managed care curriculum.

Table 23-1   Managed Care Core Concepts

1. Care over cure.[4]
2. Generalism and primary care over specialism.[4,5]
3. Outpatient rather than hospital focus.[4]
4. Population-based focus.[4,5]
5. Work is characterized by interdependence.[5]
6. Use of information to assure value.[5]
7. Service conservation over service use.[4]
8. Finance and delivery are explicitly linked.[5]
9. All participants are to be held accountable.[5]

Table 23-2   Managed Care Curriculum Principles

1. Integration: Incorporate managed care approach into existing materials.[6,7]
2. Employ teamwork, collaboration, and communication in the process of changing curriculum.[6]
3. Offer faculty development to match the pace of curricular changes.[6]
4. Include managed care practitioners or administrators as faculty.[6]
5. An interdisciplinary content will highlight the interdependence of health and human services.[7]
6. Focus on how to work within health care delivery systems.[7]
7. Use experiential learning: Aim toward the application of ideas.[6]
8. Emphasize the role of primary care in managed care.[7]
9. Case studies should ask students to "find the appropriate diagnosis" rather than "find the rare disease."[6]
10. Emphasize population-based care.[7]
11. Emphasize accountability.[7]
12. Emphasize value.[7]

Table 23-3   Competencies and Curriculum Topics—General

A. Overview
1. Define and apply concepts central to managed care systems.[6,8-10,12-14]
2. Organizational behavior.[9,15]
3. Medical legal issues.[8,10,13,14]
4. Health systems financing and economics.[6,8,10,14-16]
5. Financial incentives.[17]
6. Contracts with MCOs.[9]
7. Practice management within managed care.[9,10,14,18,19]
8. Time management.[9]
9. Understand performance evaluation mechanisms.[13]

B. Communication and teamwork
1. Communication and interpersonal skills[6,8,17-21]
2. Physician/patient relationship.[13,20,21]
3. Teamwork, leadership, and interdisciplinary collaboration.[6,8,13,14,17-20,22]

C. Primary care
1. Role of primary care provider and continuity of care.[6,13,17]
2. Assess and manage commonly encountered ambulatory problems.[10,13,18,21]
3. Recognize and address human behavior and biopsychosocial factors.[6,15,18,21]
4. Diagnose and treat affective disorders.[21]
5. Gatekeeping: Refer patients and consult appropriately and effectively.[9,12,13,17,21,22]
6. Provide cost-effective care.[13,21,22]

D. Planning and implementing patient care
1. Clinical decision making, including ethics and resource allocation.[6,8,19]
2. Ethical problem solving.[6,8,10,13,15,17,20,23]

3. Population-based care, including epidemiological thinking.[6,8,13,15,17,19,22,24]
4. Systems-based care.[10,15]
5. Use and development of (and departure from) guidelines.[6,13,17,18,20,21]
6. Working with a formulary.[18]
7. Apply evidence-based medicine.[20]
8. Alternative care options (e.g., home care, hospices).[9,13]
9. Compare roles of ambulatory setting and hospital.[10,13]
10. Negotiate patient care.[6,9,12]

E. Preventive medicine
1. Encourage health promotion and disease prevention.[6,13,17-19,21,22,25]
2. Management of health risks.[19]
3. Disease management.[6,13,17]

F. Tools
1. Informatics—computerized records and databases.[8,15,17-20]
2. Telemedicine skills.[13,17]

G. Quality and outcomes
1. Principles of utilization review and management.[6,8,13,17,18]
2. Charting and documentation to be used in utilization review.[20]
3. Outcomes measurement and patient satisfaction.[6,12,14,17]
4. Quality measurement and improvement—CQI.[6,8-10,12-15,17-20]

H. Career
1. Professional and personal growth and satisfaction.[13,18,19]
2. Research.[19]
3. Review professional literature critically.[18,21]

Teamwork has always been a concept central to the PA profession, but managed care works best when teams are truly inclusive. The ability to collaborate across disciplines—not only the medical specialties, but also branches of the social services—is prerequisite to offer complete care to the patient and engage in patient advocacy.[7,18,20] Working together or working with a patient is facilitated by effective communication, a skill that should be taught to all health care practitioners.[26]

Primary care has likewise been a historical focus of PA training. A revised approach will address the new dimension that managed care brings to even this mainstay of the profession.[6,7] Primary care in a managed system assumes the responsibility of gatekeeping, or planning care and coordinating referrals.[12,22] Those who function in the gatekeeping role need the ability to not only treat common ambulatory problems but also consult with and refer to specialists as appropriate. They must consider the implications of population-based care from an epidemiological perspective.[8,15,19,22] PAs will be called on to employ a sophisticated level of decision making that addresses managed care concerns, such as the distribution of finite resources among individuals.

Again, the goal is not to encourage PAs to withhold care that a patient needs. Most people associate the word *ethics* with managed care only in terms of deficiency. Yet managed care, applied through the filter of ethical behavior, enhances the clinician's ability to provide the highest quality of patient care.[6,8,16,23,27] At issue is the balance between the individual, population groups, practitioner time, health care resources, and MCOs that limit options through financial constraints.[6,23]

The most common means used by MCOs to influence clinical decision making is the imposition of guidelines, also called protocols or pathways. At worst, this reduces the art of medicine to a rigid, bureaucratic formula that fails to account for individual variation or independent, critical thought. If used judiciously, however, guidelines provide clinicians with a decision-making framework that can be adjusted or disregarded according to each situation.[6,20,21] Whatever view the PA or the PA program adopts toward guidelines, the fact remains that many PAs will be required to understand them, formulate them, and work with them during their careers.

One of the many areas in which the PA should be competent, in managed care in particular, is behavioral medicine. As the front-line provider in most practices, a PA must be able to recognize the complex mix of biopsychosocial factors that may underlie a presenting problem.[6] They must possess the skills to diagnose and treat common psychiatric problems and must know when to refer.[28]

In its more enlightened forms, managed care encourages PAs to address their patients' overall health by promoting health maintenance and disease prevention activities. By educating patients about healthful behavior and screening for certain cancers or other illnesses, PAs help to build both the physical and mental well-being of their patients. These activities, in turn, benefit the MCO in reduced demand for the expensive care associated with advanced disease.[6,18,21,22,25]

The use of computers to track patients facilitates the administrative tasks related to screening and preventive care.[15,18,25,29] Databases can provide reminders to both practitioners and patients when a screening procedure or follow-up is due. Streamlining the detail work in this way frees up more of the PA's time for patient care. Table 23-4 suggests topic areas for learning about information technology.

Computer programs also provide the most efficient means to track specific treatments used and the results of those treatments. These data are then used in outcomes measurement and utilization review—the most popular systems for measuring value. MCOs place a heavy emphasis on these processes, which makes PAs responsible for accurate documentation of their clinical decisions.[6,7,13,20] Indeed, PAs should be able to involve themselves in the process of utilization review and management so that they can plan better care and influence the utilization decisions being made in the MCO.[15] Table 23-5 lists desired competencies in utilization review, and Table 23-6 details key techniques to steer the course of utilization management. PAs can

Table 23-4 Curriculum—Informatics[30]

1. Use of electronic record formats.
2. Use of the Internet as a research tool.
3. Use of e-mail and groupware.
4. Database use and data analysis: Outcomes and process measures.

Table 23-5 Curriculum—Utilization Review and Management[12]

1. Complete documentation of referral requests.
2. Discuss need for specialty services with patients.
3. Communicate results of review actions to patient.
4. Use evidence-based medicine in decisions.
5. Use utilization management principles when considering treatment options.
6. Develop practice guidelines and projects for quality improvement.

Table 23-6 Curriculum—Negotiation with a Case Reviewer[31]

1. Learn utilization review and case management in different types of MCOs.
2. Be clear and confident about treatment plan.
3. Be certain that less comprehensive care is unreasonable and why.
4. Discuss how current care fits into the continuum of needed treatment.
5. Discuss appropriate treatment options.
6. Be truthful—don't exaggerate.
7. Be respectful—not argumentative or defensive.
8. Make the patient central.

Table 23-7 CME Modules

1. Concepts and principles of managed care.[17]
2. Issues in health care.[33]
3. Government and policy issues.[33]
4. Legal issues.[33]
5. Managed care economics and financial incentives.[17,33]
6. Ethics.[33]
7. Management principles.[33]
8. Leadership development.[32,33]
9. Skill in group dynamics.[22]
10. Communication and interpersonal skills.[17,33]
11. Gatekeeping and referrals.[17,22]
12. Population-based care.[22]
13. Provide cost-effective care.[22]
14. Principles of utilization and case management.[17]
15. Quality management and improvement.[17,32,33]
16. Outcomes management.[17]
17. Information systems.[17,32]
18. Patient-centered and disease-centered care.[32]
19. Foster health promotion and disease prevention.[22]

then become part of another significant activity of the practice or MCO—quality improvement.[7,15,16,18] Even when he or she is not working in a managed care setting, appreciating and applying the principles of utilization review and quality improvement will keep the PA focused on the question of how to provide the best possible care to patients.

CONTINUING MEDICAL EDUCATION

Many PAs, similar to many physicians, have entered practice with minimal or no preparation to function in a managed care setting. These clinicians often learn as they go, picking up unconnected pieces of information without obtaining comprehension of the system as a whole. In some cases, they may go to great lengths to avoid managed care and its principles for the simple reason that they do not understand it and therefore cannot discern which aspects of it will serve to enhance their practice. It is the PAs in this situation who stand to gain the most from continuing medical education (CME) in managed care.

The principles and subject areas in managed care CME do not differ greatly from those identified for PA students, but they do focus more on the concepts and processes. Of the concepts central to managed care, the most popular CME topics include managed care economic principles, communication and teamwork skills, quality improvement, and information systems (Table 23-7).[17,32,33]

EMERGING MANAGED CARE ISSUES FOR PAs

In 1998, the Center for Health Professions at the University of California, San Francisco completed a report on physician assistants in managed care for the Pew Health Professions Commission.[6] Included in the report are case studies describing PA employment issues and concerns in five actual managed care systems. These case studies are intended to provide a snapshot of PA managed care practice in the late 1990s. An example is provided in Case Study 23-1.

Although the case studies illustrate many of the key issues for PA practice in managed care organizations, several questions need to be revisited periodically as employers, policymakers, health care providers, and educators monitor the evolution of the managed care concept.

1. *Who's in charge?* In the initial formulation of the PA concept, physician assistants were closely—and exclusively—tied to physicians, often a *specific* physician. As institutional employment became more common, PAs were commonly attached to specific clinical

services with structured physician relationships. In managed care, PAs and physicians are now frequently required to have their practice reviewed, monitored, and perhaps even countermanded by an overarching structure composed of nonclinical administrators and managers. Although this structure may be intended to create efficiency, ensure consistency, and promote quality of care, clinicians are concerned that their decision-making power and their authority are declining. For PAs, this concern potentially calls into question their basic relationship with physicians and forces PAs to answer to many masters, some of whom may be administrators rather than clinicians.

2. *How can we develop and maintain our relationships with physicians in managed care settings?* In the past, physicians made decisions about hiring the PAs they worked with. Now, however, managed care physicians *and* PAs are being hired by administrative offices of managed care organizations and are then assigned to work together. This situation creates a lack of "buy-in" by supervising physicians. As a result, the PA must place a higher priority on developing a successful working relationship with the supervising physician. More attention may need to be paid to orienting the physician to the advantages of working with PAs and the importance of communication and appropriate supervision.

A further complicating factor is that a managed care system can pit physicians and PAs against each other. This is particularly true if they are not organized as team members relying on each other to maximize patient care. The less closely the physician and physician assistant are linked, the greater the danger that they will see each other as adversaries rather than as colleagues. For example, PAs who are integrated into a team—even if they have their "own" patient panel as designated primary care providers—will be more able to access their supervising physicians than if they are organized into more independent services in which physicians may consider supervision to be an interruption.

Additional tensions between physicians and PAs are created when managed care systems make the decision to decrease the physician staff and increase the number of PAs. Even if these decisions are made based on a restructuring of the primary

care–to–specialty ratio, or on performance indicators, some physicians will see these decisions as proof that PAs are competitors to physicians rather than team members who value their relationships with physician-supervisors.

3. *Are PAs and nurse practitioners (NPs) utilized any differently within managed care settings? Will this change in the future as managed care evolves? Are we (PAs) colleagues or competitors with NPs in the managed care environment?* Managed care administrators generally have a poor understanding of the similarities of and differences between PAs and NPs. Although they view both groups as physician extenders or physician substitutes, they are frequently not aware of the nuanced differences in training or licensure. The fact that scope of practice for both of these groups varies dramatically from state to state further complicates the utilization of PAs and NPs. Most PAs and NPs would agree that there are few, if any, settings in which PAs and NPs are optimally utilized.

Although initially PAs and NPs were used more or less interchangeably in managed care settings, newer graduates may be assigned different types of jobs. Nurse practitioners, for example, who now have more research and administrative hours in their coursework but fewer hours of supervised clinical practice may be most effectively utilized in managing specific patient populations rather than seeing a broad range of ambulatory care patients. PAs, on the other hand, with generally broader clinical training, may be more commonly utilized in high-volume clinics and may even be assigned time-consuming procedural responsibilities to free up physicians for more extensive oversight responsibilities. MCOs are working actively to develop models of efficient utilization of both groups.

4. *What new health occupations will emerge in the era of managed care? How will PAs relate to these new workers?* Just as PAs were created in response to a need in the health care system, it is reasonable to assume that other new health careers, occupations, and professions will arise to fill niches in the evolving health care system. Some of these new roles will be related to technology, others to administration, and still others to direct patient care. The expanded use of medical assistants rather than nurses in primary care

clinics illustrates this concept. Other examples include emerging plans by managed care systems to make greater use of patient advocates or lay health educators as a strategy for providing cost-effective health promotion services.

Some of these new patient care roles may change PA responsibilities and move them toward either supervisory or oversight roles. Other developing careers may be perceived as a direct threat to PA utilization. A driving factor may be the perception of rising salaries for PAs and NPs and the perception that new categories of health workers can more cost-effectively provide some services that had previously been seen as physician, PA, or NP tasks. The popularity of "physical therapy assistants" and the move of masters-trained physical therapists into supervisory roles with fewer direct patient care responsibilities illustrates this kind of shift. The PA profession should carefully monitor these new developments and attempt to take strategic positions that allow PAs to most effectively provide appropriate levels of health care access.

5. *How can PAs be involved most effectively in the decision making of MCOs?* All health care providers in managed care systems share the concern that they are or may be excluded from clinical decision making. There is a greater risk that this will occur if clinicians do not become well informed about managed care concepts and decision making. Articulate, committed, and knowledgeable clinicians must be willing to take on assignments that include participation in the development of evidence-based clinical guidelines, performance measures, and outcomes assessment. This is clearly an example of the important concept that "the world is run by those who show up."

6. *Who's worrying about the patients?* In all of these complex situations, it's easy to lose track of why we entered the health professions—to serve the patients. PA roles in managed care settings now include advocacy functions as a key feature of our patient care responsibilities. In addition to assessing and treating patients, we must now ensure that they have access to appropriate care and services. This advocacy may involve direct contact with the system as well as formal and informal contacts with other providers through referrals and consultations. Advocacy also includes providing patients with the knowledge and skills that allow them to use the system appropriately.

After a careful study of these issues, the Pew Commission report on PAs in managed care made a series of recommendations concerning education and practice. The practice recommendations are summarized in Table 23-8.

Text continued on p. 483.

Table 23-8   Excerpted Pew Commission Recommendations Concerning PA Practice[6]

1. The physician-PA relationship, defined by delegation and supervision, should be reaffirmed as it was created and has existed. It should not be redefined with the PA having more independent authority from the physician.
2. Physicians and physician groups should be projecting the PA into the new types of relationships that are emerging in managed care. This will create new types of relationships between PAs and physicians, all of which should maintain the traditional values and intent of the MD-PA relationship.
3. Where possible all physician residency programs should ensure that the residents have an extensive practice opportunity with a PA or an NP. This training should be carried out in a setting that encourages team practice.
4. As physician assistants move into organized practice groups and begin to work with multiple supervisors, they should be incorporated into the medical staff.
5. State practice acts should not have arbitrary practice barriers. Physician assistants should be able to practice to the full extent of their education, training, and experience, as delegated to do so by the supervising physician.
6. State practice acts and insurance payment policies should not be a barrier to the full practice of PAs under existing state laws.

INSURANCE AND MANAGED CARE GLOSSARY

AAPCC—Adjusted Average Per Capita Cost   The basis for HMO or CMP reimbursement under Medicare-risk contracts. The average monthly amount received per enrollee is currently calculated as 95% of the average costs to deliver medical care in the fee-for-service sector. The best estimate of the amount of money care costs for Medicare recipients under fee-for-service Medicare in a given area. The AAPCC is factored for age, sex, Medicaid eligibility, institutional status, and whether a person has both part A and part B of Medicare.

All-payer System   A system in which prices for health services and payment methods are the same, regardless of who is paying. For instance, in an all-payer system, federal or state government, a private insurer, a self-insured employer plan, an individual, or any other payer could pay the same rates. The uniform fee bars health care providers from shifting costs from one payer to another.

Alternate Delivery Systems   Health services provided in other than an inpatient, acute-care hospital or private practice. Examples within general health services include skilled and intermediary nursing facilities, hospice programs, and home health care. Alternate delivery systems are designed to provide needed services in a more cost-effective manner. Most of the services provided by community mental health centers fall into this category.

Any Willing Provider Laws   Laws that require managed care plans to contract with all health care providers who request it, provided that they meet the plan's terms and conditions.

Approval   A term used extensively, which implies to many the primary process of "managing" managed care. Approval usually is used to describe treatments or procedures that have been certified by utilization review. It can also refer to the status of certain hospitals or doctors as members of a plan, or it can describe benefits or services that will be covered under a plan. Generally, approval is granted by the managed care organization, the third-party administrator, or the primary care physician, depending on the circumstances.

Capitation (Capitate, Cap, Capped)   Specified amount paid periodically to health provider for a group of specified health services, regardless of quantity rendered. Amounts are determined by assessing a payment "per covered life" or per member. The method of payment in which the provider is paid a fixed amount for each person served, regardless of the actual number or nature of services delivered. The cost of providing to an individual a specific set of services over a set period of time, usually a month or a year.

Case Management   Method designed to accommodate the specific health services needed by an individual through a coordinated effort to achieve the desired health outcome in a cost-effective manner. The monitoring and coordination of treatment rendered to patients with a specific diagnosis or requiring high-cost or extensive services. The process by which all health-related matters of a case are overseen by a physician, nurse, or other designated health professional. Physician case managers coordinate designated components of health care, such as appropriate referral to consultants, specialists, hospitals, ancillary providers, and services. Case management is intended to ensure continuity of services and accessibility to overcome rigidity, fragmented services, and the misutilization of facilities and resources. It also attempts to match the appropriate intensity of services with the patient's needs over time.

Clinical or Critical Pathways (Clinical Guidelines)   A map of preferred treatment and/or intervention activities. Outline the types of information needed to make decisions, the timelines for applying that information, and what action needs to be taken by whom. Provide a way to monitor care concurrent with its provision. These pathways are developed by clinicians for specific diseases or events. Some providers are working now to develop these pathways for the majority of their interventions and are developing the software capacity to distribute and store this information.

INSURANCE AND MANAGED CARE GLOSSARY—cont'd

Decision Support Systems   Computer technologies used in health care that allow providers to collect and analyze data in sophisticated and complex ways. Activities supported include case mix, budgeting, cost accounting, clinical pathways, outcomes, and actuarial analysis.

Essential Community Provider   A provider who serves high-risk, special needs, and underserved individuals. Health plan companies must offer provider contracts to all designated ECPs in their approved service areas to serve high-risk, special needs enrollees.

Gatekeeper   A primary care physician responsible for overseeing and coordinating all aspects of a patient's medical care. In order for a patient to receive a specialty care referral or hospital admission, the gatekeeper must pre-authorize the visit unless there is an emergency.

Group-Model HMO   Health care plan involving contracts with physicians organized as a partnership, professional corporation, or other legal association. It can also refer to an HMO model in which the HMO contracts with one or more medical groups to provide services to members. In either case, the payer or health plan pays the medical group, which is, in turn, responsible for compensating physicians. The medical group may also be responsible for paying or contracting with hospitals and other providers.

Group Practice   A group of persons licensed to practice medicine in the state who engage in coordinated practice and who share common overhead expenses, medical and other records, and substantial portions of the equipment, as well as the professional, technical, and administrative staffs.

HMO—Health Maintenance Organization   HMOs offer prepaid, comprehensive health coverage for both hospital and physician services. The HMO is paid in monthly premiums or capitated rates by the payers, which include employers, insurance companies, government agencies, and other groups representing covered lives. The HMO must meet the specifications of the federal HMO act and many rules and regulations at the state level. There are four basic models: group model, individual practice association, network model, and staff model. An HMO contracts with health care providers, for example, physicians, hospitals, and other health professionals. The members of an HMO are required to use participating or approved providers for all health services, and generally all services will need to meet further approval by the HMO through its utilization program. Members are enrolled for a specified period of time. An HMO may subcapitate to other groups. For example, it may carve out certain benefit categories, such as mental health, and subcapitate these to a mental health HMO, or the HMO may subcapitate to a provider, provider group, or provider network. HMOs are the most restrictive form of managed care benefit plan because they retain control of the procedures, providers, and benefits.

Horizontal Integration   Merging of two or more firms at the same level of production in some formal, legal relationship. In hospital networks, this may refer to the grouping of several hospitals, the grouping of outpatient clinics with the hospital, or a geographic network of various health care services. Integrated systems seek to integrate both vertically with some organizations and horizontally with others. *See also* Vertical Integration.

IDS, ISN—Integrated Delivery Systems, Integrated Services Network   Many different but similar definitions exist for IDS. An IDS, as an entity, is not required to abide by strict regulations as is an HMO, but when it offers a health plan, it must then abide by the requirements of the state and federal government for health plans, insurance companies, or HMOs. Without owning a health plan product, an IDS is usually subject to the regulations that govern its separate businesses, that is, regulations governing hospitals, clinics, and physicians. An IDS can be a financial or contractual arrangement between health providers (usually hospitals and doctors) to offer a comprehensive range of health care services through a separate legal entity operating, at least

Continued

INSURANCE AND MANAGED CARE GLOSSARY—cont'd

for these purposes, as a single health care delivery system. IDS can be a network of organizations that provides or arranges to provide a coordinated continuum of services to a defined population and is held both clinically and fiscally accountable for the outcomes of the populations served. IDS can also be a health care provider organization that vertically integrates physician, hospital, and health plan businesses in some manner in order to establish a full continuum of care, seamless delivery of services, and management of care under new reimbursement arrangements. Also called delivery system, vertically integrated system, horizontally integrated system, health delivery network, and accountable health plan.

Managed Care Systems and techniques used to control the use of health care services, including a review of medical necessity, incentives to use certain providers, and case management. The body of clinical, financial, and organizational activities designed to ensure the provision of appropriate health care services in a cost-efficient manner. Managed care techniques are most often practiced by organizations and professionals that assume risk for a defined population (e.g., health maintenance organizations), but this is not always the case. Managed care is a broad term that encompasses many different types of organizations, payment mechanisms, review mechanisms, and collaborations. Managed care sometimes refers to the activity of organizing doctors, hospitals, and other providers into groups in order to enhance the quality and cost-effectiveness of health care. Managed Care Organizations (MCOs) can include health maintenance organizations (HMOs), preferred provider organizations (PPOs), point-of-service (POS), exclusive provider organizations (EPOs), physician-hospital organizations (PHOs), integrated delivery systems (IDSs), and so forth. When one speaks of a managed care organization, one is usually speaking of the entity that manages risk, contracts with providers, is paid by employers and patient groups, or handles claims processing. Managed care has effectively formed

a go-between, brokerage, or third party arrangement by existing as the gatekeeper between payers, providers, and patients. The term *managed care* is often misunderstood because it refers to numerous aspects of health care management, payment, and organization. It is best to ask the speaker to clarify what he or she means when the term "managed care" is used. In the purest sense, all people working in health care and medical insurance can be thought of as managing care.

Medical Informatics Medical informatics is the systematic study or science of the identification, collection, storage, communication, retrieval, and analysis of data on medical care services with a view to improve decisions made by physicians and managers of health care organizations.

NCQA—National Committee for Quality Assurance A nonprofit organization created to improve patient care quality and health plan performance in partnership with managed care plans, purchasers, consumers, and the public sector.

Network-Model HMO This type of HMO contracts with more than one physician group and may contract with single- or multi-specialty groups, as well as hospitals and other health care providers. A health plan that contracts with multiple physician groups to deliver health care to members. Generally limited to large single- or multi-specialty groups. This is distinct from group model plans that contract with a single medical group, IPAs that contract through an intermediary, and direct contract model plans that contract with individual physicians in the community.

Outcomes Management Systems to control the end results of medical treatment. Providers and payers alike wish to find a method of managing care in a way that would produce the best outcomes. Managed care organizations are increasingly interested in learning to manage the outcome or result of care, rather than just managing the cost of care. It is thought that through a database of outcomes experience, caregivers will know better which treatment methods result in consistently better outcomes for patients.

INSURANCE AND MANAGED CARE GLOSSARY—cont'd

Outcomes Measurement   Systems used to track clinical treatment and responses to that treatment. The methods for measuring outcomes are quite varied among providers. Much disagreement exists regarding the best practice or tools to utilize to measure outcomes. In fact, much disagreement exists in the medical field about the definition of *outcome* itself.

Outcomes Research   Research on ways to measure changes in patient outcomes, that is, patient health status and satisfaction, resulting from specific medical and health interventions. Attributing changes in outcomes to medical care requires distinguishing the effects of care from the effects of the many other factors that influence patients' health and satisfaction. With the elimination of the physician's fiduciary responsibility to the patient, outcomes data are gaining increasing importance for patient advocacy and consumer protection. Outcomes research will also be used in the future by payers to identify potential partners on the basis of good outcomes.

PCP—Primary Care Provider   A primary care provider such as a family practitioner, general internist, pediatrician, and sometimes an ob/gyn. HMOs and PPOs in particular require members to choose a PCP, and some allow members to designate midlevel practitioners as their PCP. Generally, a PCP acts as the gatekeeper, that is, he or she supervises and coordinates care, as well as providing medical care to individual members of a plan. In many cases, the PCP must approve all referrals for specialty.

Performance Standards   Standards set by the MCO or payer that the provider will need to meet in order to maintain its credentialing, renew its contract, or avoid penalty. These vary from payer to payer, and contract to contract. A set of standards that an individual provider is expected to meet, especially with respect to quality of care. The standards may define volume of care delivered per time period. Thus, performance standards for an obstetrician/gynecologist may specify some or all of the following: office hours and office visits per week or month, on-call days, deliveries per year, gynecological operations per year, and so forth.

PMPM—Per Member Per Month   The number of units of a specified cost or service divided by member months. Often used to describe premiums or capitated payments to providers, but can also refer to the revenue or cost for each enrolled member each month. Many calculations, other than cost or premium, use PMPM as a descriptor.

Population-Based Health Care   The practice of identifying the health care needs of a defined group of people—for example, those in a geographical area or those in a certain age range—as opposed to identifying needs on an individual basis. Involves the use of epidemiology, health promotion, and disease prevention.

POS—Point-of-Service   Managed care plan that allows patients to select participating or nonparticipating providers. Those who go outside the plan for services may pay more out-of-pocket expenses. A health insurance benefits program in which subscribers can select between different delivery systems (i.e., HMO, PPO, and fee-for-service) when accessing services, rather than selecting a more restrictive plan at the time of open enrollment. Typically, the costs for utilizing in-network or approved providers are less than when care is rendered by noncontracting providers. This is a method of influencing patients to use certain providers without restricting their freedom of choice too severely.

PPO—Preferred Provider Organization   Some combination of hospitals and physicians that agrees to render services, perhaps under contract with a private insurer. The services may be furnished at discounted rates, and the insured population may incur out-of-pocket expenses for covered services received outside the PPO. PPOs are a common method of managing care while still paying for services through an indemnity plan. Most PPO plans are point-of-service plans, in that they will pay a higher percentage for care provided by providers in the network. Generally PPOs offer more choice for the patient and provide higher reimbursement to the providers. *See also* POS (Point-of-Service).

Practice Parameters   Defined by the American Medical Association as strategies for patient

Continued

INSURANCE AND MANAGED CARE GLOSSARY—cont'd

management, developed to assist physicians in clinical decision making. Practice parameters may also be referred to as practice options, practice guidelines, practice policies, or practice standards.

QA—Quality Assurance   Activities and programs intended to assure the quality of care in a defined medical setting. Such programs include peer or utilization review components to identify and remedy deficiencies in quality. The program must have a mechanism for assessing its effectiveness and may measure care against pre-established standards.

QI—Quality Improvement   Concurrent systems are used to improve quality continuously, rather than reacting when certain baseline statistical thresholds are crossed. Quality improvement programs usually use tools such as cross-functional teams, task forces, statistical studies, flow charts, process charts, pareto charts, and so forth, and focus on both outcomes and the process of care.

Quality   Can be defined as a measure of the degree to which delivered health services meet established professional standards, judgments of value, and consumer satisfaction. Quality may also be seen as the degree to which actions taken or not taken maximize the probability of beneficial health outcomes and minimize risk and other untoward outcomes, given the existing state of medical science and art. Quality is frequently described as having three dimensions: (1) quality of input resources (certification and/or training of providers), (2) quality of the process of services delivery (the use of appropriate procedures for a given condition), and (3) quality of outcome of service use (actual improvement in condition or reduction of harmful effects).

Risk   The chance or possibility of loss. For example, physicians may be held at risk if hospitalization rates exceed agreed-upon thresholds. The sharing of risk is often employed as a utilization control mechanism within the HMO setting. Risk is also defined in insurance terms as the possibility of loss associated with a given population.

Safety-net Provider   Inner-city clinicians, public hospitals, and community health centers that have traditionally provided care to urban Medicaid recipients.

Section 1915(b) Medicaid Waiver   Section 1915(b) waivers allow states to require Medicaid recipients to enroll in HMOs or other managed care plans in an effort to control costs. The waivers allow states to implement a primary care case-management system, require Medicaid recipients to choose from a number of competing health plans, provide additional benefits in exchange for savings resulting from recipients' use of cost-effective providers, and limit the providers from which beneficiaries can receive non-emergency treatment. The waivers are granted for 2 years, with 2-year renewals available. Often referred to as a freedom-of-choice waiver.

Staff-Model HMO   A model in which the HMO hires its own physicians. All premiums and other revenues accrue to the HMO, which, in turn, compensates physicians. Very much like the group model, except the doctors are salaried employees of the HMO. Generally, all ambulatory health services are provided under one roof in the staff model.

UR, UM—Utilization Review, Utilization Management   Evaluation of the necessity, appropriateness, and efficiency of the use of health care services, procedures, and facilities. In a hospital, this includes review of the appropriateness of admissions, services ordered and provided, length-of-stay, and discharge practices, both on a concurrent and a retrospective basis. Utilization review can be done by a peer review group or a public agency. UR is a method of tracking, reviewing, and rendering opinions regarding care provided to patients. Usually, UR involves the use of protocols, benchmarks, or data with which to compare specific cases to an aggregate set of cases. Those cases falling outside the protocols or range of data are reviewed individually. Managed care organizations sometimes refuse to reimburse or pay for services that do not meet their own set of UR standards. UR involves primarily the review of patient records and patient bills, but it may also include telephone conversations with providers. The practices of

---

INSURANCE AND MANAGED CARE GLOSSARY—cont'd

pre-certification, re-certification, retrospective review, and concurrent review are all UR methods. UR is one of the primary tools utilized by MCOs and health plans to control overutilization, reduce costs, and manage care.

Vertical Integration   Organization of production whereby one business entity controls or owns all stages of the production and distribution of goods or services. In health care, vertical integra-

tion can take many forms, but it generally implies that physicians, hospitals, and health plans have combined their organizations or processes in some manner to increase efficiency, increase competitive strength, or improve quality of care. Generally, integrated delivery systems or health care networks are vertically integrated. *See also* IDS (Integrated Delivery Systems), Horizontal Integration.

Major portions of this glossary are excerpted and edited from: The Pohly Group. A Managed Care Glossary. Available at http//www.pohly.com/terms.shtml. Accessed July 2002.

CONCLUSION

Managed care would seem to be in a critical phase of development. There is a wide range of opinion about managed care from consumers who see it as *either* the good news *or* the bad news with few opinions in between. There is also widespread misunderstanding about the major differences between for-profit and not-for-profit managed care systems and the widely disparate decision making and incentive systems between the two models. Monitoring the evolution of managed care requires a critical eye and constant vigilance to ensure that patients truly receive access to appropriate care and services. It is often easy to lose sight of this priority amid rapid changes to systems and turf battles between clinicians and administrators.

From a policy point of view, managed care—in some iteration—often seems to be the only possible strategy for controlling health care costs, delivering care to large segments of the population, and emphasizing wellness in addition to illness. Nevertheless, we cannot yet be certain that any of these promises can be fully achieved.

CASE STUDY 23-1

In 1997 the Center for the Health Professions at the University of California, San Francisco formed a task force on PAs in managed care to create a policy document and recommend strategies for optimum utilization of PAs in managed care settings.

Their report, which was issued in 1998 as a publication of the Pew Health Professions Commission, contains five definitive case studies on PAs in managed care settings. A representative study is reprinted here. The publication, *Charting a Course for the 21st Century: Physician Assistants and Managed Care,* can be obtained from the Center for the Health Professions, 1388 Sutter Street, Suite 805, San Francisco, CA 94109. The following case study is reprinted by permission.

Physician Assistant Practice in an Underserved Urban Setting Sacramento Family Medical Clinic; Sacramento, CA

Introduction

In the late 1980s, Dr. Gil Simon, a physician in Sacramento, California, became aware of the tremendous unmet health care needs of low-income children, particularly those from families insured with Medi-Cal (California's Medicaid) in his community. In 1989, he opened a single office, the Sacramento Children's Clinic, to provide care for this underserved population. The Sacramento Family Medical Clinic today provides care for adults as well, and has expanded to six locations throughout the Sacramento area.

For a variety of reasons, costs among them, Dr. Simon employs a mix of physicians, physician assistants (PAs), nurse practitioners (NPs), and medical assistants (MAs) to provide services for the clinic's clientele. Physician assistants and supervising physicians both see the same complex mix of patients, both act as patient advocates in the frequently complicated managed care system and, with limited resources, both continually struggle to provide their patients with the best care possible.

From an outsider's perspective, little but provider name badges distinguishes experienced PAs from physicians at the Sacramento Family Medical Clinic. Both professions provide comprehensive, continuous primary care for their patients and truly act as advocates for many of their patients who are unable to navigate the complex health care system without assistance. Not surprisingly, patients often mistakenly assume that their health care provider is a physician. While some differences do exist between the roles of PAs and physicians, there seem to be more similarities than differences between the two professions in this setting.

History and Background of the Sacramento Family Clinic

Approximately 90% of the Sacramento Family Medical Clinic's clientele are Medi-Cal recipients and represent a variety of racial and ethnic backgrounds. The clinic's clientele are primarily Hmong, Russian, and Hispanic. With family incomes of no more than $583 per month* (for a family of two), those who qualify for Medi-Cal are at or well below the poverty level. As a result, the socioeconomic status of many of the clinic's patients directly impacts their ability to access health care and other services, posing significant challenges for their health care providers. Lack of

---

*Families of two must have incomes no greater than $583 a month in the state of California to qualify for Aid to Families with Dependent Children (AFDC). Medi-Cal eligibility in California is based on a number of factors, but a majority (54% in Sacramento County) of Medi-Cal recipients are eligible as a result of their enrollment in AFDC. *Source:* California Department of Social Services. A Comparison of California and National Public Assistance Statistics Through December, 1995. Information Services Bureau, 1997; and California Department of Health Services. Medi-Cal Program: Average Monthly Eligibles by County, 1995.

transportation, difficulty obtaining childcare, and limited English language skills are issues that affect many of the clinic's clientele, making clinic providers' role as patient advocates imperative.

The clinic originally began serving this population when Medi-Cal was a fee-for-service program in the late 1980s. However, in recent years, the state of California petitioned and received a federal Medicaid waiver to enroll its Medi-Cal recipients in a variety of managed care plans. As a result, the Sacramento Family Medical Clinic now contracts with several managed care organizations under California's Geographic Managed Care Plan (Omni, Foundation Health, Blue Cross, and UC Davis). Through these managed care contracts, the clinics provide care for 15,000 covered lives.

The Sacramento Clinic Today

Dr. Simon's first employee when he began the clinic in 1989 was a physician assistant. He still employs physician assistants (now numbering six), along with six physicians, two NPs, and roughly 20 MAs to provide care in the six clinics.

Each of the clinics is staffed by a team of one PA or NP and one family practice or pediatric physician. The teams are configured so that a full-time family practice or pediatric PA practices with a half-time general internist physician or pediatrician, in addition to being supported by a number of MAs. This model ideally provides a pediatric and an adult practitioner at each site. This means that the PA sees a complete panel of patients with both complex and simple needs.

Collegial relationships between PAs and supervising physicians result from frequent consultation, referrals, and an understanding of mutual boundaries and comfort levels. Nanette Patron, a PA at the 47th Street site in Sacramento, describes the relationship with her supervising physician as a close one that consists of trust, collegiality, consultation, and structured independence. She states, "Most of the doctors here let you do what you want as long as you follow basic guidelines." Brian Sharpe, a PA at the Watt Avenue Clinic in North Highlands, also explained, "I think that part of being a good PA is knowing your limitations and what you're supposed to do and what you're not supposed to do. And finding that line is something that you identify over a couple years of practice and you improve on."

The Impact of Managed Care at the Sacramento Family Clinic

When questioned about the changes that managed care has brought to the family clinic, physicians and PAs alike frequently complain of the additional paperwork and administrative headaches incurred when dealing with managed care organizations. Nearly all providers expressed concern over the amount of time spent following guidelines or gaining approval for referrals or procedures. As Nanette Patron explains, "it gets frustrating sometimes because plans constantly change their guidelines, and the specialists that we can refer to. We used to be able to send our patients out for EKGs and have them interpreted by cardiologists. But now Dr. Wilson and Dr. Gilbert interpret their own EKGs, because Omni [a managed care plan] tells us that EKGs are now part of our capitation. But what if our machine breaks down?"

Physicians and PAs also have many hopes for managed care, particularly given the relative disinterest of other providers in Medi-Cal patients during the fee-for-service era. Anne Alexis, a PA at the Rancho Cordova site, articulates her hopes for managed care: "I felt that in fee-for-service nobody wanted to see our patients for referrals and so forth. Patients would go from practice to practice, to whoever would see them. Their charts were never complete and I never knew who was seeing them or what medicines they were on. I was looking forward to managed care and having patients come to us for care with one chart and organized follow-up done as best as we could. I thought that we'd have more referral specialists available, and that we could count on the managed care organizations to provide us with the orthopedics that we need." Unfortunately, not all of Ms. Alexis' hopes have materialized with managed care: "The managed care organizations tell us, 'You find a specialist and we'll authorize it.' But we can't find them, especially the orthopedists and psychiatrists that we really need in a timely fashion," she explains.

In addition to providing medical care, many of the clinics' PAs and physicians provide their patients with a variety of other services. Brian Sharpe comments, "I was trained in medicine and in patient care, not in dealing with reams of paperwork. But I've learned to deal with a lot of other things in practice over the years." Mr. Sharpe's later comments further explained his role as a patient advocate, a particularly important role given his patient population and the advent of managed care.

Anne Alexis describes this role best when she recounts a patient encounter. "If managed care has changed anything," she begins, "it's that I find myself fighting more for my patients. I had a 2-year-old come in who wasn't speaking—the mother was congenitally deaf—and the first thing I thought was that we needed to determine if the child could hear, based on a hearing test. Well, that was denied by the managed care organization. So I had to find an audiologist through the school district to do a hearing test by special request, because they don't do hearing tests on children under age 3. After several phone calls, TDD messages, and letters, my request was denied three times by the school district. Ultimately, I had to get them to make a special exception." All told, it took Ms. Alexis a considerable amount of time and perseverance to obtain a hearing test for the child and then find appropriate resources to teach him how to speak.

PA and Physician Roles

Similarities rather than differences characterize the roles of physician assistants and their supervising physicians at the Sacramento Family Medical Clinic. Practicing side by side in close consultative relationships, PAs and physicians function well together at the clinic. Although both professions experience the same frustrations with managed care and act as patient advocates within the new system, there are some notable differences.

Brian Sharpe summarizes these differences in pay, training, and practice most succinctly when asked what advice he would give students thinking about a career as a physician assistant. "If you enjoy medicine, you get to practice medicine. And you have a little more regular job as opposed to a physician who works more than 40 hours a week and also has to run the administrative part of the practice. They have to worry about patients after they leave the clinic. Not that PAs don't worry about their patients, but at the same time, physicians have a lot of liabilities. You get paid a lot less, but your mind is a little more free." He finishes his advice for prospective PAs and reflects, "I think that now, with the glut of doctors, that physician salaries are coming down. It's a good time for physician assistants."

Study Questions†

1. To what extent are the roles of MD/PA/NP in primary care settings interchangeable?
   - ➤ Is there a way to determine the "best roles" for these providers?
2. Continuity of providers: How do long-term relationships support or develop a collaborative atmosphere?
   - ➤ What factors build collegiality among a diverse group of providers?
3. Managed Medicaid: Is Medicaid administered through managed care in your state?
   - ➤ What mechanism is used to administer managed Medicaid in your state, region, or community?
   - ➤ How are NPs/PAs included in the administration and payment structures?
   - ➤ To what extent does managed Medicaid work in your state or community?
   - ➤ What changes would be needed to make it work better for your community?
4. What new administrative skills are required for providers to function efficiently within a managed care system?
   - ➤ How do you advocate for patients within a managed system?

---

†Study questions reprinted with permission from *Shaping American Health Care: Tools for Physician Assistant Curriculum in Managed Care* (Ballweg R, Wick KH, eds. Seattle WA: MEDEX Northwest Physician Assistant Training Program, 1999).

5. Review data on members of your state or community who are below or barely above the poverty level (use U.S. Census data on-line).
   - ➤ Who are the poor and working poor?
   - ➤ Who are the people who have no access or severely restricted access to health care?

CLINICAL APPLICATIONS

1. Is there an ideal role for PAs in managed care systems? Does this role differ in primary care settings as compared with specialty settings? Are PAs and NPs interchangeable within managed care settings?
2. Compare and contrast physician/PA roles in fee-for-service as compared with capitated systems. What factors influence decisions? How are decisions made? Who has input into the decisions?
3. Are there "skills" that patients as consumers need to have within managed care systems? What is the PA's role in "training" patients to access and utilize services in managed care settings?
4. What is the appropriate function of a gatekeeper? What are the positive and negative aspects of this concept? Interview providers within an MCO to discuss their views on this issue.

REFERENCES

1. Trends and Indicators in the Changing Health Care Marketplace, 2002: Chartbook May 2002. Menlo Park, CA: The Henry J. Kaiser Family Foundation, 2002.
2. Davis A, Hawn RR, Hooker RS, et al. Managed care: the corporatization of medicine and PAs. J Am Acad Physician Assistants 1995;8:26, 33.
3. Coile RC Jr. The New Governance: Strategies for an Era of Health Reform. Ann Arbor, MI: Health Administration Press, 1994.
4. Wartman SA. Managed care and its effect on residency training in internal medicine. Arch Intern Med 1994;154:2539.
5. Brobst KL, Gunzburger L, Schwarz MR, et al. Notes on the changing face of health professions education. Joint Commission Journal on Quality Improvement 1995;21:711.
6. Phillips RR, Lee MY, Berman HA, Madoff MA. The Tufts partnership for managed care education. Acad Med 1997; 72:347.
7. Charting a Course for the 21st Century: Physician Assistants and Managed Care. The Physician Assistant Task Force on the Impact of Managed Care. San Francisco, CA: The Center for the Health Professions, University of California, 1998.

8. Meyer GS, Potter A, Gary N. A national survey to define a new core curriculum to prepare physicians for managed care practice. Acad Med 1997;72:669.

9. Guisto JA, Isikoff SJ. A proposed curriculum to teach practice management for a managed care environment. Top Emerg Med 1996;18:6.

10. Parenti CM, Moldow CF. Training internal medicine residents in the community: The Minnesota experience. Acad Med 1995;70:366.

11. Davis A, Hawn RR, Hooker RS, et al. Managed care: do corporatized medicine and PAs make a match? J Am Acad Physician Assistants 1995;8:74, 82.

12. Gomez AG, Grimm CT, Yee EF, Skootsky SA. Preparing residents for managed care practice using an experience-based curriculum. Acad Med 1997;72:959.

13. Kachur EK, Moshman EP. A managed care curriculum for primary care residents. Presented at The Continuum of the Managed Care Curriculum: Educational Objectives and Methods for Students and Residents. Key Biscayne, FL: The Robert Wood Johnson Foundation, 1997.

14. Medical College of Ohio PA Program. Health Care Teams and Systems (course syllabus), 1996.

15. Lurie N. Preparing physicians for practice in managed care environments. Acad Med 1996;71:1044.

16. Baker MD. Senior Seminar: Medical Economics (course syllabus). Philadelphia College of Textiles and Science PA Program, 1997.

17. Defino T. Educating physicians in managed care. Health System Leader 1995;2:4.

18. Cope DW, Sherman S, Robbins AS. Restructuring VA ambulatory care and medical education: the PACE model of primary care. Acad Med 1996;71:761.

19. Krause KC. Educating for patient care in the 21st century. Fam Med 1995;27:354.

20. Leshan LA. A curriculum in managed care for family medicine residents. Wisc Med J 1996;95:22.

21. Robbins AS, Cope DW, Campbell L, Vivell S. Expert ratings of primary care goals and objectives. J Gen Intern Med 1995;10:429.

22. Mainous AG, Blue AV, Griffith CH, et al. Assessing residents' readiness for working in a managed care environment. Acad Med 1997;72:385.

23. Krause KC. Ethically challenged by managed care. Fam Med 1996;28:101.

24. Behrman RE. Some unchanging values of pediatric education during a time of changing technology and practice. Pediatrics 1996;98(6 Pt 2):1249, 1289.

25. Fletcher RH, Fletcher SW. Teaching preventive medicine and health maintenance. Ann Intern Med 1992;116(12 Pt 2):1094.

26. Segal ES. Maintaining communication in a time of uncertainty. Arch Fam Med 1995;4:1066.

27. Cloutier M. Ethical issues in managed care. Paper presented at the Idaho Rural Health Conference, September 1997, Pocatello, Idaho.

28. Stoudemire A. Psychiatry in medical practice:implications for the education of primary care physicians in the era of managed care: Part 2. Psychosomatics 1997;38:1.

29. Leininger LS, Finn L, Dickey L, et al. An office system for organizing preventive services: a report by the American Cancer Society Advisory Group on Preventive Health Care Reminder Systems. Arch Fam Med 1996;5:108.

30. Faughnan JG. Informatics elements of a medical school predoctoral managed care curriculum. Available at http://dragon.labmed.umn.edu/~john/papers/inforcurr.html, 1997.

31. Ferenchick G, Simpson D, Blackman J, et al. Strategies for efficient and effective teaching in the ambulatory care setting. Acad Med 1997;72:277.

32. Pyatt RS. The role of CME and managed care. NJ Med 1997;94:55.

33. Scott HM, Tangalos EG, Blomberg RA, Bender CE. Survey of physician leadership and management education. Mayo Clin Proc 1997;72:659.

RESOURCES

Kongstvedt PR (ed). Essentials of Managed Health Care, 4th ed. Gaithersburg, MD: Aspen Publishers, 2001. *A textbook for students in health professions programs, this abbreviated edition of the author's larger work*, The Managed Health Care Handbook, *includes learning objectives and study questions illustrating managed care concepts.*

Sheldon A. Managing Doctors. Homewood, IL: Dow-Jones, Irwin, 1986. [Reprint: Washington, DC: Beard Books, 2002.] *A detailed discussion of the complex relationships between health organizations and physicians (and ultimately, PAs).*

Weldfed JA. Contracting with Managed Care Organizations: A Guide for The Health Care Provider. Chicago, IL: American Hospital Association, 1996. *A strategic approach to managed care contracting.*

Moseley GB. Managed Care Strategies: A Physician Practice Desk Reference. Gaithersburg, MD: Aspen Publishers, 1999.

CHAPTER 24

Ambulatory Services

Roderick S. Hooker

INTRODUCTION

Approximately one fourth of the noninstitutionalized civilian population in the United States had contact with providers of ambulatory care other than a physician during 2000. Such providers span a wide range of health professionals, including nurses, therapists, optometrists, chiropractors, podiatrists, psychologists, nurse practitioners, and physician assistants. Health services researchers, economists, sociologists, and managers are increasingly interested in the delegation of physician functions to these health care practitioners. The benefits of utilizing nonphysician providers include lowering overall costs, increasing accessibility of care, and improving the range of consumer choice.

In the delivery of ambulatory care, a variety of health professionals strive for legitimacy. As they do so, some of the lines that demarcated divisions of labor have become blurred. Territories once the exclusive domain of the physician have been challenged, often de facto, by gradual changes in customary practice by different types of providers other than physicians. In an effort to use a generic term for health care practitioners who provide physician-like services, medical sociologists and the federal government have adopted the term *providers* to refer to physicians and nonphysicians alike. In the present context, nonphysician providers (NPPs) refers to physician assistants (PAs), nurse practitioners (NPs), and certified nurse midwives (CNMs). This chapter focuses on ambulatory care services, how they are organized, and the role physician assistants play in the provision of these services.

Historically, the U.S. health care system has enjoyed strong, widespread public support, and between 1910 and 1970, it flowered into one of the best, if not the best, in the world. It is still superior in most areas of medicine. For those with medical insurance and unlimited access to care, this system leads the world in quality health care and adult longevity. The flaw is not in the delivery or technology, but in the lack of a national system that allows equal, unrestricted access for all Americans. What exists is a cash barrier between health care services and the people who need and cannot afford them because of the economic burden of the ever-increasingly complex and costly scientific means of providing those services. The lack of a social mandate to overcome this barrier has been partially balanced by the government enactment of Medicare and Medicaid in 1965. Unfortunately, at the time of this writing in 2002, more than 45 million Americans were either uninsured or underinsured for health coverage and did not qualify for government assistance. This group, larger than the total population of Canada, is unable to pay for the exorbitant costs of a medical office visit. As an example, Table 24-1 shows a typical case of a medical office visit in the Midwest. For a single episode of an acute illness, the cost to the patient, the insurance company, or some payer will be $126. How can the person with a limited income and no insurance pay for the nuances of life that need medical attention?

Table 24-1 Typical Costs of Medical Care	
As an example, the average cost for a minor acute episode of streptococcal pharyngitis breaks down as follows:	
Office visits (2)	$ 96
150 mL Amoxicillin suspension	15
Acetaminophen and over-the-counter medications	15
Total	$126

The demand for medical care continues to increase. Rising costs are due to many factors: public spending, insurance costs, expanding medical technology, an aging population, urbanization, and the higher price paid for the higher technical competence of our health care deliverers. It is estimated that more than $14 of every $100 of the gross domestic product was devoted to medical care (15% GDP) in 2002, and that $16 of each $100 will be spent by 2006. Nationally, health care costs are the second largest government expenditure, exceeded only by defense spending. Thus, the rising costs of health services are a major economic issue for the country as a whole.

AMBULATORY HEALTH CARE DEFINED

Ambulatory care is the personal health care service provided to someone who is not a bed patient in a hospital or other health care institution. It implies that the patient either walks in on his or her own or arrives via wheelchair, crutches, or gurney. The term *ambulatory care* covers all nonhospital health services. An *ambulatory patient* is defined as an individual seeking personal health services other than admission to a health care institution. Terms synonymous with ambulatory care are *outpatient treatment* and *medical office visit*. These visits may involve routine, scheduled, urgent, or emergent situations. Diagnoses, procedures, and various services rendered constitute a medical office visit. This is what drives the American medical system because more than 99% of contacts between providers and patients take place in an ambulatory setting.

Types of Outpatient Ambulatory Care Settings

Outpatient services range from immediate treatment for an acute and often serious illness or injury to care for a more routine matter. This care may take place in the following settings organized for ambulatory services in the United States:

➤ Fee-for-service medical practice.
➤ Prepaid group practice plans.
➤ Hospital-based ambulatory care center.
➤ Mental health centers.
➤ Community health centers.
➤ School and university health centers.
➤ Health department clinics.

➤ Home care programs.
➤ Family planning clinics.
➤ Industrial clinics.
➤ Ambulatory surgical centers.
➤ Urgency care centers.
➤ Corrections institutions.

The most important site of ambulatory care other than the hospital-based outpatient department is the practitioner's office. The hospital remains, however, the natural setting for the vertical integration of patients from outpatient departments back into the hospital. A patient enters the system from the outpatient specialty for hospitalization to the same inpatient specialty as an inpatient. After diagnosis and treatment, the patient returns to the original specialty clinic for follow-up care.

Strong economic incentives are encouraging health care systems to shift a larger portion of inpatient services, such as surgery and complex diagnostic procedures, to the outpatient setting. Physicians and administrators in group practices, hospitals, and clinics are immersed in this transition. They are in the uncomfortable position of having to devise strategies for ambulatory program activities with insufficient information, and then to make rational, cost-effective decisions while maintaining a high standard of care. Trying to establish the boundary between inpatient and outpatient care is becoming increasingly difficult because there are so many innovative programs that make the boundary difficult to define.

HISTORICAL PERSPECTIVE

Throughout history, until the advent of institutional care, all medical care was provided on an ambulatory basis. Remarkable efforts at quality medicine were made not only in Greece and Rome but in almost all societies, whether primitive or advanced, as far back as 3000 years ago. From the 16th through the mid-20th centuries, many medical services were provided to wealthy patients in their homes, while the poor were cared for in dispensaries and public clinics. Eventually, as medical care improved, more and more patients of all social classes received inpatient as well as outpatient care in hospital settings.

In the United States, ambulatory care services were traditionally provided by individual medical practitioners in their offices, in patients' homes, or in public clinics operated primarily for poor and medically indigent people. Physicians' offices were commonly located in homes, as opposed to today's medical office buildings and larger medical centers. The "typical" primary care provider before World War II was a general practitioner who made house calls, provided guidance, and offered what treatment was available, often with working knowledge and rapport spanning generations within families.

Since World War II, an explosion of medical knowledge has led to increasing specialization and more complex technology. The result has been a rapid change in how and where services are provided. Fewer physicians are able or willing to spend the time required to travel to patients' homes. Many no longer can carry with them the equipment, supplies, and other resources available in an office. Initially, this rapid growth of specialization and technology led to more frequent hospitalization. The excessive costs of hospitalization in turn led to the expansion of innovative settings for providing care, such as group practices, hospital clinics, and outpatient diagnostic and surgical centers.

For the poor, care has often been limited to public or philanthropic clinics or dispensaries. These settings eventually evolved into public hospitals and government-sponsored clinics. Efforts to integrate ambulatory care services with inpatient care were promoted in the United States and Europe through regionalization. For example, in the United Kingdom, these concepts were presented in the Dawson Report, from which eventually developed the National Health Service. In the United States, however, centralization of the health care system has not been accepted as a politically viable alternative, so there is a diverse but somewhat fractured network of providers available mostly to those who can pay.

PRIMARY CARE

Primary care service, ambulatory in nature, is the first line of contact for most patients entering the health care system. Because primary care concentrates on common problems, there is a tendency to consider it routine and as not requiring special expertise.

The goals of primary care are better served by prac-
titioners organized to provide primary care than by
practitioners trained to focus on particular illnesses,
organ systems, or pathogenic mechanisms.
Barbara Starfield, *Primary Care*
(Oxford University Press, 1992)

Starfield has formulated the key tasks of primary
care as the following:
1. First contact care.
2. Longitudinality.
3. Comprehensiveness.
4. Coordination.

In an ideal setting, primary care is delivered by an
appropriately trained health professional or team that
provides most of the preventive and curative care for
an individual or family. The role of the primary care
provider is to coordinate any services that involve
other health professionals, to integrate and explain
overall health problems, and to give attention to
psychological and social dimensions of health.
Comprehensive primary care comprises a great deal
of prevention and health promotion. Generally, primary care is provided by clinicians trained in internal
medicine, family practice, and pediatrics.

Secondary care consists of services that are usually
available at community hospitals or in offices normally found through referral or consultation following a preliminary appraisal by a primary care
practitioner. Surgery is the most typical example of
secondary care, followed by specialties such as
cardiology, gastroenterology, and radiology. Some
specialists (e.g., psychiatrists, dermatologists, obste-
tricians/gynecologists, and orthopedists) are more
accessible than others, in that they are often set up for
patient self-referral. A fee-for-service system may
even market their services. Cosmetic surgery, wellness, and weight loss clinics are classic examples of
medical services that have been actively promoted.
Newer players to this approach are physiatry (rehabilitation medicine), addiction, and oncology.

Tertiary care, at the other end of the spectrum,
tends to transcend the capabilities of the average community hospital. Tertiary care facilities, often university-based hospitals, consist of highly specialized
diagnostic, therapeutic, and rehabilitative services
requiring highly trained staff and sophisticated
equipment. These academic medical centers provide
services such as organ transplant and artery surgery,
as well as technologically complex procedures that
may still be experimental.

Use of Ambulatory Care Services

Measuring and analyzing the use of ambulatory care
resources are extremely important in defining the
scope and content of this field. To the extent that data
are available, planning for ambulatory care and analysis of patterns of use can be helpful in determining the
need for resources. Some quantitative data are available about the use of ambulatory care resources for the
nation. Although most of the data pertain to the use of
physicians, they are considered equally applicable to
other practitioners who perform in physician roles.

To understand practice patterns of clinicians in the
United States, the federal government has implemented an ongoing national study of all office-based
medical practices. This study involves a random sample of physicians, who agree to complete a data collection form for each patient they treat during a
1-week period. The data from 1999 are presented in
the sections that follow. The National Ambulatory
Medical Care Survey (hereafter also called "the
Survey") estimates that 756.7 million medical office
visits were made to non–federally employed medical
providers in the United States during 1999. The rate
of medical office visits has also held steady, at
approximately 2.8 visits per person per year. In terms
of the number, percentage, and rate of office visits,
this is an extraordinary burden on a society already
overwhelmed by spiraling medical care costs and a
maldistribution of medical providers.

Analysis by Specialty

Specialty is the type of health care service the practitioner elects to provide. Table 24-2 shows the distribution of medical office visits by specialty for the most
frequently visited specialists. General medicine and
family practice account for 23% of office visits. This
seems to parallel the proportion of general and family
physicians during the same period. Interestingly
enough, this distribution of physician specialties also
correlates well with the distribution of specialties
reported by a census of physician assistants.

Table 24-2 Percentage Distribution of Office Visits by Physician Practice Characteristics (1999)

Physician Specialty and Professional Identity	Number of Visits (x 1000)	Percentage Distribution
All Visits	697,082	100.00
BY PHYSICIAN SPECIALTY		
General and family practice	170,571	22.5
Internal medicine	135,607	17.9
Pediatrics	74,045	9.8
Obstetrics and gynecology	59,518	7.9
Ophthalmology	51,165	6.8
Orthopedic surgery	40,516	5.4
Dermatology	32,704	4.3
Psychiatry	21,174	3.0
General surgery	21,174	2.8
Otolaryngology	16,369	2.2
Cardiovascular diseases	16,566	2.2
Urology	17,415	2.3
Neurology	8,298	1.1
All other specialties	90,440	12.0
BY PROFESSIONAL IDENTITY		
Doctor of Medicine	709,071	93.7
Doctor of Osteopathy	47,663	6.3

Table 24-3 Number and Percentage of Office Visits by Patient Age and Sex

Age Group	Females (Percentage)	Males (Percentage)	Total Percentage	Total Number of Visits
<15	7.3	8.1	15.4	116,904
15-24	5.1	2.8	7.9	59,706
25-44	15.7	8.8	24.6	186,022
45-64	15.8	10.9	26.7	201,911
65-74	6.8	5.4	12.2	92,642
≥75	8.1	5.0	13.2	99,548

Analysis by Patient Characteristics

Medical office visit data according to patient age and sex are shown in Table 24-3. Females account for 59% of all office visits and for a majority of the visits in every age group except the youngest. The annual visit rate is also higher for females than for males in all age groups except the youngest. For both sexes, the visit rates increase with age after the age of 15 years. As noted earlier, the overall visit rate of 2.8 office visits per person has remained roughly the same since 1985 but ranges from 1.6 visits annually for patients aged 15 to 24 years to a high of 6.8 visits for those over age 75. This bimodal trend of a high rate of office visits for the very young and the old is characteristic of most populations and is not likely to change in the near future.

Visit characteristics data gathered for the National Ambulatory Medical Care Survey of 1999 reveal that 86% of visits were made by patients who had seen the provider before, with almost two thirds returning

Table 24-4   Distribution of Medical Office Visits by the 20 Most Common Principal Reasons for Visit, United States (1999)

Rank	Most Common Principal Reason For Visit*	Percentage
1	General medical examination	5.8
2	Progress visit, not otherwise specified	4.0
3	Postoperative visit	3.1
4	Cough	2.6
5	Routine prenatal examination	4.0
6	Symptoms referable to throat	1.9
7	Well-baby examinations	1.4
8	Vision dysfunctions	1.6
9	Knee symptoms	1.5
10	Hypertension	1.4
11	Earache or ear infection	1.2
12	Back symptoms	1.4
13	Skin rash	1.2
14	Stomach pain, cramps, and spasms	1.4
15	Fever	1.0
16	Depression	1.5
17	Medication, other and unspecified kinds	1.2
18	Low back symptoms	1.1
19	Nasal congestion	1.1
20	Headache, pain in the head	1.3
	All other reasons	60.1

From http://www.cdc.gov/nchs/about/major/ahcd/ahcd1.htm. Accessed December 2002.
*Based on *A Reason for Visit Classification for Ambulatory Care.*
Data from the National Ambulatory Medical Care Survey of 1999.

for the same problem. The 20 principal ambulatory visit reasons, complaints, or problems are listed in Table 24-4. General medical examination and upper respiratory complaints (cough, sore throat) were the most common reasons for a visit.

The principal diagnoses rendered by physicians, PAs, NPs, and nurses are presented in Table 24-5. The most common diagnoses made were primary (essential) hypertension (ranked 1st), acute upper respiratory infection (2nd), arthropathies and related disorders (3rd), routine infant or child check (4th), diabetes (5th), and back pain (6th). Collectively, these accounted for 19%, or almost one fifth, of all diagnoses in 1999.

Medication

Approximately 1.1 billion medications were prescribed or provided at ambulatory care visits in 1999.

The setting with the greatest percentage of visits with medication therapy was the emergency department, followed by medical offices. Data on the distribution of prescribed medication are listed by therapeutic class and according to frequency of prescription in Tables 24-6 and 24-7.

Cardiovascular-renal drugs (antihypertensives) constitute the largest therapeutic class, accounting for 15.6% of all drugs prescribed. The next two largest therapeutic classes of drugs are the drugs used for pain (analgesics) and the respiratory tract drugs at 10.8% and 10.4%, respectively.

Duration of visit, as defined in the survey, refers to the amount of time a provider spent in face-to-face contact with a patient. When a patient was seen by someone other than the practitioner, such as the nurse, clerk, or receptionist, the duration of the visit was

Table 24-5 Number and Distribution of Office Visits by the 20 Most Common Principal Diagnosis Groups, United States (1999)

Rank	Most Common Principal Diagnosis	Percentage
1	Essential hypertension	4.2
2	Acute upper respiratory infections, excluding pharyngitis	3.8
3	Arthropathies and related disorders	3.1
4	Routine infant or child health check	3.0
5	Diabetes mellitus	2.6
6	Dorsopathies	2.3
7	Allergic rhinitis	2.2
8	Normal pregnancy	2.2
9	Rheumatism, excluding back	2.2
10	Malignant neoplasms	2.0
11	Otitis media and eustachian tube disorders	1.9
12	Follow-up examination	1.8
13	General medical examination	1.8
14	Cataract	1.5
15	Chronic sinusitis	1.4
16	Heart disease, excluding ischemic	1.3
17	Ischemic heart disease	1.3
18	Potential health hazards related to personal and family history	1.3
19	Asthma	1.3
20	Benign and uncertain neoplasms	1.2
	All other diagnoses	57.9

Data from the National Ambulatory Medical Care Survey of 1999.

recorded as zero. More than two thirds of the visits surveyed had a duration of 15 minutes or less, whereas one third lasted longer than 15 minutes, as shown in Table 24-8. The mean duration time for all visits was 19.3 minutes.

The high rankings of routine follow-up or ongoing care as well as of relatively simple primary care problems are striking, reflecting the predominance of these types of problems in ambulatory practice. Prenatal examinations, limited examinations, hypertension, and otitis media were the most common diagnoses or services provided. More than half of the visits required a follow-up visit, initiated by either the physician or the patient.

Office-Based Practice

Most of the ambulatory care that people receive is provided in office-based practice settings. Although a significant amount of care is provided in hospital settings, the predominant source of care is the physician's office, whether individual, group (partnership), or noninstitutional clinic practices.

Two predominant private settings or forms of practice are individual and group. In an individual or solo practice, a single practitioner provides the services. Group practice is the combination of two or more practitioners in an office-based setting. In a third variation, two or more practitioners share some clerical and medical resources but function independently.

Solo Practice Ambulatory care services have been provided by physicians in individual practice since colonial times. Although individual practice still accounts for a small segment of ambulatory care, it is fading as group practice and hospital-based services are expanding dramatically. Changing lifestyles, the

Table 24-6   Number and Percentage Distribution of Drug Mentions by Therapeutic Classification, United States (1999)

Therapeutic Class*	Number of Mentions (x 1000)	Percentage Distribution
All drug mentions	1,136,686	100.0
Cardiovascular-renal drugs	176,839	15.6
Drugs used for relief of pain	122,469	10.8
Respiratory tract drugs	118,241	10.4
Hormones and agents affecting hormone mechanisms	112,902	9.9
Antimicrobial agents	106,226	9.3
Central nervous system	100,148	8.8
Metabolic and nutrient agents	74,794	6.6
Skin/mucous membrane	65,027	5.7
Gastrointestinal agents	50,526	4.4
Immunologic agents	48,310	4.3
Ophthalmic drugs	46,563	4.1
Neurologic drugs	25,222	2.2
Hematological drugs	19,189	1.7
Oncolytic agents	10,361	0.9
Anesthetic drugs	7,780	0.7
Otologics	7,032	0.6
Antiparasitics	4,828	0.4
Contrast media/radiopharmaceuticals	4,093	0.4
Other and unclassified	35,866	3.2

*Based on the standard drug classification used in the *National Drug Code Directory*, 1995 edition. Data from The National Ambulatory Medical Care Survey of 1999.

cost of establishing a practice, external pressures on practitioners, and government programs have all adversely affected the traditional dominance of individual practice. At the current rate, solo practitioners will make up one third of all practices but less than 5% of all physicians at the end of the decade.

Group Practice   Group practice is an affiliation of three or more providers, usually physicians, who share income, expenses, facilities, equipment, medical records, and support personnel in the provision of services in a formal, legally constituted organization. Traditionally, group practice has meant participation and ownership by physicians. Increasingly, dentists, optometrists, and other specialized personnel are also developing group practices. Groups may be composed only of physicians or may incorporate various other practitioners, such as PAs, NPs, podiatrists, psychologists, nurse midwives, and nurse anesthetists. Group practices may be classified as specialty (e.g., all orthopedists) or multi-specialty practices.

Prepaid Group Practice   Group practice in which health care services are reimbursed on a prepaid basis, rather than on a fee-for-service basis, is an increasingly popular form of health care delivery and is referred to as prepaid group practice. Group practices typically require that providers practice together in one organization and sometimes under one roof. The concept of prepayment has also been applied to community-based individual and small group practitioners through the development of independent practice plans, a form of health maintenance organization (HMO). More than 93% of

Table 24-7   Number and Percentage of Drug Mentions for the 20 Most Frequently Used Generic Substances, United States (1999)

Generic Substance*	Number of Mentions (x 1000)*	Percentage of Drug Mentions
All generic substances	1,325,001	—
Acetaminophen	36,343	3.2
Amoxicillin	24,125	2.1
Hydrochlorothiazide	18,534	1.6
Albuterol	17,960	1.6
Estrogens	17,777	1.6
Hydrocodone	17,155	1.5
Ibuprofen	17,071	1.5
Loratadine	15,978	1.4
Furosemide	15,413	1.4
Guaifenesin	15,059	1.3
Aspirin	15,014	1.3
Levothyroxine	14,175	1.2
Lisinopril	13,777	1.2
Prednisone	13,024	1.1
Atorvastatin calcium	12,385	1.1
Atenolol	12,025	1.1
Omeprazole	11,811	1.0
Triamcinolone	11,256	1.0
Digoxin	11,014	1.0
Fluticasone propionate	10,035	0.9

*Frequency of mention combines single-ingredient agents with mentions of the agent as an ingredient in a combination drug.
Data from the National Ambulatory Medical Care Survey of 1999.

Table 24-8   Number and Percentage Distribution of Office Visits by Duration of Visit, United States (1999)

Time Spent With Physician	Number of Visits (x 1000)	Percentage Distribution
All Visits	756,734	100.0
0*	32,377	4.3
1-5 minutes	26,156	3.6
6-10 minutes	158,163	21.8
11-15 minutes	242,530	33.5
16-30 minutes	236,888	32.7
31-60 minutes	57,068	7.9
61 minutes plus	3,550	0.5

*Represents office visits in which there was no face-to-face contact between the patient and the practitioner.
Data from the National Ambulatory Medical Care Survey of 1999.

physicians have managed care contracts. The increasing importance of prepayment has led many fee-for-service group practices to participate, at least partially, in prepayment options through insurance companies.

Practice Patterns

Since 1982, the average U.S. physician has spent 51 hours per week in patient care activities, handling 132 patient visits per week. The range in average number of visits handled is rather broad—55 visits per week for psychiatrists, 110 for surgeons, 150 for pediatricians, and 180 for general practitioners. For all specialties, rural physicians had about 35% more visits than did urban physicians. In many managed health care systems such as HMOs, military medical

facilities, and the Veterans Administration, PA and NP schedules are the same as those of the physicians, and they probably see a similar number of patients weekly.

An important aspect of the role of physician assistants is that a majority see patients primarily on an ambulatory basis, unlike physicians, who divide their time between the office and the hospital. In the United States, the PA's place in the ambulatory setting is similar to that in many foreign countries, where physicians see either ambulatory patients or hospital inpatients on a full-time basis. This division of labor has not changed appreciably over the past century. Tables 24-9 and 24-10 provide some comparative detail on office visits to physicians and mid-level providers.

Table 24-9   Average Annual Number of Office-Based Visits by Provider Type According to Primary Care Specialty (1995-1998)

	PA Visits (x 1000)	NP Visits (x 1000)	Physician Visits (x 1000)
General and family practice	4,439	2,420	183,410
Internal medicine	1,827	1,176	114,710
Pediatrics	1,547	893	87,720
Obstetrics and gynecology	573	128	64,923
Total	8,386	4,617	450,763

Table 24-10   Diagnostic, Screening and Other Services Ordered or Provided, by Provider Type (1995-1998)

	PA Visits (percentage)	NP Visits (percentage)	Physician Visits (percentage)
Diagnostic or screening services provided at visit	27.1	19.8	24.5
Pelvic examination	6.6	15.4	11.8
Breast examination	4.7	10.1	9.0
Rectal examination	2.7	*	5.4
Urinalysis	13.2	24.5	15.6
Diet	21.3	22.2	18.6
Exercise	11.1	10.4	11.6

*Figure does not meet standard of reliability or precision.

RESEARCH

Little research has been undertaken regarding what PAs actually do in practice. Although medical practice is the most important function of PAs in this sector of the U.S. health care delivery system, it is also the least studied.

Ongoing research will help to shape the delivery of medical care involving PAs by examining some of the following areas:

➤ What kind of practice arrangements they have.
➤ How many patients they see.
➤ How many office visits they handle.
➤ How often they see patients in hospitals.
➤ How many telephone calls they receive from patients.
➤ What diagnostic tests they order.
➤ What types of therapies they prescribe.
➤ What kinds of medical problems they see.
➤ What surgical procedures they participate in and what their role in the operating room is.
➤ How they spend their day.

The few studies that have been done suggest the substitution possibilities among physician assistants and nurse practitioners, for physicians. Most of the work has focused on the productivity gains possible through increased delegation of physician tasks to PAs and NPs. Estimates of the magnitude of the gains vary widely, depending on the particular setting analyzed and the constraints imposed. Virtually all of the studies have found, however, that substantial productivity is gained with increased delegation.

In this context, *delegation* refers to the types of medical problems or conditions handled by the PA in a given practice. An important component of delegation is the percentage of the practice's total office visits that those problems or conditions constitute. Most of these studies have examined some aspect of physician office visits as a measure of ability to delegate. The research consistently concludes that between 75% and 90% of primary care services can be delegated to PAs and NPs. When 100 of the most frequently seen diagnoses in a general medicine or family practice clinic are examined, the average physician assistant is comfortable treating or managing at least the first 86 of them. This 86% figure has become somewhat of an industry standard in describing what physician assistants are capable of handling solely without supervision.

These and other similar studies on PA performance were conducted in the early and middle 1970s, when the role of the PA was still developing.[1-3] Physician assistants in the aggregate are capable of handling more than 86% of the most common diagnoses. It is important to note that these percentages vary according to the practice setting and the specialty.

The extensive use of physician assistants and nurse practitioners by some HMOs indicates significant substitution possibilities. In 1971 and 1972, 79% of patient encounters in adult medicine at the Columbia Medical Plan were managed by physicians. With the gradual incorporation of PAs, that figure dropped to 38%. In 1971 and 1972, physician assistants managed 10% of initial encounters for illness and injury but conducted no long-term health management. By 1973 and 1974, PAs managed 50% of illnesses and 75% of initial injury encounters and conducted 50% of adult health care. Over the 3 years during which the Columbia Medical Plan took place, the total physician staff changed from 60% to 38%.

In 1986, Hooker[4] compared productivity rates of PAs and physicians in Kaiser Permanente in the Pacific Northwest. In this setting, which contained no triage for adult patients, physician assistants and physicians in the departments of internal medicine and family practice tended to see the same number of patients per day (20 for internal medicine, 22 in family practice). The number of patients seen annually was 30% higher for physician assistants than for the physician. This difference was attributed to the routine of the physician, who had more hospital responsibilities and time off (either as compensation or benefit). The physician and the PA managed the same types of illnesses and conditions in surprisingly similar numbers. However, patients with a diagnosis requiring hospitalization (e.g., acute myocardial infarction, cerebrovascular accident) or a progressive illness (e.g., cancer, progressive emphysema) tended to see the physician more often than they did the PA.

In the Northern California Kaiser Permanente (KP) Program, the nurse practitioners provide a health assessment program. Of the KP members who entered the health assessment program in 1976, 74%

were managed by NPs without physician referral. Two thirds of the patients referred to a physician went to a specialty clinic. In effect, the NP's visit substituted for an initial primary care physician visit. In another setting, using a mathematical model for HMO staffing patterns, Schneider and Foley[5] estimated that the substitution of one PA or NP would decrease required physician time by 53% to 60%, depending on the department.

According to a review by the Office of Technology Assessment,[6] estimates of increases in the productivity of physician practices using physician assistants range from 20% to 90% (this widely disparate range of estimates reflects different studies conducted at different times during the evolutionary phase of PA development, in the late 1960s and early 1970s). Using a relative value scale to capture home visit content, Holmes and co-workers[7] found that productivity levels in practices incorporating nurse practitioners were on average 26% higher than those in the traditional physician/nurse practice. Using activity analysis, Golladay and associates[8] estimated that a PA increased a primary care physician's productivity by 49% to 74%.

Although some of these early studies tended to find physician assistants and nurse practitioners less productive than physicians, NPP time or salary costs are much lower than a physician's time, thus producing a net gain in certain situations. In 1978, the median hourly wage for physician assistants was about $6, compared with $24 for physicians. Using these 1975 ratios, Record[9] estimated potential cost-savings (through greater task delegation in primary care) of from $500 million to more than $1 billion in 1979 dollars. This amounted to between 19% and 49% of total primary care provider costs. A congressional Office of Technology Assessment review[6] also demonstrated that employing nonphysician providers is profitable and reduces costs in the U.S. health care system.

Virtually all of the studies of physician assistants or nurse practitioners demonstrate that productivity is enhanced when they are part of the matrix of care. Their cost effectiveness stems, in part, from their lower salaries compared with physicians. The larger the organization or group practice, the more likely that incorporating a PA or an NP will enhance efficiency and cost effectiveness. Although this economy-of-scale factor has never been studied under maximal conditions, multivariate analysis suggests that the ideal ratio of PAs/NPs to physicians is 2:3. Clearly, further research is necessary in this area.

Delegation of Care

One of the stumbling blocks in maximizing the use of PAs for physician services has been the delegation issue. How much of which services can a supervising physician assume a PA or NP is capable of providing? Just as there are differences in physician approaches to providing services for any illness, there are differences in PA or NP approaches as well.

Although some of these questions deal with cost efficiency and have, at their core, the positive and negative consequences of a specific resource allocation, they also involve style and quality of care issues. Everyone hopes that the resolution of the illness will be positive and that the patient will recover with the least amount of disability. If everyone were to manage the same type of patient in the same way (for example, with 10 g of oral penicillin) and all patients recovered within 1 week, the outcome would be the same. If the PA's services fully substituted a physician's services and achieved the same outcome, the cost of that care would be less than the physician care because the PA's salary is less. In this example, the use of resources is less for the same episode of illness and the same outcome. To extend this example, a PA is capable of seeing 20 to 30 cases of acute pharyngitis on an average day. Presumably, a physician would be comfortable delegating the care of all cases of pharyngitis (or rash, or arthritis, or fractured clavicles, etc.) to the PA.

To examine the issue of delegation of care, two researchers at Kaiser Permanente in Portland, Oregon, surveyed the physician group to see what they were willing to delegate to PAs in primary care (i.e., internal medicine, family practice, and pediatrics). Johnson and colleagues[10] found that on average, physicians revealed that they thought PAs were capable of managing only 44% of frequently encountered conditions. The irony of this revelation is that the entire list of conditions was drawn from a group of the most common diagnoses PAs were already making. This gulf in understanding points to a problem prevalent in many industries: Worker competence or capabilities are underestimated. In this case, PAs not only were capable of doing more than the physicians believed they could do but were already doing it routinely.

Outcomes

In the middle 1960s, the most compelling policy question concerning health services appeared to be how to supply enough providers to meet the rising demands of health care consumers. By the middle 1970s, the dominant policy question had become how to contain the costs of health care services. By the late 1980s, the concern had shifted to outcomes of care and quality assurance. This latest question of interest has been stimulated for several reasons. First, the physician component in the cost of health care has always captured a substantial share of national health care expenditures. Second, physicians play a gate-keeping role in modern health care systems, in that they control access to hospitals, clinics, most medications, and an array of other medical care resources. It has been estimated that up to 80% of physicians' revenue arises from such self-generated activities.

Although discretion over certain courses of action in the medical care system is accepted under the legal monopoly given by societies to the medical profession, broad differences exist in the actual behavior of clinicians. Even when case mix and other patient characteristics are controlled, wide variation has been found among physicians in patterns of practice, use of outpatient services and procedures, and overall expenditures. Existing research suggests that there is little or no relationship between the intensity of resource use and the quality or outcome of care. These results have stimulated significant interest in attempts to understand the factors that account for these differences in provider behavior. Of particular interest is the extent to which factors influencing physician behavior are subject to modification by changes in training, continuing education, quality assurance mechanisms, management practices, and health policy.

Perhaps the most promising strategy for containing the costs and prices of medical services has been the development and use of physician assistants. The basic assumption is that PAs can substitute for physicians as primary care providers, system gatekeepers, or both. Because PAs are paid considerably less than physicians, costs should be less. This thinking assumes that resource use and outcomes are similar when PAs and physicians treat patients with the same problem. Most of the pivotal work on the cost-effective use of PAs and NPs has focused on acute care that involved one or a few office visits, such as pharyngitis, tendonitis, urinary tract infections, and routine physical examinations. Research is needed to determine whether NPPs are cost-effective with the same outcome in the management of chronic disease. For example, are the management and outcome the same for a 79-year-old man with congestive heart failure when he is treated by an internist as when he is treated by a family practitioner? Do internists order more tests than family practitioners do, and does their management of an episode of chronic disease cost more? What about the costs generated by a PA for the same illness?

The literature suggests that personal characteristics, professional characteristics, and setting are factors that affect physician behavior and performance. Age is the personal characteristic most consistently associated with variations in resource use; younger physicians tend to use more resources than older ones do. With regard to professional characteristics, specialty and number of years since graduation from medical school are consistent regardless of specialty or setting. As the number of years since graduation increases, the rate of resource use declines. These results hold mostly for outpatient services and procedures and probably apply to PAs as well.

Specialists and generalists differ in their practice styles and patterns of activity. Generally, specialists take more time with their patients, do more counseling, apply a more elaborate mix of resources, and use more diagnostic testing than do non–residency-trained generalists. Even when the other factors—patient characteristics and case mix—are controlled, the differences hold.

Setting-related factors constitute the other variables affecting differences in physician practice patterns and outcomes. Every work setting has its own special source of influence over the work of individual health professionals.

Group practice is the setting that has been studied extensively because of the significant increase in practitioners who have taken up this form of practice. Physicians in larger groups have higher resource use patterns and tend to order more tests than do those in smaller groups. Physicians who own their own laboratories and radiology equipment order laboratory tests and radiographic procedures more often than those who do not, when age and condition of patients are held constant.

Although numerous studies have compared the cost differences between types of physicians, only a few studies have compared physician assistants with physicians as to resource use, costs, and the quality of care. One study[11] examined the relationship between levels of medical training and direct costs for outpatient episodes of acute illness in a university family medicine clinic. Faculty, family practice (FP) residents, and PAs were studied. The average total cost per episode of illness was the same for the three provider types. This study, conducted in 1977, did, however, find significant differences in laboratory and medication costs. Faculty members and PAs generated higher costs than did FP residents for patients who tended to have bad outcomes. A similar study[12] using the same mix of providers found that functional outcomes of acute episodes that were handled by PAs were as good as or better than outcomes for those handled by physicians. No differences in patient satisfaction or mean dollar costs per episode of care were linked to provider type. Table 24-11 provides a comparison of what it would cost to see a physician or a PA for representative types of visits.

The U.S. Air Force, a major employer of PAs, examined the quality of care provided by PAs in its primary care medicine clinics. In this study,[13] quality of care judgments were based on diagnostic, therapeutic, and disposition criteria. The findings showed that PAs performed as well as physicians for 25 out of 28 nonredundant process-of-care criteria. No major differences were found between PAs and physicians in the use of laboratory, radiographic, or physical therapy procedures. Record and O'Bannon[14] examined the quality of PA performance by identifying the complication rates and the adverse drug rates for four morbidities treated by either physicians or PAs. Although PAs tended to use a greater number of diagnostic procedures, especially laboratory tests, performance was comparable to that of physicians. Hooker[4] examined

Table 24-11   Cost Comparison for Visiting a Physician or PA

Provider	N	Total Cost	Medical Office Cost	Med Cost	Image Cost	Lab Cost
BRONCHITIS						
Physician	1336	$234.74	$133.63	$96.42	$3.31	$1.37
PA	411	$224.13	$92.23	$125.74	$4.65	$1.50
TENDONITIS						
Physician	264	$183.33**	$144.77*	$30.14	$7.50	$0.93
PA	90	$149.80**	$98.77*	$40.65	$9.53	$0.84
OTITIS MEDIA						
Physician	6246	$188.39*	$140.07*	$47.77	$0.0	$0.54
PA	2008	$136.60*	$83.29*	$52.99	$0.0	$0.32
UTI						
Physician	1633	$262.17*	$142.73*	$83.91	$17.67*	$17.86**
PA	878	$210.50*	$97.70*	$91.50	$5.80*	$15.48**

Data from Hooker RS. A cost analysis of physician assistants in primary care. J Am Acad Physician Assistants. In press.
*Significant at $P < 0.001$.
**Significant at $P < 0.01$.

types of patients likely to be seen by type of provider (PA, NP, physician) in the departments of internal medicine, family practice, and pediatrics in an HMO. There was considerable overlap in the types of patients cared for and the diagnoses rendered. When patient satisfaction was examined, there were slight differences in how patients viewed their providers. Overall, these patients expressed a willingness to return to the same NP, PA, or physician in ranks of 94%, 92%, and 88%, respectively.

All of the studies on outcomes of outpatient care have a variety of limitations that affect interpretations of the findings. In general, the limited data on outcomes indicate little or no difference between physicians and PAs. The same holds for patient satisfaction.

Few of these studies have addressed the critical question of comparable resource use and costs over time. Resource use and costs have been examined mainly for acute illnesses, many of which could be interpreted as self-limited, and most analyses are based on one encounter. What is lacking is a record of how chronic morbidities are compared by various providers of primary care over the course of the condition, that is, by episodes of care. Little, if any, of the research in this area has concentrated on patients 65 years of age and older. A few studies have suggested that primary care providers may deal differently with older patients, but none has compared practice patterns and outcomes for physicians and PAs in the same setting. Finally, research needs to be conducted in settings using capitation reimbursement, in which:

1. There are no major constraints to limit patients seeking care.
2. Providers face similar incentives for resource use and quality.

Defining and Measuring Quality of Care in Ambulatory Settings

The Institute of Medicine defines quality of care as "health care that effectively betters the health status and satisfaction of the population, within the resources that society and individuals have chosen to spend for that care."[15] Any quality assessment program that evaluates the PA's overall performance should do so in relation to this definition; it should

also quantify the determinants of health care in a manner that will allow changes to be made that affect improvements in care. Some parameters used to measure quality of care are as follows.

Provider Performance Provider performance is defined as the clinician's ability to use the best available knowledge, skills, and judgment in order to produce a desired health care outcome. The parameter includes evaluation of credentials, competence, technical and interpersonal skills, and actual clinical performance.

Support Staff Performance In addition to clinical performance, support staff performance includes the education, certification, training, and experience of the support staff.

Continuity of Care Continuity denotes that the treatment plan progresses without interruption. Interruptions of care are missed appointments, omitted laboratory tests, missing radiographs, and so forth.

Medical Record System The assessment of the medical record system measures the extent to which the provider implements a system that provides timely and accurate recording of all appropriate clinical information in a way that permits easy and quick retrieval. Such a system functions as a structured framework for planning, providing, and evaluating patient care. Electronic medical records have become the norm for documenting interactions with patients in the new millennium.

Patient Risk Minimization Measures designed to reduce medical risks to a patient, such as drug profiles, allergy documentation systems, and infection control, as well as other safety measures such as fire control systems, are evaluated by this parameter.

Patient Satisfaction Patient satisfaction addresses how closely the health care services provided meet patient expectations. Levels of satisfaction with the appointment process, waiting time, financial arrangements, availability of providers, and actual care provided are evaluated.

Patient Compliance The patient compliance parameter evaluates how completely the patient assumes responsibility for following through with the health care plan. It is a measure of the mutual trust and sharing of information between providers and patients.

Access to Care The ability of patients to obtain needed health care services despite potential barriers (e.g., financial, geographical, organizational, cultural) is measured by this parameter.

Appropriateness of Services Another important indication of quality is whether a particular service provided—diagnostic procedure, therapeutic procedure, medication—was actually indicated in the care of a given patient, as well as whether a needed service was actually provided.

Cost of Services The final parameter reflects several aspects of the relationship between cost and quality of care. First, the patient's ability to pay may make needed health care less accessible. Second, cost considerations may influence whether particular services are made available to patients.

ISSUES
Supervision

By the very nature of their job description, PAs depend on physicians or physician organizations for their employment. The exception is the federal government, which hires PAs independently and then assigns them to medical units that are usually staffed with physicians.

With more than 45,000 PA graduates, PAs are spread throughout the United States and are beginning to make their presence known in a number of other countries. Unlike nurse practitioners, who maintain that they are extensions of the nursing act and can function independently, the PA is legally tied to the physician, in some form, for the basis of employment.

In some rural areas, PAs may function more or less independently at a satellite clinic, having only telephone contact with the physician. In other instances, they may be part of a large HMO and have only a perfunctory relationship with physicians in order to meet the requirements of state law. The range of relationships that PAs and supervising physicians can have is vast. For the most part, though, PAs and their supervising physicians often have close working relationships, a high level of trust, and mutual respect spanning many years.

The aging of the physician assistant profession has brought about some unanticipated changes in PA/physician relationships. First, it is not uncommon for a PA to be older and more experienced than the supervising physician. Second, the PA may be subspecialized in a certain area (e.g., gastroenterology, rheumatology, arthroscopy), and the more recently trained physician may seek the expertise of the PA to learn a procedure. Third, in a reversal of roles, the physician may even seek out the specialized PA for consultation.

Supervision is the area of PA management that tends to be interpreted with wide latitude, depending on the interpreter. Some broad definitions are as follows:

➤ *Physician assistant is* a person qualified by education, training, experience, and personal character to provide medical services under the direction and supervision of a licensed physician. License, as it applies here, is for the state or federal physician. PAs can be licensed by a state medical board by a method similar to that used for physicians. This license registers the PA with the state board of medical examiners as a practitioner of medicine. Various administrative rules, procedures, and accordances are in effect to govern the activity of the PA, depending on the jurisdiction.

➤ *Supervising physician* is the physician who directs and regularly reviews the medical services provided by the physician assistant as determined appropriate by the state regulatory agency (usually a board of medical examiners).

➤ *Agent* is the physician designated by the supervising physician and approved by the board to provide direction and regular review of the medical services of the PA when the supervising physician is unavailable.

➤ *Practice description* is the written description, submitted by the supervising physician and PA to the regulatory agency, outlining the type of medical practice and functions of the PA. A note of caution is warranted here. There is a tendency to make this practice description explicit and complete. In the long run, such detail tends to be more restrictive than helpful because the style of practice and duties tend to change over time. The PA or physician who does not follow the letter of the job description can be held in violation of the law. In writing the practice description, one does best to make it generalized, permitting as wide discretion as possible in the management of patients.

➤ *Remote supervision* describes the routine review by the supervising physician of a PA who may be in a rural area or satellite clinic. Usually, this type of clinic operation is approved for medically disadvantaged areas. In this instance, the physician supervises by telephone but is not required to be physically present at the practice site.

➤ *Scope of practice* is the legal term that defines the tasks PAs may perform. Scope of practice for the PA is determined by state laws, regulatory boards, hospitals, the PA, and the supervising physician. The scope may be restricted or expanded on the basis of a PA's training, expertise, and skill. The scope of practice is highly variable according to what is defined by the state regulatory agency.

Prescribing

Physician assistants are sanctioned to prescribe in 47 states, the District of Columbia, and most U.S. territories. They also prescribe in a variety of federal programs, including the military forces, Veterans Administration, and Bureau of Prisons, as well as Public Health Service settings.

The authorization to prescribe applies almost completely to the outpatient setting. When inpatient medications are prescribed, they are considered orders and come under a different review process.

The underlying principle of outpatient prescribing is one of delegation by a supervising physician. This means that the physician has submitted a job description of the activities the PA will perform. In some instances, the physician's name will be on the prescription alongside the PA's name. Sometimes the prescription may need to be co-signed by the associate physician, the PA may be limited by a drug formulary, or the quantities of certain drugs that the PA may prescribe may be limited.

Little is known about how well PAs prescribe. One survey found that in states where PAs are authorized to prescribe, at least 90% do so.[16] Among these same PAs, the average number of prescriptions per week was 50. From this 1990 survey, the author estimated that PAs write more than 35 million prescriptions per year.

Few studies have examined the adequacy of PA prescribing. Concerns about competence have been advanced, but there is no evidence that PAs fail to perform this role in a safe and acceptable manner. Furthermore, no study has shown that the physician is at risk if the PA inappropriately prescribes. Existing studies have compared physician and PA patterns of practice, assessing the appropriateness of the diagnosis and treatment processes or the outcome of care.

The safety issue still remains to be definitively studied. In the few litigation cases that involve physician assistants, inappropriate prescribing has not been an issue. Record and associates[14] compared the performance of PAs and physicians in a large HMO in handling four specific morbidities—streptococcal pharyngitis, upper respiratory infections, bursitis, and bronchitis. One of the outcome criteria was the rate of adverse effects from antibiotics and other drugs provided in the treatment. These researchers found no differences in rates between PAs and physicians.

Of the 47 states whose legislation allows PAs to prescribe, two thirds of these allow prescribing of federally controlled substances of different classifications (Schedules II to V). In states that do not allow prescribing by PAs, anecdotal evidence suggests that PAs influence prescribing in many ways. For instance, the PA may see the patient and then suggest a treatment to the supervising physician, who may write the prescription without seeing the patient. The physician may give the PA a number of pre-signed prescriptions to fill out as needed. The PA may act as the physician's agent and phone a prescription to a pharmacy, or the PA and physician may dispense medications from the medical office.

Progress continues to be made in the attainment of prescribing authority for PAs. Efforts by consumer groups to expand the role of the PA are under way. The federal government continues to underwrite PA education as well as to provide economic incentives to keep PAs in rural and underserved areas. These efforts, coupled with a health care system that favors the use of PAs, will expand the number of states with enabling legislation.

Legal Medicine and Risk Management

There has been a great deal of concern in recent years among health care providers, facilities, and malpractice insurance underwriters about the escalation in the number of malpractice lawsuits. Although physicians have been the primary targets of such litigation, PAs are now experiencing an increase in the number of malpractice suits being filed against them. The exact numbers are not currently known because only court cases that reach a conclusion are made available to the public, and these happen infrequently. To manage this phenomenon, hospitals, clinics, and malpractice underwriters employ the tactic of risk management. Risk managers try to develop strategies to help health care providers avoid malpractice claims by reducing potentially hazardous elements in the delivery of care. One method is to ensure that there are clear and comprehensive guidelines about the type of medical practice the clinic is engaged in and about the role the PA assumes in the delivery of this care.

Physician assistants, like physicians, are held to the standards of care provided in the community. For a plaintiff to win a malpractice suit against a health care provider, it must be shown that the applicable standard of care has been breached. Specialty areas such as orthopedics, obstetrics, neurosurgery, and emergency medicine add the peculiarities of these areas to the factors that must be considered by legal medicine managers.

The best safeguard for preventing a litigious occurrence, or for providing a solid defense in a malpractice suit, is proper documentation of what transpired during the course of a patient's care and treatment. The periodic auditing of a random number of patient records is a vital risk management function that ensures compliance with overall clinic responsibilities

and helps detect any weakness in the documentation process.

A majority of malpractice claims have alleged injury occurring in a hospital. According to the U.S. Government Accounting Office (GAO), more than 80% of the claims closed in 1984 were associated with hospital-based occurrences. Fewer than half of these resulted in an indemnity payment. In contrast, the claims for occurrences related to care in an outpatient office accounted for only about 13% of the closed claims, but half of these claims resulted in an indemnity payment. As care becomes increasingly complex in the ambulatory setting, the ratio of hospital-based to outpatient-based claims can be expected to shift accordingly. In addition, many claims that appear to originate in a hospital setting may have been a delay-in-diagnosis or failure-to-treat set of circumstances originating in the outpatient setting. Care may have been rendered in the emergency department, an urgency care unit, or a physician's private office. Determining the specific site where the problem arose may be difficult in these cases, but it is likely that the ambulatory care setting will be increasingly vulnerable.

A recurring problem is that of delays in identification and follow-up of abnormalities in test results or radiographic interpretations. Another common theme is illustrated by the patient who makes repeated visits for similar or unresolved somatic complaints and eventually files a claim alleging a failure to diagnose or a delay in the correct diagnosis of a serious medical problem.

In the third most frequently filed type of claims, the interpersonal relationship between the clinician and the patient deteriorates (or is perceived by the claimant as "unprofessional"). The relationship between the patient and the provider can also be influenced by factors outside the provider's control. For example, the patient is kept waiting too long, support staff ignores the patient or acts in a brusque manner, or the patient is unhappy with a bill.

Failure to communicate is not a recognized cause of legal action, but some risk management professionals have concluded that most medical malpractice claims arise from a communication breakdown. This potential for a breakdown in communications clearly exists in ambulatory care, where the relationship between the patient and the provider may be limited to a single encounter or series of visits, or even sustained in an ongoing pattern. In addition, there is the potential for differing perceptions of the relationship between the two parties. The patient may view the relationship as ongoing because the practitioner is the primary clinician the patient sees when in need of medical care, infrequent as visits may be. The practitioner, however, may view the relationship as episodic at best, having little recollection of the individual beyond what the medical record documentation demonstrates. Conversely, a clinician may think that there is an ongoing relationship and that the patient will follow medical recommendations, when in fact the patient has no such intention. When such a failure to communicate results in detrimental effects on the patient, his or her response may be to strike back at the clinician by filing a malpractice claim.

PRACTICE ARRANGEMENTS

Little research has been devoted to determining the effects of practice arrangements on PA productivity. Two main organizational variables are thought to affect productivity:
1. Group size.
2. Compensation in the form of a salary or a fee-for-service arrangement.

Group Size

Although the early developers of the physician assistant and Medex models envisioned a PA joining an individual or small group practice in rural America, the reality is that most PAs are in medium or large group practices, often in managed health care systems. The federal government, through the Veterans Administration system, Department of Defense, Public Health Service, and a host of other agencies that specialize in ambulatory services, employs the largest number of PAs. The next largest group practices are the health maintenance organizations, which utilize more than 2000 PAs, predominantly in outpatient services.

Group practice increases PA productivity through economies of scale that may exist for several reasons. The most important factor is that a large practice allows greater specialization and, hence, greater efficiency. This is because some investments, either machines or human assistants, are indivisible and require large patient loads to be fully utilized.

Compensation Arrangements

Physician assistants who are reimbursed by the fee-for-service method have an incentive to work longer hours and see more patients because their income depends directly on their productivity. The income of salaried PAs, on the other hand, is not tied directly to productivity, so they have little economic incentive to increase their work effort or hours beyond some minimally accepted standard. Therefore, higher productivity among fee-for-service PAs is expected.

A combination of salary and incentive bonuses can exist when a group contracts with the PA, either as a partner or as an independent provider, for a minimum amount of services. Revenues over that minimum amount, or yearly excess profits of the group, are distributed in a predetermined sharing arrangement.

Another form of PA employment, referred to as the entrepreneurial PA, is the owner or operator of a clinic. This development arises from allowing innovation to flourish in a capitalist system. An example of an entrepreneurial PA is one who joined a two-physician partnership in a rural Northeast area. One physician died, and the second physician chose retirement shortly afterward. Without a supervising physician, the PA was faced with the prospect of unemployment. Ingenuity prevailed, and the PA decided to purchase the clinic and hire two physicians to staff it. In a classic example of the tail wagging the dog, one of the physicians was employed with the stipulation that he would serve as the supervising physician for the PA, in order to meet the requirements of the state board of medical examiners. Although this example is not common, it is far from unique. Other creative practice arrangements continually emerge in which the PA owns or manages a small clinic.

Ambulatory Care Staffing Model

One concept of ambulatory medical services in managed health care settings that is gaining attention is the *medical care module*. The module consists of a group of medical personnel comprising physicians, nonphysician providers, nurses, and aides who share common resources and patients. A typical module may include an internist, a family practitioner, a pediatrician, a physician assistant, a nurse practitioner, a registered nurse, two licensed practical nurses, and two clinical assistants. Members of a health plan select (or may be assigned to) a physician or module when they first access the health care system for primary care. An example of such a scenario is illustrated in Case Study 24-1.

CASE STUDY 24-1

Sarah, a 20-year-old college sophomore, has had pharyngitis for 2 days. She calls for an appointment with her family practice physician, but the physician's schedule is booked for the day. The PA in the module has an opening. At the visit, Sarah is diagnosed as having acute suppurative pharyngitis. Penicillin is empirically prescribed, but the PA also performs a throat culture, which proves to be negative.

Sarah calls the office 2 days later, complaining that she is feeling no better. Her family practitioner is off for a few days, but the internist in the module has an opening. He agrees that the appearance of the pharyngitis seems bacterial, consistent with the first diagnosis, but judges that the duration of symptoms and resistance to antibiotics raise the possibility of mononucleosis. Results of laboratory serology are positive; the diagnosis of Epstein-Barr viremia is made, and the management program is outlined for the patient. A return appointment is recommended in 2 weeks.

Sarah now elects to see her originally assigned physician for follow-up care as well as for her annual Papanicolaou screening test and pelvic examination. Having received reports on the patient from her two colleagues, the family practitioner conducts the appropriate follow-up examination when Sarah returns in 2 weeks. Because she is recuperating normally and her female reproductive screen is normal, she is asked to return in 1 year.

Six months later, Sarah reenters the medical care system for sexual counseling and a prescription for oral contraceptives. The examination is performed and proves to be normal. She is asked to see the NP annually for prescription refills.

This module or team arrangement has maintained a feeling of continuity of care, utilized health care providers effectively, and enhanced the team concept of health care delivery. It has done so by using a diversity of medical providers, thus enhancing the delivery of care without overstaffing of physicians. The team approach is further enhanced by the sharing of a common medical record, and this is extended even further when all encounters are electronically recorded for easy retrieval.

An extension of the module is the *patient panel*. The panel of patients for each clinician is a list of patients who have either selected or been assigned to the practitioner. Because co-morbidity and disease severity increase with age, sometimes the panel is weighted by age groups to factor in the amount of care involved with certain patients. An internist's panel of patients, 15% to 20% of whom are over age 60, may include a smaller number of patients than that of the pediatrician, whose panel is skewed to the young and healthy, or that of the NP, whose panel may be predominantly middle-aged women.

Establishing Productivity

Assuming that quality care, cost containment, and quality of service are goals equally desired among physicians, management, nurses, and physician assistants of the clinic, the first step toward reaching them is establishing productivity objectives. Although standards of care are important, flexibility is an important tool in dealing with highly skilled professionals. Allocation of time by appointment types, distribution of appointments, and information systems to monitor practice parameters is important.

Generally, productivity objectives should be the same for the physician assistant as for the physician. Objectives that are negotiated rather than mandated are more likely to be accepted. In large organizations, maintaining these standards should be the responsibility of the chief of the department or the physician-manager. Once the parameters have been set, management and nursing must make commitments to support staffing to maintain this productivity goal. Organizational success depends on team effort and the partnership role that medicine, management, and nursing can and should maintain.

The first step in setting productivity objectives is to analyze appointment types as to time and resources needed. Initial and follow-up appointments are the short type that can be managed in 15 minutes. Consultations, physical examinations, and certain procedures can usually be accomplished in 30 minutes. The time needed for procedures such as minor surgery and endoscopies, and for other situations, must be negotiated with the personnel involved in performing them. Although walk-in clinics, which are structured to see the greatest number of patients in a given amount of time, are the most productive, they are also the most exhausting to clinicians and support personnel, and their employment turnover is usually high.

With the use of a primary care model mix of internal medicine, family practice, and pediatrics, a 15-minute matrix can be constructed. It is critical that the mix of appointment types be analyzed because full physical examinations and consultations require 30 minutes and must be factored into the schedule.

Another factor that must be considered in the matter of clinician scheduling is the allocation of time for the PA and supervising physician to discuss cases, as well as miscellaneous time to return telephone calls and complete paperwork. Management must also decide how much clinic time (if any) should be allocated for hospital rounds.

An example of a medical clinic schedule for a primary care clinician is as follows:

➤ 0900-1130: 15-minute office visits
➤ 1130-1200: 30-minute visit
➤ 1200-1230: Administrative time
➤ 1230-1330: Lunch
➤ 1330-1530: 15-minute visits
➤ 1530-1600: 30-minute visit
➤ 1600-1630: 15-minute visits
➤ 1630-1700: Administrative time

In this schedule, the clinician (whether PA or physician) sees 22 patients a day, a productive day by most standards. It includes 20 short-term (routine) visits; two 30-minute consultations, procedures, or physical examination time slots; and two 30-minute administrative periods to be used as buffers for consultation or physician supervision, paperwork, telephone calls, manufacturer representatives, patients over the schedule, and other duties. The day begins at 0900 to allow some preparation such as reviewing medical records; the lunch hour is an appropriate length of 1 hour; the last patient should leave by 1630. Although this model may seem unrealistic for some clinical situations, it is consistent with contemporary principles of North American management and is currently in effect in many managed health care systems around the country. The value of such a schedule is that it allows some room for overbooking but guards against role fatigue by incorporating buffer times.

This system, if all appointments are filled, produces 120 office visits per week (110 short visits and 10 intermediate visits) or 480 visits a month, which adds up to 5000 visits a year. If 90% of all visit slots are filled, the result is consistent with the productivity standard for a full-time practitioner.

Once schedules have been established with regard to appointment mix, it is critical that certain parameters be monitored because of staffing and service implications. In the area of primary care, for example, assuming that all appointments are filled, a productivity level of 3.5 patients per hour is a reasonable objective. It is incumbent upon management to develop accurate reports to monitor objective parameters such as productivity, appointment fill ratio, maximum wait times by appointment types, and types of cases seen by each clinician. Productivity can be defined in terms of:

1. Patients per hour.
2. Fill ratio (number of patients seen divided by available appointments).
3. Wait times.

Careful attention must be paid to the mix of urgent visits, walk-ins, and canceled or no-show appointments.

Regarding triage, patients should be undifferentiated and there should be no routing of patients toward or away from any one type of clinician unless some understanding is created beforehand. Experience is the best teacher, and the PA is as capable as the physician of sorting out the causes of most medical conditions. Complaints that a PA is "skimming" easy patients are less likely if all unscheduled patients have equal access to physicians or PAs, and no triage takes place.

Finally, standards of productivity need to be agreed upon by the team (manager, nurse, and clinician). If a 90% appointment fill ratio is desired, it may be necessary to overbook some patients to ensure that the ratio is maintained. It would be prudent to make sure that clinicians involved are always aware of this action and that it occurs equally among all members of the same department.

FUTURE DEVELOPMENTS IN AMBULATORY CARE

It seems safe to forecast that the health care system will continue to be affected by remarkable changes in medical technology. Some of these changes can be anticipated by a look at current developments in the research laboratories and a prediction of when they will move from the research setting into clinical use. An example of the impact of modem technology can be traced from the development and implementation of computed tomography (CT scanning) to that of magnetic resonance imaging (MRI) to that of positron emission tomography (PET scanning). All of the scanning units are expensive: CT—$800,000 to $1.1 million; MRI—$1.2 to $5 million; and PET—$2.4 to $6.5 million. Further improvements continue to be made in these scanners and image makers. Already, three-dimensional color-enhanced images are available.

Another major technological event under way is a change in the way surgery is performed. New developments in fiberoptic endoscopies, catheters, and lasers help to create new surgical techniques. In 2 short years, cholecystectomy changed from use of an open abdominal approach to use of laparoscopy in the majority of patients. Another example of developments that leapt from theory to practice in a short span is the neuroradiology techniques that allow ultrafine catheters to be placed in the center of human brain arterioles to artificially embolize tumors.

The electronic medical record has been in place for 10 years and continues to improve. For large HMOs like Kaiser Permanente, the medical record is completely paperless. This includes the outpatient encounter, prescriptions, imaging orders, laboratory studies, documenting procedures, dispensing of supplies such as a wrist support or a cane, and referrals to physical therapy or dermatology. All of these events that make up an encounter are arranged from the provider's workstation. No longer are records lost, mistakes made, or charts transferred across town. If a patient moves to another HMO, the total record can be transferred electronically with the patient's permission. The total contents of populations can be stored on a disk, or huge HMO annual records can be stored on compact disks.

"Designer drugs," which are engineered for perfect fit in human genetic makeup and have high benefit with exceptionally low side effects for a broad panoply of ills, are already in use. The Human Genome Project continues to open up unlimited areas for pharmacological management of all conditions, both common and rare. From prostaglandin analogs to granulocyte colony-stimulating factors to non-narcotic potent analgesics, new drugs consistently appear. More than 7000 drugs are available for prescription, and others continue to emerge. Technology abounds, and no practitioner can keep up with even a fraction of it.

This keyhole view of the future also includes an aging population. With the theoretical limits of human life at 120 years, the edge is already being tested. The number of centenarians rises each year, and it is estimated that there will be one million persons over 100 years old by 2010. However, this population brings a greater consumption of health services and a technology-oriented health system that prolongs life, but at a high cost. Twenty-first century gadgetry, with its high capital investment and developmental risks, faces a political system exerting tremendous pressure regarding the allocation of available resources. Another force is also at work—a public that assumes almost anything is possible and achievable. The issue then is how society will pay for all these services in the future.

One of the most significant influences on the health care system for the new millennium will be the involvement of corporations in helping to influence health system structures for the nation. This means tightening of employee health care policies, greater use of preventive medicine, and a greater number of health education programs to help employees and their families stay healthy. This involvement also means more shifting of the employer's portion of the health insurance premiums to the employee with deductibles and programs to reduce hospital use. Finally, absorbing the uninsured and underinsured is a social mandate of health reform, which means that corporations will be asked to play a bigger role.

CONCLUSION

Ambulatory care began in the physician's home and office and then moved to the inpatient setting. Now the emphasis of health care delivery is once again focused on the primary care provider in a medical office. PAs were and continue to be trained to practice high-quality care in such a setting and appear to do this well at no compromise of safety to the patient and to do it in a cost-effective manner, which makes them particularly endearing to systems that are striving to improve benefits to patients without driving up costs at the same time. The evidence is abundant that they can do this well in almost every outpatient situation.

Although the health policy landscape is littered with discarded predictions, a number of forces are functioning to allow for some optimistic forecasts. For the most part, it seems likely that health care will be characterized by a shift from an inpatient to an ambulatory focus to a greater extent than even now exists. Technological developments will allow an even greater number of procedures previously performed only in hospitals to be performed in the outpatient setting. Medical offices may cater to "drop-in" patients and may use other innovative approaches. Organized medical care, in a frenzy of competition, has already shifted from putting the patient in a queue to see the specialist to asking politely, "Do you want to be seen today?"

Without question, the organized delivery of ambulatory care will be increasingly important as society grapples with problems of costs, continuity of care, and quality. Undoubtedly, the health care system of the new century will reflect the patient's new orientation to wellness, cost control, and access. For professional PAs, the future has never seemed brighter in terms of the roles they will play in delivering ambulatory care.

CLINICAL APPLICATIONS

1. Interview physician assistants in clinics that are representative of the health care delivery systems in your communities. Find out how issues of productivity are handled in their clinic settings. Are there differences in expectations for physician assistants as compared with physicians or nurse practitioners? Discuss the interrelationships between productivity, patient care, and job satisfaction for practicing PAs.

2. In considering your ideal PA job, what expectations for productivity would be realistic? In answering this question, consider issues such as types of patients and their expectations, severity of illness, composition of the health care team in the "perfect" setting, and continuity of care. How might you work with the clinic administration to assure realistic expectations for productivity and quality?

REFERENCES

1. Rabin DL, Spector KK. Delegation potential of primary care visits by physician assistants, Medex and Primex. Med Care 1980;18:1114.
2. Zeckhauser R, Elistan M. The productivity potential of the physician assistant. J Hum Resources 1974;9:95.
3. Greenfield S, Bragg FE, McCraith DL, Blackburn J. Upper-respiratory tract complaint for physician extenders. J Fam Pract 1975;2:13.
4. Hooker RS. Medical care utilization: MD-PA/NP comparisons in an HMO. In: Zarbock SF, Harbert K (eds). Physician Assistants: Present and Future Models of Utilization. New York: Prager, 1986.
5. Schneider DP, Foley WJ. A systems analysis of the impact of physician extenders on medical cost and manpower requirements. Med Care 1977;15:277.
6. United States Congress. Office of Technology Assessment. Forecasts of Physician Supply and Requirements. Washington, DC: U.S. Government Printing Office, 1980.
7. Holmes GC, Livingston G, Bassett RE, Mills E. Nurse clinician productivity using a relative value scale. Health Serv Res 1971;12:269.
8. Golladay FL, Miller M, Smith KR. Allied health manpower strategies: estimates of the potential gains from efficient task delegation. Med Care 1973;11:457.
9. Record JC. Cost Effectiveness of Physician's Assistants in a Maximum-Substitution Model. Final Report No. HRP-0900097. Prepared under contract 231-76-0601. Phase II of a two-phase study. Washington, DC: DHEW, Health Resources and Services Administration, Bureau of Health Manpower;

Portland, OR: Kaiser Foundation Health Services Research Center, 1976.

10. Johnson RE, Freeborn DK, McCally M. Delegation of office visits in primary care to PAs and NPs: the physicians' view. Physician Assist 1985;9:159.

11. Kane RL, Olson DM, Castle CH. Effects of adding a Medex in practice costs and productivity. J Community Health 1978;3:216.

12. Nelson EC, Johnson KG, Jacobs AR. Impact of Medex on physician activities: redistribution of time after incorporating a Medex into the practice. J Fam Pract 1977;5:607.

13. Buchanan J, Hosek S. Costs, Productivity, and the Utilization of Physician's Extenders in Air Force Primary Medicine Clinics. R-2896-AF. Santa Monica, CA: Rand Corporation, 1983.

14. Record JC, O'Bannon J. Cost Effectiveness of Physician's Assistants. Final Report No. 1-MB44173(P). Prepared under contract HMEIA. Phase I of a two-phase study. Washington, DC: DHEW, Health Resources and Services Administration, Bureau of Health Resources Development; Portland, OR: Kaiser Foundation Health Services Research Center, 1976.

15. Institute of Medicine. Manpower for Health Care. Washington, DC: National Academy of Sciences, 1974.

16. Willis JB. Prescriptive practice patterns of physician assistants. J Am Acad Physician Assist 1990;3:39.

RESOURCES

Record JC, Schweitzer, SO, McCalley M, et al. Staffing Primary Care in 1990: Physician Replacement and Cost Savings. New York: Springer, 1981.

Calley F. The Cost-Effectiveness of Physician Assistants. Alexandria, VA: American Academy of Physician Assistants, 1986.

Schafft G, Cawley JF, Berk ML, Shur L. Nonphysician Health Care Providers: Use of Ambulatory Services, Expenditures, and Sources of Payment—Data, Review 22. NCHSR National Health Care Expenditures Study. U.S. Dept of Health and Human Services Publication PHS 86-3394.

Bulau M. Quality Assurance Policies and Procedures for Ambulatory Health Care. Rockville, MD: Aspen Publishers, 1990.

Kovner AR (ed). Health Care Delivery in the United States, ed 3. New York: Springer, 1990.

Inglehart JK. The administration's assault on domestic spending and the threat to health care programs. N Engl J Med 1985;312:525.

Institute for Policy Studies. Model Legislation for a National Community Health Service. Washington, DC: Community Health Alternatives Project, 1976.

C H A P T E R   2 5

Inpatient Systems

Kenneth R. Harbert

INTRODUCTION

Since the early 1980s, health care futurists have asked, "Can hospitals survive?" They raise this question because total hospital days peaked in 1975 and continue to decline, and because large hospital management firms exert increasing competitive pressure on smaller hospitals. New millennium issues, such as a market-based reimbursement era, and a paradigm shift from providers back to consumers and other purchasers of health care services will affect the survival of hospitals as we know them today.[1]

During the past decade, change has become the new paradigm of inpatient services. These dynamic changes in health care have included the following:
➤ Medicare reform.
➤ Managed care.

➤ Alternative delivery systems.
➤ Integrated delivery systems.
➤ Focus on clinical outcomes.
➤ Downsizing of facilities and staff.
➤ Shifting from inpatient to outpatient services.
➤ A trend from hospital ownership of services to nonhospital ownership of services.

According to Shortell, four dominant factors influence the future evolution of hospitals—payment, technology, workforce shifts, and consumer expectations.[2] Throughout the history of medicine, provision of inpatient services has been a fluid process of addressing changes in scientific principles and beliefs, thereby shifting practice styles from disease focus to disease prevention and wellness, and now to specific disease management.

Inpatient health care has shifted from control and maintenance of patients and providers within the hospital setting to a multiple menu of patient and provider choices, including the following:

➤ Outpatient surgery.
➤ Increased use of technologies for telemedicine.
➤ Increased networking of accessible services.
➤ Self-care.
➤ Involvement of patients and communities in decision making and strategic planning.
➤ Diversity of managed care plans.

The word *hospital* comes from the Latin word *hospitium*. In the fifth century, a hospital was a place for the reception of strangers and pilgrims.[3] Clearly, the meaning of hospital has gone through a dramatic change since then, much as our hospital system is evolving today. The specific issues for hospitals in the new millennium include those listed here[4]:

➤ Incorporation of new bio-informatics.
➤ Pharmaceutical and biotechnology for patients.
➤ Adoption and implementation of new electronic information technologies.
➤ Adjusting and adapting to new shifting patterns of disease.
➤ Meeting the increasing demands and expectations of the new global consumer movement.

In 1995, health care expenditures in the United States were estimated at $949 billion. The 1994 Health Care Financial Review by the U.S. Department of Health and Human Services[5] stated that more than 35% of health care expenditures were spent on hospital care. The Health Care Financing Administration states that total health care expenditures for hospital care in 2001 were 14% of the gross national product and estimates that national health expenditures will reach $2.8 trillion in 2011.[6]

Since 1946, the American Hospital Association (AHA) has conducted an annual survey of hospitals throughout the United States. In 1995, the AHA reported that there were 6291 registered hospitals, more than 1,080,061 inpatient beds, and an annual admission rate of 33,282,124 patients. According to the AHA, the total number of hospitals had declined to just under 5810 in 2001, and the number of beds had declined from a peak level of just over 1 million in 1983 to 830,000 in 2001. Inpatient surgeries went

from 18,000 in 1980 to 9000 in 1999. The average length of stay in 1980 was 7.6 days, which decreased to 5.9 days in 1999. Occupancy rates dropped from 75.8% in 1980 to 63.3% in 1999,[7] while the number of full-time employees in U.S. hospitals increased from 3,763,000 in 1994 to 4,454,000 in 2000, according to the U.S. Bureau of Labor Statistics. On the other hand, outpatient visits increased from 202,000 in 1980 to more than 495,000 in 1999. Outpatient surgical procedures went from 8000 in 1986 to more than 156,000 in 1999.[7]

A variety of forces have affected the performance of hospitals since 1990, including economic trends, demographic characteristics, and third party payer efforts to hold down health care costs. The AHA stated that since 1990, sharp declines in consumer and business confidence, along with a recession in the U.S. economy, have dramatically challenged hospitals' financial stability.[7] These economic factors have resulted in lower payments to hospitals and greater financial pressures.

Hospital settings are the fastest-growing area of physician assistant employment, a trend that started in the late 1980s, according to the American Academy of Physician Assistants (AAPA). In its 2001 census, the AAPA reported that more than 38% of the 40,782 practicing physician assistants in the United States were involved in inpatient hospital care, which is an increase of 8.2% since 1992.[8] Hooker and Cawley reported in 1997 that more than 8900 physician assistants (PAs) are employed full time by hospitals, with 19% working in surgical subspecialties, 19% in medical subspecialties, 15% in emergency medicine, and 10% in general surgery.[9]

Physician assistants are employed in all possible hospital settings, ranging from small rural community hospitals to large tertiary care centers. A significant number of rural and urban hospitals employ PAs as inpatient house staff within specialized departments; there they provide services through employee health and emergency departments. In a study of physician assistants employed in group practices, it was reported that more than 42% of the 300 practices surveyed utilized PAs to cover inpatient services.[10]

It is essential that PAs understand what hospital care involves. Practitioners should comprehend their roles in providing care within the inpatient setting, as well as the role of inpatient care in the new paradigm of health care in the United States.

HEALTH CARE SYSTEMS
History of Hospitals

Medicine and surgery date back to the beginning of civilization. Because early medical treatment was often identified with various religious services and ceremonies, the history of the hospital is interwoven with various religious services and ceremonies as well.

Hippocrates approached medicine with a nonreligious, rational, comprehensive approach. He was one of the early historians, with detailed records of patients and descriptions of diseases dating back to 480 BC. Hospitals in India follow principles of sanitation and offer detailed medical records that date back to 600 BC. In 600 BC, Indian physicians were appointed to serve the health care needs of a population, and regional hospitals were built by Buddha.[11] The oldest hospital in the Western world still in existence today is the Hotel Dieu in Paris, which was established around 600 AD by the Bishop of Paris—St. Landoy. Hospitals have been called the greatest medical innovation of the Middle Ages. Medieval hospitals provided comfort, nursing, and medical care, as well as charity.

The first permanent solid hospital structure on the North American continent was established in 1524 by Hernan Cortes; the Immaculate Conception Hospital is still in operation in Mexico City, Mexico. The first U.S. hospitals can be traced back to the 18th century. They were located predominantly in seaport towns and dealt with contagious diseases, which were often brought in by sailors from foreign ports. Early institutions were founded in New York, Philadelphia, Charleston, and Newport, Rhode Island; these later became almshouses, established primarily for the city poor, which were a direct result of crowding in urban areas. All of these early American hospitals were devoted to the care of the sick and were utilized by the homeless and poor.[12]

Pennsylvania Hospital, the first hospital in the American colonies, was established in Philadelphia in 1751, by Benjamin Franklin and Dr. Thomas Bond. This hospital, built to "offer relief for the sick and the miserable," housed the first medical library and the first surgical amphitheater in the colonies. Philadelphia is also home to the first college of pharmacy (Philadelphia College of Pharmacy and Science), the first medical school (University of Pennsylvania), and the first children's hospital (Children's Hospital of Philadelphia). Dr. Elizabeth Blackwell, the first woman to earn a medical degree in the United States, opened the first women's hospital in 1853, called the New York Infirmary for Women and Children. The first mental hospital was established in 1773 in Williamsburg, Virginia.[13]

Three important discoveries in the field of medicine enabled the further development of modern hospitals:

➤ William Roentgen's discovery of the x-ray.
➤ Louis Pasteur's discovery that bacteria were produced by reproduction and not spontaneously.
➤ Joseph Lister's discovery that infection could be controlled through sterile technique.

By the late 1800s, hospitals no longer were places where the sick and homeless found refuge and care; rather, they became special places for physician services aided by rapidly developing medical technology. Many hospitals that began in the late 1800s are still in existence today—Mercy Hospital and Cook County Hospital in Chicago; St. Luke's Hospital, Roosevelt Hospital, and Presbyterian Hospital in New York; Johns Hopkins Hospital in Baltimore; and Massachusetts General in Boston.[13]

Today, hospitals focus their attention on globally integrated health systems, community needs, and ever-changing federal, state, and local regulations. Health system standards have been developed by the Joint Commission on Accreditation of Healthcare Organizations (JCAHO). The Commission accredits about 84% of the nation's general hospitals as well as many long-term care facilities, psychiatric hospitals, substance abuse centers, urgent care clinics, group practices, community health centers, hospices, and home health agencies.

What Hospitals Are

The American Hospital Association defines a hospital as a licensed institution whose function is to provide diagnostic and therapeutic patient services. To be classified as a hospital under the AHA's definition, the institution must have at least six beds, an organized physician staff, and continuous nursing services. In 1995, there were 6291 hospitals in the United States, with a total of 1,080,061 beds.[7] This is a dramatic change from the late 1970s, when there were more than 7000 hospitals in the United States. Substantial changes have occurred in the role and operation of hospitals. Financially pressed hospitals have either closed or consolidated into systems or networks.

By the mid-1990s, many hospitals became part of a system or network of health care. A system is a corporate body that may own or manage health provider facilities. A network can be a group of physicians, hospitals, insurers, or community agencies that work together to deliver a broad spectrum of services in their community. An integrated delivery system is an organization or group of affiliated organizations in which hospitals and physicians combine all their activities to deliver comprehensive health care services. In 2002, many integrated delivery systems have decentralized and focus on specific specialty centers of excellence.

The types of hospitals in the United States are classified according to average length of stay, type of ownership, and primary focus of care provided. Categories include subacute, acute, tertiary, and quaternary. Types of ownership include for-profit, not-for-profit, government, and federal. *Short-stay* hospitals are those in which the average length of stay is less than 30 days. *Long-stay* hospitals usually deal with psychiatric problems, rehabilitation, and chronic illnesses, all of which require longer periods of hospitalization.

Community hospitals are defined as nonfederal short-stay general hospitals whose facilities are open to the public. Noncommunity hospitals include federal hospitals, such as military hospitals, Veterans Affairs medical centers, and Indian Health Service hospitals, as well as long-stay hospitals, as previously defined.

Voluntary hospitals are established by communities rather than by the government. They are not-for-profit organizations operated by churches, fraternal groups, and other community or charitable institutions. Voluntary hospitals can have revenue in excess of expenses, but this is usually called a surplus. Not-for-profit organizations usually do not pay income or property tax. A *proprietary* hospital is operated by individuals or corporations explicitly to make a profit, which is then returned to the investors.

Government hospitals, such as Veterans Affairs medical centers and military hospitals, can be federally funded; state funded, such as university hospitals; or supported entirely by city and county funds, such as the Cook County Hospital in Chicago and the Boston City Hospital in Boston. Government hospitals are often large institutions with more than 1000 beds.

Between 1980 and 1990, the number of community hospitals decreased by 7%—a loss of more than 446 hospitals. During this period, the number of hospitals in all bed size categories declined, with the exception of the hospitals with 200 to 300 beds, which increased by 3.4%. Large declines were recorded for hospitals at the lower end of the range of bed size with 6 to 24 beds, and at the higher end with 500 or more beds, which showed a 10% decrease since 1980.[7]

By the end of 1995, 47.8% of all urban hospitals reported joining a health care system or entering into a joint venture. Many hospitals in the late 1990s belonged to integrated regional health care systems, featuring a patient orientation; focus on efficient, high-quality care delivery; physician leadership; unified information management; and accessibility to their communities.

The trends in utilization of hospital services have varied. Declines in inpatient use and simultaneous growth in outpatient care are perhaps the most significant changes in health care delivery since 1980. Because of the shift toward increased outpatient treatment as well as technological innovations, hospitals are able to offer more types of procedures and treatments to their patients. Nearly 60% of all hospital stays are for women. Patients over 65 years of age make up about 36% of all hospital stays. With this growth in procedures and treatments for patients comes a greater need for practitioners in both outpatient and inpatient settings.

HEALTH CARE SERVICES PROVIDED BY HOSPITALS

Adult Day Care Program   A program providing supervision, medical and psychological care, and social activities for older adults who live at home or in another family setting but cannot be alone, or prefer to be with others during the day. Physician assistants may perform assessment, health monitoring, and other necessary needed medical services for the adult day care program.

Alcohol/Drug Abuse or Dependent Outpatient Services   Organized hospital services that provide medical care and/or rehabilitative treatment services to outpatients for whom the primary diagnosis is alcoholism or other chemical dependency. Physician assistants play a major role in this area.

Angioplasts   Reconstruction or restructuring of a blood vessel by operative means or by nonsurgical techniques such as balloon dilatation or laser. Physician assistants in cardiology and cardiovascular thoracic surgery are actively involved in assisting with this procedure.

Birthing Room and Labor and Delivery Patient Room   A hospital-managed combination labor and delivery unit with a homelike setting for patients who have completed specified childbirth courses and wish to participate jointly with their families in the birth of their child. Physician assistants may provide clinical services in this setting.

Blood Bank   A medical facility with the responsibility for blood procurement, blood drawing, blood processing, and/or distribution of blood supplies.

Cardiac Catheterization Laboratory   Facility for special diagnostic procedures necessary for the care of patients with cardiac conditions. Physician assistants play an active role in managing and providing clinical services in this facility.

Cardiac Rehabilitation Program   Restorative services whereby a patient is reconditioned from a state of cardiac injury or high risk to being able to resume activities of daily living at an optimal level. Physician assistants may provide administrative services, patient education about self-monitoring or cardiac conditions, stress management, and even dietary counseling.

Cardiac rehabilitation services are often used after open heart surgery, angioplasty, and acute myocardial infarction, and for patients identified as at high risk for adverse cardiovascular events.

Chronic Obstructive Pulmonary Disease Services   Services provided for the treatment of disorders such as asthma, chronic bronchitis, and emphysema, that are marked by persistent obstruction of bronchial air flow. Physician assistants may provide assessment and management, as well as instruction and education for patients with these disorders.

Community Health Promotion   Patient education program for the community regarding health promotion and disease prevention. Community health offers physician assistants many clinical, educational, and administrative potentials.

Comprehensive Geriatric Assessment   Diagnostic and evaluation services that determine elderly patients' short-term and long-term needs for health care and related services. Physician assistants provide assessment and management of medical conditions and day-to-day functional activities.

Computed Tomography (CT) Scan   Computed tomographic imaging of the head or body.

Emergency Department   Organized hospital facility for the provision of unscheduled outpatient services to patients whose conditions are considered to require immediate and acute care. Must be staffed 24 hours a day and may include a trauma center.

Extracorporeal Shock Wave Lithotripter (ESWL)   A medical device used to treat obstructions in the kidney or ureter. This device disintegrates kidney stones noninvasively through the transmission of acoustical shock waves directed at the stones. New technology is being developed to provide a similar treatment for other parts of the body.

Genetic Counseling Center   A service or center equipped with or supported by special laboratory facilities and directed by a qualified physician or physician assistant who advises parents and prospective patients of potential problems in cases of genetic defects.

HEALTH CARE SERVICES PROVIDED BY HOSPITALS—cont'd

Health Science Library   A facility that maintains an organized collection of printed and/or library materials, with a staff trained to provide and interpret such materials as required to meet informational or educational needs.

Hemodialysis   Provision of equipment and personnel for the treatment of renal insufficiency on an outpatient or an inpatient basis.

Histopathology Laboratory   A laboratory in which tissue specimens are examined by a qualified pathologist.

Home Health Services   An organized program administered by the hospital that provides medical, nursing, and other services, including social services, to patients in its own residence. The utilization of physician assistants as managers, owners, and providers of home health services continues to expand in urban and rural areas.

Hospice   A program providing palliative care, chiefly medical relief of pain, and supportive services addressing the social, emotional, financial, and legal needs of terminally ill patients and their families.

Hospital Auxiliary   A volunteer community organization formed to assist in community instruction and in carrying out the institution's purpose; serves as a link between the institution and the community.

Magnetic Resonance Imaging (MRI)   The use of a uniform magnetic field in radiofrequencies to study tissue and structure of the body.

Noninvasive Cardiac Assessment Services   Conducts cardiac studies, tests, and evaluations not performed in the cardiac catheterization laboratory or operating room, such as electrocardiography, stress test monitoring, and cardiac nuclear medicine studies.

Occupational Health Services   Often, a combined employee health and occupational health service program designed to protect the safety and health of employees from hazards, both direct and indirect, in the workplace. Physician assistants are utilized in administrative and clinical positions as members of the occupational health care team.

Occupational Therapy Services   Facilities for the provision of occupational therapy services provided by physicians and administered by or under the direction of a qualified occupational therapist.

Organ and Tissue Transplant Service   Service offering specially trained and equipped staff qualified to perform the surgical removal of viable human tissue or organs from a living donor or a deceased person immediately after death, as well as the surgical grafting of the tissue or organ into a suitably evaluated and prepared patient. Physician assistants have a long history in organ and tissue transplant clinical services. Additionally, today many physician assistants are acting as directors or assistant directors of such departments.

Organized Outpatient Services   Health care services offered by appointment on an ambulatory basis. Services may include surgery, laboratory services, and other diagnostic testing as ordered by the staff or outside physician referral. Physician assistants play a large role in providing these outpatient services; conducting pre-admission histories and physical examinations; evaluating patients for outpatient surgical, diagnostic, and therapeutic procedures; and performing diagnostic tests as ordered by the supervising physician.

Organized Social Service Department   Services that are properly directed and sufficiently staffed by qualified individuals to provide assistance and counseling to patients and their families in dealing with social, emotional, and environmental problems associated with illness or disability, often in the context of financial or discharge planning and coordination.

Health care has become a big business. Major health care corporations have developed national networks of institutions to earn a share of the 14% of the gross national product spent on health care. The Agency for Health Care Policy and Research reported that 7.3% of 19.6 million people had at least one hospital stay during 1996.[14] In 1997, the average charge for a hospital in-patient stay was $11,000, and more than 11 million children had no health insurance.[14]

Between 1980 and 1983, proprietary for-profit hospitals increased by more than 4%, while voluntary institutions increased by only 1%. In 1983, the average community hospital spent $370 per inpatient day, compared with $20 in 1950. By 2001, the average charge for a hospital stay that lasted about 3.5 days was more than $11,000. About 2.5% of all hospital stays end in death.[15]

Many factors have contributed to the trend of higher cost for hospital care:

➤ A change in demographics toward a large proportion of elderly, resulting in greater demand for medical services.
➤ Technological improvements in quality of care, adding to the cost as hospitals compete to buy the newest and latest technological advances at increased prices.
➤ A rise in the cost of health care providers, hospital employees, and medical supplies, adding to the costs passed on to the patient.[1]

In 1995, salaries, payroll, and benefits accounted for 29.5% of total hospital expenses. In 1995, the number of full-time equivalent hospital employees reached the lowest point in 15 years. Another third of hospital expenses involved medical supplies, pharmaceuticals, utilities, food, housekeeping supplies, and administration. Remaining hospital expenses included capital costs and fees paid for contracted professional and administrative services. These capital costs include the interest and depreciation on a hospital's facilities and equipment.

Hospitals are the cornerstone of the health care industry and, similar to other industries in the United States, they are going through dramatic changes.

What Hospitals Do

To understand what hospitals do, it is useful to review the criteria established by the Joint Commission on Accreditation of Healthcare Organizations (JCAHO). The Joint Commission was established to improve the quality of health care provided to the public. It develops standards of quality in collaboration with health care professionals and others and stimulates health care organizations to meet or exceed those standards through accreditation and the teaching of quality improvement concepts.[16] The JCAHO comprises many representatives of the health care industry, including the American Medical Association, American Dental Association, AHA, American College of Surgeons, American College of Physicians, and American Nursing Association. The hospital standards established by the Joint Commission are reviewed on-site during surveys performed every 3 years. In order to receive federal funds for patient care under Medicare, hospitals must be accredited by the JCAHO.

The eligibility requirements specified by the Joint Commission for Hospitals state that the hospital must be located within the United States or one of its territories or possessions, must have a current license required by governmental authorities, and must maintain facilities, beds, and services that are available 24 hours a day, 7 days a week. Additionally, the hospital must have a governing body, an organized medical staff, and a nursing care staff. The JCAHO lists the primary functions of a hospital as providing diagnosis, treatment, or rehabilitation services as follows:

➤ Diagnostic radiology services.
➤ Dietetic services.
➤ Emergency services.
➤ Infection control services.
➤ Medical records services.
➤ Nuclear medicine services.
➤ Pathology and medical laboratory services.
➤ Pharmacology services.
➤ Physical rehabilitation services.
➤ Professional library and health information services.
➤ Respiratory care services and social work services.
➤ Quality improvement and assessment programs.

Additionally, the Joint Commission states that every patient's general medical condition must be the responsibility of a qualified physician member of the medical staff who has been granted clinical privileges by the governing body and practices only within the scope of clinical privileges granted.

The purpose of the JCAHO survey is to assess the extent of a hospital's compliance with the applicable standards. A hospital must be prepared to show evidence of its compliance with each standard applicable to its operations. To be accredited, a hospital must demonstrate that it is in substantial compliance with the standards overall, not necessarily with each applicable standard.[16]

Hospitals offer a variety of services and facilities to furnish a broad range of health care services to patients who utilize the facility (see Health Care Services Provided by Hospitals box earlier in this chapter).

A physician assistant on the staff of a hospital should understand a number of terms related to hospital services. These terms are used by hospital administrators in determining the demographic base for hospitals regarding admissions, bed size, and outpatient visits. These data are provided to the American Hospital Association and other regulatory agencies. The following box provides brief definitions of the terms that administrators use to describe day-to-day operations in hospitals.

Organization of Integrated Delivery Systems

In the past, hospitals were organized in a pyramid or hierarchical form of organization, with positions in hospital departments arranged in grades or ranks, and clearly specified lines of authority from the board of governors to the chief executive officer to department heads and clinical directors of departments. The 1990s have seen the development of a matrix model of management in which personnel have input and clear lines of authority on a centralized or decentralized plane.

At the top of a hospital's organization is the governing body, usually called the board of trustees. This body is chaired by an individual who takes ultimate responsibility for the hospital's administrative operations, including the upholding of effective and effi-

cient quality standards of care throughout the institution. The board of trustees traditionally functions through committees that deal with issues such as finance, long-range planning, fundraising, and quality improvement.[17]

The head of the hospital is usually called a chief executive officer (CEO). The board usually delegates its authority to the hospital's CEO, who has the responsibility to develop the hospital's management organization. In most hospitals, the key administrators consist of the CEO, the medical director, and the board of trustees. The board holds the medical staff accountable for the delivery of a high standard of medical practice. as well as the maintenance of the professional credentials of the medical staff. As hospitals have become part of larger systems and networks, middle managers have all but disappeared.

There are five major functions within any hospital organization—nursing, finance, support services, ancillary services, and medical staff. The medical staff functions autonomously and reports directly to the medical director.[18] Many institutions find it beneficial to have one or two physicians serve as voting members of the board of trustees. In order for a hospital to be effective and efficient, clear and concise communication must occur between the board of trustees, the CEO, and the medical director. These groups clearly understand the mission, goals, and objectives of the hospital. The hospital's mission statement often includes educational, research, and health care delivery components.

Hospital Standards and Patient Bill of Rights

In the early development of hospitals, physicians were responsible for establishing standards for hospitals. In 1919, the American College of Surgeons developed minimum standards for physicians who practiced in hospitals. The American Medical Association developed standards for hospital-based internship and residency programs in the 1920s and the 1930s. These standards, together with the rise of specialty board certification organizations, increased momentum throughout U.S. institutions for the development of effective and structured medical staff organizations.

DEFINITIONS USED BY ADMINISTRATORS FOR DAY-TO-DAY HOSPITAL OPERATIONS

Adjusted Expenses per Admission Average expenses incurred by the hospital in providing care for one hospital inpatient stay. Adjusted expenses are derived by removing the expenses incurred for the provision of outpatient care from the total expense. This number represents the expenses incurred for inpatient care only; when it is divided by the total admissions, the result is the average expense for a hospital stay.

Adjusted Expenses per Inpatient Day Expenses incurred for inpatient care only. This number is derived by dividing total expenses by inpatient day equivalents.

Admissions Number of patients, excluding newborns, accepted for inpatient service during the reporting period.

Average Daily Census Average number of inpatients, excluding newborns, receiving care each day during the reporting period.

Average Length of Stay Average stay of inpatients during a reporting period. This number is derived by dividing the number of inpatient days by the number of admissions.

Bassinets The number of newborn infant bassinets set up and staffed for use at the end of the reporting period. Bassinets are not included in the bed total, and their count does not include isolettes or neonatal intensive care beds.

Beds Average number of beds, cribs, and pediatric bassinets regularly maintained for inpatients during the reporting period. Also referred to as "statistical beds." This number is derived by adding the total number of beds available each day during a hospital's reporting period and dividing this figure by the total number of days in the reporting period.

Births Total number of infants born in a hospital during the reporting period. Birth count does not include infants transferred from other institutions, and birth figures are excluded from admission and discharge figures.

Current Procedural Terminology (CPT) A set of five-digit codes that apply to medical services delivered.

Employee Benefits A component of nonpayroll expenses that includes hospital expenditures for employee Social Security, life insurance, and retirement benefits.

Diagnosis-Related Group (DRG) A code assigned to each patient discharge, based on diagnosis, surgery, patient age, discharge destination, and sex.

Expenses All costs for the reporting period, including salaries and wages, except those paid to medical and dental residents and interns and other trainees. (All professional fees and those salary expenditures excluded from payroll are defined as nonpayable expenses and are included in total expenses.)

FTE Full-time equivalent personnel.

Inpatient Days Number of adult and pediatric days of care, excluding newborn days of care, rendered during the entire reporting period.

Inpatient Day Equivalents An aggregate figure reflecting a number of days as inpatient care plus an estimate of a volume of outpatient services, which is expressed in units equivalent to an inpatient day in terms of level of effort. It is derived by multiplying the number of outpatient visits by the ratio of outpatient revenue per outpatient visit to inpatient revenue per inpatient day, and by adding the product to the number of inpatient days.

Occupancy Ratio of average daily census to the average number of beds, that is, statistical beds, maintained during the reporting period.

Outpatient Visit Visits by patients who are not lodged in the hospital and are receiving medical, dental, or other services. Each appearance of an outpatient to each unit of the hospital counts as one outpatient visit.

Revenue Inpatient and outpatient income from services rendered to patients, including payments received from or on behalf of individual patients. ***Net patient revenue*** consists of gross patient revenue minus deductions for contractual adjustments, bad debts, charity, and so forth. ***Net total revenue*** consists of net patient revenue plus all other revenue, including contributions, endowment revenue, government grants, and all other payments not made on the behalf of individual patients.

In 1952, the Joint Commission on Accreditation of Hospitals (JCAHO) was formed by a consortium of sponsors, including American College of Surgeons, American College of Physicians, American Hospital Association, and American Medical Association. The JCAHO is now the single most influential accrediting organization within the hospital industry. Although standards were originally derived from the American College of Surgeons, they have expanded to comprise the complex guidelines, policies, and procedures that largely define the current expectations of the role, function, and organization of the hospital's medical staff. These functions revolve around one basic focus—ensuring that the highest quality of care is given to its patients.[16] The medical staff's overall responsibilities include those listed here:

➤ Defining and promulgating standards of medical care.

➤ Recommending candidates for appointment to the medical staff.

➤ Granting specific practice privileges to individual members of the medical staff.

➤ Monitoring and auditing the quality of medical care services provided by hospital departments and physicians.

➤ Assessing and monitoring the ongoing process of continuing medical education for the hospital's physicians.

➤ Disciplining individual physicians whose practice patterns deviate from the norm.

It has long been established that each hospital can decide which practitioners are permitted to admit, treat, and provide services to patients within the institution. This institutional right is based on the principle that the hospital is responsible for the quality of care provided and is liable for the negligence of the physicians who are either its employees or its agents. Additionally, it is the responsibility of the hospital to screen practitioners who apply for clinical privileges and to monitor their performance in the hospital, based on the hospital's inherent duty to protect its patients.

The Health Insurance Portability and Accountability Act of 1996 (HIPAA) has proposed regulations to protect the security of electronic health information and to ensure the confidentiality and integrity of health information. These regulations apply to information that is transcribed, statements written on paper, computer records, and e-mail transmissions. PAs who use e-mail to communicate with their patients should be sure to get the patient's written consent. This is especially true when treatment is discussed or attached records are offered.

The National Committee for Quality Assurance (NCQA) is a private, not-for-profit organization dedicated to assessing and reporting on the quality of managed care plans. It is governed by a board of directors, which includes employers, consumer and labor representatives, health plan representative quality experts, regulators, and representatives from organized medicine. NCQA's mission is to provide information that enables purchasers and consumers of managed health care to distinguish among plans based on quality, thereby allowing them to make more informed health care purchasing decisions. This will encourage plans to compete based on quality and value, rather than on price and provider network. Its efforts are organized around two activities—accreditation and performance measurement—which are complementary strategies for producing information to guide choice. In the future, it plans on integrating these important activities.

NCQA began accrediting managed care organizations in 1991, in response to the need for standardized, objective information about the quality of these organizations. Since then, it has expanded the range of organizations that it accredits or certifies to include managed behavioral health care organizations, credentials verification organizations, and physician organizations (beginning in 1997). Although the managed care accreditation program is voluntary and rigorous, it has been well received by the managed care industry. More than three fourths of the health maintenance organizations (330 health care plans) in the nation are currently involved in the NCQA accreditation process.

For an organization to become accredited by NCQA, it must undergo a survey and meet certain standards designed to evaluate the health plan's clinical and administrative systems. In particular, NCQA's accreditation surveys review a health plan's efforts to continuously improve the quality of the care and service it delivers. One measure of the value of accreditation is the growing list of employers who require or request NCQA accreditation of the plans with which they do business.

The NCQA uses accreditation standards to survey health plans. These surveys are conducted by physicians and managed care experts, and standards include six broad categories:

➤ Quality improvement.
➤ Physician credentials.
➤ Members' rights and responsibilities.
➤ Preventive health services.
➤ Utilization management.
➤ Medical records.

The Patient Bill of Rights has been accepted and adopted by the American Hospital Association. This document promotes the interest and well-being of patients, and states that patients are entitled to be informed of its principles at the outset of their hospitalization. The Patient Bill of Rights in most hospitals contains the principles listed in the following box.

HOSPITAL UTILIZATION OF PAs
History of PAs in Hospitals

The concept of utilizing physician assistants within a hospital setting began when Charles L. Hudson, MD, a member of the American Medical Association's Council on Medical Services, published an article in *JAMA* in 1961, addressing the need for a greater number of medical professionals to help in hospitals.[19] Hudson described the situation in hospitals at that time as demonstrating greater population demands, larger numbers of admissions, and rising numbers of procedures. He commented that physician staff members were unable to devote sufficient time to inpatient services because of outpatient, private practice needs. Hudson suggested expanding the provision of medical professional services in hospitals by utilizing nonprofessional, non-nursing personnel. His proposal was to create an extern who would have specialized training and be an intermediary between a technician and the doctor. The extern would be able to handle many technical clinical procedures but also would have some degree of medical responsibility and medical judgment. Hudson also suggested that the role of these assistants would be carefully delineated, and the physician would assume moral and legal responsibility for their acts.

This concept was further investigated in 1964 by Eugene Stead, MD, Chairman of the Department of Medicine at Duke University. The physician assistant profession began in 1965 at the Duke University Medical Center, when four U.S. Navy–trained corpsmen began a formalized training program. Slowly but surely, other hospitals followed Duke University Medical Center in utilizing physician assistants. Montefiore Hospital in the Bronx, Yale-New Haven Medical Center in Connecticut, Marshfield Clinic in Wisconsin, Philippi Hospital in West Virginia, Geisinger Medical Center in Pennsylvania, and University of Nebraska Medical Center were early adopters of the inpatient PA role. Additionally, since the late 1960s, PAs have been utilized extensively in U.S. Veterans Affairs medical centers to provide inpatient care on medical and surgical wards.

During the 1970s, a number of changes led to greater utilization of physician assistants as inpatient health care providers. These changes included the following:

➤ Physician postgraduate medical education programs had difficulty attracting and matching physicians for major inpatient service areas, including surgery, medicine, and subspecialty areas.
➤ The number of foreign medical graduates being utilized as postgraduate physicians decreased.
➤ Federal rules and regulations regarding financial reimbursement of hospitals for physician and physician assistant services changed.

During the early 1980s, it became clear that postgraduate physicians, who historically had provided much of the care for urban and rural hospitals, were not able to keep up with the long working hours traditionally expected of them. It has been a long-standing practice that clinical skills are learned best when they are performed. Medical education on the undergraduate and graduate level is based on the premise that students and residents learn best by participating in the day-to-day care of patients, under supervision. During the 1980s and 1990s, however, inner city and urban hospitals were overwhelmed with sicker patients, an increase in victims of violence who required long-term care, increased admissions with

PATIENT BILL OF RIGHTS

Effective health care requires collaboration between a patient and his or her provider. Open and honest communication, respect for personal and professional values, and sensitivity to diversity issues are integral to optimal patient care. Hospitals and providers must provide a foundation for understanding and respecting the rights and responsibilities of patients, their families, and their health care providers. Institutions and providers must ensure a health care ethic that respects the role of patients in decision making about treatment choices and other aspects of their care. Providers must be sensitive to cultural, racial, linguistic, religious, age, sex, and other differences, as well as the needs of persons with disabilities.

The Patient's Bill of Rights was first adopted by the American Hospital Association in 1973. The latest revision, approved in 1992 by the American Hospital Association, offers the following information for patients and providers. Patients have the right to privacy. Information about their medical care is confidential. Records will not be released to anyone outside the hospital without written consent; release of information about a patient's hospitalization to the media must occur after written consent has been obtained.

1. Patients have the right to know their conditions, proposed treatments, alternative forms of treatment, and possible adverse effects.
2. Patients have the right to make decisions about the plan of care prior to and during the course of treatment, and to refuse a recommended treatment or plan of care to the extent permitted by law and hospital policy and to be informed of the medical consequences of this action.
3. Patients have the right to know the identity of their physicians, nurses, physician assistants, and other health care providers involved in their care.
4. Patients have the right to know what services are available in the hospital and the charges for those services, including charges not covered by insurance or government funding.
5. Patients have the right to know the rules and regulations of the hospital.
6. Patients have the right to an interpreter when language presents a barrier between the patient and the practitioner.
7. Patients have the right to review their records and to have the information explained or interpreted as necessary, unless access to their medical records is restricted by law.
8. Patients have the right to receive and examine detailed explanations of their bills.
9. Patients have the right to information and counseling about financial resources for health care.
10. Patients have the right to be informed, upon discharge, about continuing health care requirements and the means for meeting these requirements.
11. Patients have the right to participate in planning and to be involved in their treatment and care.
12. Patients have the right to formulate advance directives concerning treatment or designating a surrogate decision maker, with the expectation that the hospital will honor the intent of that directive to the extent permitted by law.
13. Patients have the right to be referred, transferred, or discharged.
14. Patients have the right to give informed consent prior to the start of any test, operation, medical procedure, or treatment, except in a medical emergency, particularly when a procedure or an event may have an adverse effect on them.
15. Patients have the right to give informed consent before they take part in any medical donor or organ donor program or experimental research.
16. Patients have the right to obtain consultation services with another physician by making this request known to their health care providers.
17. Patients have the right to thoughtful, courteous care provided with dignity at all times.
18. Patients have the right to receive appropriate medical care without discrimination based on race, color, age, religion, sex, sexual preference, national origin, or source of payment.

the advent of new illnesses such as AIDS, and a greater number of geriatric patients, who required more time, more attention, more procedures, and more care on a 24-hour basis. Just as the need for these services increased, the number of available residents decreased.

During the late 1970s and early 1980s, one of the first fields to utilize PAs was surgery. In 1979, Perry[20] found that more than one third of large teaching institutions with more than 400 beds employed physician assistants. By the middle of the 1980s, the role of the PA as inpatient house staff had been well established and spread from urban to rural hospitals, offering PAs expanded roles and increased employment opportunities.

Physician assistants quickly took over the role of caring for patients and other clinical functions that historically had been performed by postgraduate resident physicians within large institutions. By 1997, PAs were firmly entrenched in inpatient roles throughout hospitals in urban and rural areas in the United States. In 1997, the AAPA census reported that 50% of all PAs had some hospital responsibility, ranging from making occasional rounds to providing daily care.[9] These roles included a full range of surgery, medicine, and subspecialty areas.

When one looks at the hospitals in the United States today, it is difficult to imagine an area in which a physician assistant could not provide services. It is not uncommon for a large tertiary care center to employ well over 50 PAs in a variety of clinical departments. Nor is it uncommon for hospitals with a large staff of PAs to have administrative chief physician assistants supervising the clinical activities of other staff PAs. Current trends involve more PAs becoming hospitalists. A hospitalist is someone who specializes in the care of hospitalized managed care patients.

Inpatient Roles

Physician assistants are able to approach a patient of any age to elicit a detailed and accurate history, perform an appropriate physical examination, delineate a patient database, and record pertinent patient data, and then present those data to their supervising physician. PAs analyze health status data, formulate

medical judgments regarding this analysis, order appropriate diagnostic studies, and develop, in concert with their supervising physicians, a total management plan for the patient. As a team, the physician and PA formulate, implement, and monitor individualized treatment and management for each patient for whom they are responsible. PAs enable better communication, cooperation, and coordination of health care services for the physician, the patient, and other health care team members.

Through their primary care educational programs, PAs obtain a clear sense of clinical judgment, medical knowledge, and hands-on clinical skills and develop an understanding of the importance of humanistic attributes. PAs offer their supervising physicians the ability to manage, monitor, counsel, educate, evaluate, and refer patients with the same clinical focus that the physicians would themselves utilize in addressing the patient's medical problems and medical management.

Physician assistants are employed in all areas of the hospital inpatient setting—emergency department, ambulatory care clinics, employee health, occupational health centers, community outreach programs, and medical and surgical inpatient units. PAs also function in specialty areas such as neonatal intensive care, organ procurement, oncology, geriatrics, cardiovascular and thoracic surgery, substance abuse, and ambulatory surgery.

The typical duties and responsibilities of physician assistants in hospital and institutional settings, regardless of their bed size and urban or rural location, include the following:
- ➤ Inpatient rounds.
- ➤ Admitting new patients.
- ➤ Daily discharge summaries.
- ➤ Performing triage on ongoing patient problems as identified by nursing personnel and staff physicians.
- ➤ Inpatient afternoon chart rounds.
- ➤ Attendance at ongoing rounds with associate or house staff members.
- ➤ Performing clinical procedures, including but certainly not limited to central line placement, Foley catheterizations, lumbar punctures, thoracenteses, paracenteses, and blood gas aspiration.

➤ Issuing orders for medications and ongoing treatment.

➤ Ongoing evaluation of laboratory data.

➤ Transcription of notes.

➤ Providing continuity of care that focuses on assessment and management of all patients.

➤ Other duties as directed by the supervising physician within the particular hospital service department.

Staff PAs provide support with diagnostic and therapeutic procedures and collecting of historical and physical data, and ongoing support for attending physicians. In all areas of clinical care, the PA functions as an agent of the attending physician. Physician assistants who are providing care within a teaching service in a hospital need to develop very specific guidelines delineating what services they provide and what services the residents provide. Physician assistants can teach residents and medical students but certainly should bill for that service. Reimbursement regarding the use of physician assistants on a teaching service is an area that requires specific review by the PA, the supervising physician, and someone familiar with current reimbursement guidelines.[21]

POLICIES, PROCEDURES, AND GUIDELINES
Definitions

It is essential for the physician assistant and supervising physician to clearly delineate policies, procedures, and practice guidelines that the physician assistant will utilize while practicing within a specific service area of the hospital. These policies, procedures, and practice guidelines should be used as building blocks, along with the clinical department's specific mission, to promote group dynamics and effective, efficient team practice, recognizing that the best practice of medicine includes evidence-based decision making that ultimately offers high-quality patient care.

Guidelines (often called protocols, practice algorithms, and/or practice guidelines) allow for evidence-based recommendations from recognized medical specialty societies, other professional and scientific organizations, government health service agencies, and the medical literature. Additionally, these guidelines provide for a mechanism of constant communication between the physician assistant and the supervising physician, allowing continuous growth and improvement in the delivery of humanistic health care. With written policies, procedures, and guidelines, the physician assistant and the supervising physician can clearly delineate to nursing staff, other support staff, management staff, the general public, and regulatory agencies a concise vision regarding the utilization of PAs.

Since the late 1970s, the utilization of physician assistants in hospitals has more than doubled. How can hospitals be assured that with this increase in utilization, the physician assistant will be utilized in an effective, efficient, and safe manner? Given the diversity of inpatient duties, responsibilities, risk management issues, practice guidelines, performance measures, and other issues related to accountability and quality of care, it is essential that specific policies and procedures act as guidelines for the utilization and conduct of physician assistants. These guidelines may address issues such as credentialing, quality of care, use of evidence-based medicine recommendations, and if necessary, recruitment and internal and external salary equity.

Policies are important methods of communicating about roles, responsibilities, and functions. Policies address issues such as limits of practice, Health Insurance Portability and Accountability Act (HIPAA) regulations, appropriate supervision, methods of supervision, frequency of supervision, relaying of physician orders, on-call responsibilities, and other clinical and nonclinical functions. Procedures should be clearly defined regarding proper documentation according to American Medical Association evaluation and management guidelines that have been approved by the Office of the Inspector General.[22]

Quality indicators are items of health care quality data that can identify performance measures regarding patient care outcomes. Quality indicators are seen commonly as screening tools to provide accessible and low-cost identification of potential problems in the quality of the care being delivered by a service department within the hospital.[23]

Outcomes reflect the result of the care given and the cost of that care. Health outcomes review four major categories—health status, health-related knowledge, health-related behavior, and patient satisfaction. Quality of care hospital committees are charged with assessing health care outcomes that have relevance, are scientifically sound (evidence based), and are feasible and flexible.

A number of health care plans are using *performance measures* that indicate the strengths and opportunities for improvement in a health care plan. These measures can highlight the effectiveness of care provision, consumer satisfaction, and the most cost-effective use of resources and facilities. Physician assistants should be included in the management and/or clinical team that develops and defines performance measures for specific hospital health care plans.

Performance measures come from a variety of sources, including state or national surveys, group consensus, and quality assurance studies. The Health Plan Employer Data and Information Set (HEDIS) is a set of standardized measures designed so that health care purchasers and health care consumers have the information they need to compare health care plans' performance. HEDIS 2001 was developed with the guidance of the National Committee for Quality Assurance (NCQA) with input from more than 200 organizations representing every sector of the nation's health care industry.[24]

PAs should become familiar with the guidelines that their hospital uses to evaluate outcomes. These performance measures are vital to successful clinical practice. The Agency for Healthcare Research and Quality (AHRQ) publishes a number of findings related to performance measures and utilization and/or access to care information.[14]

Physician assistants within the hospital setting must be thoroughly familiar with the accountability and supervision provided by the attending physician, as well as with the administrative structure and the chain of command in hospitals.

Preparing for Inpatient PA Utilization

Before a physician assistant is employed by a hospital or by a group of physicians working in the hospital, a number of issues are raised regarding the justification of and need for a physician assistant. Utilization of PAs can improve accessibility to inpatient services,

increase coverage for a variety of new or old services, reinforce residency training programs, assist with and expand new technological services, and increase revenue production for the institution or the individual physician. This justification process often involves an administrator and a physician, who define and delineate parameters and issues relevant to introducing or hiring a PA.

Successful inpatient practice for PAs requires that administrators and physicians share the same vision of the PA role. Before a PA is introduced into the hospital setting, the following should be developed:

➤ A concise, clear job description that reviews the role and responsibility of the PA in providing health care services.

➤ The methodology, frequency, and accountability of supervision to be provided by the supervising physician.

➤ Delineation of clinical limitations and ongoing open communication as to how these limitations will be developed.

➤ Discussion of how the PA will interact with physicians on staff.

➤ Discussion of the practice style changes that will occur from the addition of a PA to this hospital service.

➤ Assessment of greater accessibility for patients to health care services by addition of a PA.

➤ Estimate of reimbursable services that the PA will provide within a specific department.

➤ Description of clinical procedures that will be provided by the PA.

➤ Assessment of marketing the role of the PA to patients.

➤ Determination of how nursing staff and other support staff members will interact with and respond to the addition of the PA.

➤ Establishing acceptance of specific patient populations within the service area.

The preceding issues are typically handled through negotiations between physician administrators and hospital administration. Although a PA who is considering inpatient employment should know about the results of the negotiation, the PA may or may not be part of those discussions. The PA needs to discuss the following specific issues with the supervising physician and the administrator:

➤ What responsibility will the PA have for patient coverage?

➤ Who will be accountable for supervision for the PA?

➤ Will the PA be involved in taking calls for the service?

➤ What type of clinical procedures will the PA be providing?

➤ How much supervising time will be necessary from physician staff members and house staff members?

➤ How will coverage be provided when the PA is not available or is on vacation, sick, or attending continuing medical education programs?

➤ What issues, questions, and concerns have been raised by nursing staff, secretarial staff, and other support staff members?

➤ How will patients be introduced to the services of the PA?

➤ What marketing approaches will be taken to introduce the addition of the PA to patients, clinical and technical staff members, and support staff?

A different set of issues need to be addressed by the manager/director of a clinical department that plans to hire a PA. The AAPA can provide fact sheets to supplement the PA's knowledge in these areas:

➤ Matrix liaison activities with supervising physicians, referring physicians, nursing staff, and other support staff members of the health care team.

➤ Understanding of recruitment activities necessary for sampling the national pool of physician assistants, especially activities necessary for appropriate hiring of a well-trained, well-educated physician assistant—appropriate advertising, scheduling of interviews, determination and finalization of reference checks, and queries to the National Practitioner Data Bank.

➤ Knowledge necessary for registration and licensure with the appropriate state board of medicine.

➤ Appreciation of the reimbursement issues and practices necessary to obtain reimbursement for physician assistant services.

➤ Understanding of credentialing issues relevant to physician assistants.

➤ A clear management focus concerning the role, the clinical limitations, the clinical procedures, and the method and frequency of physician supervision provided.

➤ Quality assurance and risk management issues that may be raised by support staff or physician staff members.

The key to successful utilization of physician assistants in an inpatient setting is close communication, cooperation, and coordination among supervising physicians, support staff, and management. Communication and coordination of PA services usually occur in daily hospital rounds and ongoing telephone consultations with the supervising physician. This is particularly important in the event that a patient's condition dictates a change in the ongoing management plan, or a clinical procedure becomes necessary when the supervising physician is not present. Appropriate documentation must be entered into the medical record, delineating the action taken by the PA. This process of close communication is essential to the professional rapport between the physician assistant and the supervising physician in diagnosing and developing treatment plans for ongoing inpatient care.

A standardized approach to policies, procedures, credentialing, and tracking of physician assistant productivity is vital to the ongoing utilization of physician assistants. When PAs are employed in an inpatient setting, management staff and supervising physicians must have a clear understanding of their clinical utilization. Institutional and management concerns about the utilization of physician assistants include compliance with quality improvement programs, continuing education, appropriate physician supervision, and a clear, concise understanding of the pertinent legal and regulatory requirements.

Medical Staff Bylaws

A physician assistant within a hospital setting may be an employee of a hospital, an employee of an attending physician, or an employee of a part-time salaried physician of a hospital. The scope of practice of the PA in a hospital should be carefully delineated and set forth within the Medical Staff Bylaws and should have appropriate institutional approval. Medical Staff

Bylaws identify the categories of providers eligible for medical staff membership, and usually specify uniform criteria for granting initial and continued medical staff membership. Physicians and PAs submit evidence of current state licensure, relevant training and/or education, professional experience, national certification and/or re-certification, current competence in certain procedures, evidence of stable physical and mental health status, and evidence of current and adequate professional liability insurance. Hospital privileges are not given freely to physicians, but rather are conferred by the board of trustees in conjunction with approval from an overall hospital committee or medical staff committee.

The PA's clinical privileges, which describe the activities the PA is allowed to perform, depend on favorable reaction of hospital administrators, staff physicians, hospital nurses, and other professionals. They must be informed about how, where, and when PA services will be utilized. This facilitates the amendments that will be made to the hospital bylaws for adding a physician assistant to the health care team.

Usually, the medical staff and administration develop policies and procedures and then make final recommendations to a governing body concerning the status, relationship, and function of a PA within an institution, regardless of whether that person is employed by the physician or by the institution. A general policy for employment of PAs should cover both the general overall utilization of physician assistants in a hospital situation and, more specifically, utilization of each physician assistant.

Hospitals have a responsibility to employees and others for policies that are set forth regarding the philosophy or utilization of those employees or providers. It is essential that the physician and physician assistant work as a team to obtain formal delineation of clinical privileges and any appropriate bylaw changes needed to pave the way for utilization of the physician assistant within the inpatient setting. This is particularly important when the PA is the first physician assistant to be credentialed in the facility.

The supervising physician usually bears the responsibility of gaining the necessary privileges for the physician assistant. The keys to the acceptance of the physician assistant are visible support by the chair of the specific medical or surgical hospital staff, and ongoing education of various medical, nursing, and other support staff members regarding the PA's role and responsibilities. Within a small community hospital, a useful approach is to have the physician assistant make rounds with the physician on a daily basis before formally applying for hospital privileges. During these hospital rounds, the physician should introduce the PA to support staff members, nursing staff members, and other members of the medical staff so they may understand clearly the role and responsibility of the physician assistant.

Issues often arise regarding physician assistant utilization from specific groups. Legal parameters, insurance costs, and reimbursement issues are usually questioned by hospital administrators. Medical staff members may present concerns regarding professional supervision and role delineation. Nursing staff members and nursing administration may address issues regarding relaying and transferring of medical regimens and physician orders and encroachment on professional responsibilities. Support staff and ancillary staff members may present concerns regarding interaction with and supervision by the appropriate physician assistant.

It is essential that both the physician and the physician assistant be very familiar with the intent and the specific limits of applicable state laws, the local customs of delegation and supervision by other supervising physicians, and the requirements of the state board of medicine relevant to accepting orders by physician assistants and physicians. These issues all need to be addressed so that a clear understanding can be reached regarding the style of practice that the physician and physician assistant will be providing. Additional issues that may arise include patient acceptance, quality of services, and whether a PA may see patients of other physicians when a supervising physician is not available in the hospital.

Amendment of Hospital Bylaws

It is important for the PA and the physician to develop a clearly delineated plan, so that Hospital Bylaws may be amended to allow clinical privileges for physician assistants. Hospital Bylaws should stipulate that all clinical privileges granted to physician assistants must be consistent with all applicable state laws and regulations. Bylaws should allow physician assistants to provide health care services that are within the scope of practice of their supervising physician.[25] Suggested revisions in Hospital Bylaws are provided in the box below.

Medical Staff Bylaws must stipulate that all privileges granted to a physician assistant must be consistent with applicable state laws and regulations and that a physician assistant will render patient care

---

REVISED HOSPITAL BYLAWS

- Identify the specific physician assistant who will be included under the provision of the regulations.
- Specify roles authorizing such practice.
- Identify who will be responsible for the supervision of the physician assistant.
- Define the legal responsibility between the physician assistant and the supervising physician in the hospital.
- Outline the scope of clinical practice for the physician assistant in a way that permits flexibility in the relationship between the physician assistant and the supervising physician.
- General policies can address some of the following issues:
  - Definition and classification of the scope of the function and practice of the physician assistant.
  - Identification of specific limitations, that is, specifying actions that under no circumstances should be performed by a physician assistant.
  - Responsibility of the supervising physician, whether the physician assistant is employed by the institution, by a private physician, or by a part-time physician.
  - Delineation of the responsibilities of the supervising physician.
  - Ongoing evaluation of the clinical performance of the physician assistant.

Many of these policies can be addressed in a job description pertaining to the utilization of the physician assistant within the institution.

---

services within the scope of practice of the supervising physician, and within the specific departments in which the PA is practicing as a health care provider. As has been previously mentioned, the criteria for delineating clinical privileges for the physician assistant are best spelled out as specified in the philosophy or bylaws statement. These criteria should include evidence of current state registration, relevant training and experience, compliance with state registration and licensure, and any current or past pending professional liability or disciplinary actions. The American Academy of Physician Assistants publishes guidelines for amending hospital staff bylaws.

Clinical Privileges and Job Descriptions

In order to delineate clinical privileges, many hospitals utilize a standing medical committee, which reviews and approves clinical privileges of all staff members. Members of this committee are representatives of the medical staff, administrative staff, nursing staff, physician extender department, and other ancillary support departments. Clinical departments interested in obtaining clinical privileges for their physician assistants are asked to submit a complete job description and a list of clinical privileges to the committee for its approval. The clinical privileges are developed directly from the job description for each physician assistant.

The job description for physician assistants includes the primary function in the specific department, followed by the duties and responsibilities that the physician assistant will have in concert with the supervising physician. The next part of the job description discusses organizational responsibilities and the relationship of the supervising physician and the PA. This area clearly delineates to whom the physician assistant will respond both administratively and clinically. The job description also contains qualifications that the physician assistant must meet and criteria for performance evaluation. Some examples of PA job descriptions are listed in Appendix 2.

When a physician or a hospital has made a decision to hire a physician assistant, the first step is to develop an appropriate plan for interviewing and hiring the physician assistant for the specific department and physician who will be utilizing the PA services.

After the PA has been recruited and hired, the physician assistant and the supervising physician should develop an individual checklist that will focus on specific clinical privileges for the services the physician assistant will be providing. The privileges application will be submitted to the appropriate standing medical committee for approval and will then be sent to the board of trustees for final approval.

Legal Basis of Inpatient Practice

In 1989, David Bissonette, a physician assistant employed within the department of neurosurgery at the University of Pittsburgh, wrote a comprehensive article on hospital privileges and the principles and practice of the utilization of physician assistants.[26] He identified three fundamental legal concepts that enable physicians to delegate responsibilities to physician assistants:

1. An agency relationship to the doctrine of respondeat superior (master-servant relationship).
2. The borrowed servant doctrine.
3. Liability.

These principles are central to the decisions made by a hospital's governing board, administration, and medical staff in allowing physician assistants to be utilized to deliver health care services directly to patients.

An *agency relationship* exists when three factors are present—the employer, physician, or institution consents to the relationship; the employer accrues some degree of benefit from the acts of the physician assistant; and the employer has some degree of control of, or right to control, the physician assistant. Agency principles are used to determine who is responsible for liability rather than the presence or absence of liability. If the physician assistant is considered an independent contractor rather than an employee or agent of the supervising physician, the supervising physician might not be liable for the conduct of the physician assistant.

The principle of *respondeat superior* in the law holds a person liable who is not personally negligent but is closely associated with a negligent act. In other words, the physician is liable for the activities of the physician assistant because the physician is benefiting from and controlling the physician assistant's activities and has the power and control to stop, start, or alter the performance of the physician assistant's activities.

Regarding the *borrowed servant* doctrine, the physician assistant acts at times as an agent of the institution and at other times as an agent of the physician. Likewise, the physician assistant may function as the agent of the primary supervising physician at one time and the agent of a second physician at another time.

A physician assistant is directly *liable* for his or her own negligence, just as physicians or institutions are liable for their negligent acts. A physician assistant is liable for failure to refer a patient for a problem beyond the physician assistant's competence to treat. As all PA students are taught, PAs should clearly understand their limits of practice and limits of ability to provide services. Additionally, a physician or institution is liable for negligence, selection, or supervision of a physician assistant and for deliberately directing a physician assistant to commit a wrongful act.

Bissonette[26] suggested that clinical privileges constitute permission to provide patient care services in the hospital within a defined scope of practice based on the individual's credentials, experience, ability, and competence. He also cited the American Hospital Association's policy of 1987, which recommended that nonphysician practitioners who practiced in a dependent relationship with a physician should also have their scope of practice defined by delineation of clinical privileges. The AHA policy further recommended that when a hospital-governing board has decided that nonphysician practitioners will provide patient care services in a hospital, the responsibility for reviewing credentials and for recommending privileges for individual practitioners may be delegated to the medical staff or management of the hospital. Such responsibility for physician assistants who are in a dependent relationship with a physician employer or a hospital employer may be delegated to an appropriate hospital department. The American Society of Health Care Resources Administration of the AHA[27] has suggested the following principles:

➤ The classification of a physician assistant's scope of practice should be distributed to appropriate services and staff.

➤ Services that under no circumstances may be performed by a physician assistant should be specifically described.

➤ For a PA employed by a physician or an institution, a clear responsibility of the physician should be established for identifying who the physician assistant is and who is responsible for the physician assistant in the primary supervising physician's absence.

➤ Specific occasions on which direct physical supervision by a physician may be required should be delineated.

➤ Responsibilities of the supervising physician should be delineated.

➤ The qualifications of the supervising physician and his or her ability to provide supervision, as specified by a credentialing committee, should be assessed.

➤ A mechanism for changing clinical assignment responsibilities of the physician assistant, subject to approval by the appropriate medical staff committee, should be established.

➤ A method for identifying the physician assistant to the staff and public that conforms to state law and regulations established by the federal government should be defined.

➤ Adequate professional liability coverage for the PA, either under the supervising physician or in the hospital's liability policy, should be demonstrated.

➤ Reasons and a process for termination or disciplinary action and the appropriate appeals mechanism should be delineated for the physician assistant.

The following case study provides a pioneering example of the inpatient utilization of PAs.

CASE STUDY 25-1

In 1982, the Detroit Medical Center and the Harper Hospital began utilizing a restructured residency program to provide coverage at the hospital's nonteaching inpatient service. At that time, James Frick, PA-C, calculated the need for covering 20 patients with one physician assistant.[28] Ultimately, eight physician assistants covered approximately 160 beds, mainly from 7:30 AM to 11:30 PM on weekdays. As physician assistants provided more and more services, their service was extended to include the weekends.

Working closely with the medical advisory board and the executive committee, Frick and other individuals at Harper Hospital developed an excellent credentialing process for physician extenders. This was one of the pioneer programs within the country for providing inpatient PA services. There were two modes of physician assistant utilization—one in oncology and one in general medicine wards.

The general medicine PAs followed inpatients and provided daily care for a large number of private attending physician patients. This group of PAs also provided general on-call–type coverage on afternoons and weekends for medicine and oncology patients. The oncology division employed PAs on service-based teams, allowing physician and physician assistant interaction on a one-to-one basis. PAs made rounds on patients daily in order to have a clear understanding of each patient's and physician's needs.

Frick stated that the goal of this utilization of physician assistants was to create a dynamic practice environment for PAs, making them feel an integral part of a top-notch, high-quality health care delivery system. Physician assistants within the Harper Hospital and the Detroit Medical Center provided an important service for patients and acted as a complementary, noncompetitive source of quality patient assessment.

Case Study 25-2 describes the development of a comprehensive administrative structure for PA governance within a large health system.

CASE STUDY 25-2

Geisinger Medical Center in Danville, Pennsylvania, has employed physician assistants for more than 25 years. During that time, a number of policies and procedures have been developed that allow the Geisinger Clinic, the Geisinger Medical Center, supervising physicians, and PAs to work in concert. In Geisinger's experience, PAs are best utilized when their role is clearly defined and understood by patients, administrators, physicians, nursing staff, and other support staff members, thus allowing physicians and physician assistants to act in an effective and efficient manner.

Credentialing of physician assistants was provided by the Department of Physician Extender Services until 1995. The Department was responsible for ensuring that credentialing information was obtained from staff PAs and supervising physicians. The specific criteria for credentialing were established by the State Board of Medicine of the Commonwealth of Pennsylvania, and were retained on file by the Department of Physician Extender Services. This department collected information relative to the state certification process, conferred with the appropriate human resources departments, maintained an ongoing annual audit file of personnel files, notified physician assistants of the need for biannual physician assistant re-certification, monitored State Board of Medicine activities to obtain a clear understanding of ongoing regulations pursuant to physician assistants, and operated a tracking mechanism to ensure compliance with credentialing criteria established by the State Board of Medicine.

Prior to 1995, the Department of Physician Extender Services also coordinated appropriate clinical supervision. Each PA was responsible to a supervising physician and an appropriate chief PA or clinical director for clinical services, and to an appropriate administrative director or administrative vice president for administrative duties. Physician assistants were a part of many medical staff committees and were responsible for other activities within the medical center as well.

The PAs at the Geisinger Medical Center established a quality improvement team in 1990 that focused on the following objectives:

➤ To provide a mechanism of accountability for all physician assistants.
➤ To enhance communication among physician assistants, thereby improving delivery of health care.
➤ To provide an ongoing evaluation of clinical performance and the quality and appropriateness of patient care.
➤ To provide a liaison in order to link the results of quality assurance activities with appropriate continuing medical education activities.

➤ To continue the close professional relationship between the physician assistant and the supervising physician in delivery of high-quality health care.
➤ To encourage research and publication of physician assistant quality improvement team activities.

This team consisted of PAs from a variety of departments—family practice, plastic surgery, cardiovascular and thoracic surgery, neurosurgery, employee health, obstetrics and gynecology, mental health, ophthalmology, and neonatal intensive care. In addition, representatives of the quality improvement team were asked to provide assistance, liaison, and consultation services to clinical chairs and administrators. The committee chairperson, appointed by the Director of Physician Extender Services, acted as the coordinator for quality improvement within the Department of Physician Extenders. All quality improvement activities were coordinated and integrated with ongoing hospital quality improvement activities.

From 1987 until 1994, the Geisinger Health Care System published practice guidelines for physician assistant and nurse practitioner utilization. These practice guidelines were used by more than 300 national institutions and were helpful in establishing its own guidelines. The guidelines were established by teams of physician and PAs using appropriate evidence-based recommendations from recognized medical literature sources, medical specialty practice guidelines, health service organization performance measures, and input from a variety of government quality assurance agencies. The continued cooperation and communication between the physician and physician assistant team offered a best practice model for reviewing, revising, and updating practice guidelines on a continual basis.

Other clinical guidelines for the use of physician assistants in hospitals were developed at institutions across the nation, including the first postgraduate surgical physician assistant program at Montefiore Medical Center in New York City. Dr. Marvin Gliedman was the surgeon who was instrumental in developing the postgraduate surgical training program at Montefiore; he developed specific practice guidelines for the use of surgical physician assistants in concert with federal, national, and state rules and regulations.[29]

Quality Assurance

The accountability of a quality assurance or outcomes committee should be to the appropriate medical director or the appropriate hospital-wide quality assurance committee. The dimensions of quality include the structure, process, and outcomes of the hospital service providing the delivery of care. The scope of health care activities in which most quality assurance measures are involved includes the following:

➤ Delineating scope of care.
➤ Identifying important aspects of care.
➤ Identifying appropriate indicators of quality that can be identified for important aspects of care.
➤ Establishing thresholds for evaluation.
➤ Collecting and organizing data.
➤ Taking actions to resolve or solve problems when they are identified.
➤ Assessing the actions and documenting improvement that has taken place.
➤ Providing ongoing communication relevant to well-defined performance measure variables that relate to the structure, process, or outcome of care.

When selecting performance measures, quality assurance teams will often address the following questions: Have the measures satisfied the purpose for which the analysis was intended? Are the performance measures related to the mission or objective of the department? Is it possible to collect data about the performance measure? Are these data reliable and scientifically sound? Are the data valid? Is there a method of uniformity in collecting the necessary data?

These ongoing quality assurance activities are often performed by a quality assurance team that includes a variety of health care and administrative personnel appropriately selected by the hospital for the purpose of determining how it will comply with national and/or regional standards. PAs have been and will continue to be involved in the process of assessing health care outcomes and the process of determining performance measures that the institution and/or service department uses as quality indicators.

Practice Guidelines and Protocols

Practice guidelines, protocols, and outcome measures have become a vital component of current hospital practice, as a method of providing a clear plan for the utilization of physician assistants. Their purpose is to serve as a means of close communication, cooperation, and coordination between the PA and the supervising physician in patient diagnosis and the development of treatment plans. Many PAs believe that practice guidelines and/or protocols are much too specific. Yet practice guidelines and protocols have been shown to improve the quality of care because they offer a current view of evidence-based decision making by physicians and other practitioners.

The development of protocols at the Dartmouth Hitchcock Medical Center by the Medex primary care physician assistant program led to the publication of a comprehensive textbook, which has been used by the Dartmouth medical house staff since 1983 to approach a number of medical problems in specifically evaluating defined concerns and strategies for the management of patients.

Protocols written for defined medical problems may use a variety of approaches, such as branching logic and individualized clinical data collection. According to particular characteristics of patients, protocols provide precise guidelines for arriving at a diagnostic impression and/or making specific management decisions. Protocols are usually task specific and competency oriented, facilitating the ability of the practitioner to rapidly obtain a clear, concise direction for the management of many common medical problems. Protocols allow PAs to accurately identify specific historical and physical examination data and provide guidance toward making the appropriate diagnostic and therapeutic decisions.

The most efficient practice guidelines and/or management protocols provide a framework for the utilization of the PA in performing tasks delegated by the supervising physician. These practice guidelines and/or management protocols should codify the knowledge and practices of the supervising physician and the physician assistant. Drug regimens mentioned in these guidelines should be approved by the supervising physician and by the appropriate hospital committee.

Practice guidelines and/or protocols should not be utilized as standing orders nor should they be intended as a comprehensive drug formulary. Rather, they should be a method of clarifying the communication, cooperation, and coordination of services between the PA and the supervising physician, which may consist of daily hospital rounds or ongoing telephone consultations, to allow for comprehensive management of patient problems in the inpatient unit.

Outcomes

Currently used practice guidelines provide information about prevention and performance measures. In many cases, they reflect the potential outcomes for patients. These outcomes should reflect the results of care given and if necessary the costs of that care. Not all outcome measures are pure clinical decision-making outcomes. Often they ask: Did the patient get better? Was disability reduced? Did the patient receive the highest level of care? If not, why not? This focus on health status identifies health care delivery that improves care, maintains care, or worsens care. Outcomes often compare populations across agencies or health care plans, or according to socioeconomic status.

Outcome information is often collected from medical records; satisfaction with care may be evaluated by using either consumer surveys or focus groups. Managed care organizations view outcome measures as key indicators of success. A trend toward outcomes and away from productivity is only beginning to take hold in the United States.

Productivity and Reimbursement

Physician assistants are utilized in many different areas within the hospital to provide or expand patient access to medical care. PAs can improve quality of care and redistribute workloads in inpatient units. Reimbursement for services is a key ingredient in successful inpatient PA utilization.

Physician assistant services are recognized reimbursable services and are typically billed either in the supervising physician's name or in the PA's name. In the "incident to service" billing concept, PA service is billed in the supervising physician's name and service is provided as incidental to the physician's practice of medicine. When the supervising physician is on-site (clinic or office), billing under the "incident to" provision can be done at the rate of 100% of the prevailing physician rate. The provision of "incident to" should be used only after careful examination of the Medicare carrier's manual description.[30] Medicare requires services in some locations (hospitals, operating rooms, and nursing homes) to be billed in the physician assistant's name, at 85% of the prevailing physician rate.

Physicians need not be present at all times when PAs are evaluating or treating inpatient medical problems. Physician assistants and supervising physicians should, however, be communicating routinely regarding a patient's ongoing status and treatment recommendations. It is essential that the supervisory requirements for physician assistants allow some latitude for the PA to perform the services within inpatient practice. It is through use of the physician assistant's evaluative, diagnostic, and therapeutic skills, together with ongoing communication involving the physician-supervisor's expertise, that a valued and productive service is provided.

Administrative Director

The physician assistant and the supervising physician should utilize a clear functional job description to plan the clinical privileges that the physician assistant will have within the hospital setting. A job description and delineation of clinical privileges give the supervising physician, the clinical department, and any other members of the administrative or medical staff a clear, concise tool for reviewing, approving, and documenting the activities of the PA. When clinical privileges have been approved, the PA has the assurance of the institution's endorsement for the parameters of his or her practice style. Additionally, other members of the medical and nursing staff understand the clinical role of the physician assistant within the specific department or institution.

When there is a large group of physician assistants within a hospital setting, it may be useful to appoint a senior physician assistant to be a director, manager, or administrative director of physician assistants or physician extenders. Such an individual is responsible to the medical staff and has a direct line to the medical director and appropriate senior administrator regarding recruiting, hiring, documentation of clinical privileges, certification, registration, and ongoing periodic evaluation of the hospital's PAs. As health care systems focus on downsizing, the role of a senior or administrative physician assistant is still essential if a group or department has more than five physician assistants. The senior or administrative physician assistant should be able to perform the following functions:

➤ Facilitate continuing quality improvement, medical education, and risk management assessment relevant to PA practice.

➤ Function as a liaison with the appropriate clinical and administrative directors to assist in developing policies, procedures, and protocols necessary for the best utilization of PAs within each department.

➤ Conduct ongoing recruitment activities, interacting with human resources personnel about advertising, interviewing, reference checking, and querying of the National Practitioner Data Bank for PA applicants.

➤ Assist with credentialing, including the development of specific job descriptions and clinical privileges (as well as reviewing and revising in a timely fashion when updates are necessary).

➤ Have a clear understanding of the registration process for supervising physicians and physician assistants as mandated by the State Board of Medicine.

➤ Perform time management studies, selected specific productivity studies, and ongoing quality improvement surveys to assess patient satisfaction with PA services.

➤ Manage reimbursement and productivity revenue issues regarding utilization of PAs within a specific service.

➤ Assist the medical director and the appropriate supervising physician to conduct education programs for hospital administrators, medical staff, nursing staff, and ancillary staff to enhance utilization and training of PAs. (This is particularly important when PAs are used along with house staff physicians, who may not at first understand the role of the PA.)

➤ Conduct orientation programs, both for new physician assistants to acquaint them with the hospital and for new house staff members (June and July of each year) to acquaint them with the role of PAs in the hospital.

A current excellent example of this type of function for a PA is demonstrated at Northwest Hospital Center, where Richard Rohrs, PA-C, has functioned as the Administrative Director for House Staff Services for the past 15 years. He has played a vital role in providing continuity of services in using physician assistants for this large hospital center in Baltimore, Maryland.

FUTURE OF HEALTH CARE SYSTEMS

Hospitals face a future of change unlike at any time since the 1800s. The future will focus on strategic cost-cutting practices, networking activities, integrative arrangements with physicians, and increasing local or regional community alliances. In the future, health care systems in the United States may resemble the hospitals currently in existence in Europe today. One such health care system is found in Germany, where more than 90% of the population enroll in a sickness fund through their employers, labor unions, or professional associations. This sickness fund, called Krankenkassen, reimburses local physician groups and hospitals for health care services. Hospitals are paid a capitated rate for inpatient care, and most hospital-based doctors are paid a straight salary. In the German system of health care, the government plays a major role in ownership of the hospital system. Planning in German hospital systems tends to be centralized; thus, there tends to be a higher number of hospital beds per population than in the United States. Additionally, the use of outpatient services is quite extensive, leaving only the seriously ill patient to be cared for in the hospital.

Physician assistants in hospitals provide compassionate, comprehensive services and will continue to make a difference in the future of inpatient care, not only as providers but as administrators, chief executive officers (CEOs), chief financial officers (CFOs), directors, coordinators, and advocates of health policy and public health. Current and future roles for PAs may include the following:

➤ CEO and CFO—administering the daily activities of health care systems.

➤ Administrators—administering the activities of the professional medical staff, communicating with both the clinical and the administrative elements of operational change.

➤ Directors of medical and professional services areas—administering and managing other PAs, nurse practitioners (NPs), and mid-level health practitioners who will focus on the day-to-day care of inpatients.

➤ Clinical directors of specialized departments—administering and providing clinical and administrative services within specialized areas of medical and surgical departments, such as organ transplant including xenotransplantation (transplantation of tissue and organs from animals into humans), genetic therapy combined with genetic mapping and testing, invasive and non invasive imaging centers, non invasive cardiology and neurosurgery, informatics systems, aeromedicine retrieval and transport services, and trauma services, as well as focused services, such as acting as health advocates using email and the Internet, global women's health care, infant care, geriatric care, laser surgery, and reconstructive surgery.

➤ Global health providers—meeting the increased demands and expectations of a worldwide consumer movement.

➤ Inventors and bio-informatic experts—adopting and implementing new electronic information technologies in line with the original concept of Dr. Stead when training physician assistants at Duke University in electronics, to keep pace with modern advances in medicine.

The future is ours if we act now to understand history, to empower PA students to be change agents, to learn from past mistakes and missed opportunities, and to understand professional successes. We should thank PAs who were risk takers. They challenged the systems that prevented PAs from moving forward.

Physician assistants can be key players in the future of primary care and health care in our country. We need to understand the changes in health care, and we must continue to foster the creativity, caring, compassion, and flexibility that gave birth to our profession and will forever mold its spirit. When we limit our vision of providing our services within health care, then and only then will our utilization be limited.

CLINICAL APPLICATIONS

1. What is the oldest hospital in your community? Research and describe the hospital's history. How do you think this hospital will change in the future?

2. You have been offered a position in a hospital, where you would be the first PA employed by this institution. Discuss the hospital policies and procedures that may need to be modified in order for you to function effectively. How would you suggest that your supervising physician and department chair introduce you into the hospital environment?

3. You work in a hospital system that employs 35 PAs. Although you are not the most senior PA, the position of coordinator of PA services has been offered to you. How would you write the job description for this position? How would you approach your relationship with other PAs who have been your peers, particularly those who have more seniority?

REFERENCES

1. Starr P. Health care reform and the new economy. Health Affairs, Nov/Dec 2000.
2. Shortell S. Crossing the Quality Chasm: A New Health System for the 21st Century. Washington, DC: Institute of Medicine, 2001.
3. Letourneau CV. History of hospitals, part I. Hosp Manage 1959;March:58.
4. http://sihp.brandesis.edu/council/thml/ hospitalstructure.htm. Accessed 4 March 2002.
5. Health Care Expenditures. Rockville, Md: Health Care Financing Administration, 1996.
6. http://www.hcfa.gov. Accessed 10 March 2002.
7. Hospital Statistics. Chicago: American Hospital Association, 2002.
8. 2001 Census Report, American Academy of Physician Assistants. Alexandria, VA: American Academy of Physician Assistants, 2001.
9. Hooker RS, Cawley JF. Physician Assistants in American Medicine. New York: Churchill Livingstone, 1997.
10. Synowiez PM. Utilization of physician assistants in group practice. College Rev 1986;3:57.

11. Osler W. The Evolution of Modern Medicine. New Haven-Yale: University Press, 1921.

12. Duffy J. Epidemics in America. Baton Rouge, LA: Louisiana State University Press, 1971.

13. O'Connor R. American hospital: the first 200 years. Hospitals 1976;1:58.

14. http://www.meps.ahrq.gov. Accessed 17 March 2002.

15. Elixhauser A. Hospitalization in the United States. HCUP Fact Book. AHRQ Publication. No. 00-031. Rockville, Md: Agency for Healthcare Research and Quality, 1997.

16. Accreditation Manual for Hospitals. Oakbrook Terrace, IL: Joint Commission on Accreditation of Health Care Organizations, 1995.

17. Whisler TL. Rules of the game: inside the hospital boardroom. In: Environmental Assessment 1984, Special Feature 3. Chicago: Hospital Research and Educational Trust, 1984, 3.

18. Snook DI. Opportunities in Hospital Administration. Skokie, IL: National Textbook Company, 1982.

19. Hudson CL. Expansion of medical professional services with nonprofessional personnel. JAMA 1961;176:95.

20. Perry HB, Detmer DE, Redmond EL. The current and future role of surgical PAs: report of national survey of surgical chairmen in large U.S. hospitals. Ann Surg 1983;193:132.

21. http://www.aamc.org/advocacy/issues/medicare/start.htm. Accessed 17 March 2002.

22. http://www.hcfa.gov. Accessed 17 March 2002.

23. http://www.ahcpr.gov. Accessed 17 March 2002.

24. http://www.hedis.gov. Accessed 17 March 2002.

25. American Academy of Physician Assistants. Physician Assistants in Hospital Practice. Alexandria, VA: AAPA, June 1996.

26. Bissonette D. Hospital privileges and physician assistant policies and practices. J Am Acad Physician Assist 1989;2:132.

27. American Society of Health Care Human Resources Administration. Utilization of physician assistants in health care institutions. Am Hosp Assoc Tech Adv Bull 1984;May:3.

28. Frick JC. Physician assistants as house officers: our experience. Physician Assist 1983;7:13.

29. Condit D. Dr. Marvin Gliedman, Surgical Physician Assistant. January 2002, p 9.

30. American Academy of Physician Assistants. Reimbursement Watch. Alexandria, VA: AAPA, April 2002.

RESOURCES

Essential Articles

Cooper R, Getzen T, McKee H, Laud P. Economic and demographic trends signal an impending physician shortage. Health Affairs 2002;21:140.

Walker L. Making the most of midlevel providers. Hippocrates 1999;13.

Bernstein A, Hing E, et al. Trend Data on Medical Encounters: Tracking a Moving Target. Health Affairs March/April 2001.

Committee on Quality of Health Care in America. Crossing the Quality Chasm: A New Health System for the 21st Century. Washington, DC: Institute of Medicine, 2001.

Robinson JC. The end of managed care. JAMA 2001;285:2622.

Starr P. Health care reform and the new economy. Health Affairs 2000;19:23.

Institute for the Future. Health and Health Care 2010: The Forecast and the Challenge. New York, NY: Jossey-Bass, 2000.

Fralic M, Grady R, Hegge M. Nurse Workforce: Condition Critical, Issue Brief. National Health Policy Forum, Washington, DC, June 2001.

Snyderman R, Sheldon G, Bischoff T. Gauging supply and demand: the challenging quest to predict the future physician workforce. Health Affairs 2002;21:167.

Bissonette D. Hospital privileges and physician assistant policies and practices. J Am Acad Physician Assist 1989;2:132.

Regan DM, Harbert KR. Managing the financial productivity of physician assistants. Med Group Manag J 1991;November/December:46.

Harbert K, Shipman RA, Conrad W. The utilization of physician extenders: mid-level providers in a large group practice within tertiary health care setting. Med Group Manag J 1994; 11:26.

Texts

Birembaum A. In the Shadow of Medicine: Remaking the Division of Labor and Health Care. Dix Hills, NY: General Hall, 1990. *Discusses the roles of the physician assistant, the nurse practitioner, and the clinical pharmacist. Was written by a sociologist and has a sociomedical approach to how the division of medicine has been determined for these three roles.*

Zarbock SF, Harbert KR. Physician Assistants: Present and Future Models of Utilization. New York: Praeger Publishers, 1986. *Written by a number of PAs and physicians. Discusses the various models of utilization of physician assistants in inpatient, outpatient, managed care, and military settings. Includes an excellent discussion of the variety of models utilized in the early and late 1980s.*

Hooker RS, Cawley JF. Physician Assistants in American Medicine. New York: Churchill Livingstone, 1999. *Contains vital information regarding the current role of PAs within the health care structure and health care environment. An excellent resource document about where PAs are going.*

Ludmerer K. Time to Heal. New York: Oxford University Press, 1999. *Excellent history of the American medical education system from the turn of the century to the era of managed care.*

Web Sites

➤ Disease Management: www.medscape.com.

➤ Virtual Hospital: http://vh.radiology.wiowa.edu.

➤ American Hospital Directory: http://www.ahd.com/.

➤ American Hospital Association: http://aha.org.

CHAPTER 26

Inner City Health Care

F. J. Gino Gianola and Tom Byers

"Of all forms of inequality, injustice in health is the most shocking and most inhumane."

—Dr. Martin Luther King, Jr.

INTRODUCTION

Providing health care in the neighborhoods that lie at the center of America's cities presents the physician assistant with a unique set of challenges and opportunities, demanding a special set of attitudes and skills. There is no more complex environment in which to practice, nor is there one in which there is a higher risk of heartbreak and frustration. There are few places, however, in which a dedicated practitioner can make as large a difference in the life of a community. If physician assistants and the academic institutions in which they are trained select and mentor applicants that reflect the patients cared for in the inner city, we can make a significant difference in the inner cities of this nation. We will have succeeded in affirming and understanding the cultures and lives of the citizens in the inner city.

This chapter describes the challenges and opportunities of inner city practice in the context of the unique forces that have shaped America's central cities during the past 50 years.

WHAT DO WE MEAN BY *INNER CITY*?

Inner city is a term that is used to describe the neighborhoods that lie closest to the historic center of a city, where a convergence of rivers, a deep harbor, or other natural features provided the city with a reason for being. By virtue of their location nearest the city's industrial and commercial activity, these neighborhoods had the advantage of proximity to employment but many disadvantages as well. Subject to the noise, traffic, and pollution that attend industry, these neighborhoods generally housed the working classes, while more affluent families resided in neighborhoods "uptown" or "on the other side of the tracks."

Throughout the 19th and early 20th centuries, these inner city neighborhoods played a critical role in the development of urban America. These districts provided the first homes for the numerous waves of immigrants who reshaped America's cities, and in turn provided a ready source of labor for the factories, ports, and warehouses nearby. Although many of the residents were poor and lived in terribly overcrowded conditions, many were able to use the inner city as a place to gather strength—to learn the new language, find employment, and save enough money to have better choices.

When they could afford to, many made the choice to leave the inner city for nearby neighborhoods that were less crowded. There, a little farther from the center of the city, a family might have a row house instead of an apartment, and the children might have a place to play other than the streets. Through this process, the housing in the inner cities constantly opened up again for the next wave of newcomers, while those who had succeeded remained in better neighborhoods nearby as living symbols of the reality of the American dream.

In the midst of the 20th century, a number of significant changes took place in America's cities that severely altered the role and character of the inner cities. With the end of the Great Depression and World War II, another great migration began. This time, the immigrants came not from overseas but from rural areas of the southern United States that had been devastated by the Depression. Poor whites and blacks who had suffered mightily during the 1930s and early 1940s now streamed into the inner cities of the North in search of new opportunities in the factories nearby. For a time, it appeared as if these latest newcomers would succeed in repeating the now-familiar cycle. By working hard and saving their wages, they hoped to move up and out within a generation or two. The symbiotic relationship between the inner cities, nearby industry, and middle class urban neighborhoods, however, was nearing its end.

Ironically, this change was caused in large part by the very economic boom these new residents were helping to create. The new wealth enjoyed by ordinary Americans meant that many more could afford luxuries like the automobile. Gradually, the private automobile replaced public transportation as the way in which the middle class got to work. This in turn undermined the financial health of the transit services upon which most inner city residents still had to rely. Meanwhile, new government programs were making it possible for returning servicemen to buy homes, provided the homes met certain standards that the older housing in the inner city could not meet. Both of these forces worked against the inner cities by encouraging the newly affluent to leave the city altogether for new suburban developments beyond the city's borders.

This trend accelerated dramatically in the late 1950s, as the federal government spent billions of dollars to construct a system of expressways designed to carry automobiles long distances at high speed. These new highways enabled the middle and upper classes to move even farther from their jobs in the city, and soon the lifeblood of the cities began to spill out across the countryside.

Inner city neighborhoods suffered severely from these changes. Not only were they drained of their middle class, but they also were seen as the path of least resistance for the construction of the expressways. In city after city, historic inner city neighborhoods that had nurtured generations of working-class Americans were sliced apart by highways, and hundreds of thousands of units of affordable housing were lost in the process.

As the middle-class workers abandoned the city, their jobs began to follow them. Commercial enterprises quickly followed their customers, and many industries concluded it was cheaper to build new factories in the countryside than to rebuild in the cities. Over time, this out-migration severely eroded the tax base of the cities, leaving them with few resources to heal the wounds of their inner cities.

Sadly, these demographic trends exacerbated class and racial tensions that have afflicted our nation throughout its history. For a host of reasons, ranging from discrimination in the real estate industry to fears of school busing, those who left the cities during this period were predominantly white, while those who remained were disproportionately persons of color.

As the postwar dreams of millions of American families were coming true in the suburbs, the frustration of those who had been left behind in the inner cities was growing. Beginning in Detroit in the summer of 1967, an epidemic of rioting broke out in the nation's inner cities, resulting in many deaths and the destruction of millions of dollars in property. The true extent of the damage of those riots is incalculable because they provided those with resources with one more excuse to leave the central cities.

For its part, the federal government responded to the unrest with a mix of policies that encouraged tougher law enforcement and created a wide range of social and health programs such as Model Cities and Community Health Centers. Although some of these measures initially showed positive results, the government's "War on Poverty" was short-lived. Faced with the human and economic toll of the War in Vietnam and the deaths of its most able political leaders and civil rights champions, the nation turned away from the problems of the inner cities.

A portrait of the inner cities during this period is deeply etched in America's consciousness. It is a portrait of boarded-up buildings and decrepit schools, of children left to play in alleys and men idle on the street corners, of a place where drugs and alcohol are prevalent and violence is always nearby. It is a place where there are too few choices and no good ones.

Poverty and economic hardship continue to be all too common. Today, there is still truth in this portrait, but only half-truth. It shows only the weakness of these neighborhoods and none of the resilience. It shows nothing of the spirit that knows the odds and beats them anyway, of parents who work three jobs so a child can go to college, of ministers and community leaders who keep hope alive among their followers, of women who struggle to raise children alone and do it well. In short, it is a portrait that shows all of the problems and none of the possibilities. The health care provider who chooses to practice in the inner cities today will enter a world in which both of these realities are present on the same stage, and he or she will have the opportunity to change, if ever so slightly, the balance between those forces.

HEALTH CARE IN THE INNER CITY

The population of the inner cities today is far more diverse than it was during the late 1960s, when the images of the inner city became fixed in the American psyche. New waves of immigration from every corner of the globe have brought millions of new residents to the nation's ports of entry, where many have concentrated in the inner cities. The ethnic composition of these enclaves varies widely across America. Hispanics predominate in the southern tier of major cities; the immigrant populations in northern cities are more diverse. They include large refugee populations from Southeast Asia, east Africa, and central Europe, as well as Hispanics. In Seattle, for example, the public school children speak 96 different languages at home.

This new explosion of diversity has created both challenges and opportunities for America's cities and for health care providers. In addition to the barriers to health care that grow from economic disadvantage, they must now confront barriers that grow from differences in language and culture as well. Before turning to those challenges, it may be useful to understand the character of the health care delivery system as it presently operates in most of America's inner cities. In general, that "system" differs markedly from systems of care in rural or suburban settings, and these differences have important effects on the way inner city residents use health services.

Some of the differences in health care systems can be traced to the period of out-migration from the inner cities that occurred several decades ago. As the middle class left for the suburbs, most private practitioners went with them. Some hospitals moved out of town as well, although huge past investments in their facilities made this more difficult than for doctors who simply had to relocate their offices. Those hospitals that remained faced a difficult prospect. With their base of paying patients moving farther away, they could either ally with teaching hospitals and the training subsidies they received or attempt to become specialty centers capable of attracting patients from the suburbs.

The economics drove most private hospitals to become specialty centers, which dictated policies that had the effect of shutting out those who could not afford to pay the full cost of their care. Over time, inner city populations became more and more dependent on public teaching hospitals for their care. The advent of public health insurance programs such as Medicaid and Medicare mitigated this trend for a short time, but as the rates paid by these programs began to fall behind the costs of care, the trend accelerated.

THE ROLE OF PUBLIC TEACHING HOSPITALS

The importance of America's urban public hospitals in providing care to inner city populations cannot be overstated. Simply put, if it had not been for these institutions, many millions of Americans would be without any access to care except that which private hospitals are required to provide in emergencies. In addition to the provision of care to those who could not otherwise afford it, these hospitals are major employers, often the cornerstone of the inner city's economy.

However great their contributions, urban public hospitals are also faced with severe constraints. By virtue of caring for large numbers of uninsured patients and even larger numbers whose public insurance does not cover the full cost of care, these hospitals suffer chronic budget shortages. These shortages frequently manifest themselves in overcrowding, outdated equipment, and rundown facilities.

There are also inherent contradictions in the multiple roles an urban public hospital must play. As a teaching institution, the hospital must organize services in a way that best provides instruction for the students and residents who rotate among the hospital's various departments. It must also give special emphasis to specialty care procedures the students might otherwise never have an opportunity to learn. These teaching requirements are important, but they are often at odds with the hospital's role as a community institution responsible for providing its patients with continuity of care.

Although most public teaching hospitals are extraordinarily well suited for emergent care and acute illness, they are generally less well designed for the management of chronic illness and very poorly suited to provide preventive care. When the authors of this chapter worked together in a community clinic, it was not unusual for patients to report that they had

been seen numerous times for the same health problem at the nearby public hospital, never seeing the same provider, and had been subjected to the same battery of tests repeatedly. In some cases, they had been offered markedly different diagnoses and prescriptions. One elderly man presented us with a bag of 11 different medications he had been given for hypertension, uncertain which to take.

Some public teaching hospitals have made remarkable efforts to resolve these contradictions in their roles by establishing primary care departments and satellite clinics or by working with networks of community health centers. However, these efforts have often been cut short of their full potential by funding problems, leaving the populations of the inner cities overly dependent on the emergency departments as their major source of care.

THE ROLE OF PUBLIC HEALTH DEPARTMENTS

Urban public health departments have long played a vital role in the inner cities, especially in efforts to improve environmental health and sanitation and to control the spread of communicable disease. During the short-lived "War on Poverty," some urban health departments used federal funds to expand their role to include providing new services to the inner cities. Unfortunately, most of these services were funded through "categorical grants" targeted to a specific health care problem such as sickle cell anemia or family planning, and the service delivery was also organized according to these categories. This meant that health departments might be able to provide a number of screening services and immunizations for a child but might not be able to care for the child's ear infection or other needs for which no categorical funding was available.

At times, this pattern of service delivery became absurd. In the late 1970s, for example, it was not uncommon for women to be required to visit three different health department programs and undergo three different examinations in order to piece together basic gynecological services that could easily have been provided in one primary care visit. This duplication occurred because services for sexually transmitted disease screening, birth control, and cervical cancer screening were organized categorically to make it easy to comply with federal reporting requirements.

In the most recent past, many urban health departments have de-categorized their services to more closely reflect the needs of their patients. A few have ventured into primary care either by offering services directly or through alliances with other providers. With the onset of the acquired immune deficiency syndrome (AIDS) epidemic and the increased incidence of other communicable diseases in the inner cities, health departments have also worked hard to expand their capacity to fulfill their traditional mission of protecting the public health through education, prevention, and the control of communicable diseases.

THE ROLE OF COMMUNITY HEALTH CENTERS

One of the few lasting legacies of the War on Poverty is the community health center movement, which plays a significant role in the health care of the majority of America's inner cities. Unlike public teaching hospitals and urban health departments, community health centers were expressly designed to meet the challenges of the inner cities as they existed in the late 1960s. They were intended to be governed by the communities they served, to offer relatively comprehensive preventive and primary care, and to provide services on a sliding-fee scale according to the patient's ability to pay. Community health centers were also intended to be an integral part of a larger effort to encourage community development on a much broader scale, but that larger initiative has yet to materialize.

Measured in terms of their initial goals, community health centers have had great success in many ways and have fallen short in others. They have re-established the concept of primary care in many inner city neighborhoods in which the family doctor had all but disappeared. They have cared for millions of inner city residents in a way that is generally held to be more beneficial and cost effective than other modes of care, and they have pioneered new innovations in caring for disadvantaged populations.

Like their colleagues in public teaching hospitals and urban health departments, those who practice in inner city health centers also face serious barriers to success, including chronic funding shortages and the challenges of dealing with an increasingly complex patient population (see Case Study 26-1).

CASE STUDY 26-1

The city had fallen on bad times. The major employer had just laid off thousands of employees, both blue and white collar, salaried and hourly workers. People were literally leaving their homes with unpaid mortgages. Small businesses were closing in all the neighborhoods. People who had been covered by adequate health insurance were now uncovered. The public hospitals were overwhelmed with many more visits. The working poor were now poorer, and the city services were being overwhelmed. A famous billboard sign announced to people leaving the city by the only freeway, "Would the last person leaving please turn off the lights?" It was not a good time for the city.

The Vietnam War was still being waged. There were many returning veterans and others disillusioned by the years of death and destruction to both countries. In the city that was so devastated by layoffs and a poor economy, a group of disgruntled young people aged 20 to 26 wanted to make a lasting change. With hard work and the support of the community, they built a community clinic. It was a challenge to find health care providers, especially physicians, who had time to provide care. Eventually, a small cadre of physicians was found. However, as the community clinic developed and the patient load increased, the hours needed to be expanded. Full-time staff had to be found.

The clinic had a number of medical assistants and "patient advocates" who volunteered at the clinic in the evenings. The clinic decided to train some staff to become eligible for physician assistant education. In 1976, two applicants from this clinic were accepted to the physician assistant program. The clinic provided the clinical training site, and the two graduated in 1977. They are still practicing at the same clinic, where one of the PAs is now the medical director.

This experience has been repeated over and over again in community health centers in underserved areas throughout the country. Educating people in the community in PA programs and having them return to the community is one way to keep providers in the underserved areas of inner cities.

1. This community health center appears to have had good community support. How would you get the community involved in a community health center concept? What are some of the skills taught in your PA program that would help with community work?

2. This community clinic was able to identify community members to prepare for application to a physician assistant program. How would you go about identifying potential candidates who would work and stay at a community health center? How would you assist as a graduate in identifying this type of candidate?

3. Are there any community health centers in an inner city near you? Is there a PA on staff? If yes, have you ever spoken with the PA? Have PAs ever lectured for you in your PA program? Have they lectured at your state continuing medical education program?

4. What is it that keeps a person in the inner city community clinic for an entire career?

THE INCREASING COMPLEXITY OF INNER CITY PRACTICE

The face of the inner cities has changed dramatically in the past two decades, reflecting a series of waves of immigration from all corners of the globe. Hospitals and community health centers in Seattle, for example, which once cared for patients in one or at most two languages, now routinely provide care in 10 or more languages and occasionally provide care to patients who speak dozens more. The challenges this presents begin with the need to bridge the language gap. To meet this need, inner city providers have responded in a variety of ways. Some have relied heavily on family members to translate between the doctor and the

patient, whereas others have used staff members who have other roles within the organization but are called in to translate when the need arises. As the number of patients grows, most providers begin to contract with professional interpreters, and a few hire full-time interpreters as part of the organization's staff.

The quality of medical interpretation varies widely among these methods. Even among those interpreters who are employed by health care providers on a full-time basis, there are significant gaps in their understanding of health care technology and terminology. There are certainly enormous gaps in providers' understanding of how best to use medical interpreters. Some inner city providers, like Pacific Medical Clinics and Harborview Medical Center in Seattle, have begun experimenting with ways to improve cross-cultural care through training programs for both providers and interpreters. Funding for such efforts, or even for basic medical interpretation, however, is hard to find (see Case Study 26-2).

CASE STUDY 26-2

A 24-year-old recent Vietnamese immigrant comes to the clinic with her 6-month-old son with a complaint of "constant crying." The young woman does not speak English, and her 8-year-old daughter is translating for her. You obtain a history consistent with colic. The physical examination is consistent with your diagnosis. While performing your physical examination, you note unusual linear markings on the child's skin, with erythema and discoloration of the skin surrounding the markings. You note the child has not had any immunizations.

You also note during your discussion that the child interpreting asks the mother questions and the mother responds with lengthy answers, but what the child tells you she said is a much shorter response. You ask the child when she was last seen at the clinic, and she says she has never seen an American doctor. You also find she has had no immunizations.

1. Is it appropriate to have children interpret for their parents? How common is this practice? Are there any alternatives in your community?

2. In this case, you note some unusual skin markings on the child that are bruiselike scrapes.

What do you think it is? Could there be cultural aspects to these findings? If yes, what? If you don't know, how would you find out?

3. There are many cultural norms in each ethnic community. How would you identify community resources to help you understand a specific culture?

4. Are there any other troubling issues in this case? What are they? How would you address them?

The challenge of caring for refugees and other recent immigrant communities goes well beyond the issue of interpretation. There are also enormous differences between the basic beliefs of these communities and the underlying values of American medical practice. For example, among certain Vietnamese, it is believed that if you imagine your child may become ill and it happens, you have caused it. Is it any wonder, then, that a Vietnamese mother may resist enrolling her child in a health insurance program that, in effect, requires her to imagine that her child may become ill?

The demographic change in America's inner cities is not the only change affecting the nature of health care delivery. There are also severe changes in the circumstances of the poorest members of inner city communities that make it exceedingly difficult to provide care. One such trend is the increase in homelessness. Health centers designed to serve relatively stable low-income families now find themselves caring for large numbers of homeless families, with little chance of providing continuity of care as they move from one shelter to another or from one city to another. In response, Health Care for the Homeless Projects have been created in many inner cities, providing on-site health care in shelters and sometimes in the streets.

Wood and associates[1] concluded in their 1990 Los Angeles study of 196 homeless families in 10 shelters and 194 housed poor families that "homeless children have significant child behavior and developmental problems and disorders of nutrition and growth, which are associated with multiple risk factors in their environment." Providers in the inner cities are also seeing increases in communicable diseases such as tuberculosis that seemed all but nonexistent in

urban America just a few years ago. Together with the continuing crisis of the human immunodeficiency virus (HIV) and AIDS, these infectious diseases, partly as a byproduct of immigration and homelessness, pose special challenges for the inner city.

Health care providers working in the inner city and their professional associations are addressing some of the inner city health issues. The American College of Physicians commissioned Andrulis[2] to write a paper on inner city health care. The report noted that "one in five persons in the United States live in the nation's 100 largest cities. The health care infrastructure in the inner cities often serves both urban and citizens in nearby suburbs. The fate of the inner city is therefore inseparable from the life of the nation."

Andrulis' paper brings to light Greenberg's[3] concept of the "urban health penalty." This is defined as "a condition that exists when healthier, more affluent persons leave the city and the remaining and new residents experience health problems that interact with the city's physical and economic deterioration." The description continues, "The poverty zones created by this deterioration, which include proportionately higher numbers of persons belonging to minority groups, become epicenters for economic decline, job loss and major health problems." Andrulis[2] makes another observation with which the authors of this chapter wholeheartedly agree: "The medical model is inadequate in the urban environment; multifaceted approaches are needed"[4] (see Case Study 26-2).

HEALTH AND WELFARE REFORM AND THEIR IMPACT ON THE INNER CITY

Inner city health care providers—whether they are large teaching hospitals, health departments, community health centers, or private physicians—have had to struggle against long odds to continue providing care to people in the inner cities. They have demonstrated remarkable staying power and creativity in the face of the problems we have described. Now they are faced with new challenges arising not only from changes in demographics, social conditions, and new epidemics, but from "reforms" in health care financing and the welfare system.

One can debate the motives behind these changes, but that is not our intention. Our concern is that the health care reforms that have recently been implemented with the intention of cutting costs are having serious consequences in the inner cities. They threaten not only the standard of care available to the people of the inner city but the health of the "safety-net providers" that provide those services.

In state after state, legislatures have mandated that those who are covered by Medicaid must participate in managed care plans. In many cases, the transition to managed care was not handled smoothly, and patients were not provided adequate information about the implications of the change. In Washington State, for example, more than one third of those who initially transitioned to managed care were assigned to a plan by the state rather than choosing one on their own. As a result, many inner city families with established relationships at community health centers were assigned to plans that had no providers within the neighborhood and no provisions for medical interpretation at the clinics they operate.

Fierce competition among health plans has also driven wedges among inner city providers who may not participate in the same plan. For example, the medical center that has traditionally provided most of the specialty care to patients of the community health centers in Seattle is not a full participant in the health plan organized by the community health centers, and the major urban teaching hospital has organized still another plan. As health plans compete for market share, they have purchased practices near inner city neighborhoods, sometimes "creaming" patients with health care coverage and leaving those with no coverage to the community health centers. In this environment, the pressures on the traditional providers of care in the inner city are very serious indeed.

In "Mama Might Be Better Off Dead," Abraham[4] puts a very real human face on an inner city family dealing with the multiple layers of the health bureaucracy. Abraham spent 3 years with a poor inner city family documenting the family's encounters with chronic illness and the chaos of the present health care system. Additional problems have been created by severe cutbacks in aid to refugees and by changes in federal welfare law, which are being implemented very differently from state to state. Unless new ways can be found to help the residents of the inner cities enter the economic mainstream, their problems may grow worse.

A 29-year epidemiological study conducted by Lynch, Kaplan, and Shema[5] from the University of Michigan School of Public Health stated in its conclusion, "Sustained economic hardship leads to poorer physical, psychological, and cognitive functioning." This may seem obvious to members of the communities and to health care providers working in the inner city. However, the Michigan study is able to draw a direct and clear connection between poverty and the increased incidence of illness (and not the reverse).

THE CHILDREN, THE FUTURE

A further disturbing trend in the United States is the effect of poverty on children. The National Center for Children in Poverty[6] published a study that provides persuasive data to show a significant increase in the poverty rate for children under the age of 6 years. The study states, "Evidence indicates that life in near poverty is almost as detrimental to children's health and development as living just below the poverty line,[7] and extreme poverty early in life is especially deleterious to children's future life chances."[8] Two pieces of data are included:

➤ From 1979 to 1994, the number of children under the age of 6 years living in poverty grew from 3.5 million to 6.1 million.
➤ The young child poverty rate is 3 to 12 times higher in the United States than in 12 other Western industrialized nations.

Health professionals must wrestle with these issues and become involved with their solution.

There are a few rays of hope. Buoyed by a vibrant national economy, some states are experimenting with programs that link inner city residents to the training opportunities, child care, and health services needed to find and retain employment at decent wages. Many immigrant communities seem to be successfully gaining a foothold in the mainstream economy by pooling their resources and cooperating with one another in establishing new enterprises. In some cities, new investments in the downtown commercial areas have created the prospect of new employment opportunities for inner city residents. Whether these promising trends continue to grow will depend upon the health of the economy and upon the creativity and determination of those who care about the future of inner city neighborhoods.

CONCLUSION

Ironically, the challenges of inner city health care create unique opportunities for physician assistants to take on more responsibility and accomplish greater good than might be possible in less complex environments. Regardless of which setting you choose, you will be asked to work at your full potential. You will be allowed to enter into the most intimate and important decisions of families whose language you do not speak and whose cultural beliefs you must struggle to comprehend. You will have to learn to improvise treatment regimens for patients who have neither health insurance nor shelter or decent food. You will need to learn everything there is to know about diseases that your colleagues in the suburbs may never see in their lifetime. You also will be called upon to advocate for patients who are caught in red tape in ways that Orwell himself could never have imagined.

In return, we can promise you this: It will never be dull, and at the end of many days, you will be able to truly believe that you have made a difference in the lives of your patients and in the community of which you have become a part.

CLINICAL APPLICATIONS

1. In your city, who lives in the inner city? Are there new Americans? Do you know anyone personally who lives in the inner city? Have you become involved in any community activities? If no, how will you get involved?
2. Do you know how welfare in your state works? Have you ever been in a welfare office? Do you know where the Social Security Office is in your city? Have you ever visited the office?
3. Do you know the components of case management? What are the components? Have you ever worked with a case manager? How would you find out what the case manager would need to know to help you provide the best care for your

patients? How would you discover the culture of case managers?
4. Do you know the amount of money an average person receives as assistance in your state? Could you create a budget for a family of four receiving assistance in your state?
5. Do you know how your state is moving from welfare to workfare? How would you find out how this will affect your patients and community?

REFERENCES

1. Wood DL, Valdez RB, Hayashi T, Shen A. Health of homeless children and housed, poor children. Pediatrics 1990;86:858.
2. Andrulis DP. The Urban Health Penalty: New Dimensions and Directions in Inner-City Health Care. Philadelphia, PA: American College of Physicians, 1997.
3. Greenberg M. American cities: good and bad news about public health. Bull NY Acad Med 1991;67:17.
4. Abraham LK. Mama Might Be Better Off Dead: The Future of Health Care in Urban America. Chicago, IL: University of Chicago Press, 1993.
5. Lynch JW, Kaplan GA, Shema SJ. Cumulative impact of sustained economic hardship on physical, cognitive, psychological, and social functioning. N Engl J Med 1997;337:889.
6. National Center for Children in Poverty. One in Four: America's Youngest Poor. New York: Columbia School of Public Health, 1996. (Child Poverty News and Issues, Winter 1996, Vol 6, No 2; http://cpmcnet.columbia.edu/dept/nccp/publications/newsdex.html)
7. Zill N, Moore K, Smith E, Steif T, Coiro MJ. The Life Circumstances and Development of Children in Welfare Families: A Profile Based on National Survey Data. Washington, DC: Child Trends, 1991.
8. Duncan GJ, Brooks-Gunn J. Economic deprivation and early childhood development. In: Huston AC, Coll CTG, McLoyd VC (eds). Special Issue: Children in Poverty. Child Dev 1994;65:296.

RESOURCES

Books and Articles

Rogers DE, Ginzberg E. Medical Care and Health of the Poor. Boulder, CO: Westview Press, 1993. *This book brings together eight authors who have a unique understanding and expertise in health care: Victor Fuch (economics), Mary Charlson, Doug Black, Nicole Lurie, D. Arden Miller (medicine), Paul Starr (sociology), Margaret Hamburg, and Diane Rowland (public health). The authors voice their perspectives on health care for the poor. Physician assistants thinking about working in the inner city or already working with the urban poor will benefit from reading this book.*

Abraham LK. Mama Might Be Better Off Dead: The Future of Health Care in Urban America. Chicago, IL: University of

Chicago Press, 1993. *An excellent book that puts a face on a family caught in the welfare health care system. Abraham spent 3 years with a family in Chicago as they struggled through the system with and without success. This book illustrates in detail the obstacles faced by a poor family with chronic diseases in an acute care system.*

Andrulis DP. The Urban Health Penalty: New Dimensions and Directions in Inner-City Health Care. Philadelphia, PA: American College of Physicians, 1997. *This paper, commissioned by the American College of Physicians (ACP), details many of the issues impacting health care delivery in urban areas and goes beyond just numbers. (This paper is the foundation for the ACP's position paper published in the* Annals of Internal Medicine, *1997;126:485.) In the conclusion section of his paper, Andrulis states, "Ultimately, the residents of the inner cities, their health care providers and their governments must seek to correct the current inequities and misdirections inherent in the U.S. health care system."*

Lynch JW, Kaplan GA, Shema SJ. Cumulative impact of sustained economic hardship on physical, cognitive, psychological, and social functioning. N Engl J Med 1997;337:1889. *This 29-year epidemiological study from the University of Michigan shows that poverty and economic hardship can worsen your health. In this paper, poverty and economic hardship were likened to poison—the more "doses" encountered over time, the greater the odds of major mental and physical problems. All physician assistant students should read this paper, which will contribute to some very honest debate in the classroom.*

Web Sites

http://healthlinks.washington.edu/toolkits/shikany.html. *This is a great resource pointing to many sites, including the EthnoMed home page. The EthnoMed site contains information about cultural beliefs, medical issues, and other related issues pertinent to the health care of recent immigrants to Seattle, many of whom are refugees fleeing war-torn parts of the world.*

http://statlab.stat.yale.edu/cityroom/kidlink2/health/issues.html. *A site that provides state and national information related to children. Some of the items include economic security, child welfare and safety, health, and information about other web sites.*

CHAPTER 27

Rural Health Care

David Jones and Dennis M. Bruneau

INTRODUCTION

Two centuries ago, the U.S. population of 4 million people was almost totally rural. By 1929, the industrial and agricultural movements had forced 50% of the population out of rural locations and into cities. By 1984, there were more rural Americans than ever before, but they represented only 25% of the total U.S. population.[1]

Rural residents, as defined by the U.S. Census Bureau, are those persons who live in communities of fewer than 2500 or in open country. Rural is further divided into farm and nonfarm. The Census Bureau also defines *metropolitan* and *nonmetropolitan* counties. A *metropolitan* county must have an urban population center of 50,000 or more people; adjoining

counties are usually included in the metropolitan region according to specific criteria. Any county that does not meet these criteria is classified as *nonmetropolitan*. This classification is independent of the *rural/urban* distinction, with the result that an area may be classified as both *rural* and *metropolitan* in different tables compiled from the same data.[2] Using the same raw data from the 1990 census (some statistical details are not yet available from 2000), the *nonmetropolitan* population is approximately 20%, whereas the *rural* population is approximately 25% of the U.S. total.[2] This *nonmetropolitan* definition and the resulting percentage informs other government demographic statistics on what is usually referred to as the "rural" population.

The Rural Information Center Health Service has compiled several reports on what the "rural" *(non-metropolitan)* population looks like. The 1997 figures for unemployment were 5.2% in rural areas and 4.9% in urban areas. In 1996, the rural per capita income was $18,527 compared with the urban $25,944, and rural children lived in poverty at a rate of 24% as opposed to 22% for urban areas. In 1999, the overall poverty rates were 14.3% (rural) and 11.2% (urban). Elderly Americans made up a higher percentage of the rural population (18.4%) than the urban (15%) in 1998.[3]

Frontier counties, the majority of which are in the Western states, are described as counties with very low population densities of no more than six or seven people per square mile (compared with a national average of 73).[4] The *frontier* designation is used inconsistently by the agencies that track rural populations and health, but can be useful in describing the most sparsely-populated areas of the country. Residents of these areas must often drive long distances for education, health care, and even groceries.[4,5]

STATUS OF RURAL HEALTH CARE TODAY

The health care delivery system in rural America is trying to respond to many and varied problems. Although some of these also exist in urban underserved areas, many are unique to rural America. The rural health care system is often more loosely organized than its urban counterpart and much more thinly spread. Its component parts are similar, but many of the more familiar ones are missing or are present in only skeletal form. What appears in any given system varies with the degree of remoteness and the resources of the community. Mounting evidence of the relative decline in rural health care includes the closure and deteriorating financial condition of the local hospitals and, more importantly, the shortfalls of physicians, mid-level providers (physician assistants and nurse practitioners), nurses, and other health care personnel. Large metropolitan areas have an average of more than 300 physicians per 100,000 people, compared with just 110 physicians to serve the same number of people in nonmetropolitan areas. In the smaller, more remote rural counties (under 10,000 population), the physician ratio is even lower—80 per 100,000.[6]

Since the late 1980s, medical schools have increased their emphasis on family practice residency programs. In the mid-1990s, there was a significant increase in the number of training slots in family medicine residencies, and these slots were quickly filled. By 2000, however, medical students appeared to regain their interest in specialty practice. In 2001 and 2002, some family medicine residency positions remained unfilled at the end of the matching process. This declining interest in primary care reinforces the ongoing concern about shortages of physicians in rural communities. Although physician assistants (PAs) and nurse practitioners (NPs) are one component of the rural health solution, their effective utilization requires the availability of supportive and accessible physicians as preceptors and consultants. Government agencies at the federal level have developed programs to encourage improved health care access in rural and medically underserved areas. These initiatives, which include the Health Professional Shortage Area and Medically Underserved Area designations, are discussed later in this chapter.

PAs AND RURAL MEDICINE

Census data of the American Academy of Physician Assistants (AAPA) allow us to track PA involvement in rural health. In 2001, there were 52,716 individuals eligible to practice as physician assistants. The AAPA census notes that 48.5% are in primary care (as compared with 52.7% in 1997 and 37% in 1986). Currently, 22.7% of PAs describe themselves as working in rural settings. A total of 28.3% work in communities of fewer than 50,000 (33.6% in 1997 and 30.8% in 1981). About 12% work in communities of fewer than 10,000 (down from 15.4% in 1991), with 6.5% working in areas of fewer than 5000 people.[7]

The cause of these slightly declining numbers has yet to be studied. Possible variables may include the changing balance in PA classes to include a higher proportion of women, who tend to select rural practice at a lower rate than their male counterparts. Another potential factor is the move by some institutions toward more advanced academic degrees, which may also affect rural deployment. Recommendations at the conclusion of this chapter call for maintaining the primary care emphasis in PA programs, as well as continuing to offer clinical rotations in rural locations as a strategy for recruiting new PAs to rural communities. Retention of rural PAs also needs additional study.[8] Anecdotally, rural health experts report that PAs leave rural communities when faced with the absence of an effective rural health infrastructure, which most importantly includes supportive physicians. Expansion of the number of federally designated rural health clinics has resulted in a significant growth in rural PA jobs. Details on rural health clinics are included later in this chapter.

An encouraging trend in many states has been to liberalize the PA practice act as a strategy for promoting PA practice. Often these changes have been incremental in response to concerns on the part of regulatory boards that are charged with dealing with the health and safety of the public. In Oregon, for example, the 1995 legislative session saw the ratio of supervising physicians to PAs increase to 4:1, but only in rural underserved areas. In 1997 this increased ratio was extended to all areas of the state.

MANAGED CARE

A relatively new issue for rural providers is managed care. It has been much touted as a means to cut costs. It has done so for urban areas, although—some people feel—to the detriment of the poor and disadvantaged.

Managed care in rural areas has some promise for both good and bad. If a plan allows an open choice of providers in some areas as well as a restricted list in others, it may well succeed. One of the basic tenets for a successful managed care program is a large volume of patients.[9] This allows for the economies of scale and the ability to spread risk over large numbers. Rural areas often cannot provide sufficient volume for a stand-alone plan, although flexibility in some requirements such as productivity quotas can be used to compensate. Other plans may require enrollees to travel to a select group of providers, sometimes over long distances. This travel is often not feasible for patients who may belong to such a plan as part of their participation in the Medicaid or Medicare program. As a consequence, they may delay care until they are very sick, thereby increasing costs.

In a capitated system, the providers often bear part of the financial risk. When faced with increased costs

from this type of patient, they may drop out of the program, leaving an inadequate number of providers to care for the enrollees. Plans may also discover that expanding into rural areas is unprofitable because of low numbers. They may then exercise their option to drop coverage for a given area, again leaving clients without coverage. Individual providers often choose not to participate in a plan due to low reimbursement rates and other financial risks. If a plan has been used in an area long enough to cause other nonparticipating providers to leave the area because of financial pressures, an area may be left completely without care. In the authors' own area, a plan came in and then left within 90 days because the low numbers of patients were unprofitable. Fortunately for us and the population of this area, it was not there long enough to jeopardize our clinic.

CASE STUDY 27-1

Rural hospitals and clinics in Washington State have been engaged in an adversarial relationship with managed care plans that seek to "negotiate" for rates in rural settings based on the willingness of urban clinics to "discount" their services. The third-party payers thus seek to pay significantly lower fees to providers and clinics. In rural areas, costs are often higher, based on lower volumes, and rural providers and clinics feel that their fees are truly non-negotiable. Lower fees would essentially put them out of business.

In response to this non-negotiating stance, third party payers are threatening to deny approval of care given by these rural clinics and providers, and instead require that their consumers travel long distances (sometimes farther than 60 miles and often over road systems that are impassable in severe weather conditions) to receive care that would be reimbursed by their clinic. Such a decision also puts the rural clinics and providers at risk because it decreases their volumes and thus raises their costs.

CASE STUDY 27-2

Large health care systems continue to purchase rural clinics (many of which have been small private practices with one or two physicians and one or two PAs or NPs) as a strategy for building integrated delivery systems. Purchase of these clinics also guarantees referrals into these larger health care systems at their tertiary centers and therefore significantly expands their market share.

A consequence of these buyouts has been the firing of some physicians in these outlying clinics who are deemed to practice at less than productive levels. As a result, PAs and NPs who remain in these clinics have lost valuable colleagues with whom they have had long-standing relationships. These senior physicians have been replaced by younger, less experienced physicians who are willing to work for lower salaries and higher production requirements. The PAs and NPs are concerned that they have less backup and that they may be placed in situations in which their experience may exceed that of their supervising physicians. Some of the new physicians are concerned that they have not been "trained" in how to work with PAs and NPs, and thus complain that these responsibilities add increased pressure to their already strained work environment.

On a more positive note, because the Oregon Health Plan was designed to accommodate a mix of areas with choice of providers and other areas of restricted choice, the authors are now seeing patients in their community who are able to receive the care that they had desperately needed but could not afford.

Most managed care plans that service Medicaid patients contract with state governments. There must be safeguards built into any newly designed or changed system to ensure that patients in rural areas continue to have access to care. This may require creative contracts that include, if necessary, penalty clauses for early termination. States should also require contracting organizations to include PAs and NPs in their panel of providers, something that is not done by many of the current preferred provider organizations (PPOs) and independent practice associations (IPAs). This is especially important in rural areas where PAs and NPs provide a significant proportion of primary care and may be the only providers.

There is one other related issue that affects the delivery of good primary care. Many insurance companies and managed care organizations have restricted lists of participating or preferred pharmacies, including mail-order pharmacies. Patients choosing to get their prescriptions from their local pharmacies often have to pay a significantly larger portion of their pharmacy bills. This makes it very difficult for small rural pharmacies to survive and increases the likelihood that rural patients will have to travel long distances to get urgent or emergent medications.

In our own case, the local pharmacy no longer fills any Medicaid prescriptions except those for the local assisted living facility, thereby requiring our patients to travel 70 miles to get their prescriptions filled. Medicaid patients whom we have seen after-hours must either pay cash for the after-hours medications we keep in stock or go without until they can arrange to get to another pharmacy. It is difficult to fault the pharmacies when the state Medicaid program currently reimburses them at average wholesale price minus 20%. Given the economic downturn in our state and the resultant state budget shortfall, they are proposing even lower rates of reimbursement. This translates into a worsening access problem for patients in the lower economic portion of our society.

FEDERAL AND STATE INITIATIVES
Background

There has always been a general lack of access to health care services in rural and frontier communities. Large-scale federal initiatives to deal with the problem were begun in the early 1960s, consisting of provisions for medical research, construction of health centers, and money for medical education.[1] The Rural Health Initiative followed. Its goal was to consolidate fragmented federal rural health programs, thereby avoiding duplication of services and programs and, it was hoped, making the system more efficient. Specific federal initiatives have focused on the following:

1. Personnel (the National Health Service Corps).
2. Reduction of inequities (the creation of designations for Health Professional Shortage Areas and Medically Underserved Areas).
3. Support for the actual delivery system (Rural Health Clinics and Community and Migrant Health Centers).

4. Development of infrastructure to support the rural health care delivery system (Area Health Education Centers, State Offices of Rural Health, and State Primary Care Associations).

Personnel   Multiple factors have contributed to the shortage or maldistribution of providers in rural America. These factors include the professional isolation of rural providers, cultural isolation for themselves and their families, lower salaries than those of their urban counterparts, and tenuous long-term financial viability of the practice due to low patient populations.[10] Providers at the beginning of their careers are particularly concerned about their inability to utilize the wide range of skills learned in urban training centers, and also the lack of many of the high-technology procedures physicians have come to depend on in their training.

The National Health Service Corps (NHSC), established in 1970, was designed to provide health personnel to the areas of greatest need. Initially the NHSC was a program that linked scholarships with service obligations for "payback" in medically underserved communities. Although it was initially successful in placing new physicians—and later PAs, NPs, and certified nurse midwives (CNMs)—in needy clinics, the program was criticized when many providers moved on after their time was up. Lack of retention and the resulting disruption in continuity of care became a critical issue in continued funding for the corps.

In response, the NHSC expanded its scope to include loan repayment as well as scholarship opportunities. This combination has given the NHSC more flexibility in responding to the needs of specific communities and individual providers. Over time, the NHSC has expanded the number of slots available to both PAs and NPs, and has also periodically supported the training of dentists and mental health providers. Since its beginning, over 22,000 individuals have provided service as members of the National Health Service Corps. Currently, more than 2300 NHSC clinicians are serving 3.6 million people in America's rural and urban underserved communities.[11]

Parallel to the development of the NHSC, the federal government began investing directly in the training of primary care providers, including family medicine residencies and physician assistant and nurse practitioner educational training programs. Funding formulas for these programs provided incentives for the development and support of rural training opportunities. Many PA programs specifically received support for the recruitment of individuals from rural communities to be trained for rural practice. In the 2002 grant cycle, PA programs with strong track records of graduate placement in rural and medically underserved areas receive additional funding points in the grant review process.

Reduction of Inequity Through "Designations"

Originally created in 1965 (through Public Law 89-290), the first shortage area designations were initially utilized as a tool to implement health professional loan repayment programs.[12] Today's designations—Health Professional Shortage Areas (HPSAs), Medically Underserved Areas (MUAs), and Medically Underserved Populations (MUPs)—are used to direct scarce public moneys to areas of greatest need.

HPSAs are rural or urban and take into account a number of issues, including access barriers—such as language difference—that prevent a specific population group from using the area's existing providers, the percentage of the population with incomes below the poverty level, and those eligible for Medicaid. The most critical component of the designation is the ratio of the number of people in the population group to the number of primary care physicians serving the group. Interestingly, physician assistants and nurse practitioners are not currently included in the formula that determines eligibility for this designation. In addition to HPSA designations for primary care providers, there are specific HPSA designations for dental and mental health services.

MUAs were originally used to determine the basis of need for the development of community health centers.[13] State agencies apply to the federal office of Shortage Designations and provide the following data:

1. Infant mortality rate.
2. Proportion of the population over 65.
3. Proportion of the population with incomes below the poverty level.
4. Ratio of population to primary care providers.

Based on the concern that these federal designations were not always sensitive enough for state-level concerns, Public Law 99-280 enabled state governors to further designate state-specific MUPs in areas of unique need. State criteria are generally seen as more lenient and more responsive to local needs.[12]

Although all three types of designation have been helpful in bringing more resources to rural America, they have also generated significant controversy. Some of the dissatisfaction has been with specific formulas—and cut-off points—in use at any given time. There has been a more general dissatisfaction with the cumbersome process involved in achieving these designations.

The sad fact is that none of these designations gives a clear picture of the level of the "underservedness" that exists in this country. The granting of each of these designations involves a fairly high level of sophistication, the prior existence of an administrative infrastructure, and the availability of complex data sets. Thus, some of our most underserved areas have difficulty in meeting the administrative criteria for these designations even though they are clearly "eligible."

Rural Health Clinics and Community Health Centers

Another attempt to meet rural health needs was the passage in 1977 of PL 95-210, the Rural Health Clinics Act. This act provides for the cost-based reimbursement of services to Medicare patients by mid-level providers who practice in communities that are both "rural" and "underserved." See Figure 27-1 for an overview of Rural Health Clinic (RHC) requirements.

Initially, the RHC qualification process under PL 95-210 was onerous and excessively cumbersome. Congress had expected several thousand clinics to apply, but by 1990, there were only about 600. In the late 1980s and early 1990s, Congress reviewed the program to see why there were so many fewer clinics than expected. This resulted in a number of changes that improved the certification process, so that by 1997, more than 3000 clinics were certified. The creation of the National Association of Rural Health Clinics has resulted in the availability of valuable technical assistance and networking support among clinics and clinicians.[14] This association has also been very effective in promoting rural health clinics at the state and community levels.

Reimbursement for RHCs is determined by the federal government's Centers for Medicare and Medicaid Services (CMS), which reviews submitted cost reports annually to adjust the reimbursement rates as needed. These rates were established with a cap (currently approximately $65 per visit). PL 95-210 makes it feasible for mid-level providers to staff a facility by assuring a guaranteed level of reimbursement. This is particularly critical in clinics with a high percentage of Medicare and Medicaid patients.

Medicaid cost-based reimbursement is not without controversy and is currently under fire as states are granted waivers by the federal government to try new and innovative strategies to serve this population. One example is the Oregon Health Plan, in which diagnoses were ranked as to their threat to life or potential for creating permanent sequelae. A line was then drawn through the list (corresponding to the amount of money available). Diagnoses above the line are covered, and those below are not. Oregon tried to eliminate the cost-based reimbursement to RHCs under this plan, but strong efforts of the Oregon Rural Health Association and Oregon Primary Care Association prevented this. If states succeed in eliminating the cost-based reimbursement for RHCs, it will make it much more difficult for them to survive financially.

Another clinical service strategy for improving access to rural health care has been the development and expansion of federally funded clinics such as Community Health Centers and Migrant Health Centers. Administered through the federal government's Bureau of Primary Health Care, these clinics have been identified for a threefold expansion by the Bush administration as a strategy for improving health care access to the underserved.[15] An estimated 10% of the U.S. uninsured population receive care in the community health center system. Community Health Centers have proved to be satisfying employment settings for both physician assistants and nurse practitioners. Many PA programs have strong links with community health centers where strong and effective PA role models have served as excellent preceptors (and potential recruiters) for PA students.

Purpose: To encourage and stabilize the provision of out-patient primary care in underserved areas through the use of physicians, physician assistants, and nurse practitioners. Requirements for designation include the following elements.

- Location: Rural health clinics must be located in communities that are both "rural" and "underserved"

- Staffing:
  - One or more physicians
  - One or more PAs, NPs, or CNMs
  - PA, NP, or CNM must be on site and available to see patients 50% of the time the clinic is open for patient care

- Clinic must be able to deliver direct out-patient primary care services (including basic laboratory tests)
  Clinics must be able to provide first response to common life-threatening injuries and acute illnesses

- Clinics must have links to provide for:
  - Inpatient hospital care
  - Specialized physician services
  - Specialized diagnostic and laboratory services
  - Interpreters and assistive communication devices

- Administrative infrastructure including:
  - Written patient care policies
  - Guidelines for medical management
  - Medical Record System with written policies and procedures, a designated responsible individual, and
  - policies on confidentiality and the release of information

Figure 27-1 Rural Health Clinics Act—PL 95-210. Modified from the National Association of Rural Health Clinics web site.[14]

Infrastructure   Federal support has also created several new categories of organizations at the state level, which have been designed to increase and support health care access. These include Area Health Education Centers (AHECs), Primary Care Associations, and State Offices of Rural Health.

In their start-up phase, AHECs must be housed primarily in medical schools. Over time—and with diminishing federal funding—the expectation is that the AHEC would gain state legislative support. The AHEC's goals are further delineated in the box on p. 555.

Primary Care Associations are networks of community health centers that provide support (e.g., training, continuing medical education, provider recruitment) and technical assistance to strengthen community health centers at the state level. Similarly, state Offices of Rural Health promote rural health at the state level.

AREA HEALTH EDUCATION CENTER FUNCTIONS

- Form links between health care delivery systems and educational resources in underserved communities.
- Create collaborative, community-based education and training opportunities for health professionals, students, and primary care resident physicians.
- Increase the number of individuals from minority and underserved communities who enter health careers.
- Create systems for learning and networks for information dissemination.
- Support multidisciplinary and interdisciplinary training in response to community needs.
- Promote health, prevent disease, and provide cost-efficient primary health care services.
- Respond to emerging needs and priorities.
- Provide technical assistance to educators and others.

Modified from AHEC web site.[16]

Typically, offices of rural health have worked to create links between providers and educational institutions, to promote recruitment and retention activities for rural providers, and to serve as a liaison between the state government and federal agencies.

State Initiatives Despite federal policies and initiatives, there is a general understanding that many solutions to rural health issues should be managed at the state or community level. This attitude reflects the rural population's general distrust of "big government."

One example of a state initiative for rural health improvement is Oregon's state income tax credit of up to $5000 for qualified rural health care providers and matching funding for AHECs. Oregon also has a state-funded loan repayment program that can retire a significant portion of the educational debt incurred for qualified physicians, PAs, and NPs. Eligible practitioners can get up to $25,000 in debt forgiveness per year of service in an underserved area for up to 4 years. Other states are considering similar legislative relief.

RURAL AND FRONTIER HOSPITALS

With many economic, demographic, geographic, and health policy stresses on the rural health delivery system, most rural communities are experiencing great difficulty maintaining local health services. During the past two decades, while urban and suburban medical systems have been responding to the changes of managed care, specialty care, and centralized

medicine, rural health systems have remained in turmoil with few alternatives. The most profound change in the rural medical landscape is the looming extinction of the rural and frontier hospital.

It is well known that one component of the problem rural Americans encounter is the shortage of health care providers. The other is the vanishing rural hospital. They are dependent on each other to be a viable presence in rural settings. According to the Office of the Inspector General, there were 2489 rural hospitals in 1987. By 2001, the number had declined to 2000, a 20% decrease. The rate of closure has slowed during the past recent years, although smaller hospitals often operate at a loss and must rely on Medicare payments for their survival.[17,18] Such hospitals function under the shadow of possible closure.

The closing of a rural hospital has a much greater impact on the rural community than the closing of a hospital in urban and suburban communities. It is almost certain that a rural hospital closure will leave its residents with no other choice but to travel long distances to the nearest care. When a rural hospital closes, it weakens the local economy, social well-being and vitality, and political strength of the population it has served.

The Limited-Service Rural Hospital

The Medical Assistant Facility (MAF) in Montana was the first nationally demonstrated program of the limited-service hospital concept. The MAF concept was particularly well suited to Montana, given its relative size (the fourth largest state) and its sparse and aging population. Of Montana's 56 counties, 44 are considered frontier. Since 1980, the frontier counties of Montana have lost significant numbers of the younger population to the lure of urban attractions. As a result, this not only has reduced the total population but has increased the median age. In addition, Montana residents have to contend not only with the state's size but also with the most severe weather conditions in a winter that may last as long as 6 months of the year.

Relying almost exclusively on physician assistants and nurse practitioners for coverage, the MAF model incorporated the following features:

➤ MAF facilities were limited to a 96-hour admission. Longer stays required discharging patients or transferring them to a full-service hospital.

➤ MAFs had to be located in a county with fewer than six residents per square mile, or the MAF could be located more than 35 miles from the nearest hospital.

➤ MAFs had to provide emergency services and basic laboratory services. More complex diagnostic services could be available by contract.

➤ There had to be a provider on-call at all times who was able to respond within 1 hour to the MAF site.

➤ All MAFs were required to have formal agreements with hospitals, skilled nursing facilities, and home health agencies for services the MAF could not provide.[19,20]

➤ Where there was a physician assistant or nurse practitioner working as the sole provider at an MAF hospital, the rules required that a physician must review all admissions by telecommunication within 24 hours of admission and visit the facility every 30 days.[19]

The MAF concept depended on the full utilization of a variety of community resources. Typically the support staff and area nursing personnel from nursing homes, assisted living, and home health agencies shared duties serving an MAF unit when there was an admission. In at least one Montana county, the MAF, nursing home, home health, dental, mental health, substance abuse counseling, family planning, WIC program, and outpatient clinical services were grouped under one administration and one budget. Incorporating services and sharing support staff affords fuller employment opportunities and is cost-efficient. The flexibility of multidisciplined employee staffing and of their working hours helped to reduce overhead. In some counties, the MAF project became a key employer for rural residents, helping the local economy significantly.

After Montana created laws for the MAF concept in 1987, it was then presented to the Health Care Financing Administration (HCFA) to demonstrate the efficacy of the MAF model. Finding the MAF model promising, HCFA funded a multilayered demonstration project. The project was dependent on the issuance of a Medicare waiver by HCFA. The waiver conditions were these:

1. To accept the MAF licensure rules in lieu of the Medicare Hospital Conditions of Participation.
2. To waive those conditions not applicable to the MAF program.
3. To reimburse Medicare services on the basis of reasonable cost.
4. To allow the state's peer review organization to provide utilization review services for all patients.

The objectives of the MAF project were as follows:

➤ To demonstrate that as a result of the MAF option, frontier communities in Montana could prevent the permanent loss of institutional health care services that would ordinarily result from hospital closure.

➤ To demonstrate that Medicare and Medicaid program patients in Montana's frontier areas would accept the MAF as a satisfactory alternative to the traditional full-service hospital.

➤ To demonstrate that the MAF could provide low-intensity health care services equal in quality to those provided by full-service hospitals located in other frontier areas.

➤ To demonstrate that the MAF model had the potential for implementation in frontier areas elsewhere in the United States.

The MAF demonstration project ultimately required congressional authorization, and in December of 1990, a Medicare waiver was granted. Several days later, the first MAF site received licensure.[21]

In the ensuing 10 years, the MAF project was instrumental in creating new models of health care delivery in rural hospitals. Proponents of the MAF model pointed out that the rules imposed less service restriction and focused on saving a small hospital without the complex formal networking and restructuring of local health systems that were required by some other models.

EACH/RPCH

Begun in seven states by congressional authority, the Essential Access Community Hospital/Rural Primary Care Hospital (EACH/RPCH) program was a second model to allow rural and frontier communities to have a limited-service hospital. The program also relied on the use of physician assistants and nurse practitioners in the models. A key feature of the program was the provision of a higher cost-based Medicare reimbursement rate for the RPCH facilities, and recognition of the larger EACH hospitals as sole community providers, thus raising their Medicare reimbursement rates. Sole community provider rates are based more on historical costs than is normally allowed under Medicare's prospective payment system.[22]

The program was started in early 1990 in California, Colorado, Kansas, New York, North Carolina, South Dakota, and West Virginia. Much like the MAF model, the duration of admission was held to an average of 72 hours for all admissions on an annual basis. As the EACH/RPCH program demonstrated early success in helping rural communities build local networks of providers beyond the hospital-to-hospital link, researchers found that networking had generally been challenging for rural facilities. Some of the factors making it difficult to create a viable network include local politics, changes in personnel, variable interest at the larger referral hospital, community concerns related to historical rivalries or control, and a situation wherein the designated referral facility was not historically the facility with a previous strong relationship with the community.[22,23]

Critical Access Hospitals

In October of 1999, all MAF and EACH/RPCH programs were grandfathered to the federally designated Critical Access Hospital (CAH). There are a total of 600 active Critical Access Hospitals in 47 states overseen by the Federal Office of Rural Health Policy.

There is some concern that the CAH program may not be appropriate for very small and frontier communities. Mr. Kip Smith, the current director of the Montana CAH program, noted that there are currently 24 CAH facilities in Montana, and all are serving their rural and frontier communities under the new policies.[24] Under the federal policy, all CAHs must have a practitioner on-site 24 hours every day. Many of the much smaller frontier communities with limited financial and manpower capability have a difficult time meeting the 24/7 policy. The financial demands could force frontier CAHs to close down over time.

The MAF program allowed the use of nurse triage as a first line of health advice and care,[24,25] a system no longer accepted under CAH. This issue is one example of the generalized approach by well-meaning federal policymakers who are not cognizant of the differences between rural and frontier communities. In the East, many federally designated rural communities have large percentages of low-income citizens. In the West, frontier towns are poor and are also geographically isolated from emergency medicine and hospital services. For residents of Jordan, Montana, for example, the nearest medical facility beyond its CAH is in Miles City—85 miles away.[25] One can imagine the experience of having to drive 85 miles in one of Montana's frequent winter blizzards. Many counties in Montana are larger in area than some eastern states. Perhaps with a process of education and awareness, policies can be modified to meet needs based on economic and geographic barriers.

The authors have experienced, when discussing frontier medicine with federal policymakers or legislators, that a useful description includes the fact that the nearest McDonald's and Subway are 70 miles from Condon, Oregon. We also remark that the most influential people in frontier regions are the UPS and Federal Express agents. Frontier towns have unique isolation problems that should be addressed effectively when it comes to federal and state health policymaking. A flexible policy would help financially weak and isolated communities to have some health care rather than none at all.

Others might argue that quality of care and legal issues arise when dual policies are authorized. Those concerned policymakers have an obligation to assure that the standards of the medical community are being fulfilled. Western folk living on the edge of nowhere feel that they have a right to set their standards accordingly, and they do accept the fact of not living near a full-service hospital. Something is better than nothing. It is part of what a Western culture and a pioneering nature have been since the days of homesteading.

The hope is that frontier medicine can be seen as a unique issue, and that solutions can be designed to provide access to quality care by reasonable and prudent collaboration.

RURAL PRIMARY CARE WITHOUT PHYSICIANS: TWO DECADES OF SUCCESS

High on an expansive treeless plateau in eastern Oregon, a rancher and his wife live 8 miles away from a town of fewer than 750 people. On a cold and windy day, the rancher was stricken with palpitations, severe shortness of breath, and weakness. His wife rushed him to the local clinic, where a diagnosis of supraventricular tachycardia was made. He was given medication to successfully abort the dysrhythmia, was observed, and was transported via ambulance to the nearest full-service hospital 70 miles away. He most likely would not have survived had the community still been without their successful clinic, staffed by two PAs. Prior to the arrival of the PAs in late 1980, this rancher would simply have been loaded into the ambulance, provided with basic life support, and transported the full 70 miles before receiving any definitive care.

The town of Condon, Oregon (population 800), had experienced the periodic loss of health care since 1968, when the last regular physician left town. The situation was partially alleviated in 1972, when an NHSC physician came to town for 2 years. He was followed by an NP, also employed by the NHSC. After a year, the NP resigned from the NHSC in favor of private practice. A combination of unfavorable state regulations, particularly with regard to prescriptive privileges, and local political problems forced him to quit in 1978. When he left, he recommended

that the people of Condon form a special taxing district (a health district) to support the clinic and isolate the provider from political pressures.

The residents were determined to have local health care available (it is a 70-mile drive to the nearest full-service hospital and a full range of specialists). They also wanted care to be available on a 24-hour basis. Realizing that the local patient base of 1200 did not permit a freestanding clinic, they determined to form a health district as recommended. (Oregon is one of five states that permit this, the others being Illinois, Arizona, Utah, and Washington.[26]) Working with the Oregon Office of Rural Health (established by the legislature in 1979), they determined that their needs would best be served by hiring *two* mid-level practitioners. This arrangement would enable round-the-clock care, yet help insulate against provider burnout by limiting call duty to every other night and every other weekend instead of all the time.

Two PAs (the authors of this discussion) started in November 1980 and are still practicing in the town. In the first few years of the practice, the tax subsidy constituted nearly 50% of the budget. It currently is 30% to 35%, with the rest being generated from patient revenues, including Medicare and Medicaid. As an incentive to both providers and taxpayers, any excess income at the end of each year is divided between the providers and the health district as a return on subsidy. This promotes good will and encourages local patients to use the facility. It does require reminding the population that they still need to pay for services in order to keep the tax subsidy at a manageable level. Another long-term funding strategy developed in Condon was the establishment of a foundation. Its goal is to build the principal to an amount whose annual interest earned would be enough to offset the yearly tax subsidy, thus reducing and conceivably eliminating the subsidy at some point in the future.

Although the patient census in Condon did not justify two providers, the on-call schedule did. It encouraged the providers to stay for a longer time. If a facility has a high turnover of providers, patients are reluctant to patronize it because they have no continuity of care. They would rather suffer the inconvenience of travel to another community if they believe they can start and remain with one provider.

In many respects, places like Condon are the reason PAs were developed. The practice situation often does not warrant the presence of a physician. In fact, the placing of a physician in such sites is not cost effective. PAs in sites such as Condon and the MAF and CAH models utilize the full range of their skills, from preventive medicine and family practice to emergency cardiac and trauma care. One of the basic tenets of the PA profession, which has led to their wide acceptance by both patients and the public at large, is the fact that PAs increase access to health care in areas where it has been at a premium.[27]

REQUISITES FOR A RURAL PA

Attributes needed for practicing in a rural setting include more than just the obvious medical skills. Although few if any health professional training programs include business classes, it is vital that someone in a rural practice have good business skills. In addition, rural providers need time management skills to help avoid some of the common family stresses. They also need to have a thorough knowledge of their own skills and limitations and enough self-confidence to function comfortably within these confines.

Business Management

Most rural practices operate on the edges of profitability. The more remote the practice site, the more this tenuousness is a reality of everyday life. Good business management skills can turn a marginal practice into a profitable and sustainable one, as long as there are no adverse outside forces, such as a large decrease in the patient base. The abilities to build a budget and operate within it, to manage accounts receivable and avoid a large burden of uncollectable debt, and to arrange timely purchase of necessary supplies (having enough on hand to allow proper functioning, but avoiding tying up a large amount of capital in unnecessary inventory) all contribute to a successful practice.

Health care practices are more commonly turning to computers to help manage the business side of the operation. There are reasonably priced medical software programs (MediSoft is one example) that do all

the necessary accounting, including printing the bills and aging the account balances (to avoid carrying bad accounts too long), and that can also generate a variety of reports. One can summarize patient visits by provider, insurance coverage, diagnoses, and demographics. These data are often quite useful for making various state and federal reports (including the Medicare cost reports required under PL 95-210, the Rural Health Clinic Act), as well as for applying for grants to fund specific programs or equipment purchases. The provider profiles are statistical summaries that reveal the mix of charges a given provider generates (office services based on the time spent and complexity of the management decisions required) and compare them with what would be expected for a given patient mix. Several studies show that all medical providers, but especially rural providers, routinely undervalue the time they spend with patients. They consistently select a lower-value charge than they should, thus shortchanging themselves and their practices. Use of provider profiles can help monitor charges and ensure that revenues generated are commensurate with the care provided.

Medicare and Medicaid reimbursement gives a large boost to the financial stability of rural clinics; however, reimbursement from other insurance companies and third-party payers can also have a substantial impact. If the policies of the major insurance carriers in a state or an area do not allow for reimbursement for PA services, it can be very difficult for a clinic to survive. Many clinics therefore bill for PA services under the name of the physician. This practice, however, simply disguises the amount of service that is provided by PAs and delays appropriate recognition of it. Without such recognition, it is hard to generate enough pressure at either the corporate or the state regulatory level to foster any changes in policy. Clinics must ascertain the policies of the insurance companies active in their areas and work to change those that are unfavorable. For instance, Blue Cross of Oregon reimburses the PAs in Condon, but the Blue Cross policies held by federal workers do not because they are federal policies and are not state regulated. We would encourage all PAs to bill under their own names and to work with their clinic business managers to identify and work with companies that resist PA reimbursement.

Clinics must maintain an accurate and up-to-date listing of supplies and their costs. It is then incumbent upon all staff, especially providers, to keep a detailed count of supplies used for any given patient so that they may be charged out accordingly. The exception to this is for procedures (such as laceration repair or lesion removal) for which there is a set charge regardless of code. Although this approach may seem overly detailed, costs for supplies add up rapidly if not controlled. In a practice in which the financial margins are cut very fine, such details can mean the difference between survival and closure. Because of the multiple costs involved in maintaining a workable inventory of supplies, it is necessary to charge them out at a rate that is higher than the acquisition cost. In most cases, using the base price plus 75% to 100% of this value determines the patient cost fairly. Although it is still important to track supplies used and to bill them accordingly, this is gradually becoming less meaningful because various third-party payers disallow the charges; they are considered to be part of the overall bundled service for the procedure done. For instance, we can no longer charge out for the sterile suture packs used for laceration repairs.

Self-Knowledge and Self-Confidence

PAs in rural settings learn quickly that they must know themselves and their skills thoroughly. It does not take long to find out where one is lacking. Sometimes such concerns can be easily addressed; at other times one merely needs to acknowledge limits and stay within them. If training has exposed one to many of the highly technological aspects of medicine, one must learn to do without most of them. Providers need to learn their skills in history taking and physical examination because these will often lead to the diagnosis, which will then be confirmed by the limited laboratory evaluations available locally.

In addition, all providers are finding that laboratory evaluations are more limited than they have been due to a federal law, the Clinical Laboratory Improvement Act of 1988 (CLIA). Under this act, laboratory techniques were divided into waived, moderate complexity, high complexity, and physician provider microscopy (PPM), which includes urine sediments, KOH, and saline preparations. After lobbying by the AAPA and others, the PPM was modified to include PAs and NPs among the providers who could perform the designated tests. For the waived and PPM categories, a facility must have a license as a laboratory, but no proficiency testing is required. The classification depends on the perceived immediate impact on patients and their care. The more likely a test is to have an immediate life-threatening impact on a patient, the higher in complexity it is judged to be. The more tests a facility offers, the more expensive the certification and quality assurance (QA) process becomes. It often becomes a choice between abandoning a test procedure and investing several thousand dollars for a new machine, followed by several hundred dollars a year to maintain required QA controls.

Some of the CLIA categorizations of tests are unarguable, but others seem haphazard. A urine pregnancy test with built-in controls falls into the waived category, but a strep screening test, also with built-in controls, is considered moderate complexity. Some strep screening tests are in the waived category, whereas others by different manufacturers are in the moderate complexity category, even though both have built-in controls. As providers find fewer tests available on-site, management decisions have to be made before test results can be obtained on specimens that must be mailed away for analysis.

Time Management

PAs in rural settings, similar to those everywhere, have to learn to pace themselves, not only with the daily patient schedule but also with on-call time, vacations, and continuing medical education (CME) conferences. One of the biggest problems facing rural providers is how to arrange for coverage while they are away. It is often difficult and expensive to bring someone in to cover for even a few days. The chance to take some relaxation time is critical to avoiding burnout. The ability to get away for CME helps the PA to upgrade knowledge and allows some interaction with peers to relieve the professional isolation that rural providers often feel.

Computer Skills

As has been noted, one of the problems facing rural practitioners is the difficulty in arranging coverage while one is absent to attend CME meetings. Others are the availability of up-to-date reference materials to research new treatments and side effects and the ability to communicate with peers for suggestions about a particular patient. Most, if not all, PA education programs use computers extensively throughout the clinical portions of their training. This experience stands the students in very good stead should they choose to practice in a rural or frontier setting. The Internet has a vast array of medical sites that include full-text journal articles and information on poison control and complementary medicine, as well as sites that deal with both the clinical and professional sides of being a PA. Several journals also have an on-line option to earn CME credits. It is now possible (and, in fact, will soon be required by the National Commission on Certification of Physician Assistants [NCCPA]) to log one's CME on-line. Several universities now offer advanced degrees on-line, most of which are at the master's level. Access to on-line resources is available to almost any location through a variety of set-up options, including the local cable TV company, the local phone company via various Internet service providers, or satellite Internet services. A small dish can be set up that provides data transfer speeds faster than those offered by cable modems or DSL connections. The downside to these faster services is that the costs involved usually escalate in direct proportion to the speed of the connection. These costs do tend to be higher in rural areas to the point where satellite services become the most viable option at a cost of around $80 per month (in the local Oregon market as of 2002).

Medical Skills

The medical skills that the rural PA must have are built on the basic primary care skills taught in all training programs. Some become rusty with disuse, and others are sharpened considerably. Some skills that are not taught by many PA programs, and that may be new to the provider but may also be essential patient care skills in a rural environment, include the ability to take limited x-rays (chest, extremities, and flat plate and upright abdomen for free air) and to perform basic laboratory tests and electrocardiograms (ECGs). If these are done, an excellent (and to our

minds almost mandatory) risk-reduction strategy is to have the x-rays and ECGs reviewed by an appropriate specialist.

In many areas, surgical skills other than those needed for repair of lacerations or removal of small lesions may lie dormant. Inpatient skills may become less useful as one locates in a progressively more rural area. In many rural areas, no hospitals are available. In those areas that do have hospitals, a provider's obstetrical and surgical skills may be unused simply because small rural hospitals cannot afford to make such services available, owing to either high insurance costs or the prohibitive costs of maintaining fully staffed and equipped surgical suites. Many rural PAs who currently have hospital privileges may lose them in the future, not through any fault of their own or pressure from other providers, but simply because the economics of rural areas will force many more rural hospitals to close their doors.

Emergency Skills

Specific medical skills will also include those involving trauma and cardiac emergency care. Attaining and maintaining Advanced Cardiac Life Support (ACLS) certification may well be essential, both for the provision of quality patient care and the comfort of the provider. Similarly, an Advanced Trauma Life Support (ATLS) course may prove beneficial.

PAs in rural areas will find it critical that they work closely with the local emergency medical service (EMS) system and emergency medical technicians (EMTs). This will help ensure that the preferred protocols of the supervising physician, the PA, and the receiving hospital are clearly understood and followed by all concerned. The PA must be involved in the training and continuing education of local EMTs. This gives the PA intimate knowledge of the capabilities and limitations of the personnel available and helps to build trust between the PA and the EMTs.

For those familiar with trauma treatment in urban areas, the care available in rural areas may sometimes seem primitive by comparison. The "golden hour of trauma" in a rural area may be the time needed for emergency personnel to arrive at the accident scene and start rendering care. Although EMS philosophy in urban areas has shifted from "scoop and run" to stabilization in the streets and then back to "scoop and run to the nearest trauma center," rural areas have continued with stabilization at the location. For the severely injured patient, the primary job for the EMTs and PAs may be stabilization and packaging for transport. In recognition of the need for emergency care, many states including Oregon have developed levels of EMT education and certification that allow the use of automatic or semiautomatic external defibrillators down to the basic or first-responder levels. The use of some emergent cardiac medications is also allowed at the EMT-intermediate level. This allows for needed definitive care during the sometimes lengthy transport times.

The method of transportation may vary with the type of injury or problem found. When a ground ambulance would take 2.5 hours to reach the nearest neurosurgeon, helicopter ambulance transport may become the vehicle of choice. Transport times may vary with the time of year. What may take a little more than an hour in the spring or summer may take 2 hours or longer in the winter. If a patient has an acute medical problem such as an unstable acute myocardial infarction, the PA may have to travel in the ambulance. This requires either another PA for coverage in town or an understanding by the community that there may be periods when no care is available because the PA has gone with the ambulance.

With acute illnesses, PAs in rural areas may find themselves providing treatments that would push the envelope in an urban setting. For example, under classic protocols, a febrile patient with acute pyelonephritis may well be hospitalized. In rural areas, this same patient may be treated aggressively with fluids and antibiotics and then watched for 24 hours to check for improvement or the need for inpatient therapy. This decision may be made electively, or it may be forced on the provider by adverse weather conditions. Another example is peritonsillar abscess, which may be an automatic ear, nose, and throat (ENT) referral in the city but might be handled by a rural PA through consultation and then aspiration, with appropriate follow-up care.

How much is handled in the manner just described depends on the relationships the PA develops with the supervising physician and consultants. As these relationships progress, the amount of care entrusted to the PA may increase or decrease according to past experiences. Each PA must remain individually comfortable, however, with what he or she is asked to do by supervisors and consultants.

CHALLENGES AND REWARDS OF RURAL PRACTICE

Many rural providers find that the salaries available to them do not approach those of their urban counterparts. Rural areas need health care but often do not have the resources to meet the salary and benefit packages offered in larger centers. The PA then needs to look for other factors that can compensate for this loss. These may include a safer environment in which to raise a family, often a more relaxed lifestyle (except for on-call time), and accessibility to superb recreational facilities. It is critical that a PA contemplating a rural position find some way to experience the realities of a rural existence *with the family,* so that everyone in the family understands what is and is not available. If, for example, easy access to live theater is important to a PA or spouse, they will probably not survive in a rural area unless they can make do with local school or community productions, in which they also may have to participate to fill out a cast.

Some of the professional rewards that one finds in a rural setting include the ability to use most, if not all, of one's training. The most common exceptions to this are obstetrical and surgical skills. Rural PAs usually have a much greater degree of independence (often regulatory as well as actual) than they would have in an urban setting, although this can be a two-edged sword because of the temptation to overstep limits. In rural practice, one can take pleasure in the fact that one can have a tremendous impact on the well-being of patients and can be involved in all aspects of their lives, from taking care of a newborn and reinforcing parenting skills to helping ease the pain of an elderly patient who is dying. Every community has an honest appreciation of its provider's skills. Rural PAs also find that they truly are meeting a need, one that might well go unmet if they were not present. Medical needs in underserved rural and inner city areas are what PAs were originally created to meet. The PA profession has consistently shown that it can do an excellent job of meeting them.

MEDICAL PRACTICE ACTS FOR PA UTILIZATION

There is no question that well-qualified PAs should be allowed to provide direct medical care as well as to prescribe and, in many cases, administer and dispense medications. This privilege, however, must always come under the supervision of an approved supervising physician. Most importantly, all utilization laws controlling PAs must observe the highest standards for public safety and the principles of correct patient care.

In the rural setting, PAs should be allowed greater flexibility to accomplish the multidisciplinary problems they will encounter when a physician is not immediately or remotely available. The law should be designed to enhance physician supervision without impeding PA practice in remote locations. State laws and agencies should not dissuade cross-training or the performance of accessory procedures such as taking radiographs and performing certain basic laboratory tests. Medical practice acts should also include provisions for locum tenens, language to promote reimbursement for services rendered by a PA, a system to provide peer review, networking among several providers, and a database information service for rural providers.

It is imperative that any regulating committee or board have significant PA representation, including an active rural PA practitioner, to ensure comprehensive policies. We recommend that rural PAs get involved at the regulatory level because all too often participation by urban counterparts is easier, more widespread, and more influential when laws and policies are created "for the good of all." Oregon and Washington are two examples of states in which active involvement by the PA community in the regulatory process has enhanced PA practice significantly over the past 5 to 10 years.

FUTURE DIRECTIONS AND RECOMMENDATIONS

The future of PAs in rural medicine is effectively as open as the profession wishes to make it. The trend in PA practice seems to be toward specialization. The more specialized PAs become as a profession, the more they are likely to duplicate the maldistribution of physicians—the very problem that PAs were designed to alleviate. Another hazard of specialization is that the voice of the profession tends to become more fragmented because each subgroup feels that the rest of the group does not speak for them. As PAs relocate to urban areas to take advantage of the more lucrative job offers there, the maldistribution problem becomes more pronounced, and we run the risk that another, alternate provider class must be developed to fill the niche for which PAs were designed.

Rural health care access will continue to be burdened by barriers and deficiencies. This discussion is not intended to show why one should avoid rural health service, but rather simply to ensure that anyone considering rural practice will be aware of all its satisfactions, challenges, and rewards. Certainly, the problems at hand are difficult. Some of the more uniquely rural ones may never be resolved. However, we believe that there is a rewarding and satisfying future for PAs in rural medicine. We wanted to give an overview of many of the health care issues that rural Americans and rural practitioners face. Our hope is that many of these problems will be addressed by a consortium of informed policymakers, educators, practitioners, and—perhaps most importantly—informed citizenry, representing rural localities. We wish to put forth the following recommendations, which we believe are vital to improved rural access to health care:

➤ Federal and state health policies must demonstrate that all urban and rural Americans are equally entitled to appropriate primary health care.

➤ PA education programs should emphasize primary care training with a strong orientation to selecting and educating appropriate candidates for rural or other underserved populations.

➤ Financial incentives should be available, including scholarships for PA students, CME and income tax credits (both federal and state), and liability insurance relief for PAs and other practitioners electing to work in underserved areas.

➤ State laws and regulations should be composed to authorize PAs to provide adequate primary care, including the ability to prescribe, administer, and dispense medications without direct physician supervision. Without flexibility in the laws governing the scope of PA practice, rural communities cannot seek innovative ways to bring health care to their locales. The laws must also include provisions for locum tenens coverage to allow for CME and vacation relief.

➤ A reasonable reimbursement rate or value for PA services should be made available by all public and private insurers.

➤ PAs need to consider, in selecting practice sites, that rural health service in HPSAs is a basic tenet of the PA profession.

➤ AHECs, rural providers, state PA academies, and PA programs should cooperate to organize rural clerkships or preceptorships. They should also research and develop funding resources to enable PA students to participate in a meaningful rural health experience involving exposure of their families to rural living.

➤ Rural PAs should always be active in the training process of the EMS personnel in their communities.

➤ Everyone concerned with health care in rural or other underserved areas must be active in a campaign to establish a firm financial base for rural clinics. Whether it involves developing strategies for increased utilization, subsidizing local care with tax dollars, ensuring that federal and state programs offer an adequate reimbursement rate for services rendered, or any combination of these, it is imperative that a firm financial base be maintained.

➤ All personnel of a rural clinic must understand methods of efficient operations to help keep costs down. PA program curricula should include some classes on business and personnel management issues and should teach the concept that networking of administrative and health care services in rural and frontier medicine is often necessary for those services to survive.

➤ Solo provision of health care services is very stressful. Staffing a rural clinic with at least two PAs helps overcome the major obstacle of provider burnout. The patient encounter numbers alone at many rural clinics do not justify two practitioners. However, having two providers available reduces on-call stress and increases each provider's time off to attend CME or relax. It also helps reduce the stress in their personal and family lives.

➤ Anyone in rural medicine should be aware of the rural health associations on the state and national levels. Joining one or both will provide the member with current information on issues and trends pertaining to rural health care policy and delivery of care. In addition, state and national offices of rural health, as well as the AAPA, can provide technical assistance to PAs, rural clinics, and hospitals on all aspects of rural health care delivery.

CONCLUSION

Rural medicine is more complex than it first appears and requires great versatility on the part of the practitioner. It can be incredibly fulfilling and unimaginably wearing. PAs and PA students who are contemplating rural health care as a career must make an honest evaluation of their motivations, skills, and adaptability before committing themselves to it. They must consider the needs of their spouses and families, including any current or expected financial obligations. One of the hard facts of rural practice is that the need is great but the resources are often not sufficient to compensate practitioners accordingly. PAs were designed to meet health care needs in areas like this. We must, as a profession, ensure that this goal is not relinquished in the pursuit of financial gratification.

CLINICAL APPLICATIONS

1. Contact the rural health constituencies in your state or region (e.g., offices of rural health, primary care associations, AHECs) and determine whether there are major changes occurring in rural health care delivery in your area. How are these changes affecting the following areas?
   ➤ Access to care.
   ➤ Retention of primary care providers in rural communities.
   ➤ Utilization of PAs and NPs.

➤ Development of new health care delivery models.

➤ Viability of rural hospitals.

➤ Reimbursement policies for PAs and NPs.

2. Interview three rural PAs. Find out which aspects of their physician assistant training best prepared them for their current clinical role. What additional training would they now seek if they had the opportunity? In their opinion, what are the most effective methods (e.g., CME, Internet access, telemedicine, other venues and activities) for decreasing isolation and maintaining the most up-to-date clinical competence?

3. What is "rural"? Apply the various formal and informal definitions of "rural" to your state or region using census and demographic data obtained from state and national databases currently available on the Internet.

Acknowledgments

The authors would like to thank Keren H. Wick, PhD (MEDEX Northwest Physician Assistant Program, University of Washington), for extensive revision and updating on this chapter for the 3rd edition.

REFERENCES

1. AAPA position paper: physician assistants and rural health care. J Am Acad Physician Assist 1990;3:414.
2. United States Census Bureau. American FactFinder on-line (including data tables and glossary). Available at http://factfinder.census.gov/servlet/BasicFactsServlet. Accessed 3 July 2002.
3. Rural Information Center Health Service. Rural health statistics. Available at http://www.nal.usda.gov/ric/richs/stats.htm. Accessed 3 July 2002.
4. Ciarolo JA, Wackwitz JH, Wagenfeld MO, Mohatt DF. Focusing on "frontier": isolated rural America. Boulder, CO: WICHE Mental Health Program, 1996. Available at http://www.Wiche.edu/MentalHealth/Frontier/letter2.html. Accessed 3 July 2002.
5. Frontier Education Center. The geography of frontier America: the view at the turn of the century. Ojo Sarco, NM: Frontier Education Center, 2000. Available at http://www.nal.usda.gov/ric/richs/frontierinventory.htm. Accessed 3 July 2002.
6. Centers for Disease Control and Prevention. Health, United States, 2001. Urban and Rural Chartbook. Washington DC: Department of Health and Human Services, 2002.
7. AAPA Census Reports. Alexandria, VA: American Academy of Physician Assistants. Last updated May 2002. Available at http://www.aapa.org/research/index.html. Accessed 5 July 2002.
8. Larson EH, Hart LG, Goodwin MK, Geller J, Andrilla C. Dimensions of retention: a national study of the locational histories of physician assistants. J Rural Health 1999; 15:391.
9. AAPA Policy Brief: Managed Health Care and Rural America. Alexandria, VA: AAPA, 1997. Available on-line at http://www.aapa.org/gandp/mhc-rural.html. Accessed 8 July 2002.
10. Robinson J, Guidry JJ. Recruiting, training, and retaining rural health professionals. In: Loue S, Quill BE (eds). Handbook of Rural Health. New York, NY: Kluwer Academic/Plenum Publishers, 2001:337.
11. National Health Service Corps web site. Available at http://nhsc.bhpr.hrsa.gov. Accessed 5 July 2002.
12. U.S. Congress, Office of Technology Assessment. Health Care in Rural America. Washington, DC: U.S. Congress, Office of Technology Assessment, 1990.
13. Aday LA, Quill BE, Reyes-Gibby CC. Equity in rural health and health care. In: Loue S, Quill BE (eds). Handbook of Rural Health. New York, NY: Kluwer Academic/Plenum Publishers, 2001:45.
14. National Association of Rural Health Clinics. Rural Health Clinics Act PL 95-210. An overview. Available at: http://www.narhc.org/Program%20Overview.htm. Accessed 5 July 2002.
15. Mueller KJ. Rural health policy: past as a prelude to the future. In: Loue S, Quill BE (eds). Handbook of Rural Health. New York, NY: Kluwer Academic/Plenum Publishers, 2001:1.
16. Area Health Education Centers. Bureau of Health Professions web site. Available at http://bhpr.hrsa.gov/interdisciplinary/ahec.html. Accessed 5 July 2002.
17. Human J, Director, Office of Rural Health Policy, Health Resources and Services Administration. Prepared statement before the House Committee on Ways and Means, Health Subcommittee. Federal News Service Congressional Hearing Testimonies, September 12, 1996.
18. Office of Rural Health Policy web site. Available at http://www.ruralhealth.hrsa.gov. Accessed 8 July 2002.
19. McCarty K, MAF Director, Helena, MT. Telephone conversation with authors, 16 December 1997 and 6 January 1998.
20. Sider K, Administrator, Dahl Memorial MAF Hospital, Ekalaka, MT. Telephone conversation with authors, 5 January 1998.
21. McCarty K. Hospitals on the frontier: health progress. J Catholic Health Assoc USA 1992;May:42.
22. HCFA Finalizes Rule to Improve Hospital, Emergency Treatment Access: Health Care Policy Report. Washington, DC: Bureau of National Affairs, May 31, 1993.
23. Wright G, Felt S, Wellever AL, et al. Limited Service Hospital Pioneers: Challenges and Successes of the Essential Access Community Hospital/Rural Primary Care Hospital (EACH/RPCH) Program and Medical Assistance Facility

(MAF) Demonstration. Draft Final Report. Washington, DC: Mathematica Policy Research, Inc., March 28, 1995.

24. Smith K, Director, Montana Critical Access Hospitals, Helena, MT. Telephone conversation with authors, 29 April 2002.

25. Hegeman W, Garfield County CAH, Jordan, MT. Telephone conversation with authors, 29 April 2002.

26. Lopes P, Nichols A. Special Tax Supported Ambulatory Care Health Districts. Monograph #15. Tucson, AZ: The Southwest Border Rural Health Research Center, University of Arizona College of Medicine, 1990.

27. Willis J. Is the PA supply in rural America dwindling? J Am Acad Physician Assist 1990;3:433.

CHAPTER 28

Alternative Delivery Sites

Sarah F. Zarbock

INTRODUCTION

Physician assistants practice in a wide range of settings, with more than half of the clinically practicing respondents (53.7%) to the American Academy of Physician Assistants (AAPA) 2001 national census survey reporting that they practice in a primary care specialty (family practice, general internal medicine, emergency medicine, general pediatrics).[1] When the census data were broken down by primary work setting, however, only 0.9% stated that they worked in a nursing home or long-term care facility, and only six individuals indicated that their primary work setting was the patient's home. These figures are essentially similar to the findings of the AAPA's 1997 census survey (55.7% and 0.9%, respectively).[2]

This chapter focuses on a small sector of clinical practice for PAs—the home, nursing home, and hospice. Before each practice setting is discussed individually, it is important to provide some basic background demographic information about the patients seen, collectively, in these alternative practice settings.

With the aging of America, increased numbers of older patients will be cared for in settings other than the outpatient clinic or hospital. Although people older than 65 years constitute only around 13% of the U.S. population, they consume about one third of health care dollars.[3] In July 1994, there were 33.2 million elderly (aged 65 or older), representing one eighth of the total population. Among the elderly, 18.7 million were ages 65 to 74, 11.0 million were ages 75 to 84, and 3.5 million were age 85 or older. The elderly population increased 11-fold from 1900 to 1994, compared with only a 3-fold increase for those under age 65.[4] With the advent of the aging baby boomers, these numbers will only increase. People aged 65 or older have a tremendous need for services at home; 5% of them live in nursing homes, but 15% live at home and require assistance. Of those over age 85, 22% reside in nursing homes, and 35% live at home and require assistance.[5]

More than any other identifiable group, the elderly receive care in a variety of health care settings and often move between settings over time. These settings include the office, outpatient clinic, hospital, home, residential care facility, nursing home, and hospital. Coupled with the need for elder care, the recent national emphasis on controlling the rising cost of health care, particularly among the elderly, has focused attention on the potentially increased role of physician assistants (PAs) and other nonphysician providers in caring for the elderly.[3] It is generally assumed that at least two thirds of the care given to persons older than 65 years will continue to be provided by family practitioners and internists. Similar to findings of the 1997 AAPA census, the 2001 AAPA census shows that 34.5% of PAs will be in a family or general medicine practice, and 8.5% will be in general internal medicine.[1] Therefore, it follows that PAs can continue to make an important contribution in caring for geriatric patients in all settings.

A role for PAs in providing geriatric health care was recognized early in the development of the profession.[3] Because a significant portion of PA education is focused on the management of chronic diseases, PAs have found themselves in the position of being especially knowledgeable about caring for elderly patients.

The role of the PA who works only in a practice with geriatric patients is very similar to the role of a PA in the primary care setting. PAs use the same core skills—taking the history, performing the physical examination, making an assessment, and developing and carrying out an appropriate treatment plan. Thus, PAs are well suited for a role in practice settings in which a majority of patients are elderly.[3]

The most recent change that has affected PA practice, and the health care landscape overall, is the advent of managed care and its role in shaping health care access and financing. With an increasing emphasis on cost effectiveness and with PAs being able to perform approximately 80% of the tasks that physicians perform in the primary care setting,[6] the PA is a less costly provider for much of the routine care required by older patients.

Another important piece of the financial puzzle is the reimbursement for services provided by a PA while under the supervision of the physician-employer. Since the expansion of Medicare reimbursement in 1987 to include PA services in nursing homes and skilled nursing facilities, care provided by PAs in these settings has been reimbursable at 85% of the physician reimbursement rate. As a result of the Balanced Budget Act (BBA) of 1997, which went

into effect on January 1, 1998, Medicare pays the PA's employer for medical services provided by PAs in all settings at 85% of the physician's fee schedule. This includes hospitals (inpatient, outpatient, and emergency departments), nursing facilities, offices and clinics, the patient's residence, and first-assisting at surgery. Assignment is mandatory and state law determines supervision and scope of practice.

HOME CARE

Home care in the United States is a diverse and dynamic service industry. The 1998 Home and Hospice Care Survey findings indicate that more than 20,000 providers delivered home care services to some 7.6 million individuals because of acute illness, long-term health conditions, permanent disability, or terminal illness.[7] This figure represents roughly 2.8% of the U.S. Bureau of Census estimated U.S. population. Annual expenditures for home health care were projected to be $41.3 billion in 2001.[7] American health care service is expanding rapidly into the home. Three key factors are the pressure on physicians by third party payers to discharge patients earlier from hospitals, the growing elderly population, and the breakthrough in life-saving technologies.[8]

The re-emergence of the home as a site of health care in the past decade is a trend that is expected to continue.[3] This increase is a consequence of the advent of diagnosis-related groups (DRGs)—a reimbursement system introduced by Medicare in the early 1980s to reduce costs and length of patient stays associated with hospitalization. One outcome of DRGs was the early discharge from hospitals of patients who still required acute care. Having left the hospital, a patient's only options were to enter a nursing home or intermediate care facility, or to obtain services at home. Nursing home placement may not be a viable option for many Medicare patients because of a shortage of nursing home beds and limited Medicare coverage of nursing home costs. Thus, patients increasingly have needed health services provided in their homes.

Approximately 44% of all patients discharged from the hospital by primary care physicians require posthospital medical or nursing care that cannot be provided by family or friends alone.[9] According to the

American Medical Association (AMA) *Guidelines for the Medical Management of the Home Care Patient,*[9] between 5% and 10% of all patients in a medical practice receive home care services. The AMA also found that for every patient in a nursing home, three more severely impaired patients are cared for in their own homes. An estimated 20% of patients over age 65 have functional impairments with related home care needs. Of recipients of home care, nearly half are over the age of 65, and the amount of home care they use tends to increase with age. Age and functional disability are likely predictors of the need for home care services. Estimates indicate that as many as 9 to 11 million Americans need home care services.[9] Most will receive services from so-called informal caregivers, family members, friends, or others who provide uncompensated care.

The National Association for Home Care (NAHC) found that of the total home care organizations as of December 1995, approximately 9100 were Medicare-certified home health agencies, 1850 were Medicare-certified hospices, and 7800 were home health agencies, home care aide organizations, and hospices that do not participate in Medicare. More recently, the number of Medicare-certified home health agencies declined to 7512. NAHC believes the 31.5% decline in agencies since 1997 is the direct result of changes in Medicare home health reimbursement enacted as part of the Balanced Budget Act of 1997. Hospital-based and proprietary agencies have grown faster than any other type of certified agency.[10]

Total home care spending is difficult to estimate. In August of 1995, the Congressional Budget Office projected home care expenditures would be $36 billion in 1996 and estimated they would grow an average of 13% for the period 1996 to 2005.[7] Medicare is the largest single payer of home care services; in 1992, it accounted for more than one third of total home care expenditures.

The elderly experience both the normal progression of aging and various pathological states that medicine and technology alone cannot rectify. Because of these changes, the elderly are often not capable of providing for their activities of daily living or transporting themselves to a physician's office, a hospital, or a clinic.

An interesting survey, conducted by the National Center for Health Statistics (NCHS), gathered valuable information on what diseases or conditions accounted for the need for home care in the elderly. Close to 30% of home care patients admitted to home health agencies in 1994 had conditions related to diseases of the circulatory system. Persons with heart disease, including congestive heart failure, made up 20% of this group. Stroke, diabetes, and hypertension were also frequent admission diagnoses for home care patients.[7]

In 1998, 33.5% of Medicare home health patients had conditions related to diseases of the circulatory system as their principal diagnosis. People with heart disease, including congestive heart failure, made up about half of this group. Injury and poisoning, diseases of the musculoskeletal system and connective tissue, and diseases of the respiratory system were also frequent principal diagnoses for Medical home health patients. Medicare home health patients with neoplasms accounted for 7.0%, and diabetes accounted for 7.9%.[7]

Many hospital patients are discharged to home care services for continued rehabilitative care. Again, as hospital stays have shortened, the percentage of patients requiring these services has increased. The five most common hospital discharge diagnoses to home care are hip and femur procedures, major joint procedures, heart failure, chronic obstructive pulmonary disease, and stroke.[7]

Physicians in Home Care

There are a variety of reasons why few physicians visit patients in their homes, some of them related to the realities of today's health care environment. It is an inefficient use of a physician's time, provides inadequate financial reimbursement, and does not use all of the diagnostic capabilities (laboratory and radiological evaluations) routinely available in the office.[10] Home care has some inherent inefficiencies in cost per visit because of the travel time involved. Thus, the efficiency of home care must instead be assessed against the cost of the same care provided in other medical settings. Other major barriers include conflicting regulatory and legal requirements and lack of physician education in home care.[10]

Less quantifiable and more difficult to address, although just as influential in affecting care provided in the home, may be the biases and discomfort associated with providing care in the home setting. Medical care is customarily provided in clean, well-lit offices, with a group of nurses and administrative staff to assist the physicians. Patients are scheduled to allow for maximum utilization of the physician's time, often every 15 minutes in busy practices. There is usually on-site diagnostic equipment, results from tests are immediately available, and physician colleagues may be nearby for consultation.

Clearly, not all patient evaluations may be managed in the home setting. More than just the practicalities of the physician-patient encounter influence why physicians are reluctant to make house calls. Most people feel more comfortable and confident on their own "turf," and certainly physicians should be no exception. Nonetheless, visiting a patient at home serves two major purposes: It provides a wealth of information about the environment in which the care is provided, and it facilitates a closer relationship between the physician and the patient and family. When visiting, one can see the physical setup, such as where the patient's bed is in relationship to the rest of the household. Special problems may be identified such as poor living conditions, including inadequate heating. Seeing where and how the patient lives provides insight into the financial situation of family members and how that may influence their ability to provide care. How do family members interact and communicate with each other? These factors affect the development of the most individualized plan of care.

In addition, because the home visit is an invitation into the life of the family, there is less of the hierarchical order that occurs in the traditional office or hospital setting. The relationship is more as equals, or as friends. The unexpected bonus that many physicians experience once they overcome their reluctance to make a house call is that they have seen a whole new facet of their patient's life. They appreciate the special bond that may develop—a bond that could not occur in any other setting.[10]

Over time, the home has become more prominent as the site of acute, intermediate, and long-term care for patients of all ages with or without requirements for medical technology.[11] A 1992 survey of home visiting practices and attitudes of family physicians and internists showed that the mean number of house calls for family physicians was 21.2 visits per year and for internists was 15.7 per year, despite an unfavorable reimbursement climate for home care provided by physicians.[11] Another survey of internists and family physicians revealed that about one half of respondents had made a house call over the past year, but few had done so more than five times.[12]

The role of the physician includes many tasks that could be managed by the PA. The primary task, of course, is management of medical problems. The patient in need of home care usually has multiple, complex medical problems. The crux of appropriate medical management in the home is to optimize the patient's independence and minimize the effects of illness and disability. The PA can play a critical role in identifying home care needs and developing, in conjunction with members of an interdisciplinary team, a plan based on both short- and long-term goals. As part of this plan, it is necessary that any new, acute, or emergent medical problems be evaluated and findings communicated to the patient, family members, and team members. The PA can also assist with the reassessment of the care plan, outcomes of care, and quality of care.

In establishing a close working relationship with the home care patient, the PA in conjunction with the supervising physician will participate in a variety of discussions with the patient. Topics should include the disease process and treatment options; the effect of the disease and its treatment on the patient's daily functioning and lifestyle; the expected course of the illness, both over the short and the long term; tasks that the patient and caregiver will be expected to perform; and the stress and burdens arising from chronic illness and methods for relieving such stress for both the patient and caregivers. It is always wise to discuss the patient's potential for rehabilitation; the need for monitoring of conditions by both patient and caregiver; the early signs of instability or deterioration, which should be reported to the physician; and, finally, improvements in function or condition, which also should be reported to the physician.[9]

Specifically, a series of assessments are generally required in order to evaluate the patient's and caregiver's ability to implement the care plan. One important aspect of the evaluation is the patient's ability to perform activities of daily living (ambulating, toileting, feeding, bathing, dressing, continence) and the more complex instrumental activities of daily living, such as taking medications appropriately, arranging transportation, using the telephone, preparing meals, shopping, doing housework, and handling finances. A screening functional assessment should include both a subjective report from the patient and family and the PA's observations during the physical examination, as well as a vision and hearing screening. The goal is to assess not only the severity of the functional disability but also the cause and what might help overcome it.[9]

Mental/cognitive, psychosocial, and nutritional assessments should also be conducted along with an evaluation of medication use and compliance. Other items that need to be evaluated are the caregiver burden and ability to participate in the home care plan, as well as the home environment, the resources available in the community, and the financial status of the patient and family.[9]

Reimbursement for PA-provided services in the home underwent an important change as a result of the Balanced Budget Act that came into effect on January 1, 1998. Prior to this, although PA services in the home were reimbursable at 85% of the physician charge, the physician had to be on-site when the services were provided, thus negating the benefit of PA-provided services. As of 1998, PAs could provide medical services in the home with the stipulation that the supervising physician could be reached, even if only by electronic communication. At this time, there are no data on PAs working in the home setting, but it would be reasonable to assume that home care could be a part of any primary care services already reimbursed.

Interdisciplinary Team

One of the unique aspects of home care is the nature of the collaborative team effort. In the home care setting, individual professional roles overlap in a set of shared tasks. Because usually only one member of the team is in the home at a time, that member must be aware of the total home care plan of treatment and must be able to evaluate, advise, or assist the patient and the caregiver as needed. In addition to the seven services covered under the Medicare home health benefit (skilled nursing; home health aide; physical, occupational, and speech therapy; nutritional guidance; and medical social services), many other health professionals and paraprofessionals provide services for home care patients. A short, incomplete list might include respiratory therapists, pharmacists, podiatrists, dentists, volunteers, and friendly visitors.

Because many of the health problems of the elderly living at home are not purely medical, the PA needs to be familiar with local resources. This multidimensional approach underscores what some believe to be the best argument for home care[7]: "It is the humane and compassionate way to deliver health care and supportive services. It reinforces and supplements the care provided by family members and friends and maintains the recipient's dignity and independence, qualities that are all too often lost in even the best institutions. Furthermore, home care allows patients to take an active role in their care and become members of the multidisciplinary health care team."

HOSPICE CARE

Hospices provide palliative care, as opposed to curative care.[13] Hospice services include supportive, social, emotional, and spiritual services provided to the terminally ill, as well as support for the patient's family. Care is primarily provided in the patient's home to maintain peace, comfort, and dignity. As stated by the Hospice Association of America[13]: "Hospice care relies on the combined knowledge and skill of an interdisciplinary team of professionals—physicians, nurses, medical social workers, therapists, and counselors, in addition to volunteers—who coordinate an individualized plan of care for each patient and family. Hospice reaffirms the right of every person and family to participate fully in the final stage of life."

Connecticut Hospice in Branford was the first hospice in the United States; it began providing services in March of 1974. The Medicare program identified 2273 hospices as of January 2001.[7] There were also an estimated 200 volunteer hospices in the United

States. In 1998, hospices served nearly 400,000 patients.[7] Less is known about the hospices that do not participate in the Medicare or Medicaid program because the rules and regulations for licensure vary by state.

Congress enacted legislation in 1982 creating a Medicare hospice benefit. Medicare hospice participation increased dramatically, largely as a result of a 1989 Congressional mandate that increased rates by 20%. From 1984 to January 2001, the total number of hospices participating in Medicare rose from 31 to 2273—a greater than 73-fold increase.[7] Of these hospices, 960 are freestanding, 739 are home health agency based, 554 are hospital based, and 20 are skilled nursing facility based.[7]

An admission criterion for most hospice programs is that the patient has a life expectancy of 6 months or less. In addition, patients have a desire both to remain at home and to forego life-sustaining treatments, including resuscitation. Data show that 57.4% of hospice enrollees in 1998 had conditions related to neoplasms as their first-listed diagnosis as opposed to 75.6% in 1992.[7] Cancer of the lungs, prostate, and breast accounted for most of the malignancies. All noncancer diagnoses went from 24.4% in 1992 to 42.6% in 1998. These diagnoses primarily included congestive heart failure, chronic obstructive pulmonary disease, stroke, and Alzheimer's disease.[7]

The home is the predominant site of hospice care throughout the patient's illness until death, intermittently over time, or for most of the final days but with death occurring in the hospital. As such, hospice care from the clinician's standpoint is a variant of home care and incorporates many of the same issues—physical assessment, psychosocial support, disease and symptom management, use of a multidisciplinary team, and patient and family education.[14]

Crucial to the concept of hospice care is an unequivocal, aggressive effort to provide relief of pain and symptoms during the patient's final stages of life.[15] The overall goal is to allow the patient to function as normally as possible while alleviating pain and other symptoms. Pain experts have noted that because pain is a subjective experience, it is often difficult to evaluate, and clinicians do not have objective signs to enable them to quantify the severity of pain.

The patient's subjective report is the basis for successful management of pain: "Pain is whatever the person experiencing it says it is and it exists whenever he says it does."[15]

Perhaps the greatest contribution that a clinician can make when taking care of hospice patients is to be as knowledgeable as possible about pain assessment and management. As part of this process, rigorous attention to the patient history and physical assessment, similar to all other clinical evaluations, continues to provide the most valuable clues as to the pain's cause and location. Furthermore, all approaches to pain therapy must include not only the cause but also its psychological and social consequences. Pain does not exist strictly as a physiological phenomenon but incorporates the individual patient's beliefs and the social context in which he or she lives. Pain is a *total* experience that also encompasses family relationships, cultural background, religious tenets, and social support systems and activities. Some believe that nowhere else in medicine is it more important to have a holistic approach to caring than in the management of pain in the terminally ill patient.[15]

Very few PAs are involved in the provision of hospice care, but that may change with time as more dying patients choose to be cared for at home. The number of hospice patients continues to grow. By definition, as interdependent colleagues with physicians, PAs' clinical practice mirrors that of their physician-employers and supervisors. This is especially true in family practice and primary care settings, where patients are taken care of on a continuum, culminating for some with hospice care. As was mentioned previously, part of the reason for this trend is that services provided by PAs in the home are now partially covered by Medicare. Caring for terminally ill patients involves a very special kind of relationship in which a bond can develop—a bond that could not occur in any other setting. Some hospice providers believe that physicians should not participate in hospice care if they are unwilling to make a home visit.[15] Hospice, home care staff, and PAs can help facilitate the physician visit; in the case of the PA, he or she can be the visitor who works closely with the physician in providing, coordinating, and managing care in this unique setting. Case Study 28-1 is an example of home hospice care provided for an acquired immune deficiency syndrome (AIDS) patient.

CASE STUDY 28-1

Mr. B was a 33-year-old patient with AIDS. After his life partner died 4 years earlier of AIDS, Mr. B became active in the local human immunodeficiency virus (HIV) community. He did many speaking engagements for schools and health professions groups. As Mr. B's health deteriorated, he moved back to his mother's home. Mr. B discussed his feelings about his impending death with his PA, particularly his fear of dying in a hospital like his partner, "hooked to all those machines and out of it or in pain." The PA educated Mr. B and his mother about hospice care, including the option for self-regulated pain medicine.

When Mr. B entered the terminal phase, he and his mother asked for home hospice care. Mr. B's primary physician and PA coordinated the care, and the PA made home visits periodically. After one visit, the PA remarked to his supervising physician, "It's like a constant open house for Mr. B and his mother. There's almost always a group of friends around, who bring food and help with housework. Mr. B has been planning his memorial service and telling each of his friends and relatives what he wants done, including music and poetry. He is such a remarkable man. People come to help take care of him, and they leave feeling cared for by him. Me included."

The physician and PA made sure that Mr. B was adequately medicated for pain with self-regulated delivery methods. He needed less medication than was expected and was comfortable most of the time. Mr. B died at home, surrounded by family and friends, pain-free, and mentally clear until the end. Mr. B's memorial service was the celebration of his life that he had planned.

NURSING HOME

The nursing home remains an underserved area where physician involvement in care is minimal.[3] Despite the complex medical needs of nursing home residents, only 35% of primary care physicians spend time working in a long-term care facility.[16] The

opportunity for PAs to work in nursing homes increased when Medicare expanded its reimbursement in 1987 to include PA services in nursing homes and skilled nursing facilities.

Medicare coverage for medical services performed by PAs in nursing or skilled nursing facilities is provided at 85% of the physician's fee schedule. In general, Medicare reimburses services provided by a PA if those same services are covered when performed by a physician.[16] Although the physician must supervise the overall medical care of the nursing home patient, the physician may delegate some nursing home visits to the PA, after the patient has been admitted to the facility. After the patient has been admitted to the facility, Medicare requires that the patient be seen at least once every 30 days for the first 90 days and every 60 days thereafter. The physician must make the first visit. Under Medicare guidelines, PAs may alternate required routine visits (at 30- or 60-day intervals) with their supervisor and may provide acute care. (Acute care visits are unlimited but must be medically necessary.) Additional visits beyond what is required are covered if warranted by the patient's medical condition. The PA can exclusively perform these additional visits; Medicare generally will pay for a total of 18 visits a year.[17]

According to the 2001 AAPA Census, 66 PAs (0.4%) cite a nursing home or long-term care facility as their primary *employer* and 158 (0.9%) cite it as their primary work *setting*. For those PAs who work at least 32 hours per week at a primary clinical job, 757 (7.1%) see some nursing home patients, and 9906 (92.9%) do not (data represent only respondents who reported complete information about both hours and visits for all patient types). According to the 1997 AAPA Census, 54 PAs (0.4%) and 122 PAs (0.9%) cite a nursing home or long-term care facility as their primary employer and work setting, respectively—essentially indicating no change between 1997 and 2001.[1,2]

Case Study 28-2 illustrates the contribution of a PA to the care of a patient in a nursing home.

CASE STUDY 28-2

Mr. L was an 83-year-old retired engineer with Alzheimer's dementia who had been in a nursing home for 3 years. During the previous 6 months, he became more hostile and combative, requiring sedation or restraints on some occasions. The PA became acquainted with Mr. L through yearly physical examinations and noticed that Mr. L often mumbled about church and prayers.

One day, the PA found Mr. L strapped into a chair in the hall because he had been very agitated and had struck at an aide. The PA had a portable tape player in her backpack, which she decided to try. She placed the headphones in Mr. L's ears and started a tape of church hymns. Mr. L relaxed in his chair and smiled. The aide who had been threatened by Mr. L walked by, stopped, and said, "You know, that's the first time I've seen that man smile."

When Mr. L's family was told about his response to the music, they brought in a tape player and a supply of audiotapes. Although Mr. L's condition continued to deteriorate, his behavior was much less of a problem for the nursing home staff to manage.

CONCLUSION

Closer evaluation of the most effective ways to use PAs will be undertaken now that Medicare reimbursement has been extended to PAs in all settings. Certainly for home care, and to a lesser extent for hospice care, the opportunities for PAs will increase because more and more patients are being taken care of in their homes and reimbursement is available. The utilization of PAs in nursing homes is also expected to increase as supervising physicians explore ways in which to have PAs supplement their care in this setting. There are clear financial incentives for PAs to be involved in these alternative sites of care. Equally important is the challenge and reward of working with patients and their families. PAs need to be open-minded about these opportunities and must be able to expand their locus of practice.

CLINICAL APPLICATIONS

1. If you were to conduct home visits, what equipment and materials would you assemble in order to effectively assess and manage the problems of a variety of patients?

2. How would you conduct an evaluation of sight, hearing, and activities of daily living during a home visit?

3. You are following a 68-year-old woman with terminal colon cancer. She is living with her son and daughter-in-law and is enrolled in a hospice program. On a home visit, the patient's son confides in you that he is, "worried about all the pain medicine my mother gets. I think she'll get addicted." How do you respond?

4. Some health care workers find the nursing home environment difficult because patients generally do not experience improvements in their health status. If you had a nursing home position as a PA, how would you maintain your ability to care for each resident as an individual and avoid discouragement? What do you think the rewards would be for you in working in this health care setting?

REFERENCES

1. 2001 AAPA Physician Assistant Census Report. Alexandria, VA: American Academy of Physician Assistants, 2001.
2. 1997 AAPA Physician Assistant Census Report. Alexandria, VA: American Academy of Physician Assistants, 1997.
3. Segal-Gidan FI. The role of PAs in caring for the elderly. J Am Acad Physician Assist 1997;10:27.
4. U.S. Department of Commerce. U.S. Census Bureau, 2001. Available at www.census.gov/.
5. Slotkin JP, Jacques PF. Home health care. In: Ballweg R, Stolberg S, Sullivan EM (eds). Physician Assistant: A Guide to Clinical Practice. Philadelphia: WB Saunders, 1994.
6. Hooker RS. Ambulatory services. In: Ballweg R, Stolberg S, Sullivan EM (eds). Physician Assistant: A Guide to Clinical Practice. Philadelphia: WB Saunders, 1994.
7. Basic Statistics About Home Care 2001. Washington, DC: National Association of Home Care, 2001.
8. American Academy of Home Care Physicians [brochure]. Columbia, MD: American Academy of Home Care Physicians, 1997.
9. Guidelines for the Medical Management of the Home Care Patient. Chicago, IL: American Medical Association, 1992.
10. Zarbock SF. Home care: an opportunity for physicians. Home Care Provider 1996;1:100.
11. Goldberg AI. Home healthcare: the role of the primary care physician. Compr Ther 1995;21:633.
12. Ratner ER. Home care for the '90s. Med J Allina 1997;6. Available at http://www.allina.com/Allina_Journal/Summer1997/ratner.html.
13. Hospice Facts and Statistics. Washington, DC: Hospice Association of America, 1997.

14. Goltzer SZ. Hospice: compassionate care for dying patients. AAPA Recertification Update 1992;3:1.

15. Pain. Springhouse, PA: Nursing Now Books, 1985.

16. Kemle KA. Common medical problems in the nursing home population. J Am Acad Physician Assist 1997;10:39.

17. Basic Statistics About Home Care 1996. Washington, DC: National Association of Home Care, 1996.

18. Powe ML. Medicare reimbursement for PAs: Know what is covered. J Am Acad Physician Assist 1997;10:65.

RESOURCES

Geriatrics: special issue. J Am Acad Physician Assist 1997;10. *Provides a wealth of information about caring for geriatric patients, including the role of PAs, common medical problems in the nursing home population, the status of Medicare reimbursement for PAs, types of community resources available to the elderly, and the value of the periodic health examination.*

American Academy of Home Care Physicians (AAHCP), 10480 Little Patuxent Parkway, Suite 760, Columbia, MD 21044; (410) 730-1623, 740-4572 fax. *Professional organization that provides network and technical assistance, a quarterly publication, and educational programs.*

Physicians and Home Care: Guidelines for the Medical Management of the Home Care Patient. Chicago, IL: American Medical Association, 1992. *In February of 1987, the American Medical Association (AMA) first convened the Home Care Advisory Panel to consider educational efforts that would assist physicians to better understand their role in the delivery of medical care in the home. The panel developed these guidelines for the practice of medicine in the home setting, including sections about the role of the physician, the physician/patient relationship, medical management in home care, patients' rights and responsibilities, coordination of care and case management, and community resources. Provides the location of state aging services and resources. Available from the AAHCP.*

Goldberg AI. Home healthcare: the role of the primary care physician. Compr Ther 1995;21:633. *Valuable article that summarizes the findings of a major study conducted by the AMA's Department of Geriatric Medicine and the University of Minnesota's Department of Family Practice, which was designed to determine house call attitudes of both generalists and specialists. Outlines specific criteria for successful home care.*

CHAPTER 29

Family Practice and Internal Medicine

Lynda White and Nelson Herlihy

INTRODUCTION

Family practice, primary care internal medicine (general internal medicine), and pediatrics are the medical fields in which practitioners treat patients with a broad spectrum of medical problems. Family physicians treat more outpatients than hospitalized patients; general internists treat more hospitalized patients than do family physicians but also treat patients on an outpatient basis. Both emphasize lifetime continuity of care, with health promotion, disease prevention, and strong attention to psychosocial issues.

The training of family practice physicians is broad, whereas training in internal medicine is focused on in-depth adult medicine. Family physicians treat patients of all ages, diagnose, and treat problems in all the organ systems, including gynecology and in some practices obstetrics. General internists, in contrast, diagnose and treat adult patients with problems in many of the organ systems, varying according to the breadth of knowledge and interest of the practitioner. Both treat the patient as a whole person.

These generalists are much in demand, and jobs in both family practice and internal medicine abound. Job opportunities are predicted to increase in the future owing to cost containment and expansion of the health services industry. Physician assistants (PAs) work under the supervision of these primary care physicians in a variety of settings such as multispecialty clinics, private offices, county clinics, urgent care clinics, and hospitals. Sometimes the PA's practice setting is geographically remote from the physician, and supervision is provided by telephone and/or electronic means.

HISTORY OF FAMILY PRACTICE

Through the early 1940s, the realm of generalist medicine included general practitioners who did not complete a residency, as well as graduates of the few general practice residency programs. Members of both of these groups constituted the membership of the American Academy of General Practice (AAGP). Following World War II, the number of general practitioners fell steadily as the number of specialists grew, fueled by a technological explosion in the United States. However, public demand and the need for well-trained generalists who could treat common medical problems in all age groups, including obstetrics, led to a resurgence of generalists in the late 1960s. In 1969, the specialty of family practice began with a radical restructuring of the old AAGP to form the American Academy of Family Practice (AAFP). The AAFP implemented new standards for a 3-year residency, board certification and re-certification examinations (the first specialty to do so), and a fundamental redefinition of the profession to include emphasis on continuity of care, disease prevention, family dynamics, counseling, and psychology. Simultaneously, more medical schools began departments of family practice, inspiring students to enter family practice. During the 1970s, the number of family practice residency training programs in the United States increased from 12 to more than 350. Because the 1970s was an era of social consciousness, many medical students selected family practice as a way to make a contribution to society through medicine.

In the 1980s, the general focus of the country's consciousness gradually shifted away from a social justice perspective. This shift was reflected in medical schools, and medical training focused on the subspecialties. Because the fee-for-service system emphasized payment for procedures, procedure-oriented specialists began earning four to five times more than family physicians. The specialists' increased earning potential turned many individuals away from primary care (family practice, general internal medicine, pediatrics, obstetrics and gynecology). Although 13% of medical students nationwide chose family practice in 1982, by 1991 that number had decreased to 10%.[1] In 1996-1997, 16.6% of medical students chose family practice. In 1999-2000, that percentage had fallen to 12.8%.[2]

Many hospitals, health systems, and health maintenance organization (HMO) plans continue to have positions available in family practice. Family physicians generate lower costs than do subspecialists because they can treat medical problems in all age groups and in all organ systems. Table 29-1 indicates the characteristics of the family physician practice as of May 2000. These primary care physicians not only treat their patients in the outpatient setting but also treat them when hospitalized. In 2000, it was determined that approximately 25% of family practice

Table 29-1 Profile of Family Physicians (May 2000)

Characteristics	Average Per Week
Office visits	94.7
Hospital visits	10.6
Nursing home visits	3.0
House calls	0.4
Hours of patient care–related services in urban area	40.7 hours
Hours of patient care–related services in rural area	41.5 hours
Total hours in practice	50.8 hours

Data from American Academy of Family Physicians. *2001 Facts about family physicians*, Tables 14 and 15, AAFP Practice Profile I Survey. Retrieved from http://www.aafp.org/facts/FactsIndex.xml 24 May 2002.

physicians aided in routine obstetrical deliveries, 51.4% managed their patients in intensive care, 48% managed patients in coronary care settings, and 36% performed minor surgery in the hospital. The salary for family physicians in 1999, as reported in the last survey by the American Academy of Family Practice, indicated a mean of $133,900/year with a range of $113,400 to $152,100.[2]

HISTORY OF INTERNAL MEDICINE

After the Flexner Report was published in 1910, medicine and its specialties evolved rapidly into the system we know today. In 1932, the Commission on Medical Education advised: "A particular identification for those who profess to be specialists should be created." As a result, a number of specialty boards were incorporated between 1932 and 1940. Internal medicine became a board certified specialty with the incorporation of the American Board of Internal Medicine (ABIM) in 1936. The move to specialize quickly found support.[3]

Originally, internists considered all of medicine (except pediatrics and obstetrics and gynecology) their domain. However, as various specialties and subspecialties formed their own boards, the focus of internal medicine narrowed. The ABIM's purpose was to set high standards for the certification of a few internists who would be outstanding consultants ready to receive the referrals of general practice physicians. However, during and after World War II, the incentives (in terms of both prestige and finances) for physicians to become board certified were considerable. Certification soon became the norm.

WHAT IS FAMILY PRACTICE?

Because family physicians exclusively manage more than 90% of the problems they encounter, family practice demands a knowledge base that is greater in breadth than any other specialty. The required broad knowledge base is focused on the most common diagnoses and management, rather than on the less common ones, which may require referral. Family practice physicians are trained to diagnose and treat common problems thoroughly and to recognize an unusual or complex diagnosis at its undifferentiated stage.

Family physicians perform histories and physical examinations, and treat chronic and acute illnesses and conditions in patients of all ages. Additionally, women are seen for their general gynecological problems, annual pelvic examinations, birth control, and prenatal care. Some family physicians do obstetrical deliveries.

Family physicians treat the whole family and focus on the patient as a whole person. They are ideally as much concerned with patients' feelings, family lives, and jobs as they are with patients' presenting complaints or illnesses. The family physician often counsels a patient for the common problems and stresses of living. Some family physicians also counsel couples, perform crisis intervention, and even manage psychotic patients on medications.

Because the family physician provides continuity of care, the patient is able to see the *same* physician on each visit. This enables physicians to know their patients more completely and to develop a deeper healing relationship. When a patient's problems are beyond the scope of the family physician, the patient is referred to one or more subspecialists and care is coordinated by the family physician.

Health care maintenance is an important component of family practice. This includes immunizations and other preventive measures that are age- and disease-specific, including diet, exercise, and relaxation. Providing techniques for handling stress and for expressing sorrow and resentment are very important parts of health maintenance because these unexpressed and unresolved feelings can contribute to the source of an illness.[4]

These key ingredients of continuity of care and health care maintenance allow family physicians to provide less costly health care to their patients. Healthy lifestyles and appropriate screening examinations maintain the health of the patient or allow discovery of the illness in its early stages, when it is less costly to treat. Continuity of care allows the physician to know the patient well and to follow the patient's lifestyle changes or chronic illnesses closely, so that problems are less likely to become out of control and therefore more costly to manage.

WHAT IS INTERNAL MEDICINE?

Although internists are board certified, the specialty is best defined by its approach to medical problems. All practitioners use the history and physical examination to point to the diagnosis. A treatment plan is initiated and followed up so results can be assessed. The internal medicine practitioner's approach is the same as the approach of family practitioners except that each step along the way is more in-depth, with a focus on adult illnesses. The internist's method is to work with a differential diagnosis that begins with the chief complaint and enlarges to account for the various details of the history. The physical examination narrows the differential somewhat and usually helps to rank-order the possibilities. Diagnostic laboratory and radiology further narrow the logical choices. However, with complex problems, a diagnosis may be advanced only tentatively while the patient is followed to observe the cause of the disease. Treatment is often withheld until the diagnosis can be sorted out of the differential with some assurance.

In large measure, the attitudes and methods of internal medicine were created by the "fathers" of medicine, such as William Osler. Many of the "pearls" (e.g., Osler's nodes) now associated with particular diseases were originally "found" in the careful observations of these physicians. In general, internists are slower to reach a diagnosis and are more given to deliberation over the details of the case—more like the methodical detective than the cop on the beat.

Many of the patients followed by an internist have chronic diseases or multiple diseases. Some of these diseases, such as diabetes, need not only treatment but also monitoring for the complications of the disease. Diseases such as rheumatoid arthritis cannot be cured. Much of the art of dealing with patients who have such chronic or multiple diseases is a commitment to the patient during the vagaries of disease. Understanding the natural history and variability of these chronic diseases is important in anticipating the patient's course. Emotional reassurance, a hopeful attitude, negotiating the level of treatment, practical solutions to degrees of disability, and an understanding of the effects on other family members are tools of the successful internist.

PAs EMPLOYED IN FAMILY PRACTICE AND INTERNAL MEDICINE
Historical Perspectives

The PA movement began in the United States in 1965, when the priority for improvement in health care was for the old, the poor, and rural and inner city residents who lacked access to care. The number of physicians in primary care was too low to accommodate all the patients who lacked access to care. One strategy was to increase the number of medical students, but that would not solve the immediate problem.

The PA movement was started in response to this need for access to medical care. All early graduates were trained in primary care, and most worked in primary care practices upon graduation. These early graduates practiced in rural clinics, public health clinics, institutions, prisons, and general and family medicine practices in small communities.[5]

Practice Characteristics of Recent PA Graduates

Over the past 16 years, a mean of 55.8% of new PA graduates entered positions in primary care (family practice, general internal medicine, and general pediatrics) (Table 29-2). In 2000, 53.9% of new graduates entered primary care.[6]

Since 1985, new graduates who have chosen primary care have continued to select family and internal medicine as their top choices. Over the 10 years from 1991 to 2000, an average of 73% of the new graduates who chose to work in primary care chose family medicine and 16% chose general internal medicine. From 1999 to 2000, new graduates entering primary care in family practice have declined from 74.9% to 67.3%, and those entering primary care in internal medicine for the same time period have increased from 14.8% to 21.5% (Table 29-3). Family practice continues to be the most popular specialty in all geographic regions, with the highest percentage of new graduates choosing family practice in the Heartland and the Western regions (Table 29-4).[6]

Salary Range for PAs Working in Family Practice and Internal Medicine

The salary range for PAs graduating in 2000 and working in all specialties indicated a mean of $59,839

Table 29-2 Employment of Recent PA Graduates in Primary and Non-Primary Care Medicine, 1985 through 2000

Academic Year	Primary Care		Non-Primary Care		Total	
	N	%	N	%	N	%
1985-86	399	59.9%	278	41.1%	677	100%
1986-87	404	55.6%	322	44.4%	726	100%
1987-88	418	56.4%	323	43.6%	741	100%
1988-89	422	52.2%	387	47.8%	809	100%
1989-90	398	48.2%	427	51.8%	825	100%
1990-91	508	58.1%	367	41.9%	875	100%
1991-92	511	53.5%	444	46.5%	955	100%
1992-93	674	55.7%	537	44.3%	1211	100%
1993-94	826	58.0%	597	42.0%	1423	100%
1994-95	852	55.5%	684	44.5%	1536	100%
1995-96	817	52.2%	702	44.8%	1566	100%
1996-97	970	62.3%	588	37.7%	1558	100%
1997-98	1046	56.9%	792	43.1%	1838	100%
1998-99	1113	54.5%	928	45.5%	2041	100%
1999-2000	1176	53.7%	1015	46.3%	2191	100%
2000-2001	1143	53.9%	977	46.1%	2120	100%
16-year mean	716	55.8%	570	44.2%	1286	100%

Data from Simon A. Seventeenth Annual Report on Physician Assistant Education in the United States, 2000-2001. Alexandria, VA: Association of Physician Assistant Programs, 2001.

Table 29-3 Trends in the Primary Care Medical Specialty Selection of Recent Graduates, 1991 through 2000

Clinical Specialty	1991 (47)* %	1992 (51)* %	1993 (53)* %	1994 (48)* %	1995 (56)* %	1996 (57)* %	1997 (68)* %	1998 (74)* %	1999 (77)* %	2000 (76)* %
Family medicine	72.2	71.1	71.0	76.0	75.4	73.1	73.2	75.1	74.9	67.3
Internal medicine	14.3	16.3	15.1	16.0	15.4	16.9	17.7	16.3	14.8	21.5
General pediatrics	5.9	5.9	8.4	4.6	5.2	6.4	5.3	5.6	6.8	5.5
Obstetrics and gynecology	7.6	6.7	5.5	3.4	3.1	3.6	3.8	3.0	3.4	5.7

Data from Simon A. Seventeenth Annual Report on Physician Assistant Education in the United States, 2000-2001. Alexandria, VA: Association of Physician Assistant Programs, 2001.
*Number of programs supplying data.

Table 29-4   Medical Specialties Selection by 2000 PA Graduates by Consortia Region

Consortia Region	N†	Family Medicine		Internal Medicine*		Surgery*	
		Mean	(%)	Mean	(%)	Mean	(%)
Northeastern	19	6.9	43.1%	5.0	31.3%	4.1	25.6%
Eastern	10	9.0	54.5%	4.3	26.1%	3.2	19.4%
Southeastern	12	8.3	52.2%	4.2	26.4%	3.4	21.4%
Midwestern	17	13.6	68.0%	3.5	17.5%	2.9	14.5%
Heartland	6	28.8	78.9%	4.9	13.4%	2.8	7.7%
Western	12	13.5	75.8%	3.1	17.4%	1.2	6.7%
Total	76	12.4	62.3%	4.5	22.6%	3.0	15.1%

Data from Simon A. Seventeenth Annual Report on Physician Assistant Education in the United States, 2000-2001. Alexandria, VA: Association of Physician Assistant Programs, 2001.
*Includes subspecialties.
†Number of programs providing data.

Table 29-5   Mean Salary Range for Physician Assistants by Specialty in 2000

Specialty	Mean Salary Range ($)
Emergency medicine	78,898
Family practice without urgent care	65,493-68,191
Family practice with urgent care	68,191
General internal medicine	66,850
Internal medicine (subspecialties)	63,237-79,370
Obstetrics and gynecology	63,690
Occupational medicine	73,879
General pediatrics	67,723
Pediatrics (includes subspecialties)	57,062-76,329
General surgery	70,779
Surgery (subspecialties)	69,004-88,586

Data Services and Statistics. Alexandria, VA: American Academy of Physician Assistants, 2002.

with a standard deviation of $11,063. The mean salary for all practicing PAs responding to a survey of the membership of the American Academy of Physician Assistants (N=13,383) indicated a mean salary of $71,224, with a standard deviation of $18,438. The specialty in which a PA works has an impact on the salary received. Those working in primary care (family practice, general internal medicine, general pediatrics, and obstetrics and gynecology) have mean incomes below the overall mean. The mean yearly salary for PAs working in general surgery is $2588 above the salary for PAs working in family practice with urgent care, and $3929 more than those working in general internal medicine. Table 29-5 depicts an overview of salaries by specialty. This table does not correct for the number of years in practice, for sex, or for geographic region.[7]

In addition to salary, overall financial compensation may include bonuses and a percentage of revenue from patients seen by the PA. In a few cases, the PA is a partner in the practice, although managed care has markedly reduced these situations. Compensation in many settings includes such benefits as professional liability insurance, individual health insurance, disability insurance, term life insurance, state license fees, dues to the American Academy of Physician Assistants, reimbursement for continuing medical education course fees, re-certification fees, and state PA chapter dues.

CHALLENGES AND REWARDS IN FAMILY PRACTICE

PAs in family practice often have their own panel of patients who continually return to them each time they are seen for a medical problem. This affords the patient continuity of care. It also allows the PA the greatest opportunity to know the patient and understand the psychosocial impact of that patient's health.

PAs also treat patients in the context of the family, often treating the children, the parents, and the grandparents in the same family. The opportunity to observe individuals and families as they develop, change, and grow is one of the rewards unique to family practice. Also, identification of stressors in one family member that affect other family members provides insight into the forces contributing to health or illness of the individual. For the clinician, having such a comprehensive picture of the patient is rewarding, in that it removes much of the mystery in discovering the cause of the individual's disease.

Because PAs in family practice treat patients in all age groups, of both sexes, and regarding all organ systems, their care can be very comprehensive and consequently very rewarding. The focus on health maintenance and disease prevention allows PAs in family practice to feel they are making major contributions to the patient's health.

PAs are able to manage 80% to 90% of the outpatients seen in a family practice and consult the physician-supervisor if confronted with an unfamiliar problem. They might also consult if the patient's problem is complicated. PAs in family practice are often involved in the team approach as they work with psychologists, social workers, teachers, medical and surgical specialists, nutritionists, occupational, speech, and physical therapists, and clergy.

Some PAs are involved in the ongoing care of hospitalized patients and many are the major communication link between patients and their families. They may make rounds, write orders on patients, and review cases on a daily basis with the physician. When the patient is ready for discharge, the PA may be involved in discharge planning.

The challenge of working in family practice is its breadth. Maintaining such a large database requires constant discipline. One must also become comfortable with "not knowing all there is to know," acknowledging one's own limits, and requesting guidance.

The case histories that follow provide examples of a typical day for a PA working in family practice. Cases have been chosen that would be treated in family practice and probably would not be treated in internal medicine. If these cases were treated by a subspecialist, health care maintenance and other age-specific patient education might not routinely be discussed.

CASE STUDY 29-1

The first patient, Joan, is a 32-year-old woman with a green malodorous vaginal discharge. She has had the same sexual partner for the past 6 months. She does not think he has any other partners, and he is asymptomatic, as far as she knows. She first noticed this discharge 3 days ago and finds it to be unlike the yeast infections she has had in the past. There has been no itching. For the past 2 days, she has been douching with water. Intercourse last night was too painful to complete.

Joan's last menstrual period was 2 weeks ago and was normal for her. She has never been pregnant. Her method of birth control is "the pill"; her partner does not wear condoms. The patient denies abdominal pain, fever, or chills. She is basically healthy and was feeling well prior to the onset of the vaginal discharge. She has had no surgeries or hospitalizations, takes no medications other than the oral contraceptives, and has no allergies.

She does not appear ill, and her vital signs are normal. On pelvic examination, Bartholin's glands, the urethra, and Skene's glands are normal. The vaginal vault reveals a greenish discharge, which is applied to two slides—one with saline added, and one with KOH. On bimanual examination, no cervical motion tenderness is noted. The uterus is small, firm, and midline. No tenderness or masses are found in the adnexa. The saline slide reveals active trichomonads; the KOH slide is without evidence of yeast.

The diagnosis is *Trichomonas* vaginitis. Joan is treated and cautioned not to drink alcohol while on the medication. She is told *Trichomonas* vaginitis is a sexually transmitted disease. She may have contracted it from her current partner, or it may have been dormant and contracted from a previous relationship. The partner will need to be treated also and cautioned about alcohol. The use of condoms and "safe sex" are discussed. She wants to think about a human immunodeficiency virus (HIV) test and will be tested for syphilis today. *Neisseria gonorrhoeae* and *Chlamydia trachomatis* cultures are also sent to the laboratory.

The patient is surprised that she has a sexually transmitted disease and is concerned about her relationship. She and her partner have been having problems for some time, and she wants to talk with him about this new development. A nonjudgmental approach is discussed.

Because Joan is due for her annual examination, she will make an appointment after her next period. The patient does not need to return for a recheck if the discharge is resolved after she completes the medication. She will call for recommendations if she feels a counselor is needed to help resolve her problems with her partner.

CASE STUDY 29-2

The next patient is John, a 54-year-old man who wants a sebaceous cyst removed from his back because it itches and periodically becomes infected. He is obese, has hypertension, and smokes. He takes an antihypertensive but is not working on the other two health problems. John has never been hospitalized, has had no surgeries, and has no known allergies.

The area of the cyst is cleaned with disinfectant and infiltrated with an anesthetic. The cyst is removed in total. The area is sutured closed, an antibiotic ointment is applied, and the wound is dressed. The patient is educated about signs of infection and is asked to return in 7 days for suture removal.

This patient wants to quit smoking and has had several failed attempts. The attending PA discusses the nicotine skin patch with him, and the patient expresses interest in trying it. When he comes back for the removal of his sutures, diet and exercise will be discussed.

John is lonely since his divorce, and his progress in resolving these issues will also be discussed at the next visit. Often patients do not need counseling as much as they need a neutral person to offer a perspective different from their own. Frequently, patients solve their own problems if they are encouraged to verbalize them.

CASE STUDY 29-3

The next patient, Martin, is a 6-month-old male brought in by his mother for a well-child checkup and immunizations. His mother has no problems to discuss concerning her son. Her pregnancy and labor were uneventful, and she delivered vaginally at 39 weeks. Martin's weight was 7 pounds 13 ounces at birth. He is healthy and awakens every 3.5 hours for a feeding of iron-fortified formula. There are no problems with his feeding, urinating, or defecating.

The PA conducts a review of his developmental milestones. Martin can now roll from back to front, sits well alone, turns to voices, reaches for objects, and passes them from hand to hand. All are appropriate skills for 6 months. This is the third child for this mother, so she is experienced in raising children. The patient's physical examination is normal, with height, weight, and head circumference at the 50th percentile. He is uncircumcised; his foreskin does not retract, and the mother is discouraged from forcibly retracting it. The mother is instructed to observe the foreskin and is told that it usually becomes retractable before 2 years of age.

His immunizations are up-to-date, so today Martin will receive his third set of immunizations. Because there are no problems and Martin is growing well, he will return at 1 year of age for a tuberculin (TB) skin test and hematocrit. The mother is reminded that all electrical outlets need to be plugged, cabinet doors latched, and cleaning solutions put up out of Martin's reach. Martin is not to be left unattended on a bed because he might roll off. The mother is using a car seat and has an emetic at home for accidental poisonings.

CASE STUDY 29-4

The next patient is a 17-year-old high school senior and basketball player who complains of an ankle sprained 2 hours ago. Frank jumped for a basket and came down on the lateral aspect of his left foot. He has applied ice and has been elevating his foot. Frank has had no previous injuries and wonders if his ankle is broken. Although the ankle is swollen, the patient heard no popping when he came down on his foot. He has no other medical problems and no allergies.

The patient hobbles to the examination table. The left ankle is swollen, with point tenderness over the calcaneofibular ligament. The range of motion is restricted by pain, and the patient is able to bear minimal weight on his left foot. There is no reason to think this 17-year-old has fractured his ankle, so it will not be radiographed. The patient is sent home with an elastic wrap on his ankle and on crutches. He will return in 10 days for reevaluation.

On his return visit, some patient education and health maintenance will be done. Frank will be taught to examine his testicles for masses because his age group is most at risk for this form of cancer. His immunizations will be brought up-to-date. Sexuality, smoking, drinking, drugs, and driving will also be discussed. Because adolescents rarely see a health care provider, as much as possible must be done at each visit. With a painful ankle, the patient cannot hear much now, but on his return visit, he will be more comfortable and better able to absorb the information.

Some unhealthful habits are begun in this age group, so it is important to continue education that optimally was begun at a young age. Homicide and suicide are the major causes of death at this age, so

looking for signs of depression or aggression is important. Adolescents resist preaching, and the wording of the message is important.

An internist probably would have referred this patient directly to an orthopedist, who would have treated only his ankle. The pediatrician or family practice clinician is responsible for health maintenance, but he or she can address it only if the opportunity is provided by the patient presenting with an illness or injury.

CASE STUDY 29-5

The next patient, Joseph, is a 27-year-old man who comes in with pain in his right eye. He has been cutting wood with his chain saw and thinks a wood chip hit his eye. He irrigated the eye well with water but feels there is still something in it. His vision is intermittently blurred in that eye. He attributes this condition to the tearing. There are no other injuries. His last tetanus immunization was 2 years ago. Joseph has no medical problems and no known allergies.

The patient's vision will be tested prior to the examination of his eye, so it will be clear that the examination itself does not cause loss of vision. Today his vision is 20/20 in the right eye, the left eye, and both eyes together. His right eye is tearing and red. With fluorescein dye in the eye, a corneal abrasion is observed. The eye is examined for a foreign body and none is found. The patient is told to apply antibiotic drops at home and to return in 2 days for the eye to be checked for infection. At that time, when Joseph is feeling more like listening, abstinence and safe sex will be discussed, and he will be taught to examine his testicles. As with the last patient, homicide and motor vehicle accidents are among the greatest causes of death in this age group, so depression, aggression, drinking, drugs, and driving will be discussed.

CASE STUDY 29-6

The next patient is a 26-year-old woman, Annie, who presents with atopic dermatitis on her hands. She has had this condition for 8 years, and it has improved with the use of a 1% hydrocortisone cream. The affected area has enlarged, and she wants a different treatment because the hydrocortisone is no longer effective. She also has an allergy to penicillin and has hay fever and asthma, but no other medical problems. She is taking birth control pills and has one sexual partner. Her last pelvic examination was 11.5 months ago; her Papanicolaou smear was normal.

On observation, her skin problem appears to be atopic dermatitis and is limited to her hands. Because Annie has no other problems today, the condition will be treated with a stronger steroid cream, and she will be scheduled for an annual examination of her thyroid, heart, lungs, breasts, abdomen, and pelvis and a Pap smear. At that time, her PA will discuss with her safe sex, birth control, breast self-examination, nutrition, drugs, and exercise.

CASE STUDY 29-7

The last patient, Maria, is a 57-year-old obese Hispanic woman complaining of increased thirst and urination without dysuria. She has hypertension, for which she takes an antihypertensive, and has a family history of diabetes. Her husband died 3 months ago, and she is still feeling "down."

Besides her hypertension, Maria is basically healthy. She has lost 10 pounds since her husband's death. Her appetite has improved a little, but she continues to awaken at 2:00 AM and cannot return to sleep. She always feels fatigued and has little interest in seeing her friends. The patient does continue to go to church. She has one son in the area, who is an attorney for the state and is very busy, so Maria does not see him as often as she would like.

Her random blood sugar today is 363 mg%, blood pressure is 140/85, pulse is 82, and respirations are 16; her height is 5 feet, 4 inches, and her weight is 180 pounds. Her heartbeat is regular without murmurs, her pulses are good, and her lungs are clear. She has no lesions on her feet.

During this visit, an oral diabetic agent is prescribed, and the importance of diet and weight loss is discussed. The patient is encouraged to undertake an exercise program of walking 20 minutes 5 days per week. She has not modified her salt

intake and eats a high-cholesterol diet with much pork, refried beans, and tortillas. The impact of her diet on both hypertension and diabetes is explained. In the future, she will be sent to a dietitian for a culturally relevant diet.

The next visit will include a discussion of the importance of keeping her toenails trimmed and noticing if sores on her feet resist healing. Sometimes the health educator rather than the PA does this teaching.

Maria has been encouraged to attend a community support group on grieving and loss, but she has not done so. Is Maria fatigued from lack of sleep or because of her diabetes, or is she depressed? Her appointment will be a long one, and the PA or the family physician will talk to her about grieving. The provider will discuss with Maria her feelings about her husband and his death, so she can express some of her grief. The grieving process itself will also be discussed again. During this visit, her blood sugar will be checked. On the third visit, home monitoring of the patient's blood glucose levels will be discussed, and her diet and exercise will again be evaluated. Her psychological well-being will also be discussed on this visit.

CHALLENGES AND REWARDS IN INTERNAL MEDICINE

The PA in internal medicine works in the same collegial relationship that is found in other branches of medicine. The routine day includes seeing patients, taking histories, performing examinations, ordering diagnostic aids, prescribing courses of treatment, and arranging follow-up. Additionally, the internal medicine PA may make nursing home visits or hospital rounds or may perform special procedures such as treadmill tests or flexible sigmoidoscopies. However, internal medicine PAs generally see fewer patients per day than do PAs in other specialties. Many of the patients are in the age range of 50 to 100 years. Histories are taken more slowly and are often augmented with history from a spouse or caretaker. Examinations are thorough, with a search for subtle clues to subacute or uncommon chronic diseases. More time is taken to educate the patient about the possibilities, the workup, and the various potential outcomes. Treatment plans are often not so clear-cut. The benefits and risks of a treatment plan are discussed, and the choice is negotiated.

Many internal medicine PAs develop areas of special knowledge or skill such as treadmill testing, diabetic education, or arthritis management. The outlook for internal medicine PAs is generally excellent. Many group practices and multi-specialty clinics are finding PAs a welcome addition. Because PAs share the load of routine cases, internists are free to spend more time at the hospital or on more difficult cases.

A typical day for a PA in an internal medicine practice might include the following cases:

CASE STUDY 29-8

Joyce, a 34-year-old woman with non–insulin-dependent diabetes, comes in with a 3-day history of profuse rhinorrhea, sinus congestion, irritated throat, and dry cough. She has had fevers to 101.2° F. She reports no facial pain, stiff neck, chest pain, shortness of breath, joint pain, rash, or wheezing. Physical examination reveals postnasal drainage but little else. Her blood sugars, usually well controlled, have been running in the low- to mid-200s during her illness. A diagnosis of viral upper respiratory tract infection is entered in her chart, and she is given advice for symptomatic treatment at home. She is further instructed to increase her glyburide from 5 mg twice a day (bid) to 10 mg bid until her sugars return to levels below 140 mg.

CASE STUDY 29-9

Randy, a 37-year-old male, is scheduled for a complaint of palpitations. He has noted episodes of skipped beats occurring randomly, but more and more frequently over the past 3 weeks. He was diagnosed 3 years earlier with mitral valve prolapse. He has no history of hypertension, chest pain, shortness of breath, exercise intolerance, or edema. He is a nonsmoker, consumes little or no caffeine, and has not consumed over-the-counter stimulants.

On examination, the only positive finding is a midsystolic click without a murmur. An electrocardiogram demonstrates a normal sinus rhythm of 68 and no extrasystole. The patient is reassured. Further discussion reveals that the patient has been under considerable stress while interviewing for and beginning a new job. A brief counseling session on the effects of and methods for ameliorating stress ensues. He is advised to return in 10 days with the assurance that he may return sooner if symptoms continue. Chart review notes a normal thyroid-stimulating hormone (TSH) done with his yearly examination 2 months ago.

CASE STUDY 29-10

The next patient, Carter, 55 years old, is returning for the results of laboratory and x-ray tests ordered the previous week. He was seen for a painless lump in the right axilla measuring 2.5 × 2 × 4 cm. Two nontender lymph nodes, one in each axilla, were also noted. There were no cervical, epitrochlear, supraclavicular, or inguinal nodes. The liver and spleen were not palpable. He had had no history of weight loss, rashes, joint pain, fevers, or night sweats. His chest x-ray showed no adenopathy or bony or lung lesions. The complete blood count (CBC) gave no evidence of anemia, infection, or eosinophilia. Reexamination confirmed a subcutaneous, slightly firm mass with the "slipping" sign, indicating a lipoma. Reassurance is given along with an explanation of the benign nature of lipomas.

CASE STUDY 29-11

The patient with an 11:00 AM appointment is a new patient, Emerson, 52 years old, who comes in because of concern about a lingering dry cough. An antecedent upper respiratory infection resolved after a few days, but a mild dry cough continued. More importantly, the patient's blood pressure is 170/100. The patient's father died of myocardial infarction at age 49. Emerson had been told on several occasions that his blood pressure was elevated, but he had not been diagnosed as having hypertension.

Over the past 2 years, he has gained 40 pounds. The patient has no regular exercise habits, although he plays softball occasionally on the weekends.

He admits to considerable job stress and a smoking habit that has gone from one pack per day to two over the past year. Further questioning reveals that the patient has been consuming a fifth of vodka per week.

The remainder of the visit is dedicated to counseling regarding alcohol abuse and cardiovascular risk factors. The patient acknowledges a "drinking problem" and his desire to stop. He is referred to Alcoholics Anonymous and is scheduled to return in 1 week for a follow-up blood pressure check and discussion of his alcohol use. Smoking cessation will be addressed in later visits because Emerson says that he can't conceive of not smoking while trying to quit drinking.

CASE STUDY 29-12

The first afternoon patient is a 77-year-old woman, Dora, with a 3-day history of nausea and vomiting, once or twice a day. Her diagnoses include non–insulin-dependent diabetes, hypertension, hypothyroidism, and recent aortic and mitral valve replacements. The patient reached the on-call physician over the weekend and was prescribed an antiemetic. She believes that she has the "flu" but is concerned because she is not getting better. She reports no fever, chills, joint pain, diarrhea, constipation, hematemesis, chest pain, shortness of breath, cough, PND, abdominal pain, or peripheral edema. The medications, some prescribed by the cardiac surgeon, include antihypertensives, digoxin, Lasix, hypoglycemics, thyroxine, and potassium.

Initial examination reveals a blood pressure of 108/66 and a pulse of 48. An electrocardiogram shows new ST and T wave changes in I, aVL, and V_3 through V_6. The supervising physician is notified, and the patient is admitted to the hospital for suspicion of myocardial infarction and possible digitalis toxicity. The history and physical examination findings are dictated by the PA.

CASE STUDY 29-13

Somewhat behind schedule because of arranging the admission of the previous patient, the PA goes on to the next room to see a 28-year-old man, Jarvis, who has burning epigastric pain. He has several first-degree relatives with peptic ulcer disease. Sheepishly, he admits to taking their Tagamet on and off over the past few months. The pattern of his history is consistent with acid peptic disease. Fortunately, he does not smoke.

A review of his past history is remarkable for partial small-bowel resection 5 years earlier from Crohn's disease. He has done well since his surgery and has not returned to his gastroenterologist for more than 3 years. After a brief examination, the majority of the visit is spent discussing the importance of follow-up for Crohn's disease, given its indolent nature and possible serious sequelae.

CASE STUDY 29-14

Several patients are seen with the upper respiratory tract "virus-of-the-month" infections. They are known to the practice and are otherwise medically stable. They need only reassurance that signs of sinusitis, bronchitis, and pneumonia are absent.

The last patient of the day is a 62-year-old man, Alan, with complaints of "blood in the urine" and burning on urination. His symptoms have been intermittent for 2 days without fever, chills, rash, or abdominal or back pain. He denies a history of new sexual contact or local trauma. He has no prior history of urinary tract infections, prostatic enlargement, or symptoms of prostatic hypertrophy.

Examination of the back, abdomen, genitals, and prostate is unrevealing. Cultures for *Neisseria gonorrhoeae* and *Chlamydia trachomatis* are taken. A urinalysis is requested. The patient is given doxycycline on a suspicion of *Chlamydia* infection. Results of the urinalysis, available after the patient leaves, demonstrate motile trichomonads. A note to call the patient with the additional results and Rx for metronidazole is placed in the patient's chart, as is a note to further discuss possible treatment for his sexual partner.

THE FUTURE FOR PAs IN FAMILY PRACTICE AND GENERAL INTERNAL MEDICINE

Using the standard developed by the Council on Graduate Medical Education (COGME) for optimum generalist physician–to–population requirement (80 generalist physicians for a population of 100,000),

Lurie and associates predict the generalist optimum physician current supply of 69/100,000 will grow to 85/100,000 by 2025 if the number of medical school graduates choosing primary care continues at current levels.[8]

These calculations are contradicted by other groups. In 1999, COGME commissioned several papers for the purpose of exploring the need for generalist providers by 2005. Libby and colleagues found that based on the lowest COGME standards for adequate generalist physicians per 100,000 population (60/100,000), regardless of type of third party payer, and considering the doubling of nonphysician providers, there will be a deficit of generalist physicians in 2005.[9]

In another paper commissioned by COGME, Colwill and co-workers projected that if family practice residents graduate at the current rate, there would be 34.4 generalists/100,000 population in 2020, still short of the lowest COGME standard of 60 generalists per 100,000 population.[10]

With the exception of the paper by Libby and associates, these predictions do not include in their calculations the nonphysician clinicians. Seventy five hundred nurse practitioners (NPs) graduated in 1999. By 2005, there will be more than 115,000 NPs in clinical practice, a number similar to that of the family physician. By 2015, the number of NPs will reach 170,000. Most NPs are trained and practice in various areas of primary care. Other potential generalist providers include PAs. It is projected that the number of practicing PAs will grow to 62,000 by 2005 and to 100,000 by 2015.[11] If the current trend continues, at least half of these will choose primary care.

Regardless of the accuracy of predictions of undersupply or oversupply of generalist health care providers, the lack of availability of such providers will likely continue in medically underserved geographic areas and with underserved populations of the inner city and rural areas.[12] Every state continues to have state and federally designated underserved sites, populations, and areas. Some of the underserved sites and areas include the following:

➤ Community health centers.
➤ Migrant health centers.
➤ Health care for the homeless grantees.
➤ Public housing primary care grantees.
➤ Certified rural health clinics.
➤ National Health Service Corps sites.
➤ Indian Health Service sites.
➤ Federally qualified health centers.
➤ Primary medical care health professional shortage areas (HPSAs).
➤ State or local health departments.
➤ Ambulatory practice sites designated by state governors.

Albert Simon,[13] Director of the Department of Physician Assistant Sciences at Saint Francis University, points out that in order to have a job in the new job market, a PA will need to be:

1. Technically competent, which will include functioning as a case manager and overseeing a large group of patients who may be monitored by in-home devices.
2. Oriented toward consumer satisfaction. Consumers have many choices and will leave the health plan if they are not satisfied.
3. Flexible. Generalist training is more important than ever. PAs need to be able to adapt to changing assignments throughout their careers.
4. Excellent communicators. Communication with patients will be all-important, including communication through video and electronic media.
5. Innovative. PAs need to constantly monitor their performance, working to be more time-efficient while providing quality care as judged by the consumer. The consumer, not the provider, will be the determiner of quality.
6. Multi-skilled. PAs need to bring not only their generalist training but additional skills to the practice.
7. Technologically competent. PAs need to constantly adapt to new technologies.
8. Visionary. PAs need to be able to look into the future and predict what will be needed to compete well in a few years, in 5 years, and in 10 years. The health care system is not going to be static. This is a very difficult task that requires PAs to be constantly observing and staying informed.

In addition, PAs in the 21st century must be lifelong learners and must be able to critically evaluate the medical literature.

CONCLUSION

With the advancing technology of the computer, handheld personal digital assistants, and telemedicine, many more diagnoses will be managed by protocols prepared by experts. These technologies will be of great assistance to PAs in rural areas and other sites with physician backup great distances away. Because it is less difficult to entice PAs to live in these areas than it is family practice doctors or general internists, these technological advancements will bring an improvement in care to the patients in these areas.

Access to continuing education for clinicians in the very rural areas, especially when there is only one provider in the community, can be problematic. However, Internet-delivered continuing medical education and computer-assisted information retrieval systems will allow even rural practitioners to practice high-quality medicine. Regardless of which prediction for future numbers of generalist providers becomes a reality, new graduates would do well to focus on primary care and on serving underserved and rural populations.

CLINICAL APPLICATIONS

1. If you worked in family practice or general internal medicine, how would you formulate a plan to stay current with the medical knowledge needed for these practice settings?
2. How would you work on improving your counseling skills to help patients with a variety of mental health problems and life adjustment issues? For example, how would you counsel the patient, Randy, in Case Study 29-9 and Emerson in Case Study 29-11?
3. What do you think you would find most challenging and most satisfying about working as a PA in family medicine and in internal medicine?

REFERENCES

1. Schmittling G, Graham R, Hejduk G. Entry of U.S. medical school graduates into family practice residencies: 1990- 1991, and ten-year summary. Fam Med 1991;23:297.
2. American Academy of Family Physicians. Facts about Family Practice 2001. Available at http://www.aafp.org/facts.xml. Accessed 15 July 2002.
3. Howell JD. The invention and development of American internal medicine. J Gen Intern Med 1989;4:127.
4. Siegel B. Love, Medicine and Miracles. New York: Harper & Row, 1986.
5. Schafft GE, Cawley JF. The Physician Assistant in a Changing Health Care Environment. Rockville, MD: Aspen Publishers, 1987.
6. Simon A. Seventeenth Annual Report on Physician Assistant Education in the United States, 2000-2001. Alexandria, VA: Association of Physician Assistant Programs, 2001.
7. American Academy of Physician Assistants Data Services and Statistics. Unpublished raw data. Alexandria, VA: Association of Physician Assistant Programs, 2001.
8. Lurie JD, Goodman DC, Wennberg JE. Benchmarking the future generalist workforce. Eff Clin Pract 2002;5:95.
9. Libby D, Kindig D. Estimates of physicians needed to supply underserved Americans adequately until universal coverage. In Council on Graduate Medical Education, Resource Paper Compendium: Update on the physician workforce. Washington, DC: U.S. Department of Health and Human Services Health Resources and Services Administration, August 2000.
10. Colwill JM, Cultice J. Increasing numbers of family physicians—implications for rural America. In Council on Graduate Medical Education, Resource Paper Compendium: Update on the physician workforce. Washington, DC: U.S. Department of Health and Human Services Health Resources and Services Administration, August 2000.
11. Cooper RA. Health care workforce for the twenty-first century: the impact of nonphysician clinicians. Annu Rev Med 2001;52:51.
12. Bureau of Health Professions, Health Resources and Services Administration, Public Health Service of the U.S. Department of Health and Human Services. Market forces: are they working for the nation's vulnerable? Newslink 1997;3:1.
13. Simon A. A glimpse of the future. In: Proceedings from Defining the Future Characteristics of Physician Assistant Education. Alexandria, VA: Association of Physician Assistant Programs, 1996.

RESOURCES

American Academy of Family Physicians. Facts About Family Practice 2001. Available at http://www.aafp.org/facts.xml. Accessed 15 July 2002. *"Facts about Family Practice" delineates various aspects of family practice as presented by the American Academy of Family Practice.*

Simon A. Seventeenth Annual Report on Physician Assistant Education in the United States, 2000-2001. Alexandria, VA: Association of Physician Assistant Programs, 2001. *This yearly report is based on information from PA programs and includes demographics of the clinical practice of new graduates.*

American Academy of Physician Assistants Web Site Data and Statistics Section. Available at http://www.aapa.org/research/index.html. Accessed 15 July 2002. *Data from the annual survey of PAs in clinical practice who are members of the American Academy of Physician Assistants are reported on this web site.*

CHAPTER 30

Emergency Medicine

David J. Pillow, Jr. and Edward M. Sullivan

INTRODUCTION

Many people can relate a vivid story involving themselves or a family member in an emergency room (ER). From personal experience to syndicated TV programs, the stories of life and death drama that take place in a busy ER can be both exhilarating and traumatic for patients and providers alike. Health care providers will experience a high level of anxiety from their own personal experiences as well as from the stories they have heard from their co-workers. Patients seeking treatment in an ER usually expect the worst, and each visit can be terrifying. Expectations are always high for both, and striving for a good outcome is always the main objective. It is the purpose of this chapter to give the ER provider some basic information that will help dissipate some of the concerns and fears and will provide some explanations for the stories that circulate through the medical ER circle.

With the formation of the American College of Emergency Physicians (ACEP) in 1968, the ER gained recognition not only as a clinical specialty but also as an academic discipline. As such, some 10 years later, the word "room" was dropped and the discipline matured into a full "academic department."

The first emergency medicine residency training program was established at the University of Cincinnati in 1970, and 12 years later, specific requirements for emergency medicine training programs were approved by the Accreditation Council for Graduate Medical Education. In keeping with this philosophy, the PA profession has, from its inception, required emergency medicine education as part of the curriculum. Additionally, postgraduate residency programs for those PAs who desire more training in this specialty have been developed.

The emergency department (ED) health care philosophy has changed over the past 30 years. The ED is now viewed more as the property of the community at large than as a for-profit medical facility providing a specifically designed service. Some patients view the ED as an outpatient or family practice walk-in clinic rather than a true emergency department. Because of this attitude, some patients may perceive their problem as urgent and feel that their very presence in the ED is sufficient to categorize their complaint as an emergency. Additionally, ED personnel adhere to an unwritten law that "the patient defines the emergency," regardless of the true nature of the illness or injury. To accommodate these attitudes and to take care not to injure a patient, EDs are open 24 hours a day, 7 days a week, 365 days a year.

In view of this changing attitude, ED personnel have had to adjust their treatment philosophy to handle the increased patient load. To meet this increased demand, hospital-based EDs began to employ full-time emergency medicine physicians to staff their EDs. As this practice became more prevalent, a few visionary physicians formed organizations to provide emergency services on a contract basis and began to hire physicians to support these contracts.

One such organization is the Metroplex Emergency Physicians Association (MEPA) based in Dallas, Texas. MEPA was founded in 1979 by Dr. Ron Hellstern, an emergency medicine physician, to provide competent health care for five area hospitals.[1] His guiding principle is to provide high-quality, patient-friendly, cost-effective, and convenient urgent and emergent medical care. He established the team concept, with communication and coordination among all the members as a high priority. Members of the team vary but usually consist of an emergency medicine physician, a mid-level practitioner (physician assistant [PA]) or nurse practitioner (NP), staff nurses, technicians, and administrative/clerical staff. The MEPA policy manual states, "The goal of the MEPA physicians and mid-level practitioners must be committed to the service ethic. This means that each health care provider will voluntarily accept responsibility for making medical care understandable and reassuring for the patients, and that all MEPA employees will strive to deliver the needed medical care in a warm and supportive manner."[2] MEPA currently employs 150 physicians and 30 mid-level practitioners, and supports 22 contracts in a five-state area, 14 of which are in the Dallas–Fort Worth area alone.

PRINCIPLES OF EMERGENCY MEDICINE

The emergency medicine approach to patient care is an important concept to understand because it is unique within the health care system. It is primarily a *complaint-oriented* rather than a *disease-specific* specialty. The objective is to focus on the single most important reason the patient has reported to the ED. This philosophy may, at times, seem uncaring, but it is necessary for quick, correct treatment and the smooth functioning of the ED. The provider must be able to get to the "bottom line" as quickly as possible, rule out life- or limb-threatening conditions, and complete the patient's stay in the ED in a timely fashion.

To aid in decision making, the American College of Emergency Physicians and the emergency medical system (EMS) established some general principles governing the practice of emergency medicine. This set of principles can be found in some form or another in all the classic emergency medicine texts.[3] Practitioners and students alike routinely exercise these principles in developing a foundation in emergency medicine that will aid in their approach to all patients seen in the ED.

Triage

Triage is the sorting of patients according to their specific health care needs and matching those needs with the ability of a specific ED to provide that care. Most EDs are equipped to treat any patients regardless of their complaint. However, those who cannot be treated in a given ED are stabilized and transferred, usually by ambulance or helicopter, to a medical center that can better serve their condition.

General Emergency Department Principles

Unfortunately, many of the patients seen in the ED do not conform to established algorithms, which usually leaves the health care provider frustrated and confused. The following general principles were established to give the provider some basis to start the evaluation when a patient enters the ED. These principles should be used as *guidelines only*.

1. **Identify a life-threatening condition.** The moment the patient presents to the ED, the possibility of a life-threatening condition must be ruled out. This attitude is deliberately cultivated by health care providers in emergency medicine. The patient is considered unstable until demonstrated otherwise, usually by history, physical examination, and laboratory evaluation (e.g., electrocardiography [ECG], x-rays, and blood studies). Health care providers in the ED must be able to identify those patients in need of immediate lifesaving intervention, must be able to initiate those measures, and must solicit the assistance of all ED staff in stabilizing the patient to reverse a life-threatening condition.

2. **Stabilize a life-threatening condition.** This is the mandate for prehospital care through the

EMS as well as all ED personnel. How this is done is usually as individual as the patients themselves. Stabilizing measures are the subject of courses in advanced cardiac life support (ACLS) and advanced trauma life support (ATLS), and of the paramedic manual and the first third of most ED textbooks. ACLS and ATLS courses are open to most mid-level practitioners and play a leading role in initial life-saving management of an unstable patient. The role of the mid-level practitioner in this setting can vary from one ED to another and from one supervising physician to another, but the learned life-saving measures are standard and reliable with any unstable patient. All ED health care providers should be certified in ACLS at the minimum.

3. **Find an explanation for the life-threatening condition.** Once the patient is stable, the health care provider should develop a differential diagnosis for the condition and coexistent disease that may still result in a life-threatening consequence. Once this has been initiated, the health care provider can then consider other medical needs of the patient. When this phase begins, the patient can be considered truly stable.

4. **Recognize coexistent pathology.** This may be related to the original complaint, or it may be an incidental finding during the history and physical examination. For example, the patient who has been seen in the ED on numerous occasions for alcohol abuse may have other alcohol-related disease that will need follow-up after the patient has been discharged from the ED.

5. **Determine why the patient has presented *now* rather than earlier or later.** The answer to this question may reveal a great deal about the course of the patient's pathology and may present important information about the patient's mental, physical, emotional, and social reserves for dealing with illness. Consider the following examples.

CASE STUDY 30-1

A patient with known coronary artery disease experiences daily angina and presents by ambulance to the ED. The usual questions on character of pain, location, radiation, and duration fail to reveal any difference in this episode of chest pain from the patient's usual experience of angina. Further questioning reveals that the patient has experienced three episodes of numbness and weakness of the right arm over the past 2 hours. The review of systems may have revealed these new symptoms, but direct questions such as "What is different now?" and "What made you call the ambulance?" can give the patient an avenue for short-circuiting the usual pattern of questions.

CASE STUDY 30-2

A woman who has had a vaginal discharge for 2 weeks reports to the ED because "that's when she could get a babysitter for her children and a ride to the hospital."

CASE STUDY 30-3

Another patient reports to the ED with difficulty breathing. When questioned, he relates that he has lost his job and has run out of his seizure medication and cannot afford a refill.

In each case, the health care provider should be able to follow a clear sequence of events that logically led the patient to the ED door. If this is not clear, the provider should ask, "Why now?"

6. **Address the patient's symptoms.** Every effort should be made to relieve the patient's complaint whether by medication or by treatment (e.g., suturing a laceration or simple reassurance). If, however, the patient's symptoms cannot be relieved in the ED, the patient may need hospitalization or referral to another physician whose specialty may include the patient's findings. *Every patient leaving the ED should have the name of a physician who has been identified to follow up his or her complaint.*

7. **Consider the necessity for determining a diagnosis before the patient leaves the ED.** To the disappointment of patients as well as the health care provider, some patients leave the ED with no definitive diagnosis. The health care provider can make every effort to find the cause of the patient's complaint, but in some cases, it is just impossible. What the patient should

receive in these cases is an explanation of the diseases and conditions that have been ruled out. Consider the patient with painless vaginal bleeding. She may leave the ED knowing that she is not pregnant, she is not anemic, she does not have a readily identifiable disease, and she has a follow-up appointment the next day with a gynecologist, but no definitive diagnosis. Each ED patient should be informed of what has been discovered about his or her condition and what remains to be investigated; he or she should be reassured that the condition is not life threatening and should be told what can be done for the symptoms, and where the patient should go to pursue a diagnosis if one has not been rendered.

8. **Decide on the patient's disposition.** Can hospitalization provide more of the patient's needs at this time than an outpatient setting? How will follow-up be accomplished? Does the ED have the resources for the necessary follow-up? What is the worst case scenario of the patient's condition if the patient is lost to follow-up? These questions should have answers, and the patient or the patient's family must have a clear understanding of "where to go from here," if necessary.

9. **Discuss the ED course and the plan for follow-up with the patient and his or her family.** What are the patient's expectations? Have they been met? Patients need to know that the health care provider has understood their concerns and expectations. Each patient should be given the opportunity to ask questions and participate in his or her own health care. The patient should be told what to anticipate from the therapy prescribed, what type of adverse effects to expect, if any, and when and where to obtain needed follow-up.

10. **Record the entire visit in the patient's record.** Document *all* the information gathered during the patient's stay in the ED. Remember, the health care provider is responsible for knowing the information in the nursing record as well.

It is quickly obvious that patients' reasons for coming to the ED are many and varied. Although patients may label their medical problems as "emergencies," only a small percentage of visits to an ED fit that medical definition. Medical emergencies fall into three commonly recognized categories—*critical, acute,* and *urgent.*

➤ *Critical* or life-threatening emergencies are those that require reversal of the pathologic state within minutes in order to prevent the patient's death, for example, cardiac arrest, airway obstruction, or severe hemorrhage.

➤ *Acute* emergencies are conditions that will deteriorate into critical emergencies if therapy is not instituted within the first hour of the patient's presenting to the ED, for example, pulmonary edema, acute asthma, or ruptured ectopic pregnancy.

➤ *Urgent* emergencies can be described as disease processes or injuries that have the potential to progress to life-threatening conditions, if untreated. This category includes pneumonia with hypoxia, small-bowel obstruction, testicular torsion, acetaminophen overdose, acute glaucoma, and periorbital cellulitis. The provider who is geared psychologically and educationally only to take care of "emergencies" will be at odds with the patient who comes to the ED with a non-emergent complaint.

The Role of Mid-Level Health Care Providers in the Emergency Department

Mid-level practitioners—PAs, and NPs—work not only with a variety of patients but with a combination of other physician-supervisors, nurses, clerks, and consultants. They must possess a great deal of tact and skill in communicating and in coordinating patients' care with these other caregivers and providers. In emergency medicine, as in medicine in general, there may be several ways to treat a given disease process. Because the patient is always referred to another physician for follow-up, the patient's care becomes the responsibility of more than one provider. The emergency department PA must be able to balance a variety of therapeutics and referring physicians' preferences and remain an advocate for the individual patient's circumstances. Also, the PA should become familiar with each physician on the referral list so that when the patient reports for follow-up, all pertinent information (i.e., history, physical examination, laboratory tests, x-ray results plus any specific tests unique to the referred physician) is present in the patient's record.

One of the attractions of ED work for PAs is the lack of predictability. Not only is the flow of patients variable, but the diagnoses and complaints are equally challenging. The PA is in the unique position to learn from everyone, especially the patients. The following examples illustrate this axiom. A patient who speaks only Russian may be on adequate therapy for gastritis despite the fact that the tablets are unfamiliar and the writing on the bottle is in Russian. The sickle cell patient who knows his disease and symptoms reports that morphine and not Demerol (meperidine) works better for a painful crisis. If a patient's chief complaint is chest pain, regardless of the patient's age, cardiac disease must be ruled out. Making a diagnosis may be only part of the job; discovering the patient's "agenda" is equally important.

The role of the PA in emergency medicine is evolving, and practice will continue to vary from academic, urban-based emergency medicine to rural, single-coverage sites. In 1990, the American College of Emergency Physicians published the following position statement on the use of PAs in emergency medicine: "The PA is called on to be flexible as well as in his or her role in the ED. Sometimes a leader, but always a member of the health care team, a PA needs to communicate well on all levels."[4] The PA who continues to work in emergency medicine will grow in clinical knowledge and find variations in treatment modalities for each individual patient. At each level, from student to experienced emergency clinician, the PA needs to identify resources within and outside the department to complement his or her skills.

PAs are currently providing services in a variety of positions within emergency departments, including those in prehospital patient care, patient triage, and patient care within the ED, as well as selective administrative functions. To further assist its members, ACEP has developed the following guidelines regarding the role of PAs in emergency departments that are open and staffed 24 hours a day by emergency physicians.[5] These guidelines should not be interpreted as mandatory by legislative, judicial, or regulatory bodies or by the ACEP.

1. PAs should be placed in clinical and administrative situations where they will supplement, but not replace, the medical expertise and patient care provided by emergency physicians.

2. PAs should work clinically under the supervision of an emergency physician who is physically present in the ED, who evaluates the care of each patient, and who assumes ultimate responsibility for the patient. The number of PAs whose clinical work can be simultaneously supervised by one emergency physician must be defined.

3. The PA's scope of practice must be clearly delineated. Minimally, this delineation should include:
   a. A description of the PA's role and responsibilities in the ED.
   b. A listing of the types of patients and conditions the PA has credentials to treat.
   c. A listing of the types of patients and conditions the PA may not treat.
   d. A listing of the types of patients and conditions that require immediate consultation with the supervising emergency physician.
   e. A listing of the procedures the PA may perform prior to or after consultation with the emergency physician, and those he or she may perform only under the direct supervision of the emergency physician.

4. Credentialing procedures must be specifically stated and should be similar to those required of other allied health professionals. All emergency department PAs should be nationally certified or should meet the requirements of the state or federal jurisdiction in which they function.

5. The medical director of the ED or a designee has the responsibility for providing the overall direction of the activities of the PA in the ED.

6. PAs working in EDs should have or acquire specific experience or specialty training in emergency medicine. They should receive a supervised orientation program preferably by the medical director of the ED and appropriate training and continuing education in emergency medicine. They should also acquire knowledge of specific ED policies and procedures. Additionally, PAs must be aware of and participate in the quality assurance activities of the ED.

7. There should be a written contract that clearly addresses all of the items previously listed and other standard contractual issues.

Fast Track

In order to meet the increasing demands of the community and to accommodate the changing philosophies of emergency medicine, many of the busiest EDs have created an "Urgent Care Clinic" or a "Fast Track" within the physical confines of the ED. These areas are specifically designed for the treatment of minor injuries or illnesses that do not require the full services of the ED. EDs that are treating more than 2000 patients a month have discovered that setting aside one or two beds that are used solely for this designation can greatly relieve the congestion in waiting rooms where patients have had to wait sometimes 4 to 6 hours for treatment of a simple laceration.

The fast track area has traditionally been located in a region of the ED that previously was used only for overflow on busy nights, or a back room or a wide hallway converted to a treatment area by adding a few beds and some curtains. In newer EDs, this area may be physically set apart from the regular ED and occasionally may even have its own entrances and waiting rooms. This fast track area has become the domain of the PA for the treatment of minor, uncomplicated diseases and injuries.

The types of patients seen and treated in a fast track vary, but some of the more common diagnoses are sprains, simple fractures, simple lacerations, uncomplicated otitis media, colds, cough, sore throat, bronchitis, ingrown toenails, foreign body in the foot or hand, low back pain, abscessed tooth, uncomplicated urinary tract infection, rashes, minor cellulitis, uncomplicated diarrhea, insect bites, minor dog bites, first- and second degree burns, simple abscesses, poison ivy rash, motor vehicle accident with minor injuries brought to the ED for evaluation, and aches and pains from shoulders to feet.

In all of these cases, the PA in the fast track has the ability to upgrade a patient from fast track to full ED if the patient's condition should warrant more complicated treatment or additional evaluation. The most valuable asset to the ED with a fast track is a good triage nurse who can spot a potentially bad situation and route that patient to the main ED for appropriate treatment.

The PA Student in the Emergency Department

The emergency medicine rotation is usually one of the most enjoyable for the PA student, regardless of the intended future direction of his or her career. The student is very likely to see a variety of patients and diseases. Additionally, the student learns by being available to listen to the many presentations made by other team members to the supervising physician. Typically in an academic institution, the PA student has more contact with the staff physician and the senior emergency resident than on any other inpatient service. This is a distinct advantage when performing procedures, correlating laboratory results with clinical presentation, confirming physical findings, and interpreting imaging studies. The staff physician and the senior resident provide guidance and suggestions unavailable in textbooks, especially during treatment, and referral options based on their accumulated clinical experience.

As a PA student gains skill in the practice of emergency medicine, it may help to identify staff members who will encourage and support the development of the PA's clinical judgment and who will also endorse the expansion of his or her responsibilities in the ED. The relationship between the emergency medicine physician and the emergency medicine PA must be based on mutual trust of each other's integrity and abilities.

It is impossible to generalize about the role of the PA student in a particular ED. However, the following suggestions may help make the experience smoother and more meaningful:
1. Identify the immediate supervisor.
2. Are there protocols restricting the type of patients PA students can or cannot see?
3. At what point in the workup should the student present the case to the supervisor?
4. What are the protocols for unstable patients?
5. What laboratory studies is the PA student able to order without first consulting the supervisor?
6. When do PA student orders have to be co-signed?
7. At the end of the shift, to whom does the PA student report?

The PA student should keep in mind that each rotation is not just an opportunity to learn a different branch of medicine but a chance to evaluate each field for possible employment. It is also a time to reflect on that specialty's approach to the patient, the pace and rhythm of the discipline's work, and its present and potential utilization of PAs.

Who's Who in the Emergency Department

Personnel in Table 30-1 might be found in a hospital-based ED with a level I trauma center and an associated residency training program with elaborate social services support.

The ED in a small rural community will have a completely different makeup, that is, minimal staffing of a physician or mid-level practitioner and a nurse. Most EDs fall somewhere between these two extremes.

The role and functions of a PA in the ED are affected by the types and numbers of other providers. The PA may work with a single physician and split the patients according to severity, or he or she may be required to see all patients and then present the findings to a staff physician whose only function is to consult and advise.

Residents The presence of physician residents adds another dimension to an ED practice. A full-time emergency department PA can provide consistency and stability in a department that is in constant change with rotating interns and residents. The PA who has been employed in an academic ED for any length of time must now take on the additional task of teacher.

Primary Care Providers Community primary care providers and specialists play a significant role in the smooth functioning of all EDs. Ideally, each patient should have a primary care physician or clinic where they usually seek their first medical treatment. Additionally, every primary care physician expects to see his or her patients after an ED visit. Specialists, on the other hand, depend on consults from the ED staff. All of this requires a tremendous amount of communication. Regardless of the care given in the ED, it is important that the ED professional staff stress the continuing role of the primary care physician and encourage the patient to return to his or her primary care physician as soon as possible after an ED visit.

Table 30-1 Emergency Department Personnel

Providers	Caregivers	
Staff physicians who supervise	Charge nurses	
Residents	Primary RN supervisor	
Mid-levels	Nursing assistants	
Medical and PA students	Nursing students	
CONSULTANTS		
Private primary care providers		
Physician specialists		
Nonphysician therapists		
ANCILLARY PERSONNEL		
Prehospital	**In-hospital**	**Post-hospital**
EMS personnel*	Unit clerks	Chemical dependency units
Security	Social services	Shelters
Poison control	Translators	
Chaplains		

*EMS, emergency medical service.

Specialists The determination of when to consult a specialist and who presents the patient to the specialist is not clearly delineated in most EDs. Some specialists want to talk only to the ED physician; others want to talk to the provider who has done the workup on the patient. There are many unwritten protocols that the emergency care provider must be made aware of as he or she learns the resources and habits of physicians in the practice community, most of which will be learned on the job.

Nursing Staff The ED does not run without its nursing staff. They are vital to the smooth functioning of the department. Nurses usually spend more time with the patient than anyone else, including the provider. They are one of the few constants in a department in which provider turnover is the rule. ED nurses have a wealth of knowledge and experience that can be useful to all providers. Occasionally, the technical functions of the PA and a nurse overlap. This is probably truer in small EDs. Because of this, communication within the team is essential. The PA who works closely with the nursing staff in providing patient care will maintain a good productive relationship that contributes to the smooth running of the ED.

THE PROBLEM-ORIENTED HISTORY AND PHYSICAL EXAMINATION

The ED history and physical examination are reviewed and refined to support the overall concept of the ED. Because of this, most ED charts have a very small space reserved for the admitting problem and physical findings associated with that problem. Brevity, without compromise of important facts and findings, is the rule.

History

There is nothing intrinsically difficult or different about obtaining a history from a patient in the ED. It is important to discern early what the determining factor was that required the patient to seek treatment in the ED. The importance of the chief complaint (CC) takes on a new meaning because that is the problem that will be addressed by the ED staff. Those patients with multiple problems or chronic diseases who have acute exacerbation of their symptoms (e.g.,

sickle cell crises) are usually referred to their primary care physician once it has been determined that the ED has addressed and treated any immediate complication to their chronic existing problems.

The initial interview concerning the patient's CC should take place as soon as possible after the patient reports to the ED. It must be determined early in the patient's workup whether the complaint is a new problem or an exacerbation of an old illness. If this is an old complaint, the previous history regarding any prior diagnosis, treatment, and its effectiveness must be documented. The importance of this information should be emphasized to avoid the possibility of additional blood tests, x-rays, or a hospital admission. Too often, a patient waits until discharge and announces, "That's what the last doctor did and it didn't help."

There are some significant differences between the history of an injury and the history of a medical complaint. The cause of an injury may be as significant as the injury itself. Consider the following: A patient presenting with a broken wrist from a fall on the ice is treated differently than a patient who fainted, fell on the ice, and broke his or her wrist. In the second case, the injury to the wrist becomes secondary until the cause of the syncope episode is investigated. Patients who cannot give a history of an injury because of intoxication or decreased level of consciousness must be suspected of having occult serious pathology.

The time elapsed after an injury is another important factor, especially in cases of lacerations or fractures. Some wounds are left to heal secondarily if too much time has elapsed between the injury and the patient's reporting to the ED.

The mechanism of injury as well as a description of the instrument causing the injury should be recorded whenever possible. This information may help in selection of initial treatment by revealing the amount of tissue damage and the potential for infection at a later date.

Additional pertinent information that is dependent on the chief complaint is equally important to ascertain (e.g., Which is the dominant extremity of a patient with an injury to an arm or hand? Does the patient with bronchitis smoke? In the case of a dog bite, how was the dog acting at the time the patient was bitten? Has the dog bitten more than one person? Where is the dog now?) The patient also needs a tetanus immunization. Other crucial information includes a history of allergies, chronic diseases such as diabetes, chronic renal failure, hypertension, or peptic ulcer disease; anything that may have an implication or that might cloud the issue of the patient's chief complaint should be recorded.

The emergency department PA must often rely on sources of information other than the patient to obtain an entire history. Non–English-speaking patients need a translator. The patient with altered mental status needs additional sources for information on the family—primary care provider, an old chart, or any other hospitals or medical agencies where the patient may have been treated. In some instances, ED personnel may know the patient and can provide valuable input regarding their condition.

Occasionally, simultaneous treatment and obtaining a history may take place. For example, a patient with an acute exacerbation of asthma may feel more comfortable answering questions while receiving a breathing treatment.

Physical Examination

The first data recorded in the physical examination are the patient's vital signs. The supervising physician in the ED should be made aware of all patients with significantly abnormal vital signs as soon as they are obtained. What constitutes significantly abnormal vital signs occupies chapters in emergency medicine textbooks and encompasses 90% of the course of study of emergency medical technicians (EMTs) and paramedics. Serial vital signs, those taken every 5 to 10 minutes, are an important indicator of the patient's response to treatment. These, plus the patient's general appearance, may provide an overall picture of the patient's medical condition.

The next statement should include the patient's level of awareness and orientation. "Alert and oriented times three" means patients are aware of:

➤ Who they are.
➤ Where they are.
➤ What has happened to them.

Additionally, a general psychological statement using well-defined phrases such as cooperative, anxious, or hostile may set the tone for the patient's

examination. The speech pattern or content, the manner of dress, and the patient's personal hygiene should all be documented.

The following two examples illustrate what may appear in the patient's chart during workup.

CASE STUDY 30-4

Mrs. Jones is a 42-year-old woman appearing older than her stated age who smells unwashed, looks disheveled, and is wearing multiple layers of filthy clothing, including a parka in the month of August. She stated she was homeless and living on the street. After initial observation, the health care provider assesses the patient's mental, physical, and emotional capacity and how well she is dealing with her environment. Her chief complaint is observed as a mild cellulitis of the left foot. Determining that she is not diabetic and that her tetanus is up-to-date, the health care provider prescribes the appropriate treatment for her cellulitis and advises her to elevate her foot for 3 days. The health care provider then addresses the circumstance that put the patient at risk for this illness and determines that it may be impossible for her to comply with the treatment because she is homeless.

For children, the provider must substitute interactions, verbalizations, and spontaneous activities for the mental status and psychiatric examinations normally obtained in an adult.

CASE STUDY 30-5

The second patient is a 3-year-old girl who enters the ED with her mother and baby sister. The patient smells unwashed, looks disheveled, and is dressed in dirty shorts, tee shirt, and no shoes. It is August and the ED is located in a small town. The mother reports that the child has a fever and is complaining of ear pain. The mother is neatly and appropriately dressed for the weather. The second child, a baby, is clean, dressed in diapers, and asleep on the mother's shoulder. Meanwhile, the 3-year-old spends time alternating between whining and resting her head on the mother's knee or actively tearing up the waiting room. The health care provider should not have the same concerns with the appearance of this patient as he or she would have for the patient in Case Study 30-4. Unkempt and dirty can be considered the natural state of a 3-year-old during the summer months. The presence of the mother and the other sibling, as well as the patient's interaction with the mother, gives invaluable clues on the coping mechanisms and relationships of this patient to the family.

Another area of pertinent information about patients in the ED is their comfort or pain level. Some phrases that are commonly used to describe this include the following: no distress, no pain with normal gait and stance, moderate respiratory distress, uncomfortable with movement, writhing during examination.

Finally, the hydration and nutritional status of the patient should be assessed. This is especially important in geriatric and pediatric populations. Neither elderly nor very young patients tolerate dehydration well; prompt intervention with intravenous (IV) fluids may be needed before a full assessment can take place. IV fluids may be initiated in the early phase of any ED visit while other causes for the patient's condition are being considered.

The remainder of the physical examination is based on the differential diagnosis generated during the history. A thorough examination of the system within which the chief complaint originated must be performed. "Abdominal pain," for instance, demands an examination of all contiguous areas, including the chest, the pelvis, and the back. There are many causes for abdominal pain, and if the answer is not forthcoming in the routine examination, the diagnosis may be found in remote areas (e.g., the thyroid gland or a spider bite on an extremity). A chief complaint of dizziness requires examination of the cardiovascular system, the neurological system, the visual system, and the vestibular system.

Once the history and physical examination have been completed, a differential diagnosis or working diagnosis is established. Constant reassessment and reexamination may change the working diagnosis or may confirm the original diagnosis; studies usually aid in this determination.

Laboratory Tests

The health care provider must remain cognizant of the need for a diagnosis when ordering laboratory tests and medical imaging studies. A minimum amount of testing combined with the history and physical examination may offer the diagnosis. However, some questions need to be considered before any laboratory testing is ordered.

➤ **Will the test results provide additional information for determining the patient's diagnosis and treatment?** For example, an otherwise healthy 4-year-old child is brought to the ED with a temperature of 101.8° F (38.8° C) and is pulling at his ear. Physical examination reveals a bulging, red tympanic membrane. The diagnosis is made by history and physical examination. A complete blood count (CBC) shows a mildly elevated white blood cell count (WBC), which does not alter the diagnosis or the treatment.

➤ **Will laboratory test results alter the workup or treatment of the patient?** The same patient with a minimally elevated WBC count may not need antibiotics, and the patient with a markedly higher WBC count may need to be admitted to the hospital for IV antibiotic therapy.

➤ **Will the results of the tests be back before the patient leaves the ED?** Consider the following.

CASE STUDY 30-6

A 21-year-old man reports to the ED with a simple, uncomplicated laceration to his forearm. During the history, the patient reveals that he has had a 15-lb weight loss over the past 6 months and occasionally some bloody diarrhea. He requests a human immunodeficiency virus (HIV) test. Should this be considered part of the treatment for his laceration? It seems clinically indicated by his history. The facility has the ability to do an HIV test, but the results will not be back before the patient is discharged. Is it the ED's responsibility to act on the results? Is there a mechanism within the ED for follow-up of a patient with serious pathologic laboratory test results? In this case, the patient could be better served in an outpatient setting by a primary care provider.

➤ **Do the laboratory test results need interpretation that the ED cannot provide?** The ED physician is responsible for the initial interpretation of x-rays. However, the overall interpretation of the entire x-ray study for liability issues should be performed by a licensed radiologist. Most ED physicians will overread an x-ray and treat the patient conservatively rather than wait for an interpretation by the radiologist the next day.

➤ **Will the laboratory test results aid in the patient's follow-up care?** ED health care providers make it a priority to know each individual consultant and the specific laboratory tests they may favor. Additionally, the ED provider often orders these tests and will have the results before the consultant sees the patient. Community practices vary widely in mechanisms and protocol for obtaining outpatient imaging studies from the ED. However, acting in the patient's best interest and efficiently with the local system may dictate that the laboratory test should be initiated in the ED.

The ED record is a chronological summary of the patient from the occurrence of the injury or start of the illness to the patient's discharge or release from the ED. It should contain a complete history of the activity of the patient while in the ED. A good format to follow is the SOAP note described in Chapter 8.

Many laboratory tests are available to most hospital-based EDs. However, only a few of these tests are commonly performed in EDs. The following list indicates those tests that have proved to be the most cost-effective in revealing the broadest range of relevant information in the shortest amount of time.

Diagnostic Tests Commonly Ordered in the Emergency Department

➤ CBC with differential and indices.
➤ Electrolytes, including blood urea nitrogen, creatinine, and Ca^{2+}.
➤ Arterial blood gas with O_2 saturation.
➤ Carbon monoxide level.
➤ Urinalysis.
➤ Pregnancy test (urine or serum).
➤ Lipase and amylase.
➤ Wet prep and KOH of vaginal secretions.

➤ Serum levels of drugs (e.g., acetaminophen, theophylline, phenytoin).
➤ Gram's stain and cell count of various body fluids (e.g., cerebrospinal fluid, joint fluid).

THE COMMUNITY

It is extremely useful for the health care provider in the ED to know the community in which the ED is located and the specific population it serves. Occasionally, the ED provider may be unable to address some of the patient's complaints because of a lack of understanding concerning the culture and background in which the patient resides.

A knowledge of the community allows the health care provider to appreciate disease patterns and predilections with regard to race, geography, and socioeconomic status. This type of preparation expands the differential diagnosis of patients to include those diseases that are more prevalent in each distinct community.

Another significant factor affecting both the types of diseases and the volume of patients using the ED for their primary health care is the fluctuation of the local economy. Health insurance plays a major role for these patients. Any loss of benefits may result in an increased number of patients who cannot afford to visit a family physician. Even worse, such a loss may cause the patient to delay seeking medical treatment until illness is much more advanced, placing an even greater stress on the health care system. A number of studies have been done to attempt to correlate various economic factors with ED use. Brunette and co-workers investigated the timing of the volume of 911 calls to the distribution of the welfare checks in Hennepin County, Minnesota.[6] They also looked at the numbers of patients served in the Hennepin County Medical Center ED, the numbers of patients admitted to the county alcohol receiving center (ARC), and the admissions to the Hennepin County jail around the time of the check dispersal. This study revealed a significant drop in these volumes of patients as the number of days elapsed after the checks were distributed. The authors noted that the largest volume recorded was an increase in ARC admissions. ED volume and the number of Hennepin County ambulance runs were also significantly increased at check dispersal and tapered off as time elapsed. The authors were careful to point out, however, that a cause-and-effect relationship had not been established with these data, and they could only speculate on the possible relationship of increased cash flow with an increased consumption of alcohol.

Some of the major factors affecting a health care provider's understanding of the cultural attitudes toward health, disease, and therapeutics are:

➤ Economic status.
➤ Religious beliefs.
➤ Ethnic and racial background.
➤ Social differences.

An appreciation of what sickness is and how it relates to these factors in each different group can aid the ED provider in prescribing those therapies that will result in the successful treatment of each individual patient.

THE ROLE OF THE EMERGENCY DEPARTMENT WITHIN THE HEALTH CARE SYSTEM

Regardless of the size of the ED or the type of hospital it serves, the ED usually functions as an independent clinic where patients are admitted and discharged by ED personnel alone. Other departments of the hospital depend on the ED to properly triage sick and injured patients and stabilize those patients who may require further hospitalization. Each department usually has an agreement or a protocol for the joint management of the patient in the ED. These protocols are as individual as the hospital, and the provider must make every effort to stabilize the patient according to established protocols before transferring the patient to the hospital ward. Certain types of patients, such as major trauma victims, unstable pediatric patients, or pregnant women with other medical conditions, may be best handled by those specific departments, and communication with that department is the most important factor in the initial management of those patients.

The ED operates under both internally and externally imposed mandates. ED providers can serve as gatekeepers to admittance of patients to the rest of the hospital. They are expected to handle an ever-changing set of circumstances and a random stream of patients exhibiting a random set of medical illnesses that may or may not result in specific diagnosis and treatment. They protect vulnerable patients, act as the medical witness in matters of litigious personal injury, and assume leadership in disaster management. The ED is responsible for maintaining acceptable standards of quality assurance in patient care. If the hospital participates in training programs, the ED may also be required to provide an education for physicians, PAs, nurses, EMTs, and paramedics.

Most hospitals that support the ED have plans for dealing with unstable medical or major trauma patients. Often hospitals use a "code team" to respond to cardiac arrests within the institution; this may mean that physicians from the ED participate in those codes. Specified members of this team are alerted when patients requiring stabilization or resuscitation are identified.

Ideally, the PA is part of a code team. In a busy ED where more than one resuscitation may be conducted at a time, the PA may be called on to "run" the code. All PAs working in emergency medicine should be ACLS-certified and must be able to direct a code according to those protocols. Most PAs, however, will find themselves working in a department with experienced physicians, nurses, and paramedics. They will have the opportunity to participate in numerous resuscitations and learn the variations on the ACLS theme before they are asked to run a code.

The principles taught in advanced trauma life support (ATLS) are invaluable in the organized approach to a critically injured patient. Certification in ATLS is not available to PAs; however, all PAs working in an emergency setting are strongly encouraged to take advantage of this course. ATLS principles and skills are an invaluable tool for recognizing physical findings and initiating proper treatment to help stabilize the patient.

It has been the experience of many PAs working in the ED that their skills in managing minor trauma (e.g., simple lacerations) are extremely valuable. If there is a niche for PAs in the ED, this seems to be it. Here, PAs tend to shine clinically. They provide a high degree of quality care with speed and accuracy. This ability is extremely desirable in many health care settings, from busy metropolitan EDs with multiple-provider coverage to rural health care clinics where the PA may work alone. Consequently, this allows the physician the latitude to concentrate on other tasks.

Disaster management from earthquake preparedness to toxic decontamination control is an important aspect of today's industrialized world. Disaster management is already a structured entity within most towns and urban centers. In place are designated disaster offices and volunteer teams and protocols that involve many different community service organizations such as fire, civil defense, hazardous waste management, and search and rescue teams. It is inevitable that the ED, including the prehospital team, will be an intrinsic part of a disaster response separate from the emergency management of individual patients. The PA may well have a place on the team, especially if he or she is willing to play a very different role than in the ED. If the PA develops an interest in these areas, he or she might be in a position to provide a unique service to the community in conjunction with the disaster relief team. A member of such a team can expect instruction in disaster management principles and an orientation to the highly choreographed response to various possible disaster scenarios.

The ED that hosts an emergency medicine residency program is ripe with opportunities for the experienced PA in teaching and conducting and participating in clinical research. Students, interns, and emergency medicine residents enter the department yearly with widely varying experience in ED procedures. An experienced PA working in an emergency setting is in an ideal position to teach procedures such as suturing, IV access techniques, immobilization and casting techniques, orthopedic procedures, abscess and wound care management, and use of specialized equipment. The PA has the opportunity to acquaint new residents and students with the accepted standards of practice regarding the techniques and supervision of ED procedures. More importantly, the PA has the obligation to educate these new health care providers to the PA concept, PA practice, and the role of the PA in emergency medicine.

Patient follow-up is traditionally a weak link in emergency medicine. Once the patient leaves the ED, the emergency clinician usually hears from or about the patient again only if there is a complication. Because EDs were originally conceived of for a one-time visit for an unstable patient, follow-up was an unaccustomed bonus for a physician wishing to see the final result of his or her treatment. Today, many patients depend on the ED for their primary health care, and follow-up has become a legal and practical dilemma for all EDs. The use of PAs for patient follow-up and call-back is widening. Occasionally, PAs are employed in EDs strictly for follow-up of abnormal laboratory values or x-ray–reading discrepancies. Some departments use mid-level providers to review charts for completeness and adherence to predetermined protocols. Different EDs have different follow-up needs, but again, because of their temporal stability and familiarity with department protocols, procedures, and resources, PAs are excellent candidates for organizing and staffing a follow-up program.

In 1990, Beth Israel Medical Center published an overview of its 8-year experience with PAs in the ED.[7] One of the unique features of the Beth Israel ED was the emphasis on patient follow-up. All the PAs employed in the ED participated in quality assurance chart reviews and in re-contacting a statistically select group of patients for a follow-up phone call and revisit if indicated.

Ideally, the ED should function as the patient's health care source for only a short period of time. That often means that the ED provider may not know what happens to the patient when he or she leaves the department. Even with the best intentions and best follow-up instructions, the ED loses track of patients. Because the ED staff does not establish an ongoing relationship with the patients they treat, they must be able to tolerate a lack of closure both intellectually and emotionally.

The next section of this chapter is designed to give a new provider in the ED some practical information and "how to" tools for evaluating some of the more common complaints that are seen in most busy EDs today. These are meant as guidelines only. For treatment of wounds and specifics on laceration repair, please refer to Chapter 13.

GENERAL APPROACH TO THE EVALUATION OF ABDOMINAL PAIN

The approach to the patient with abdominal pain involves a directed history, a complete physical examination, selected laboratory tests, and selected radiographic (x-ray) procedures.

History The history should include the following:

➤ Description of the pain—onset, duration, quality, radiation, exacerbating and relieving factors.

➤ Prior similar pain.

➤ Gastrointestinal symptoms, including vomiting, diarrhea, last normal bowel movement, appetite, food intolerance.

➤ Urinary tract symptoms—dysuria, frequency, hematuria.

➤ Gynecological review—last normal menstrual period, gravida and para status, number of abortions and miscarriages, discharge, dyspareunia.

➤ Prior abdominal surgery.

➤ Prior diagnostic evaluations—upper gastrointestinal series, barium enema, intravenous pyelogram (IVP), ultrasound, computed tomography (CT).

Physical Examination The physical examination should be head to toe and should include a rectal examination with a stool guaiac and a pelvic examination for women with lower abdominal pain.

Laboratory Studies The laboratory evaluation involves selection from a menu of laboratory and x-ray studies depending on clinical impressions from the history and physical examination. The laboratory menu includes CBC, urinalysis (UA), SMA-7, aspartate transaminase (AST), alanine aminotransferase (ALT), bilirubin (total, direct, indirect), alkaline phosphatase (AP), amylase, and lipase. The x-ray menu includes flat plate abdomen, upright film abdomen, upright posteroanterior (PA) chest film for free air, ultrasound of the gallbladder and pelvis, and IVP and CT scan with double contrast (IVP dye and oral contrast).

Acute Cholecystitis

History The patient presents with pain in the right upper quadrant that is of rapid onset and variable in character. The pain may be described as sharp, aching, or cramplike. It often radiates to the back and is usually accompanied by nausea with or without vomiting. Patients may have a history of similar episodes for some time in the past that lasted minutes to hours and often left them tender to touch for a few days. The pain may be brought on by eating fatty or greasy food.

Physical Examination The hallmark is the physical examination, which reveals tenderness to palpation in the right upper quadrant of the abdomen. The tenderness may increase when the PA has the patient take a deep breath while palpating the right upper quadrant (Murphy's sign). The patient may also have epigastric tenderness, particularly if there is concomitant pancreatitis. The patient may be febrile.

Laboratory Studies Laboratory evaluation should include CBC, UA, amylase and lipase, AP, bilirubin, AST, and ALT. Gallbladder disease is a leading cause of pancreatitis, the other common cause being alcohol. Eighty percent of gallstones are radiolucent, so a flat plate of the abdomen will show gallstones only 20% of the time. Ultrasound identifies gallstones very reliably and is noninvasive. The definitive test for cholecystitis is the nuclear hepatoiminodiacetic acid (HIDA) scan. If the common bile duct becomes visible and the gallbladder does not, there is a functional obstruction in the cystic duct. Although ultrasound can detect gallstones, it does not detect obstruction of the cystic duct. The HIDA scan is particularly useful in differentiating appendicitis from cholecystitis.

Treatment Patients with fever, complicating pancreatitis, or unremitting pain require admission to the hospital for IV fluids and parenteral antibiotics and analgesics. Patients who have normal laboratory studies, no fever, and bearable pain can be sent home with oral pain medication, next-day follow-up with a surgeon, and instructions to return immediately if the pain intensifies or fever occurs.

Ureteral Colic

History Patients with ureteral colic present with a spectrum of pain. At one end is the patient who presents with severe pain in the right lower quadrant that is sharp and constant and may radiate to the costovertebral angle (CVA) area or the testicle on the same side. At the other end of the spectrum, the patient exhibits mild pain somewhere in the area stretching from the kidney down to the lower abdomen and into the testicle or vagina on the affected side.

Physical Examination   The patient is in marked distress—pale, diaphoretic, nauseated, and writhing on the examination table with pain. The hallmark of a stone is that in spite of the severe pain, tenderness is usually minimal. It may require careful questioning to establish that palpation really is not increasing the severity of the pain the patient is experiencing.

Laboratory Studies   Laboratory evaluation usually consists of a CBC, SMA-7, and routine UA with culture and sensitivity if indicated. UA usually shows microscopic hematuria, unless the stone is completely blocking the ureter. An IVP is obtained to definitively diagnose the problem and guide management. All urine should be strained while the patient is undergoing evaluation in the ED, and any stone passed should be sent to the pathology laboratory for analysis.

Treatment   When the provider is confident from the patient's history and physical examination that he or she has a stone, an IV infusion with Ringer's lactate should be started. The patient may be given morphine sulfate IV in increments of 5 mg every 3 to 5 minutes or until the pain can be tolerated. The patient should also be given an IV antiemetic such as prochlorperazine (Compazine) 5 mg, or promethazine (Phenergan) 25 mg. IV ketorolac tromethamine (Toradol) 30 mg, is also effective in pain relief.

Indications for Admission   The indications for admission include the following:
1. Stone greater than 5 mm in size.
2. Accompanying urinary tract infection requiring emergency urological consultation for decompressive procedure.
3. High-grade obstruction on IVP.
4. Intractable pain (often accompanies high-grade obstruction).

The patient with a stone less than 5 mm in size without high-grade obstruction or accompanying infection, and without intractable pain, may go home. The patient should be given a urine strainer and should be instructed to strain all urine and save for analysis any stone passed regardless of size. The patient should also be given a potent oral analgesic (Lorcet 10 [hydrocodone 10 mg plus 650 mg of acetaminophen]) and should be told to return immediately if severe pain or fever develops. The patient should also be instructed to force fluids and to follow up with a urologist in 2 to 3 days with x-rays, laboratory results, and a copy of the ED record.

Appendicitis

History   Patients with appendicitis can be very easy or very difficult to diagnose. The patient who is easy to diagnose presents with a history of pain that was initially periumbilical and crampy but within 12 to 24 hours, the pain localized in the right lower quadrant. The pain is worse with movement and is accompanied by nausea and anorexia. Unfortunately, many patients with appendicitis have atypical histories and their laboratory and x-ray findings do not fit the classic picture. The hallmark in these difficult cases is the consistent presence of tenderness in the right lower quadrant. Temperature can be normal, the patient can be hungry, and WBC counts can be normal. If the patient has consistent right lower quadrant tenderness and if a ureteral stone as well as gynecological pathology has been ruled out, a surgical consult is warranted.

In many cases, the patient will have nonspecific abdominal pain with no clues for the diagnosis of appendicitis in the workup and still may turn out to have this problem. In any patient with abdominal pain of unknown cause whom the provider is electing to send home without a baseline examination by a surgeon, a follow-up examination in 6 to 12 hours is mandated. The patient should be instructed to return to the ED immediately if the pain worsens or localizes to the right lower quadrant.

Physical Examination   On physical examination, the patient has a mild fever and localized tenderness in the right lower quadrant at McBurney's point.

Pressing deeply on the left side of the abdomen, which causes the patient to experience pain in the right lower quadrant, is a positive Rovsing's sign. Coughing intensifies right lower quadrant pain. A tap on the patient's heel also intensifies the pain and the patient is tender on the right side on rectal examination.

Laboratory Studies The patient's WBC count is usually over 10,000/mm^3 but less than 15,000/mm^3 with a left shift. The abdominal film reveals a fecalith in the right lower quadrant, and a few air-fluid levels in the small bowel in the right lower quadrant may be visible.

Treatment The treatment for suspected appendicitis is surgery.

Diverticulitis

History The patient presents to the ED with pain in the left lower quadrant. However, the diagnosis of diverticulitis in the ED is a clinical one.

Physical Examination The hallmark of the physical examination is localized tenderness in the area of the inflamed diverticulum. Patients exhibit rebound tenderness and fever.

Laboratory Studies Leukocytosis is found on the CBC.

Treatment These patients should be admitted for IV fluids, parenteral antibiotics, analgesics, and frequent reexamination. In cases in which there is no rebound tenderness and no significant fever, and the patient is able to keep fluids down, the patient may be discharged from the ED. If this is the case, an oral antibiotic should be prescribed as well as bedrest, a low-residue diet, and next-day follow-up examination.

Cystitis

History The diagnosis of cystitis is usually straightforward. The patient complains of frequency and dysuria.

Physical Examination The physical examination is usually unremarkable with only mild suprapubic tenderness. In cases that are not clear-cut, there is the possibility that the bladder irritative symptoms are coming from an adjacent inflammatory condition such as pelvic inflammatory disease (PID), diverticulitis, or appendicitis. However, the tenderness on palpation is much more prominent in these other conditions than would be expected for cystitis. Sometimes a stone lodged at the ureterovesical junction will cause irritative bladder symptoms, but the pain from a stone is usually much more intense and the urine has no WBCs unless there is a complicating infection.

Laboratory Studies Urinalysis shows variable numbers of WBCs and red blood cells (RBCs). The patient may have a positive nitrite and leukocyte esterase on urine dipstick test. A urine culture and sensitivity should be sent in all patients with impaired defenses, history of recurrent infections, or past surgery of the urinary tract.

Treatment Treatment regimens seem to change frequently. One of the best sources for antibiotic therapy is *Sanford's Guide to Antimicrobial Therapy*.[8] This booklet is updated yearly and currently suggests 3-day therapy with a number of different antibiotics, depending on the specific needs of the patient.

Pyelonephritis

History Pyelonephritis is usually a straightforward diagnosis. The patient may complain of a few days of urinary frequency and dysuria followed by fever, chills, myalgia, nausea, and back pain. The patient may also complain of nonspecific abdominal pain and have nonspecific abdominal tenderness on examination.

Physical Examination The hallmark is CVA tenderness, especially reliable if it is unilateral. This can be demonstrated most reliably by sliding the hand under the supine patient and pressing upward into the CVA area. Occasionally, pyelonephritis can be extremely difficult to diagnose. Consider it in young children, usually girls, who present to the ED with fever and no identifiable source evident after history and physical examination. Also consider pyelonephritis in adults with nonspecific abdominal pain, low-grade fever, and mild unilateral CVA tenderness.

Males with pyelonephritis usually fit into one of the following groups:

1. Very young with a congenital malformation of the urinary system.
2. Older patients with obstruction due to prostatic hypertrophy.
3. Any patient with an indwelling catheter.

Laboratory Studies   A urine culture and sensitivity should always be ordered on all patients suspected of having this problem. Blood cultures at two sites are indicated in all febrile patients. These patients should be admitted unless they exhibit a very mild case without significant fever or vomiting.

Treatment   If the patient is admitted, IV antibiotics should be given. If the patient is discharged, oral antibiotics should be given with 24-hour follow-up instructions.

THE FEMALE WITH LOWER ABDOMINAL PAIN AND VAGINAL BLEEDING
General

History   The history should include the pertinent information (either positive or negative) about any of the following:

➤ Pain—onset, duration, character, radiation, exacerbating and relieving factors.
➤ Prior similar episodes.
➤ Last normal menstrual period, gravida and para status, number of abortions and miscarriages.
➤ Gastrointestinal symptoms—vomiting, diarrhea, last normal bowel movement.
➤ Urinary tract symptoms—dysuria, frequency, hematuria.
➤ Gynecological symptoms—vaginal discharge, dyspareunia.
➤ Prior gynecological problems—pelvic infection, ovarian cyst, endometriosis.
➤ Prior abdominal surgery.

Physical Examination   A complete physical examination should be done to record tenderness or masses on the abdominal examination, any discharge, the appearance of the cervix on pelvic examination, and tenderness on rectal examination. A tilt test should be done routinely on all female patients with vaginal bleeding and lower abdominal pain.

Laboratory Studies   A CBC, UA, and urine pregnancy test should be done on all women of childbearing age. In addition, during the pelvic examination, cultures for *Gonorrhoea* and *Chlamydia* should be collected. A blood type and Rh factor should be done in all women who are diagnosed with an abortion or an ectopic pregnancy. If the Rh factor is negative, the patient should receive a RhoGAM [Rh_0 (D) immune globulin] injection.

Pelvic Ultrasonography   A patient with abdominal pain, tenderness on pelvic examination, and a positive pregnancy test will need a pelvic sonogram. In order to definitively diagnose an ectopic pregnancy, the fetal heartbeat must be visualized in an adnexal mass. However, the unusual report shows the uterus to be empty, some free fluid in the cul-de-sac, and a suggestion of an adnexal mass. An elevated quantitative beta-human chorionic gonadotropin (β-hCG) will correlate with a lower abdominal mass noted on sonography for the diagnosis of an ectopic pregnancy. By the fifth week of gestation, a gestational sac should be detectable in the uterus. By 6 weeks, a fetal pole can be seen, and by 7 weeks a fetal heartbeat can be observed. The quantitative β-hCG level is around 1500 IU/L at 5 weeks. A β-hHCG level greater than 1500 IU/L with an empty uterus on sonography is very suspicious of an ectopic pregnancy. Pelvic sonography is also very helpful in the pregnant patient with vaginal bleeding in whom the viability of the fetus is of concern. In this situation, the lack of significant pain is not suspicious of an ectopic pregnancy, and a sonogram should not be considered as part of an ED workup. However, a sonogram should be obtained as soon as possible during normal working hours.

Pelvic Inflammatory Disease

History   Patients with pelvic inflammatory disease (PID) present with a spectrum of pain ranging from a mild-to-moderate constant aching pain to severe constant pain with fever. The latter patient often walks into the ED with a slow shuffling gait, bent over, and clutching her lower abdomen with both hands. This presentation is characteristic and common enough to be dubbed "the PID shuffle." Patients with PID are frequently menstruating or have recently finished a period.

Physical Examination   The hallmark of PID is pain with cervical motion tenderness and diffuse pelvic tenderness on bimanual examination. Fever may or may not be present.

Laboratory Studies   The patient's WBC count may or may not be elevated. Ectopic pregnancy must be ruled out by a urine pregnancy test. It is cost-effective to add a screening test for syphilis in any patient with a clinical diagnosis of PID.

Treatment   With the information gained in the evaluation, patients can be sorted into three categories using the following criteria:

1. Patients who need admission: Temperature of 101° F (38.3° C) or higher, WBC count of 15,000/mm^3 or higher, and rebound tenderness on examination of the abdomen. These patients should be treated with cefoxitin 2 g IV every 6 hours coupled with doxycycline 100 mg IV every 12 hours until the patient has responded clinically and the WBC count returns to normal. Patients treated as outpatients should get a ceftriaxone (Rocephin 250 mg) injection intramuscularly followed by a 10-day course of doxycycline 100 mg twice daily.
2. Patients who can be treated with antibiotics as outpatients: Temperature less than 101° F (38.3° C), WBC count less than 15,000/mm^3, and no rebound tenderness.
3. Patients who can be treated symptomatically pending the results of cervical cultures: Reliable patients who are afebrile with minimal tenderness.

Tubal Pregnancy

A female of childbearing age with lower abdominal pain is considered to have an ectopic pregnancy until proved otherwise.

History   A patient with tubal pregnancy usually presents 6 to 8 weeks past her last menstrual period with fairly sudden onset of unilateral sharp pain that becomes constant and is exacerbated with motion. If bleeding is massive, she may have fainted or may complain of dizziness on standing. Pain may radiate to the shoulder if blood is irritating the diaphragm. There may be a history of prior PID or a previous ectopic pregnancy.

Physical Examination   Physical examination demonstrates a spectrum of findings based on the underlying pathophysiology. At one end of the spectrum, the patient exhibits severe pain, shock, and an abdomen distended with blood. At the other end, the patient complains of mild aggravating unilateral pain, and mild-to-moderate tenderness on examination.

Laboratory Studies   These patients require a urine pregnancy test. Patients with pain and a positive pregnancy test need an emergency pelvic sonogram and an immediate Ob-Gyn consultation. As has been mentioned previously, the quantitative β-hCG is very useful to correlate with sonographic findings in arriving at a presumptive diagnosis.

Treatment   The treatment for a tubal pregnancy is emergency surgery. The patient can very rapidly develop life-threatening complications, mainly internal hemorrhage.

Threatened Abortion

History   It is useful to consider vaginal bleeding a complication of a pregnancy until it can be ruled out by a urine pregnancy test. In patients who are pregnant and bleeding, it must be determined whether they are threatening to have a miscarriage, are in the process of having a miscarriage, or have completed having a miscarriage.

Physical Examination   Usually the assessment of the cervical os enables the PA to differentiate these possibilities. The patient who presents with slight bleeding, mild or no cramps, a closed os, and no significant tenderness on pelvic examination can be diagnosed as having a threatened abortion. The patient with significant bleeding and cramps in which the os admits a ring forceps is in the process of miscarrying. It is more difficult to diagnose threatened abortion in multiparous patients because the os is often stretched from previous childbirth and may appear open on casual visualization.

Laboratory Studies A quantitative β-hCG is helpful as a baseline test in these patients because in normal pregnancies, the quantitative β-hCG doubles every 2 days during the first trimester. Sonography is an extremely helpful adjunct in cases that are questionable. It is wise to do an emergent pelvic sonogram to make the differentiation.

Treatment Occasionally, the patient is bleeding profusely and tissue may be noted protruding from the cervical os. Removing the tissue with a ring forceps should be done immediately and often results in a marked decrease in bleeding. If the patient is having a miscarriage, an immediate Ob-Gyn consultation should be obtained. If the patient has a closed os and a normal hematocrit, and is not bleeding massively, she may be discharged from the ED with instructions to go home and rest. She should return to the ED if the bleeding increases, or if she has any tissue loss. Refer the patient for follow-up the next day to her regular Ob-Gyn physician.

Vaginitis

The patient who complains of a vaginal discharge requires a pelvic examination, a cervical culture for *Gonorrhoea* and *Chlamydia,* and a wet prep for yeast and *Trichomonas.*

The diagnosis is often very straightforward from the history and physical examination.

Yeast Vaginitis Yeast vaginitis usually causes intense itching and the patient complains of the characteristic white "cottage cheese" discharge. The vulva may be inflamed.

Treatment of yeast vaginitis is accomplished by any number of antiyeast regimens.

Trichomonas Vaginitis *Trichomonas* vaginitis causes a copious malodorous discharge that is yellow-green in color and often frothy. Itching may be present but is much less prominent than in yeast infections.

Treatment of *Trichomonas* vaginitis is metronidazole (Flagyl) in a single 2-g dose administered to the patient and her sexual partner. If the patient is in the first trimester of pregnancy, a 20% saline douche or clotrimazole may be used.

Bacterial Vaginosis

Bacterial vaginosis usually presents with a grayish white discharge that is malodorous but not frothy, and itching is not prominent. The wet prep may show "clue cells," which are desquamated epithelial cells with clusters of bacilli clinging to their surfaces, giving them a stippled appearance. *Gardnerella vaginalis, Peptococcus,* and non-*fragilis Bacteroides* have all been implicated as etiologic.

Bacterial vaginosis is treated with metronidazole 500 mg twice daily for 7 days with no treatment of the sexual partner. Because treatments change from year to year, the reader should consult *Sanford's Guide to Antimicrobial Therapy* for the latest recommendations.[8]

MANAGEMENT OF THE FEBRILE CHILD YOUNGER THAN 2 YEARS OF AGE
A Child Younger than 3 Months of Age

The child younger than 3 months of age with a temperature greater than or equal to 100.4° F (38° C) should undergo a full septic workup, be placed on parenteral antibiotics, and be admitted to the hospital. A full septic workup includes a CBC, SMA-7, blood cultures at two sites, routine UA and culture (preferably obtained by suprapubic aspiration), stool for fecal leukocytes and culture (if diarrhea is present), lumbar puncture, and chest x-ray. The reader should refer to the current issue of *Sanford's Guide to Antimicrobial Therapy* for the latest antibiotic recommendations.[8]

A Child 3 Months to 4 Years of Age

Regardless of the level of temperature, if the child appears acutely ill, he or she must be admitted for treatment. If the child does not appear acutely ill and has a focus of infection on examination that most likely is the source of the fever, the infection should be treated and the parents asked to contact their pediatrician within the next 24 hours. For example, the child who has bilateral otitis media with a temperature of 102° F (38.8° C) but is taking fluids well and does not appear toxic can be treated and discharged from the ED.

If the child is not toxic in appearance, has a temperature of 102° F (38.8° C) or higher, and has no focus of infection on examination, the child is at risk for bacteremia. A WBC and differential should be obtained. If the WBC is greater than 15,000/mm³, blood culture should be done along with a UA and chest x-ray. The child should be treated with a parenteral antibiotic, and instructions should be given to the parents to contact their pediatrician in 12 to 24 hours.

If the child is not toxic in appearance and has a temperature of 102° F (38.8° C) or higher, no focus of infection on examination, and a WBC less than 15,0000/mm³, he or she should be treated symptomatically with reexamination in 12 to 24 hours.

EYE EMERGENCIES
Initial Evaluation

All persons with eye complaints should have a *visual acuity* recorded on their chart as the first step in evaluation. This should be done with the patient wearing his or her glasses or contacts if possible. If glasses or contacts are not available, use a piece of cardboard with a pinhole to correct refractive errors. The Snellen eye chart is a satisfactory method for assessing visual acuity in most cases.

In many cases, the patient will be having so much discomfort that a *topical anesthetic* will need to be instilled in the eye before the visual acuity testing can be done. The skin should be gently pinched under the lower lid and the lid pulled outward to form a small pouch. Warn the patient that the medication will sting, and place a drop or two of the anesthetic into the pouch; have the patient gently close his or her eye for a few seconds. This pouch technique is much more comfortable to the patient than is dropping eyedrops directly onto the surface of the cornea.

Direct inspection with a light source directed onto the eye from the side will show obvious abnormalities and is a good way to evaluate the depth of the anterior chamber. Usually, the entire anterior chamber will be illuminated, but in the case of a shallow anterior chamber, only the lateral half illuminates and the medial half remains in a shadow. Eyes with shallow anterior chambers should not be dilated because glaucoma can be precipitated.

If there is any suggestion in the patient's history of a problem that might involve a disrupted corneal epithelium (e.g., foreign body sensation, eye pain, or chemicals in the eye), it is helpful to add *fluorescein dye* to the eye before the slit lamp or Wood's lamp examination. Fluorescein-impregnated paper strips are moistened with ophthalmic irrigating solution and are touched lightly to the lower palpebral conjunctival surface to instill the dye. Excess dye is rinsed away with the ophthalmic irrigating solution if needed, and the eye is viewed under a black light. Areas of disrupted corneal epithelium fluoresce brightly.

Slit lamp examination should be learned by direct demonstration and hands-on instruction.

Lid eversion is necessary to evaluate foreign body sensations in the eye, or when corneal examination reveals vertical linear abrasions. The patient is asked to look down and the upper lid eyebrows are grasped gently between the thumb and index finger and pulled outward. A cotton-tipped swab is used as a fulcrum behind the tarsal plate over which the lid is everted. The swab is then removed and the lid held everted with the thumb. It is very helpful to keep the patient looking down during this maneuver because if the patient looks up, the lid spontaneously reverts to its normal position. This maneuver can be done at the slit lamp and allows the provider to scan the undersurface of the lid with the slit lamp, searching for any foreign body.

Funduscopic examination with the direct ophthalmoscope is part of every standard eye examination. This can usually be accomplished without dilating the pupil.

Tonometry with the Shiøtz tonometer should be done on any eye in which the history and eye examination suggest glaucoma. With the patient supine, the eye is anesthetized topically, the lids are gently retracted with caution not to touch the globe, and the tonometer is placed on the cornea. It is helpful to have an assistant place a finger 3 feet over the patient's face so the patient can fixate on it to help hold the eye still. The scale reading on the tonometer is converted to millimeters of mercury (mm Hg) by a chart that accompanies the tonometer. Normal intraocular pressure is 16.1 ± 2.8 mm Hg. In acute glaucoma, intraocular pressure is usually markedly elevated (40 to 50 mm Hg), and in iritis, the intraocular pressure may decrease. Application tonometry using the slit lamp and the new Tonopen are more advanced ways to measure intraocular pressure.

If the history suggests possible penetrating ocular injury, x-rays of the orbit for foreign body should be obtained. A Waters view of the orbits is helpful in the evaluation of possible fractures associated with blunt trauma to the eye. Tomograms of the orbital floor or a CT scan may be necessary to diagnose a blowout fracture of the orbital floor, if clinical suspicion is high and routine x-rays fail to show the fracture.

Common Eye Infections

Stye A stye (external hordeolum) is a staphylococcal infection of small glands along the external lid margin. A red swelling appears in the lash line of the lid margin, accompanied by pain, tenderness, and often considerable edema of the lid. Eventually, a yellow summit appears, indicating suppuration. Treatment consists of hot compresses to hasten suppuration and a local antibiotic instilled into the eye. Incision is usually not indicated and systemic antibiotics should be withheld unless the infection is spreading into the eyelid with poor localization. A stye may also occur on the inside of the lid (internal hordeolum), and the treatment is identical.

Conjunctivitis Conjunctivitis is inflammation of the conjunctival surfaces of the eye. Conjunctivitis has diverse causes, including bacterial infection, viral infection, allergy, ultraviolet light exposure, and trauma. In most cases, the patient presents with eye discharge, redness, and mild pain. In simple cases, it is standard practice to treat with a local antibiotic and refer to an ophthalmologist if the patient fails to respond to treatment. Conjunctivitis in newborns and infants requires special considerations that are beyond the scope of this discussion.

1. *Acute purulent conjunctivitis* is characterized by a profuse purulent eye discharge. Causative bacteria include pneumococci, streptococci, *Haemophilus influenzae* (Koch-Weeks bacillus), *Haemophilus conjunctivitis,* staphylococci, and *Neisseria catarrhalis.* Mixed infections are common. Treatment is started empirically with an antibiotic eyedrop or ointment, and Gram's stain and cultures are reserved for resistant cases.

2. *Viral conjunctivitis* is also characterized by an eye discharge. It differs from bacterial conjunctivitis in that the discharge is less profuse and preauricular lymph node enlargement is often present. Gram's stain shows a preponderance of lymphocytes and mononuclear cells without bacteria. However, because routine Gram's stains are not recommended, treat with an antibiotic eyedrop or ointment, and reserve Gram's stain and cultures for resistant cases.

3. *Allergic conjunctivitis* is distinguished by itching, watering, redness, and mucoid discharge. Edematous swelling is noted in which the bulbar conjunctival surface may protrude out of the eye or overlap the cornea in ballooning folds. The clinical picture is distinct, and treatment is with an antihistamine vasoconstrictor eyedrop (Vasocon-A).

4. *Traumatic conjunctivitis* is an acute purulent conjunctivitis induced by traumatic contamination.

5. *Ultraviolet keratoconjunctivitis* is caused by exposure to ultraviolet radiation. Common sources include welders' electric arcs, sunlamps, or sunlight reflected by snow. Around 12 hours after exposure, the patient develops severe bilateral eye pain, watering, and photophobia. The pain is usually so intense that the eyes cannot be opened until a drop of topical anesthetic is instilled. Slit lamp examination with fluorescein stain reveals a diffuse stippled uptake of dye over the surface of the cornea, and the conjunctival surfaces are diffusely injected. Treatment is an antibiotic eyedrop, a cycloplegic, and patching of both eyes. Systemic analgesia is usually required.

Orbital Cellulitis Orbital cellulitis is a serious infection of bacterial origin. The patient has high fever, eye pain, redness and swelling of orbital tissues, and ophthalmoplegia in severe cases. Infection may extend from an infected sinus or tooth, or there may be a primary site of infection. In children, orbital cellulitis is usually a primary infection. In either case, treatment is immediate referral for hospitalization and IV antibiotics.

Corneal Infections

Corneal infections may be primary or may arise after trauma has broken the corneal epithelium. Bacterial ulcers are frequently associated with purulent conjunctivitis and have a grayish appearance. Immediate ophthalmologic consult should be obtained. Any corneal abrasion may become secondarily infected with bacteria, fungi, or herpesvirus. When the fluorescein-stained cornea is examined under the slit lamp, a characteristic dendritic pattern is often seen with herpesvirus infection. An ophthalmologic consult should be obtained immediately and antiviral eyedrops prescribed.

> Placing topical steroids in an eye with a herpesvirus infection has resulted in rapid progression of the infection with corneal destruction. This danger is one of the main reasons for the dictum that under no circumstances should a non-ophthalmologist ever prescribe topical steroids for eye problems.

Ocular Foreign Bodies

Conjunctival Foreign Bodies

Conjunctival foreign bodies cause pain and a sensation that something is in the eye. Those in the lower conjunctival sac are easily removed with a moistened cotton-tipped applicator after topical anesthesia. Foreign bodies under the upper lid are exposed by everting the lid, as discussed earlier. They usually are found 2 to 3 mm from the lid margin and are also easily removed with a moistened cotton-tipped applicator. The cornea must be examined carefully under the slit lamp with fluorescein staining to search for multiple vertical corneal abrasions. These scratches are caused by the motion of the foreign body back and forth across the cornea each time the patient blinks. If abrasions are present, instill a topical antibiotic, a cycloplegic, and double-patch the eye for 24 hours. If no abrasion is present,

prescribe a topical antibiotic eyedrop to instill four times daily for 2 to 3 days to prevent traumatic conjunctivitis. If the eye is patched, it should be reexamined in 24 hours. Patching is for comfort only and is optional.

Corneal Foreign Bodies

Corneal foreign bodies also cause pain and a sensation that something is in the eye. The foreign body is usually easily seen by direct vision or slit lamp examination after topical anesthesia. Removal is accomplished with an eye spud, a 25-gauge needle attached to a cotton-tipped applicator, or the special ophthalmologic corneal burr attached to a battery-operated drill. The latter technique is especially efficient if there is a metallic corneal foreign body because a *rust ring* usually remains in the cornea after removal of the metal. It is important to use the drill to remove these rust rings as completely as possible. Any residual rust increases the healing time of the abrasion and the inflammatory response of the eye. After removal of the foreign body and any residual rust, instill an antibiotic eyedrop, a cycloplegic, and double-patch the eye. Patching is for comfort only and is optional. Reexamination is necessary in 24 hours. Avoid placing steroids in the eye because these reduce the resistance of the cornea to infection. Do not use an antibiotic ointment unless the abrasion is very superficial (there have been instances in which a drop of ointment has been epithelialized in the abrasion, with formation of an ointment "cyst" that later requires operative removal).

Intraocular Foreign Bodies

Intraocular foreign bodies are easily overlooked if the index of suspicion is not high. Obtain orbital films any time the patient gives a history of striking a hammer on a piece of metal, or similar activity in which a small foreign body could be projected into the eye with enough force to penetrate the eye. If the x-ray is positive for a foreign body, immediate ophthalmology consultation is required.

Eye Injuries Arising from Direct Trauma

Hyphema

A hyphema may result from blunt trauma to the eye that causes bleeding into the anterior chamber. The bleeding may completely fill the anterior chamber, resulting in an "eight-ball" appearance. More commonly, the anterior chamber is partially filled with blood layering out inferiorly. Immediate ophthalmology consultation is required.

Iritis Iritis may follow trauma to the eye. The patient complains of pain and photophobia. The bulbar conjunctivae are diffusely injected, especially in the perilimbal region. The pupil is miotic and visual acuity is decreased. On slit lamp examination, WBCs are seen in the anterior chamber. Ophthalmology consultation should be obtained.

Traumatic Mydriasis Traumatic mydriasis may occur occasionally following blunt trauma to the eye. Usually, the dilated, fixed pupil reverts to normal in a few days without specific treatment. Rarely, the dilatation may be permanent.

Retinal Detachment Retinal detachment is heralded by a decrease in vision often described as light flashes followed by a "curtain" type of field defect. The fundus appears gray and rippled or undulating, and the retinal vessels are elevated and abnormally tortuous. If the retina is detached only peripherally, it may not be visible on direct ophthalmoscopy and vision may be normal. For this reason, it is prudent to refer patients with significant blunt trauma for ophthalmologic examination if any suspicious history is present (i.e., light flashes, black spots, film or cloud over vision, curtain coming down).

Orbital Blowout Fracture Orbital blowout fracture may occur when an object larger than the orbital rim strikes the eye, compressing the orbital contents. The increased intraorbital pressure "blows out" the thin and weak orbital floor. The inferior rectus and inferior oblique muscles may prolapse into the defect, causing diplopia on upward gaze. Plain x-rays may not reveal the fracture. A CT scan or tomograms of the orbital floor may be necessary to demonstrate the fracture.

Differential Diagnosis of the Red Eye

Conjunctivitis In conjunctivitis, the eye is diffusely injected. There is no change in visual acuity, intraocular pressure, or pupillary size and reaction.

Iritis In iritis, the injection is concentrated in the perilimbal area. The visual acuity and intraocular pressure are decreased. The pupil is miotic and cells are present in the anterior chamber.

Acute Glaucoma In acute glaucoma, the eye is diffusely injected. The visual acuity is decreased and the intraocular pressure is markedly elevated. The pupil is dilated and frequently reacts sluggishly or not at all. The cornea often has a hazy appearance.

Chemicals in the Eye The first thing that should be done is to immediately instill a topical anesthetic and irrigate the eye profusely. Hang a 1000-mL bag of normal saline and run the entire amount over the surface of the eye. Any particles of material should be removed with a moistened cotton-tipped applicator. Assessment of the eye is then done in standard fashion. Superficial corneal injuries are treated in the same way as abrasions from other causes with a topical antibiotic, a short-acting cycloplegic, and patching, with reevaluation in 24 hours. The patch is for comfort only and is optional. Severe corneal burns or alkali burns require ophthalmologic consultation.

EAR, NOSE, AND THROAT EMERGENCIES
Epistaxis

The first step in the treatment of epistaxis is to have the patient squeeze the nose firmly between the thumb and index finger and not let go for at least 10 minutes. However, if the patient is in shock or has uncontrolled hypertension, immediately give the usual treatment for those entities while the patient holds his or her nose.

History In the vast majority of cases, patients are stable. The history is taken while focusing on the common causes of epistaxis—trauma, respiratory infection, hypertension, or underlying hemostatic defect.

Physical Examination Examination of the nose is accomplished with an ear, nose, and throat (ENT) headlight, a nasal spectrum, a metal tip attached to suction, a pair of bayonet forceps, a small medicine cup, cotton balls, and 4% cocaine solution.

Laboratory Studies Consider laboratory studies in patients who have unstable vital signs or a history of hemostatic defect. A CBC, platelet count, prothrombin time, partial thromboplastin time, SMA-7, and type and crossmatch are the tests selected according to the clinical picture. Again, a vast majority of patients do not require laboratory work.

Treatment The provider should place a gown over his or her clothes and give the patient an emesis basin to catch any bleeding. An attempt should be made to visualize the site of bleeding. First, remove clots from the patient's nose with the forceps or by having the patient blow the clots into the emesis basin. If active bleeding is occurring, have the patient lean forward and let the blood run into the basin. The goal is to differentiate anterior from posterior epistaxis and to visually identify the bleeding site if it is anterior.

Anterior Epistaxis The most common site for epistaxis is anterior. A small pumping blood vessel can be located on the anterior inferior portion of the nasal septum. It often appears to be a tiny worm sticking out of the ground and waving in the breeze.

Once the site has been identified, take the bayonet forceps and wrap part of a cottonball around the forceps, making a pledget of cotton. Soak the pledget in cocaine, squeeze out the excess, and insert it into the nose. Leave it in place for 10 minutes, remove it, and cauterize the bleeder with a silver nitrate stick. Hold the silver nitrate stick in place for 10 seconds, and then observe for cessation of bleeding. Once the bleeding has been controlled, place a small anterior petroleum jelly gauze pack and a Band-Aid with a space for the nostril cut out on the side that does not have the packing. Instruct the patient not to do any physical exertion and to keep the head elevated above heart level for 48 hours. Give the patient a referral for removal of the packing in 48 hours and instructions to return immediately if bleeding recurs.

Posterior Epistaxis Patients with posterior epistaxis need a nasal pack and may need admission to the hospital. Insertion of a nasal pack is extremely uncomfortable. Anesthetize the whole nasal passageway using cocaine-soaked cotton pledgets inserted deeply into the nose and layered to fill the cavity. Consider premedicating the patient with an injectable analgesic.

A useful first step is to insert a Merocel foam nasal pack after coating it with antibiotic ointment. Drip saline from a 10-mL syringe on the packing and it will expand into a spongelike pack that fills the nasal cavity. It should be removed in 48 hours and must be remoistened before removal.

The Nasostat is a commercially available device that can be inserted into the nose and inflated carefully by following the directions that come with the device. It has an anterior and a posterior balloon that can be filled with saline.

In a patient whose hemorrhage cannot be controlled with the measures above, a No. 10 or a No. 12 Foley catheter with a 30-mL balloon can be inserted into the nose until it can be seen in the posterior pharynx. Inflate the balloon with water and pull it snugly against the posterior aspect of the nares. Take petroleum jelly gauze and pack it in with bayonet forceps, starting along the bottom of the nasal passageway and layering it upward to fill the nose. An assistant is needed to hold traction on the Foley catheter as the pack is placed in the nose against the balloon. A small square of sponge cast padding with a slit in it is used as a pad between the nose and a small C-clamp. If this fails to control the hemorrhage, get an ENT specialist to help. These patients all need admission to the hospital.

Removal of Intranasal Foreign Body

The usual patient is a child who has put some small object up his or her nose and comes into the ED with the mother. These patients rarely present with a unilateral purulent nasal drainage. Phenylephrine (Neo-Synephrine) nasal spray often works in trying to coax the child to blow the foreign body out of the nose.

The easiest way to remove most foreign bodies from the nose is with an ear curette. The child should be restrained in a papoose board with an assistant positioned to control the patient's head. Gently slide the curette over the top of the foreign body and then drag it out. This succeeds in nearly all cases. If the object is suitable for grabbing, remove it with a small pair of alligator forceps. No special treatment is needed after removal.

Septal Hematoma

It is very important in any case that involves trauma to the nose to look for a septal hematoma and to document on the chart its presence or absence. Failure to diagnose a septal hematoma can be disastrous for the patient. The septal hematoma may become infected, leading to destruction of the cartilage of the nasal septum and subsequent collapse of the nose with saddle deformity. Immediate ENT consult is indicated, for drainage of the hematoma and packing of the nose.

Ruptured Eardrum

History   Usually, the patient presents complaining of ear pain following trauma. Most commonly, the patient may have been slapped on the ear or may have fallen while water-skiing and slapped the ear on the water. Rarely, the trauma is due to an object introduced into the ear in an attempt to remove earwax.

Physical Examination   The physical examination reveals a defect in the eardrum that is clearly evident.

Treatment   Treatment consists of keeping the ear dry and administering an oral analgesic and a systemic antibiotic appropriate for otitis media. Patients seem to feel better if they place a small, dry cottonball in the ear. These small perforations heal in nearly all instances, and the patient can simply be reassured. It should be recommended that the patient follow up with an ENT specialist or the family doctor in 2 weeks, or immediately if increased pain, fever, or purulent ear drainage occurs.

NECK PAIN AND LOW BACK PAIN

When dealing with a patient who is complaining of neck or low back pain in the ED, the following questions should be answered:
➤ Is there a fracture or other abnormality of the bones?
➤ Is there a radiculopathy (diseased condition of roots of spinal nerves)?
➤ Is there a muscle or ligament abnormality?

History   An accurate history includes every episode of this pain both past and present.

Physical Examination   The physical examination is the key to detecting signs of radiculopathy.

Neck

1. Palpate areas of tenderness.
2. Check and record the *range of motion.* Have the patient turn the neck to the right as far as he or she can until the pain begins, and record the rotation in degrees. Then have the patient turn to the left.
3. Do a nerve root–directed *motor and sensory examination* (Table 30-2).

Radiculopathy can usually be detected with the motor and sensory examination. Reflexes are not as helpful because multiple nerve roots are reflected by reflexes in the arms.

Laboratory Studies   Obtain x-rays, which show bony abnormalities. Disk space narrowing, spur formation, congenital abnormalities, and postsurgical changes (prior fusions) are most common. There may be a straightening of the normal C-shaped curve of

Table 30-2 Motor and Sensory Examination of Nerve Roots–Neck

Nerve Root	Motor	Sensory	Reflex
C5	Deltoid	Lateral shoulder	—
C6	Biceps	Thumb	Biceps
C7	Wrist extensors	Long finger	Triceps
C8	Finger flexors	Little finger	—
T1	Finger abductors	Inner upper arm	—

the cervical (C) spine. This is due to spasm of the surrounding muscles. Of course, if the patient is presenting with neck pain following recent trauma, the first step is to get a full C-spine series to rule out fracture before performing the physical examination.

Using the previously described format, an example of the patient's chart would be as follows.

CASE STUDY 30-7

History   A 40-year-old man with a 3-week history of increasing pain in the posterior neck that radiates into the right arm and has a burning quality. No prior similar pain, no history of injury.

Physical Examination
- ➤ Pain to palpation of right paraspinous muscles.
- ➤ Right rotation, 30 degrees; left rotation, 60 degrees.
- ➤ Motor, C5-T1: Weakness in right biceps; otherwise normal.
- ➤ Sensory, C5-T1: Decreased sensation to touch and pinprick in right thumb; otherwise normal.
- ➤ Triceps reflex normal; biceps reflex decreased.

Laboratory Studies   X-rays reveal disk space narrowing with large hypertrophic spurs at the C5-C6 level.

Diagnosis   C6 radiculopathy (herniated disk vs. pressure from spur).

Treatment   In this case, treatment can be selected from muscle relaxants, analgesics, anti-inflammatory drugs, and physical therapy. Patients who do not respond to conservative therapy need orthopedic or neurosurgical referral for consideration of surgery.

Lower Back
1. Palpate areas of tenderness.
2. Check and record the range of motion. Have the patient bend forward as far as he or she comfortably can, as if doing a "toe touch," and record where the fingertips rest (floor, knees, midthigh, etc.).
3. Do a nerve root–directed motor and sensory examination (Table 30-3).

Straight Leg Raising
Straight leg raising (SLR) should be tested and recorded. Raise the patient's straightened leg slowly from the table until a point is reached that intensifies the pain in the back. Record it as, for example, "SLR positive at 30 degrees" or "SLR negative to 90 degrees." If the patient experiences pain in the opposite side of the back and the opposite leg, this is very suggestive of a ruptured disk. This phenomenon is called *crossed straight leg raise,* and in some studies, it is 90% correlated with a ruptured disk.

The patient's chart may read as follows.

CASE STUDY 30-8

History   A 35-year-old man with a history of sudden onset of pain in the left lower back 2 weeks ago while lifting a 50-lb box at work. The pain now radiates into the left leg, and he occasionally feels numbness in his foot. Several milder episodes of pain have occurred over the past 3 years, none severe enough for a physician visit.

Examination
- ➤ Pain to palpation of left paraspinous muscles, left sacroiliac joint, and left buttock over the sciatic nerve.
- ➤ Forward flexion: Fingertips to knees.

Table 30-3   Motor and Sensory Examination of Nerve Roots—Lower Back

Nerve Root	Motor	Sensory	Reflex
L4	Quadriceps	Above knee	Knee jerk
L5	Great toe extensor	Medial foot	–
S1	Calf	Lateral foot	Ankle jerk

➤ Motor, L4-S1: Subjective weakness in left calf with toe raises; otherwise normal.
➤ Sensory, L4-S1: Decreased sensation over the lateral foot; otherwise normal.
➤ Knee jerk: Normal.
➤ Ankle jerk: Normal, right; absent, left.
➤ SLR L to 30 degrees; crossed SLR R to L to 60 degrees.

Laboratory Studies X-rays reveal disk space narrowing of L5-S1.

Diagnosis Acute low back pain with herniated disk and S1 radiculopathy.

Treatment In this case, treatment can be again selected from muscle relaxants, analgesics, and anti-inflammatory drugs. Recent studies have shown that patients with low back pain do better with "activity within the limits of pain" than with bedrest or physical therapy. Patients who do not respond to conservative treatment need orthopedic or neurosurgical referral for consideration of surgery.

SPRAINS
Differentiating Sprains

A ligament is a tough fibrous structure that runs from bone to bone. Sprains are ligamentous injuries, and it is essential to divide them into three categories for treatment purposes.

First-Degree (Mild) Some fibers of the ligament have been torn, but there is no loss of function and no loss in the strength of the ligament.

History Historically, one finds only mild disability. Indeed, the disability may be so mild that the patient does not even seek the advice of a physician.

Physical Examination Physical examination reveals mild tenderness and swelling over the injured ligament, with no instability.

Treatment The treatment is *RICE* (rest, ice, compression, and elevation). In this case, the ligament is not weakened and a cast or a brace is not needed.

Second-Degree (Moderate) A larger portion of the ligament is torn, enough to weaken it functionally. It is difficult to determine clinically the extent of the damage and just how much of the ligament is torn.

History Historically, there is some degree of immediate disability. The patient is unable to continue to use the joint normally.

Physical Examination The physical examination reveals a moderate amount of local tenderness and swelling over the injured ligament, but no instability.

Treatment Treatment consists of immobilizing and protecting the injured ligament while it heals. In this case, the ligament is only partially torn, and wide retraction of the ends of the torn ligament is not part of the injury process. Therefore, satisfactory healing should occur provided the joint is adequately immobilized and protected. The specific method of immobilization depends on the joint involved and is discussed later.

Third-Degree (Severe) The entire ligament is torn with complete functional loss.

History Historically, there is immediate and complete loss of function of the affected joint. Severe second- and third-degree sprains cannot be separated on the basis of the history alone because loss of function occurs in both.

Physical Examination The physical examination reveals marked tenderness and swelling over the torn ligament.

Laboratory Studies The diagnosis depends on demonstrating abnormal motion of the involved joint by x-ray, with stress on the joint, or both.

Treatment Treatment is usually surgical. Efficient repair is dependent on the apposition of the torn ends of the ligament, which may be widely separated. A less satisfactory alternative is to treat third-degree sprains with immobilization, with the hope that the ends are close enough together to heal. A secondary surgical procedure is then done if subsequent instability occurs.

Specific Sprains

Metacarpophalangeal Joint of the Thumb

The metacarpophalangeal joint of the thumb (Figure 30-1) has collateral ligaments and a strong palmar ligament (volar plate).

History The history reveals that the patient's thumb has been subjected to a hyperabduction stress. This occurs most commonly from the steering wheel in deceleration accidents, from the ski pole in falls while snow-skiing (ski-pole thumb), and from other injuries in which the thumb is hyperabducted.

Physical Examination The physical examination reveals swelling and tenderness at the metacarpophalangeal joint. Gentle hyperabduction stress reveals instability if a complete tear of the ulnar collateral ligament is present.

Laboratory Studies X-rays are normal.

Treatment An immediate orthopedic consultation is needed. There is controversy about the best way to treat this injury. If the ligament ends are in apposition, a satisfactory result can be obtained by immobilization in a thumb spica cast. A grade III rupture of the ulnar collateral ligament is exhibited by an interposition of the adductor aponeurosis and a "turning back" of the proximal end of the ligament (Figure 30-2). A second-degree sprain would be treated with a thumb spica splint for 3 weeks. A first-degree sprain would be treated symptomatically.

Occasionally, the adductor pollicis brevis aponeurosis interposes itself between the torn ends of the ligament. In this situation, surgical intervention is mandated to repair the instability and avoid a rapidly progressive degenerative arthritis in the joint (Figure 30-3).

Metacarpophalangeal Joint of the Fifth Finger

History The history reveals an injury that puts a hyperabduction stress on the radial collateral ligament of the metacarpophalangeal joint of the fifth finger.

Physical Examination The physical examination reveals tenderness and swelling in the joint. If the ligament is completely ruptured, it will be unstable with

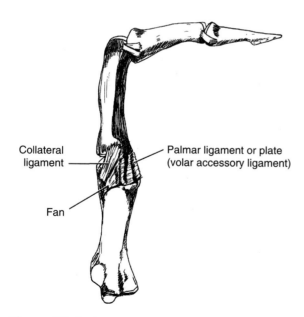

Collateral ligament

Palmar ligament or plate (volar accessory ligament)

Fan

Figure 30-1 The metacarpophalangeal joint of the thumb has collateral ligaments and a strong palmar ligament (volar plate).

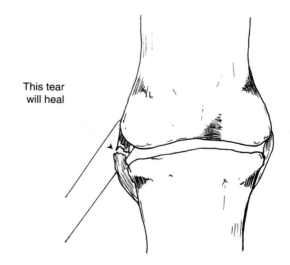

This tear will heal

Figure 30-2 Grade III rupture of the ulnar collateral ligament with the ligament ends in apposition.

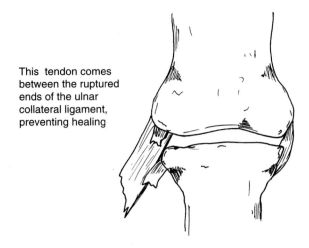

This tendon comes between the ruptured ends of the ulnar collateral ligament, preventing healing

Figure 30-3 Grade III rupture of the ulnar collateral ligament with interposition of the adductor aponeurosis and turnback of the proximal end of the ligament.

stress, and sometimes the short abductor pulls the finger into ulnar deviation.

Treatment   Treatment for first-degree sprains is symptomatic. Second-degree sprains can be treated by taping the fourth finger to the fifth finger; immediate orthopedic referral is provided for complete ruptures. Ruptures of the collateral ligaments of other metacarpophalangeal joints are rare, and do not need operative repair owing to the stability provided by surrounding structures.

Proximal Interphalangeal Joint

The proximal interphalangeal joint has collateral ligaments and a thick volar plate as does the metacarpophalangeal joint. These ligaments may rupture with or without an associated dislocation.

History   The history reveals an injury to the finger. Sometimes the patient describes a dislocation that was self-reduced or was reduced by a friend before arrival in the ED.

Physical Examination   The physical examination reveals tenderness and swelling, and the x-ray is negative for fractures. Gentle stress of the collateral ligaments reveals instability if a complete rupture is present. The volar plate is tested by gently hyperextending the joint.

Treatment   Treatment is immediate orthopedic referral if collateral ligament instability is found. Some orthopedists treat with surgical repair, whereas others treat conservatively with splinting. Second-degree sprains can be immobilized for 3 weeks by buddy-taping the injured finger to the adjacent finger and encouraging active range of motion. First-degree sprains are treated symptomatically.

Wrist Sprains

Wrist sprains are very uncommon. Most wrist sprains are actually strains of tendon attachments or bony injuries. Navicular fractures in the wrist are notorious for not appearing on x-ray initially. Additionally, they have a high incidence of avascular necrosis of the proximal fragment. When this occurs, the patient requires surgery to remove the devascularized portion of the bone. It is a good practice to splint any significant wrist injury and have the patient follow up with an orthopedist. A thumb spica splint should be used if a navicular fracture is suspected.

Elbow Sprains

The ulnar collateral ligament of the elbow is attached to the humerus superiorly and the ulna inferiorly on the medial aspect of the joint (Figure 30-4).

The elbow also has a lateral ligament known as the radial collateral ligament, which extends over the radial head as the annular ligament of the radius (Figure 30-5). A ligamentous injury here is relatively uncommon. The ligaments may be torn by hyperextension or by lateral motion (forced abduction of the extended arm). If x-ray studies are negative, it is not necessary to stress-test for instability. The elbow joint has inherent bony stability and is a non–weight-bearing joint. A good result is obtained regardless of the degree of sprain by using a protective sling and gradually increasing the motion within the limits of pain until the joint is pain-free.

Ankle Sprains

The lateral side of the ankle is supported by the anterior talofibular, calcaneofibular, and posterior talofibular ligaments. Anterior and posterior

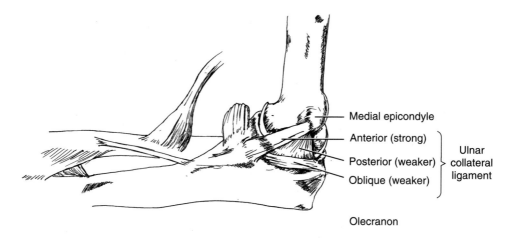

Figure 30-4 Ulnar collateral ligament of the elbow.

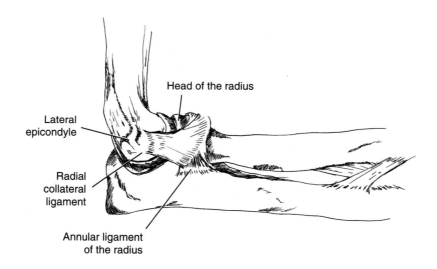

Figure 30-5 Radial collateral ligament of the elbow.

tibiofibular ligaments bind the fibula to the tibia (Figure 30-6).

The medial side of the ankle is supported by the multiple components of the thick deltoid ligament (Figure 30-7).

Eighty-five percent of all ankle sprains are inversion injuries. This force is usually an internal rotation and plantar flexion of the foot in relation to the leg. The anterior talofibular ligament is always injured first, followed by the calcaneofibular ligament, and in

very severe cases with dislocation, the posterior talofibular ligament. It is very difficult to clinically differentiate a severe second-degree sprain from a third-degree sprain of the ankle.

Some physicians recommend local or IV regional anesthesia followed by stress x-rays to demonstrate instability and also recommend surgical repair of complete ligament ruptures, especially in competitive athletes. Other physicians recommend treating both second- and third-degree sprains by cast or brace

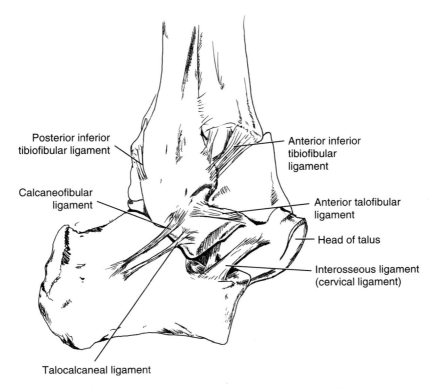

Posterior inferior tibiofibular ligament

Calcaneofibular ligament

Anterior inferior tibiofibular ligament

Anterior talofibular ligament

Head of talus

Interosseous ligament (cervical ligament)

Talocalcaneal ligament

Figure 30-6 Lateral view of the ligaments of the ankle.

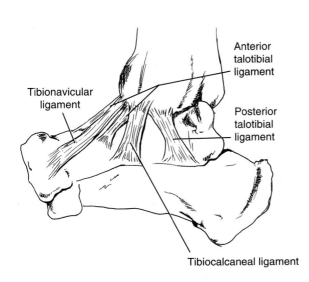

Anterior talotibial ligament

Tibionavicular ligament

Posterior talotibial ligament

Tibiocalcaneal ligament

Figure 30-7 Medial view of the ligaments of the ankle.

immobilization and reserve surgery for patients who demonstrate an unstable joint after the conservative treatment has been completed and the ankle has healed. The following treatment, from the *Manual of Acute Orthopaedic Therapeutics* by Iversen and Swiontkowski,[9] is a useful approach for the nonorthopedist for this type of injury.

HISTORY The history should focus on the mechanism of injury and the amount of functional disability for grading the sprain. Find out if there have been prior injuries to the ankle and if so, how they were treated.

PHYSICAL EXAMINATION Inspection will reveal ecchymosis and swelling of the ankle. Palpate carefully over the posterior talofibular ligament, calcaneofibular ligament, anterior talofibular ligament, deltoid ligament, and the anterior capsule to define the areas of injury. In addition, check for instability by performing the anterior drawer test. This is performed by holding the leg with one hand and grasping the heel with the other. Pull forward gently on the heel, attempting to subluxate the talus anteriorly within the ankle mortise. A positive anterior drawer test indicates complete rupture of the anterior talofibular ligament. In addition, significant tenderness and swelling over the deltoid ligament or anterior capsule indicate that a severe sprain has occurred.

LABORATORY STUDIES   X-rays should be taken provided the patient meets the criteria outlined in each individual ED.

TREATMENT   Treatment consists of synthesizing information from the history and physical examination to determine the severity of the sprain and diagnosing it as first, second, or third degree.

First-Degree Sprain
HISTORY   The patient sustains an injury but there is little functional disability. The patient may even have been able to finish the activity and can bear weight without much discomfort.

PHYSICAL EXAMINATION   Physical examination reveals mild tenderness and swelling, usually confined to the anterior talofibular ligament.

TREATMENT   RICE.

Second-Degree Sprain
HISTORY   The patient usually has functional disability immediately after the injury and is unable to continue activity. The patient bears weight poorly or not at all.

PHYSICAL EXAMINATION   Physical examination reveals moderate-to-severe swelling and tenderness over both the anterior talofibular and calcaneofibular ligaments. There is usually no significant tenderness over the deltoid ligament or the anterior capsule, and the anterior drawer test is negative.

TREATMENT   Treatment consists of immobilizing the ankle, placing the patient on crutches, and referring the patient to an orthopedist in 24 to 48 hours for reevaluation. Immobilize by cast or splint. The ankle

can be wrapped in two 4-inch rolls of cast padding followed by an Ace bandage or by using a plaster stirrup splint.

Third-Degree Sprain
HISTORY   The patient experiences immediate loss of function of the injured ankle and may relate that the ankle "feels" unstable with any attempt at weight bearing.

PHYSICAL EXAMINATION   Physical examination reveals severe swelling and tenderness over the anterior talofibular ligament, the calcaneofibular ligament, and occasionally, the posterior talofibular ligament. There is also tenderness over the deltoid ligament and the anterior capsule, and the anterior drawer test is positive.

TREATMENT   The orthopedist should be contacted immediately. This allows the orthopedist the option of obtaining stress films and treating the injury surgically. It also gives the orthopedist the option of conservative treatment (i.e., soft roll, Ace bandage, ice, elevation, non–weight-bearing with crutches for a few days, followed by a short leg walking cast or ankle fracture splint for 6 weeks). If long-term lateral instability results from nonoperative treatment, surgical repair will be necessary.

Ankle sprains have a high associated morbidity. The average duration of disability has been reported to be between 4 and 26 weeks, and only 25% to 60% of patients are symptom-free 1 to 4 years after injury. These so-called minor injuries, therefore, deserve careful diagnosis and treatment.

Knee Sprains   The medial side of the knee is supported by the tibial collateral ligament. The following diagrams picture the tibial collateral ligament and bony attachments to the femur and tibia (Figure 30-8, A and B).

The lateral side of the knee is supported by the fibular collateral ligament and the iliotibial band (Figure 30-9, A and B).

The anterior and posterior cruciate ligaments provide anterior and posterior stability (Figures 30-10, A and B and 30-11).

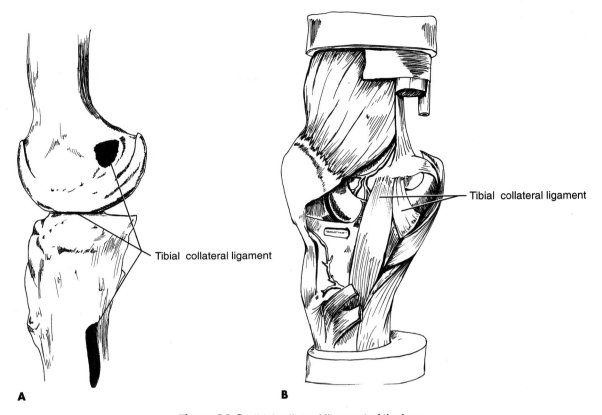

A   B

Figure 30-8 Tibial collateral ligament of the knee.

HISTORY The history of injury provides important clues concerning which structures may have been damaged. Most injuries occur while the patient is weight-bearing with the foot fixed. A blow from the lateral side is likely to produce a tear of the medial collateral ligament, the anterior or posterior cruciate ligament, and the medial meniscus. Blows from the medial side, although rare, produce tears of the lateral collateral ligament, the iliotibial band, and the lateral meniscus. A hyperextension injury either forward or backward may produce tears of the cruciate ligaments.

PHYSICAL EXAMINATION The physical examination begins with gentle palpation for areas of tenderness. The presence or absence of an effusion (fluid in the joint) should be noted. Record the range of motion and check for ligamentous instability. Lay the patient down with the knee extended, and gently apply varus and valgus stress.

LABORATORY STUDIES The knee is x-rayed to rule out a fracture (Figure 30-12), if the patient meets criteria for x-rays.

Valgus Stress Instability in this position indicates rupture of both the collateral and cruciate ligaments. If the knee is stable in extension, flex the knee 25 to 30 degrees to relax the cruciate ligaments, and repeat the examination. Instability in this position indicates medial or collateral ligament tears (Figure 30-13, *A*).

Anterior Drawer Sign Have the patient flex the injured knee to 60 to 90 degrees and place the foot firmly on the table. It is easy to fix the foot in this

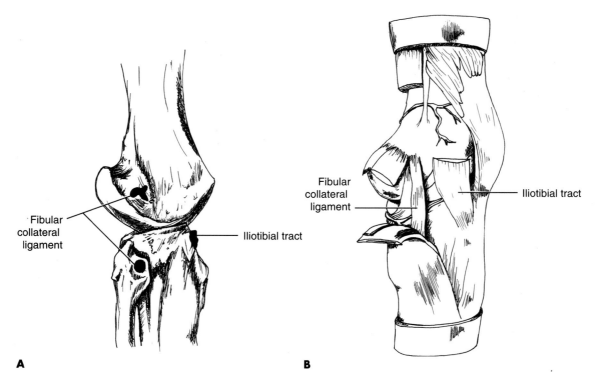

Figure 30-9 Fibular collateral ligament and iliotibial band.

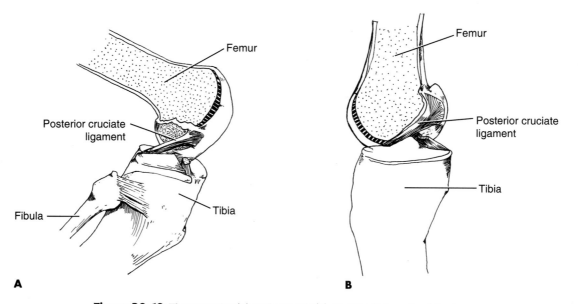

Figure 30-10 The posterior (**A**) and anterior (**B**) cruciate ligaments of the knee.

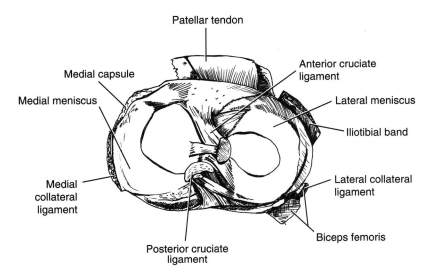

Figure 30-11 Cross section showing the ligaments of the knee.

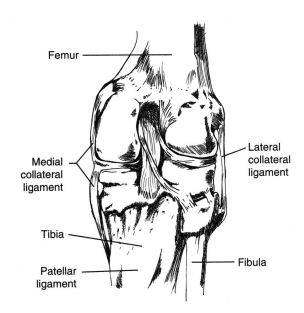

Figure 30-12 The knee from the front with the superficial structures removed.

position simply by sitting on it, which leaves both hands free to examine the knee (Figure 30-13, *B*).

Pull the lower leg forward and backward, looking for any movement or instability in the joint. Any movement forward is positive for a tear of the anterior cruciate ligament and any movement backward is positive for a tear of the posterior cruciate ligament.

An alternative way to test the anterior cruciate ligament is to have the patient sit on the side of the examination table with the knee flexed 90 degrees. Gently pull forward on the proximal lower leg, looking for forward displacement of the tibia on the femur. If motion is present, this is a positive anterior drawer sign and indicates a complete rupture of the anterior cruciate ligament (Figure 30-14, *A* and *B*).

Lachman Test The Lachman test is also very helpful for demonstrating anterior cruciate ligament instability. With the knee flexed 30 degrees, gently pull the lower leg forward on the femur, again looking for abnormal anterior motion. Assessment of the stability of the ligaments is difficult if the examiner is rough. Pain will cause the patient to contract the powerful thigh muscles, which may mask significant instability. Additionally, it is extremely important to examine both the patient's knees, comparing the injured knee with the normal knee. This should be done because of the considerable variation from patient to patient in normal ligamentous laxity. Knee sprains are divided into first, second, and third degree for treatment purposes.

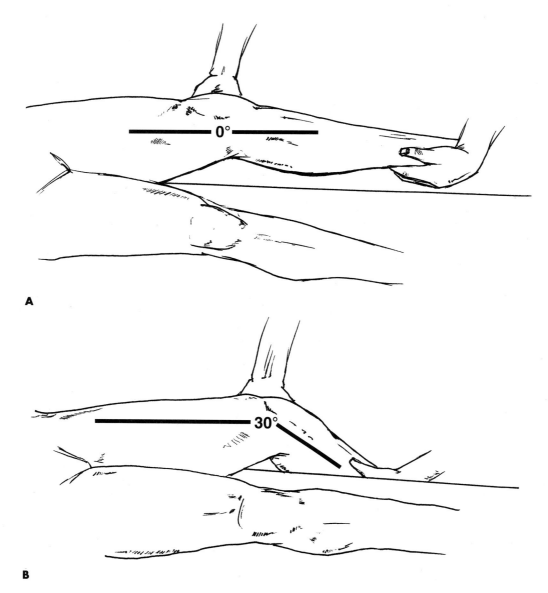

Figure 30-13 Negative movement **(A)** and instability **(B)** of the knee under valgus stress.

First Degree

HISTORY   The patient experiences mild or no immediate loss of function.

PHYSICAL EXAMINATION   Physical examination reveals tenderness and mild swelling over the involved ligament. An effusion is not present. Gentle passive movement of the joint reveals a normal or near-normal range of motion. Stressing the ligaments may cause pain, but no instability is evident.

TREATMENT   Treatment is RICE: Rest with activity within the limits of pain, ice, compression with an Ace bandage, and elevation.

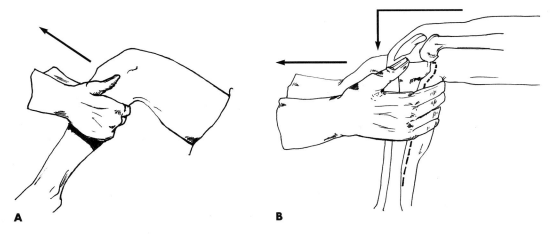

Figure 30-14 Anterior **(A)** and alternative **(B)** drawer signs.

Second Degree

HISTORY   The patient usually has some immediate loss of function.

PHYSICAL EXAMINATION   Physical examination reveals more swelling and tenderness over the involved ligament, and an effusion is often present. Range of motion is decreased. Stress testing reveals mild or no instability.

TREATMENT   In this case, the treatment is protection and referral. A useful approach follows:

➤ Aspirate the joint if a large effusion is present and is causing severe pain.
➤ Wrap the knee with an Ace bandage, starting at the foot and wrapping to above the knee to avoid a tourniquet effect.
➤ Apply a prefabricated posterior knee splint.
➤ Place the patient on crutches.
➤ Instruct the patient to apply ice for 20 minutes every 2 hours while awake.
➤ Prescribe a nonsteroidal anti-inflammatory drug as an analgesic.
➤ Have the patient perform ten 7- to 10-second isometric quadriceps contractions every hour while awake.
➤ Refer the patient to an orthopedist for follow-up in 24 to 48 hours.

Third Degree

HISTORY   The patient has immediate loss of function and may report that the knee feels unstable with attempted weight bearing.

PHYSICAL EXAMINATION   Severe tenderness and swelling are usually present over the involved ligaments. An effusion is usually present, although if the joint capsule is torn, the blood may leak out into the surrounding tissues. Range of motion is severely decreased and stress testing reveals instability, which is the hallmark of a third-degree sprain.

TREATMENT   Immediate orthopedic consultation is indicated if instability is demonstrated.

It is very important not to diagnose a second-degree sprain if a third-degree sprain is really present because the treatment for a third-degree sprain is usually surgical. Therefore, if the examination is inadequate because the patient is experiencing too much pain to relax the knee, consult an orthopedist immediately. The orthopedist may wish to examine the patient under anesthesia.

About 85% of patients who sustain a hyperextension injury of the knee and have a bloody effusion on examination have an anterior cruciate ligament tear. In light of this fact, it is prudent to obtain a next-day orthopedic consultation, even if instability could not be demonstrated on examination. The classic example of this type of injury in football is the punter whose down leg is hyperextended by a defender attempting to block the kick.

It is very difficult to diagnose a cartilage injury in an acutely injured knee unless the knee is "locked." This occurs when the torn cartilage blocks full extension of the knee and the patient reports that something is preventing him or her from straightening the knee. The knee is usually locked in 20 to 30 degrees of flexion. Consult the orthopedist immediately and follow the treatment regimen for second-degree knee sprains.

Patellar Dislocation   A common injury easily confused with a sprain is a patellar dislocation.

History   The patient relates that the knee went out of joint or dislocated. Complete loss of function is present if spontaneous reduction has not occurred.

Physical Examination   Physical examination reveals that the patella dislocated laterally and the patient is holding the knee at around 30 degrees of flexion. If the patella has spontaneously reduced, an effusion is usually present and tenderness is marked along the medial aspect of the patella, where supporting tissues were torn when it dislocated. Bending the knee slightly and applying a gentle force to the medial aspect of the patella with the fingers may demonstrate the instability of the tendon and re-dislocate the patella. Usually the patient apprehensively stops the examination at this point.

Treatment   If the dislocation is still present, it can easily be reduced by straightening the knee and pulling the patella toward the midline. Often, the dislocation has spontaneously reduced before examination. Although x-ray results are usually negative, occasionally a thin sliver of patella may appear medially to the patella. This sliver was avulsed as the kneecap dislocated laterally out of the femoral groove. A sunrise view of the patella is helpful in ruling out this fracture (Figures 30-15 and 30-16).

Shoulder Sprains and Strains   Patients reporting to the ED with shoulder pain frequently have negative results on standard x-rays. However, many have

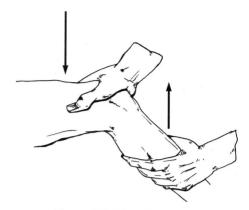

Figure 30-15 Lachman test.

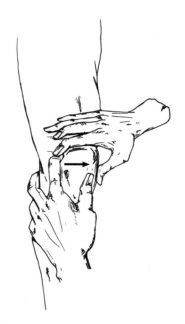

Figure 30-16 Patellar apprehension test.

significant injuries that require specialized care. Always helpful are a good understanding of the anatomy of the shoulder and an awareness of the clinical presentations of dislocations, acromioclavicular sprains, rotator cuff tears, and ruptures of the long head of the biceps tendon.

A fibrous capsule holds the humeral head in the glenoid cavity. Any sprain of the shoulder injures this capsule. The tendons of the muscles of the shoulder, which make up the rotator cuff, blend with this capsule, making it very difficult to differentiate sprains from strains, but it is not important from the standpoint of treatment.

Figure 30-17 shows the posterior portion of the rotator cuff, which is made up of the infraspinatus and teres minor tendons. The infraspinatus has been cut and lifted to show the fibrous capsule underneath. The axillary nerve, which supplies motor power to the deltoid muscle and sensation to the lateral upper arm, is also visible. The tendons of the supraspinatus and subscapularis muscles form the superior and anterior portions of the rotator cuff. The long head of the biceps tendon enters the shoulder joint and is attached to the superior rim of the glenoid (Figure 30-18).

Anterior Dislocation of the Shoulder

HISTORY   The patient gives a history of sustaining a force that caused a combination of abduction, extension, and external rotation of the shoulder. The capsule of the shoulder joint is torn from the glenoid, and the humeral head rests inferiorly and anteriorly in a subcoracoid position.

PHYSICAL EXAMINATION   The physical examination finds the patient holding the arm in slight abduction. The acromion will be prominent and the deltoid will be flattened. Exclude neurovascular injury by feeling pulses, checking the function of the axillary nerve (most commonly injured), and checking the function of the musculocutaneous nerve. The axillary nerve provides sensation to the lateral upper arm and motor power to the deltoid, which abducts the shoulder. The

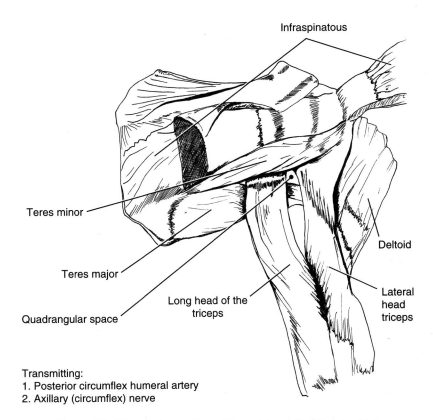

Transmitting:
1. Posterior circumflex humeral artery
2. Axillary (circumflex) nerve

Figure 30-17 Posterior portion of the rotator cuff of the shoulder.

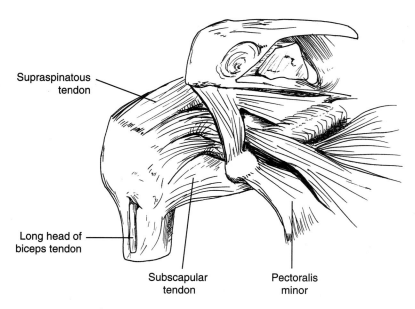

Supraspinatous tendon

Long head of biceps tendon

Subscapular tendon

Pectoralis minor

Figure 30-18 Anterior portion of the shoulder.

musculocutaneous nerve provides sensation to the volar radial side of the forearm and motor power to the biceps muscle. Loss of function is usually due to a contusion of one of these nerves and usually resolves spontaneously in a few weeks to 3 to 4 months.

Before examination, an analgesic should be administered parenterally and x-rays taken. If a fracture is revealed, especially one involving the greater tuberosity or humeral head, immediate orthopedic consultation should be obtained.

TREATMENT If no fracture is present, the shoulder reduction can be accomplished in several ways; however, only the countertraction method is discussed here. With the patient supine, an assistant should position himself at the head of the bed on the side opposite the dislocated shoulder. A sheet should be looped over the patient's chest through the axilla, on the injured side, returning the sheet under the patient's back to exit near the assistant. The assistant stabilizes the patient and applies countertraction as the shoulder is reduced. The operator, using both hands to grasp the wrist on the arm with the injured shoulder, applies gentle traction, straightening the arm to 20 to 40 degrees of abduction. The operator

can then lean back slowly, allowing his or her own body weight to apply even and steady traction and encouraging the patient to let the shoulder muscles relax and "turn into jelly." It is helpful to coach the patient in letting the muscles relax more and more with each exhalation. If reduction is not achieved in 2 to 3 minutes, midazolam (Versed) should be administered through an IV line at 1 milligram every 30 to 60 seconds until relocation occurs or a maximum dose of 10 mg is reached. Follow the conscious sedation protocol for the ED when using IV midazolam. After reduction, the arm is placed in a shoulder immobilizer and the patient is referred to an orthopedist within the next 7 days.

Posterior Dislocation of the Shoulder Posterior dislocations of the shoulder are rare and may be easily missed.

HISTORY The mechanism of injury is usually a direct driving force against the lower end of the humerus while the arm is flexed forward. These injuries usually occur during a seizure with convulsions or from severe trauma. The force is transmitted up the arm, driving the humeral head posteriorly behind the glenoid. The patient experiences intense pain and is unable to move the arm, while the outward appearance of the shoulder is deceivingly normal. The patient holds the arm fixed to his or her side, usually with the forearm across the abdomen.

PHYSICAL EXAMINATION　The patient resists any attempt to examine or externally rotate the arm or shoulder.

LABORATORY STUDIES　The AP x-ray appears normal because the head of the humerus moves almost straight backward and is not displaced inferiorly to any significant extent. An oblique x-ray must be taken with the patient erect and facing the cassette. This allows the central beam of the x-ray to correspond to the plane of the body of the scapula. In difficult cases, a transaxillary view taken while the arm is abducted under general anesthesia is diagnostic.

TREATMENT　Orthopedic referral is indicated immediately.

Rotator Cuff Tears

HISTORY　Rotator cuff tears may accompany shoulder dislocations and severe shoulder strains. They are difficult to diagnose unless massive.

PHYSICAL EXAMINATION　On physical examination, the patient is unable to initiate abduction and the arm falls to the patient's side when passively abducted to 30 degrees and dropped (drop arm test). If the patient can actively abduct the arm as little as 15 to 20 degrees, a complete rotator cuff tear can be ruled out.

LABORATORY STUDIES　The tear can be confirmed with an arthrogram and surgical repair is necessary, especially in athletes.

TREATMENT　Orthopedic consultation should be obtained if this complication is diagnosed.

Acromioclavicular Joint Sprains　The clavicle is connected to the acromion process of the scapula by the acromioclavicular (AC) ligament (AC joint). The AC ligament is weak and is easily ruptured with mild

trauma. The clavicle is anchored to the coracoid process of the scapula by the strong coracoclavicular ligament.

HISTORY　The mechanism of injury is a downward force over the superior acromion process, resulting in varying degrees of sprain to the AC joint. The most common example of this is a fall on the point of the shoulder, as from a horse or a motorcycle.

It is critical to diagnose the degree of sprain in a shoulder injury. A first-degree sprain exhibits an incomplete tear of the AC ligament without subluxation of the joint. A second-degree sprain is more severe and demonstrates a disruption of the AC ligament that allows partial separation of the AC joint, while the coracoclavicular ligaments remain intact. A third-degree AC sprain (complete shoulder separation) is a complete tear of the AC and coracoclavicular ligaments with a complete dislocation of the AC joint (Figures 30-19 through 30-21).

PHYSICAL EXAMINATION　In a first- or second-degree sprain, the patient has point tenderness and swelling over the AC joint. Deformity is not present or is negligible.

LABORATORY STUDIES　If standard shoulder x-rays are negative, stress x-rays should be taken. A single view of both AC joints is made with a 5- to 10-lb weight attached to the wrists of a standing patient. The patient must be educated not to take the strain off the AC joint by contracting the biceps muscles, or a false-negative result may occur. A *first-degree* sprain has a normal stress film. A *second-degree* sprain shows widening of the AC joint but no increased distance between the coracoid and the clavicle. The upward displacement of the distal clavicle should not be more than the full diameter of the clavicle. These injuries may be treated symptomatically with pain relievers and immobilization with a sling for 10 days to 3 weeks, followed by a rehabilitative exercise program.

The patient with a *third-degree* sprain has an obvious deformity with the skin tented by the distal end of the clavicle and the shoulder dropped down. Routine views of the shoulder usually show the clavicle to be riding

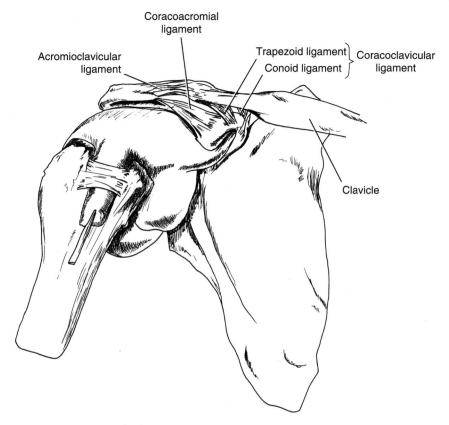

Figure 30-19 Ligaments of the shoulder.

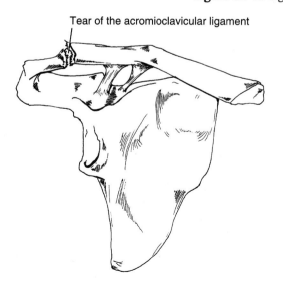

Figure 30-20 Second-degree sprain of the shoulder, with tear of the acromioclavicular ligament.

high, completely out of the AC joint with a widened space between the clavicle and the coracoid. Third-degree sprains require orthopedic referral. At the current time, most orthopedic surgeons advocate surgical repair, especially in athletes (see Figure 30-21).

Rupture of the Long Head of the Biceps Tendon
The biceps tendon runs in the intertubercular groove of the humerus through the shoulder joint to attach to the posterior superior aspect of the glenoid.

HISTORY   This injury is most commonly found in the elderly, usually as a result of attrition due to chronic bicipital tenosynovitis. Under these circumstances, it acquires a secondary attachment to the intertubercular groove and is discovered at autopsy. Clinically, this would be an elderly patient with a chronically painful shoulder that suddenly quits hurting when the rupture

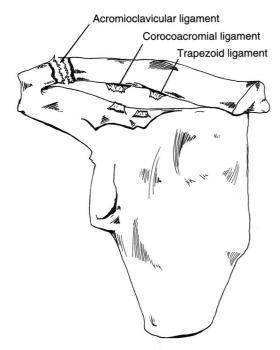

Figure 30-21 Third-degree sprain of the shoulder, with complete shoulder separation.

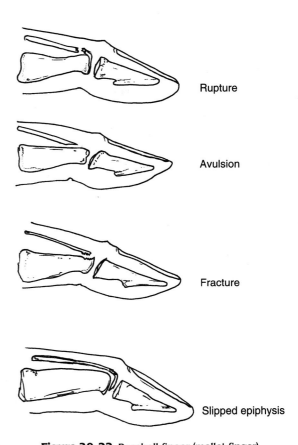

Figure 30-22 Baseball finger (mallet finger).

is complete. The muscle belly bunches up and appears prominent in the distal arm; however, surgical repair is generally not indicated in this group of patients.

Acute rupture in a younger person occurs as a result of forceful contraction of the biceps muscle, or forceful downward movement of the arm with the biceps contracted. The diagnosis is readily apparent when the patient contracts his or her biceps with the arm abducted 90 degrees and externally rotated.

TREATMENT Treatment is always surgical, whereby the long head of the biceps tendon is fastened into the intertubercular groove of the humerus.

MISCELLANEOUS CONDITIONS
Baseball Finger

Also known as *mallet finger*, the pathology is pictured in Figure 30-22.

History The patient presents with a history of blunt trauma to the end of the finger.

Physical Examination Physical examination reveals tenderness, swelling, and inability to extend the distal interphalangeal (DIP) joint. The DIP joint is pulled into flexion by the unopposed flexor digitorum longus tendon.

Laboratory Studies X-rays range from normal to an avulsion fracture or may reveal an epiphyseal fracture.

Treatment If the extensor tendon is avulsed from its attachment to the distal phalanx with no fracture or a small avulsion fracture, treatment consists of immobilizing the distal phalanx in hyperextension. A commercially available STACK finger splint is excellent (Figure 30-23).

If the STACK splint is not available, peel the foam off a piece of padded aluminum splint material and construct a small metal dorsal mallet finger splint (Figure 30-24).

If the avulsed fragment involves one third or more of the articular surface, immediate orthopedic consultation is indicated for surgical repair.

Ruptured Central Slip of the Extensor Tendon

The central slip of the extensor tendon attaches to the base of the middle phalanx. The lateral bands converge and attach to the base of the distal phalanx (Figure 30-25).

History The patient who ruptures the central slip presents with a jamming injury to the finger.

Physical Examination Physical examination reveals tenderness and swelling over the dorsum of the

proximal interphalangeal (PIP) joint. The patient is unable to extend the PIP joint or extends it weakly. Careful testing of extensor function must be done with every PIP joint sprain or this injury is easily missed.

If it is missed, over time the lateral bands will slip below the axis of motion of the PIP joint and pull the PIP joint into flexion and the DIP joint into hyperextension. This is called the boutonnière deformity and the patient ends up with a serious problem requiring surgical correction (Figure 30-26).

Laboratory Studies X-ray results are negative.

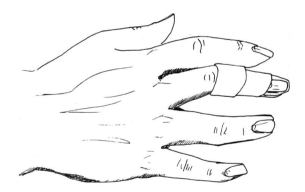

Figure 30-23 STACK finger splint.

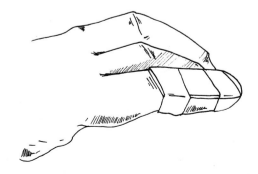

Figure 30-24 Metal mallet finger splint.

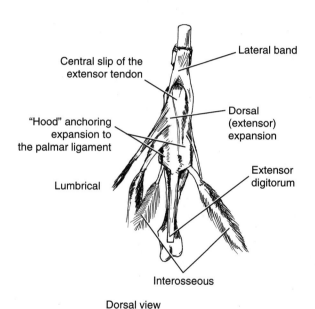

Dorsal view

Figure 30-25 Dorsal view of the middle phalanx, showing the central slip of the extensor tendon.

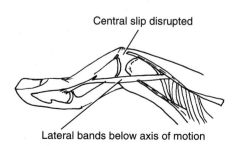

Figure 30-26 Central slip disrupted.

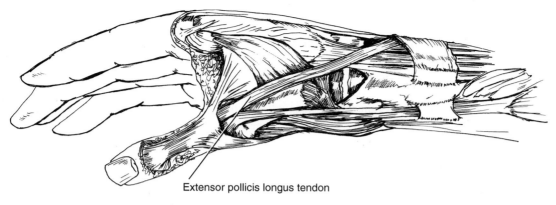

Extensor pollicis longus tendon

Figure 30-27 Extensor pollicis longus tendon.

Treatment If injury is detected early, splinting in extension for 3 weeks usually results in adequate healing.

Rupture of the Extensor Pollicis Longus

The extensor pollicis longus tendon is the sole extender of the interphalangeal (IP) joint of the thumb (Figure 30-27).

History The patient presents with a history of blunt trauma to the thumb, or with a spontaneous inability to extend the distal phalanx of the thumb some time after a fracture of the distal radius. It also occurs occasionally in people who have occupations that require continuous motion with the wrist in dorsal flexion and radial deviation (drummers). The tendon runs obliquely across the dorsum of the radius and is gradually destroyed from friction.

Dislocation of the Extensor Tendon at the Metacarpophalangeal Joint
History Here the radial aspect of the joint capsule of the metacarpophalangeal (MP) joint will rupture, usually following a blunt trauma.

Physical Examination When the patient tries to extend the finger actively, the tendon will slip off to the ulnar side at the MP joint. Passive extension of the finger "pops" it back into place.

Treatment An orthopedic consultation for surgical repair is indicated.

Rupture of the Flexor Digitorum Profundus
The flexor digitorum profundus tendon attaches to the base of the distal phalanx and flexes the DIP (Figure 30-28).

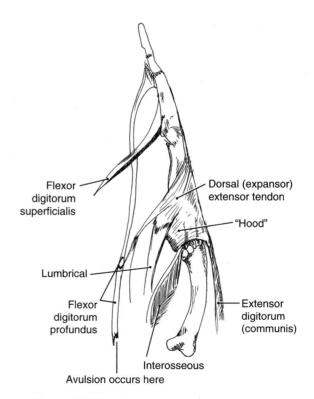

Flexor digitorum superficialis

Dorsal (expansor) extensor tendon

"Hood"

Lumbrical

Flexor digitorum profundus

Extensor digitorum (communis)

Interosseous

Avulsion occurs here

Figure 30-28 Flexor digitorum profundus tendon.

History The patient sustains some blunt trauma, which results in disinsertion of the profundus tendon from its attachment on the volar aspect of the base of the distal phalanx.

Physical Examination Physical examination reveals inability to flex the distal phalanx.

Laboratory Studies This may occur with or without a tiny bone chip being evident on x-ray.

Treatment Referral for surgery is indicated.

NEUROLOGICAL AND TENDON EVALUATION OF THE FOREARM, WRIST, AND HAND
Median Nerve

Motor function is tested by having the patient touch the tip of the thumb to the tip of the fifth finger. Sensory function is tested on the volar aspect of the distal phalanx of the index finger.

Ulnar Nerve

Motor function of the ulnar nerve is tested by having the patient pinch the thumb against the index finger while the examiner palpates the dorsal interosseous muscle for contraction. An alternative method is to have the patient lay his or her hand palm-down flat on the table and adduct and abduct all the fingers.

Sensory function is tested on the volar aspect of the distal phalanx of the fifth finger.

Radial Nerve

Motor function is tested by having the patient dorsiflex the wrist.

Sensory function is checked on the dorsum of the hand in the web space between the index finger and the thumb.

Distribution of Nerves of the Hand

The standard distribution of the cutaneous nerves to the palm and dorsum of the hand is shown in Figure 30-29, *A* and *B*. There are many variations in this

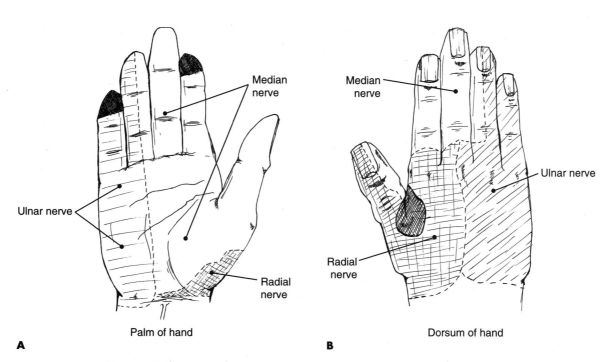

Figure 30-29 A, Sensory nerve distribution of the hand. **B**, Anatomy of the hand.

pattern, and it is helpful to know the areas of the hand that are supplied by this nerve. These areas are called the autonomous zones and are shaded darkly within each dermatome.

Testing for sensation can be done in several ways:

➤ *Sharp-dull:* A sterile 18-gauge needle can be used to touch the patient in various places over a specific dermatome, using both the point and the hub of the needle to determine if the patient can differentiate between the two.

➤ *Light touch:* The examiner touches the area to be examined lightly with his or her finger, comparing the sensation with the uninjured extremity.

➤ *Two-point discrimination:* Using a straightened paper clip bent into a U shape, the patient is asked to determine whether two points are felt or just one. The examiner positions himself or herself in such a way that the patient cannot observe the area being tested. The patient should be relaxed and comfortable. The examiner simultaneously applies the two blunted ends of the paper clip lightly to the area being tested. A normal finger pulp can discriminate points 2 to 4 mm apart. On areas of skin that are calloused and tough, this area widens to 4 to 6 mm apart. On the dorsum of the hand, the patient should be able to determine a normal distance of about 8 to 10 mm. Another useful point is that sweating will be absent from the skin when sensory innervation has been interrupted.

Tendon Laceration Injuries

A laceration on the dorsum of the distal forearm, wrist, and hand can cause tendon injuries that are difficult to diagnose if one does not have a thorough knowledge of the anatomy. Evaluating these types of injuries involves testing the function of the tendon both actively and actively against resistance while directly visualizing the wound, with bleeding controlled by a tourniquet.

This is important, for if the common extensor to the middle finger is lacerated proximal to the intercommunicating slips from the other extensor tendons, the patient will still be able to actively extend the middle finger. Also, a laceration of the extensor pollicis brevis is easily missed because the extensor

pollicis longus is capable of extending both the MP joint and the IP joint. The extensor carpi radialis longus can be bisected and the patient could still be able to extend the wrist with the extensor carpi radialis brevis, and vice versa. For these reasons, it is critical to evaluate the tendons not only functionally but also under tourniquet control to directly visualize any tendon injury. This is the only way to reliably diagnose complete and partial tendon ruptures.

Testing Tendon Function To test *extensor digitorum communis* tendon function, have the patient actively extend each finger and hold it extended against resistance. Significant pain or weakness may indicate a partial laceration of the tendon. Have the patient extend the thumb against resistance while the *extensor pollicis longus* and the *extensor pollicis brevis* tendons are palpated. These tendons will be tense if they are intact. Test wrist extension against resistance using the other hand to palpate over the *extensor carpi radialis longus, the extensor carpi radialis brevis,* and the *extensor carpi ulnaris* tendons. Intact tendons should feel tense and be strong.

The volar aspect of the forearm, wrist, and hand is equally treacherous. A knowledge of the anatomy and how to test each tendon is required to avoid morbidity.

The *flexor digitorum superficialis* functions to flex the PIP joint of the fingers. Because the flexor digitorum profundus can also flex the PIP joint, its influence must be eliminated during the examination. This can be accomplished by holding all the fingers in extension except the finger to be tested. Have the patient rest his or her hand on a flat surface palm-up and stabilize all the fingers in extension, except the finger to be tested. The patient should then flex the remaining finger at the PIP joint actively and actively against resistance. Pain and weakness may indicate a partial laceration. If the tendon is completely transected, there will be no flexion.

The *flexor digitorum profundus* is tested by holding the PIP joint in extension and checking for flexion of the DIP joint actively and actively against resistance.

The *flexor pollicis longus* flexes the IP joint of the thumb and can be tested in like manner.

The *flexor carpi radialis* and *flexor carpi ulnaris* flex the wrist and are tested by having the patient flex the wrist against resistance while palpating each of the tendons in turn.

The *palmaris longus* tendon has no essential function and may be left alone or repaired at the physician's and the patient's discretion. Any laceration of this tendon can be diagnosed only by direct visualization under tourniquet control.

Tourniquet control of bleeding can be achieved by inflating a blood pressure cuff on the upper arm. With the patient in a supine position, have him or her point the injured extremity toward the ceiling while straightening the arm and holding it there for a couple of minutes, to allow as much venous blood to drain as possible. With the arm still elevated, the blood pressure cuff should be inflated to 250 mm Hg and held there during the examination. This procedure provides the examiner a bloodless field and, although it is uncomfortable for patients, most can tolerate it for up to 15 minutes.

MISCELLANEOUS CONDITIONS
Insect in the Ear

The patient presents to the ED in distress with a history of awakening from sleep with pain and motion in the ear. The usual culprit is a roach that has crawled into the ear canal while the patient was asleep. Occasionally, and less commonly, the patient relates that something flew into his or her ear. To kill the insect, fill the ear canal with Auralgan eardrops, alcohol, or 2% lidocaine. After the insect is dead, it can be removed by flushing the ear with a Water-Pik or a 20-mL syringe with a 14-gauge angiocath attached. Only lukewarm water should be used. If this method fails, the insect will have to be removed piece by piece with a small pair of alligator forceps, using an otoscope for direct visualization.

Fishhook Removal

The most common and effective way to remove a fishhook is first to anesthetize the entire area surrounding the hook. Push the hook barb through the skin. Cut off the barb with a small pair of wire cutters. Withdraw the hook by reversing it through the original puncture site. Note: While cutting off the barb, catch it before it flies away by placing a 4 × 4 gauze over the hook barb before clipping it with the wire cutters.

Ingrown Toenail

Patients often present to the ED with an infected ingrown toenail, usually on the big toe. The standard treatment is to remove the ingrown portion of the nail, thereby releasing pressure on the surrounding tissue. This is best accomplished by a digital block with 0.5% bupivacaine (Marcaine) and removal of the lateral one fourth of the nail on the affected side. Once adequate anesthesia has been achieved, slide one half of an opened hemostat under the edge of the nail from the top to the cuticle margin. Close it and roll the edge of the nail toward the center, pulling it from beneath the inflamed nail fold. The hemostat can then be removed and the freed edge of the nail cut off with a pair of scissors. Dressing the toe should include antibiotic salve, Adaptic, and a small roller gauze. Systemic antibiotic and analgesic should be prescribed, and the patient should be instructed to follow up with the regular family physician for a wound check in 48 hours.

DRUG AND ALCOHOL POISONING IN THE EMERGENCY DEPARTMENT

Alcohol and drugs are estimated to be involved in more than 50% of all visits to the ED. This is true from small suburban EDs to large county trauma centers. Recognizing the physical and physiological patterns of intoxication will help the ED provider with the early management of these patients and may predict other concurrent pathology, any possible sequelae, and their eventual disposition.

There are several factors that work against the health care provider when he or she is attempting to treat a patient in the ED who is under the influence of alcohol or drugs. These patients are often unwilling or unable to give a clear history of the events that led to the ED visit. There are considerable consequences involved both legally and socially with substance abuse, and patients often consider it in their best interest to prevaricate. Despite this, the ED provider is asked to distinguish the differences between the patient with an acute intoxication and a patient with preexistent pathology. Additionally, the ED provider may be confronted by a patient with both a preexistent illness and an acute intoxication. In this case, the past medical history will help to determine specific management.

Alcohol creates a myriad of pathologies. It leaves no system untouched and remains a difficult addiction to treat. A complete discussion on alcohol and its associated complications is beyond the scope of this chapter; however, a brief explanation of the additional history needed for the completeness of the treatment of an intoxicated patient admitted to the ED is warranted.

Considering that what looks, smells, and tastes like alcohol is not always alcohol, and conversely, that ethanol is an ingredient in many substances, it is imperative that the cause of the patient's condition be identified before any medical intervention is initiated. Additionally, its presence is not always readily appreciated by the history. A breathalyzer is a quick, cheap method for confirming the presence of alcohol in a patient, but it is not sufficient to rule out other ingestions. If the patient arrives by ambulance, EMS personnel who were first to treat the patient may provide valuable information about the circumstances and condition. Questions should be asked, such as: Who called the ambulance? Where was the patient picked up? What containers or paraphernalia were apparent at the scene? Were there any witnesses and what did they report? Was there any trauma? Do the paramedics know this patient from previous runs? At this point, it is extremely important to know this patient's drinking habits. The patient's drinking pattern may predict withdrawal complications, and the health care provider has the ability to plan for the patient's recovery in a safe environment.

Alcoholism is a physiologically global addiction that affects all the major organ systems. A comprehensive physical examination must be part of the treatment. The vital signs and a complete visual examination of the skin are two of the most important steps that can be accomplished when evaluating the patient. Completely undress the patient and take care to look for obvious trauma. This information should correlate directly with the history. Keep in mind that intoxication can historically and physically mask signs and symptoms of trauma. Laboratory tests should be judiciously guided by the history and physical examination.

A few simple laboratory tests should be considered for all intoxicated patients. These patients are frequently hypoglycemic and a blood glucose level should be determined as soon as the patient is stable. Alcoholics are prone to metabolic and electrolyte imbalances as well as dehydration. Pulse oximeters should be initiated soon after the patient reports to the ED for determination of the patient's oxygen saturation level; cardiac monitors will provide reassurance during the treatment of the patient.

The provider should know what resources within the hospital and community are available to patients with alcohol-related problems. Before the patient leaves the ED, two questions should be answered: Is this an opportunity to offer the patient and family assistance with alcoholism? Does this patient have medical follow-up?

Alcohol is not the only recreational drug with medical complications. Cocaine is probably the most often used and most commonly encountered recreational drug nationwide. Narcotics, hallucinogens, benzodiazepines, and the ever-changing designer drugs are popular and all carry health risks. These classes of drugs can often be recognized by their characteristic physical signs, and it is imperative that the PA know the pattern, complications, and treatment for these drugs.

The distinction between a drug of abuse and a medication is largely a legal definition rather than a medical one. Any patient with an overdose is considered to be the responsibility of the ED to evaluate and manage. Fortunately, there is an extensive network of poison control centers around the nation to assist in identifying and isolating the toxic substance and recommending appropriate therapy.

Following are some general principles for treating the patient with an acute overdose:
1. Identify the patient and get an accurate history about the ingestion as soon as possible. Details may tend to blur or be forgotten altogether as time elapses after an ingestion. Inquire about the amount of the drug ingested, its strength, and over what period of time the drug was taken. Was the drug combined with any other medications? Is this a regularly prescribed medication or an over-the-counter medication? Has the patient eaten, or is there any alcohol involved? Did the patient vomit? If so, when and how many times, and what was in the vomitus? What was the

maximum number of milligrams that the patient could have taken, based on the historical evidence and the scene? What did the patient say about the ingestion during transport? Does the patient have any medical problems? Again, the family and the prehospital personnel are good sources of information. Question the EMT about the condition of the scene. The unintentional overdose is most often by its nature a single-agent ingestion. The suicide attempt, however, must always be suspected to be a multidrug ingestion. Commonly available and potentially lethal substances such as aspirin and acetaminophen may complicate the picture of an overdosed patient. Additionally, these medications are clinically undetectable.

2. Monitor the patient while gathering information about the overdose and while considering the treatment options. In addition to monitoring of vital signs, a stable patient should be placed on a cardiac monitor and a pulse oximeter. An IV line will allow quick intervention in the patient who is unstable. Monitoring for expected signs and symptoms of the drug's toxicity is inexpensive and offers immediate intervention as soon as the drug(s) is identified. There are relatively few specific antidotes to most of the available drugs; however, oxygen, glucose, and naloxone (Narcan) are commonly used and are standard drugs for paramedics to administer to patients in the field. These three medications should not be neglected in the ED. Other antidotes require specific clinical or laboratory evidence of ingestion and toxicity before their use, and the descriptions are found in most standard ED texts. In the majority of overdoses, patients who are clinically stable receive activated charcoal to absorb any drug remaining in the gastrointestinal tract.

3. The patient admitted to the ED with a deliberate overdose activates a special and unique set of guidelines. The health care provider is obliged to treat this patient, regardless of the circumstances and occasionally with full knowledge that the patient may make another attempt as soon as he or she leaves the facility. It may be impossible to sort patients with a deliberate overdose from those experiencing an accidental overdose. Initially, the health care provider must assume all overdoses are intentional and that all patients need to be protected from themselves. The precautions taken to ensure the patient's safety while in the ED vary from community to community, and most EDs are very aware of the ramifications of holding a patient against his or her will. Patients cannot be restrained or detained without cause, and usually this is delineated in a document called a "hold." Each state has specific guidelines that must be met when providers are attempting to hold a patient, and in most cases, PAs are not authorized to sign and initiate the hold. A hold initiates a cascade of events that should include informing the patient and family that a hold has been signed, why it was thought necessary, what restrictions will be placed on the patient's movements, and how and when the patient will be released from the hold. Holds, although necessary, should not be initiated thoughtlessly and should be frequently reevaluated for their continued necessity.

Some key questions in evaluating the intoxicated patient include the following:

1. How did the patient come to the attention of the ED?
2. Is trauma involved? Can the patient protect his or her own airway?
3. Is alcohol intoxication confirmed? How?
4. Is ethanol alone responsible for the patient's clinical state?
5. Is the patient progressing as expected in his or her detoxification? If not, have other pathologies been considered?
6. Has the patient's disposition been planned, and how will he or she be kept safe until then?

LEGAL AND ETHICAL DECISIONS IN EMERGENCY MEDICINE

The emergency arena presents some unique ethical and legal choices to the medical practitioner. The issues of treatment of minors, resuscitation of the terminally ill, elder abuse, attempted suicide, mental illness, and determination of incompetence are just a few examples. Providers in some branches of medicine may work with one or more of these issues on a regular basis. In this case, the patient is known and the clinician has access to the medical chart for completeness. The ED clinician is at a considerable disadvantage in attempting to treat a patient because of this lack of knowledge; therefore, the physician or PA must proceed with the belief that the treatment given to the patient in the ED is desired. In retrospect, the treatment may be resented, contraindicated, unnecessary, or controversial.

Some of these cases have been litigated so extensively that formal guidelines covering the permutations and combinations of a situation have been established. Decisions to act or not act, to investigate or not investigate, and to uphold the rights of one party over the wishes of another are less clearly defined. The outcome depends on the practitioner's willingness to accept responsibility for these moral questions as part of the job. Few clinicians relish this kind of unhappy controversy and may use the situation as an opportunity to educate a patient and family about the options and consequences of each procedure and to empower them to participate in the decision-making process. Allowing the patient and family this freedom creates a jointly shared responsibility and is more likely to result in a more favorable outcome for all involved.

One of the least acknowledged but most frequently encountered ethical decisions in emergency medicine is the decision to treat the sickest patient first. The long-cherished belief in "first come, first served" is frequently disregarded from the time the patient enters the ED and remains throughout the stay. Although the concept is not new to most patients, it still causes protests at the triage desk.

Privacy, both physical and informational, is a concern of all branches of medicine. Because of the physical layout of most EDs, privacy is a difficult commodity to ensure. Patients and families themselves often forget that their conversations can be overheard by the patient in the next cubicle. PAs should avoid contributing to this unrestrained exchange of information by presenting their patients quietly when on rounds, refraining from discussing a conscious, competent patient's condition with family or friends without the expressed consent of the patient, and ensuring the privacy of the physical examination. When in doubt about how the patient wants the examination conducted or his or her test results discussed, it is prudent to discuss everything with the patient first. Questions from a patient about other patients in the ED often reflect the inquirer's anxiety about his or her own medical problem. Reasonable curiosity and human concern can be met with reasonable replies. The PA should deflect with tact and compassion the questions that pry into another patient's private business.

Information regarding the patient's visits to other hospitals is protected under the right to privacy act. The patient must sign a consent form authorizing the release of these records to another facility. All states have exceptions to the privacy of information act and require reporting of cases in one or more of the following areas: Communicable diseases; victims of violence, including child and elder abuse; animal bites; venereal diseases; poisonings; and unexplained death. The patient must be informed that this information will be reported to the public health services, social services, or the appropriate law enforcement agency.

The medical system's obligation in treating minors (those under the age of 18) has always been a gray area. The law provides the following guidelines:

1. If an emergency exists, treat.
2. If the patient is a minor who presents for evaluation of pregnancy-related problems, venereal disease, or substance abuse problems, most states provide for treatment of the condition without prior consent or reporting to the parent or guardian.
3. If the patient presents for a nonurgent condition, obtain consent of the legal guardian before the patient is treated.
4. If a legal guardian is unavailable, a court may appoint a guardian.

Regardless of the law involved, remember that these children are still entitled to participate in their own care and to be informed of their diagnoses and possible treatments.

ED personnel are often in the position of evaluating patients whose mental competence is in doubt. Indeed, people are sometimes brought in from the community solely for the purpose of having the ED physician determine their mental competence. The elements of competence should be reviewed in advance. People are judged to be competent if they:

1. Have the ability to understand options.
2. Can understand the consequences of choosing each of those options.
3. Can evaluate the relative merits of those options with regard to their value system.
4. Can communicate their wishes.

Occasionally, patients are admitted to the ED from nursing homes or a psychiatric facility with their mental competence and legally appointed guardian previously determined. This is usually documented in the forms that accompany patients from their residences. Frequently, these patients have a terminal condition. The legal guardians appointed to make decisions will have been consulted and will have signed forms attesting to how they believe the patient would wish to be treated or not treated as they approach death. Do-not-resuscitate (DNR) means that in the event of cardiac arrest, cardiopulmonary resuscitation and ACLS measures to restart the heart should not be used. Do-not-intubate (DNI) would seem to be a fairly self-explanatory order but actually has some important and common exceptions that need to be considered before the patient has respiratory compromise. The intent of the DNI order is to prevent a terminally ill patient from being intubated and becoming ventilator-dependent with no hope for regaining independent respiratory function. On the other hand, elderly patients or patients with eventually terminal diseases can suffer temporary respiratory complications such as pneumonia from which they could fully recover if they were temporarily assisted by intubation and ventilation. When this circumstance is explained to the patient or family, they can appreciate the distinction between the two anticipated outcomes and may well suspend the DNI order.

DNR and DNI do not mean that patients cannot be treated. The patient who is admitted to the ED with these standing orders should still be treated for reversible conditions. This may include IV fluids, antibiotics, diuretics, antiarrythmics, oxygen, Foley catheter, or whatever is clinically indicated to relieve the presenting complaint. In addition to the DNR or DNI order, the patient may have written orders further limiting care (e.g., no IV antibiotics or no hyperalimentation). Laws vary from state to state concerning advance directives and decision making for incompetent patients. In the absence of clear, written documentation of the patient's wishes, the department is obliged to proceed with resuscitation.

SPECIAL CONSIDERATIONS

The ED is also the repository for a heterogeneous group of patients with a chief complaint of "bizarre behavior." During the initial evaluation of these patients, it is imperative that the cause of their behavior be considered organic and correctable. Unlike most of the other patients in the ED, these patients usually do not author their own chief complaint and are often denying it vigorously. These patients generally have a difficult time understanding why they have been detained in the ED to begin with. "Bizarre behavior" or "altered mental status" encompasses a wide range of disease processes. The diagnosis of a psychiatric disorder may precede the true cause and relationship of an intracranial bleed. Patients who appear "high" act bizarre, as do patients who are hypoxic. Delusional patients may view the health care provider as a threat and strike out. They may have a violent psychotic personality or they may be hypoglycemic. Patients who won't answer questions may be stubborn and angry, or they may be recent stroke victims. The ability to triage these patients appropriately takes a special appreciation of all the possibilities.

Occasionally, some of these patients may exhibit violent behavior. The first rule for the provider in attempting to treat these patients is to protect himself or herself. The second rule is to protect the other patients in the ED, and the third rule is to protect the patient in question. The patient in police custody and restrained is usually the accompanying officer's responsibility. However, if the patient is not under arrest, it is up to the ED personnel to appropriately restrain and/or isolate the patient. The ED provider is now in the delicate position of making a judgment about the potential for a patient to become violent based solely on the history provided by others relating to the patient's behavior before arrival in the ED.

When patients are considered to be at risk for harming themselves or others, the ED is obliged by law to ensure that this does not happen. If the ED provider elects to use physical restraints, he or she must ensure the patient's safety by frequent and periodic reassessments. The evolution of these events may be a relatively rare occurrence in certain EDs and may be a daily routine in others.

There are many legal and ethical questions involved in restraining patients against their will. The law provides for medical "holds" on patients if:

➤ The patient is considered to be a danger to himself or herself.
➤ The patient is considered to be a danger to others.
➤ The patient is considered to be unable to care for or make decisions for himself or herself.

Although the PA may initiate a hold on a patient by virtue of being the first to evaluate the patient, the physician of record is responsible for signing the hold. There is no correct answer, only a weighing of the risks and benefits of restraining patients and placing them on hold and the importance of an accurate history and physical examination as soon as a patient reports to the ED.

When a provider is confronted by a patient who is acting strangely and cannot give a history regarding the illness, the physical and mental assessment may be inadequate. There are available in most EDs four quick diagnostic screens that may identify a life-threatening condition in these types of patients:

➤ Oxygen saturation.
➤ Serum glucose level.
➤ Electrocardiogram.
➤ Blood alcohol level.

Other valuable diagnostic tests that may be considered but for which the results will take longer to obtain are:

➤ Serum electrolytes.
➤ Blood urea nitrogen.
➤ Arterial blood gases.
➤ Urinalysis.

Drug or medication overdose should always be a consideration in evaluation of the patient with an altered mental status or abnormal behavior pattern. Medications prescribed and taken in overdoses may be the problem, and any indication of a specific substance that may be found in the patient's blood should be relayed to the laboratory. This information can often direct the laboratory in deciding which test should be conducted. However, the laboratory should not be solely depended on for providing a diagnosis. The history and physical examination along with the laboratory findings will reveal the most appropriate treatment for the patient. It is imperative that each health care provider in the ED be familiar with the categories of chemicals that laboratories may screen for, what type of specimen that laboratory may need, and the time it takes to report the results. Additionally, the PA must be aware of what prescriptive and nonprescriptive drugs commonly cause behavioral changes, and how to counteract them. Considering these questions may save valuable time when one is confronted with an uncooperative patient with an inadequate history.

Patients with psychological illness are sometimes identifiable by their typical patterns of behavior; however, organic pathology in a patient with a known psychological illness still must be considered. This is especially true for the patient presenting to the ED with a significant change in behavioral routine. In this case, the old chart may be a most helpful clue to the patient's illness and may reveal an identifiable profile or characteristic that the patient is not exhibiting at the present time.

Most ED providers are not well versed in the evaluation of patients with psychological illness, and the activity in a typical ED is not an ideal environment for a comprehensive psychological workup. First, all medications and their prescribed dosages must be reviewed. The patient may be in the ER because of a medication change or a dosage change, or because of an interaction of a medication with another drug, or the patient for some reason has been unable to take a scheduled medication. Psychotropic medications are well known for side effects, abnormal interactions with other drugs, and individually narrow therapeutic windows. If the evaluation of a patient with a known psychiatric illness fails to reveal any physical cause of this ED visit, then reevaluation by a psychiatrist or other specialists in mental health must be initiated.

More than in any other medical setting, the ED is confronted with patients and families in crisis. Providers here experience firsthand how families with different cultural and religious beliefs deal with unexpected medical emergencies. The reaction of patients with a minor illness and their family may demand more flexibility on the part of the ED personnel than the responsibility incurred at the time of another patient's death within the department.

The ED is one of the few socially acceptable public places where people tend to "let their hair down," and the emotions expressed may reflect a reaction to much more than the patient's medical emergency. Individual patients vary in their reactions to the loss of control, to pain, or to the uncertainty of a medical illness, as do their families. Sometimes the behavior of the patient and his or her family seems totally inappropriate and disproportionate to the patient's situation. This may be a culturally comfortable way for the patient and the family to react, but it may not be comfortable for the ED staff. It is important for each provider to recognize this and allow the patient some latitude, thus giving back to the patient some of the control lost when his or her life was interrupted by the event that necessitated the ED visit.

However, when one patient's method of coping is total decompensation, it is time for the ED staff to step in. If the department is big enough and empty enough, this may simply be a matter of moving the patient to a more secluded area. When this isn't possible, the ED provider must impress on the patient that moderating his or her behavior is mandatory, to the extent of threatening to expel the patient from the ED if the behavior does not change. It is preferable to give the options and allow the patient to suggest a resolution, but most importantly, the patient, family, friends, and anyone else in the ED must realize that the ED provider is in command and that he or she has the authority to maintain control by whatever means necessary within the law.

ED personnel are confronted with patients in pain, fearful of a serious diagnosis, hostile, distrustful, worried, anxious, humiliated at the loss of privacy, and angry at their incapacity. These predominantly negative emotions inevitably surface in some patients and occasionally may be directed at a provider. The provider experiences similar emotions when confronted by a hostile, angry patient. Pain may arouse fear. Fear can create anxiety. Anxiety begets anger and hostility. *The alleviation of pain may be the single most important act a provider can perform in the ED.* Additionally, this simple understanding may short-circuit the cascade from pain to hostility and avoid serious confrontations.

CLINICAL PEARLS IN EMERGENCY MEDICINE

The following is a list of selected clinical pearls gathered by the authors of the textbook, *Emergency Medicine: An Approach to Clinical Problem-Solving,* by Hamilton and co-workers,[3*] reprinted here with permission from W.B. Saunders Company. Many of these pearls apply to everyday care in the ED. Many will stand the test of time; others will be forgotten as research proves them obsolete. At the present time, they offer an insight into the hazards and rewards of the specialty. Reviewing them before each tour of duty is a worthwhile exercise. Although many others are worth learning, these are some of the best.

A. The New Job
    1. Respect is earned.
    2. Befriend, through a show of respect, the nursing staff.
B. Maximizing Patient Satisfaction With Your Care
    1. Avoid medical jargon.
    2. Learn how to tell a patient you don't know what's wrong.
    3. Let the patient know he or she is always welcome to return.
C. Minimizing Patient Dissatisfaction
    1. One hour feels like three behind a curtain.
    2. A companion makes the wait less unbearable.
    3. Give the patient an estimate of the time needed to complete the evaluation. Significant delays require an honest accounting.
D. You Are the Patient's Advocate
    1. If you must, err on the side of helping the patient.
    2. Respect the patient's need for privacy.

---

* From Hamilton G, Sanders A, Stange G, et al. Emergency Medicine: An Approach to Clinical Problem-Solving. Philadelphia, WB Saunders, 1991, pp 16-18.

3. Always consider the "costs" of your interventions.

4. Don't negotiate any medically important decision with a patient with an altered sensorium, particularly if it is due to alcohol or other substance abuse.

5. If a patient is a source of potential harm to himself or others, or cannot take care of himself, he must stay for observation or admission.

6. Physical restraint may be necessary and appropriate to protect the patient or ED staff.

7. Do not discharge a now "sobered" patient who has recovered from acute alcoholism without performing a repeat history and physical examination.

8. Anxiety and hysteria are diagnoses of exclusion.

E. Clinical Judgment

1. When the clinical impression does not fit with the history, physical examination results, or laboratory evaluation, STOP! Rethink and expand the differential diagnosis.

2. If the patient can't walk, he can't go home.

3. If the ancillary data do not fit the clinical picture, reconfirm the accuracy of the data before making treatment and disposition decisions.

4. If you seriously consider a specific diagnosis when working through a differential diagnosis, then you should rule it out with the appropriate tests.

5. "If you don't know what to do—do nothing." Observe the patient closely for the evolution of the disease process instead of gambling on a marginally indicated therapeutic intervention.

6. Always assume that females of childbearing age might be pregnant and act accordingly.

7. The patient who returns to the ED on an unscheduled basis is first assumed to be at high risk for a serious illness.

8. Abnormal vital signs must be repeated and explained.

9. A patient who won't look at you during the history and physical examination is usually either depressed or manipulative. Almost never is such a person shy.

10. Patients usually have one major medical problem for each decade of life after the age of 60.

11. Never completely trust a younger child, a geriatric patient, an alcoholic, or a drug abuser. That is, corroborate the history and carefully interpret the physical findings in each of these patients.

12. Listen closely to the suggestions of patients and their families about what is wrong and how they should be treated.

F. Specific Clinical Situations

1. During the winter months, if the whole family has "the flu," be sure to consider carbon monoxide poisoning.

2. Ask what caused the trauma in the patient you are treating. Trauma is often considered the only problem and not potentially the result of another problem.

3. Consider the diagnosis of ruptured (or expanding) abdominal aortic aneurysm in all patients over 60 years old who appear to have renal colic.

4. Because the eye is to see, record its acuity.

5. Always confirm a field or bedside glucose oxidase strip reading in the ED with a blood glucose level.

6. Multiple drug allergies often correlate highly with functional or psychogenic complaints.

7. Chest pain radiating below the umbilicus or above the maxilla is seldom cardiac in origin.

G. The Pediatric Encounter

1. Speak to children in language they can understand.

2. Allow the parent(s) to stay in the room. Observing the child's interaction with his or her parents is an important part of the evaluation.

3. Children are rarely hypochondriacs.

4. Examine neurovascular and motor integrity before focusing on the injured area.

H. Communicating With the Attending or Consulting Physician
   1. Confirm admission or discharge with the primary physician before committing yourself to the patient.
   2. When in doubt, a second opinion to confirm a clinical impression is always appropriate.
I. Avoid Supporting the Legal Profession
   1. Don't think you are going to win just because you are in the "right."
   2. Protect yourself by protecting the patient.
   3. A printed form never saved anyone.
   4. One of the most hazardous moments in emergency medicine is "signing out" patients to a colleague at the end of one's shift. A complete and accurate exchange of information and impression is necessary.
J. Destroying Your Credibility
   1. Subvert the call schedule or be chronically late.
   2. Yell at someone.
   3. Give an opinion before looking at the patient.
   4. Treat a number, not the patient.
K. Your Mental Health
   1. Every physician/PA/student has moments of self-doubt.
   2. There is always a disposition.
   3. When you find yourself becoming angry with a patient ("positive personal hypertension sign") during history taking, you must step away momentarily. The patient may be malingering and withholding or providing misleading information, or you may be fatigued or have lost your perspective in your role. In any case, the emotion and its origin must not be allowed to influence or impair your judgment.
L. Do's
   1. Meet every patient turned over to you at the change of shift.
   2. Order soft tissue radiographs to rule out suspected soft tissue foreign bodies.
   3. Respond to complaints by private attendings immediately to avoid irreparable damage.
   4. Always see and interpret the diagnostic studies you have ordered.
M. Don'ts
   1. Never say: "There is nothing wrong with you."
   2. Do not expect patients to remember verbal information.
   3. Do not try to weasel out of accepting responsibility when you blew it. Admit the error, apologize, and get on with life.

CLINICAL APPLICATIONS

1. Describe how the perceptions of emergency medicine by patients and clinicians have changed over the past 30 years.
2. Identify 10 general principles that guide the practice of emergency medicine.
3. Define the following categories of medical emergencies—critical, acute, and urgent.
4. Describe the typical role of a PA in an emergency department.
5. If you accepted a position in an ED, how would you update your knowledge base and clinical skills for this practice specialty? What might you expect to be the challenges and satisfactions that you would experience as a PA in emergency medicine?

REFERENCES

1. Mengert T, Eisenberg M, Copass M. Emergency Medical Therapy, ed 4. Philadelphia: WB Saunders, 1996.
2. Metroplex Emergency Physicians Association Policy Manual. Dallas, Texas, 1995.
3. Hamilton G, Sanders A, Strange G, et al. Emergency Medicine: An Approach to Clinical Problem-Solving. Philadelphia: WB Saunders, 1991.
4. ACEP, 1990.
5. ACEP, 1990.
6. Brunette and coworkers.
7. Beth Israel Medical Center, 1990.
8. Sanford's Guide to Antimicrobial Therapy, 1998.
9. Iversen LD, Swiontkowski MF. Manual of Acute Orthopaedic Therapeutics, ed 4. Philadelphia: Lippincott Raven, 1994.

RESOURCES

Cain H. Flint's Emergency Treatment and Management, ed 7. Philadelphia: WB Saunders, 1985.

Dunmire S, Paris P. Atlas of Emergency Procedures. Philadelphia: WB Saunders, 1994.

Jastremski M, Dumas M, Penalver L. Emergency Procedures. Philadelphia: WB Saunders, 1992.

Salyer S. The Physician Assistant Emergency Medicine Handbook. Philadelphia: WB Saunders, 1997.

CHAPTER 31

Pediatrics

Linda M. Dale

INTRODUCTION

The skills of the physician assistant (PA) involve both the art and the science of medicine. The role of the PA in pediatrics is to be a resource and guardian for the physical, emotional, and mental health of infants, children, and adolescents as they evolve along a continuum of growth and development. Helping parents with the anxieties of the awesome responsibility of a new life, seeing the tangible effects of using healing skills on behalf of a child, working with special needs children to grant them the dignified life they are entitled to, and getting to know families and watching their children mature are just a few of the rewards. As in the practice of medicine in any other realm, there are also tragedies and losses that require commitment and compassion if the physician assistant is to be of

true service to children and families. The privilege of working with young people as they grow and mature cannot be underestimated.

This chapter reviews the history of the practice of pediatrics in the United States, the role of physician assistants in pediatrics, issues in pediatric medicine as they help define pediatric practice, settings and areas of specialization in which physician assistants work within pediatrics, and challenges for the future.

HISTORICAL PERSPECTIVE

In the United States, pediatrics did not emerge as a distinct area of medicine until the late 1800s. The first infant mortality studies were done in Philadelphia in 1871. The Society for the Prevention of Cruelty to Children was founded in 1876. Public health efforts on behalf of children began in 1897, when the New York state legislature mandated that New York City hire doctors and nurses to work with families in an attempt to alleviate the suffering of infants dying of "summer diarrhea." White House Conferences on Children began in 1910 during the administration of Theodore Roosevelt. Subsequent conferences have been held every decade since then. The Child Labor Law was passed in 1916. In 1930, the American Academy of Pediatrics was founded. The Shepard-Towner Act, passed in 1921, authorized health care funds for mothers during childbearing years and for infants. This act served as the foundation for Title V programs that mandated health services for indigent mothers and children to be administered by health agencies in states and territories. Services for crippled children were also provided. In the 1960s, services for children were expanded with the Maternal and Child Health, Crippled Children, Head Start, Job Corps, and Medicaid programs.[1,2] There have been numerous advances and losses in the provision of health care on behalf of children. Experience has proved that in periods of economic uncertainty, programs for children are among the most vulnerable to governmental cutbacks.

The contributions of physician assistants to pediatric health care began in 1969, with Henry K. Silver, MD, and the innovative Child Health Associate Program at the University of Colorado School of Medicine. The 3-year Master of Science program was designed to create new professionals able to provide comprehensive health services to children in an era when it was anticipated that resources for children would continue to be strained. As envisioned by Silver, child health associates are trained to work with physicians as colleagues and associates. They provide a wide range of diagnostic, preventive, and therapeutic services for children as well as parent and patient education, support, and counseling.[3]

Although the Child Health Associate Program was designed to offer specialized training in pediatrics, all current physician assistant training programs that emphasize primary care provide pediatric training. Graduates of many programs may choose pediatrics as an area of focus. Physician assistants identifying pediatrics or pediatric subspecialties as

their areas of practice represent 4.0% of the members of the American Academy of Physician Assistants (AAPA).[4]

ISSUES IN PEDIATRICS

Pediatric practice encompasses the care of patients from birth through adolescence. One way to define the scope of pediatric practice is to look at the risks to health and development that affect children and adolescents. Health supervision and attention to both acute and chronic illness should be provided to all children as they mature.

Table 31-1 ranks the causes of infant (<1 year of age) mortality in the United States.[5] The statistic of 6.9 infant deaths per 1000 live births in 2000 (preliminary data) is the lowest ever recorded.[5] However, the infant mortality rate is higher in the United States than in many other developed countries. In 1998, the United States ranked 23rd in infant mortality among countries with a population of at least 2.5 million.[5] Many of the deaths in this age group could be prevented by provision of adequate health services to pregnant women. The risks of prematurity, low birth weight, and perinatal infection can in many cases be minimized by appropriate intervention.

In the postneonatal period (28 days to 11 months), the mortality rate has also declined. Much of the mortality in this age group reflects the postponement of death from neonatal conditions. Although sudden infant death syndrome (SIDS) is a significant cause of death in this age group, the rate of SIDS deaths has fallen since 1992, when the American Academy of Pediatrics recommended putting infants to sleep on their backs or sides.[6]

The death rate for black infants during the first year of life is 2.3 times greater than for white infants. The higher number of deaths among black infants reflects the higher percentages of infants born in low and very low birth weight categories. Although access to health care and socioeconomic status partially explain this discrepancy, other factors may contribute to the disparity. Efforts at prevention continue to challenge health care providers.[5]

Table 31-2 reviews the major causes of death among children in the United States older than age 1 year.[5] Unintentional injuries rank first for all age

Table 31-1 Percentage of Infant Deaths, United States, 2000*

Rank Order	Cause of Death	Percent
1	Congenital anomalies	20.7
2	Disorders relating to short gestation and unspecified low birth weight	15.4
3	Sudden infant death syndrome	7.7
4	Newborn affected by maternal complications of pregnancy	4.9
5	Newborn affected by complications of placenta, cord, and membranes	3.7
6	Respiratory distress syndrome	3.6
7	Accidents (unintentional injuries)	3.0
8	Bacterial sepsis of newborn	2.6
9	Intrauterine hypoxia and birth asphyxia	2.3
10	Diseases of the circulatory system	2.3
	All other causes	33.8
Total		100.0

Modified from Hoyert D, Freedman M, Strobino D, Guyer B. Annual summary of vital statistics: 2000. Pediatrics 2001;108:1250. Reproduced with permission from American Academy of Pediatrics.
*The 10 leading causes of death before age 1 year, per 100,00 live births.

Table 31-2 Major Causes of Death by Age, United States, Ages 1-19 Years, 2000

Causes of Death	Age (Years)*			
	1-4	**5-9**	**10-14**	**15-19**
Accidents (unintentional injuries)	36.0	41.1	37.7	48.8
Congenital anomalies	9.5	6.1	4.6	0.0
Malignant neoplasms	8.0	15.4	12.6	5.4
Assault (homicide)	6.4	4.4	5.4	13.8
Diseases of the heart	3.4	3.1	0.0	2.8
Intentional self-harm (suicide)	0.0	0.0	7.2	11.7
All other causes	36.7	29.9	32.5	17.5
Total	100.0	100.0	100.0	100.0

Modified from Hoyert D, Freedman M, Strobino D, Guyer B. Annual summary of vital statistics: 2000. Pediatrics 2001;108:1252. Reproduced with permission from American Academy of Pediatrics.
*Percentage of all deaths.

groups. Suicide and homicide are prominent in the teen years.

When assessing risks to children's health, one should note that many of the conditions affecting children are avoidable. A major component of pediatric care focuses on health promotion and disease prevention. The goals of the American Academy of Pediatrics for child health supervision include the following:

1. Lowered child mortality.
2. Reduced disability and morbidity.
3. Promotion of optimum growth and development.
4. Help for children to achieve longer, fuller, and more productive lives.[7]

The status of children in the United States today illustrates some of the problems encountered in the provision of health care. National crises such as inadequate health care services, poverty, and homelessness take their toll on children. Ten to 12 million children are among those Americans who lack health insurance. Millions more are considered underinsured. Health insurance currently is designed to cover events such as hospital and surgical care, which fortunately occur infrequently for most children.[8] Families with health insurance may find the cost of preventive care (i.e., immunizations) or outpatient care for acute illnesses prohibitive. These services may not be covered or may not be sought because of high deductibles. Health care reform has occurred in the marketplace, if not in public policy. What remains in many instances is managed care, in which options have been curtailed and care has been rationed. Among the populations most threatened by this free-market approach are children, particularly those with special needs.

The result of the medical neglect of children is readily apparent when one examines the problems facing youth today. Threats to children's health are exacerbated by lack of access to health care and by poverty.[8] Poor children are much more susceptible to the effects of prematurity, perinatal infections, infectious diseases of early childhood, child abuse, accidents, homicide, suicide, teen pregnancy, and school failure.[9] Poor, inner city children are much less likely to receive required immunizations by age 2.[10]

Some of these issues may be resistant to easy solutions. It is tempting to be overwhelmed by the magnitude of problems facing our youth. Individual contributions by committed health professionals, however, often make an enormous difference in the lives of specific children and their families. Resourceful, innovative approaches allow individual PAs to make a difference with both families facing multiple problems and families blessed with stability and healthy children. Giving advice about topics as mundane as teething, pacifiers, sleep habits, and picky eating is one of the ways that a PA may help break a family deadlock and enable a child and parents to focus more on positive issues than on the inevitable struggles involved in child-rearing.

WHAT IS THE PRACTICE OF PEDIATRICS?

CASE STUDY 31-1

Parents of healthy 6-month-old twins bring the babies in for a routine checkup. The mother has several questions about the boy, Thomas, who still wants to eat every hour, is irritable, and cries for hours in the evening. The girl, Theresa, is an "easy baby," who smiles readily, eats every 3 to 4 hours during the day, and settles down to sleep without difficulty.

The realm of pediatric care includes the monitoring of health and of the normal progression of growth and development of the child. Care provided to children encompasses visits for periodic health supervision, acute illness, and chronic illness, and case management for children with special needs. The psychosocial arena in which children function has an impact on their ability to meet and adapt to challenges to optimal growth. All of these areas offer the physician assistant the opportunity to contribute in a meaningful way to children and families. Figure 31-1 provides a format for the content and tasks of periodic child health supervision visits.[11]

The Pediatric Interview

The first part of any medical encounter focuses on the medical history. For many encounters in pediatrics, the history is related by a third party (caregiver), not the patient. The level of concern expressed by the parent or caregiver should never be underestimated. A parent's concerns and suspicions are often the most accurate. It is important to keep in mind that parents might not implement a treatment plan if they feel that their concerns were not heard. The practitioner needs to hone observation skills about normal child development and behavior in order to augment and interpret the information given by the parent.

Appropriate methods of inquiry always are open ended, allowing the people with the concerns to delineate their worries in their own words and to elaborate on their own observations. Frequently, it is important for the PA to clarify these concerns by following up with questions such as these: "What worried you

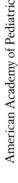

Figure 31-1 Recommendations for preventive pediatric health care from the American Academy of Pediatrics Committee on Practice and Ambulatory Medicine. (*Reproduced by permission of Pediatrics 2000;105:645. Copyright © 2000.*)

most about her?" "Why did that worry you?" and "What were you hoping we could do for her today?" These questions often are useful in sorting out underlying fears and concerns that parents have about their children.[12] Examples of questions that parents might not be able to ask directly include the following: "Will allowing my baby to sleep on her stomach cause SIDS?" "Will this cold turn into asthma?" "Will flying on a plane with this ear infection burst my child's eardrum?"

When the clinician is assessing developmental milestones, it is often the quality of the child's interaction that gives clues about the capacity of the child to develop skills necessary to interact with, manipulate, and master tasks for learning, language, and movement. Gentle but thorough inquiry gives the clinician a complete database, which is critical toward reaching the appropriate diagnosis and treatment plan.

The interview with an adolescent can be more complex and challenging for some practitioners. However, it can be immensely rewarding to observe and participate as teens define themselves as separate and distinct from their family. Parents of teens also want to talk with the PA and to have their concerns heard. It is essential that the adolescent be allowed the opportunity to be interviewed independently, providing the possibility of discussing issues of a confidential nature. This practice encourages teens to take responsibility for their own health behaviors. Often a young person may have an apparently superficial concern that serves as a means of asking about bigger worries, such as the possibility of an unwanted pregnancy or a sexually transmitted disease, or the means of obtaining a safe, effective, birth control method. These types of concerns illustrate the need for the adolescent to feel assured that confidentiality will be preserved and that the practitioner can be trusted. The physician assistant, the teen, and the parent(s) should meet at the end of the visit in a joint conference to review the health status of the adolescent and to go over the information shared with the teen that is not of a confidential nature.

Most states offer specific legal protection to health care providers who provide services to a teen that are confidential. Examples of confidential visits include counseling about birth control, sexually transmitted disease, drug and alcohol use or abuse, and mental health issues.[13] It is also important for the provider to be honest about the limits of confidentiality. In general, when the PA judges that the topics discussed by the teen arouse apprehension about the safety of that teen or others, for instance remarks that seem suicidal or homicidal, confidentiality should not be protected. Being up front and honest with the teen about these concerns will often protect the professional relationship between the provider and the teen.

The Physical Examination

The physical examination in pediatrics requires a thorough and comprehensive approach. Many findings on physical examination need to be tied to age-specific norms. For example, vital signs demonstrate wide variation from infancy through adolescence. Appropriate approach to the patient requires techniques that are age-related.

When the patient is an infant, it is very reassuring to a parent to observe that the PA handles the baby with confidence and with sensitivity. A particularly irritable infant may be exquisitely sensitive to touch and handling. Sometimes it is helpful to parents to validate their observations by demonstrating specifically how an infant responds to the stimulation of the physical examination. The spectrum of temperamental style is often readily apparent during the newborn period, and coping strategies might be discussed during the first visit.

As a baby grows and develops, stranger anxiety may make a physical examination more difficult because the infant reacts to the unfamiliar health care provider. An active, curious infant often will want to inspect and handle diagnostic equipment. At this age, it is wise to have toys in one's "bag of tricks" with which to distract the infant. A toddler approaching independence may perceive the physical examination both as invasive and as an enforced limiting of activity. From the age of 9 months to about 3 years, it is often helpful to do much of the examination with the child in the parent's lap. This may reassure the anxious child, and the parent may provide a helpful extra set of hands as the examiner interacts with the child. It is wise to set up the examination to proceed from least invasive (i.e., inspecting fingers and toes, testing extraocular movements with a finger puppet) to most invasive procedures (i.e., pneumatic otoscopy, looking at the back of the throat) in order to maximize the cooperation of the child.

At about 3 to 5 years of age, children are usually delightful, cooperative, anxious-to-please, and genuinely interested in what the examiner is doing. If, at this age, a child is still extremely anxious about getting a physical examination, further investigation is warranted. Perhaps the child has been very ill and has undergone some traumatizing procedures. Sometimes messages from elsewhere intimidate the child with threats about "shots." It is always important for the PA to be alert to extreme anxiety or indifference so as to be attuned to these symptoms as potential manifestations of reactions to child abuse. For a child who is temperamentally more anxious without specific cause, playing with a "doctor kit" or reading books about going to the doctor can help the child feel some mastery of the experience of a medical visit.

As a child approaches the early school-age years, his or her need for modesty becomes more evident during the physical examination. Appropriate gowns and drapes may help alleviate the child's discomfort. During the course of the physical examination, the physician assistant may take the opportunity to focus exclusively on the child and engage him or her independently in conversation.

In a child who is approaching the end of the latency period, the clinician must be attuned to signs of the development of secondary sexual characteristics. Again, concerns about modesty and normalcy can be paramount for the patient. It is not uncommon for clinicians to feel some discomfort in working with teens as they go through the physical process of sexual maturation. Frequently, working with patients in this age group provides a stimulus for health care providers to consider feelings and issues about their own adolescent experience. Potentially, this stimulus may enable the clinician to be more genuinely attuned to the teen's experience, serving to enhance the overall rapport.

Care of Patients

Growth   Assessment of growth is one of the most important indicators of overall health in childhood. Measurements of morphological growth give evidence of underlying biochemical, organic, and developmental competencies.[14] There are noticeable differences in the rates of growth and maturation of organ systems. In neural, lymphoid, general, and genital development, different age-specific phases of accelerated development can be noted.

From infancy through age 3 years, height, weight, and head circumference are measured at every health supervision visit. After age 3 through adolescence, weight and stature measurements are obtained. These parameters are plotted on growth charts (Figure 31-2) compiled by the National Center for Health Statistics. These charts provide norms of growth from a cross section of children from the United States representing various ethnic and economic groups. As norms, the growth curves provide a background against which to assess the growth of an individual child. It is important to realize that once a child has established a pattern and velocity of growth, evidence of continuation of that pattern indicates the integrity and ability of the child to attain overall growth potential. Variations in normal patterns may reflect nutritional problems, physical illness, and psychosocial disruptions. Concerns arise with disproportionate acceleration or deceleration in growth.

CASE STUDY 31-2

Ericka is 15. She is petite and will be competing in gymnastics again this year. She needs a physical examination in order to participate in her sport. In taking the history, the PA learns that Ericka has not started menstruating yet. Her mother started her periods when she was 12, and her older sister started in "seventh grade." Ericka's parents are both small: Mom is 5 feet, 3 inches, and Dad is 5 feet, 7 inches.

In adolescence, an estimate of sexual maturity rating (SMR) is added. This is helpful in determining how a teen is progressing through the period of rapid growth and in assessing the rate and pattern of sexual development. The Tanner (SMR) scale presents ranges of normal development with descriptions for each stage of growth for penis, testes, and pubic hair development in males and pubic hair and breast development in females. This is useful clinically in helping the clinician to predict height spurt for both

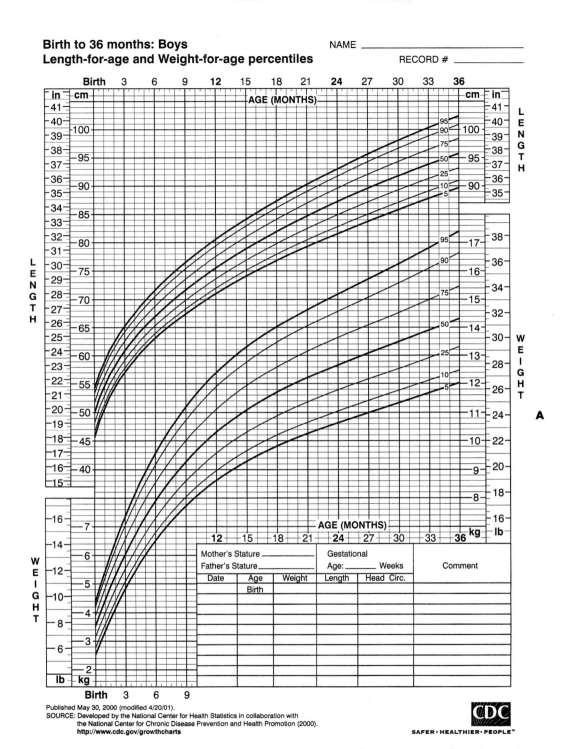

Birth to 36 months: Boys
Length-for-age and Weight-for-age percentiles

NAME _____

RECORD # _____

Published May 30, 2000 (modified 4/20/01).
SOURCE: Developed by the National Center for Health Statistics in collaboration with
the National Center for Chronic Disease Prevention and Health Promotion (2000).
http://www.cdc.gov/growthcharts

Figure 31-2 Physical growth charts from the National Center for Health Statistics (NCHS). **A** and **B**, Boys: birth to age 36 months. **C**, Boys: ages 2 to 18 years. *(Developed by the National Center for Health Statistics in collaboration with the National Center for Chronic Disease Prevention and Health Promotion [2000]. Available at http://www.cdc.gov/growthcharts.)*

Continued

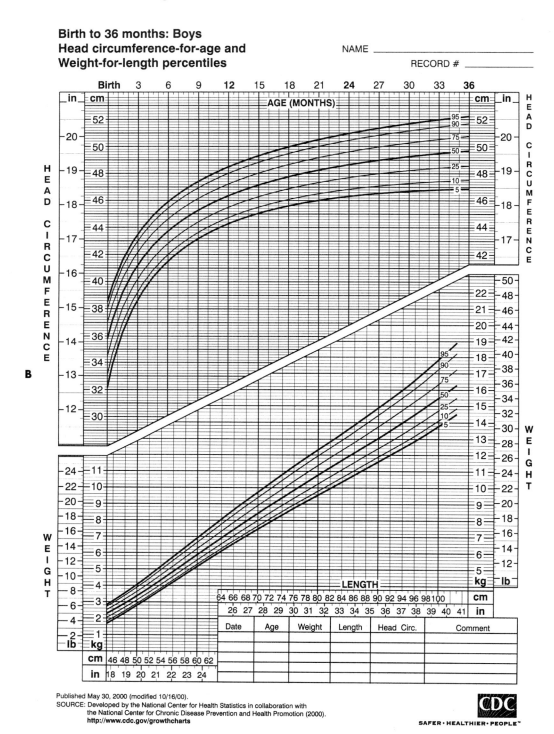

Birth to 36 months: Boys
Head circumference-for-age and
Weight-for-length percentiles

NAME _____

RECORD # _____

Published May 30, 2000 (modified 10/16/00).
SOURCE: Developed by the National Center for Health Statistics in collaboration with
the National Center for Chronic Disease Prevention and Health Promotion (2000).
http://www.cdc.gov/growthcharts

Figure 31-2, cont'd For legend see p. 655.

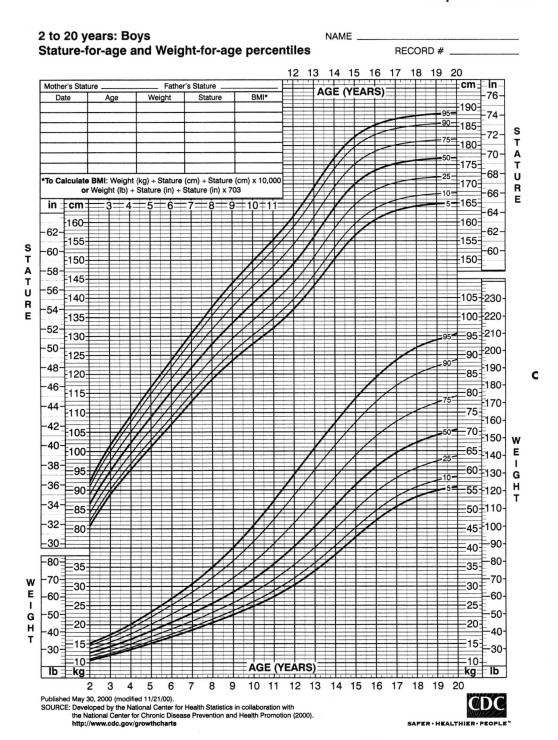

Figure 31-2, cont'd For legend see p. 655.

sexes and menarche for females. These norms also alert the clinician to precocious or delayed puberty.

Nutrition Concerns about feeding are common in pediatrics. Adequacy of the diet influences overall health status and growth of the child. Nutritional habits from childhood carry over to adulthood and therefore potentially have consequences for health risks throughout life.

Questions about feeding are initiated when parents make choices about breast-feeding or bottle-feeding. Although breast-feeding is recognized as preferable, physician assistants in primary care pediatrics should be able to discuss the advantages and disadvantages of both breast-feeding and bottle-feeding and should be sensitive to the parents' feelings as they make the decision for the child. The ideal is to promote a feeding style that provides the optimal nutritional status and feeding relationship for the child and family.

After early infancy, parents may seek advice about the initiation of solid food and about the quality and balance of the child's diet. The clinician needs to have a working knowledge of food sources that supply adequate calories, protein, vitamins, and minerals in order to assess the nutritive value of the child's diet. It is also necessary to be attuned to normal fluctuations in the child's appetite. Feeding problems include difficulties with the feeding interaction, overfeeding, and underfeeding. The complications of failure to thrive, obesity, attitudes toward food, and unusual eating behaviors, such as anorexia or binging and purging, may have lifelong repercussions.

Laboratory Screening Routine laboratory screening is also a part of the pediatric health supervision examination. All children should be screened in the newborn period for metabolic diseases and hemoglobinopathies. Vision, hearing, and blood pressure determinations are also performed routinely. Utilization of tuberculosis, cholesterol, anemia, urine, and lead screens is subject to an assessment of prevalence and risk factors for individual patients and communities.

Immunizations As recently as 1900, 53% of children died in childhood from infectious diseases.[15] The treatment of infectious diseases has dramatically improved, but many serious or fatal infectious diseases of childhood are preventable through vaccination. Immunization remains a cornerstone of pediatrics. Figure 31-3 lists the recommendations for childhood vaccinations.[16] Current vaccine guidelines include immunization against diphtheria, pertussis, and tetanus (DPT); poliovirus (IPV); measles, mumps, and rubella (MMR); *Haemophilus influenzae* b; hepatitis B virus (HBV); and pneumococcus (PCV or PPV).

In recent years, vaccine recommendations have been revised. These revisions have been prompted by the development of new vaccines such as the *H. influenzae* b conjugate vaccine (HbCV), pneumococcal conjugate vaccine (PCV), pneumococcal polysaccharide vaccine (PPV), and the varicella vaccine. The resurgence of measles and the rising rates of hepatitis B and pneumococcal infection have also influenced these changes.

CASE STUDY 31-3

Three-year-old Katie's father brings her to the emergency department for evaluation of fever and irritability. She has been ill for 2 days with a cold and has not been eating well. In talking with the father and by reviewing the medical records, the PA ascertains that Katie has not had a routine checkup since she was 6 months old. The family has no consistent source of health care. The father does not think Katie has had shots since she was 6 months old.

Because access to and utilization of health care greatly influence the chance that a child will be fully immunized, the physician assistant should take advantage of every opportunity to bring a child up-to-date on immunization by reviewing the record of immunization at each encounter. It is imperative that the expected and more serious adverse reactions to immunizations be discussed with parents as a part of the informed consent process. Significant adverse reactions should be reported. The National Childhood Vaccine Injury Act allows for compensation to families for significant events following vaccination.

Interruption of the routine immunization schedule can cause some confusion about how to bring a

Recommended Childhood Immunization Schedule
United States, 2002

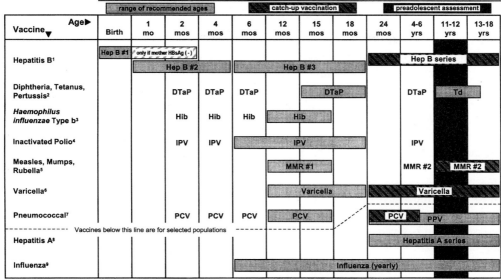

This schedule indicates the recommended ages for routine administration of currently licensed childhood vaccines, as of December 1, 2001, for children through age 18 years. Any dose not given at the recommended age should be given at any subsequent visit when indicated and feasible. ▓▓▓ Indicates age groups that warrant special effort to administer those vaccines not previously given. Additional vaccines may be licensed and recommended during the year. Licensed combination vaccines may be used whenever any components of the combination are indicated and the vaccine's other components are not contraindicated. Providers should consult the manufacturers' package inserts for detailed recommendations.

1. Hepatitis B vaccine (Hep B). All infants should receive the first dose of hepatitis B vaccine soon after birth and before hospital discharge; the first dose may also be given by age 2 months if the infant's mother is HBsAg-negative. Only monovalent hepatitis B vaccine can be used for the birth dose. Monovalent or combination vaccine containing Hep B may be used to complete the series; four doses of vaccine may be administered if combination vaccine is used. The second dose should be given at least 4 weeks after the first dose, except for Hib-containing vaccine which cannot be administered before age 6 weeks. The third dose should be given at least 16 weeks after the first dose and at least 8 weeks after the second dose. The last dose in the vaccination series (third or fourth dose) should not be administered before age 6 months.

Infants born to HBsAg-positive mothers should receive hepatitis B vaccine and 0.5 mL hepatitis B immune globulin (HBIG) within 12 hours of birth at separate sites. The second dose is recommended at age 1-2 months and the vaccination series should be completed (third or fourth dose) at age 6 months.

Infants born to mothers whose HBsAg status is unknown should receive the first dose of the hepatitis B vaccine series within 12 hours of birth. Maternal blood should be drawn at the time of delivery to determine the mother's HBsAg status; if the HBsAg test is positive, the infant should receive HBIG as soon as possible (no later than age 1 week).

2. Diphtheria and tetanus toxoids and acellular pertussis vaccine (DTaP). The fourth dose of DTaP may be administered as early as age 12 months, provided 6 months have elapsed since the third dose and the child is unlikely to return at age 15-18 months. **Tetanus and diphtheria toxoids (Td)** is recommended at age 11-12 years if at least 5 years have elapsed since the last dose of tetanus and diphtheria toxoid-containing vaccine. Subsequent routine Td boosters are recommended every 10 years.

3. *Haemophilus influenzae* **type b (Hib) conjugate vaccine.** Three Hib conjugate vaccines are licensed for infant use. If PRP-OMP (PedvaxHIB® or ComVax® [Merck]) is administered at ages 2 and 4 months, a dose at age 6 months is not required. DTaP/Hib combination products should not be used for primary immunization in infants at age 2, 4 or 6 months, but can be used as boosters following any Hib vaccine.

4. Inactivated poliovirus vaccine (IPV). An all-IPV schedule is recommended for routine childhood poliovirus vaccination in the United States. All children should receive four doses of IPV at age 2 months, 4 months, 6-18 months, and 4-6 years.

5. Measles, mumps, and rubella vaccine (MMR). The second dose of MMR is recommended routinely at age 4-6 years but may be administered during any visit, provided at least 4 weeks have elapsed since the first dose and that both doses are administered beginning at or after age 12 months. Those who have not previously received the second dose should complete the schedule by the visit at 11-12 years.

6. Varicella vaccine. Varicella vaccine is recommended at any visit at or after age 12 months for susceptible children (i.e. those who lack a reliable history of chickenpox). Susceptible persons aged >13 years should receive two doses, given at least 4 weeks apart.

7. Pneumococcal vaccine. The heptavalent **pneumococcal conjugate vaccine (PCV)** is recommended for all children aged 2-23 months and for certain children aged 24-59 months. **Pneumococcal polysaccharide vaccine (PPV)** is recommended in addition to PCV for certain high-risk groups. See *MMWR* 2000;49(RR-9);1-37.

8. Hepatitis A vaccine. Hepatitis A vaccine is recommended for use in selected states and regions, and for certain high-risk groups; consult your local public health authority. See *MMWR* 1999;48(RR-12);1-37.

9. Influenza vaccine. Influenza vaccine is recommended annually for children age ≥ 6 months with certain risk factors (including but not limited to asthma, cardiac disease, sickle cell disease, HIV, and diabetes; see *MMWR* 2001;50(RR-4);1-44), and can be administered to all others wishing to obtain immunity. Children aged ≤12 years should receive vaccine in a dosage appropriate for their age (0.25 mL if aged 6-35 months or 0.5 mL if aged ≥ 3 years). Children aged ≤ 8 years who are receiving influenza vaccine for the first time should receive two doses separated by at least 4 weeks.

For additional information about vaccines, vaccine supply, and contraindications for immunization, please visit the National Immunization Program Website at www.cdc.gov/nip or call the National Immunization Hotline at 800-232-2522 (English) or 800-232-0233 (Spanish).

Approved by the Advisory Committee on Immunization Practices (www.cdc.gov/nip/acip), the American Academy of Pediatrics (www.aap.org), and the American Academy of Family Physicians (www.aafp.org).

Figure 31-3 Recommended childhood immunization schedule for the United States, 2002. *(Approved by the Advisory Committee on Immunization Practices. Available at http://www.cdc.gov/nip/acip.)*

child's immunization status up-to-date. If a child comes in with lapses in DPT, HbCV, IPV, and HBV schedules, the next doses should be given as if the interval were usual. Missed immunizations do not require that the entire series be reinstituted. The schedule is shown in Table 31-3.[17]

Sometimes clinicians are hesitant to immunize a child because of concerns about contraindications or reactions. This reluctance contributes to the unacceptable number of children in the United States who are not fully immunized. Afebrile minor illnesses, such as colds and diarrheal illnesses, in a child who is otherwise in good health are not contraindications to immunization. Vaccination should be deferred if an illness could be potentially exacerbated by an adverse effect or an adverse reaction to the vaccine.

Special consideration is given to immunization of immunocompromised patients and of preterm infants. Alterations in immune function can result from immunosuppressive therapy such as corticosteroids, chemotherapeutic agents, and that given to transplant recipients. Patients with congenital disorders of immune function are also more susceptible to adverse outcomes from immunizations, especially with live viral vaccines. Live bacterial and viral vaccines (oral polio, MMR, and varicella) and bacillus Calmette-Guérin (BCG) are contraindicated for patients with congenital disorders of immune function.[17] The inactivated polio vaccine (IPV) can be used safely. Patients on immunosuppressive therapy require a thorough evaluation of the underlying disease, the type of therapy as well as its schedule and dose, previous infectious disease, and immunization history. Patients with symptomatic human immunodeficiency virus (HIV) infection should not receive live viral vaccines. Because of the risk of complications from measles, however, it is recommended that MMR be given regardless of symptoms.[18]

Preterm infants can be immunized safely at the usual chronological age. If a baby is still in the nursery, DPT and HbCV can be given.[18] Under new guidelines approved by the Advisory Committee on Immunization Practices and the American Academy of Pediatrics, IPV is the poliovirus vaccination recommended for routine immunizations; it can be given safely to hospitalized infants. See Figure 31-3.

A thorough discussion of immunization practices and policies is available in the *Red Book: Report of the Committee on Infectious Diseases,* of the American Academy of Pediatrics; this is an excellent reference for practicing PAs.[17]

Development and Behavior

CASE STUDY 31-4

Three-month-old Angela is brought in by her mother for shots. During the visit, the mother tells the PA that she is worried about the baby because the grandmother doesn't think that the baby is "acting right." Grandma has noticed that the baby doesn't look around and watch when people walk into the room and talk to her. Further review of the family history reveals that the mother has two other children who have been removed from the home because of suspicion of child abuse.

A cornerstone of pediatrics is an appreciation of how children progress through normal development. Components of this process include the cognitive, affective, motor, and language skills that a child attains throughout normal maturation. Because none of these processes happens in a vacuum, an understanding of the circumstances of the home and community in which the child functions is important.

Freud, Erickson, Piaget, and Mahler have influenced the assessment of childhood development. The observations and theories established by these and other analysts of human behavior have allowed the formulation of general principles, many of which are included in developmental screening tests. The following basic principles apply to human development:

➤ Development is a continuous and dynamic process.
➤ The sequence of development is generally the same for all individuals.
➤ The pace or rate of development is variable for each child.[14]
➤ Development is affected by the overall health of the child. Acute and chronic illness may adversely affect the performance of a child on a screening test.

Table 31-3   Recommended Immunization Schedules for Children Not Immunized in the First Year of Life*

Recommended Time/Age	Immunization(s)[†]	Comments
YOUNGER THAN 7 YEARS		
First visit	DTaP, Hib,[‡] HBV, MMR	If indicated, tuberculin testing may be done at same visit.
		If child is 5 y of age or older, Hib is not indicated in most circumstances.
Interval after first visit		
1 mo (4 wk)	DTaP, IPV, HBV, Var[§]	The second dose of IPV may be given if accelerated poliomyelitis immunization is necessary, such as for travelers to areas where polio is endemic.
2 mo	DTaP, Hib,[‡] IPV	Second dose of Hib is indicated only if the first dose was received when younger than 15 mo.
≥8 mo	DTaP, HBV, IPV	IPV and HBV are not given if the third doses were given earlier.
Age 4-6 y (at or before school entry)	DTaP, IPV, MMR[‖]	DTaP is not necessary if the fourth dose was given after the fourth birthday; IPV is not necessary if the third dose was given after the fourth birthday.
Age 11-12 y	See Figure 1-1, p. 22	
7-12 YEARS		
First visit	HBV, MMR, dT, IPV	
Interval after first visit		
2 mo (8 wk)	HBV, MMR,[‖] Var,[§] dT, IPV	IPV also may be given 1 mo after the first visit if accelerated poliomyelitis immunization is necessary.
8-14 mo	HBV,[¶] dT, IPV	IPV is not given if the third dose was given earlier.
Age 11-12 y	See Figure 1-1, p. 22	

*Used with permission of the American Academy of Pediatrics. 2000 Red Book: Report of the Committee on Infectious Disases, ed 25. Elk Grove Village, IL: American Academy of Pediatrics, 2000. Table is not completely consistent with all package inserts. For products used, also consult manufacturer's package insert for instructions on storage, handling, dosage, and administration. Biologics prepared by different manufacturers may vary, and package inserts of the same manufacturer may change. Therefore, the physician should be aware of the contents of the current package insert. Vaccine abbreviations: HBV indicates hepatitis B virus; Var, varicella; DTaP, diphtheria and tetanus toxoids and acellular pertussis; Hib, *Haemophilus influenzae* type b conjugate; IPV, inactivated poliovirus; MMR, live measles-mumps-rubella; dT, adult tetanus toxoid (full dose) and diphtheria toxoid (reduced dose), for children 7 years of age or older and adults.

[†]If all needed vaccines cannot be administered simultaneously, priority should be given to protecting the child against the diseases that pose the greatest immediate risk. In the United States, these diseases for children younger than 2 years usually are measles and *Haemophilus influenzae* type b infection; for children older than 7 years, they are measles, mumps, and rubella. Before 13 years of age, immunity against hepatitis B and varicella should be ensured. DTaP, HBV, Hib, MMR, and Var can be given simultaneously at separate sites if failure of the patient to return for future immunizations is a concern. For further information on pertussis and poliomyelitis immunization, see the respective chapters (Pertussis, p. 435, and Poliovirus Infections, p 465).

[‡]See *Haemophilus influenzae* Infections, p. 262, and Table 3-11 (p. 268).

[§]Varicella vaccine can be administered to susceptible children any time after 12 months of age. Unimmunized children who lack a reliable history of varicella should be immunized before their 13th birthday.

[‖]Minimal interval between doses of MMR is 1 month (4 wk).

[¶]HBV may be given earlier in a 0-, 2-, and 4-month schedule.

➤ Major events in the child's milieu may also alter the performance of the child on developmental screening. Examples of potentially stressful events are deaths, separations, moves, and the illness of a family member.[15]

For physician assistants working with families, attention to development during infancy and early childhood is a necessity. The timing and frequency of health supervision visits enable the PA to take on the roles of family advisor and advocate for the child. Periodic screening with developmental tests such as the Denver II and Bayley Infant Development Scales allows for measurement against norms for age. Marked deviation from norms mandates a more intensive and specific developmental evaluation. Many readily available checklists of developmental milestones may facilitate developmental screening.

CASE STUDY 31-5

Seven-year-old Brett is brought in by his parents. They have just attended a school conference, at which the teachers reported noticing that Brett has a lot of difficulty staying "on task." He is up and out of his seat, frequently disturbing other children. He is about 6 months behind the other children in reading. At home, he is "creative" and loves Nintendo, but "forgets" and loses things, talks loudly, and interrupts at meals. He needs frequent reminders to do simple things like getting ready for school in the morning. Any chores he must do require constant supervision.

Although early childhood is a period of rapid acquisition of new skills, developmental issues continue to be evaluated in patients through adolescence. During the school years, it is important to be cognizant of the child's capacity for learning, social interaction, and motor skills. With teenagers, topics address how a patient is managing in school, at work, with peers, and with family. It is reassuring to both patients and families to know that the issues that arise in the process of maturation are normal and expected. Discerning when patterns and progression through development are not consistent, either for the patient or in comparison with norms, is critical.

The individuality of each child manifests itself throughout the child's life. These stylistic characteristics are often apparent in infancy. Temperamental styles influence how the child reacts to stimuli and how he or she is perceived by the family as well as by teachers, peers, and co-workers. Qualities such as shyness, adaptability, and creativity are among the many traits to which others in the child's environment respond. The perception of and value placed on these traits play a role in the child's integration of self and development of self-esteem. Coping skills and stylistic traits influence the child's adaptation to stressful events such as changes in schools, moves, losses, and divorce. Because no child is protected completely from difficulties while growing up, it may be helpful to the family for the clinician to recognize how the child responds to these events.

Health care providers are in a unique position to observe a child and family throughout the child's growth to maturity and are frequently solicited for advice about behaviors. Sometimes this advice focuses on suggestions about setting limits and applying discipline as the family strives to live harmoniously. When conflicts arise, interactions may reflect the inability of family members to recognize temperamental patterns and to develop mutually acceptable alternative behaviors that are complementary. Physician assistants can be helpful by communicating their observations to the family and offering alternatives for management of these issues. Many of the issues come under the heading of "parenting." Some of the problems for children, however, are a predictable part of developmental and maturation processes and should be addressed routinely through anticipatory guidance during health supervision visits.

Physician assistants must also be attuned to deviations from expected difference in behavior. Children are not immune to serious psychiatric disturbances. Although it is important for the PA to appreciate normal behavior, it is equally important that he or she be aware of symptoms of underlying psychopathology. Appropriate referral for therapeutic intervention may be essential in helping the child and family.

Anticipatory Guidance

Eleven-year-old Jason is in for a routine camp physical. In reviewing his general health and activities, the PA finds that Jason enjoys riding his bike, rollerblading, and skateboarding. He has had two trips to the emergency department this year—one for stitches and one for a possible concussion. He does not wear a bicycle helmet or use pads when rollerblading or skateboarding. He does not use seat belts while riding in the car, and neither do his parents.

Preparing parents for expected milestones in a child's health and development is an integral part of the practice of pediatrics. Information about growth, development, behavior, day care, nutrition, family functioning, television use, injury prevention, and management of illnesses is a part of every visit. Discussion of these topics by PAs builds alliances with parents by offering support and acknowledging the parents' competency to provide for the child. Anticipatory guidance should be timed for age-appropriate tasks and skills.

As a child approaches adolescence, the health care visit includes topics about which the young person will have to make decisions. Discussions about risk-taking behavior, peer pressure, smoking, alcohol, drugs, sexuality, and safe sex are all relevant.

Because accidents are the leading cause of death in childhood after infancy, a discussion of safety and injury prevention should be a component of every health maintenance visit. The list of topics should be adapted to the risks associated with the child's age. The American Academy of Pediatrics' Injury Prevention Program (TIPP) provides a questionnaire that assesses hazards and offers information to parents. Subjects for discussion range from use of car seats to avoidance of burns, falls, head injuries, drowning, choking, and poisoning. Home safety topics must include the availability of a working smoke alarm. As the child grows, possible further topics include bicycle safety, use of helmets and seat belts, and firearms in the home.[19]

Acute Illnesses

His mother brings in 2½-year-old Matthew with concerns about persistent diarrhea. The diarrhea started 10 days ago, maybe with a "low-grade" fever. Although the stools were initially quite frequent (8 to 10 per day), the diarrhea has now tapered off to about four "really mushy," foul-smelling stools each day. Matthew was almost potty-trained but is now back in diapers. The mother thinks Matthew is beginning to look like he has lost weight. Workers at his day care center are also concerned.

While caring for their ill child, parents interpret symptoms and make judgments about their severity. With a preverbal infant, it is sometimes difficult for parents to decide how ill the child is. Sometimes, the first provider contact with the family will occur over the telephone, helping the family determine whether the child needs to be seen by the provider. In the outpatient setting, the physician assistant will evaluate information from the history, perform a thorough physical examination, decide on diagnostic studies, make the diagnosis, offer appropriate therapy, and discuss with the family the nature and course of the illness and the means of making the child comfortable. The physician assistant's supervising physician is always available for consultation on difficult cases.

Elements of appropriate patient management include telephone and office triage skills and decisions about home management versus hospitalization. It is essential to keep access to care and transportation in mind when planning for follow-up.[19] During the physical examination, subtle clues such as whether the child is playful and smiling often help the physician assistant ascertain important features about the severity of illness.

Anticipatory guidance also occurs during an illness visit. It is important to discuss with the parent the signs of worsening illness and when to call or bring the child in for reevaluation. Parents frequently have questions about contagion, return to day care or school, and timing and adverse effects of medications. Addressing all of these issues facilitates satisfying the family's needs and helps ensure compliance with therapy. It also helps build the parents' confidence and ultimately enables the PA to feel at ease with the reliability of the family.

Chronic Disease Visits

> ### CASE STUDY 31-8
>
> Three-year-old Felicia, who has spina bifida, comes into the clinic for her biannual evaluation. She is an only child, and her parents do not want to have any other children. She is still in diapers. Both parents work, and although an aunt has been able to provide day care until now, the aunt is moving away. Felicia's last hospitalization was 3 months ago for foot surgery. She had a bad bladder infection a month ago and is still on antibiotics. Felicia's parents want to know when she will be potty-trained and also think she has outgrown her leg braces.

The spectrum of afflictions that affect children chronically is broad and includes entities such as recurrent otitis media, asthma, abdominal pain, congenital anomalies, sequelae of prematurity, developmental delays, and mental retardation. Current estimates are that about 7.5% of pediatric patients are affected by chronic illness or disability.[19] Some of these conditions are limited to one organ system and respond well to interventions. Others are multifocal, and their impact on the child's life pervades many layers of functioning.

Physician assistants are increasingly assuming the important role of case manager.[20] Because patients with chronic illnesses need ongoing follow-up and evaluation, a multidisciplinary team approach is commonly used in providing their care. The team includes various medical and surgical specialists, a nutritionist, a physical or occupational therapist, a speech and language therapist, a social worker or psychologist, and a teacher. The case manager facilitates a coordinated approach to address the child's needs. Ideally, all those involved in the child's care meet on a regular basis to assess the child's progress, establish goals, and work with the parents to implement a realistic treatment plan. The child's and family's processes of adjustment to the illness or disability are ongoing. With each developmental stage, new issues arise. The ultimate goal is to maximize the child's potential through early intervention and to support family members as they work with the child's special needs.

Care of the Hospitalized Patient

Physician assistants are also increasingly involved in the management of hospitalized patients. In some settings, the PA will have primary responsibility for ongoing patient care and will review cases with an attending physician on a daily basis. Physician assistants make daily rounds on patients, write progress notes, evaluate laboratory data, and write orders for patient care. The type and severity of illnesses the PA follows vary among settings.

Skills for appropriate patient management ultimately are the same as for office practice. They include the ability to take a complete history that comprises essential elements to reveal the correct diagnosis; in addition, a thorough physical examination must be performed, laboratory or diagnostic studies must be used judiciously, and the information obtained must be critically analyzed. The utilization of observation skills in evaluating and reevaluating the patient as the illness takes its course, arranging discharge, and formulating follow-up plans are also components of comprehensive hospital care. The PA is involved in helping the family understand the illness and is often very aware of the psychosocial aspects of case management. It is in this interface with the family that the PA provides the "care" for the patient that is most highly valued.

CHOICES FOR PRACTICE

The opportunities available to a PA who wishes to practice in pediatrics are ample. Physician assistants are used as a vital part of health care teams providing service to children. Physical settings include ambulatory clinics for children and adolescents in both private and public sectors. Sites include health maintenance organizations, private offices, public health facilities, migrant and inner city clinics, and emergency departments. PAs also provide inpatient health care services in hospitals and facilities for the chronically ill and disabled.

Specialization within the field of pediatrics is also increasingly available. Physician assistants work as specialists or subspecialists in neonatology, pediatric asthma and allergy, endocrinology, hematology and oncology, orthopedics, child abuse and neglect, and adolescent medicine, to name just a few. The opportunity and availability of other settings continue to grow because of the interest and ability of well-trained physician assistants to bridge gaps in pediatric care.

Challenges in Pediatrics

The image of childhood is accompanied by the promise of hope and opportunity. That image, coupled with the dictum of medicine that in order to care for a patient one begins by caring about the patient, presents the pediatric PA with many challenges.

Provision of comprehensive and compassionate health care to children sometimes leads one to question expectations of what life should be like in childhood. Some children are not blessed with a carefree and safe existence. It may be very difficult to deal with a child and family who are forced to relinquish expectations and to grieve when a child is diagnosed with a debilitating birth defect, chronic disease, or terminal illness. Some children are victimized by gruesome acts of maltreatment at the hands of adults through either neglect or outright abuse. Abject poverty does not seem fair in a country with so many resources.

Despite these injustices, every child is in need of care and advocacy by committed professionals. Putting aside strong feelings in order to move through a difficult situation requires dedication, reflection, a supportive team, and the ability to see that growth occurs even in the midst of sadness. The patient needs the PA's talents. Difficult as these occasions are, they are ultimately opportunities for true service and often yield meaningful professional and personal lessons.

Rewards and Satisfactions

The practice of pediatrics offers numerous professional opportunities for pleasure and affirmation. Children frequently are delightful and charming. They are always spontaneous and guileless. It is from opportunities to interact with children in a helpful and productive way that many rewards come. As a PA,

one has the chance to observe growth and evolution, not just as children mature physically but also as they develop personality and character.

The intellectual challenge of understanding the disease processes of childhood and providing appropriate diagnoses is also rewarding. For the most part, children are readily healed. Medical care given to children is very affirming, because in most instances, their physical resilience is exceptional.

The provision of empathetic listening and appropriate reassurance from an individual removed from the immediacy of problems is highly valued by parents as the pace of society becomes more frenetic and mobility interrupts important connections to the extended family. Parents want to do the best they can for their children, even in the most difficult circumstances. It is a genuine privilege for the PA to be able to provide guidance to families and young children. The role offers the opportunity to help families build on inherent strengths and maximize their confidence in their ability to provide appropriate support and nurturing.

Pediatrics, like other primary care subspecialties, is filled with variety. A day in a pediatric office can be filled with many "routine" visits for which the intervention is relatively simple. There are many times, however, when diagnostic acumen and the ability to appreciate subtleties make a difference in the life of a particular child and family. The niche of a pediatric PA requires a knowledgeable and experienced view of what to expect from normal processes in childhood as well as expertise in pathological processes in children.

CONCLUSION

There is no doubt that physician assistants will continue to be in demand for their ability to provide high-quality health care to pediatric patients. Traditionally, PAs have augmented and amplified the availability and quality of health care for children.

Crises in provision of health care services for children will, unfortunately, continue to expand the areas for contribution. In the United States, as a result of chemoprophylaxis of HIV-infected pregnant women, transmission of the acquired immunodeficiency syndrome (AIDS) virus is estimated to occur in fewer than 500 newborns per year. However, pediatric

AIDS is a leading cause of death in children throughout the world and it was estimated at the end of 2000 that there were 2.0 million children living with HIV/AIDS.[21] Infants are also subject to the ravages of intrauterine exposure to drugs and alcohol. Lack of prenatal care directly influences the number of infants born prematurely and with congenital problems. Poor access to health care exacerbates complications from illnesses and disabilities. Children who are homeless face a multitude of health and psychosocial problems. Domestic violence affects children from the perinatal period through adolescence. Teen pregnancy remains an ongoing problem in the United States.

Although this litany may seem like a cry of despair, *all* children in the United States are in need of care. Physician assistants are uniquely able to provide this care and meet children's health care needs. As Osler[22] wrote, "Useful your lives must be, as you will care for those who cannot care for themselves, and who need about them, in the day of tribulation, gentle hands and tender hearts."

CLINICAL APPLICATIONS

Case 1

It is February. The McCarthys have brought 9-month-old Robert in because of a cough. He is in the third day of this illness and has not run a fever. They state that this is "really weird" because he seems fine during the day—coughs occasionally and is hoarse, but is eating great and playful. He was up most of last night with a dry, barky ("almost honking") cough. The McCarthys live in a small rural community in the mountains, 45 minutes away when the roads aren't snowy.

1. What would be your differential diagnosis for this illness?
2. How would the family's access to care affect your treatment decisions?
3. How would the child's age affect your treatment decisions?

Case 2

Ms. Tannenbaum is here for an ear recheck with 16-month-old Rebecca. It is her fourth ear infection since she started day care 6 months ago. Ms. Tannenbaum is almost in tears because she can't take any more time off from her job and wants to know what to do to prevent Rebecca from getting any more infections.

1. What questions would you ask to help her think through Rebecca's risk for ear infections?
2. Would you advise her to take her child out of day care? Why or why not?
3. What about the day care center's contribution to Rebecca getting ear infections? Are there other options for child care? What would you recommend?

Case 3

Mr. Fletcher brings in 10-year-old Jeff to the HMO you are working in. The family is on their way out of town to Disneyland for a long-awaited family vacation. Jeff announced last night that he had a sore throat, and he seems to have the sniffles this morning. Mr. Fletcher seems rushed and lets you know that their old family doctor treated any sore throat with antibiotics. They really want to start him on penicillin today before their 4:00 PM flight. Jeff has a 3-year-old sister, and his grandmother is joining them on this trip. Mr. Fletcher is concerned that the whole family will end up sick if Jeff doesn't start on antibiotics.

1. What additional history would you take about Jeff's symptoms?
2. What are the risks and benefits of starting Jeff on antibiotics?
3. What are your options for laboratory diagnosis, and how reliable are they for predicting whether this is an infection that requires antibiotics?

GENERAL CLINICAL APPLICATION QUESTIONS

1. If you accepted a position as a PA in pediatrics, how would you update your knowledge base and clinical skills?
2. What do you think you would find personally challenging and rewarding about working in pediatrics?

REFERENCES

1. Rudolph A. The health care system. In: Rudolph R, Oglesby A (eds). Pediatrics. New York: Appleton-Century-Crofts, 1977.

2. Rudolph A. Pediatric health supervision. In: Overby K (ed). Rudolph's Pediatrics. Norwalk, CT: Appleton Lange, 1991.

3. Silver H, Ott J. The child health associate: a new health care professional to provide comprehensive health care to children. Pediatrics 1973;51:1.

4. American Academy of Physician Assistants. 2001 AAPA Physician Assistant Census Report. Alexandria, VA: American Academy of Physician Assistants, 2001.

5. Hoyert D, Freedman M, Strobino D, Guyer B. Summary of vital statistics: 2000. Pediatrics 2001;108:1241.

6. Guyer B. Annual summary of vital statistics, 1996. Pediatrics 1997;100:905.

7. American Academy of Pediatrics. Statement of child health supervision. Bull Pediatr Pract 1972;6:3.

8. Harvey B. Special report: a proposal to provide health insurance to all children and all pregnant women. N Engl J Med 1990;323:1216.

9. Kohl S. The challenge of care for the poor child. Am J Dis Child 1991;145:542.

10. Hinman A. What will it take to fully protect all American children with vaccines? Am J Dis Child 1991;145:559.

11. American Academy of Pediatrics. Recommendations for preventive pediatric health care. Pediatrics 2000;105:645.

12. Korsch B, Freemon B, Negrete V. Practical implications of doctor-patient interaction analysis for pediatric practice. Am J Dis Child 1971;121:110.

13. Sayvetz A. Consent to treatment and access to minors' medical records. Colorado Lawyer 1988;17:1323.

14. Silver H, Kempe C, Bruyn H. Development and growth. In: Handbook of Pediatrics. Los Altos, CA: Lange Medical Publications, 1977.

15. Mortimer EA Jr. Preventive pediatrics and epidemiology. In: Behrman RE (ed). Nelson Textbook of Pediatrics, ed 14. Philadelphia: WB Saunders, 1992:147.

16. Center for Disease Control. Recommended childhood immunization schedule, United States, 2002. Available at http://www.cdc.gov/nip/recs/child-schedule.htm. Accessed 8 April 2002.

17. American Academy of Pediatrics. Recommended Immunization Schedules for Children Not Immunized in the First Year of Life. In: Pickering LK (ed). 2000 Red Book: Report of the Committee on Infectious Diseases, ed 25. Elk Grove Village, IL: American Academy of Pediatrics, 2000.

18. Peter G (ed). Active and passive immunization. In: Report of the Committee on Infectious Diseases, ed 24. Elk Grove Village, IL: American Academy of Pediatrics, 1997.

19. Schmitt B. Ambulatory pediatrics. In: Hathaway WE (ed). Current Pediatric Diagnosis and Treatment, ed 10. Norwalk, CT: Appleton Lange, 1991.

20. American Academy of Pediatrics. Report on the future role of the pediatrician in the delivery of health care. Pediatrics 1991;87:401.

21. Huttenlocher A, Wara D. Immunologic disorders. In: Rudolph A, Kamei R, Overby K (eds). Rudolph's Fundamentals of Pediatrics, ed 3. New York: McGraw-Hill, 2002.

22. Osler W. Doctor and nurse. In: Aequanimatas with Other Addresses to Medical Students, Nurses and Practitioners of Medicine. Philadelphia: The Blakiston Company, 1932.

RESOURCES

Barone M. The Harriet Lane Handbook: A Manual for Pediatric House Officers, Children's Medical and Surgical Center of The Johns Hopkins Hospital, ed 14. St. Louis: Mosby, 1996. *Great reference for procedures, drug dosages, and emergency treatment.*

Behrman R. Nelson Textbook of Pediatrics, ed 15. Philadelphia: WB Saunders, 1995. *A classic textbook containing detailed discussion of disease entities.*

Hay W. Current Pediatric Diagnosis and Treatment, ed 13. Stamford, CT: Appleton Lange, 1997. *An excellent, readable general reference.*

Pickering LK (ed). 2000 Red Book: Report of the Committee on Infectious Diseases, ed 25. Elk Grove Village, IL: American Academy of Pediatrics, 2000. *Best reference on immunizations and infectious diseases in childhood.*

Rudolph A (ed). Rudolph's Fundamentals of Pediatrics, ed 3. Stamford, CT: McGraw-Hill, 2002. *A classic textbook with excellent chapters on psychosocial issues and diseases.*

Schmitt B. Pediatric Telephone Advice. Boston: Little, Brown, 1980 (new edition pending). *Indispensable guide for practitioners and office staff.*

Schwartz M. The 5-Minute Pediatric Consult. Baltimore: Williams & Wilkins, 1997. *Quick synopses and algorithms for pediatrics.*

CHAPTER 32

Obstetrics and Gynecology

J. Kirkland Grant and Edward M. Sullivan

INTRODUCTION

Mid-level providers have long been involved in the practice of obstetrics and gynecology (OB-GYN), dating back to early midwifery. Certified nurse midwives (CNMs) play a large role in some OB-GYN practices, performing all uncomplicated vaginal deliveries, with the doctor called in for complicated vaginal deliveries or cesarean sections. Most OB-GYN physicians, however, do not have much experience with any sort of mid-level provider, particularly physician assistants (PAs). The practice of medicine has changed considerably over the past few years, with OB-GYN physicians taking on increasing primary care roles and reimbursement steadily declining with the growth of managed care and discounted fees. This offers an ideal opportunity for the

growth of PAs in the field of obstetrics and gynecology. The broad primary care training of physician assistants allows them to fit into this niche and make a substantial contribution. The PA can pick up abnormal findings on physical examination and has a broad understanding of other disease processes as they relate to obstetrics and gynecology and to primary care. The fact that PAs are trained by physicians gives PAs a point of view parallel to that of their OB-GYN supervisors.

A majority of mid-level clinicians working in obstetrics and gynecology are women and have been easily accepted by both physicians and patients. Some women feel more comfortable being examined by a woman clinician and actively seek out an OB-GYN practice where female clinicians are available. If the clinician is a caring individual with a willingness to listen and puts the patient at ease, however, that woman will become a long-term patient no matter the sex of the clinician.

One attribute of obstetrics is a uniquely hectic schedule. In large practices, one physician may be scheduled out of the office all day to cover deliveries. Smaller practices do not have this luxury, and often a physician is called away from a busy office to deliver a baby or attend other surgical emergencies. PAs can provide an ideal solution to such problems. Through planning of enough flexibility into the office schedule, the PA can cover many of these absences and minimize patient rescheduling. Although some patients may still choose to reschedule for a physician's appointment, most would prefer to be seen in a timely fashion. Utilization of a PA to provide backup and allow flexibility in scheduling also gives peace of mind to the physician, who can be assured that patients will be seen in his or her absence and that rescheduling or lengthy waiting room stays can be avoided.

A physician assistant is ideally suited to assist the supervising physician in surgery. In most hospitals, PAs can first-assist on all minor and major surgeries. Familiarity with the physician's technique can allow the PA to anticipate the physician's needs. This can help the procedure go more smoothly because often the scrub techs are different for each case and may not be accustomed to working with that physician and anticipating his or her needs.

COUNSELING

The daily routine of an OB-GYN clinician includes extensive and intensive opportunities for counseling of patients. Although it would be generally inappropriate for the OB-GYN physician to delegate all counseling tasks to the PA, it is equally true that the PA can provide these services cost-effectively, particularly for patients with extensive and complicated concerns. Although many patient education videos are available for patients to watch, these sometimes raise questions that a PA can help put in perspective and individualize for each patient. The patient about to undergo a surgical procedure benefits from multiple visits to ensure that she understands the scope of

the procedure and its benefits as well as its potential limitations.

By seeing a PA as well as a physician, the patient can be counseled thoroughly regarding her goals and expectations. Any specific concerns can be referred back to the physician for further consultation if necessary. Preventive care is one of the most important services health care providers can offer their patients and is most effectively achieved through patient education, counseling, and consistent follow-up. PAs working in obstetrics and gynecology are particularly proud of the relationships they develop with their patients throughout pregnancies and other transitions in their lives.

PAs must take care not to assume that their women patients are heterosexual. During the initial history, asking patients whether their sex partners are male, female, or both can elicit valuable information with a nonjudgmental approach. The differential diagnosis of a medical problem, as well as appropriate education and counseling, may be influenced by the patient's sexual orientation. For example, right lower quadrant pain in a lesbian patient would be less likely to be caused by pelvic inflammatory disease than in the heterosexual population. PAs who acknowledge the sexual orientation of lesbian, bisexual, and heterosexual women will be better able to develop positive relationships with their patients.

Patient Concerns

The PA has the opportunity to provide in-depth counseling and information about female anatomy and physiology, contraception, the menstrual cycle, sexually transmitted diseases (STDs), sexual problems and concerns, infertility, premenstrual syndrome, conception, prenatal care, breast-feeding, sterilization, breast self-examinations and mammograms, menopausal symptoms, hormone replacement, and a multitude of other reproductive and general health concerns. Despite the increasing availability of women's health information, women have many questions about reproductive concerns and problems. They often turn to the Internet for guidance, but some of the information posted on the Internet is false or misleading. It is important that the PA review this information carefully with the patient and put it in proper perspective for the individual that he or she is counseling. Similarly, information is often released by the press before it is available for review by health care providers. A thorough understanding of these issues can help the clinician to put the information in perspective for the patient.

Women may not know when they ovulate and are therefore more likely to get pregnant unintentionally. Some women think that the birth control pill can also protect against sexually transmitted diseases. Although it is true that the hormone effect causes thickening of the cervical mucus and may help retard the upward spread of chlamydia or gonorrhea into the fallopian tubes, this offers no protection against herpes, acquired immunodeficiency syndrome (AIDS), trichomonas, or condyloma. Many women are also misinformed about their own anatomy. A common question, especially among teenage girls, is whether a tampon or diaphragm can "get lost." Education and counseling are essential parts of the role of PAs in obstetrics and gynecology.

The First Pelvic Examination

CASE STUDY 32-1

A 16-year-old high school student comes to the office for her first pelvic examination and Papanicolaou (Pap) smear. She is accompanied by her mother. The patient appears apprehensive, showing little eye contact with the PA. After a focused history and physical examination, the PA performs the pelvic examination using the techniques described in the text Box. The PA offers the patient a mirror to view her cervix. After seeing her cervix, the patient becomes more animated and asks several questions about the examination, providing the PA an opportunity to educate the patient about normal female anatomy and physiology.

The first pelvic examination illustrates the importance of taking time for patient education and discussion. A woman coming in for her first examination may be apprehensive and afraid. Her friends and relatives may have shared with her detailed descriptions of painful and humiliating pelvic examination experiences. Some women are virgins and are concerned

PELVIC EXAMINATION PROCEDURE

- Show the patient the speculum and how it works.
- If the patient is virginal, smaller speculums should be available. Make sure they are ready before the patient is placed in a lithotomy position (in stirrups). Assure the patient that the hymen will remain intact.
- Describe the process for obtaining a Papanicolaou smear, reassuring the patient that it generally takes more time to describe the process than to perform it.
- Describe the bimanual examination and tell her how to relax. Instruct the patient to keep her bottom on the table and allow her knees to fall apart. If her knees are together, this tightens the introitus and makes the speculum examination and bimanual examination more difficult. She should try to keep her face and neck relaxed, focusing on a relaxing poster placed on the ceiling above the examination table. Remind her not to hold her breath, but to continue slow, deep breathing in through her nose and out through her mouth. An experienced nursing assistant in the room can help the PA and talk with the patient.
- Elevate the head of the examination table to give her a sense of greater participation and control.
- Have a mirror available to let her see her cervix.
- When the patient has her legs in stirrups, drape a sheet discreetly over her knees. Gently touch the inner part of her thigh, then slowly slide your gloved hand down to the vulva, so as not to startle the patient.
- Explain that you will first examine the external glands and urethra. Then gently insert a finger into the vagina and gauge the opening for selection of a speculum of proper size.

that they cannot be examined without tearing of their hymen. This situation requires a sensitive, caring clinician who will take the time to explain clearly what a pelvic examination involves in order to alleviate the patient's anxiety. This explanation should be presented by a clinician who has performed many pelvic examinations and has developed techniques to make the examination more comfortable. The procedure described in the text box can be applied to a first pelvic examination or any pelvic examination when appropriate.

After the pelvic examination has been performed, the clinician can spend time talking with the patient about sexually transmitted diseases, contraception, anatomy, the menstrual cycle, and other issues she may raise.

A teenager may be accompanied to her examination by a parent, usually her mother. Although this can be beneficial to the patient, sometimes the parent's presence can cause the patient to be inhibited, and she may not want to talk about some of her concerns. The clinician must be very sensitive to this and must know when to discreetly remove the parent from the examination room and ask the patient whether there are any issues she would like to discuss in private. Any issues of confidentiality she may have should be met with reassurance that information from her medical record, including topics of discussion, is not available to other individuals, including her parents, without her permission.

Often, a teenager may have scheduled the appointment to obtain birth control. It is important that the clinician discuss all the available methods, along with their risks, benefits, and possible adverse effects, to help her make an informed decision. Once she has selected a method of birth control, she needs further careful instruction on how to use the method correctly. It is especially important that a clinician be available to a teen for questions and to deal with any potential problems that could cause her to stop using her chosen method. The patient should understand that the clinician is available by telephone and that makers of oral contraceptive pills (OCPs) have toll-free lines that offer answers to many questions about the OCP. The patient should be advised to call before discontinuing the use of any method because of a problem or uncertainty. Minor adverse effects often will resolve within the first 2 or 3 months of use. Any major adverse effects should be reported immediately.

Teens also are often unaware of the types of sexually transmitted diseases (STDs) to which they can be exposed and the possible consequences of these diseases. Every patient encounter should include review and reinforcement of this information. It is important for the clinician to emphasize that although the birth control pill may prevent pregnancy, it will not protect her from STDs.

Sexual Issues

Many women have questions and concerns about sexuality but are uncertain and embarrassed about expressing them to the clinician. PAs in OB-GYN need to be knowledgeable about and comfortable in discussing with patients sexual concerns and problems. Skill in taking a detailed history of a sexual encounter is a required competency for the OB-GYN clinician, as is knowledge of appropriate treatment interventions and resources. Most patients will not volunteer any information about sexual problems. If they perceive that the clinician is hurried or uncaring, they will not mention the problem even if they are asked if they have any questions or anything else they wish to discuss.

Open-ended questions can be very helpful in drawing out the patient. It is essential that the clinician maintain a nonjudgmental attitude. Often the patient simply needs to be reassured that what she is experiencing is normal or common among other women. Documentation of items discussed is important to refresh the PA's memory when the patient returns for future visits but need not be extremely detailed unless such detail is pertinent to the patient's problem. More information about taking a sexual history is included in Chapter 10, "Interviewing and Communication Skills."

Premenstrual Syndrome

Many women experience premenstrual syndrome (PMS) with its many psychological and physical symptoms. Unfortunately, the exact cause of PMS remains unknown, which hampers clinicians' ability to counsel and treat women. Sometimes PMS is blamed for symptoms that are actually the result of other problems. The PA should be familiar with PMS, including its signs and symptoms and their timing in the cycle; he or she must also be attuned to other possible causes of a patient's symptoms. Having the patient keep a detailed monthly chart of her periods and note the timing and severity of her symptoms can help the clinician determine if the condition is PMS and can help in identification of the primary symptoms. Recently, severe PMS has been categorized as PMDD (Premenstrual Dysphoric Disorder). A lot of information is available on the Internet, which provides a good resource for patients.

Many treatment modalities have been recommended for PMS. Because no single treatment or combination of treatments is effective for all women, it is best that the treatment plan be tailored to fit the individual complaints. All women benefit from exercise, diet modification, and vitamin and mineral supplementation. Extra vitamins C, E, and B complex as well as calcium and magnesium may benefit the patient. Hormone supplementation, diuretics, antidepressants, anxiolytics, and antiprostaglandin agents (nonsteroidal anti-inflammatory drugs [NSAIDs]) all have roles in the treatment of specific complaints. In some cases, biofeedback or professional counseling may be needed. In every case, thorough discussion of the treatment plan and close follow-up are part of successful treatment. The most effective treatment in studies to date has been the selective serotonin reuptake inhibitors (SSRIs) and related drugs. Some studies have shown up to a 70% response. Prozac has been marketed under the label Sarafem for the targeting of PMDD. Some women have responded to the medication after taking it for only 7 to 10 days before their expected menses, even though peak effects of the drug are not usually noted until after 6 weeks of continuous use. For those with more severe PMDD or for those who do not respond to the premenstrual regimen, daily doses should be offered.

Conception

Unfortunately, many women do not seek medical advice when they are planning to get pregnant. Often, so much emphasis is placed on preventing unplanned pregnancies that when a couple is ready for a pregnancy, they can be unaware of the need for preconception planning. Studies now indicate that taking vitamins (particularly folic acid) before conception can reduce the incidence of certain birth defects, such as spina bifida and anencephaly, and may lower the incidence of spontaneous abortion. It is important for a couple to verify immunity to rubella before planning a pregnancy; those patients who are not immune should be immunized. Rubella vaccine (or measles, mumps, rubella [MMR]) should not be given to a pregnant woman, and pregnancy should be delayed 3 months after immunization. If the woman is diabetic, strict control of her blood sugar before conception can reduce the incidence of birth defects. Certain medications that women may be taking such as antihypertensive, antiepileptic, or antiacne medications, are contraindicated during pregnancy and should be changed before pregnancy is attempted, or immediately upon discovery of a pregnancy. Overweight women should be instructed about diet, and the effects of tobacco, alcohol, drug, and caffeine use before and during pregnancy should be reviewed.

Information about the normal menstrual cycle and ovulation and the optimal timing and frequency of intercourse can be of help. If patients are taking the OCP, they should be advised to wait at least two cycles after discontinuing the pill. If they do conceive before that time, they can be reassured that the pregnancy will most likely proceed without complication. Patients using Depo-Provera should know that it may take up to a year for their menstrual cycle to return to normal and for ovulation to resume. Any other health issues should be addressed before conception if possible.

Infertility

Infertility often requires extensive counseling by the clinician. Couples who have problems conceiving often are very anxious and frustrated. They usually have friends who have conceived very easily or who have had rapid success with infertility workups and cannot understand why they are unable to conceive. Many feel pressured by family and colleagues to produce offspring, and this compounds the anxiety. Although most causes of infertility fall into three major categories (anovulation, tubal blockage, and low sperm count), there are hundreds of potential causes for infertility, and only a systematic investigation may uncover them.

Some women come in wanting a single test to see if they can get pregnant. The only such test is a positive pregnancy test. Other patients come in seeking a "fertility pill," thinking that it will help them get pregnant no matter what the cause of their infertility may be. Education and explanation of various tests, their results and meaning, and the implications of those results for future pregnancy need to be provided in great detail. Patients need to understand that there is only one chance a month to get pregnant, and even if everything is in working order, the chances of getting pregnant during any one cycle may be only 20%. Therefore, some infertility workups can last for years. Both the patient and her spouse should be encouraged to come to office appointments whenever possible so they can be updated on the status of the workup, because it is often difficult for the patient to adequately understand detailed and complicated findings. Certain laboratory assessments or tests must be done on specific days of the menstrual cycle, so detailed instructions must be given. Some OB-GYN practices are hiring PAs to work exclusively in the area of infertility because it is such a labor-intensive aspect of practice.

Pregnancy

A pregnant woman experiences many hormonal and physical changes and sometimes is uncertain whether what she is feeling is normal or abnormal. Even if she has been pregnant before, each pregnancy is different and may bring new questions and concerns not previously raised. Adequate counseling and education can help prevent anxiety. Couples want to know about the growth and development of the fetus, changes in the mother's body throughout the pregnancy, and when quickening (first time fetal movement is felt) occurs. The fetal heartbeat usually can first be detected at 5 to 6 weeks by sonogram (depending on the machine), at 10 weeks by Doppler, at 15 weeks by fetoscope, and at 20 to 22 weeks by regular stethoscope. Numerous good reference books are geared toward pregnant women, and prenatal classes should be encouraged, but these sometimes raise other questions that the clinician should be prepared to answer.

Pregnant women should be counseled about which over-the-counter (OTC) preparations are safe. If they have questions about any medications that they are currently taking or that have been prescribed by other physicians during their pregnancy, they should call before initiating the medicine. The *Physician's Desk Reference (PDR)* and other drug-prescribing handbooks list the pregnancy category of each drug. Generally speaking, Category A and B drugs can be used safely during pregnancy, although some are contraindicated in the first trimester and others in the third trimester. Category C drugs can be used if the benefits outweigh the risks. Drugs such as phenytoin (Dilantin), which is known to cause an increased incidence of birth defects, may need to be continued despite the risks. Consultation with appropriate specialists will help the patient decide if the medication should be discontinued or changed.

Warning signs to be discussed with the pregnant patient differ with each trimester. Bleeding in the first trimester may be indicative of a threatened abortion, an ectopic pregnancy, or just cervical irritation. Severe vaginitis may at times cause bleeding as well as cervical polyps or vaginal lacerations. In the third trimester, placenta previa or abruptio placentae needs to be ruled out. Discharge in the third trimester might occur with premature rupture of the membranes (PROM), but infections that could precipitate PROM should be identified and treated. Braxton Hicks contractions begin at the start of the third trimester, but if they are strong and regular, premature labor must be ruled out. Cystitis may be the cause of uterine irritability; if untreated, it may progress to premature labor. A patient should be instructed to call if contractions are more frequent than 10 minutes apart and she is less than 37 weeks, but to wait until the contractions are strong and regular if 37 weeks or over.

When diabetes or another high-risk factor is identified, patients need extensive education to help prevent possible complications. Counseling and education of the pregnant woman constitute a major part of good prenatal care. Special considerations for teen pregnancies, single mothers-to-be, elderly gravidas, and other conditions should be incorporated into the patient education. Consultation with other specialists or with a perinatologist for complications should be done in a timely fashion. Depending on the scope of the physician's practice, these patients may be referred to a high-risk center, or they may be followed in conjunction with the specialist.

Postpartum Concerns

Once a woman has delivered, she often has questions and concerns about the postpartum period and breast-feeding. Postpartum depression is common and must be evaluated so the clinician can judge whether medication or counseling may be necessary. Couples will have questions about when they can resume sexual intercourse, how soon after delivery they might get pregnant again, and how contraceptives should be used in the postpartum period. Progestogen-only contraceptive pills have been used in breast-feeding women, but they are not as reliable and usually are not used in other situations.

A woman must make many adjustments to her life with a newborn baby. The lack of sleep and emphasis on the baby may leave her tired and disinterested in sex, while her partner may begin to feel unloved or left out. She must be encouraged to occasionally take some time out for herself, and her partner should be educated about normal postpartum conditions. If the partner is supportive and helps with the care of the baby, their relationship will be strengthened.

Menopause

Women have questions from their mid-30s on about the onset of menopause. This is an area of misinformation and often-unfounded concerns. Many women believe that the current cultural preoccupation with youth devalues women as they leave their childbearing years. Women in the perimenopausal period may experience mood swings, hot flashes, sleep disturbance, and changes in their body habitus. Postmenopausal women can have vaginal dryness, breast atrophy, and other physical changes. The challenge to the clinician is to provide information on menopause as a normal developmental phase rather than an illness. Prevention of osteoporosis and cardiovascular disease and consideration of hormone replacement must be discussed. Reports of a possible association between breast cancer and estrogen replacement must be put into perspective. The long-term benefits of preventive care must be emphasized, especially for women who are already postmenopausal and may not be having any menopausal symptoms.

CASE STUDY 32-2

A 49-year-old paralegal visits her OB-GYN office after 6 months of amenorrhea. During the preceding year, she experienced irregular menstrual periods with slightly lighter flow, sometimes skipping a month. During the 6 months since her last period, she has experienced fatigue. The fatigue seems to be due to waking up several times at night with sweating and hot flashes. She has also noticed less interest in sex with her long-term partner and some decrease in lubrication when having sex. The physical examination and pelvic examination are normal except for atrophic-appearing vaginal mucosa.

The PA discusses the risks and benefits of hormone replacement therapy with the patient. Because she has no medical history that would contraindicate hormone replacement and because she is at risk for osteoporosis, the patient decides to start replacement therapy. A combination of estrogen and progesterone is initiated with good results. The patient's symptoms abate and her sexual activity and enjoyment increase. The patient is educated about the importance of breast self-examination and regular follow-up with the PA for breast and pelvic examinations and Pap smears.

The continued need for annual pelvic examinations and regular Pap smears must be explained because women often feel they no longer need this care after they have completed their childbearing years. After age 50, annual mammograms are recommended. Although they may be uncomfortable, newer mammogram units and experienced technicians can minimize discomfort. New bone density measurements can be obtained to gauge the degree of osteoporosis when appropriate. The need for continued exercise, diet modifications, and increased calcium intake must be explained. The clinician must be sure to obtain a sexual history in menopausal women and must not assume that they are no longer sexually active. If the patient experiences dyspareunia (painful intercourse), a careful history and examination can determine whether this is due to atrophic vaginitis, inadequate lubrication, infection, or possible anatomical changes.

TASKS AND PROCEDURES
Annual Examinations

The most routine activity for OB-GYN clinicians is the performance of annual examinations. Every woman coming in for her yearly examination needs a history update or a complete history if she is a new patient; a complete physical examination, including breast and pelvic examinations; a Papanicolaou (Pap) smear; appropriate laboratory studies for routine screening and any identified problems; and counseling for expressed concerns. This is also the time to teach or reinforce proper technique and timing of the breast self-examination and the indications and timing for mammography. It is not uncommon for an astute clinician to pick up previously unnoticed problems, such as an enlarged thyroid, a heart murmur, or a pelvic mass in a patient who presents for a yearly examination without any problems or complaints.

Patients often will not volunteer information about problems, either out of embarrassment or because they think a symptom is normal. Women with endometriosis may have severe dysmenorrhea but may think that all women have severe cramps. Patients may not know that NSAIDs are generally superior to acetaminophen in helping to alleviate menstrual cramps. In some cases, laparoscopy may be warranted to diagnose the problem and treat the symptoms. Many women are reluctant to volunteer information about bladder control problems. Even young women may lose urine with coughing, sneezing, or jumping up and down. Questions about incontinence should always be asked of each patient during history taking. It can also be helpful to put a poster in the restroom that may prompt reticent women to ask about treatment options. A routine examination is also the time to provide counseling about anatomy, physiology, the normal menstrual cycle, nutrition, contraception, STDs, sexual problems and concerns, and normal developmental changes.

Contraception

Most women of childbearing age come to an OB-GYN practice at some time for the provision of a prescribed method of birth control. It is important for the clinician to review all options to help the patient select the optimal method for her use. It is also important to take a detailed history, including a sexual history, to help determine which method to recommend.

The oral contraceptive pill (OCP) is still the favorite choice for most women. Its safety record, effectiveness, and relatively low incidence of adverse effects cannot be overlooked. Studies have also shown that the OCP lowers the incidence of endometrial cancer and ovarian cancer. Most women will have some relief of dysmenorrhea, and there is even an OCP with a Food and Drug Administration (FDA) indication for the treatment of acne. Teenagers often have trouble remembering to take the pill at the same time each day. Although there are ways to help them remember, such as placing the pill pack next to a toothbrush, this still remains a challenge. Women smokers over age 35 or women with a history of thrombosis, hypertension, or other medical problems are not candidates for the OCP.

Careful instruction on when to begin and how to take the OCP is essential. If a woman forgets to take a pill, she should be instructed to take the missed pill as soon as possible or to take two the next day. If she forgets for 2 days, she should take two pills each day for the next 2 days. If she forgets for longer than 2 days, she should discontinue that pack and begin a new pack the following week. Patients must be reminded that the OCP may not be effective if pills are missed and that they may experience breakthrough bleeding.

Depo-Provera (a preparation of medroxyprogesterone acetate) has been approved for contraceptive use in the United States after decades of use in other countries. Depo-Provera is a slow-release, long-acting progestin that is given as an injection every 3 months. This works very well for women who have trouble remembering to take a pill every day. Depo-Provera is even more effective than the OCP in preventing pregnancy. The drawbacks include a greater number of adverse effects than the OCP, including weight gain, hair loss, and menstrual disruption. After long-term use, most patients will experience amenorrhea, and it may take up to 1 year before they can conceive after discontinuing the use of Depo-Provera. It can offer an alternative for the smoker over 35 years of age who desires to use a hormonal contraceptive method.

Intrauterine devices (IUDs) are undergoing a resurgence after litigation troubles in the mid-1980s. Currently, three IUDs are available in the United States—the Progestasert, the ParaGard, and a newer IUD, which is like a marriage of the other two. The Progestasert is filled with progesterone hormone, which is supposed to decrease vaginal bleeding. The hormone is gradually consumed and the IUD must be replaced every year. It offers a good choice for women who want relatively short-term contraception. The ParaGard consists of a T-shaped, copper-wrapped device that has now been approved for 10 years. The Mirena is a copper-wrapped IUD that also contains a progestogen, which has been used extensively in contraceptive pills. It can be left in place for 5 years and has the advantage of decreasing menstrual flow. Many women will become amenorrheic while using this device. This property has led to an indication for its use for treatment of menorrhagia, outside of its contraceptive benefits. IUDs are contraindicated in women with a history of pelvic inflammatory disease (PID) and are a poor choice for women who have multiple sex partners and are likely to be exposed to STDs such as gonorrhea and chlamydia. Effectiveness is similar to that of the OCP, although in the clinical trials for Mirena in the United States, there were zero pregnancies. The IUD also may offer a good alternative for the smoker or for the woman who is not ready for permanent sterilization but desires long-term contraception. Insertion of an IUD is a simple office procedure, taking less than 5 minutes, that any PA can learn to perform. (see Box).

A diaphragm fitting must include teaching the patient how to insert and remove the diaphragm, as well as how to use and care for it. The patient should be allowed time to insert and remove the diaphragm herself under supervision. Omission of this important step is linked to noncompliance. The patient who is uncertain about her ability to correctly place her diaphragm is unlikely to use it consistently. A major advantage of the diaphragm is its lack of any hormonal adverse effects. Studies of certain cohorts of women using the diaphragm for contraception have shown very respectable success rates. One complaint about the diaphragm is the lack of spontaneity involved in having to insert it just before intercourse. Patients should be counseled that they can insert the diaphragm several hours in advance, and if longer than 2 hours has elapsed, an applicator for spermicide can be inserted into the vagina without the need to replace the diaphragm. It should not be removed before 6 hours after intercourse.

Rhythm and withdrawal are relatively ineffective methods that some couples practice. Spermicides alone offer slightly better protection. Although a condom is not as effective as the other methods detailed here, it does offer the benefit of protection from many STDs. Women who are not in a long-term, mutually monogamous relationship should be counseled to use a condom even if they are using one of the other contraceptives.

Over the past several years, a full array of new contraceptive techniques have been developed. Some of these have been immensely popular, and in others, the popularity has waned. The Norplant is one of these. The Norplant system consists of three to six polymeric silicone (Silastic) implants containing a progestogen that are inserted into the upper arm. Training and practice are required to make insertion of Norplant smooth and correct. The manufacturer of the Norplant system provides training materials and workshops to teach the technique, which involves making a small incision in the upper arm and using a trocar to insert the capsules. Its 5-year life span makes it attractive to patients who want long-term contraception. Adverse effects are relatively common, including menstrual disruption, bloating, weight gain, and hair thinning. Counseling is particularly important for determining whether Norplant is a good choice for the patient and for providing education about its adverse effects. Norplant is currently involved in extensive litigation, prompting many practices to discontinue inserting the device until this situation resolves. A modification is in the works.

The contraceptive patch is a recent development that should prove to be very popular. This is essentially the birth control pill that can be taken

DR. GRANT'S PARAGARD IUD INSERTION TECHNIQUE

- Prior to insertion, the patient should have been counseled about the IUD and the technique for insertion, and given the brochure for review. Because of past litigation problems with the IUD, the information can be a little frightening and must be put in its proper perspective.
- An NSAID taken 30 minutes before insertion can reduce the discomfort.
- Lay out the instruments you will need for insertion—the proper IUD, a tenaculum, a sound, scissors, and sterile gloves—and pour an antiseptic (Betadyne, if the patient is not allergic) into a medicine cup. A nonsterile speculum and large swabs should be available.
- With the patient in lithotomy position, perform a pelvic examination with disposable gloves to ascertain the size and position of the uterus (midposition, anteverted, retroverted, etc.).
- Change gloves, insert the speculum, and swab off the cervix with the antiseptic solution.
- Carefully open the sterile IUD package, apply the sterile gloves, and prepare the IUD for insertion by folding the arms of the T and inserting them into the introducer. Insert the plunger into the opposite end.
- I have found that unless the uterus is sharply anteflexed or retroflexed, or the cervical os is very narrow, a tenaculum is often not necessary, and thus the procedure is much less uncomfortable.
- Gently insert the IUD with a slight curve, matching the uterine position, until resistance is met. If the IUD has been inserted 7 to 8 cm, you have reached the fundus. While keeping pressure on the plunger, withdraw the introducer, which will allow the arms of the T to reextend.
- If the IUD does not go past the internal os, have an assistant open the sterile tenaculum, grasp the anterior lip of the cervix, and place gentle traction on the uterus, which will straighten the uterus and usually will allow the IUD to be inserted. If you still have difficulty, sound the uterus to identify the canal.
- Trim the two strings with scissors. Have the patient feel the strings so she knows what they feel like.
- Give the patient a prescription for an antibiotic and stress that it is important she fill it right away. One or two doses is usually sufficient for prophylaxis. (Give samples if available.)
- Instruct the patient to check periodically that the strings are in place. If she cannot feel them, she should recheck after her next menses. If she still cannot find the strings, she should come in to be checked to see if the IUD is still in its proper place. Sometimes the strings can curl up in the os and can easily be removed with a cotton-tipped swab.
- Have the patient follow up in 6 weeks to ensure that the IUD is in place.
- The technique for the newer Mirena is somewhat different, and I recommend that you attend one of the training sessions to gain proficiency in its insertion. The Progestasert insertion is essentially the same as the ParaGard.

(applied) once a week, 3 weeks on, 1 week off. Patch technology has matured to yield a patch that is well tolerated and associated with minimal loss, although a replacement patch is available at the pharmacy should a patch fall off prematurely.

Lunelle is a once-a-month injection that is similar to taking a pill-pack at a time. The patient will continue to have regular menses, unlike with Depo-Provera, and generally has fewer adverse effects than with Depo-Provera. Finally, a self-inserted contraceptive ring is left in place for a week.

Regardless of the type of birth control method chosen by the patient, the clinician's role is to recognize any problems associated with the selected method of birth control and to manage those problems appropriately. Because many OB-GYN physicians feel that their time can be most effectively spent performing deliveries and surgery or dealing with complicated patients, the PA can assume an essential role in addressing the patient's contraceptive needs.

Prenatal Care

Pregnant women are seen in the office numerous times during their pregnancy, which offers a unique opportunity for PAs to develop close rapport with their patients. Every prenatal visit should include assessment of weight and blood pressure, urine checks for glucose and protein, measurement of fundal height, auscultation of fetal heart tones after 10 weeks, evaluation of any new signs and symptoms, discussion about patient concerns, and education appropriate to the stage of pregnancy. Initial laboratory work during pregnancy includes a complete blood count (CBC); a blood type Rh and antibody screen; screening for rapid plasma reagin, hepatitis B antigen, human immunodeficiency virus (HIV), and rubella; and a Pap smear. Abnormal findings should be reviewed with the patient, and tests should be repeated as necessary.

After 14 weeks, a maternal serum alpha-fetoprotein level should be obtained. When this result is abnormal, the patient is understandably fearful, and the clinician must appropriately counsel the patient. The patient should be reassured that there are often false-positive results, but the possibility of a serious problem cannot be totally discounted. An ultrasound or sometimes an amniocentesis may be necessary to determine the cause of an abnormal value. All pregnant women have a disruption of their glucose metabolism, and hypoglycemia is a frequent cause of dizziness and fainting that patients usually do not recognize as hypoglycemia. Instruction on proper diet will usually relieve these symptoms.

When entering the third trimester, the patient may develop hyperglycemia, and screening should be done on all patients. This usually consists of a blood glucose drawn 60 minutes following a 50-g glucose load. If elevated, further studies should be done to confirm gestational diabetes. If gestational diabetes is diagnosed, the patient needs to understand the need for very tight glucose control to prevent macrosomia and to reduce the incidence of stillbirth, birth trauma, and neonatal metabolic problems. Fetal well-being tests should be instituted, such as nonstress tests, which in some cases can be performed in the office under supervision by a PA.

Some OB-GYN practices alternate a patient's prenatal visits between the physician and the PA. Others may designate specific visits to specific providers. Some physicians prefer to have the PA complete the initial history and physical. Others prefer to use this longer visit as an opportunity to bond with the patient. In some clinics, PAs provide prenatal care for low-risk patients, and physician services are reserved for high-risk cases. At any visit, if the PA detects potential problems or complications, he or she is able to refer the patient to the physician for immediate evaluation.

Common Problems and Complaints

Frequently, patients come to an OB-GYN practice for evaluation of specific problems and complaints. The PA should be able to initiate evaluation of these common problems and should know when to refer the patient to the physician. Common problems include vaginitis, urinary tract infection, symptoms of STD, pelvic pain, pelvic infection, abnormal bleeding, abnormal menses, infertility, and abnormal Papanicolaou smear.

The PA should be able to diagnose and appropriately treat the simpler problems without physician consultation. When the patient complains of vaginal itching or discharge, diagnosis can often be made via a wet prep. *Trichomonas* are easily diagnosed, and yeast can be seen under the microscope. The presence of clue cells indicates bacterial vaginosis. Vaginal pH can also be helpful, and newer deoxyribonucleic acid (DNA) probes are now available to diagnose the more common pathogens. Less commonly, beta streptococcus, *Escherichia coli,* or other bacteria may be causing the symptoms and can be detected by culture.

A purulent cervical discharge may be seen with *Chlamydia,* gonorrhea, or other less common pathogens, some sexually transmitted and others not. Cultures and DNA probes are available to make the diagnosis. If an STD is suspected, appropriate tests should be obtained. Because a definitive diagnosis cannot be made without the culture results, the clinician should inform the patient that cultures are being taken to cover all bases, so the patient does not accuse her partner of being unfaithful only to have the tests later come back negative.

A urinalysis can easily be performed in the office with the aid of simple dipsticks and a centrifuge to spin down the urine. The presence of leukocytes or bacteria in the urine alerts the clinician to the possibility of a urinary tract infection (UTI). Red blood cells may be seen with a severe, acute UTI but may also be seen with urolithiasis or other kidney disease.

With a more involved problem, the PA can assist the physician by taking a careful history of the problem, performing a careful and thorough physical examination, and ordering appropriate laboratory work before referring the patient to the physician. Thus, the physician is saved the time and effort of the initial work and is able to use the information gathered by the PA to make a diagnosis and recommend an appropriate treatment plan more quickly.

Obstetrical and Gynecological Emergencies

A clinician must always be alert to the possibility of overlooking a serious problem. The signs and symptoms that a patient presents with do not always mirror those described in the textbook. A perfect example of this is a woman presenting with an ectopic pregnancy. The classical symptoms are unilateral pelvic pain, spotting, and a pelvic mass. The pain may be intermittent at first, becoming severe only when the ectopic begins to rupture. The patient may have had what she describes as a normal menstrual period only 2 weeks before the time she presents to the office. A positive pregnancy test may be the only thing that alerts the clinician to the lurking danger. Ectopic pregnancy is still one of the leading causes of pregnancy-related death. If diagnosed early, an unruptured tube can often be salvaged. Appendicitis in pregnancy can be very difficult to diagnose because of the physiological changes of pregnancy and the upward displacement of the appendix by the enlarged uterus. A strong index of suspicion is the key to timely diagnosis of these and other potentially life-threatening conditions.

PRACTICE CHOICES IN OBSTETRICS AND GYNECOLOGY

Practice settings for PAs in OB-GYN range from strictly outpatient to strictly inpatient settings. Some PAs move back and forth between the hospital and the clinic as part of their daily routine. Some practices are based on the assumption that the PA is best used in providing continuity in the office during the frequent and unplanned absences of the physician for deliveries and surgeries. Other practices with a large proportion of hospitalized patients may choose to assign the PA exclusively to the performance of hospital tasks, including managing patients in labor, assisting at surgery, and providing preoperative and postoperative care.

It is common for OB-GYN PAs in an outpatient clinic to have their own schedules of patients to see each day. Because physician schedules may be full for weeks in advance, the PA's schedule may include a number of patients with complicated problems that cannot wait (e.g., bleeding problems, possible infections, pelvic pain). In addition, the PA's daily schedule might include several routine annual examinations, follow-up visits with previously treated patients, and overflow patients from physicians called away from the office.

Many OB-GYN PAs report that the variety of patients they see on a daily basis is one of the most rewarding aspects of their practices. This variety also gives the PA the opportunity to perform a wide range of procedures in evaluating problems. PAs routinely perform cervical biopsies, vulvar biopsies, endometrial biopsies, and destruction of genital warts using chemicals or cryosurgery. Some PAs are actively involved in the evaluation and treatment of breast disease. Although some clinicians may choose to restrict their practice to routine visits, PAs working in any specialty over time generally expand their clinical and procedural expertise. A professional development plan for any clinical job should ideally include active planning for the acquisition of further skills and expanded responsibilities.

CONCLUSION

Growing concerns for women's health issues as well as health care reform plans that increase access to OB-GYN services are resulting in greater utilization of PAs. Many clinics are making the decision to expand the mix of providers (PAs, nurse practitioners [NPs], and CNMs) rather than adding physicians to OB-GYN practices. Some primary care clinics are hiring PAs with OB-GYN backgrounds specifically to provide family planning and prenatal services to their patients. Health maintenance organizations (HMOs) increase access to all OB-GYN services through the utilization of PAs and NPs. Research projects investigating women's health issues actively seek PAs and NPs to conduct the clinical components. Clinics serving

HIV-positive women utilize PAs and NPs to provide evaluation and treatment services. OB-GYN clinics in small communities are choosing PAs to expand services when they are unable to economically support additional physicians. In all of these situations, PAs are filling important niches in the health care system and are increasing patient access to OB-GYN services.

CLINICAL APPLICATIONS

1. Identify the steps in performing a pelvic examination.

2. Describe common symptoms of premenstrual syndrome and appropriate treatment approaches.

3. Discuss an approach to screening and preventive measures for the best outcomes of pregnancy for mother and child.

4. Identify typical symptoms of perimenopause and the risks and benefits of hormone replacement therapy.

5. Discuss typical roles of PAs working in OB-GYN. What would you find challenging and rewarding about practicing in OB-GYN?

C H A P T E R 3 3

Surgery

Timothy J. King and Edward M. Sullivan

"Experience is best borrowed and not learned."

—**Anonymous**

Continued

INTRODUCTION

The advent of the physician assistant (PA) profession in 1965 created a uniquely skilled clinician who bridged the gap between the medical and the nursing professions. Initially, a majority of PAs chose to practice in general and family medicine, with a few migrating to the surgical theater and the care of the surgical patient. According to the American Academy of Physician Assistants 2001 membership survey, PAs in general surgery and the surgical subspecialties represented 20.9% of all practicing PAs. As a group, this was second only to those PAs practicing family or general medicine (34.5%). Overall, 25.7% of PAs in the 2001 survey indicated that they assist in surgery as part of their job description.[1]

Most PAs, by virtue of their broad clinical training and on-the-job experience, exhibit significant versatility and work in surgery without additional formal training beyond PA school. However, a handful of PA surgery residency programs offer advanced training for graduate PAs, illustrating a continued demand for surgically trained PAs. These residencies allow PAs to learn and perform surgical house staff functions. In addition to postgraduate surgical training programs, three surgical assistant (SA) programs weave extensive surgical training into a parallel curriculum modeled on the traditional PA paradigm.

Surgical PAs and SAs work in both inpatient and outpatient settings, often augmenting resident staff or substituting for resident coverage in hospitals not using resident staff. Working within a team model with the surgeon as "captain of the ship," they are employed by university-based academic hospitals, community hospitals, individual and group surgical practices, and health maintenance organizations (HMOs), as well as preferred provider organizations (PPOs) and institutions representing all areas of surgery and surgical subspecialties, including general and vascular, orthopedic, transplantation, pediatric, cardiothoracic and thoracic, neurosurgical, plastic and reconstructive, otolaryngological, urological, trauma, obstetrics-gynecology, and surgical critical care. The roles assumed by surgical PAs reflect the flexibility and high quality of training demonstrated by performance of surgical house staff functions traditionally delegated to the surgeon-in-training. The PA provides a reliable standard of care for the teaching surgical staff; becomes a liaison with the surgeons, medical staff, and allied health professionals; and, most importantly, provides continuity of care for the team as the surgery resident staff rotates through the various surgical services. Both patient and family benefit from increased contact with a surgical staff member who can provide advocacy and prompt evaluation and education when required.

The American College of Surgeons recognizes PAs as valuable members of the first-assistant team, even though the tasks performed by PAs on a surgical service encompass the entire spectrum of care. PA surgical duties also involve initial patient evaluations (history and physical), admission orders, and preoperative preparation; first- and second-assisting in the operating room (OR), including independent procedures (e.g., harvesting of saphenous vein, insertion of invasive monitoring lines and assist devices, incision closure); providing postoperative care through discharge from the hospital; and evaluating and treating patients during postoperative visits in an outpatient setting. Thoracentesis and chest tube insertion, lumbar puncture, central venous catheter placement, paracentesis, and advanced cardiac and trauma life support are within the expertise of, and are common practice for, most surgical PAs. Many surgical PAs provide formal instruction to residents, medical students, other PAs, and team members. PAs may also be involved in clinical research and publication. Most third party payers cover PA services in surgery, and payment is provided to the PA's employer. Law mandates Medicare coverage with a PA first-assistant at surgery at a reimbursement rate of 85% of that allowed for a physician providing the same services. Detailed information on third party reimbursement for PAs may be obtained from the American Academy of Physician Assistants in Alexandria, Virginia.

> *"We should always let our judgments and recommendations be guided by the fact that we operate on patients, not on diseases."*
>
> **Stanley O. Hoerr**
> *American Journal of Surgery* **(1962)**

Today, more than 20% of all PA graduates enter the workforce in surgery and the surgical specialties, and all PA students are required to participate in a minimum of one surgical rotation as part of their training program. This chapter is constructed to serve as a practical primer of surgical principles and routine tasks, in the hope that it will alleviate some of the anxiety a PA student may feel when introduced to a busy surgical service. The spectrum of surgical practice is exceedingly broad, and no single chapter can present a comprehensive guide for each student's educational requirements. Therefore, a general surgery perspective is used to illustrate this overview and to emphasize the basic skills that are universally used in surgical practice. The "Clinical Procedure" sections are highlighted to emphasize key elements of performance. Other areas offer only brief overviews, with the hope that the student will pursue a detailed study of these areas as he or she continues training.

Much of this chapter concentrates on the specific actions required of the PA in the OR, where technical demands allow few mistakes. The remainder of the chapter discusses the appropriate preoperative evaluation of the patient in preparation for surgery, routines and requirements important to bringing the patient safely through surgery to discharge, and a few of the more common postoperative problems and complications.

GENERAL OVERVIEW

Practice and repetition are the essential elements of successful surgery, particularly when one is developing and refining manual dexterity; thus, one can comprehend the lengthy period required to train a surgeon. The PA should focus on this simple understanding when approaching surgical rotations or a new postgraduate position: sustained effort brings maximum reward.

Surgical PAs must remember that they are part of a team and that the patient is the ultimate benefactor of the team's efforts. To form a cohesive unit, each member should understand the others' roles, and personality conflicts should be identified early and resolved in a manner that optimizes patient care. Surgery requires stamina and emotional stability. Many long hours are spent at the operating table during lengthy procedures, and a strong constitution is needed to meet the demands experienced by the tense situations that may be encountered by the team. A good sense of humor, solid interpersonal skills, and a steady sense of self are necessary assets for keeping the team working toward a common goal with élan and efficiency, resulting in effective patient care.

To be an effective team member in this milieu, one must learn self-control and self-discipline. These strengths are often learned by observing senior, experienced team members and should be consciously cultivated, for they are equally as important as knot-tying and suturing. PAs are often called on in critical situations to perform highly technical tasks with little margin for error and to make decisions that may directly and quickly affect the health of a patient. Self-control and disciplined behavior are major assets enabling the PA to provide quality surgical care.

LEARNING THE ROPES

The practice of surgery comprises an enormous scope of patient physiology and care conditions. It can be as uncomplicated as suturing a clean superficial finger laceration in the emergency department or as complex as caring for a neutropenic cancer patient who must undergo major chest surgery that requires an extended ventilator-dependent period and postoperative total parenteral nutrition. Therefore, the practice of surgery requires an intimate and detailed understanding of anatomy and pathophysiology.

Most PAs learn anatomy in the context of what is joined to what, and where structures are located. The surgeon, on the other hand, is concerned with how each structure interrelates with the adjacent and adjoining structures in its vicinity, and how altering the anatomy and function of each structure affects the individual patient. Three-dimensional, spatial understanding of this concept is critical to the safe and effective performance of any surgical or invasive procedure. This concept can be illustrated by considering the insertion of a subclavian central venous catheter, a common surgical task. An iatrogenic disaster can occur if one does not understand the position of the subclavian vein and artery beneath the clavicle relative to that of the lung. A pneumothorax or an undetected subclavian artery cannulation may occur as a result of deep probing beneath the clavicle during this procedure.

Sound knowledge of the methods of accurate diagnosis, through the history and physical examination (PE), understanding of normal body physiology and adaptation to stressors, and a detailed comprehension of the pathogenesis and natural history of surgically treatable diseases allow the preservation and manipulation of the patient's physiological processes during surgical care. This concept is aptly demonstrated during cardiac surgery, during which an artificial physiological state is created when the native circulation is manually bypassed and the heart is stopped with a cardioplegic solution. Oxygenation, electrolyte and acid-base balance, and vascular volume are all controlled extracorporeally by the perfusionist. Postoperatively, the patient's cardiac preload, afterload, and inotropic efficiency are manipulated pharmacologically to optimize tissue perfusion and adequate cardiac output, and the heart rate is controlled by an external, computer-controlled pacemaker. Pulmonary function is controlled by ventilator respiration.

Many textbooks are available for learning techniques of surgical diagnosis, indications for surgery, specific treatment regimens, surgical procedures, and complications. They are elemental to acquiring essential surgical knowledge and serve as invaluable guides for the novice and the experienced surgical PA alike. The surgical resident should be able to suggest one or two textbooks recognized as standards for the care, treatment, and evaluation of diseases germane to their particular surgical specialty. Many texts are available that present guidelines for the routine care of the surgical patient. These provide capsulated, practical information on writing orders, treating common problems, and so forth.

Surgical anatomy texts and operative atlases are available for each of the commonly performed surgical procedures. Atlases detail each important step of a procedure, emphasizing anatomical landmarks, routine surgical maneuvers, and the use of important specialty instruments and techniques. Anatomical plates feature detailed dissections of pertinent tissues.

Surgical intensive care manuals and surgery physiology texts, coupled with physician guidance and practical experience, are useful means of mastering the preoperative and postoperative aspects of patient care. This approach is especially fitting for patients requiring complex physiological support.

ASSISTANT IN SURGERY

Historically, the roles of first- and second-assistant in surgery have been filled by experienced surgeons, nurses, and certified surgical technicians. The proliferation of qualified PAs and SAs trained in surgical assisting now brings the skills of another practitioner, trained in the medical model, to the operating suite.

The *first-assistant* is the person directly opposite the surgeon at the OR table, who actively participates in the conduct of the procedure. Most PA surgical rotations are dominated by members of the surgical residency and by fellows, who seek practical hands-on experience in the OR. The educational opportunity available within a group of surgical patients for first-assisting is limited, and often the roles of second- and even third-assistant are relegated to PAs and medical students. This may displace the student from the operative field, thereby diminishing his or her ability to adequately practice the harmonized and educated movements of an experienced surgical team.

In these instances, however, the student has a unique opportunity to learn many of the subtleties and nuances that will serve well when the opportunity to actively first-assist arises. Although tugging at the end of a retractor may seem like an interminable task, it enables one to observe and appreciate the practiced movements and coordinated efforts of the surgeon and first-assistant without peril of poor performance from lack of experience. The basic techniques of incision creation, appropriate tissue retraction, gentle tissue handling, hemostasis, knot-tying, and wound closure can all be gleaned from keen observation at the table.

JUDGMENT, HANDS, TOOLS, AND DEVICES

Surgical procedures are composed of a series of physical motions centering on tissue dissection and manipulation, with experienced judgment directing the action. All operations are memorized step by step, including common intraoperative alternatives, in order to achieve the optimum result. The proper use of surgical instruments must be mastered, but more importantly, the PA must learn to use each one efficiently, effectively, and safely. Maneuvers such as the use of the scalpel, suturing, knot-tying, tissue retraction, and intravenous (IV) and chest tube insertion require learned manual dexterity and hand-eye spatial coordination that are mastered with study and practice. An assistant's hands are the most valuable tools he or she brings to the table, next to sound surgical decision-making skills.

Surgical judgment is the ability to recognize what should or should not be done during an operation or during the care of a surgical patient. This judgment can be acquired only through active immersion in the surgical environment. The frequently touted axiom "See one, do one, teach one" does not embody the value of experience to the surgical PA. The appropriate when's and how's for manipulating a nerve, holding the large bowel, using electrocautery, or adjusting a ventilator's settings come with time and demonstration, not with trial and error. This is why the chapter's motto is so poignant.

Academicians often refer to the concept of the "practice" of surgery. This state of constant renewal and relearning must occur as new techniques and modifications, materials, and devices are applied to care for the surgical patient. The OR and intensive care unit (ICU) are replete with devices requiring electrical input and computer control; all essential personnel are required to be skilled in their use and maintenance, and many require attention and oversight from PAs. It is extremely important for the clinician to know completely each device's operation and to be able to troubleshoot that device if an emergency arises from its malfunction. Intraoperatively, such malfunctions may account for an inordinate rise in total anesthetic time and an increase in morbidity.

Each instrument, retractor, and needle has inherent properties of action that, in the hands of an experienced user, become direct extensions of the hands and fingers. Spending time in the instrument cleansing and sterilization area is an excellent opportunity for the PA to handle instruments and practice their use without the pressure of timed performance in the OR. The staff can aid in instrument identification, and the novice PA can handle each of the commonly used instruments of the specialty and practice proper hand position and control of the instrument with the goal of understanding its actions and precise use. A short time spent practicing outside the OR can prevent fumbling and uncoordinated movements during the actual operation.

WHO'S WHO IN THE OPERATING ROOM
The Surgical Team

The surgical team may consist of all or a combination of the following people: attending surgeon, fellow, fifth-year resident, junior resident, intern, and student(s).

Attending Surgeon   In most academic centers, the attending surgeon is an experienced staff member who has the ultimate responsibility for the surgical team's patients. He or she is responsible for the training of the fellows and fifth-year surgical residents, and frequently teaches the more difficult and complex surgical techniques and decision making to this group. Attending surgeons often have particular areas of clinical interest (e.g., oncology, intensive care, trauma, burns, gastrointestinal disorders) and are commonly involved in research. The attending surgeon participates in the training of students on the surgical rotation as well, and is called on to personally operate on the more difficult surgical cases that require experienced judgment.

Fellow   A graduate of a surgical residency, a fellow has elected to continue studies in a specific subspecialty (e.g., vascular, trauma, cardiac, neurosurgery). Each fellowship lasts between 1 and 3 years, during which an intense training regimen prepares the fellow to practice in the chosen specialty. Much of this training is spent in the OR, learning and performing specific specialty procedures. Many fellowships include a specified opportunity to conduct research activities.

Fifth-Year Resident   The fifth is the last year of residency for most general surgery programs, although some extend to 7 years. The fifth-year resident is responsible for the overall day-to-day patient care provided by the team. He or she performs the most complicated operations with the attending surgeon, instructs junior residents in the OR, and provides consultation on the care of newly admitted patients and complicated cases.

Junior Resident   The junior resident is the workhorse of the residency staff. This person is responsible for the minute-to-minute care of the patient as provided by the surgical team. The junior resident does a large volume of the service's operating and is responsible for the training of the second-year resident and intern. A resident in the second year of training along with the intern does much of the admitting and discharging of the service's patients. Additionally, the second-year resident usually serves extended rotations in the emergency room and ICU to hone emergency care, triage, and surgical intensive care unit (SICU) skills.

The Intern   The first-year resident, or intern, is a recently graduated medical student, and a new arrival on the surgical service. He or she is responsible for the brunt of the everyday tasks required for patient care—routine orders, admissions, discharges, consults, night call, IV lines, tubes, laboratory tests, and radiological studies. Interns are engaged in learning the basic surgical skills and techniques required for general patient care. They are excellent sources of information for PA students, and because of the great burden of tasks thrust on them, interns commonly allow PA students to learn by doing.

The Student   Medical and PA students are a valuable part of the surgical team in that students provide the additional staff required to efficiently operate a large-volume service. While constantly observing, students help manage the day-to-day needs of their assigned patients—history and PE, beginning IVs, drawing blood specimens, inserting chest tubes, casting, wound care, emergency department duties, patient assessment, patient transport, dressing changes and wound care, and monitoring response to treatment. In addition, PA and medical students learn basic surgical techniques such as suturing and knot-tying, inserting monitoring lines, and first-, second-, and third-assisting in surgery. After adequate observation and performance of techniques monitored by senior team members, the student's motto should be, "I will do that for you."

The Anesthesia Team

The anesthesiologist is responsible for evaluating the patient for anesthesia and, in coordination with the operating team, for providing safe conduct of the patient through the chosen anesthetic technique. Anesthesiologists care for the patient throughout the recovery room period and into the SICU if required. Many have particular expertise in pain management.

Certified registered nurse anesthetists (CRNAs) train in nurse residency programs to perform many of the same tasks as a physician or a doctor of osteopathy (DO) anesthesiologist. Deeply versed in anesthetic practice, CRNAs provide quality care, often without the direct supervision of an anesthesiologist, and are used by many surgeons for uncomplicated surgical procedures. Limitations on CRNA practice are dictated by hospital and state regulations and vary from institution to institution and from state to state.

Anesthesiology assistants (AAs) are individuals who attend a training program to conduct anesthesia, but who are not physicians or CRNAs. Several training programs are available in the United States, although only a handful of states have regulations or laws that allow administration of anesthesia by AAs. AAs perform anesthesia practice under the supervision of a licensed anesthesiologist and are valued members of the anesthesia team, on which they are utilized.

Operating Room and Recovery Team

Postanesthesia Recovery Unit (PARU)/Recovery Room Nurse The PARU nurse is trained in assessing and treating the patient in the immediate postoperative period, including maintenance of hemodynamic and cardiopulmonary stability, pain management, and crisis intervention when necessary. Such professionals are invaluable sources of guidance and information on postanesthesia patient care.

OR Director Usually a veteran registered nurse (RN), the director controls the overall activity of the OR and is responsible to the chief of surgery (a surgeon) and the hospital's director of nursing. The OR director represents the OR to other hospital departments, manages the department's fiscal requirements, and oversees the management of OR personnel. He or she can set the tone for a favorable climate for PAs in the OR.

OR Supervisor Also usually an RN, the OR supervisor manages the day-to-day activities in the OR and makes important policy decisions in conjunction with the OR director. The supervisor is responsible for problem solving, overall procedure and OR staff scheduling, instrument purchases, and staff training.

Control Room Supervisor As the title implies, the control room supervisor controls the scheduling of surgery and personnel assignments on a daily basis. He or she checks for the proper availability of equipment for each case and acts as a traffic coordinator for busy surgery departments.

Head Nurse There is usually one head nurse per shift. He or she helps micromanage the OR environment for smooth and efficient daily operations. Often, the head nurse is a very experienced nurse with good problem-solving abilities and adaptability. He or she is a liaison between the OR staff and the surgeon.

Staff Nurse Staff nurses are usually RNs and licensed practical nurses (LPNs). They have two overlapping roles—circulating nurse and scrub technician or scrub nurse.

Circulating Nurse (Circulator) The circulator supervises the general activity of each individual in the OR, including assessing the patient in the holding area before bringing him or her into the OR and transporting the patient to the recovery area after surgery. Patient safety, also the responsibility of the circulator, centers on appropriate positioning of the patient on the OR table and preparation of the patient by scrub preparation of the skin before the incision. The circulator assists the scrub nurse in assembling the supplies and instruments required for the operation and in accounting for all sponges, needles, and instruments before and after each operation. Circulators provide additional supplies for the operative field when required. They receive and connect the various tubes and wires coming from the sterile field (e.g., suction tubes, laparoscopic equipment, and electrocautery wires) to the appropriate devices. They operate and troubleshoot nonsterile equipment and prepare tissue specimens received from the surgeon for transport to the pathologist for analysis.

Scrub Nurse Scrub nurses assist the surgeon by providing all instruments, sutures, and supplies required for the smooth execution of each procedure. Scrub nurses anticipate the needs of the surgeon and first-assistant by understanding each step of a procedure and by monitoring the progress of the operation, often handing the appropriate instrument to the surgeon without prior request. In addition, the scrub nurse occasionally assists in retracting tissues, cutting sutures, sponging blood from the field, and operating the suction. A well-trained and experienced scrub nurse often performs certain portions of the procedure without direct supervision by the surgeon. One of the scrub nurse's primary responsibilities is knowing the location and count of all items in the sterile operative field before, during, and after surgery, ensuring that nothing has been left in the wound. The scrub nurse is an invaluable source of information on the conduct expected of the PA or medical student in the OR and the skills required at the OR table. Also, a scrub nurse who has worked frequently with a given surgeon may have invaluable information regarding that surgeon's preferences and dislikes in the OR.

Certified Surgical Technologist (CST) Although not an RN or LPN, the CST is trained by an American Medical Association (AMA)–approved center and meets rigid certification examination criteria to perform a wide variety of functions in the OR. Many of these responsibilities parallel those of the scrub nurse, although many large institutions do not allow CSTs to circulate during surgery. CSTs often assist the surgeon while scrubbed and fill an important position in the operating suite.

PREOPERATIVE PATIENT EVALUATION

"For us, an operation is an incident in the day's work, but for our patients, it may be and no doubt it often is the sternest and most dreadful of all trials, for the mysteries of life and death surround it, and it must be faced alone."

Sir Berkeley Moynihan (1865-1936)

The most important portion of the evaluation of surgical patients (after stabilization in emergencies) is assessing their ability to safely undergo the proposed surgical procedure. This assessment concentrates on the patient's replies to questions derived from the past medical history and systems review. Information gained from past medical records and family members is equally as important as PE findings, diagnostic laboratory results, and radiology reports.

Obtaining a comprehensive history is critical and is discussed in Chapter 9. The portions pertinent to surgical patient are briefly reviewed for emphasis (see Boxes). Most surgeons do not assess all physiological systems before surgery, often relegating this task to the PA. This is a prime opportunity for the PA to establish a trusting relationship with the patient and family. It is during this initial contact that the PA can explain the usual preoperative preparations, the planned surgical procedure, its risks and benefits, and the expected postoperative course.

SAMPLE ADMISSION ORDERS

- Admit to
- Diagnosis
- Condition
- Vital signs
- Allergies
- Nursing (tubes, wound care, respiratory care, oxygen, etc.)
- Diet
- IV fluids
- I/O (fluids into and out of patient), daily weights
- Medications
- Studies (chest x-ray, electrocardiogram, pulmonary function tests, etc.)
- Laboratory tests
- Call House Officer for (limits of temperature, vital signs, urine output, drain output, etc.)

THE FIVE Ps OF MEDICATIONS

Pain:	Oral or parenteral pain meds (scheduled or as needed [prn]). Consider patient-initiated pain pump.
Pillow:	Sleeping pill (prn).
Poop:	Stool softener or cathartic (scheduled or prn).
Pus:	Antibiotics; topical agents for skin or wound care.
Previous:	Long-term medications the patient has been using; may need to be changed postoperatively.

The History

Each type of surgery demands different information about the history of present illness. In acute, life-threatening emergencies, a paucity of information may be available. In acute surgical cases (allowing several hours before surgical intervention), the history of present illness should detail the type, severity, and duration of symptoms; associated symptoms (e.g., pain, nausea, vomiting, syncope); previous similar episodes; previous evaluation, if any; previous treatments; family history of similar problems or anesthesia complications; and last oral intake. A detailed history should center on past operations, particularly those that may have a bearing on the present illness. Electively scheduled surgery allows a more leisurely but thorough patient evaluation.

Detecting "co-morbidity" by eliciting information on co-existing diseases that could lead to complications before, during, or after surgery is a prime focus in taking the history of a surgical patient. Co-morbid disease can increase the risk of complications, which could be ameliorated or prevented with preoperative medication or treatment. Early identification allows appropriate consultation with other services and pre-emptive treatment of expected postoperative problems. Table 33-1 lists diseases and conditions that must be detected and evaluated before surgery.

Table 33-1   Major Diseases or Conditions Requiring Evaluation Before Surgery

- Diabetes mellitus and other endocrine diseases
- Cardiac disease
  Rheumatic heart disease
  Valvular disease
  Arrhythmias
  Prior myocardial infarction
  Angina
  Severe hypertension
  Congestive heart failure
- Pulmonary disorders
  Moderate to heavy smoking
  COPD
  Asthma
  Obesity
- Hematological diseases
  Bleeding disorders
    Thrombocytopenia and hemophilia
    Moderate to severe anemia (sickle cell, iron deficiency, etc.)
    Thromboembolic disease (deep vein thrombosis, pulmonary embolism)
- Thyroid disease
  Hyperthyroidism
  Hypothyroidism
- Adrenal dysfunction
- Liver disease
  Hepatitis (drug-induced, viral, cholestasis)
  Cirrhosis
- Electrolyte disorders
  Calcium, potassium, phosphorus, sodium, magnesium
- Acute or chronic renal failure
- Neurological diseases
  Seizures
  History of stroke or transient ischemic attacks
  Myasthenia gravis
    Multiple sclerosis
- Pregnancy
- Peripheral vascular disease
- Rheumatological diseases
  Rheumatoid arthritis
  Systemic lupus erythematosus
  Gout
  Sarcoidosis
- Psychiatric disease
  Heavy alcohol use, schizophrenia, bipolar disorder
- Risk factors for HIV and hepatitis
- IV or other street drug use/abuse

COPD, Chronic obstructive pulmonary disease; *HIV,* human immunodeficiency virus.

In general, the information required during the preoperative evaluation is as follows:

➤ An assessment of the general state of health, including exercise tolerance, recent weight gains or losses, usual state of emotional health, and frequency of routine medical care.

➤ A review of the patient's current drug use, which should alert the PA to underlying pathophysiological diseases that may affect the course of surgery (e.g., digitalis as a clue to heart disease). Obtain a history of drug use, both prescribed and over-the-counter, including tobacco, aspirin, nonsteroidal anti-inflammatory drugs, street drugs, and herbs or other alternative or complementary medications used. The quantity and duration of use of tobacco products should be identified and chronicled in the chart and discussed with the surgical team.

➤ An identification of all medication and food allergies, including type and severity of reaction (e.g., pruritus, respiratory distress).

➤ A thorough menstrual and obstetrical history from female patients, including any anesthetic complications that occurred during childbirth. Menstrual history is especially important for patients who may not suspect that they are pregnant, or for patients who could be anemic from heavy menstrual blood loss.

➤ Previous hospital charts, when possible, to review the patient's past surgical performance (e.g., type of surgery and anesthesia, complications, anesthetic problems, blood transfusions, and extended ICU admissions).

The review of systems (ROS) is especially useful in determining the patient's overall health status. Regardless of the schedule of the patient's usual health care, important problems may have developed in the interim that need evaluation before surgery. Attention should be given to detecting risk factors for communicable viral diseases such as hepatitis and the human immunodeficiency virus (HIV).

In the ROS, questions should be directed toward problems involving the cardiopulmonary and endocrine systems because these systems account for a majority of postoperative deaths and morbidity. Sample ROS questions are listed in the Box.

SAMPLE ROS QUESTIONS FOR PREOPERATIVE EVALUATION

These sample pertinent questions are not a comprehensive guide to ROS questioning but are useful as a basis for review of each system during the preoperative evaluation.

General
How is your general health?
If emergent surgery required—When was your last meal?
Have you been sick lately, or are you under the care of a doctor for any problems?
What are the names of any other physicians providing care for you?
Any history of cancer?
Tell me about your weight and appetite.
How is your energy level?
When was your last tetanus immunization?
Have you had a pneumovax immunization? (splenectomy or over age 65)

Drugs
Ask the patient to bring all home medications to the hospital or office for evaluation.
Do you take any prescription medications? Which ones? Do you take them on a regular basis?

SAMPLE ROS QUESTIONS FOR PREOPERATIVE EVALUATION—cont'd

Have you taken, or are you now taking, oral or injected steroids?

Do you take any over-the-counter medications, including vitamins and cold medicines (antihistamines and ephedrine-like medications)? Have you used any aspirin, Advil, Motrin, or other anti-inflammatory medications over the past 10 to 14 days?

Do you take any herbs or home remedies?

Do you use marijuana, heroin, cocaine or crack, methamphetamines, opioids, or barbiturates? Any other street drugs?

Do you drink alcohol? How much per day or week and for how many years? Have you ever been admitted or evaluated for alcohol problems?

Use the answers to these questions to investigate specific systems affected by the medications cited (e.g., ask diabetes/endocrine questions if patient is taking oral antihyperglycemic agents).

Respiratory
When was your last chest x-ray?

Do you smoke? If yes, how many packs a day and for how long?

Have you been diagnosed with asthma, bronchitis, emphysema?

Have you ever been hospitalized for pneumonia, bronchitis, or asthma?

Have you ever been on a ventilator after surgery or for any other reason?

Do you cough every morning or on some mornings? Do you ever cough up anything? Describe it. Have you had a recent cough or cold?

Have you ever been exposed to or had tuberculosis? If so, which treatment did you receive and for how long?

Are you prone to sinus infections?

What medications do you take for your respiratory problems?

Do you need oxygen at home to breathe?

Cardiac
What heart medications are you taking?

Do you have high blood pressure? How long have you had it?

What was your last measured blood pressure?

Do you have high cholesterol or triglycerides?

When was your last electrocardiogram?

Have you ever had a stress test or a cardiac echo or catheterization?

Have you ever been told you have a heart murmur?

Have you ever had a heart attack or rheumatic fever? When was your heart attack?

Do you have an irregular heart rhythm? Do you have an implanted pacemaker?

Have you ever had heart surgery?

Cardiac
Do you ever get chest pain? How often? Related to what activity?

Are you ever short of breath, or do you ever wake up at night short of breath?

How many pillows do you need to sleep on? If you have climbed any stairs recently or walked around the block, how far did you go before becoming short of breath?

What is the hardest work you've done in the last couple of weeks and how did you tolerate that?

Do you have pain in your legs when you walk? Does it subside with rest?

Do you have any swelling in your feet or your hands?

Continued

SAMPLE ROS QUESTIONS FOR PREOPERATIVE EVALUATION—cont'd

Endocrine
Do you have diabetes or thyroid disease? For how long? Which medications do you use?
Have you had any complications/problems related to your diabetes/thyroid disease?
Have you ever had any problems with your adrenal glands?
Have you taken any steroids in the past year? Do you have heat or cold intolerance?
Do you get up at night to urinate? If so, how many times?
Do you urinate very frequently?
How well do you sleep?
Are you nervous?
Have you had any weight gain or weight loss lately?
Are you frequently thirsty?

Hematological
Do you bleed easily?
When you cut yourself, do you quickly stop bleeding?
Do you have frequent nosebleeds?
Does anybody in your family bleed easily?
Has anyone in your family been told they have von Willebrand's disease or hemophilia?
Do you bleed when you brush your teeth?
Have you ever been told that you are anemic?
Have you been told you have too much blood (polycythemia)?
Do you have any history of thrombophlebitis or blood clots in the lungs or legs?
Have you had any blood transfusions in the past? If yes, how many units or what kind? Any problems associated with them?

Gastrointestinal/Nutrition
How is your appetite?
Have you had any weight gain or loss?
Are you nauseated or do you have vomiting? Have you had any abdominal or pelvic operations?
Have you ever vomited up blood?
Have you ever had bloody or tarry stools?
Have you ever had an ulcer?
Do you have abdominal pain (type, location, relation to foods, treatment)?
What are your bowel habits like?
Have you ever been jaundiced?
Have you had hepatitis in the past?
Are there any foods that you cannot eat?
If diabetes or neurological disease, have you ever been told that you have trouble with emptying your stomach (delayed gastric emptying)?
Have you ever had an upper or lower endoscopy?

Genitourinary
Have you ever had any kidney or renal diseases? Are you prone to bladder infection or prostate infection?

SAMPLE ROS QUESTIONS FOR PREOPERATIVE EVALUATION—cont'd

Do you have a history of kidney stones or blood in your urine?
Do you have any problems with urinary incontinence?
Do you have difficulty with urination?
Do you get up at night to urinate?

Neurological and Psychiatric
Have you ever had a seizure or a convulsion? Do you take any medications for this? Which ones and for
   how long?
Do you have history of a stroke or transient ischemic attacks?
Have you ever had an arm or leg go dead, or have you ever been paralyzed or had a numb limb?
Have you ever had trouble with your vision, either loss in one eye or seeing double?
Do you have frequent headaches?
Do you have any impairment of your memory or speech?
Do you have any difficulty with your motor coordination?
Do you have any problems with vertigo (dizziness)?
Have you seen a psychiatrist or psychologist?
Do you have any anxiety or nervous disorders?
Do you have a history of depression?

Gynecological/Obstetrical
Have you been pregnant? How many times? What were the results of those pregnancies?
Did you have any complications?
Do you think you could be pregnant now? When was your last menstrual period?
Are you using birth control pills or another type of birth control?
What is your usual menstrual flow?
Do you have any trouble with your menstrual period, especially significant bleeding?

Anesthesia
Have you or has anyone in your family had problems with anesthesia?
Have you or has anyone taken a long time to wake up from anesthesia (antipseudocholinesterase
   deficiency)?
Have you or has anyone in your family had a high temperature as a result of anesthesia (malignant
   hyperthermia)?
Have you ever had to stay on the ventilator after surgery? (Important question for chronic obstructive
   pulmonary disease [COPD] patients.)

Musculoskeletal
Do you have arthritis of any kind?
Are any of your joints frozen or hard to move?
Do you have any back problems?
Do you have any muscle diseases?
Do you have any artificial joints?

The Physical Examination

A complete physical examination (PE) should be performed on each patient if time permits. The value of a complete PE in identifying possible sources of complications that can be managed expectantly cannot be overestimated. Preoperative physical findings are often used in the postoperative period to explain new signs and symptoms, as evidenced by the following example.

CASE STUDY 33-1

A 45-year-old man admitted with acute gastrointestinal bleeding from a perforated duodenal ulcer undergoes a successful 2-hour operation through a mid-line incision under general anesthesia. He is transferred to the PARU extubated and in good condition. The PARU nurse notes that the patient is unable to move the fourth and fifth fingers of his right hand and is too groggy to appropriately answer questions relating to this alarming finding. The anesthesia staff is concerned that the patient was improperly positioned on the OR table and may have experienced pressure on the ulnar nerve at the elbow or from inordinate traction on the brachial plexus at the shoulder during the surgical procedure.

If a thorough history and PE had been performed on admission, the patient's previous trauma-related ulnar nerve injury would have been detected, eliminating needless panic among the staff.

Although a complete PE should be performed, its focus should be on the state of the patient's cardiopulmonary and vascular systems, where many surgical complications may arise. Full vital signs, with the blood pressure measured in both lying and standing positions, may reveal orthostatic changes. Thorough examination of the vascular system, including the carotid, aortic, and femoral arteries for bruits, may indicate vascular or cerebrovascular disease. A peripheral vascular examination is useful in assessing edema, signs of superficial or deep phlebitis, varicose veins, or distal limb perfusion problems. Shiny atrophic skin, thick ridged nails, and ulcers on the foot may be signs of chronic arterial insufficiency. Edema may be a sign of congestive heart failure or serum protein insufficiency of liver disease or malnutrition. The limbs and neck should be examined for adequacy of IV or arterial vascular access and evidence of IV drug abuse.

The remainder of the examination should focus on the detection of physical signs of co-morbid diseases or factors that may affect postoperative recovery such as ambulatory difficulties; visual, hearing, or coordination impairment; diminished pulmonary reserve; and easy fatigability due to congestive heart failure or chronic obstructive pulmonary disease.

Laboratory and Radiological Evaluations

The approach to the preoperative laboratory examination has undergone revision over the past 10 years and is reduced to a minimum for most patients. The underlying methodology for ordering laboratory tests should be based on a thorough history and PE and not on a routine testing template. A significant amount of a patient's hospital bill is accumulated by laboratory and diagnostic testing. The PA can play an important role in cost containment.

Most hospitals require all patients to have a complete blood count (CBC) with differential and a chemistry panel, including electrolytes, glucose, blood urea nitrogen, and serum creatinine before surgery. Chest radiography is performed only when an abnormality is suspected on the basis of history or physical findings, or when preexisting cardiopulmonary disease is present. A history of tobacco use should be elicited in all patients. Electrocardiograms are recommended for patients older than 40 years if review of the cardiac system reveals any positive findings, or if the patient is known to have cardiac disease.

The history and physical findings should provide justification for other laboratory studies that may be indicated before surgery. Prothrombin time (PT) and partial thromboplastin (PTT) tests are ordered for patients who give a specific personal or family history of coagulopathies, or who are taking warfarin or heparin. A bleeding time may also be ordered for patients taking platelet aggregation inhibitors (e.g., aspirin, ibuprofen, dipyridamole [Persantine], other nonsteroidal anti-inflammatory drugs, or coagulation inhibitors). Patients with known risk factors for liver disease should undergo liver function testing, and a history of genitourinary disease or symptoms should prompt urinalysis or 24-hour urine collections for creatinine clearance. Patients taking medications such as digoxin, quinidine, theophylline, or antiepileptics may require evaluation of serum drug levels before surgery.

A history of significant pulmonary disease or suspected pulmonary dysfunction (e.g., in heavy smokers) requires pulmonary function testing and arterial blood gas sampling before surgery. Echocardiograms and exercise stress testing are usually indicated for patients with a history of untreated angina, previous myocardial infarction, or significant hypertension.

A rational approach to identifying those patients with infectious viral diseases, notably HIV and hepatitis, should involve asking questions about risk factors associated with acquiring these diseases, even though all patients should be treated with the use of universal precautions.

Guidelines for mandatory testing of such patients vary by state and are controlled by hospital policies. Check with the hospital's infection control committee to obtain this information.

A final note on preoperative evaluation: The examiner should use PA and physician medical and surgical consultations to further evaluate patients when he or she is unsure of the severity or importance of a particular disease process. Consultants can often suggest methods by which the patient's ability to tolerate surgery can be assisted with an emphasis on postoperative care in difficult cases.

Preoperative Evaluation of Elderly Patients

As the U.S. population of patients 65 years and older increases over the next 20 to 25 years, PAs should expect to be an integral part of their care. The elderly are at higher risk of morbidity and mortality in the perioperative or postoperative period because of their age-altered physiology. The American Society of Anesthesiologists categorizes individuals as high operative risks solely because of an age greater than 75 years, acknowledging the problems related to the care of the elderly surgical patient.

The overall effect of aging is a decrease in the physiological reserve of the elderly individual as a consequence of normal changes in various organ systems. Cardiovascular system changes are related to decreases in cardiac output and are a response to exogenous stressors. The heart undergoes ventricular hypertrophy, often with calcification of the mitral and aortic annuli. Vascular tree resilience decreases, and peripheral vascular resistance increases. The final result is a higher risk of developing additional problems such as fluid overload, septic shock, and renal failure, all of which can be iatrogenically induced.

The renal system undergoes a marked reduction in number of nephrons, and the glomerular filtration rate slows with age. Importantly, these changes are not often reflected in the serum creatinine level because of the dependence of this measurement on muscle mass. Because muscle mass is decreased in elderly patients, reliance on serum creatinine level as a predictor is inaccurate.

In the nervous system, there is a decrease in cerebral blood flow in coordination with variable age-related changes in problem-solving skills and short-term memory. Elderly patients may have significant declines in vision and hearing. In the postoperative period, these losses, coupled with sensory deprivation in the foreign environment of the hospital room, recovery area, or ICU, can cause confusion and agitation. Delirium is a more common finding in postoperative elderly patients, secondary to the altered pharmacodynamic and pharmacokinetic processing of anesthetic and analgesic agents. This alteration is primarily a result of the changes in volume, distribution, and reservoir for deposition of such drugs.

The pulmonary system undergoes significant changes secondary to age, with smaller thoracic cage volume and greater thoracic rigidity. Respiratory muscle strength and endurance both decline. Measurements of pulmonary function may show larger functional residual capacity and dead space, as well as a decrease in the forced expiratory volume and peak expiratory flow rate. These changes contribute to the elderly patient's sensitivity to the effects of general anesthetics and increase the risk of postoperative pneumonia and atelectasis.

The geriatric patient population may present with a broad spectrum of disease processes inherent to their advancing age. Myocardial infarctions, hypertension and hyperlipidemia, cancers, neurological disorders such as Parkinson's disease or dementia, diabetes mellitus, and rheumatic disorders occur more often among the elderly.

For patients with evidence of malnutrition, a nutritional analysis will be helpful in evaluating total protein, albumin, prealbumin, transferrin, calcium, phosphorus, magnesium, vitamin B_{12}, and folic acid levels. Pulmonary function testing with the addition of arterial blood gas values may be ordered for patients undergoing thoracic or upper abdominal procedures, to furnish baseline values in the event of postoperative pulmonary problems. Pulmonary artery catheterization and echocardiography may be indicated in patients with significant murmurs, congestive heart failure, or significant preexisting pulmonary disease.

The most common postoperative and perioperative complications for elderly patients are myocardial infarction, heart failure, fluid overload, pneumonia, and pulmonary embolus. Other complications include urinary tract infection (UTI), septic complications, renal failure, and metabolic problems. Common diseases, such as pneumonia and dehydration, do not manifest in the typical manner; the patient who has a UTI, pneumonia, or a myocardial infarction may become confused rather than present with the typical manifestations of these conditions.

Postoperative rehabilitation is important for all patients, but greater emphasis is required for the older patient. Patients who spend extended periods in bed are at increased risk for thrombophlebitis, pulmonary embolus, and atelectasis proceeding to pneumonia.

A final area of preoperative importance for the geriatric surgical patient regards provision of prophylaxis against common postoperative complications. These include encouraging smoking cessation, ordering preoperative and postoperative use of bronchodilators in patients with bronchospastic pulmonary disease, and providing preoperative and postoperative chest physiotherapy, including incentive spirometry, coughing, and deep breathing. Prophylaxis also involves preoperative treatment of pulmonary infection and infected sputum, as well as early postoperative ambulation.

Discharge Planning   Planning for home care and discharge should begin when the patient is first admitted to the hospital. It is critical that each elderly patient's current level of physical, mental, and emotional functioning be assessed, along with their ability to care for themselves after discharge. Interviews with the family, nursing home workers, and the patient will provide a baseline assessment of the patient's ability to manage activities of daily living (ADLs). Questions should be directed toward assessing the patient's level of independence and needs for assistance with feeding, bathing, and self-cleansing, as well as his or her ability to ambulate, sit, stand, and walk. It is very useful in this instance to enlist the aid of a medical social worker, a discharge planner, or a geriatric clinician to obtain an in-depth analysis of the patient's and family's ability to provide care and resume ADLs.

BLOOD AND BLOOD PRODUCTS

Few deaths per year occur among the 4 million transfusions received each year in the United States, but the recognition and identification of the acquired immunodeficiency syndrome (AIDS) and hepatitis C as blood-borne diseases have led to a national effort to rethink transfusion requirements for surgical patients. Historically, patients undergoing surgery were thought to require transfusion if their hemoglobin fell below 10 mg/dL. Currently, patients with healthy cardiovascular, neurological, and pulmonary systems are often closely evaluated for hemodynamic instability during and after surgery before the ordering of blood transfusions. Hemoglobin values of 7 to 8 mg/dL are now thought to be acceptable for a healthy group of select patients.

Often the PA must explain to the patient and family the potential need for blood and blood product transfusion during surgery. Reports of HIV, hepatitis C, and other blood-borne infections linked to blood transfusions have elevated public fears. Legally, every patient should be informed of the possible need for blood transfusion before surgery, when applicable. Many institutions ask all surgical patients to sign consent for transfusion. The fundamentals of informed consent for homologous transfusion (of community-acquired banked blood) include the following:

1. Explaining the risks, benefits, and alternatives.
2. Allowing an opportunity for the patient to ask questions.
3. Obtaining a signed consent.

The patient undergoing an operation in which blood transfusion may be needed should understand that the American Association of Blood Banks (AABB) has instituted regulations that exclude high-risk individuals from the donor pool for blood and blood products. Self-exclusion is promoted to potential donors, and lengthy questioning of all potential donors screens other high-risk individuals from donation. Assays for the HIV antibody and hepatitis C are used to screen for seropositive blood products; very few donors who are infected with these diseases, and who are not seropositive, are missed by these methods. Patients found to be seropositive for hepatitis and HIV are permanently excluded from donating blood or blood products in the future.

The viral agent most commonly transmitted by transfusion is cytomegalovirus (CMV). Harbored in leukocytes, CMV is not a significant problem for non-immunocompromised patients. However, blood specifically screened for CMV is required for immunocompromised patients (including bone marrow and solid organ transplant recipients), CMV-seronegative pregnant women who require blood, premature infants, and HIV-positive patients who are CMV-negative.

Less life-threatening complications related to homologous blood transfusion include febrile reactions and urticaria. Fever is the most common problem occurring in transfusion. It appears in approximately 5% of all transfusions and manifests as a transient elevation in basal body temperature of 1° C to 2° C, although serious cardiopulmonary compromise can occur on rare occasions. Antipyretics or antihistamines frequently are given prophylactically to blood recipient patients. Urticaria is easily managed with antihistamines and antipyretics.

More serious symptoms associated with transfusion are rare (<1%). They include pulmonary edema, renal failure, anaphylaxis, bacterial contamination, and death.

Alternatives to Blood Transfusion

The following techniques have gained increased utilization as alternatives to homologous banked blood. These can be considered when religious beliefs (e.g., some Jehovah's Witnesses) or fears regarding blood-borne contagious diseases lead patients to refuse banked blood transfusion.

Autologous Blood Donation The patient's own blood is preoperatively collected for storage and eventual transfusion. This gives the patient the comfort of knowing that his or her own blood will be used to replace the amount lost during surgery. Preoperatively, donation is scheduled as frequently as 1 unit of blood every 72 hours, provided that the hematocrit remains greater than or equal to 33%. Patients are routinely given iron supplementation to spur erythropoiesis; the number of units obtained depends on the patient's erythropoietin response and increase in blood cell production. This blood can be stored a maximum of 30 to 42 days. Planning and foresight are required to enroll the patient in an autologous deposit program.

Designated Blood Transfusion Patients often ask whether donors known to them can deposit blood for use in homologous blood transfusion. There have been blood supply shortages in the United States, and encouraging individuals to donate blood products benefits all patients. However, there is no evidence to date indicating that this type of blood transfusion is safer than the homologous blood from the general population. In addition, family members who are at high risk for HIV or hepatitis may be forced to reveal this status when they must decline to participate in designated donation. A patient who makes such a request should be made to understand that there are no guarantees for an exact match between donor and recipient, even if they have the same blood type. Educating the patient and family about the safety of the blood supply in general and informing them of other alternatives should be part of all presurgical counseling.

Autologous Blood Salvage (Autotransfusion) Intraoperative blood salvage from the sterile surgical field entails passing the recovered blood through a cell saver via washing and centrifugation. This procedure removes the active products of coagulation and the heparin anticoagulant used in the collection system. Of great benefit during orthopedic and cardiac operations, autologous cell salvage has reduced homologous blood transfusions significantly over the past several years for selected procedures. This concentrated collection is primarily composed of red blood cells with a hematocrit of approximately 55%. Total recovery of cells is approximately one half to two thirds of the initially collected volume, possibly eliminating the need for transfusion.

Transfusion Adjuncts

Several pharmacological agents provide alternatives for the patient who requires autologous blood transfusion. Recombinant erythropoietin is used in patients with renal failure to increase red blood cell (RBC) mass. Another agent is desmopressin, a synthetic analog of vasopressin (antidiuretic hormone). It has no important vasomotor effects and has been shown to increase levels of factor VIII and von Willebrand factor.

Hemodilution   Preoperative hemodilution consists of a one-for-one exchange of whole blood with a crystalloid or colloid IV solution after anesthesia induction but before skin incision. Patients can be hemodiluted to a hematocrit of 22% to 25%. As blood loss commences and the hematocrit drops below 20% to 22%, it is replaced with the collected blood.

Hemoglobin Substitutes (Artificial Blood)   Intensive research efforts continue to search for a safe but inexpensive solution containing synthetic hemoglobin molecules for use in humans. Several models exist for this technology, but their applicability outside research institutions has not been established.

Ordering and Administering Blood and Blood Products

Type and Crossmatch (T&C)   The patient's blood is matched for A, B, O, and Rh type against specific donor units. When a T&C is ordered, the number of units that may be required should be specified on the request form. These units will be held in reserve for approximately 24 hours. If it is anticipated that the blood will not be required during or after surgery, the T&C order should be canceled, freeing the blood for other patients.

Type and Hold (Type and Screen)   The patient's A, B, O, and Rh type are established and screened for antibodies. *No blood is available for this patient until further ordered by crossmatch!*

Blood Bank Products

Whole Blood   All blood elements are available in this blood. One unit equals approximately 450 mL. This form is not often used.

Packed Red Blood Cells (PRBCs)   Almost all plasma is removed. One unit equals approximately 250 to 300 mL. This is the most commonly used red blood cell replacement product.

Platelets   Platelets are supplied in packs equal to 1 unit of whole blood. They may be collected from a single donor but are usually pooled from many donors. One pack is approximately 50 mL. Platelets are usually given in multiples of 6 to 10 packs per patient.

Cryoprecipitate (Cryo)   This pack contains factors VIII and XIII, von Willebrand factor, and fibrinogen. Cryoprecipitate is used in patients with bleeding disorders, particularly secondary to von Willebrand's disease and fibrinogen deficiency.

Fresh Frozen Plasma (FFP)   FFP contains coagulation cascade factors II, IV, VII, IX, X, XI, XII, and XIV. It is used primarily for patients with an undiagnosed bleeding condition or when large quantities of packed RBCs (usually more than 10 units of blood) may be required. FFP comes in packs of approximately 150 to 250 mL per unit.

Washed RBCs   Almost all white blood cells (WBCs) are removed from blood products given to decrease the antigenicity of this fluid. Washed RBCs are used in patients who are to undergo renal or other transplantation, who are severely immunocompromised, and who have a history of previous transfusion reactions.

Leukocyte-Poor Blood Cells   Most of the WBCs are removed to make the compound less antigenic.

Leukocyte-poor blood cells are less pure than washed RBCs, and one unit equals 200 to 250 mL.

Transfusion Procedures   A large-bore needle of 18 gauge or larger must be used for blood transfusion. Any patient receiving blood is first identified with a wrist bracelet containing specific information about blood type and Rh compatibility. It is mandatory that the patient's identification information from the ID bracelet be verified by comparison with the identification information contained on the label on the matched donor blood unit. Typically, two individuals cross-check each other before blood is administered to the patient.

Blood products are transfused only with isotonic saline. Mixing of blood products with other IV solutions may cause cell agglutination or lysis. Blood is frequently given quickly through pressure IV bags that accelerate administration. Additionally, cold blood is infused through a blood warmer to prevent cooling of the patient's core temperature.

After transfusion, all of the empty blood packs are banded together and sent back to the laboratory. In the event of a febrile transfusion reaction, small quantities of the blood left in the bags are used to determine antigenic status and to investigate possible pathogenic contamination of the blood administered to the patient.

DOCUMENTATION

"If it was not written down, it has not been done."

Specific entries are placed into every patient's chart for tracking and documenting care. Absence of these entries may delay or even cause the cancellation of a surgical procedure.

Consent

This includes explaining the proposed procedure to the patient and family or legal guardian, including the benefits and risks, and available alternatives. This explanation must always include the possibility of bleeding complications, infections, allergic reactions to medications or anesthesia, the possibilities of blood clot, possible damage to adjacent organs, lung or heart problems, and even death.

Other risks specific to the proposed procedure should be disclosed. Consents for photography and observers in the OR may be appropriate as well. A witness who is not directly part of the surgical team (e.g., a staff nurse) should witness the explanation and sign the consent along with the patient and the PA. A skilled translator must be used to obtain consent from a patient whose native language is not English. A physician member of the team obtains most surgical consents.

Implied consent is used for patients with life- or limb-threatening emergencies who are incapable of understanding the implications of the proposed operation. Patients who are in shock or who are unconscious are often treated under this category. Attempts should always be made to locate a family member or guardian, and any efforts to do so should be documented.

The Preoperative Note

The preoperative note is documented on the patient's chart in paragraph or list form before surgery to reiterate and substantiate important issues about the patient's preparation for surgery. It contains a statement regarding the patient's need for surgery, a basic review of the patient's preoperative condition, and the type of procedure proposed. Results of a brief PE are also included. This note reviews only the pertinent laboratory values and important radiographic findings. The consent status is documented, noting whether the patient, family, or other decision maker (e.g., legal guardian) has signed the consent, or if implied consent is in effect. Risks and possible complications are listed for medical legal documentation, particularly if the patient is undergoing a difficult surgical procedure (e.g., possible loss of finger function for repair of a crushed hand injury, or risk of cerebrovascular accident after carotid endarterectomy).

The expected disposition of the patient (e.g., admission to ICU or rehabilitation unit after surgery) is included to notify and prepare other services for future patient arrivals (see Box).

The Postoperative Note

The operative note, handwritten into the chart directly after surgery, records the intraoperative findings and conduct of the patient's surgery. This note is

---

PREOPERATIVE NOTE

To be written the afternoon before the planned procedure; serves as checklist, and to document that someone actually checked labs, studies, and availability of blood products.
- Date
- Preoperative diagnosis
- Procedure planned
- Laboratory results
- CXR
- ECG
- Other preoperative diagnostic studies (angiography results,CT/MRI findings, etc.)
- Risks and possible complications
- Consent signed
- Expected patient disposition

---

particularly valuable to other practitioners who are following the patient postoperatively, especially in light of the fact that the typed operative note, which is a complete description of all events that occurred during the course of surgery and is dictated by the surgeon after surgery, may not be transcribed and available on the chart for 2 or 3 days postoperatively.

The postoperative note contains the following information in list form:

➤ Preoperative diagnosis(es).

➤ Postoperative diagnosis(es). May well be different from the preoperative diagnosis (e.g., suspected malignant mass found benign by intraoperative pathology analysis).

➤ Name of the procedure. If multiple procedures were performed, they are named either sequentially or in decreasing order of "severity."

➤ Surgeon's name. Occasionally, a co-surgeon is also listed.

➤ Name(s) of assistant(s). All those assisting in surgery, including students, are listed here.

➤ Anesthesiologist's and/or anesthetist's name.

➤ Type of anesthesia administered (e.g., regional, general, spinal, local).

➤ Important intraoperative findings. Describes what was anatomically and clinically discovered during the procedure; may include the results of frozen section specimens sent to the pathologist, intraoperative radiological examinations, foreign objects found, and organs affected.

➤ Estimated amount of blood loss (EBL). This is an estimation of the amount of blood measured in the suction reservoirs combined with an approximation of the amount of blood soaked into the sponges used and an estimation of the loss of blood intraoperatively onto the drapes. Blood loss is usually established by consensus between the anesthesiologist and the surgeon.

➤ Urine output during the operation. Usually measured by an indwelling urinary catheter.

➤ Intraoperative IV fluids. Types and amounts of fluids given to the patient during surgery. IV fluid replacement often necessitates the use of multiple agents, including crystalloid and colloid solutions, blood and blood products, and, in some cases, medications that require large amounts of IV fluids as a vehicle for delivery (e.g., mannitol, sodium bicarbonate).

➤ Specimens sent to pathology. Can be a useful paper trail if specimens are misplaced.

➤ Drains. Each drain is listed by type(s), location(s), and type of collection reservoir.

➤ Tubes and lines. Lists all tubes and IV lines, including those inserted preoperatively and during the course of the procedure. Chest tubes, arterial lines, bladder catheters, nasogastric (NG) tubes, or pulmonary artery lines may be inserted. The author must be sure to include the size and location of each one (e.g., "18-gauge right radial arterial line").

➤ Implants. Lists any artificial materials implanted into the patient, such as joints, penile or breast prostheses, mesh materials, heart valves, and dialysis conduits. Includes the manufacturer's name, type of prosthesis, and registration number for each. Any registration stickers or cards should be stamped with the patient's identification information and mailed to the registration agency of the manufacturer, after copies have been placed in the chart.

➤ Complications. Accurately describes what occurred, with specifics as to what was done to correct the problem, as well as the status of the patient on delivery to the recovery room.

➤ Disposition of patient. Should note how and for what destination the patient left the operating suite (e.g., to the PARU, extubated and in satisfactory condition, or to the ICU intubated and in poor condition).

➤ *(See Box for a summary of the contents of the postoperative note.)*

POSTOPERATIVE NOTE

- Preop Dx
- Postop Dx
- Procedure(s)
- Surgeon(s)
- Assistant(s)
- Anesthesiologist/CRNA/AA
- Intraoperative findings
- Type of anesthesia
- EBL (estimated blood loss)
- Urine output
- IV fluids
- Specimens
- Drains
- Tubes and lines
- Implants
- Complications
- Disposition

PREPARATION FOR SURGERY

A significant portion of the surgical PA's responsibility outside the OR involves preparing the patient, the patient's family, and the hospital staff for surgery. This includes identifying the patient's diagnosis and need for surgery but also requires establishing the patient's ability to tolerate the proposed surgical procedure, while fully educating the patient and family and orchestrating the many details required to safely lead the patient through the upcoming ordeal. The PA may act as the team coordinator before surgery, a role that is invaluable to most surgeons.

Patient and Family Education

The patient should be well versed about what is about to take place. The patient and family should understand the need for surgery, the routines required for preoperative evaluation and preparation, and the usual preoperative and postoperative courses of events. This education also includes a complete explanation of the risks and benefits of the proposed procedure. All consents should be signed and witnessed, including consents for the specific type of procedure(s) and for the administration of blood and blood products. The patient's apprehension should be expected because of anticipated future pain, possible loss of function, the question of ability to continue working, and the general environment of the hospital. The PA has the ability and the time to sit down with the patient and family to explain upcoming events from the admission process through the postoperative course and must allow time for the patient and his or her family to vocalize their concerns and fears. Patients who have received education regarding the expected level of pain and the activities they will be required to perform after surgery have been shown to require fewer analgesics, cooperate more willingly after surgery, and have less protracted recoveries. By providing preoperative instruction on the value of deep breathing and early ambulation after the procedure, along with an explanation of the probable tubes and lines remaining after surgery, of where the patient may be for a short period (i.e., ICU), and of the known efficacy of prescribed analgesics, the PA can ensure better patient compliance and cooperation during postoperative convalescence.

Many patients have concerns and fears because of previous difficulties with surgery and anesthesia. Older anesthesia practices may have caused prolonged nausea and vomiting or severe headaches from spinal anesthesia. In addition, patients recall "horror stories" from family and friends about their surgical experiences, which are usually embellished by time. Each patient should be prompted to voice these concerns so they may be discussed and alleviated as much as possible before surgery.

Excluding the family from the education process eliminates an informed source of support for the patient in times of crisis and may propagate unwarranted tension between the staff and family. An explanation of the facilities and services available for the family's support should include access to the medical social worker and chaplain, sleeping accommodations, meals, and visiting hours. Hospitals often have staff members responsible for such education, but supplying it during the early phases of care encourages trust and exhibits compassion.

The PA should be readily available when the family needs information and can serve as a liaison between the family, hospital staff, and surgeon. This role includes interpreting medical jargon, explaining the ramifications of laboratory or radiological results, personally performing routine procedures if the family asks, and sending progress reports to the family from the OR during long procedures.

Preparing Hospital Staff

The OR staff should be informed about the type and anticipated length of the procedure and should be promptly notified of unanticipated changes or special requirements.

If the patient requires preoperative antibiotics for a procedure that has a high risk of infection (e.g., gastrointestinal, genitourinary, or gynecological procedure, infected wound, endocarditis prophylaxis), these should be administered 30 minutes before skin incision to ensure adequate tissue drug levels. The PA should review all laboratory, radiological, electrocardiographic, and other preoperative test results before the operation and should immediately investigate and report any abnormalities. If a frozen section examination of tissue is required, the pathology department should be informed of the approximate time the specimen will be available to ensure the presence of a pathologist to process the specimen. The PA should also inform radiology if any intraoperative radiographs are anticipated (e.g., arteriograms, cholangiograms, bone fixation, post–joint replacement films).

Other preparations include ascertaining the availability of special items specifically required for the planned procedure. When a special tissue or device is needed, the matter should be brought to the attention of the OR staff as soon as possible before surgery to facilitate the ordering and arrival of these materials.

Pertinent radiographs, computed tomography (CT) scans, and magnetic resonance imaging (MRI) scans should always be available in the room for intraoperative reference and surgical planning.

Before the procedure begins, the PA should work with the team to make certain the patient is correctly and safely positioned on the OR table, with all bony prominences cushioned, and that the security straps are in place. Invasive monitoring lines and tubes should be inserted after the patient has been sedated or anesthetized, if prudent, to avoid undue patient discomfort and anxiety.

A Note on Deep Vein Thrombosis and Pulmonary Embolism

The severe morbidity and mortality of postoperative deep vein thrombosis (DVT) and pulmonary embolism require routine prophylaxis for all high-risk surgical patients. DVT and pulmonary embolism may occur because of the venous stasis created by various patient positions on the OR table (e.g., lithotomy with pressure on the calves) or by low-flow states occurring during hypotension. Risk factors for these postoperative complications include age over 40 years, obesity, history of malignancy, previous history of DVT or pulmonary embolism, and long or complicated surgical procedures.

Two methods may be used, in addition to early postoperative ambulation, to prevent DVT and pulmonary embolism. Either low-dose heparin or a heparin analog may be used as pharmacological prevention. Externally applied pneumatic compression and pressure gradient elastic stockings are effective mechanical means of preventing DVT (Figure 33-1). These can be applied at the time of surgery and can remain in place until the patient is ambulatory.

ASEPSIS AND INFECTION CONTROL IN THE OPERATING ROOM

By advocating a controlled OR environment with sterile OR attire and precision housekeeping methods, surgeons can safely perform deeply invasive procedures and care for traumatic and dirty wounds with confidence to avoid surgical infection. Methods of controlling iatrogenic contamination, in conjunction with the development of heat and chemical

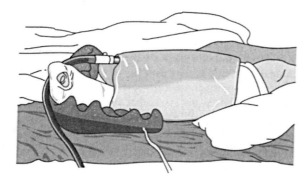

Figure 33-1 External pneumatic gradient antiembolism-stocking.

sterilization processes to effectively kill microorganisms, ensure that modern surgery is now practiced in an environment that is maintained in as clean and sterile a state as possible.

The concept of aseptic technique is simple. Sources of contamination should be isolated from the area where surgery is being performed. All procedures should be done in a field devoid of living microorganisms, including patient skin flora, to decrease the morbidity and mortality associated with wound infections. Asepsis also involves recognizing and alleviating conditions advantageous to the growth of bacteria (e.g., removal of dead tissue, serum, and blood from the wound or incision) and avoiding gaps or "dead space" between wound tissues, which might result in hematoma formation. It also comprises the use of preoperative antibiotics.

Operating Suite Geography

To protect the actual OR from contamination by outside microorganisms, the surgery department is divided into several geographic zones to promote isolation. Entry into the *periphery* of the operating suite, where patients are delivered and received in preparation for surgery, is unrestricted. Family members may be allowed in this area with staff permission, and hospital personnel are not required to wear specific clothing here. The *intermediate zone,* clearly marked by signs and closed doors, is restricted to persons appropriately dressed in hospital scrub clothes; street clothes are forbidden in this area. Finally, the *sterile*

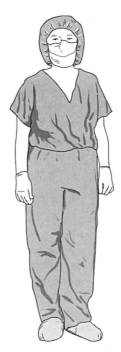

Figure 33-2 *Typical surgical garment.* Note cap, mask, and shoe covers. The shirt is tucked into the pants, and no jewelry is worn.

OR itself, including the scrub rooms and the areas immediately adjacent to the actual operating suite, is limited to those personnel prepared to work in an aseptic or sterile environment. Personnel in the OR suites must have clean scrubs, shoe covers, a hat or a cap, and a facial mask (Figure 33-2).

Dress and Hygiene

To promote good aseptic technique, OR staff must adhere to strict personnel hygiene regimens to reduce iatrogenic contamination of the OR. Major areas of microbial burden are the head, neck, axilla, hands, groin, perineum, legs, and feet. Hair is an excellent place for bacteria to reside, and hair proteins can cause significant foreign body reactions during the healing process. Personnel must cover all head hair with a hat or a hair bonnet. Those with beards should wear a hood that covers the sides of the face and chin.

Anyone entering the intermediate zone of the suite must wear appropriately laundered scrub attire as provided by the hospital. Scrubs laundered at home should not be worn in surgery. Shoes worn in the OR are not worn outside the OR unless they are covered by "clean" shoe covers to remove the risk of trailing blood and body fluids through the hospital. Any scrub attire worn outside the OR suite should be covered with a long, buttoned laboratory coat.

Universal Precautions and Surgery

Proper OR attire also gives personnel protection from inadvertent exposure to infectious agents. Although asepsis protects the patient from iatrogenic infection, sterile clothing also insulates the health care provider from diseases transmitted by the patient. Both the Centers for Disease Control (CDC) and the Occupational Safety and Health Administration (OSHA) have established standards for the prevention of transmission of infectious diseases, including HIV, in health care settings. Universal precautions mandate that all human body fluids, blood, and tissues be considered potentially contaminated and containing viral pathogens. PA students are required to receive hepatitis B immunization several months before exposure to direct patient care.

Surgical Garments

Surgical garments are considered barriers against patient-borne diseases as well as iatrogenic transmission of infection to patients.

Masks and Goggles   Respiratory droplet infection from the oral and nasal pharynx has been identified as a major source of contamination. Therefore, an impermeable mask must be worn in the OR to cover the nose and mouth. The least effective mask is the molded, preshaped mask with an elastic string, because of its poor conformance to most facial contours. Its preformed dimensions allow escape of excess droplets from the mask's sides.

To be efficacious, a surgical mask must be worn over both nose and mouth, so that air passes only through the filtering system. It should be firmly molded around the nose, with the upper strings tied at the back of the head and the lower strings tied behind the neck. Crossing the strings across the back of the head distorts the compliance of the mask along the cheek, resulting in leakage of expired air. This is problematic for health care providers who wear glasses, because when the expired warm air mixes with cold OR air, lenses are fogged. Some masks contain adhesive strips across the nose to prevent this problem. A strip of surgical tape may also be used to seal the top of the mask. Additionally, it may be necessary to apply a defogger to glasses before entering the OR to prevent this nuisance.

Masks also protect the wearer from patient-borne pathogens. Gerberding and colleagues[3] found that a high percentage of OR personnel were exposed to blood through facial mucocutaneous splashes and identified several variables associated with increased risk of blood exposure—loss of more than 300 mL of blood, procedure lasting longer than 3 hours, emergency procedures, major surgical procedures, procedures required for trauma or fracture, laparotomies, intra-abdominal gynecological procedures, vascular procedures, otolaryngological procedures, and cutaneous abscess drainage.

All personnel at the operating table, including anesthesia staff, must wear goggles, glasses with specifically designed splash guards attached to the sides, or masks with splash guards attached to decrease the transmission of communicable diseases. These precautions prevent contamination from splashes on odd trajectories from the operative field. Glasses alone are not adequate to prevent splashes from the side or between the glasses and the cheek.

Some masks are designed to filter microorganisms transmissible to the wearer. These are effective for procedures during which voluminous smoke plumes containing viral agents (as small as 0.3 μm) are generated, such as laser ablation of lesions containing human papillomavirus from genital or rectal lesions. High-filtration masks should be used for these procedures.

Masks should be changed between cases and whenever saturated by moisture from respiration.

Gloves   Sterile gloves are designed to provide maximum sensitivity for the user while providing a sterile barrier to disease transmission. A discussion of the appropriate choice of glove size and type is not within the scope of this chapter. Glove allergies, caused by the talc used to lubricate the hand for entry into the glove or by the latex materials used in manufacturing, can cause severe dermatitis in a small number of wearers. For such persons, some gloves are designed to be hypoallergenic. In severe cases, a dermatologist may prescribe a topical steroid cream until the irritation subsides.

Double Gloving   Wright and associates[4] showed that 27% of the glove tears from sharp instrumentation occurred on hands that were retracting tissues during surgery. Of that group, 67% were caused by needles, 10% by scalpels, and 23% by other instruments, such as cautery tips, wire, skin staples, bone cutters, and bone chisels. An additional 15% of glove tears occurred on hands holding instruments, and a small subset occurred during hand-typing of sutures ("suture cuts"). Other mechanisms of glove tears occurred during the passing of sharp instruments between individuals at the table and contact with sharps (e.g., needles, scalpels) laid on the table during activities such as suture-tying. Bleeding occurred in more than 80% of sharps injuries in this study. A majority of glove tears occurred on the fingertips. Quebbeman and co-workers[5] demonstrated the inadequacy of single-gloving practices among surgical personnel, documenting a glove failure rate of approximately 51%, glove failure being defined as tears in the glove after surgery, or when there is blood on the hand after glove removal without known trauma or penetration of the gloved hand by a sharp instrument.

Both studies advocated the use of double gloves by OR personnel to reduce risks of blood-borne contamination. Additionally, these reports demonstrate a significant decrease in finger contamination rate, from 51% to 7%, for those who wore double gloves. Of 130 participants in the Quebbeman study,[5] 7% found that two gloves were too tight and caused numbness and 1% found them too baggy. Almost 88% were in favor of wearing two gloves, however. Finally, 82% of the participants indicated that they would wear double gloves routinely, and an additional 2% said that they would wear double gloves when operating on high-risk patients. Eighty-eight percent of these participants remarked that tactile sensation and comfort were satisfactory with double gloves.

Gowns and Shoe Covers   The surgical gown is a principal barrier against disease transmission. High-risk procedures, as previously noted, should probably mandate the addition of a sterile sleeve over the gown's arms to prevent strike-through (i.e., penetration of moisture through protection, resulting in possible microbial transmission).

The shoe cover is an overlooked place of potential disease transmission. Most personnel in surgery wear lightweight shoes with cloth or synthetic material shoe covers. Particularly during urological and arthroscopic irrigation procedures or trauma resuscitation, large quantities of fluid may accumulate on the floor, saturating the wearer's shoes. All OR personnel should be aware of this mechanism of blood exposure and should don lightweight, knee-high disposable boots in situations with potential for exposure to this problem. These procedures may also require that personnel wear a plastic "cook's apron," which slips over the head and ties behind the back, protecting the front of the wearer from seepage through the front of the gown.

The following precautions should be taken by persons performing surgical procedures:
1. Goggles, glasses with side guards, face masks, knee-high shoe covers, waterproof aprons, and additional sleeves should be worn, depending on the type of surgery expected.
2. Double gloving reduces blood-borne contamination.
3. Extreme care should be exercised when sharps are present on the table. Instruments should be passed via an intermediary table or tray, if possible. *The assistant's immobile, retracting hand should be safeguarded while sharps are in use.*
4. During suturing, the needle should not be kept in the hand while knots are being tied. Optimally, the needle should be cut from the suture as soon as the suture is in place. If this is not possible, the point of the needle should be clamped within the needle holder and placed on the sterile field away from the hands. The needle should always be grasped with forceps immediately after it pierces the tissue and should be transferred back to the needle holder without direct touching of the needle with the gloved hand.

5. All scalpel blades should be placed onto and removed from the knife handle by a hemostat. Hypodermic needles should not be recapped.

6. Some glove tears and finger cuts result from hand-tying of sutures. The distal or proximal interphalangeal crease should not be used as a fulcrum for tying knots. The pads of the fingers should be used to tighten knots to prevent "suture cuts."

7. Gloves should always be worn when there is a risk of contacting a patient's body fluids. Even the seemingly innocuous tasks of phlebotomy, cleansing of the patient after surgery, dressing changes, and insertion of NG tubes can result in inadvertent pathogenic exposure of the health care provider.

8. All accidental mucocutaneous inoculation, needlesticks, cuts, and so forth, should be reported to the surgical team and OR staff to ensure proper serological evaluation of the patient in the postoperative period.

9. Operative personnel with open lesions, weeping dermatitis, and so forth, should refrain from close contact with patients. This precaution can be a problem for operative personnel who experience "washing trauma" from frequent hand washings, which may cause cuts, abrasions, and minor lesions. Keeping the skin of the hands well moistened helps prevent such trauma.

SKIN PREPARATION

Remember: Handwashing between patient PEs eliminates the leading cause of nosocomial infection.

Appropriate attire, preparation of the hands at the scrub sink, shaving and preparing the patient's skin for incision, erecting barriers against microbial contamination, meticulous tissue handling, and an expeditious work ethic during surgery contribute to maintaining low patient morbidity and mortality. Complete elimination of all skin flora and of all microorganisms from the operative field is preferable, although an altogether aseptic operative field is not possible. However, appropriate skin preparation can reduce the numbers of microorganisms to an absolute minimum.

Resident flora is removed from the skin on and around the operative site with a combination of mechanical scrubbing with an antibacterial soap and application of an antibacterial solution after the scrub. Although some operative areas, such as the eye, ear, nose, throat, mouth, and perineal and perianal regions, cannot be adequately sterilized, aseptic techniques are used to prevent further contamination of the surrounding field.

The operative area is shaved to remove only the hair that may interfere with the incision and surrounding region. Wet shaving with a safety razor is preferred to dry shaving, which can cause razor drag, leaving abrasions, tiny lacerations, and greater postoperative discomfort.

Agents Commonly Used for Operative Site Skin Preparation and Surgical Hand Washing

Povidone-iodine or iodophor products are supplied in two distinct liquid versions. For the operative site preparation, a detergent *scrub* is first applied with sponges to mechanically remove gross dirt and oils from the skin. After the skin has been blotted with a sterile towel, a nondetergent *solution* is "painted" onto the area. This thin film of povidone-iodine continues to have bactericidal action for up to 8 hours after application. The solution's brown color also effectively outlines the borders of the surgical scrub, allowing accurate placement of the towels and drapes before incision. Patients and OR staff who have a history of sensitivity or allergic reaction to iodine should refrain from the use of either of these preparations for surgical scrubs.

Chlorhexidine gluconate, when used in a 4% concentration, is bactericidal and has persistent antimicrobial activity after application. Repeated scrubbing throughout the day enhances its activity. Because this agent is nonirritating for a majority of the patient population, it is commonly used for hand washing and preparation of the operative site. Chlorhexidine gluconate scrub soap adequately prepares the skin, and no solution is required after the scrub.

Parachlorometaxylenol (PCMX) is a useful skin preparation agent, particularly for those allergic to iodine-containing preparations. This agent is often combined with an emollient to reduce skin drying.

Hexachlorophene, although used infrequently, is an effective skin preparation solution for those patients and staff allergic to povidone-iodine and chlorhexidine gluconate. It accumulates on the skin after several days of use, causing an overall decrease in skin flora.

CLINICAL PROCEDURE

During skin preparation of the operative site, personnel must make sure that the solution does not pool beneath the patient. Such a pool might serve as an electrical ground to the table during the use of electrocautery or, if unnoticed during postoperative skin cleansing, may lead to chemical skin burns. In addition, the PA should always check the safety profile for use of these agents in sensitive areas such as the eye, ear, vagina, and rectum.

THE SURGICAL HAND SCRUB

Agents commonly used for hand scrubbing often come in sterile prepackaged brush and sponge units. Alternatively, brushes are packaged separately, and the scrub soap is kept at the scrub sink in containers with foot-operated dispensing controls.

CLINICAL PROCEDURE

Povidone-iodine solutions tend to be drying, and multiple scrubs throughout the day can produce drying and cracking of the cuticles and hands. Personnel who frequently scrub for surgery should take care to apply emollients and non–oil-based lotions to their hands several times during the day, if possible, to prevent the occurrence of these potential conduits for bacteria. Chlorhexidine gluconate, PCMX, and hexachlorophene are often combined with emollient lathering agents and may be less drying than the povidone-iodine solutions for those who scrub frequently.

General Preparations

The PA should inform the scrub nurse before scrubbing, so a gown and appropriate gloves will be ready. The skin should be kept clean and in good condition. *Anyone with open wounds or weeping dermatitis evident on the hands or arms should not scrub for surgery.* Fingernails should not reach beyond the fingertips, to reduce trauma to the patient and inadvertent glove punctures. All hand and wrist jewelry should be removed. A cap and mask should be in place, glasses or goggles should be adjusted, and all neck jewelry should be covered or removed before scrubbing. Shoe covers should be worn at all times within the OR, and the ties from surgical scrubs and shoelaces should be tucked inside the waistband or shoe cover.

The 5-Minute Scrub

1. A scrub brush impregnated with the choice of antiseptic agent is chosen. The package is opened and saturated with solution from the foot-controlled dispenser.
2. The water temperature is adjusted to a comfortable level.
3. The hands are passed beneath the running water with one or two motions, allowing the water to flow from fingertips to elbow and wetting to 3 inches above the elbow. The hands are kept above the waist.
4. The soap solution is used to wash the hands and arms and to remove the gross dirt and dead skin.
5. The hands and brush are rinsed.
6. The brush is again saturated with soap.
7. Under running water, the fingernails of one hand are cleaned with a sterile pick to remove subungual debris (the brush is kept in the hand holding the nail pick) and rinsed.
8. The process is repeated for the other hand.
9. The time should be noted. The fingers are scrubbed with a circular motion for 1½ minutes, including the nails, knuckles, and web spaces. The fingers and hand are regarded as having four sides for the purpose of the scrub.
10. Circular scrubbing is continued for 1 minute on the arm, roughly dividing it into thirds and scrubbing to 3 inches above the elbow (Figure 33-3).
11. The brush is transferred to the scrubbed hand, and the process is repeated on the unscrubbed arm and hand.
12. When 5 minutes have elapsed, the brush is discarded, and the hands and arms are rinsed of lather by passing them through the water

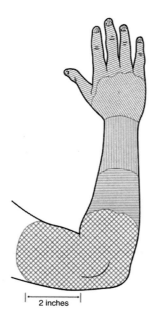

Figure 33-3 Divide your hands and arms into sections for the surgical scrub.

stream, allowing the water to cascade from fingertips to elbow—never in the reverse direction. One or two passes should be sufficient to remove the lather.

13. The water is turned off with the knee.
14. The arms are held above the waist so that any residual water drips from the fingers to the elbows.

All subsequent scrubs of the day should last 5 minutes.

GOWNING AND GLOVING
Drying Hands and Arms

Hands and arms must be dried thoroughly before gowning and gloving. The towel is passed from the sterile table by the scrub nurse, or it is taken from the sterile instrument table, with care taken not to drip any water onto the table. The towel is opened to its fullest length and is kept well away from the scrub clothes. Only one end of the towel is used to dry the first hand and arm. A blotting and twisting motion is used as the fingers and arms are rotated. Each finger is dried individually; then the process is completed, working from wrist to elbow. Once the first arm has

been dried, *the opposite end of the same side of the towel is used to dry the other hand and arm in a similar manner.* The towel is then discarded by being given to a waiting circulating nurse or dropped into a soiled cloth receptacle.

Donning Gown and Gloves

Donning the sterile gown depends on the method used to place gloves on the hands. When the gloves are donned without assistance (closed-glove technique), the hands and fingers are kept within the gown sleeve. Partial finger extrusion is needed when someone else (i.e., the scrub nurse) applies the gloves (Figure 33-4).

For the *closed-glove method,* the gown is carefully removed from the sterile field (without dripping water

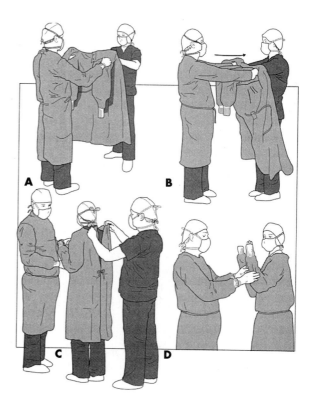

Figure 33-4 *Being gowned.* Place your outstretched arms into the armholes (**A**). The circulator will pull the gown onto your shoulders (**B**) and fasten the ties (**C**). The scrub nurse will adjust the sleeves before gloving (**D**).

onto the field) and is gently shaken, well above the floor, to loosen the folds and fully extend the gown. The hands are placed into the armholes, and the circulating nurse, who is unsterile, pulls the gown onto the wearer's shoulders and fastens the gown from behind. The hands are not placed through the wrist cuffs but remain within the sleeve of the gown itself. The gown's cuffs may be used like mittens to manipulate the fingers and hands into the first glove, without touching the glove with the bare hand (Figure 33-5).

The *open-glove method* requires assistance from a sterile team member. The gown may be donned as previously described or may be placed by the scrub nurse. The arms are extended at a 90-degree angle in front of the body, and the gown is placed over the

shoulders by the scrub nurse. The fingers are partially extruded through the wrist cuffs so the cuff end rests just below the thumb.

The right glove is placed first. The fingers are slightly abducted, and the hand is gently inserted into the glove as the scrub nurse circumferentially expands the wrist cuff. The scrub nurse then expands the left glove's wrist cuff. With the right hand, the wearer gently pulls the edge of the cuff toward the body and places the left hand into the glove (Figure 33-6).

Even appropriately sized gloves can cause distal hand paresthesias if the gown's cuff is bunched over the median nerve at the volar wrist. The mid-arm section of the gown is held stationary with the opposite hand during the open-glove method, and the cuff is adjusted after the closed-glove method.

Occasionally, a glove becomes contaminated or sustains a puncture or tear during surgery and must be changed. If this occurs, step back from the sterile field and extend the wrist of the contaminated hand

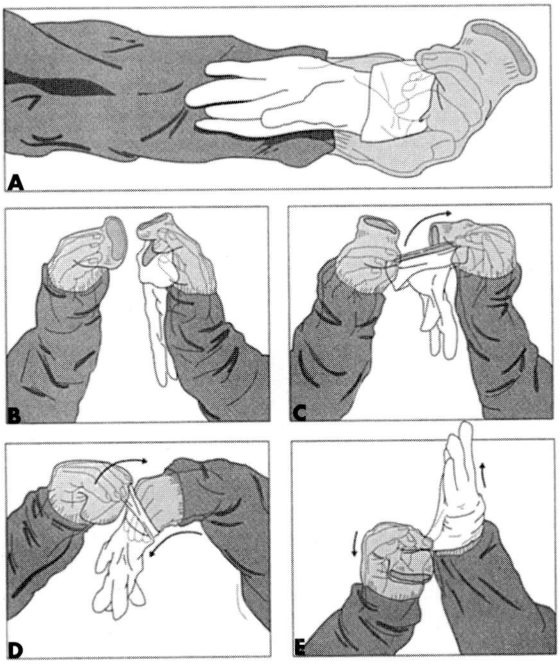

Figure 33-5 *Gloving yourself.* **A,** Keep the fingers within the gown's cuff, and use the cuff as a mitten to manipulate the fingers into the glove. **B,** Place the glove's thumb-side down onto your hand and wrist, with the fingers pointing toward your elbow. **C** and **D,** After grasping the edge of the cuff between your thumb and index finger, flip the glove over while using your other hand to pull the glove onto your hand. **E,** Adjust the gown cuff for comfort. Repeat for the other hand.

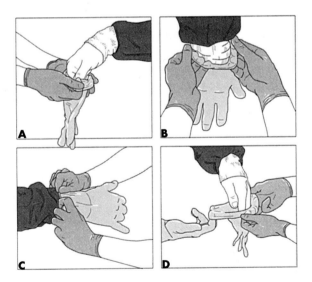

Figure 33-6 *Being gloved by another.* Insert your right hand into the opened glove held by the scrub nurse (**A** and **B**), pushing deeply into the glove to seat your fingertips (**C**). Grasp the left cuff's edge with your right hand and insert fingers (**D**). Adjust cuffs for comfort.

up to the circulating nurse, who will pull the glove from the contaminated hand. The scrub nurse assists with a new glove placement by the open-glove method. Care must be taken to keep the exposed hand away from any portion of the sterile field.

All surgical gowns have a wraparound tie at the waist that prevents the back of the gown from becoming unfastened. On disposable gowns, the paper "handle" is carefully handed to the circulating nurse while the person donning the gown turns in a circle or pirouette. The tie is gently pulled from the paper handle, with no touching of the contaminated handle, and is secured to the front tie of the gown. For nondisposable gowns, the wraparound tie must be given to a sterile person. Alternatively, the tie may be wrapped in an empty sterile glove wrapper, which is handed to a nonsterile person as the turn is made. If the tie is dropped, an unsterile team member may fasten the back of the gown with a hemostat or other instrument. The wearer must remember not to discard the instrument into the trash or soiled cloth receptacle at the end of the procedure.

Removing Gown and Gloves

The gown is always removed before the gloves by pulling it forward across the shoulders and down onto the arms after the rear ties have been released. The gloved hands are then removed from the gown cuffs. The gown is rolled into a ball, with all contaminated surfaces kept in the interior of the ball, and is discarded into the appropriate receptacle. The gloves are removed by grasping the outside of one glove near the wrist with the other hand and turning the glove inside out as it is removed. This glove is held in the palm of the remaining gloved hand. The ungloved hand then reaches inside the cuff of the remaining glove and pulls it from the hand, inside out, encompassing the glove previously removed. The gloves are discarded into the appropriate receptacle. This method internalizes all fluid-contaminated portions of the gown and gloves and prevents accidental contamination of the skin (Figure 33-7).

MAINTAINING A STERILE FIELD

The area immediately surrounding the operative site, the sterile instrument tables, and any open sterile

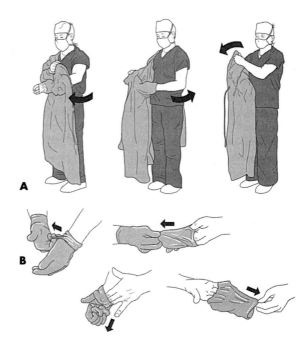

Figure 33-7 *Removing gown and gloves.* **A,** With gloves on, and after the front and back ties are loosened, pull the gown from your shoulders, rolling the soiled exterior into a ball. **B,** Grasp the outside of the first glove's cuff and pull from your hand. Hold the removed glove in the remaining glove. Grasp the inside of the remaining glove, removing it inside out while enveloping the previously removed glove.

instrument packs is designated as the "sterile field" (Figure 33-8). There are no intermediates between sterile areas in the operating suite and the unsterile areas.

All personnel in the operating suite are responsible for the maintenance of the sterile environment. The cardinal rule is to replace any item *suspected* of contamination, even if contamination was not directly observed.

In most institutions, students are encouraged to approach the sterile field to observe the conduct of surgery. The student should do the following:

1. Use a short step platform to see over the operating staff's shoulders.
2. Ask anesthesia personnel for a position near the head of the table to observe over the drapes.

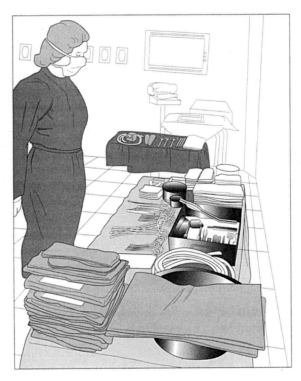

Figure 33-8 *A typical sterile field.* See text for explanation.

CLINICAL PROCEDURE

Although it seems redundant to say that only sterile items are used within sterile fields, this axiom is of paramount importance. Use the following "rules" for maintaining the sterile field in the OR:

➤ Only the front of the gown is considered sterile in the areas from the axilla to the waist and from the fingertips to approximately 3 inches above the sleeves.

➤ Hands should be kept in front, in sight, and above waist level at all times. They should never touch the face or be folded beneath the axilla.

➤ If some portion of the arm or elbow becomes contaminated, a sterile "sleeve" can be placed by the scrub nurse or CST to cover that area and eliminate the need for a complete gown change.

Nonsterile persons reaching across a sterile field contaminate the entire area. A wide margin of safety should be maintained by those working around a sterile area. Nonsterile persons should always pass behind those who are scrubbed and in sterile attire for surgery.

All those involved in draping the patient should stand an arm's length from the OR table to prevent gown contamination. Sterile persons should pass each other back to back so their unsterile areas are facing each other. A sterile person should face a sterile area to pass it. In addition, sterile persons should stay within the sterile field and should not walk around the OR suite or go outside the room unless absolutely necessary. Those considered sterile should keep contact with the sterile area to a minimum by not leaning on the instrument tables or the draped patient. Sitting or leaning on a nonsterile surface is considered a break in technique unless the operating team must be seated to perform a specific procedure.

Tables are sterile only at tabletop level; any part of the sterile drape that falls over the edge is considered contaminated. The table height should be appropriately adjusted to maintain a maximally sterile field. Any items that drop below waist level are considered contaminated and should be discarded from the field.

Disease transmission may occur as a result of strike-through, or penetration of moisture in whatever form, through the protection of gown or drapes. This can occur when sterile packages are laid onto wet areas or when the drying cycle of heat sterilizers does not completely dry the enveloping package wrapping. It may also result when blood or other fluids penetrate the gown of the assistant or surgeon. Choosing gowns with waterproof front panels, wearing oversleeves, and using waterproof coverings on instrument tables can prevent iatrogenic transmission of infectious agents via strike-through.

CLINICAL PROCEDURE

Drape placement usually requires monitoring by the circulating nurse and/or anesthesia staff, who ensure adherence to sterile technique. The following guidelines should be used:

➤ Drapes should be held high enough above the table to prevent contamination from the unsterile table and patient, but not high enough

➤ Walk around the table to complete the draping procedure when necessary, and never reach across the table.

➤ When a drape is placed near a nonsterile area or is handed to the anesthesia team to create the sterile barrier between them and the operating team, the drape should form a cuff over the gloved hand of the sterile person, who offers it to the unsterile area in that manner. This technique prevents drape contamination as the anesthesiologist or other nonsterile person pulls a portion of the drape into position.

➤ Sterile personnel should touch no part of the draping material that falls into a nonsterile area. If a portion of the draping material becomes contaminated and needs replacement, the circulating nurse will grab its edge and slowly pull it off the table. It then can be replaced with a new drape.

Handling Tubes and Lines

After the patient has been draped, the tubes, wires, and cords required for the procedure will be passed from the sterile field to a waiting nonsterile person. These may include electrocautery pencil wires, suction tubing of various sorts, cardiopulmonary bypass tubing, cell-saving equipment, laparoscopy cords, and ultrasound transducers. They are usually contained on the scrub nurse's back table until needed. The ends are handed to the circulating nurse or anesthesia staff.

CLINICAL PROCEDURE

The equipment tubes are tightly clipped to a fold of drape with a nonpenetrating towel clip or Allis clamp, to prevent the weight of the tubing from pulling them off the sterile field. A fold of the drape is gathered to encompass the tube and wire and is tightly clamped shut with the Allis clamp or towel clip.

PATIENT POSITIONING

Patients receiving anesthesia, whether general or regional, are at great risk for injury caused by improper physical movement or improper placement on the OR table. Abnormal pressure on nerves for extended periods may result in palsy or irreversible paralysis of muscle innervation or sensory

distribution of that nerve. Stretching the brachial plexus by abducting the arms more than 90 degrees during a breast or chest procedure can result in hand dysfunction, as can pressure on the ulnar nerve by the hard table surface (Figure 33-9). Pressure on the proximal calf and the peroneal nerve in the lithotomy position can cause footdrop or venous stasis in the calf deep veins, with subsequent deep vein thrombosis and pulmonary embolus.

The surgeon and/or assistant guides the positioning with the anesthesia team. Other members of the operative team assist the process. Proper patient positioning facilitates access to the operative site and provides maximum patient safety. The chosen position is decided by the patient's age, height, weight, cardiopulmonary status, and preexisting diseases, such as rheumatic disorders. For example, the extremely obese patient is positioned with a slightly elevated head and thorax to facilitate mechanical ventilation during surgery.

Most OR tables are manually or electrically controlled through hydraulic lifts and gears that allow a table to be manipulated into various positions, including lateral inclines and Trendelenburg or reverse Trendelenburg tilts. The head and feet can be independently controlled or removed from the main table, and a middle portion of the table (the "kidney rest") allows elevation of the central portion of the body. Parallel side rails allow the attachment of retractor

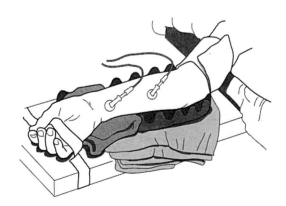

Figure 33-9 *Safety padding for the patient's wrist and elbow to prevent nerve or vessel injury.* Note the proper anatomical alignment of the wrist.

devices and arm supports. The PA should become familiar with all these functions and should be able to manipulate a table into all of its positions. Additionally, the PA should understand how to remove the various table segments as required to position the patient for surgery and should be competent in attaching devices such as retraction systems and arm boards to the table.

Common Patient Positions (Figure 33-10)

Supine   The patient is placed flat on the back with arms either outstretched at less than 90 degrees or placed at the sides. This position is used for access to any anterior body part, particularly the chest, abdomen, pelvis, and extremities.

Prone   The patient is placed face down. If general anesthesia with endotracheal intubation is planned, the patient is first placed in the supine position. Anesthesia is induced, the endotracheal tube is placed, and the patient is turned over. This position is useful for access to the posterior portions of the body.

Jackknife   The torso and legs are lowered slightly after the patient is placed in the prone position. This position is useful for lower spine and rectal procedures.

Lithotomy   The legs are positioned slightly flexed above the table and are supported in slings or stirrups with the patient lying supine. The table portion beneath the legs is then removed from the upper table or is lowered to hang perpendicularly. The patient's buttocks can then be positioned at the edge of the table, allowing access to the genitals, perineum, and anorectal anatomy. This position is used primarily for obstetrical, gynecological, urological, and anorectal operations.

CLINICAL PROCEDURE

Several important considerations for proper patient positioning are given here. The PA should assist the anesthesia team and the circulating nurse in safely positioning the patient on the table and during the induction of anesthesia. All staff should keep in mind that inadvertent injury may occur beneath the drapes as a result of poor positioning and may remain unnoticed until the end of the operation. Such an injury may not respond to therapeutic treatment and may result in permanent paralysis or dysfunction.

➤ Wheels on both the table and the transport stretcher should be locked before transfer of the patient to or from the OR table.

➤ Anatomical alignment of the patient on the OR table should be maintained as close to normal as possible. This prevents overstretching of, or pressure on, nerves and blood vessels. Proper anatomical alignment can be facilitated by inserting pillows between the legs of a patient in the lateral position or behind the knees of a patient in the supine position.

➤ Pad all bony prominences to prevent nerve or vessel injury. The thorax of a prone patient should be supported with foam pillows to facilitate chest wall excursion and adequate ventilation.

➤ Never cross the patient's legs in the supine position.

➤ Give careful consideration to the patient's joints during transfer or positioning so they are not moved past their normal range of motion. This is especially important for positioning the legs and hips in the lithotomy position. Older patients with osteoarthritis or rheumatological diseases require careful padding and positioning to avoid iatrogenic injury.

➤ All fixed appliances or instrumentation that come into contact with the patient's skin must be adequately padded (e.g., leg slings or stirrups for lithotomy, sleighs or sheets to keep arms tucked at the patient's side, foam pads on wrists or elbows on arm boards, foam heel pads).

➤ Every patient is secured to the table with straps or tape to prevent accidents. Patients under the influence of sedative, narcotic, and anesthetic agents are prone to confusion and agitation, especially when awakening from general anesthesia, and often attempt to sit up or get off the table before they are fully awake and competent.

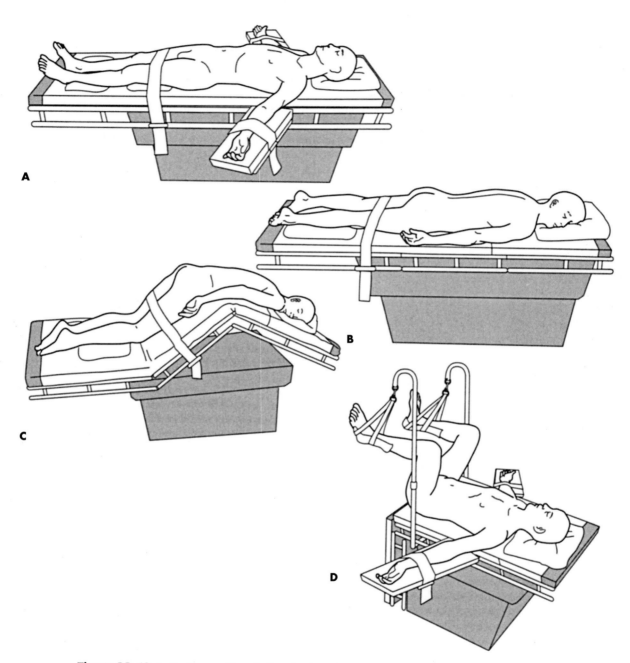

Figure 33-10 A, Supine position. Patient is placed on back with arms at sides or extended to 90 degrees and head in alignment with body. Legs are uncrossed, with a safety strap placed above knees. **B,** Prone position. Patient is usually anesthetized while supine, and then turned. Arms are placed at sides, with rolls beneath axilla to facilitate respiration. **C,** Jackknife position. Patient is usually anesthetized while supine, and then turned. Knees are flexed slightly to reduce lumbosacral stress. **D,** Lithotomy position. Patient is on back, and foot section of operating table is removed or lowered to 90-degree angle. Buttocks are moved to table's edge. Feet are suspended in straps to flex knees. Legs are placed into or removed from the stirrups simultaneously to avoid hip injuries.

OPERATIVE SITE DRAPING AND EQUIPMENT

One of the most important steps in preparing the operative site is appropriate draping of the patient to create a sterile area around the incision. Several layers of materials are used for this purpose, and each surgical specialty has special draping procedures and drape material specifically designed for each procedure.

After aseptic preparation of the skin by application of the appropriate agent, as was previously discussed, the operative site should be rectangularly draped with folded cotton towels held in place with towel clips. Because these towel clips pass through the towels into a nonsterile area, they are always considered contaminated after placement. If the clips need to be removed, they are discarded from the sterile field, and the area where they penetrated the drapes should be overlaid with additional sterile draping material.

A large sterile sheet containing a fenestration, or central opening, is placed over the field, allowing access to the operative site. Fenestration size is chosen to allow sufficient access to the area of incision and to allow a large enough area for use of the appropriate equipment (e.g., retractors) for limb manipulation, and so forth.

CLINICAL PROCEDURE

Personnel should always drape with cotton towels an area wider and longer than the planned incision. Incisions may need to be lengthened during the course of the procedure (Figure 33-11). After placement of the towels, nonwoven fabric or disposable paper drapes are used to completely isolate the remainder of the exposed patient from the incision site. These drapes are called quarter-, half-, or three-quarter sheets according to their size. They are placed over the patient's feet, torso, limbs, and head as required for each procedure (Figure 33-12). Occasionally, a limb will be draped in a sterile plastic tunnel with one closed end if that limb requires manipulation by the surgeon or assistant.

SURGICAL ASSISTING AND INSTRUMENTATION

The principal means of preparing to assist at an operation is to study the proposed operation before the

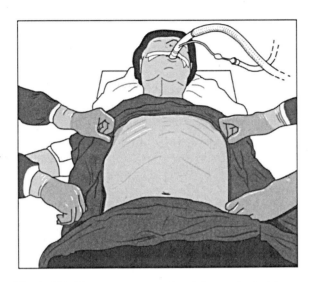

Figure 33-11 Widely draping the abdomen for incision.

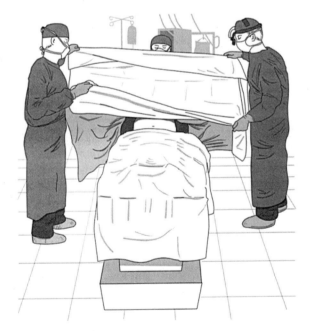

Figure 33-12 Placing the drapes between the anesthesia area and the surgical team.

procedure. All assistants should be prepared to answer questions regarding the current indications for the planned procedure, its attendant complications and expected results, and possible alternative procedures. Review of the pertinent regional anatomy and the steps of the operation is required so that a minimum of instruction is required from the surgeon during the operation, excluding those instructions needed to direct the assistant's hands or for discussion of intraoperative decisions.

SAs must be intimately familiar with the instrumentation used to extend the functions of their hands. After mastering the use of basic surgical equipment and instrumentation, the surgical PA can progress to understanding the nuances of the surgical procedure itself. Many eponyms are used to describe similar instruments; therefore, descriptive names are used here to avoid confusion.

Retraction Devices

Many kinds of retractors are used to provide exposure. Some are manually controlled extensions of the assistant's hands, as in the Senn, Army-Navy, Richardson, Deaver, and Harrington retractors. Others are self-retaining locking devices, such as the Weitlaner, Balfour, Bookwalter, and Iron Intern retractors. Only a handful are used with any frequency, despite the many types available for each surgical specialty.

Handheld Retractors (Figures 33-13 and 33-14)

Army-Navy and Senn Retractors   Of the smaller retractors, the Army-Navy and Senn are used to retract small amounts of superficial tissue. The Army-Navy retractor (Figure 33-13, *A*) has two flat blades of different lengths. The Senn retractor (Figure 33-13, *B*) has a rake on one end and a flat blade on the other.

Richardson Retractor   The Richardson retractor (Figure 33-14, *A*) is manufactured with blade widths from small to large and often has two different blade widths on opposite ends for quick size changes. It is used primarily for retracting tissues within cavities (abdomen and pelvis) and for deep incisions.

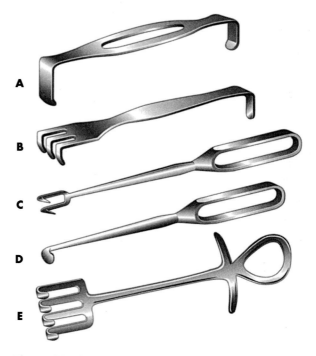

Figure 33-13 *Handheld retractors.* **A,** Army-Navy retractor. **B,** Senn retractor. **C,** Skin hook. **D,** Vein retractor. **E,** Rake.

Deaver and Harrington Retractors   The Deaver retractor (Figure 33-14, *B*) is a curved instrument with a narrow to wide, flat blade. It is used for viscera and abdominal wall retraction. The Harrington or "sweetheart" retractor (Figure 33-14, *C*), so named because of its characteristic heart-shaped shovel, provides deep retraction within a cavity without disturbance of more superficial structures. This instrument is also used for delicate organs such as the lobes of the liver.

Ribbon or Malleable Retractor   Another commonly used retractor is the ribbon or malleable retractor (Figure 33-14, *D*). It has a flat blade and can easily be formed into different useful shapes where preformed retractors prove inadequate. The ribbon retractor is also used to keep the viscera within the confines of the abdomen during closure of an abdominal incision.

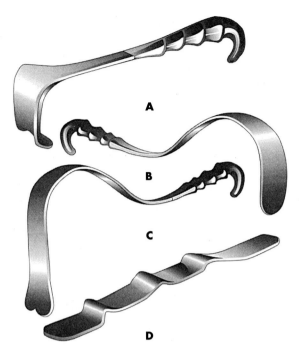

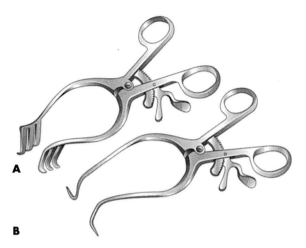

Figure 33-15 *Self-retaining retractors.* **A,** Weitlaner. **B,** Gelpie.

Figure 33-14 *Handheld retractors.* The blades of these retractors should be padded with moistened gauze pads to prevent injury to the viscera. **A,** Richardson. **B,** Deaver. **C,** Harrington. **D,** Ribbon or malleable.

CLINICAL PROCEDURE

A retractor used on delicate tissues or that will be held in one place for an extended period should be padded with a wet saline gauze pad to prevent tissue desiccation or trauma. Because students frequently find themselves attached to a retractor, learning some simple tips can aid the process.

➤ Flat-bladed instruments without rounded handles should be padded with a sponge pad to ease the holder's hand pain.

➤ Retraction can be a tedious affair, resulting in fatigue and fidgeting. The student should use retraction time to observe how the surgeons work as a team and how tissues are handled. The best method of becoming a good first-assistant is to observe and copy accomplished assistants.

➤ The retractor holder must be especially aware of the tissues against which he or she is pulling. Care should be taken with delicate tissues, such

as the liver, nerves, lungs, or blood vessels, which could be permanently damaged by overaggressive retraction. Usually, the surgeon positions the retractor and adjusts the amount of tension required from the assistant to facilitate tissue exposure. The student should constantly monitor the retraction instrument and strive to maintain the appropriate amount of exposure required. If asked to reapproximate the retractor, ask for specific instructions. Some instructions may entail "towing in," which means to lift up on the handle of the retractor while pulling downward with the tip of the retractor, or "towing out," which means precisely the opposite actions.

Self-Retaining Retractors Self-retaining retractors have locking mechanisms that keep the blades apart and in place while spreading the edges of the incision and holding other tissue in place, thus freeing the surgeon's and assistant's hands for other tasks.

Weitlaner and Gelpie Retractors Two of the most commonly used self-retaining retractors are the Weitlaner and Gelpie retractors (Figure 33-15). These are used to retract skin edges for superficial procedures. Care must be taken not to puncture vital tissues or oneself with the sharp points of these retractors.

Balfour and Bookwalter Retractors The Balfour and the Bookwalter are self-retaining abdominal wall retractors with various deep and shallow blades that can be attached and removed as needed. The Balfour retractor is placed within the incision, spread apart as needed, and locked in place by tightening of a wing nut (Figure 33-16). The Bookwalter retractor has a single post that attaches to the table's side rail. This attachment takes some practice to master. A crossbar mounted on the post holds an oval or round ring to which various sizes of Richardson, malleable, and Deaver-like blades may be attached with adjustable, ratcheted "clips."

Goligher Retractor and Iron Intern The Goligher retractor (Figure 33-17, *A*) is used for abdominal operations in the superior regions of the peritoneal cavity, particularly for gallbladder, liver, and stomach procedures. It is easily attached to a crossbar placed onto the head of the OR table. The Iron Intern (Figure 33-17, *B*) uses a series of locking arms and joints to position retractors within the abdomen or pelvis.

Learning to Use Retractors It should be noted that each specialty has its own specifically designed retraction devices that must be mastered as the student rotates to each surgical service. The student should not experiment with these instruments directly before or during the surgical procedure because of the risk of accidental instrument contamination; however, when the patient has been successfully delivered to the recovery area and the instruments have been transferred to the instrument washing room, there is an excellent opportunity for hands-on experience and for learning how to use these devices.

Cutting Instruments

Scalpels The single most common cutting instrument in the OR is the scalpel (occasionally called a knife). The four most-utilized scalpel blades are the No. 10, No. 11, No. 15, and No. 20. A medium No. 3 scalpel handle is used with all blades except the No. 20 blade, which requires a larger (No. 4) handle. The No. 10 and No. 20 blades are general-purpose blades used to create most large incisions. For safe practice,

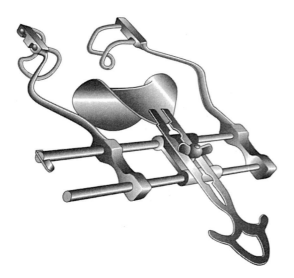

Figure 33-16 The Balfour self-retaining retractor uses deep and shallow blades to separate the abdominal incision. The perpendicularly placed bladder blade can keep the bladder out of the operative field. Place a hand between the viscera and the abdominal wall to prevent inadvertent trapping of viscera while opening this retractor.

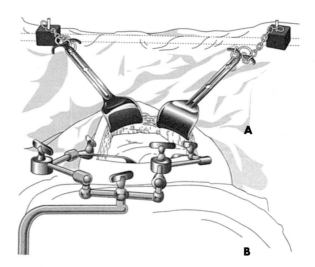

Figure 33-17 A, The Goligher retractor (shown elevating the upper abdomen) is attached to a bar crossing the head of the table. It is useful for liver, biliary, stomach, diaphragm, and lower esophageal surgeries. **B,** The Iron Intern (shown retracting the lower abdomen) has multiple arms and can be adjusted to hold a variety of differently shaped retractor blades.

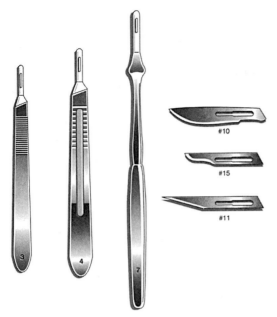

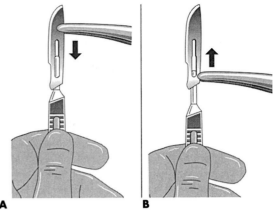

A   **B**

Figure 33-19 **A,** The scalpel blade is placed by use of a hemostat. The key-shaped groove is inserted into the side grooves of the handle and slowly snapped into place. **B,** The heel of the blade is lifted with a hemostat and is slid away from the assistant to remove it.

Figure 33-18 Scalpels and scalpel blades. Note the shapes of the No. 10, No. 11, and No. 15 blades. They are frequently used with the No. 3 or medium handle. A No. 7 or small handle can be used for precise blade control. The No. 4 handle, slightly larger than the No. 3, may be used by individuals with large hands or for indelicate incisions.

the scalpel should be engaged and removed from the handle with a ratcheted, locking hemostat to prevent injury (Figures 33-18 and 33-19).

For large incisions, the scalpel is held in the palm of the hand so that the belly of the blade is used to make the incision (Figure 33-20, *A* and *B*). Scalpels require minimal downward pressure from the operator to incise the skin. The skin should be held firmly under retraction with the other hand to provide a smooth surface upon which to cut. The entire arm of the operator is moved from the shoulder as the scalpel is held perpendicular to the skin and pulled toward the operator.

Finer, more intricate incisions are created with the No. 15 blade with the scalpel handle held like a pencil. This allows maximum accuracy, especially when incisions other than straight lines are made. Placing the middle, fourth, and fifth fingers of the hand on the patient's skin provides a point of stabil-

ity for more accurate control of the point of the scalpel (Figure 33-20, *C*).

The pointed No. 11 blade has several uses. It often is used for incising abscesses; the sharp edge of the blade tip is thrust up into the abscess and pulled outward with a sawing movement to incise the skin.

Most scalpel incisions are made precisely perpendicular to the skin. An angled or beveled cut undermines the dermis and epidermis, possibly resulting in necrosis of the skin secondary to circulatory impairment. This yields a less cosmetic scar in the best of circumstances and wound infection from devitalized skin tissue in the worst cases.

Scissors   Scissors come in various sizes and models—straight or curved, heavy or delicate; short, medium, or long. The Metzenbaum and Mayo scissors are most frequently used. The Metzenbaum scissors are thin-tipped dissecting scissors, whereas the Mayo scissors are heavy, blunt-bladed scissors used for cutting heavy structures, especially sutures (Figure 33-21). Scissors should be held with the points following the natural curve of the hand. However, for cutting along tissues curved toward the hand, the scissors should be turned over for proper usage.

Assistants are frequently asked to cut sutures; although this in itself is a simple maneuver, a few words of advice are warranted. Use heavy scissors to cut sutures; delicate scissors are more expensive and can be dulled if they are used to cut suture material. A steady hand held palm-down against your other arm or hand, or against the patient, gives excellent control of the tips of the scissors, which is the only portion that should be used for cutting sutures. The slightly open blades of the scissors should be placed on the upheld suture and slid down the sutures until the knot is felt against the blades of the scissors. The blades of the scissors should be rotated 45 degrees and closed

to cut the suture. Care must be taken to ensure that the scissors do not cut anything but the suture and that the suture does not get caught within the blades. Otherwise, the scissors may pull the suture from the tied tissue, causing bleeding or other adverse effects.

When absorbable sutures such as chromic and plain gut are cut, a tag of 3 to 4 mm is left to prevent the knot from unwinding. Synthetic nonabsorbable sutures, such as nylon and Prolene, have a springlike memory and require a tag of 7 to 10 mm to prevent unwinding. Nonabsorbable sutures such as silk and surgical cotton usually do not require a tag and may be cut on the knot. The tails of a closely placed series of sutures can be easily controlled and cut using the maneuver illustrated in Figure 33-22.

A

B

C

Figure 33-20 A, The balance grip. The scalpel is allowed to pivot against the middle finger while the lateral movements are controlled with a gentle pinch between the index finger and the thumb. The end of the handle rests within the palm. Only a slight downward pressure is needed to cut through the dermis. **B,** The index finger can be placed on top of the knife handle to further control unwanted lateral blade movement. **C,** Holding the scalpel in the pencil or precision grip exercises maximum control on the blade's movement. The hand is usually rested on the tissue for further stability. This grip should be used only for short incisions.

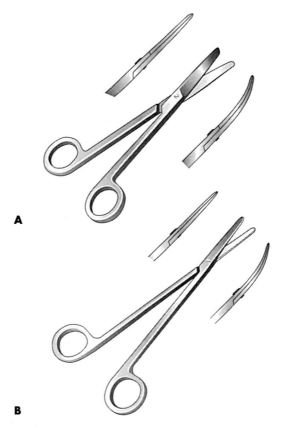

A

B

Figure 33-21 A, Mayo scissors are used for cutting thick structures and sutures. **B,** Metzenbaum scissors are used for dissecting, transecting vessels, and opening viscera.

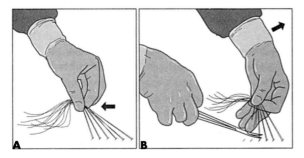

Figure 33-22 A, Rows of tied sutures can easily be cut by gathering all the suture ends into one hand and pulling the ends toward you, graduating the suture tail lengths. **B,** Apply upward tension while cutting the suture closest to you, to keep previously cut tails out of the scissors' blades.

CLINICAL PROCEDURE

"Pass pointing" occurs when the tips of the scissors extend past the structure or suture chosen for cutting and accidentally sever an unintended structure on the other side. Keep the tips of the scissors in your direct line of vision to avoid this complication. If there is any question, another team member should be asked to make the cut.

Surgical Sponges and Pads

Removing blood from the wound allows exposure and examination of the anatomy. Dabbing the wound with absorbent gauze pads or sponges of various sizes is usually sufficient, but with copious bleeding, suction devices are important for clearing the operative field of fluids. Sponges are designated with various eponyms: 4 × 8-inch coarse-weave sponges ("4 × 4s," "Raytecs") are used for minimal bleeding in smaller areas. Larger, tightly woven laparotomy sponges ("laps," "lap pads") are used to absorb many times their weight in blood and fluids.

CLINICAL PROCEDURE

All surgical gauze pads have a blue radiopaque thread either woven into their substance or attached as a loop. These blue threads are readily located on radiography if a sponge has been inadvertently left within a body cavity after surgery. All sponges used during surgery must be accounted for by OR personnel and

therefore should not be used for bandages or wound dressings.

Suction Devices

The *Yankauer tip (tonsil tip)* is one of the most commonly used suction tips. It allows for aspiration of large volumes of fluid, although it has the disadvantage of easily clogging or occluding when the tip is brought into close approximation with tissues or large blood clots. Placing a gauze sponge over the tip and suctioning fluid through the gauze may prevent clogging. The Poole tip has an inner canal surrounded by a fenestrated outer sleeve containing smaller holes that prevent inadvertent occlusion. For use in delicate procedures, a *neuro* or *Frazier* suction device uses a 3- to 5-mm cannula opening with a vented side port on the handle to control the suction force applied at the tip (Figure 33-23).

CLINICAL PROCEDURE

Use a pencil grip to hold suction tips. This allows defined, precision control of the instrument, which is

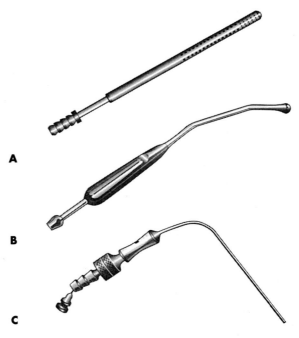

Figure 33-23 *Suction tips.* **A,** Poole tip. **B,** Yankauer or tonsil tip. **C,** Frazier or neuro tip.

especially important for delicate vascular and micro-surgical procedures.

Forceps, Clamps, and Needle Holders

Forceps are divided into two categories: those with teeth and those without teeth. Thumb forceps require finger apposition in the form of a pencil grip to handle tissues. Ratcheted forceps (clamps) can be locked onto tissues and left in place, freeing the hands for other efforts.

Thumb Forceps   Toothed thumb forceps (Figure 33-24, *D*) are used on tissues that require a firm grip, such as fascia, or for abdominal wall closure. *Bonney* and *rat-tooth* forceps are good examples of heavy-toothed thumb forceps. Small *Adson* forceps (Figure 33-24, *B*) are ideal for everting the skin edges when staples are placed for incision closure. One should never use toothed forceps on nerves, blood vessels, bowel, or other viscera.

Smooth forceps are used for handling delicate structures. *DeBakey* forceps (Figure 33-24, *C*), a useful variant of the smooth forceps, were originally designed for vascular surgery. Their unique, interpolating, smooth tooth design causes minimal tissue crushing by distributing the grasping forces equally throughout the tips. *Cushing* (Figure 33-24, *E*) and *Potts* forceps are smooth, finely tipped forceps used for similar purposes.

Smooth forceps should not be used to handle fascia or skin because the excessive force required will damage these instruments.

CLINICAL PROCEDURE

Knowing how much tension to apply to each type of tissue is a key element of tissue preservation. Grasping the tissue closest to the site of action imparts the greatest control over the tissue's movement. Only a minimal amount of pressure is then required to move the tissue. For nerves and blood vessels, the enveloping adventitia should be grasped to prevent vessel-crushing injuries. Manipulate the skin by grasping the dermis located beneath the epidermis or by using a skin hook (see Figure 33-13, *C*).

Locking (Ratcheted) Forceps   Ratcheted or locking forceps ("clamps") are instruments known by

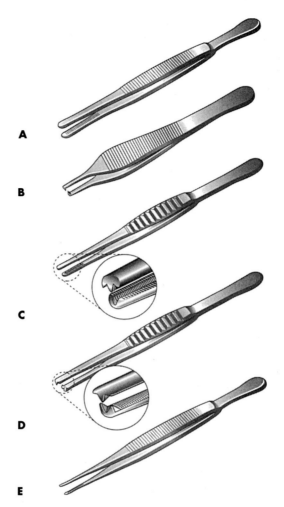

Figure 33-24 *Thumb forceps.* **A**, Plain. **B**, Adson with teeth. **C**, DeBakey. **D**, Toothed. **E**, Cushing.

many eponyms (Figure 33-25). The *hemostat* clamp (Figure 33-25, *A*) may be straight or curved and may have serration on all or part of the blade length. Smaller hemostats, called *mosquito* clamps, have very fine tips. *Crile* and *Kelly* clamps are larger versions of the hemostat. Even larger are the *Peán* and *Carmalt* clamps, which are used to clamp large blood vessels before transection and tying. *Right-angle* clamps (Figure 33-25, *C*) can be used to dissect around veins or arteries or to pass suture material around tubular structures.

The *Kocher* clamp (Figure 33-25, *G*) is a traumatic toothed clamp applied to hold structures that will be removed or will not undergo harm from severe crushing, such as the rectus sheath fascia. *Allis* clamps (Figure 33-25, *I*) have perpendicular teeth along their edges but by design are less traumatic than Kocher clamps and can be used on structures for retraction or for apposition of tissue edges. A *Babcock* clamp (Figure 33-25, *H*) is used to gently hold delicate viscera or to encircle tubular structures for gentle retraction.

Needle Holders   Needle holders ("needle drivers") are designed with fine, medium, and heavy tips with a variety of handle lengths (Figure 33-25, *F*). The driver's tip size is determined by the delicacy of the needle used for suturing. The depth at which the suturing occurs determines the length of the handles. Generally, the shorter lengths are easier to guide and are used for suturing with precise control. Using a delicate needle holder for a heavy needle destroys the integrity and locking ability of the instrument.

CLINICAL PROCEDURES

Unfortunately, ringed instruments (such as clamps, needle holders, and scissors) are designed for right-handed individuals. All surgeons and assistants should be proficient in the use of these tools with either hand because frequently, the instrument will be used in the nondominant hand. The left-handed assistant may have to practice using these instruments more than the right-handed person. It takes precisely the opposite motions and movements to control these instruments with the left hand, particularly for opening ratcheted clamps or cutting with scissors. Perfection requires concerted effort and practice. Several guidelines follow.

Do not allow your fingers to protrude through the rings past the distal interphalangeal joint. Placing the proximal interphalangeal joint through the rings severely restricts the ability to quickly disengage the instrument from the hand. The thumb ring should be controlled with the thumb's pad only. Occasionally, it is useful to place the ring and little finger into the other ring for control. The index finger can be placed onto the shaft or middle of the instrument, to provide better control, in the "tripod grip" (Figure 33-26). At best, lack of proficiency with these instruments may cause delay; at worst, finger fumbling with an instrument may avulse a vessel, causing unnecessary bleeding.

The clamp's locking ratchets allow a mechanism to release the instrument from the hand while continuing to grip the tissue. To disengage a ratcheted clamp in the right hand, the thumb pushes outward and the remaining fingers pull inward to release the locking

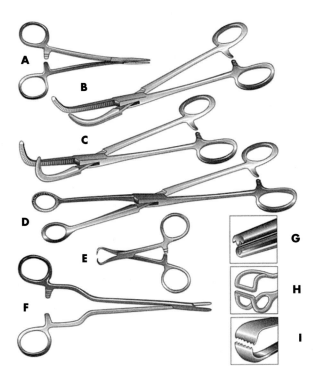

Figure 33-25 *Ratcheted locking forceps (clamps)* **A,** Straight hemostat. **B,** Large clamp. **C,** Right angle. **D,** Ring (sponge). **E,** Towel clip. **F,** Needle holder. **G,** Kocher. **H,** Babcock. **I,** Allis.

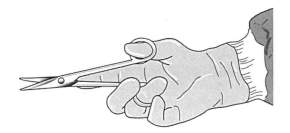

Figure 33-26 The tripod grip can be used with a ringed forceps to optimize control of the instrument's tips. The index finger helps guide and stabilize the instrument, thereby reducing hand tremor. Rotate the hand palm-down for the best hand muscle control and strength.

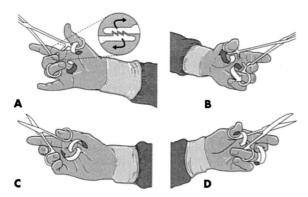

Figure 33-27 Control of ratcheted instruments takes practice, particularly with the nondominant hand. **A,** To open locking ratcheted forceps with the right hand, the thumb is pushed toward the body and upward while the other fingers are pulled toward the palm. **B,** The reverse relationship holds for the left hand. **C,** Creating close contact of the blades during closure allows scissors to cut rather than tear tissues. In the right hand, the thumb moves away from the palm and body as the other fingers pull toward the palm. **D,** Again, the opposite holds for the left hand.

mechanism. The opposite movements are needed for the left hand (Figure 33-27, *A* and *B*). Practice using these instruments with both hands, with the curved tip pointing up and then with the tip pointing down. Similar finger motions are required for proper cutting action with scissors (Figure 33-27, *C* and *D*).

As with thumb forceps, ratcheted forceps should encase only enough tissue in the tips of the instrument to enable a firm grip. For instance, blood vessels should be grasped without trapping surrounding structures. Finally, although blunt by design, the forceps' ratchets can tear gloves or accidentally entrap other tissues or sutures. Caution should always be used when applying and disengaging these instruments.

Drains and Tubes

Drains are placed *prophylactically,* to prevent accumulation of fluids and to encourage the obliteration of dead space, or *therapeutically,* to promote escape of fluids that have already accumulated.

General Precautions

➤ Drains act as two-way conduits. The benefits of a drain must be weighed against the risk of introducing infection.

➤ Because a drain permits bacterial ingress and prevents full closure of a wound, it should never be brought out through the operative incision.

➤ A drain should always be fixed to the skin with sutures.

➤ A drain that is too hard or stiff may cause pressure necrosis of surrounding tissues, especially if placed near a large blood vessel, tendon, nerve, or solid organ.

Types of Drains and Tubes   Drains may be classified into four basic categories: sump drains, self-suction drains, straight drains, and chest tubes.

Sump Drains   Sump drains have two parallel lumina leading to a multiholed distal tip. One lumen is used to aspirate fluid, and the second lumen allows air to enter the cavity being aspirated, thus preventing undue suction from pulling of tissues into the aspiration ports and clogging of the holes. Salem sump NG tubes are characteristic of this drain type.

Self-Suction Drains   A self-suction or closed-suction drain is attached to a vacuum device, bulb, or wall suction to provide continuous drainage of a wound site or cavity. Bulbs are usually hand-charged (squeezed) to initiate suction. Hemovac, Jackson-Pratt (Figure 33-28, *C*), and Blake (Figure 33-28, *D*) drains are self-suction drains.

Straight Drains   Straight drains do not use suction; rather, gravity is used to facilitate fluid movement. The Penrose drain (Figure 33-28, *A*), a flat latex tube, is a good example of a straight drain. This category also includes gastric and jejunal tubes (tubes placed directly through the skin into the stomach or jejunum), which may be used to drain the gastrointestinal tract or to provide infusion of enteral nutrition.

Chest Tubes   Chest tubes inserted through the chest wall into the thorax are suction drains designed to help maintain lung inflation and drain fluids or blood from the pleural space. They are connected to a water seal and then to a suction source. The water pressure prevents an accidental lung collapse if the suction source is intentionally or accidentally discontinued.

A seal is maintained at the chest wall to prevent air leaks by wrapping a petroleum jelly–impregnated gauze strip around the skin entrance of the tube.

CLINICAL PROCEDURE

A Penrose drain is secured to the skin with a simple suture or a large safety pin designed to keep the drain

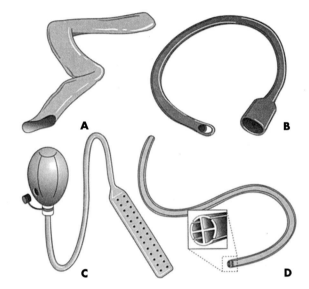

Figure 33-28 Four frequently used drains. **A,** Penrose. **B,** Red rubber catheter. **C,** Jackson-Pratt. **D,** Blake. *Inset,* Cross section of Blake drain, showing channels that run its entire length.

from slipping out of the exit site or back into the body. A Salem sump tube is taped to the nose or face to secure its position. Chest tubes and self-suctioning drains are secured with a suture tied to the tube and sewn to the skin. Figure 33-29 illustrates how to sew a drain to the skin.

Removal of Drains   Drains should be removed as soon as drainage has subsided.
1. Warn the patient that there will be some pain; consider pre-medication for anxious patients.
2. Remove surrounding bandages and cut attaching skin suture.
3. *Always release suction before pulling.*
4. Be prepared for leaks and drips.

MINIMALLY INVASIVE SURGERY

In the late 1980s, Eddie Jo Reddick, MD, brought advanced technology into general surgery when he published several reports regarding the first laparoscopic cholecystectomies performed in the United States. Endoscopy and laparoscopy techniques date back to the early 1800s, but Reddick and surgeons in France working at the same time can be credited with introducing surgeons from all disciplines to the concept of performing surgery with minimal incisions and decreased recovery times (minimally invasive surgery [MIS]). For many diseases requiring surgical evaluation, intervention, or treatment, a laparoscopic or endoscopic procedure may be considered the first line approach (Figure 33-30).

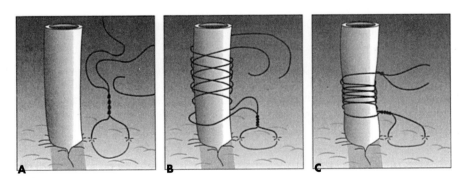

Figure 33-29 Sewing a drain to the skin. **A,** Create a loop by driving the needle through the skin. Pull the two suture ends to equal lengths, cut off the needle, and tie four or five half-knots above the skin, leaving room for postoperative tissue edema and to prevent the suture from cutting through the skin. **B,** Sandal-lace the suture ends loosely around the tube three or four times. **C,** Gently push the sandal lacing together while tightening the loops. Do this firmly but not too tightly to avoid strangulating the flow of fluid within the tube.

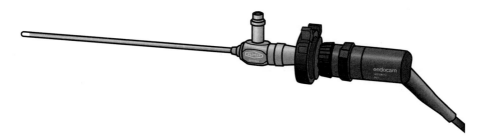

Figure 33-30 Laparoscope and camera head.

MIS includes the realm of arthroscopy employed by orthopedists worldwide. A large number of procedures are performed intraluminally via endoscopes through bronchoscopy, colonoscopy, and esophagogastroduodenoscopy. This section concentrates on general MIS in the abdomen and thorax (Figure 33-31).

An entire culture blossomed around MIS in which much of the equipment is disposable. Equipment manufacturers developed MIS forceps, needle holders, suturing devices and ligatures, irrigation and suction, biopsy devices, retractors, and hemorrhage control methods (Figure 33-32, *A* and *B*). One of the major advances allowing safe performance of laparoscopic cholecystectomy was the development of a preloaded device to apply titanium clips to close the cystic duct and control blood vessels via the laparoscope. It is safe to say all American hospitals performing surgery have MIS equipment. Approximately 85% of cholecystectomies and a majority of kidneys removed from living donors for transplant in the United States are performed with the use of MIS.[6]

Minimally invasive surgical techniques reduce cosmetic deformity and essentially minimize damage to the patient during surgery. Laparoscopy can be defined as insufflation of the abdomen, leading to MIS. Thoracoscopy (or video-assisted thoracic surgery [VATS]) entails deflating the lung and introducing the camera through the chest wall. Other MIS procedures are performed beneath the skin, as seen in endoscopic saphenous vein harvesting for coronary artery bypass grafting. A thoracotomy may be replaced by VATS through several small punctures in the intercostal spaces, and the 8-inch incision from a traditional cholecystectomy is replaced with four, 1- to 2-cm punctures in the anterior abdomen from a

laparoscopic approach, with patient recovery measured in days and not weeks. The list of procedures performed via minimally invasive techniques has grown significantly since the late 1980s (Table 33-2) and will continue to expand as techniques are perfected and data analysis demonstrates which procedures offer the best outcomes for the patient. The complete value of MIS has not been proved in all

---

Table 33-2   MIS Procedures

- Laparoscopic cholecystectomy
- Laparoscopic appendectomy
- Laparoscopic colon resection or colostomy formation
- Laparoscopic inguinal and umbilical herniorrhaphy
- Laparoscopic Nissen fundoplication
- Laparoscopic kidney harvesting for donation
- Laparoscopic adhesiolysis
- Laparoscopic Heller's myotomy
- Laparoscopic nephrectomy
- Laparoscopic gastrostomy and jejunostomy feeding tube insertion
- Laparoscopic adrenalectomy
- Laparoscopic bladder and gynecological procedures
  - Hysterectomy
  - Bladder suspension
- Thoracoscopic bleb resection, lung and pleural biopsy
- Thoracoscopic sympathectomy
- Thoracoscopic lung volume reduction
- Thoracoscopic esophagectomy
- MIS harvesting of the internal mammary artery
- MIS harvesting of the saphenous vein

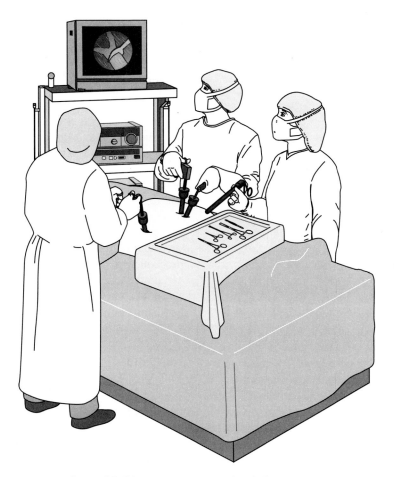

Figure 33-31 Typical OR layout for cholecystectomy.

cases, and some procedures are best left to classical open surgical approaches.

MIS typically involves replacement of human binocular three-dimensional vision by the use of a small video camera that projects two-dimensional images onto monitors posted around the OR table. Some advanced systems use dual cameras to mimic a three-dimensional surgical field, but these are not in common use. The surgeon makes a 1-cm incision to blindly introduce a needle used to introduce CO_2 into the abdomen to raise the anterior abdominal wall away from underlying viscera (Figure 33-33). The surgeon pushes a sharp trocar through another small incision and slides the camera down the hollow

sleeve or "port" left after the inner trocar obturator is removed. Ports have valves that trap gas within the abdomen while allowing instrument passage down the inner lumen. Side valves allow attachment of tubing for gas insufflation (Figure 33-34). Twelve- to 15-inch-long instruments are then used to perform the surgery. Electrocautery may be used for dissection and hemorrhage control. An ultrasonic dissecting device, the Harmonic Scalpel, can be used to avoid inadvertent burns from cautery use.

Laparoscopic video images are confined to the immediate field of vision directly in front of the camera, and the loss of the three-dimensional spatial relationships ordinarily seen with binocular vision requires careful instrument use, judicious use of electrocautery, and meticulous control of bleeding. MIS eliminates the familiar tactile sensations associated with open surgery tissue handling, and suturing can be extremely frustrating in a two-dimensional environment. American College of Surgery data show that the learning curve for MIS procedures is steep, and an average of 25 to 30 procedures is required before a surgeon is considered skilled in that particular procedure.

Surgical PAs are often asked to assist with MIS procedures. Most MIS requires at least a camera holder, while many such procedures require active participation by the first-assistant. The best method of acquiring the skills necessary for MIS proficiency is to spend time in an MIS lab within your training institution or hospital. There, trocar insertion, camera manipulation, and acquiring an understanding of the operating characteristics of the various instruments and devices can be practiced without risk of patient morbidity.

The references that follow this chapter contain several excellent sources of information on MIS procedures and instruments that are not mentioned or adequately detailed in this section. We advise students to spend time with the laparoscope, CO_2 gas insufflator, videoscope light source, and associated instruments to gain understanding of their use at the operating table and to learn techniques for troubleshooting this high-tech equipment during surgery.

CLINICAL PROCEDURE

The field of view is often reversed on the video monitor from what you do with your hands for instrument manipulation. For example, the port acts as a fulcrum through the abdominal wall. Pushing down on the handle of the instrument outside the body causes the tip of the instrument to move up within the abdominal cavity. Rightward movements of the handle cause leftward movement of the instrument tip.

Depth perception on the video monitor comes with practice. Watching your hands outside the abdomen and estimating how deeply the instrument is inserted within the patient can assist with acquiring an under-

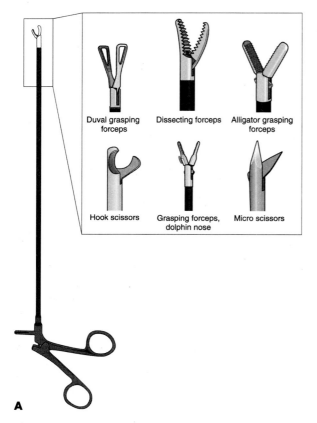

Duval grasping forceps

Dissecting forceps

Alligator grasping forceps

Hook scissors

Grasping forceps, dolphin nose

Micro scissors

A

Figure 33-32 A, Laparoscopic instruments with a variety of heads.

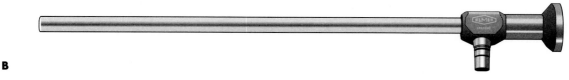

B

Figure 33-32 B, Laparoscope.

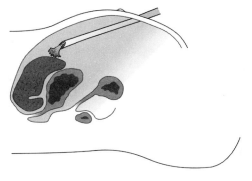

Figure 33-33 Abdominal wall separated from viscera by CO_2 gas.

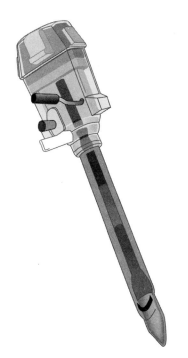

Figure 33-34 Trocar.

standing of how to safely move instruments within the abdomen or chest. Observe for shadows, the position of other instruments, and the relationship of your instruments to the anatomy to gain confidence with tissue and instrument control.

The camera operator becomes the surgeon's eyes. The only important field of view is where the surgeon

is working; therefore, keep the camera focused on the surgeon's working instruments and the anatomy under scrutiny. Try to avoid tissue spray during dissection and irrigation splashes onto the camera lens. Lens fogging can be problematic and is best addressed before surgery by wiping a commercial antifogging agent onto the lens and warming the scope before introducing it into warm humid tissue. Dabbing the lens onto the liver or other relatively fat-free tissue can also wipe the lens clean. A well-directed stream from an irrigation device is also helpful.

Electrocautery energy can arc within a body cavity or ground to an adjoining metal instrument, thereby transferring energy to a distant site and causing a serious injury or an occult burn that is not obvious until 1 or 2 days postoperatively. Use extreme care when using electrocautery and examine surrounding tissues at the end of the procedure to look for signs of electrothermal injury.

Anatomy identification is critical to success with MIS. The most common intra-abdominal injuries for MIS include visceral perforation (bladder, bowel, intestine) and damage to tubular structures such as the ureter, common bile and cystic ducts, and blood vessels.

All MIS procedures carry risks. Each procedure should be treated as if it could be converted into a traditional open operation if difficult anatomy, uncontrollable bleeding, or a complication warrants improved access to the surgical field. A good assistant must know the surgical conduct required for both MIS and open approaches and must expect that some procedures will be converted. The OR staff should have full traditional instrumentation immediately available in the OR for such unanticipated events.

SURGICAL BLEEDING

The secret of controlling intraoperative hemorrhage lies in its prevention. There are several reliable methods to control surgical bleeding. Some take advantage of the body's intrinsic clotting mechanisms (e.g., direct pressure) and some are artificially applied (e.g., topical thrombin). Bleeding compounded by coagulation defects is a broad topic beyond the scope of this chapter.

Direct Pressure

The easiest way to stop bleeding from small vessels is to apply gentle manual pressure. The systolic pressure in small vessels (between 5 and 10 mm Hg) is easily controlled in this manner. Direct pressure can be achieved by gently pushing the vessel against the underlying tissue with a finger or with the tip of a hemostat, sponge, scalpel, suction unit, or sponge attached to a long-handled clamp (ring forceps). Squeezing the vessel with forceps or between the fingers also is effective. Normal clotting for small vessels takes place within 15 to 30 seconds and may be all that is required for control. Direct pressure also gives the surgeon time to control bleeding in larger, high-pressure vessels with a hemostatic clamp or ligature if needed (see later).

During some procedures, diffuse bleeding may require pressure for extended periods; for example, a large sponge may be packed against the bleeding surface and held in place by the assistant's hand or with a retractor while some other portion of the procedure is completed. This is especially efficient for areas that have innumerable small or pinpoint "bleeders" that would be time-consuming to control individually.

CLINICAL PROCEDURE

When sponging blood from an area, do not aggressively drag or scrape the sponge across the tissue. This action removes coagulated blood products from the ends of blood vessels and allows bleeding to resume. Blotting is the safest method. Large amounts of clot can be removed by irrigating the area with saline and using suction, or by scooping them by hand into a basin.

Electrocautery

The electrocautery unit (Bovie, cautery, or electrosurgical unit) (Figure 33-35, *A*) uses high-frequency electrical energy to cut tissue or coagulate bleeding. The preferential conduction of electrical energy by blood vessels facilitates coagulation. It is crucial to remove pooled blood and irrigation fluids from the operative field that may act as an insulator or disperse the cautery's energy, thereby diminishing its effectiveness.

Electrocautery may be used in two different ways. In the bipolar mode, a tweezers-tip instrument is used to control bleeding vessels when the two tips complete the electrical circuit at the point of application (Figure 33-35, *C*). The advantage of bipolar cautery is its precise application of energy to small and delicate areas. This is particularly efficacious for microvascular surgery, microneurosurgery, and plastic surgery procedures. Most bipolar units are operated by the surgeon through a foot-controlled switch.

In the monopolar mode, a grounding pad is attached to the patient from the electrocautery unit, and an electrosurgical "pencil" is used to complete a circuit through the patient when it touches bleeding tissues (Figure 33-35, *B*). This "pencil" has a rocker switch or two buttons on its shaft that activate either a continuous application of electrical energy for cutting through tissue, or pulses that can coagulate specific sources of bleeding. Most units can produce a blend of cut and coagulation waveforms to combine the desired features of each.

The cut mode easily cleaves most tissue and does not penetrate very deeply into the surrounding tissue. It is not effective for coagulating bleeding.

In the coagulation mode, the metal blade or needle tip can be directly applied to the tissue or to an intermediary instrument, such as a clamp or forceps, that has been placed onto a bleeding vessel. It can also be used to coagulate a small blood vessel along its visible length before the vessel is transected. The coagulation mode penetrates deeply into the surrounding tissues and can cause thermal damage to unseen arteries, nerves, and other delicate tissues surrounding the cautery tip and vessel surface.

CLINICAL PROCEDURE

Judgment involving the practical use of this instrument comes only with experience, through which one learns which vessels will respond to electrocautery coagulation. Great care must be taken when touching an intermediary instrument such as a clamp or forceps for coagulation because it will burn all tissues it comes in contact with. Before engaging the coagulation mode, be sure the grasping instrument is not touching the skin or other

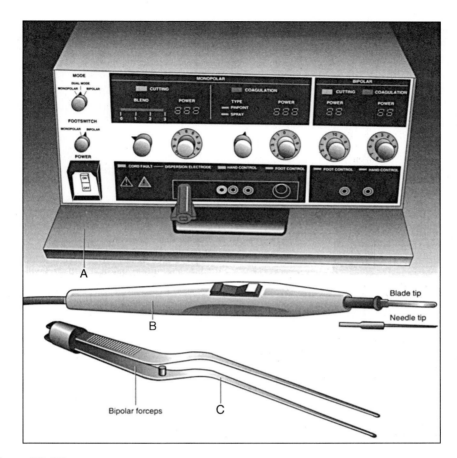

Figure 33-35 A, Typical electrocautery unit. **B,** The monopolar electrosurgical "pencil" can cut or provide hemostasis through activation of the handle switch. **C,** Bipolar tips provide precise application of energy to the tissues.

important tissues in the vicinity of the vessel being coagulated.

Although there is little risk from this technology, holes in gloves can allow burns through electrical conduction to the hands or fingers, and loose grounding pads can cause severe electrical burns to the patient. The grounding pad should be in full contact with the chosen skin site and should not be placed on a bony prominence or over an implanted metal prosthesis (e.g., hip prosthesis). This is just one aspect of OR safety, and PAs should become familiar with the correct and safe use of this device. The manufacturer of the specific electrocautery machine in use in the OR can provide in-service instruction to OR staff and students.

Clamps, Clips, Ligatures, and Sutures

Larger hemorrhaging blood vessels are not safely controlled by direct pressure, packing, or electrocautery, and a wide variety of clamps, ligatures, sutures, and clips are available for this purpose.

Clamps   Bleeding from larger blood vessels may be controlled by the application of a clamp or ratcheted forceps appropriate to the size of the vessel's diameter.

If the vessel is already cut and bleeding, grasp it with smooth thumb forceps to temporarily control the flow, and then apply the ratcheted forceps. A vessel to be clamped before cutting should be held in place with thumb forceps and carefully isolated from the surrounding tissues with blunt dissection with a small hemostat. To accomplish this maneuver, gently advance the clamp parallel to the vessel while opening and closing the jaws to create a tunnel under and around the vessel (Figure 33-36). Both sides require dissection. Place two hemostats, tips facing each other, on opposite ends of the vessel. A small overhang of each tip around which to wrap the suture should extend past the vessel. Close the clamps and transect the vessel with Metzenbaum scissors. Only the vessel

itself should be included in the jaws of the clamp. Frequently, the surgeon or assistant will tie a suture beneath these clamps to achieve hemostasis. Very small vessels may be coagulated with electrocautery.

Often, the student or new assistant will be asked to control the clamp when the surgeon ties a suture around the vessel. Give the surgeon a clear view of the vessel. Provide adequate exposure by keeping your hands out of the surgeon's line of sight and by retracting surrounding tissue away from the vessel being tied.

"Rock" the clamp away from the underlying tissue as the tie passes around the back of the clamp. Then gently rock the clamp in the opposite direction, elevating the tip so the suture may be passed completely around the vessel (Figure 33-37). The vessel end with the highest pressure should be tied first. Do not pull the clamped vessel up during this maneuver; pulling might avulse vessels, resulting in the retraction of the open bleeding vessel deep into the surrounding tissue with resultant hemorrhage that is difficult to control.

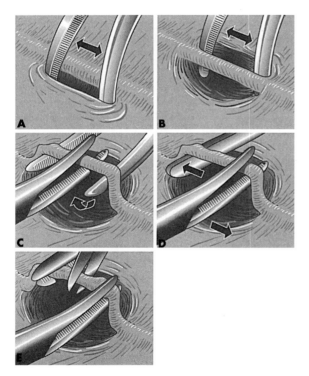

Figure 33-36 A and **B,** Clamps can be used to dissect the loose areolar tissues surrounding blood vessels. Small movements of the tips during spreading prevent tearing of unseen adjacent blood vessels. **C** and **D,** After a clear tunnel is developed, hemostats are placed on both ends of the vessel, which is then divided with scissors **(E).** The end closer to the main circulation is tied first to prevent hemorrhage if the vessel slips from the clamp.

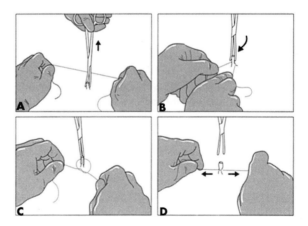

Figure 33-37 Tying a vessel held within a clamp. **A,** The heel of the instrument is raised to allow passage of the suture behind the clamp. **B,** The clamp nose is then slightly lifted to allow circumferential wrapping of the suture. **C** and **D,** The clamp is released when instructed, or when the first half-knot is securely tightened. Note the position of the tying fingers parallel to the vessel during knot-tightening to prevent accidental avulsion from shearing forces. Withdraw the clamp parallel from the vessel to avoid entangling the suture ends. This maneuver takes coordination and communication with the person tying the suture.

CLINICAL PROCEDURE

After the surgeon has tightened the first throw of the knot, slowly open the clamp and withdraw it from the wound. Occasionally, the surgeon asks the assistant to "flash" the clamp during tightening of the first throw of the knot. To do this, slowly release the clamp *while keeping tension on the tissue within its jaws. Do not let go of the vessel.* As the surgeon tightens the first throw, firmly reapply the clamp and hold steady while the remainder of the knot is completed. "Flashing" is especially useful for controlling vessels that have the potential to retract deeply into the surrounding tissue, where they would be inaccessible for further hemostasis. Flashing is also useful when a large-diameter vessel must be "bunched up" to allow more tissue to be encompassed within the knot and when another tie, clip, or ligature is required for complete control of the vessel.

When sutures are tied to replace a series of clamps, the clamp closest to the person tying the sutures should be tied first. This prevents snagging of the suture on adjacent clamps.

Clips   Titanium clips are used to control bleeding and occasionally serve as radiopaque markers in cancer patients who are expected to have postoperative radiation therapy. Clips are easy to apply and take less time than tying sutures, a characteristic advantage in many situations. Long-handled applicators are used to place clips in narrow or deep spaces where suture-tying is difficult. Clips are significantly more expensive than sutures, however, and can obscure the surrounding anatomy through signal scatter during computed tomography.

Clips are placed on bleeding vessels in the same manner as sutures. A clamp or forceps is used to occlude the end of the vessel, and the vessel is clipped before division. Clips are applied by firm squeezing of the handles of the applicator.

CLINICAL PROCEDURE

Clips must completely encompass the vessel to provide reliable hemostasis. If this is not possible, a suture tie or ligature must be used. Clips loaded onto nondisposable applicators are tricky to use. If the clip handle is slightly squeezed and released before the clip is applied, the clip will fall from the applicator tip and another will need to be reloaded, wasting valuable time. This is not the case with preloaded, multiclip, disposable instruments.

Suture Ligatures   Suture ligatures are used to attain hemostasis of larger veins and arteries when simple suture ties or clips are deemed inadequate or inappropriate. They are particularly useful on vessels of larger caliber and close to the higher systolic pressure of the central circulation, which have the potential to dislodge a simple suture tie or a clip over time.

A figure-eight suture ligature can be used to control vessels that retract deep into the surrounding tissues and cannot be located for clamping and do not respond to the application of electrocautery. This ligature encompasses surrounding tissues and directly compresses the bleeding vessel (Figure 33-38, *A*). Care must be demonstrated to avoid inclusion of valuable structures in the suture ligature and to avoid narrowing the lumen of adjacent tubular structures.

Another variation of the suture ligature enables hemostasis of large vessels. The suture is passed *through the middle* of the vessel being held within the jaws of a hemostat; then the ends are brought around the clamp from opposite directions before being tied (Figure 33-38, *B*).

Absorbable Hemostatic Agents

Several agents are used to control bleeding by promoting the formation of an artificial clot or by providing a matrix framework for a clot to form. They are designed to control oozing in instances of hemorrhage from multiple tiny vessels. Hemorrhaging from solid organs with enveloping capsule damage (e.g., small spleen or liver tears) can be controlled in this manner. Occasionally, such agents can be applied to a vascular anastomosis to control needle-hole bleeding.

Thrombin   Thrombin applied topically as a powder or solution is particularly useful for capillary oozing. In its liquid form, it can be used in conjunction with an absorbable gelatin sponge to form a bulky

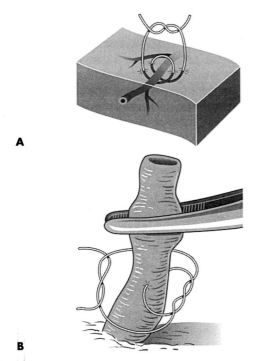

A

B

Figure 33-38 **A**, Vessels hidden beneath enveloping tissues that cannot be readily located or are diffusely bleeding may be controlled with the figure-eight suture shown here. Care must be taken not to ligate important surrounding structures. **B**, The suture ligature prevents suture slippage on large or high-pressure vessels.

hemostatic plug for highly vascular regions such as the liver or spleen.

Absorbable Gelatin Sponge (Gelfoam) Gelfoam helps form a bulky artificial clot in vascular areas, as mentioned previously. It is usually wetted with thrombin or isotonic saline to allow pliability (saline) or greater clot formation (thrombin). It can be left in the surgical site and will be absorbed in 4 to 6 weeks. The diffuse but copious bleeding frequently encountered in liver surgery, including biopsies, can often be controlled with this agent.

Oxidized Cellulose (Surgicel) A treated surgical gauze, oxidized cellulose acts as a physical matrix for clot formation and does not actively cause any alteration of the clotting cascade. It is produced in several forms, including strips, gauze pads, and pledgets. Pledgets can be sewn into place with sutures to seal needle punctures created during vascular or cardiac procedures. Oxidized cellulose can be left in the surgical site, but it is commonly removed after coagulation has taken place.

Microfibrillar Collagen Hemostat (Avitene, Angiostat) This agent is packaged as a friable, flat pad that works through adhesion to the bleeding site by platelet aggregation. This agent is very efficacious for spleen or liver tears and for diffuse bleeding from multiple small vessels.

CONCEPTS FOR SURGICAL ASSISTING
Suturing, Knot-Tying, and Staples

Understanding suture and needle construction, their handling characteristics, the differences between absorbable and nonabsorbable sutures, the probable rate of absorption for each type of suture, and surgical knot-tying is a key element of surgical practice. When an improperly tied suture fails, serious hemorrhage, wound dehiscence, or incisional hernias may occur. It is beyond the scope of this chapter and it would be unreasonable to duplicate the excellent efforts of preexisting instruction manuals to adequately address this topic, with the exception of several pieces of advice (see also Chapter 14).

Student should obtain a manual for knot-tying techniques and a knot-tying board. These items can be obtained through the PA training program or from one of the major suture manufacturers (USS/Davis and Geck or Ethicon—see References). The student should begin practicing *before* the first surgical rotation. Like playing a musical instrument with accomplishment, knot-tying requires dedicated practice.

The speed at which knots are tied is not as important as accurate placement of a reliable series of knots ("throws") with the suture material. Creating a tight knot without *strangulating* the tissue takes practice and avoids unnecessary ischemia that may impede tissue healing.

Wearing a pair of gloves and wetting the suture can approximate the in vivo environment. Use the pads of the fingers when tightening knots to prevent cuts in gloves and fingers.

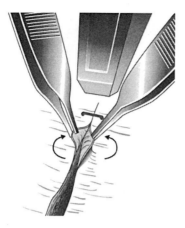

Figure 33-39 Use Adson's forceps with teeth to evert the skin edges when placing skin staples. Center the stapler head on the incision, and gently push downward before pulling the stapler handle. Pull backward after setting the staple to disengage the skin. Occasionally, keeping the handle squeezed after firing the staple stabilizes the skin, allowing easier relocation of Adson's forceps for the placement of the next staple.

Stainless steel staples can be used to close the skin incision in lieu of sutures. They are less likely than sutures to leave scars tied across the skin, which may leave "railroad tracks" perpendicular to the incision (Figure 33-39). Staples are usually not used on the face or on very thin skin.

Tissue Preservation

Preserving exposed tissues is essential to promoting postoperative healing and involves preventing desiccation, minimizing fluid loss, and handling tissues gently. Exposed tissues should be kept moist with saline-soaked gauze or repeated irrigation when possible. The gauze-padded blades of locking retractors should also be kept moist. Gentle handling of tissues with forceps and hands is paramount, and a minimum amount of force should be used to accomplish tissue movement. For instance, tearing of the spleen's capsule during retraction or laceration of the short gastric vessels has caused many bleeding injuries during manipulation of the left or transverse colon.

Facilitating the Procedure

Anticipation of the surgeon's movement through thorough knowledge of the procedure allows a system of teamwork to develop between the surgeon and assistant. It also decreases the length of both operative and anesthesia time. The assistant can become intimately familiar with the nuances and preferences of each surgeon, further facilitating the team approach. The alert assistant should be one step ahead of the surgeon in anticipating the next phase of the procedure and should know what instruments and maneuvers are required to accomplish that step. For example, as the surgeon makes an abdominal incision, the assistant should place proper countertraction opposite the surgeon's hand to facilitate the scalpel's penetration of tissue planes. Additionally, when a blood vessel is to be ligated, it is dissected free of the surrounding tissue and clamped with two hemostats—usually one placed by the surgeon and the other by the assistant.

Providing adequate exposure and visibility is a mainstay task of assisting. An old surgery axiom holds: "If the surgeon is struggling, then the exposure is inadequate." If the first-assistant adjusts the overhead surgical lights to illuminate the central operative field and controls the retraction devices, including directing the hands of the second-assistant, the surgeon can concentrate on the operation without distraction. Understanding what the surgeon needs to see comes with experience and knowledge of the steps involved in the procedure. Use instruments that are long enough to keep fingers out of the line of the surgeon's sight. Once good exposure is achieved, hand movements and retractors should remain in place unless a more refined move will benefit the surgeon. For routine operations, the team eventually uses fewer moves and needs little discussion to complete the procedure.

CLINICAL PROCEDURE

Surgery is a two-handed act. Each hand should be doing something, whether retracting, suctioning, or sponging. Good combinations include the suction tip or sponge and a retractor; forceps and suction tip; or forceps and needle holder. Some instruments, such as the thumb and ratcheted forceps, can be "palmed" in the

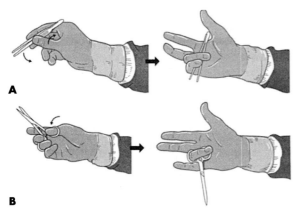

Figure 33-40 A, Hold the thumb forceps in a balanced grip similar to the precision grip described earlier, and "palm" it into the hand, leaving the thumb and index and middle fingers free for other tasks. **B,** Ringed instruments can also be palmed to free the fingers for other tasks. One ring is held on the second interphalangeal segment of the ring finger and is supported in place by the fifth finger. The instrument is flipped into position, and the thumb is inserted into the ring for use.

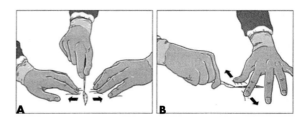

Figure 33-41 Traction placed onto both sides of the incision and during dissection allows visualization of underlying structures and the application of less force to cleave through tissue. **A,** Two-handed traction during abdominal incision. **B,** One-handed traction.

hand to free the fingers for other tasks (Figure 33-40). This maneuver eliminates the need to frequently regrasp the same instrument if a task such as suctioning blood from the field requires attention for a brief moment.

Traction

Surgical exposure requires the judicious use of tissue traction. Not to be confused with retraction, tissue traction allows continuous exposure of underlying structures during the cleavage of tissues with scissors, scalpel, forceps, or electrocautery by gentle pulling of joined tissues in opposite directions. The initial use of traction occurs during the skin incision, as the surgeon or assistant uses the scalpel to divide the skin. Both the surgeon and the assistant pull on opposite sides of a line created by the scalpel to spread the tissue as it is cleaved (Figure 33-41, *A*). Alternatively, a finger can be placed on either side of the incision to be made by the scalpel, if the incision is being accomplished without assistance (Figure 33-41, *B*). Forceful traction, however, can cause immense harm by

injuring delicate nerves, tearing arteries and veins, and causing uncontrolled hemorrhage, or by tearing organs, particularly the liver and spleen.

Dissection

Tissue dissection should always follow anatomical planes when possible, many of which are defined by the surrounding loose areolar tissues. Gentle traction helps separate and expose structures so less force may be needed during *sharp* dissection with the scissors or scalpel. In addition to opening and closing scissors blades to cut tissues, long cuts can be accomplished by enclosing fascial tissues into the crotch of the partially open blades of a pair of scissors and pushing the scissors along the intended cut without further moving of the blades. This is particularly helpful when dissecting adventitia away from arteries and veins. The closed blades can also be pushed gently into tissue planes, gently spread, and then removed to dissect with minimal trauma. The closed blades can be gently used to elevate structures before dividing them. A cardinal rule for surgeons and assistants alike is this: *Never dissect or cut tissue that cannot be seen.* Experienced surgeons understand that this maneuver is very dangerous and that use of knowledge, judgment, and extreme caution is needed.

Blunt dissection, less refined and controlled, is accomplished with instruments that are not considered sharp. It can be useful for separating sheets of loose areolar tissue but should be confined to places where vessel, nerve, or organ tearing is unlikely.

Dissection is truly learned through experience, which has no substitute.

POSTOPERATIVE CARE

With normal postoperative recovery, the patient should demonstrate each day objective evidence of improvement, and postoperative care is directed toward promoting healing and resuming the normal ADLs. The goals of postoperative care are to anticipate and avoid common problems and to discover problems early so prompt intervention can prevent serious complications. Because the realm of postoperative complications is broad, a cursory overview is provided here to guide the student toward further learning.

Postoperative Notes

All postoperative patients should be evaluated soon after surgery. These checks are an excellent opportunity for a student to learn how a postoperative patient should look and are the times at which many acute postoperative problems are detected (see following Box).

POSTOPERATIVE CHECK

To be made after the patient leaves the recovery room and before the PA leaves for the day.
- Time and date
- Vital signs
- Verbalized complaints, if any
- Physical findings
  Neurological (alertness, any gross deficits)
  Lungs
  Heart
  Abdomen (be extremely gentle after abdominal operation)
  Incision/dressing (do not remove dressings unless severe bleeding is noted)
  Extremities (lesions, swelling)
- I/O (urine output, emesis, NG and drain output)
- Postoperative laboratory findings or other diagnostic studies
- Assessment
- Treatment plan

The first postoperative note documents how well the patient has done since leaving the OR. Subsequent notes document the patient's recovery process and response to treatment. The first note includes the patient's subjective comments, mental status, and vital signs, a note on hemodynamic stability, IV fluid volume infused since surgery, oral intake if any, urinary and drain outputs per hour or per 8-hour shift, current medications, ventilator settings, and so forth. It should also include results of a relevant problem-oriented PE. The assessment of the patient's status is noted in the chart, as are therapeutic plans until the next evaluation.

Morning Rounds

A PA surgical assistant's day begins early, with evaluation of assigned patients *before* the surgical team meets for formal morning rounds. The nursing staff that follows the patient through the night should be consulted often and should be encouraged to discuss their assessment of the patient's progress. A clipboard, personal digital assistant (PDA), or index card system can help maintain an updated log on each patient's serial laboratory findings and serum drug levels, radiological and diagnostic evaluations, vital signs and daily weights, and intake and output records. A reliable system will help alert the team to any abnormal trends. The team should know the medications and dosages of each patient, including the number of days the patient has been taking critical medications such as antibiotics.

Formal rounds involve seeing the patients with the rest of the team. The previous day's notes should be reread, and the PA or PA student should anticipate questions from the attending, residents, or intern, which could range from "What were the patient's intake and output?" to "What are the most common etiologies of this patient's disease process?" A textbook is a good source for gaining understanding of the patient's disease and should be read as soon as the patient is assigned to the team and a free moment occurs in the PA student's schedule.

Present the patient to the team with the following information: name, number of days after operation, procedure performed, important co-morbid diseases, the overnight course, vital signs, input and output

(I&O), pertinent lab and x-ray data, and weight (noting any change up or down). A list of the pertinent positive findings on PE, any problems noted, and what should be done for the patient that day, such as advancing the diet, removing tubes, ordering laboratory or radiological studies, discharge, and preoperative preparation, should be compiled. The presentation should be concise.

The orders and notes may have been written or will need writing after rounds. Postoperative chart documentation is an important part of the medical legal record (Table 33-3). Surgeons are prone to writing abbreviated notes to save time. Brevity may be efficient for charting in surgery, but remember that all patient complaints need to be fully evaluated and documented in the chart.

Postoperative notes (aside from the brief note written for the first postoperative check) or daily progress notes always contain two important accounting dates at the top of each note: the number of days since surgery (POD; day 1 is the day *after* surgery), and the number of days of antibiotic therapy and the names of antibiotics (see Box at right). Patient status after whichever procedure (status post or "S/P") follows. The postoperative note follows the typical SOAP format described in other chapters and briefly reviewed here. Emphasis should be given to the patient's pain control, diet, nausea or vomiting, bowel function, ambulatory status, and vital signs, which can all be used as indicators of the patient's progress.

SOAP Format for Postoperative Notes

Subjective Patient comments may include passing flatus, eating well/ready to eat, nauseated, pain medications insufficient, feel good, feel bad, and so forth. The note should always include patient complaints. The examiner should also include any subjective observations of the patient; for instance, "Looks better."

Observation The vital signs, total I&O (which includes an accurate accounting of oral intake), IV fluids, medications, drains, urine and stool, and daily weight should be recorded.

Record a general description of the patient (e.g., awake and alert, intubated, in bed, sedated).

CONTENTS OF POSTOPERATIVE (DAILY PROGRESS) NOTE

POSTOPERATIVE DAY (POD) # X; TYPE OF ANTIBIOTIC(S) AND NUMBER OF DAYS PATIENT HAS RECEIVED THEM

S(ubjective)
- Patient comments (include all complaints)
- Family and allied health observations
- General observations, e.g., "Looks better"

O(bservation)
- Vital signs
- Daily weight
- General
- I&Os
  - Oral
  - Drains
  - IVF
  - NG tube
  - Urine (since surgery if immediately postoperative; otherwise, per 24 hours)
- Important medications
- Laboratory test results
- X-ray findings
- Other (ventilation/pacemaker settings, etc., as applicable)
- Physical findings (mental status, surgical site, heart, lungs, abdomen, extremities, other as needed)

A(ssessment)
- How is the patient progressing? Any complications? Recommendations from consultants?

P(lan)
- What should be done for the patient (stop IV, increase dietary level, increase ambulation, dressing change, etc.)?

The PE consists of auscultation of the heart and lungs and palpation of the abdomen. The extremities should also be checked for signs of DVT. The operative site and wound should be observed under aseptic or sterile conditions. The appearance of the wound (erythematous, dry, presence of bleeding or exudate,

Table 33-3	Charting Tips
Purpose of chart notes	Daily checklist for writer Communication with other members of team Communication with other health care teams Documentation for historical reference
Important items to include	Legal document Give laboratory, x-ray, and other results in objective section, and use the assessment section to say whether values are normal, abnormal, etc. Date and time of EVERY note and order Signature; printed last name; title of writer; pager number may be useful to nursing staff Co-signature for student notes and orders

Important items to exclude	1. Editorial comments
	  a. Would you want the patient to read what you have written?
	  b. Would you want it read out loud in court?
	2. Use of "VSS" (vital signs stable) or "stable" is not good documentation of patient status
	3. Any mention of exact discharge date. Instead say "Discharge when..." *or* "Discharge if..."

intactness of staples or sutures) should be recorded. All IV lines, tubes, and drains should be examined for signs of infection. The patient's mental status should also be noted (e.g., awake, confused, easily aroused).

Laboratory and other *diagnostic test results* are also reported here.

Assessment   A number of terms and phrases can be used to describe the patient's progress through recovery—stable, improved, worse, nauseated, pain well managed, diet progressing adequately; IV fluid volume and urine output are sufficient. All the patient's complaints should be addressed here as well, and conclusions should be drawn as to what may be the cause of each complaint. Evidence must be provided for any conclusions.

Plan   Actions or investigations needed to address any patient complaints are recorded here. Questions and suggestions for plans should be part of the verbal presentation to the team. However, no changes should be made until a senior team member has cleared the new orders.

Daily Considerations in Patient Care

Basic questions that need to be answered each day concerning the patient are as follows:

➤ Can the dietary level be advanced? Most patients proceed from nothing by mouth (NPO) to clear liquids to regular diet. Feeding usually resumes once the patient has bowel sounds, is passing flatus or has bowel movements, and mentions being hungry.

➤ Can the patient ambulate? Get up to sit in a chair? Use the bathroom or shower?

➤ Can any of the IV medications be given by mouth or stopped entirely?

➤ Can oxygen therapy be cut back or discontinued?

➤ Can any tubes be removed? NG tubes should be removed before feeding resumes. Urinary catheters are usually removed when accurate measurement of I&O is no longer necessary and the patient is able to take care of this function without assistance.

➤ Can the sutures or staples be removed?

➤ Can the drain(s) be removed? Wound drains are usually removed when the output is less then 30 mL per day.

➤ Are any laboratory, radiological, or other diagnostic studies needed?

➤ Does the patient need respiratory, physical, or occupational therapy?

➤ Does the patient need a social worker or discharge planner to help arrange home care after discharge?

Notes on Wound Care

The initial operative dressing or bandage should stay in place for 2 to 4 days. If blood continues to soak through a dressing, fever appears, or wound pain increases, the wound should be examined promptly. Circling the shape of blood soaking through the bandage and observing further spread can indicate how brisk the bleeding is.

Wounds that are left to heal by secondary intention should be packed with moist, isotonic saline–soaked gauze pads that are replaced every 8 hours. This process mechanically débrides the wound, allowing the removal of necrotic tissue and providing a clean bed for healing.

Common Postoperative Problems

There is no substitute for experience, but preparation and suspicion can assist in early detection of postoperative problems. PA students interested in surgery should find time during their surgical rotation, or should request a separate elective rotation, to care for patients in the surgical ICU. Encountering the spectrum and severity of SICU problems is an excellent means of learning about complex IV fluid infusion therapy, acid-base imbalance, electrolyte abnormalities, and physiological monitoring systems. It also provides an opportunity to better understand and practice the techniques and theory of pulmonary ventilation, polypharmacy, and insertion and monitoring of invasive lines and devices.

Postoperative complications can be divided into two categories—those occurring as a result of altered physiology and preexisting disease, and those created by the staff (iatrogenic). Complications can range from simple postoperative fever to bleeding and shock requiring resuscitation and reoperation.

Postoperative Fever   Fever is probably the most common postoperative dilemma the student will encounter on the surgical service. Fever is not normal in the postoperative patient, and any significantly elevated temperature must be evaluated. Febrile patients should receive a thorough PE, a chest x-ray, a urinalysis with culture and sensitivity, and a CBC with differential. Fever secondary to an infection or inflammation that is subsequently resolved by surgery (e.g., cholecystitis) should defervesce within several days after surgery. The patient with an oral temperature of 99.5° F probably can be watched for several hours in lieu of initiating a full diagnostic battery. However, high fever (>101.5° F [38.6° C]), tachycardia, decreased blood pressure, or diminished urinary output should be evaluated emergently by the senior staff and will require a full workup comprising the previously listed diagnostic tests with blood cultures to rule out sepsis.

Most postoperative fevers fall into the following etiological categories (the "Four Ws"): wind, wound, water, and walk.

Wind   Temperature elevations during the first 48 hours are usually of pulmonary origin. Thus, the value of the cough, deep breathing, and incentive spirometry exercises should be taught preoperatively to all patients undergoing major surgery. The lungs are predisposed to be a source of fever because of the following:

1. Hypoventilation from general endotracheal anesthesia or the effects of narcotics.
2. The tendency to avoid coughing, secondary to pain (of note with abdominal and chest incisions).
3. Simply sedation.

A chest radiograph is obtained to evaluate for pneumonia and atelectasis due to alveolar collapse. Purulent sputum should be sent to the laboratory for Gram's stain and culture and sensitivity testing, including anaerobe identification.

Atelectasis is treated by encouraging the patient to cough and take deep breaths and by the use of incentive spirometry. Early patient mobilization and ambulation with assistance from physical therapy also helps prevent postoperative fever from a pulmonary source. Pneumonia can occur at any time during the postoperative course and should always be a part of the differential diagnosis for fever.

Wound Wound infections, including intra-abdominal abscesses, usually declare themselves on the fourth through seventh postoperative days. In general, the sooner an infection manifests, the more virulent the pathogen and the more serious the sequelae. The dressing should be removed and the wound examined for purulent drainage, expanding erythema or induration, and, most importantly, increasing pain and tenderness at the operative site. The first indication of wound infection is increasing pain. Dark discoloration, blisters, and foul-smelling exudates are grim signs and should be evaluated by a senior team member. Removal of a single stitch or staple may allow the escape of trapped pus and introduction of a sterile swab into the wound to gently search for pockets of infection. Aerobic organisms cause most wound infections, but all exudates should be sent to the laboratory for aerobic and anaerobic microbial culture and sensitivity testing. Fungal infections occur, albeit rarely, and immunocompromised patients are at highest risk. Grossly infected wounds must be reopened and drained. Superficial infections may be managed with oral antibiotics after drainage, but most nosocomial infections demand parenteral antibiotics.

If no other source for a fever can be located, a CT scan or MRI may reveal the source. An intra-abdominal abscess may be difficult to diagnose. Abdominal trauma, undergoing a contaminated abdominal procedure (e.g., ruptured diverticulitis or appendix), a history of peritonitis, and the creation of an intestinal suture line (e.g., bowel resection with reanastomosis) are all potential sources of intra-abdominal abscess. CT-guided drainage or reoperation may be necessary.

Water Indwelling urinary catheters cause most UTIs. They rarely cause sepsis unless the upper tract is involved. Upper UTI can manifest as fever, chills, and flank pain. A urine sample should be sent for a urinalysis along with aerobic and anaerobic culture and for sensitivity testing. Patients may complain of dysuria or frequency after an indwelling catheter has been removed; however, the results of the urinalysis should guide treatment. Elderly patients may have had a UTI before admission; this is more prevalent in men with bladder outlet obstruction and urostasis secondary to prostatic hypertrophy. Such patients may

benefit from the insertion of a urinary catheter to drain the infected region.

Walk Deep vein thrombosis usually occurs around the 5th to 14th postoperative days. The best method of treating DVT and the subsequent catastrophic possibility of pulmonary embolism is prophylactic therapy through the use of intermittent external compression devices, gradient pressure leg stockings (see Figure 33-1), or pharmacological agents such as subcutaneous heparin or heparin analogs. The index of suspicion should always be high for this disease because the physical findings may be unreliable. The patient's leg may be tender, hot, edematous, or indurated, but more commonly, no abnormalities are noted. Homans' sign (pain in the calf when the foot is dorsiflexed) is rarely present.

The gold standard for diagnosis is the injection of radiopaque contrast material into a foot vein after application of a tourniquet on the proximal leg, which forces contrast material into the deep venous system. Complete blockage or irregularities of the normally smooth vein wall are diagnostic of DVT. Duplex scanning combines both Doppler and B-mode ultrasound imaging and is the quickest method by which to diagnose DVT. A positive duplex scan is grounds for instituting anticoagulation with heparin. Phlebography can be used to diagnose cases in which patients' results of duplex scans are equivocal. Patients with DVT should be considered for admission to the SICU for observation. All patients will require heparinization.

Other Causes of Fever Abrupt, high, spiking fevers should lead to the evaluation of existing indwelling devices. All intravascular devices can cause fever if they become infected. Heart valves, IV catheters, central venous catheters, arterial lines, pulmonary artery catheters, and NG tubes (which may cause sinusitis) can be sources of infection. The physical findings may be subtle (mild erythema or cellulitis at the catheter entry site) or completely nonexistent. Heart valves can be evaluated by echocardiography and blood culture; a cardiology consultation should be requested if an infected valve is possible. *The possibility that the fever is caused by one of these devices should be strongly considered when the blood culture yields* Staphylococcus aureus.

Treatment dictates that the device be removed, and that 7 to 10 days of antistaphylococcal antibiotic coverage be initiated. An infectious disease consult may be warranted. Fevers from Gram-negative infections usually defervesce quickly after removal of the foreign device, unless florid Gram-negative sepsis has developed.

Avoiding Iatrogenic Problems   *A final word on a practical topic.* Many postoperative problems occur as a result of forgetting of the organized routine in the rush of managing a busy surgical service. Iatrogenic complications are almost always preventable with forethought and the development of a system for approaching every patient and his or her management. It is beyond this discussion to consider all iatrogenic omissions in the detailed context they deserve. The student is encouraged to address the evaluation and treatment of common postoperative problems through reading one of the texts listed in the Resources list and by gaining experience under the guidance of a senior surgical mentor.

These are a few pearls of wisdom for avoiding the common pitfalls of routine postoperative care:

➤ Know the I&O status of each patient and the IV solution's base composition, additives, and rate. *Vascular volume overload from inappropriate or overaggressive IV therapy is preventable.*

➤ Potassium is easily lost through the urine, NG tube, diarrhea, or vomitus, and intravascular potassium can be diluted by IV fluid replacement. IV fluids should include potassium to account for those losses. Even mild hypokalemia can cause prolonged bowel immotility (ileus) or cardiac arrhythmias in patients receiving digitalis.

➤ Tubes should be removed promptly when no longer needed. UTIs often result from urinary catheters left in place too long.

➤ All intravascular devices, incisions, and wounds should be inspected daily.

➤ Early ambulation and mobilization should be encouraged.

➤ Medication dosages for elderly patients and patients with renal or liver failure should be titrated. Drug levels for aminoglycosides, vancomycin, or cardiopulmonary medications (e.g.,

digitalis, theophylline) should be monitored when appropriate.

➤ A thorough PE should be performed each day and with each call to evaluate a sick patient. Every attempt should be made to discover problems early in their evolution (e.g., congestive heart failure, sepsis, respiratory distress). Pulmonary embolism, myocardial infarction, or cerebrovascular accident should always be considered in patients with shortness of breath, chest pain, or unexplained hypotension.

CONCLUSION

The future of PAs in the health care arena is not only secure but expanding within all aspects of medicine, including new and existing roles in the surgical theater. The ingenuity and resourcefulness of individual PAs will shape and expand the existing roles for the surgical PA. This responsibility lies not only in the hands of the PA but also in the hands of the supervising physician and the institutions that employ surgical PAs. As teaching hospitals cut back on the numbers of residency slots in surgery and try to meet restrictions on the number of hours worked by residents each week, it is very conceivable that PAs will be expected to fill these vacant positions (see Box). PAs are well suited for these tasks, and with proper supervision and direction from the surgical house staff and faculty, the PA can make the transition from physician resident to PA house staff smooth and uncomplicated for both the institution and the surgical teams involved. The cost-effectiveness and excellence in patient care exhibited by PAs in all aspects of medicine have been repeatedly verified and are emphasized by the dramatic increase in applications to, and the number of, PA programs across the nation. PA education must meet this challenge by incorporating into the curriculum options for PA students in surgical education and allowing students some aspect of freedom in choosing their clinical experiences. There is a demonstrated need for PAs in surgical health care today, and the program curriculum that meets this need will stand at the forefront of PA education and provide a strong and viable future that is versatile enough to meet changing health care environment demands.

RESPONSIBILITIES OF THE PA STUDENT ON SURGICAL ROTATION

I. Give total care to each patient.
  A. Preoperative.
    1. Admission history and PE.
    2. Admission orders.
    3. Preoperative orders.
    4. Preoperative note.
    5. Insert IVs, tubes, or catheters, if asked.
  B. Perioperative.
    1. Accompany patient to OR; first-assist or second-assist at procedure.
    2. Operative note.
    3. Postoperative orders.
    4. Postoperative check.
  C. Postoperative.
    1. Daily patient care.
      a. Early morning evaluation, assessment, plans for day, orders.
      b. Morning rounds with patient progress reports.
      c. Accompany patient to diagnostic procedures when feasible.
      d. Perform diagnostic and therapeutic procedures when feasible (NG intubation, arterial blood gases, venipuncture for laboratory studies, venous catheterization, spinal tap, thoracentesis, etc.).
      e. Write daily progress notes.
      f. Quick afternoon assessment.
      g. Evening rounds with report of daily activities, laboratory results, diagnostic study results, etc.
      h. Check final pathology results (24-48 hours postoperatively).
      i. Speak with the patient's family.
    2. Assist with writing of discharge orders, prescriptions, and other discharge paperwork.
    3. Date and time on all notes and orders.
II. Read about the patient's specific disease processes and planned procedure before surgery.
III. Attend all rounds, conferences, and lectures pertaining to the surgical service and surgical rotation.
IV. Be the patients' and families' advocate. Find answers to their questions; do not be afraid to say, "I don't know, but I'll find out."
V. Ask questions.

CLINICAL APPLICATIONS

1. Identify the members of a typical surgical team and describe their functions.
2. Identify the members of a typical OR and recovery team and describe their functions.
3. Discuss the key elements of an admitting history and PE for a surgical patient.
4. Identify the elements and format of a preoperative and an operative note.
5. List three "rules" for maintaining the sterile field in the OR.
6. Identify the elements and format of a postoperative check and a postoperative daily progress note.
7. What do you think you would find personally challenging and rewarding about practice as a PA in surgery?

REFERENCES

1. 2001 AAPA Physician Assistant Census Report. Alexandria, VA: American Academy of Physician Assistants, 2001. Available at http://www.aapa.org/research/01census-intro.html.
2. American College of Surgeons. Statements on Principles. Qualification of the first assistant in the operating room.

Available at www.facs.org/fellows_info/statements/stonprin.html#2b.

3. Gerberding JL, Littell C, Tarkington A, et al. Risk of exposure of surgical personnel to patients' blood during surgery at San Francisco Hospital. N Engl J Med 1990;322:1788.

4. Wright JG, McGeer AJ, Chyatte D, Ransohoff DF. Mechanisms of glove tears and sharp injuries among surgical personnel. JAMA 1991;266:1668.

5. Quebbeman EJ, Telford GL, Hubbard S, et al. Risk of blood contamination and injury to operating room personnel. Ann Surg 1991;214:614.

6. Comaro A. Tiny holes, big surgery. Minimal surgery hurts less and scars less—but is it right for you? U.S. News and World Report, Volume 133, Issue 3, Section: America's Best Hospitals 2002, Special Report.

RESOURCES

Eubanks S, Swanstrom LL, Soper NJ, Eubanks WS. Mastery of Endoscopic and Laparoscopic Surgery. Philadelphia: Lippincott, Williams & Wilkins, 2000 (ISBN: 0316268658). *A complete textbook for those working in the minimally invasive surgical environment.*

Lederman RJ. Tarascon Internal Medicine & Critical Care Pocketbook, 2nd ed. Tarascon Press, 2000 (ISBN: 1882742206). *The newly updated Tarascon Internal Medicine & Critical Care Pocketbook, 2nd edition, is a concise pocket guide with quickly identifiable clinical information.*

Zollinger RM. Atlas of Surgical Operations. New York: McGraw-Hill, 2002 (ISBN 0071363785). *One of the best "how-to" general surgery atlases with clear line drawings of many common general surgical procedures. Probably not an affordable student purchase but should be regularly consulted in the medical library before one assists with general surgery cases.*

Doherty GM, Meko JB, Olson JA. The Washington Manual of Surgery (CD-ROM for PDA), 3rd ed. Philadelphia: Lippincott, Williams & Wilkins, 2002 (ISBN 0781738776). *Practical hands-on reference for general surgical patient care.*

Blackbourne L. Surgical Recall, 3rd ed. Philadelphia: Lippincott, Williams & Wilkins, 2002 (ISBN 0781729734). *Good study book for rounds and conferences.*

Cameron JL. Current Surgical Therapy, 7th ed. Chicago: Mosby, 2001 (ISBN: 0323014283). *Another comprehensive clinical textbook of surgery well worth acquiring as a general reference work.*

Clary BM, Milano CA. The Handbook of Surgical Intensive Care: Practices of the Surgical Residents at Duke University Medical Center, 5th ed. Chicago: Mosby, 2000 (ISBN: 0323011063). *An excellent pocket reference for patient care in the surgical ICU.*

Gomella LG, Lefor AT. Surgery on Call, 3rd ed. New York: Appleton & Lange, 2001 (ISBN: 0838588174). *Handy book to have on rounds on the floors, in the critical care unit, and in the emergency department. A practical pocket guide to specific inpatient surgical problems.*

Deitch EA, Fisher HR. Tools of the Trade and Rules of the Road: A Surgical Guide. Philadelphia: Lippincott Williams & Wilkins, 1997 (ISBN: 0397513933). *This practical, portable handbook is designed to teach surgical residents the basic tasks they are often not formally taught, but are expected to know.*

Schwartz SI, Galloway AC, Shires GT. Principles of Surgery, 7th ed. New York: McGraw-Hill, 1998 (ISBN: 007912318X). *One of the most definitive surgery texts covering plastic through vascular surgery. It has several companion handbooks and review texts that facilitate studies for examinations and the PA certification examination.*

Ethicon Knot tying Manual. Available at http://www.jnjgateway.com/public/USENG/ 5256ETHICON_Encyclopedia_of_Knots.pdf. *A web site pdf file containing an e-text on sutures and knot-tying.*

U.S. Surgical Davis and Geck Knot Tying Manual. Available at http://www.ussdgsutures.com/knot-tying/index.html. *A web site pdf file containing an e-text on sutures and knot-tying.*

CHAPTER 34

Orthopedics

Patrick Auth

INTRODUCTION

Orthopedics is the surgical specialty dealing with musculoskeletal disorders, including trauma. Physician assistants (PAs) who work in orthopedic surgery appreciate the mixture of office-based practice and the opportunity to participate in surgical procedures. PAs with backgrounds as athletic trainers or physical therapist assistants find orthopedic practice a particularly appealing employment niche. This chapter explores the utilization of PAs in orthopedics, presents an overview of the approach to the orthopedic patient, reviews selected common problems, and discusses the challenges and rewards of orthopedics for PAs.

PAs IN ORTHOPEDICS

According to the 2001 Census of the American Academy of Physician Assistants, 8.2% of PAs

nationwide work in orthopedic surgery, compared with 48.5% in primary care.[1] Orthopedics is the largest of the surgical subspecialties, employing almost twice as many PAs as the next most frequent choice—cardiovascular surgery—which employs 4.4% of PAs nationwide.

The utilization of PAs in orthopedic surgery is increasing, by both percentage of the job market and absolute numbers. Compared with 1998, when 921 PAs (6.9%) worked in orthopedics, 1416 PAs (8.2%) were employed in orthopedics in 2001.[1,2] By comparison, during the same period, PAs in cardiovascular surgery retained the same segment of national employment—4.4%—although the number of PAs increased from 588 in 1998 to 760 in 2001.

Orthopedic PA roles vary from strictly office-based to primarily hospital-based, although the most typical role includes both outpatient and inpatient responsibilities. In the office, PAs evaluate patients and initiate treatment, including splints, casts and other orthopedic devices. Typical outpatient problems include activity-related injuries, degenerative or chronic use conditions, and follow-up after surgical procedures. Orthopedic PAs may first-assist at surgery and may follow orthopedic patients through the course of their hospitalizations.

The foundation of evaluating any patient with an orthopedic problem is the history and physical examination because these result in the diagnosis of up to 90% of orthopedic conditions. The core competencies of orthopedic history, musculoskeletal physical examination, and special orthopedic tests are discussed in the following sections.

ORTHOPEDIC HISTORY

A thorough and accurate orthopedic history provides the necessary information for the clinician to make an accurate preliminary diagnosis. Physician assistants use the orthopedic history for important information about the disorder, its prognosis, and treatment.

The orthopedic history includes the following[3,4]:

➤ The patient's age and lifestyle.
➤ Work history.
➤ Sports and training habits.
➤ Hobbies.
➤ Dominant hand.
➤ Past joint disorders.
➤ Past medical history, including previous injuries, surgeries, and treatments.
➤ Current medications and allergies.

The chief complaint must be thoroughly explored according to the PQRST format. The following questions also provide invaluable information in the diagnosis of orthopedic conditions[3,4]:

➤ *What is the patient's age?* Many orthopedic conditions are age-related. For example, congenital hip dysplasia, Osgood-Schlatter, and Legg-Calvé-Perthes are diseases known to occur in a younger patient population. Arthritic conditions such as degenerative joint disease and osteoarthritis are noted more often in an older patient population.
➤ *What is the occupation of the patient?* Occupations that involve repetitive activities such as lifting, typing, reaching, grasping, and pulling predispose the joints and spine to injuries. As a result of poor body mechanics and repetitive use, muscles and joints become overstressed, which can result in overuse injuries such as carpal tunnel syndrome, low back sprain/strains, rotator cuff tendonitis, and DeQuervain's tenosynovitis.

➤ *What was the patient doing at the time pain first started?* Information surrounding the onset of the pain helps the physician assistant understand the mechanism of injury and if there was a specific episode in which a body part was injured.

➤ *Has the patient experienced the pain before?* An answer to this question helps the physician assistant determine if this is a new or recurrent injury. If the pain is recurrent, the PA will explore the site of the original pain and radiation, duration and frequency of the symptoms, previous diagnostic studies, recovery time, and treatment that alleviated the symptoms. This information will help the PA determine if the condition is acute or chronic and allows assessment of the patient's tolerance to pain.

➤ *Is the pain associated with activities, rest, time of day, and posture?* Insidious onset of morning pain, fatigue, and polyarthritis is associated with rheumatoid arthritis. Peripheral nerve entrapments and thoracic outlet syndrome are typically worse at night. Chronic pain is often associated with posture, fatigue, and activity. Pain in only one joint suggests bursitis, tendonitis, or injury.

➤ *Is the pain associated with symptoms elsewhere in the body?* A butterfly rash on the cheek is associated with systemic lupus erythematosus. A scaly rash and pitted nails of psoriasis are associated with psoriatic arthritis, and red, burning, and itchy eyes are associated with Reiter's syndrome.

➤ *How does the patient describe the pain?* Muscle pain is typically dull and aching, aggravated by a particular joint or spine range of motion; nerve pain is sharp and burning and radiates in a specific nerve distribution. Bone pain is described as deep and boring. Vascular pain is diffuse and aching and is referred to other parts of the body.

➤ *Does the patient experience a "locking," "clicking," or "giving way," or a "pop" or "shift" in the joint?* A history of "locking" or "clicking" sensation is associated with a meniscal tear or loose body. A history of "giving way" is associated with a patellar dislocation, and "pop" or "shift" is associated with a cruciate or collateral ligament knee rupture.

➤ *Is the patient experiencing any life, work/school-related, or economic stressors?* Job security, academic issues, and martial and financial problems can all contribute to increasing pain because of psychological stress.

MUSCULOSKELETAL PHYSICAL EXAMINATION

The musculoskeletal physical examination is similar to the evaluation of other organ systems. The examination is systematic and includes inspection, palpation of bony landmarks, assessment of range of motion, muscle testing, sensory evaluation, and special maneuvers.

During inspection, the physician assistant looks for symmetry of joints, joint deformities, or malalignment of bones. During inspection and palpation, the joint, surrounding tissues, and bony landmarks are assessed for swelling, ecchymosis, muscular atrophy, skin changes, subcutaneous nodules, and crepitus, which is an audible and/or palpable crunching during movement of tendons or ligaments over bone.[5]

The next step in the physical examination is to assess the range of motion of the joint so as to demonstrate limitations in range of motion or increased mobility and joint instability from ligamentous laxity. Measuring joint motion provides an index for limitations, as well as important information concerning the results of treatment.[5]

Muscle testing provides a semiquantitative measurement of muscle strength (Table 34-1). A sensory evaluation must be done if the patient presents with a motor and/or sensory deficit. Evaluation of peripheral nerves is outlined in Table 34-2.

SPECIAL ORTHOPEDIC TESTS

Once the physician assistant has completed the history and physical examination, special orthopedic tests can be performed to assess a disease or condition in a particular joint. The results of orthopedic test(s) are used in combination with a thorough history, physical examination, and diagnostic studies to arrive at a diagnosis. Table 34-3 lists some of the more common orthopedic tests.[5,6]

COMMON ORTHOPEDIC PROBLEMS

This section of the chapter addresses selected common orthopedic problems, with discussion of typical patient presentation, preferred diagnostic studies, treatment goals, and approach to treatment.

Shoulder

Impingement Syndrome An impingement syndrome results from compression of the rotator cuff tendons and the subacromial bursa between the

---

Table 34-1   Grading of Manual Muscle Testing

Numeric Grade	Descriptive Grade	Description
5	Normal	Complete range of motion against gravity with full or normal resistance
4	Good	Complete range of motion against gravity with some resistance
3	Fair	Complete range of motion against gravity
2	Poor	Complete range of motion with gravity eliminated
1	Trace	Muscle contraction but no or very limited joint motion
0	Zero	No evidence of muscle function

From American Academy of Orthopaedic Surgeons. *Essentials of Musculoskeletal Care*, Section 1, General Orthopaedics, Table 1.

Table 34-2   Evaluation of Peripheral Nerves

Nerve	Muscle	Sensory
UPPER EXTREMITY		
Axillary	Deltoid shoulder abduction	Lateral aspect of arm
Musculocutaneous	Biceps-elbow flexion	Lateral proximal forearm
Median	Flexor pollicis longus–thumb flexion	Tip of thumb, volar aspect
Ulnar	First dorsal interosseous abduction	Tip of little finger, volar aspect
Radial	Extensor pollicis longus–thumb extension	Dorsum of thumb web space
LOWER EXTREMITY		
Obturator	Adductors-hip adduction	Medial aspect, midthigh
Femoral	Quadriceps-knee extension	Proximal to medial malleolus
Peroneal		
Deep branch	Extensor hallucis longus–great toe extension	Dorsum of first web space
Superficial branch	Peroneus brevis–foot eversion	Dorsum of lateral foot
Tibial	Flexor hallucis longus–great toe flexion	Plantar aspect of foot

From American Academy of Orthopaedic Surgeons. Essentials of Musculoskeletal Care, Section 1, General Orthopaedics, Table 42.

greater tubercle of the humeral head and the undersurface of the acromial process.[7] The patient's symptoms include shoulder pain aggravated by overhead motions and/or inability to move the shoulder because of pain. The hallmark physical examination finding is pain reproduced by the painful arc maneuver.[8] There is also subacromial tenderness and a positive impingement test, and no physical examination signs of tendon inflammation. Magnetic resonance imaging (MRI) is indicated for chronic cases to rule out a rotator cuff tear. Treatment goals include increasing the subacromial space to reduce the degree of impingement and prevent the development of tendonitis and tendon rupture. Pendulum stretching exercise combined with prescription of a nonsteroidal anti-inflammatory drug (NSAID), restrictions on overhead reaching and positioning, and physical therapy for toning exercise are the treatments of choice.[8,9]

Biceps Tendonitis   Biceps tendonitis refers to inflammation of the long head of the tendon as it passes through the bicipital groove of the anterior humerus. The patient reports shoulder pain aggravated by lifting or overhead reaching. Physical examination reveals local tenderness in the bicep groove,

pain aggravated by flexion of the elbow isometrically, positive Yergason's test, and a painful arc maneuver.[7] MRI is indicated if concurrent rotator cuff tendon tear is suggested by examination. The treatment goal is to reduce inflammation and swelling in the bicep tendon through restriction of lifting and reaching, application of ice, phonophoresis, weighted pendulum stretching, and toning exercise for the short heat biceps and brachioradialis tendon.

Glenohumeral Osteoarthritis   Glenohumeral osteoarthritis is wear and tear of the articular cartilage of the glenoid labrum and humeral head. It is often preceded by trauma. Injuries associated with the development of osteoarthritis include rotator cuff tear, shoulder dislocation, humeral fracture, and rheumatoid arthritis. The patient complains of gradual onset of shoulder pain and stiffness. Physical examination reveals local tenderness under the coracoid process, restricted abduction and external rotation range of motion, crepitation with range of motion, swelling of the infraclavicular fossa, and/or general fullness to the shoulder. Radiographs reveal osteophyte formation at the inferior humeral head, flattening and sclerosis of the humeral head, narrowing of the articular

Table 34-3   Common Orthopedic Tests

Structure Tested	Orthopedic Test	Procedure	Rationale
Cervical spine	Foraminal compression (Spurling's test)	Patient bends head to one side; examiner carefully presses straight down on the head.	Pain that radiates into the arm toward which the head is flexed during compression indicates pressure on a nerve root.
	Valsalva maneuver	Patient seated, instruct patient to bear down as if moving his bowels.	Localized pain of the spine indicates a space-occupying lesion (herniated disk protrusion, tumor).
	Jackson's compression test	The patient rotates the head to one side; examiner exerts downward pressure on the head. Performed bilaterally.	The test is positive if on testing, pain radiates into the arm, which is indicative of pressure on the nerve root.
Shoulder	Adson's maneuver	Patient seated, establish radial pulse, instruct patient to rotate head and elevate chin to the side being tested. Examiner laterally rotates and extends patient's shoulder. Patient instructed to take a deep breath and hold it.	Decrease or absence of the radial pulse—a positive test for thoracic outlet syndrome.
	Yergason's test	Patient's elbow flexed to 90 degrees and stabilized, against the thorax, forearm pronated. Examiner resists supination, while the patient also laterally rotates the arm against resistance.	Tenderness of the bicipital groove, or tendon may pop out of the groove—indicative of bicipital tendonitis.
	Impingement test	Patient's arm is forcibly elevated through forward flexion by the examiner.	The patient's face shows pain, reflecting a positive test result. This is indicative of overuse of the supraspinatus muscles.
Elbow	Cozen's test	Patient seated, examiner stabilizes the patient's forearm. Patient is instructed to make a fist and extend it. Examiner forces extended arm into flexion against resistance.	Pain in the area of the lateral epicondyle—indicative of lateral epicondylitis.
	Golfer's elbow	Examiner palpates the patient's medial epicondyle, the patient's forearm is supinated, and the elbow and wrist are extended by the examiner.	Pain in the area of the medial epicondyle—indicative of medial epicondylitis.

Continued

Table 34-3   Common Orthopedic Tests—cont'd

Structure Tested	Orthopedic Test	Procedure	Rationale
Elbow—cont'd	Tinel's sign	Patient seated, examiner taps the groove between the olecranon process and the medial epicondyle with a reflex hammer.	Tingling sensation in the ulnar nerve distribution is a positive sign—indicates neuritis or neuroma of the ulnar nerve.
Wrist	Tinel's sign	Examiner taps over the palmar surface of the wrist.	Paresthesia in the median nerve distribution—indicative of carpal tunnel syndrome.
	Phalen's test	Examiner flexes the patient's wrists and holds this position for 1 minute.	Paresthesias in the median nerve distribution—indicative of carpal tunnel syndrome.
	Finkelstein's test	Patient instructed to make a fist with the thumb across the palmar surface of the hand and then to stress the wrist ulnarward.	Pain distal to the styloid process of the radius—indicative of DeQuervain's disease.
Hip	Ortolani's click test	Pediatric patient is supine, examiner grasps both thighs, thumbs on the lesser trochanters, and flexes and abducts the thighs bilaterally.	A palpable and/or audible click—positive signs for a displacement of the femoral head into or out of the acetabular cavity.
	Patrick's test (Faber)	Patient is supine, the examiner places the patient's test foot and leg on top of the knee of the opposite leg; the examiner lowers the test in abduction.	A positive test is indicated by the test leg's remaining above the opposite leg—indicative of hip disease.
	Trendelenburg's test	Patient is standing, the examiner grasps the patient's waist and places his thumbs on the posterior superior iliac spine on each ilium. The examiner instructs the patient to flex one leg at a time.	This test assesses the stability of the hip and the ability of the hip abductors to stabilize the pelvis on the femur. If the posterior superior iliac spine of either side fails to rise when the leg is flexed indicative of a weak gluteus medius on the opposite side of flexion.
Lumbar spine	Straight leg raising test	Patient is supine, examiner raises the patient's leg to point of pain or 90 degrees, drops the leg slightly until there is no pain; examiner then dorsiflexes the patient's foot.	Radiating pain with ankle dorsiflexion—stretching of the dura mater of the spinal cord (disk lesion, sciatic).

Table 34-3   Common Orthopedic Tests—cont'd

Structure Tested	Orthopedic Test	Procedure	Rationale
Lumbar spine —cont'd	Yeoman's test	Patient prone, the examiner stabilizes the pelvis and flexes the patient's leg and extends the thigh.	Deep sacroiliac pain indicates a sprain of the anterior sacroiliac ligaments; lumbar pain indicates lumbar involvement.
	Bowstring test	Patient supine, examiner places the patient's leg atop of his shoulder. Firm pressure from the examiner's thumb is applied to the popliteal area.	Pain in the lumbar region or radiculopathy—indicative of tension or pressure on the sciatic nerve.
Knee	McMurray's test	Patient supine, knee flexed at 90 degrees, examiner externally rotates the leg as examiners extend the leg; repeat for internal rotation.	A palpable or audible click— indicative of a meniscal tear.
	Anterior/posterior drawer sign	Patient supine, hip flexed to 45 degrees, knee flexed to 90 degrees, patient's foot on table held in place with examiner sitting on the foot; examiner grasps behind flexed knee and exerts pulling and pushing pressure on the leg.	Gapping when the leg is pulled is indicative of anterior cruciate ligament laxity; gapping when the leg is pushed is indicative of posterior cruciate ligament laxity.
	Abduction (valgus stress) and adduction (varus stress) tests	Patient is in supine position, examiner applies valgus stress at the knee, ankle is stabilized in slight lateral rotation; repeat with examiner applying varus stress.	Laxity with valgus stress is indicative of medial collateral ligament instability; laxity with varus stress is indicative of lateral collateral ligament instability.
Ankle	Anterior drawer sign	Patient supine, examiner grasps the foot and exerts a pulling and pressure on talus; tibia and fibula are stabilized with examiner's hand.	Laxity when the tibia is pushed is indicative of anterior talofibular ligament instability. Laxity when the tibia is pulled is indicative of posterior talofibular ligament tear.
	Tinel's sign	Examiner taps over the posterior tibial nerve.	Paresthesias radiating to the foot—indicative of tarsal tunnel syndrome.
	Lateral and medial stability test	Patient in supine position, examiner grasps the patient's foot and passively inverts; repeat with eversion.	Laxity with inversion indicative of anterior talofibular and/or calcaneofibular ligament instability; laxity with eversion indicative of deltoid ligament instability.

cartilage, irregularities at the inferior glenoid fossa, and spurring of the humeral head. Treatment combines exercise to improve range of motion and muscular support with ice applications and the use of an NSAID to reduce the inflammation.

Elbow

Olecranon Bursitis
Olecranon bursitis is inflammation of the bursal sac located between the olecranon process of the ulna and the overlying skin. Most cases are caused by repetitive trauma in the form of pressure.[7] The patient complains of pain and swelling behind the elbow. Physical examination reveals swelling, heat, and redness over the olecranon process, but range of motion is not affected. Diagnosis is confirmed by bursal fluid analysis to differentiate acute traumatic bursitis from gout and infection. The goals of treatment are to reduce swelling and inflammation and to prevent chronic bursitis. Treatment includes aspiration, drainage, and laboratory analysis of bursa fluid, neoprene elbow sleeve, corticosteroid injection, and antibiotics for infection.

Wrist

DeQuervain's Tenosynovitis
DeQuervain's tenosynovitis is an inflammation of the extensor and flexor tendons of the thumb. The tenosynovitis develops as a result of repetitive or unaccustomed use of the thumb (gripping and grasping), which leads to friction of the tendons as they pass over distal radial styloid. The patient complains of wrist pain and difficulty with grasping. Physical examination reveals tenderness and swelling at the radial styloid process; inflammation and swelling of the extensor pollicis longus, extensor pollicis brevis, and abductor pollicis longus tendons; and decreased range of motion of the thumb. Tenderness is noted over the distal portion of the radial styloid; pain is aggravated by resisting thumb extension and abduction and by a positive Finkelstein's maneuver. Treatment goals include reducing inflammation in the tenosynovial sac, thereby preventing adhesions from forming and tendonitis from recurring. Treatment includes a thumb spica splint, physical therapy (ice, phonophoresis with hydrocortisone gel, stretching exercises), and NSAIDs. Corticosteroid injections may be indicated for patients experiencing symptoms for longer than 6 weeks.[7,10]

Carpal Tunnel Syndrome
Carpal tunnel syndrome is a neuropathy of the median nerve that results from compression under the transverse carpal ligament at the wrist. The patient complains of a loss of sensation in the median nerve distribution (thumb, index, and medial one half of the long fingers). Physical examination reveals decreased sensation (light touch, sharp/dull) of the median nerve distribution, a positive Tinel's sign, and a positive Phalen sign. Thenar muscle atrophy is a late finding. The nerve conduction velocity test is the test of choice to confirm median nerve compression. The goal of treatment is to reduce compression of the median nerve and prevent recurrence of carpal tunnel syndrome through improved ergonomics. The treatment includes wrist splint, reduce repetitive wrist motion, NSAIDs, ergonomics, physical therapy (stretching exercises for the flexor tendons), and corticosteroid injection. Surgical release is considered if motor symptoms have developed or symptoms fail to improve.[7]

▓▓ CASE STUDY 34-1

History
A 44-year-old female secretary presents to the primary care office with an 8-week history of increasing right hand pain. The pain is associated with numbness of the right thumb and index and long fingers, and is worse after an 8-hour day at work. The patient reports that she frequently drops objects and is having difficulty opening doors with her right hand. Recently, the patient has awakened at night with the numbness and needs to shake her hand to get relief from the numbness.

Physical examination
The patient is right hand dominant.

Inspection: Hand reveals no thenar atrophy, skin is warm and moist.

Sensation: Decreased sensation to light touch of the median nerve distribution of the hand. Two-point discrimination and vibratory sensation of the hands are intact bilaterally.

Motor: Thumb opposition against resistance reveals no weakness of the thenar muscles.

Peripheral pulses: radial, ulnar, and brachial pulses are strong and equal bilaterally.

Special tests: Positive Phalen and Tinel's tests.

Diagnostic tests

Radiographs of the wrist are normal. Electromyogram (EMG) and nerve conduction velocity (NCV) studies confirm carpal tunnel syndrome.

Diagnosis

Carpal tunnel syndrome.

Treatment

Carpal tunnel syndrome is the most common compression neuropathy in the upper extremity; it affects adults of all ages, women more than men. It is common during the last trimester of pregnancy and often resolves after childbirth. When associated with distal radius fractures, it must be recognized and treated emergently with carpal tunnel release. In this case, the patient should be treated conservatively with splinting of the wrist in neutral position, a course of NSAIDs, and avoidance of repetitive activities of the right hand and wrist. The patient should wear the splint all day and while sleeping. Work-related carpal tunnel may be improved with ergonomic modifications, such as using keyboard supports and antivibration padded gloves, repositioning the wrist at the keyboard or assembly line, and avoiding holding the wrist in a flex position. Corticosteroid injection into the carpal ligament is used as an adjunct treatment. Decompressive surgery is considered with persistent hand pain that does not resolve with nocturnal splinting, when conservative therapy fails, or with rapidly developing motor or sensory deficits.

Dorsal Ganglion Dorsal ganglion is an overproduction of synovial or tenosynovial fluid and its accumulation into the subcutaneous tissue from abnormalities in the wrist or the extensor tendon sheath. The patient complains of a painless lump at the wrist. Physical examination reveals a highly mobile, fluctuant cyst overlying the wrist, with minimal tenderness and full range of motion of the wrist. The goals of treatment are to reassure the patient that it is not cancer, and then to aspirate the cyst to prevent recurrence. Treatment includes aspiration, reassurance and education of the patient, a wrist brace to limit repetitive motions, and surgical excision of the cyst and sinus if treatment is refractory.[7]

Hand

Trigger Finger Trigger finger is an inflammation of the flexor tendons of the finger as they cross the metacarpophalangeal (MCP) head in the palm. As a result of repetitive gripping, pressure over the palm causes swelling and inflammation of the flexor tendons. As the swelling and inflammation increase, the flexor tendons lose their smooth motion under the A1 pulley, the specialized ligament that anchors the tendon to the bone. The patient complains of a painful finger and a loss of smooth motion of the finger when gripping.[11] Physical examination reveals tenderness at the base of the finger, increased pain with tendon extension, and clicking or locking with active flexion of the proximal interphalangeal (PIP) joint (fingers) and the interphalangeal (IP) joint (thumb). Treatment goals involve reduction of swelling and inflammation in the flexor tendon sheath, which allows smoother movement of the tendon under the A1 pulley, and the prevention of recurrence. Treatment includes ice, restricted gripping, buddy-taping or metal finger splint, and corticosteroid injection for persistent cases. Surgical release is considered if symptoms are not relieved with injection.[7,11]

Chest

Costochondritis Costochondritis is inflammation of the cartilage at the junction of the rib and the costal cartilage. Patients complain of anterior chest pain. Physical examination reveals local tenderness either 1″ from the midline of the sternum or at the costochondral junctions and reproducible pain by chest wall compression. Radiographs of the chest are normal. The goals of treatment are to reassure the patient that this is not a cardiac condition and to reduce inflammation. Treatment includes reassurance, restriction of strenuous activity, NSAIDs, and local anesthetic injection.[7]

Hip

Trochanteric Bursitis Trochanteric bursitis is an inflammation of the lubricating sac located between the midportion of the trochanteric process of the femur and the gluteus medius tendon/iliotibial tract, caused by repetitive flexing of the hip. A disturbance in gait is the most common cause of a trochanteric bursitis. The patient complains of hip pain over the outer thigh or difficulty upon walking. Physical examination reveals local tenderness of the greater trochanter, increased hip pain at the extremes of internal and external rotation and with resisted hip abduction, and normal range of motion of the hip. Findings of underlying lumbosacral or sacroiliac diseases, gait disturbance, or leg length discrepancy may also be noted.

Radiographs of the hip are recommended to evaluate for underlying disease. The goals of treatment are to reduce inflammation of the bursa, correct disturbances of gait, and prevent recurrence with hip and back stretching exercises. Treatment includes application of heat; passive stretching of the gluteus medius tendon, lumbosacral spine, and sacroiliac joint; and the use of NSAIDs, therapeutic ultrasound, and the transcutaneous electrical nerve stimulation (TENS) unit for chronic bursitis, as well as corticosteroid injection.[7,11,12]

Knee

Chondromalacia Patella
Chondromalacia patella is the pathological entity of cartilage softening on the underside of the kneecap. Typically, this condition is an overuse syndrome. Poor muscle tone, overdeveloped vastus lateralis, flexibility deficits, pes planus, and blunt trauma to the knee predispose to the condition. The patient complains of anterior knee pain and a "noisy" or "clicking" or "catching" sensation of the knee, infrequently associated with swelling. The patient may complain of the knee "locking." Physical examination reveals painful retropatellar crepitation, the patella may be visibly subluxed, and a palpable patellar click and positive apprehension sign may be noted. Radiographs of the knee should include a sunrise view to evaluate for lateral subluxation, narrowing of the patellofemoral articular cartilage, and osteoarthritic changes. Treatment goals are to improve patellofemoral tracking and alignment, reduce pain, and slow down the development of arthritis. Treatment includes NSAIDs to improve quadriceps strength and endurance, knee sleeve for

pelvic muscle strength, and for persistent cases, local corticosteroid injection.[7]

Prepatellar Bursitis
Prepatellar bursitis is an inflammation of the bursal sac located between the patella and the overlying skin. The most common cause is blunt trauma resulting from a fall. The patient complains of swelling of the knee and pain in front of the knee. Physical examination reveals swelling and inflammation over the inferior portion of the patella, bursal sac tenderness, and normal range of motion. Chronic prepatellar bursitis has a cobblestone-like roughness or a palpable thickening. Treatment goals are to identify the cause of the bursitis and reduce the inflammation. Treatment approaches include padding and protection of the bursa, and aspiration and drainage for diagnostic studies.[7,12]

Baker's Cyst
Baker's cyst is an abnormal collection of synovial fluid in the fatty layers of the popliteal fossa. The fluid escapes from the synovial lining, resulting in a fibrotic reaction in the subcutaneous tissue and cyst formation. The patient complains of tightness behind the knee. Physical examination reveals a palpable cystic mass in the medial aspect of the popliteal fossa. No signs of peripheral vascular insufficiency are noted. A large cyst may impair knee flexion. Diagnostic ultrasound can assess the size of the cyst, but definitive diagnosis requires aspiration. The goal of treatment is to correct the abnormal accumulation of fluid. Treatment includes advising that the cyst may resolve on its own; restricting squatting, kneeling, and repetitive bending; applying a knee sleeve; and providing local aspiration and corticosteroid injection. Surgical removal may be advised if the cyst interferes with full function of the knee.[7]

Meniscal Tear of the Knee
A torn meniscus is a disruption of the fibrocartilage pads between the femoral condyles and the tibial plateaus. The main function of the menisci is shock absorbency of the knee joint. The mechanism of injury involves rotatory stress on a weight-bearing knee. The patient complains of the knee "locking," "clicking," or "giving way." Physical examination reveals: joint line tenderness, a positive McMurray's test, joint effusion,

decreased passive range of motion, and inability to squat or kneel. Radiographs of the knee may show degenerative changes. MRI confirms the presence of a meniscal tear. Goals of treatment are to define the type and extent of the tear, strengthen the muscular support of the knee, and determine the need for surgery. Treatment includes ice, elevation, and physical therapy to strengthen the knee. Isolated meniscal tear in a repairable zone in a young patient should be repaired; symptomatic meniscal tear in a nonrepairable zone or a complex meniscal tear should be arthroscopically débrided.[7,11,12]

CASE STUDY 34-2

History

A 25-year-old female soccer player presents to the primary care physician with a sudden onset of left knee pain while playing soccer. The patient states that she twisted her left knee while playing soccer and heard a "pop"; the knee suddenly gave way. The patient states the knee immediately swelled and she was not able to continue in the game. She has no past medical history of knee injury.

Physical examination

Inspection: Swelling of the left knee.

Palpation: No tenderness of the meniscus or patellofemoral and collateral ligaments.

Sensory: Intact sensation to light touch and sharp/dull.

Peripheral pulses: Femoral, popliteal, dorsalis pedis, and posterior pulses strong and equal bilaterally.

Range of motion: Passive and active motion of the left knee decreased with flexion and extension.

Special tests: Positive bulge sign, positive patellar ballottement test; positive Lachman's test and anterior drawer sign, negative posterior drawer sign; negative McMurray's sign and varus and valgus stressing.

Diagnostic tests

Anteroposterior and lateral radiographs of the knee are negative.

MRI positive for anterior cruciate ligament tear.

Diagnosis

Anterior cruciate ligament tear.

Treatment

The anterior cruciate ligament (ACL) is a primary stabilizer of the knee, and a tear of the ACL results from a twisting or hyperextension force applied to the knee joint. Initial treatment includes rest, ice, knee immobilization, NSAIDs, and crutches. An arthrocentesis in this case will most likely reveal hemarthrosis of the knee. In the absence of a distended knee joint, there is no need for aspiration of an acutely injured knee. Definitive treatment of an ACL tear for a young, active patient is reconstruction and referral to the physical therapy department for rehabilitation. Female athletes, particularly those playing soccer, gymnastics, and basketball, are at the highest risk for ACL injury. Older or less active patients can be treated more conservatively with physical therapy with the goal to control instability.

Ankle

Plantar Fasciitis   Plantar fasciitis is inflammation of the origin of the longitudinal ligament that forms the arch of the foot. Predisposing conditions include obesity, flatfeet (pes planus), working on concrete, poorly fitted shoes, and prolonged standing. The patient complains of heel pain aggravated by weight bearing. Physical examination reveals tenderness of the plantar fascia, pain with calcaneal compression, and limited flexibility of the Achilles tendon. Radiographs and bone scan are indicated to rule out stress fractures. Radiographs are indicated to rule out pressure-aggravated heel spur. Treatment goals are to reduce inflammation and increase the flexibility of the heel and ankle. Treatment includes reduction of weight bearing, padded arch supports, NSAIDs, stretching exercises, corticosteroid injection, and surgery for recurrent fasciitis.[7,11]

Foot

Bunion   Bunion is a bony prominence and valgus deformity of the great toe. Asymmetrical pressure over the articular cartilage caused by narrow shoes occurs over years. The patient complains of abnormal-looking toes, pain of the great toe, and shoes that do not fit. Physical examination reveals metatarsophalangeal (MTP) joint tenderness and enlargement, hallux valgus deformity of the great toe, crepitation of the joint, and limited range of motion. Radiographs assess the valgus angle and degree of arthritic changes. Treatment goals are to reduce joint inflammation and prevent arthritic deterioration and further valgus deformity. Treatment includes advising the patient to wear loose-fitting shoes and prescribing NSAIDs. Bunionectomy may be considered to improve alignment, reduce medial joint line pressure, and improve function.[7,11]

Hammer Toe   Hammer toe describes the toe deformity caused by contracted extensor tendons of the foot. The hammer toe deformity is a result of years of tight, inflexible extensor tendons. The patient complains of pain over the ball of the foot, calluses, or abnormal-looking toes. Physical examination reveals tight extensor tendons, tenderness directly over the MTP joint, corns, and calluses. Treatment goals are to stretch the dorsal extensor tendons and reestablish normal toe alignment. Treatment includes loose-fitting shoes, padding for corns and calluses, stretching exercises, and flexor tenotomy or arthroplasty if symptoms and deformity are persistent.[7]

Fractures

A significant portion of the physician assistant's scope of care in an orthopedics practice involves the evaluation, diagnosis, and management of fractures. A fracture refers to a broken bone and is a result of direct or indirect violence to the bone. Table 34-4 lists definitions of fractures. The history should included a detailed account of the mechanism of injury, the position of the joint at the time of injury, the motion of the joint that exacerbates or relieves pain, neurological symptoms, previous musculoskeletal injuries, past illness (e.g., asthma, heart disease, peripheral vascular disease, diabetes mellitus, bleeding disorders), last meal, medications taken (e.g., steroids, anticoagulants), and history of smoking.[11]

Physical examination must comprise a meticulous head-to-toe examination that includes the following:
➤ The joint above and below the injured joint.
➤ Neurological examination (range of motion, sensory, motor).
➤ Peripheral vascular.

The emergent treatment of the patient with potential injury to more than one organ system is handled by a team of specialists, including an orthopedic practitioner. Treatment is organized in three stages: primary survey, secondary survey, and definitive management. The *primary survey* is concerned with the ABCs (airway, breathing, and circulation). The *secondary survey* includes a careful account of the accident, a description of the mechanism of injury, a thorough physical examination, and radiological studies. Radiographs of the joint above and below the injury site and comparison views should be considered. Special views may be ordered after consultation with the radiologist.[11]

The *definitive management* of fractures, after serious injuries to the head, abdomen, and chest have been stabilized, includes the following:
➤ Elevation of the extremity.
➤ Cold compress to reduce swelling.
➤ Immobilization (splinting, cast).
➤ Analgesics.
➤ Manual or surgical reduction.

Table 34-5 lists some of the most common orthopedic fractures seen in a primary care office.

Pediatric Orthopedics

This section provides an overview of selected problems in pediatric orthopedics, including etiology, patient presentation, diagnostic studies, treatment goals, and approach to treatment.

Osteochondritis Dissecans   Osteochondritis dissecans of the knee results from repetitive stress that causes osteonecrosis of the underlying bone and ultimately a subchondral stress fracture. The most common location is the medial femoral condyle. Symptoms usually present during childhood, including pain and stiffness after running and sport activities. Physical examination may be unremarkable or may reveal mild effusion or quadriceps atrophy. Management involves modifying activity to prevent symptoms. The patient may not be involved in sports for 3 to 12 months. Indications for operative treatment include an unstable knee, a loose body, or persistent symptoms after nonoperative management has been implemented.[13]

Table 34-4 Definitions of Fractures

Closed	Fracture site does not communicate with the exterior of the body
Open	Fracture site communicates with the exterior of the body
Articular	Fracture that involves the joint surfaces
Undisplaced	Hairline fracture without loss of normal anatomic configuration
Displaced	Separation of fracture fragments has occurred with loss of anatomic configuration
Angulated	Fracture with a bending or angular deformity (Figure 34-1)
Comminuted	Fracture involved bone fragment in more than two pieces
Avulsed	Bone fragment pulled off by attached ligaments (Figure 34-2, *A*)
Oblique	The fracture line site runs obliquely to the axis of the bone
Compression	The fracture is common in cancellous flat bones because of the spongy consistency (Figure 34-2, *B*)
Impacted	Fracture that is produced by severe violence that drives the bone fragment firmly together (Figure 34-2, *C*)
Spiral	Fracture produced by a twisting or rotatory force
Segmental	Fracture with a single, large, free-floating segment of bone between two well-defined fracture lines
Stress	The bone may undergo a "fatigue" fracture from repetitive forces
Pathological	Fractures that occur from relatively minor trauma to diseased bones (Figure 34-2, *D*)

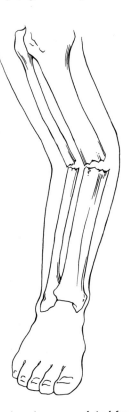

Figure 34-1 Fracture type, angulated fracture. *(From Eiff MP, Calmbach WL, Hatch R, Higgins MK. Fracture Management for Primary Care. Philadelphia: WB Saunders, 1998:12.)*

Continued

Table 34-4   Definitions of Fractures—cont'd

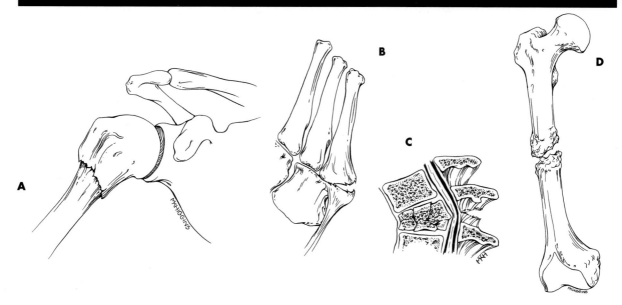

Figure 34-2 Fracture types. **A**, Impacted. **B**, Avulsion. **C**, Compression. **D**, Pathologic. *(From Eiff MP, Calmbach WL, Hatch R, Higgins MK. Fracture Management for Primary Care. Philadelphia: WB Saunders, 1998:9.)*

Salter-Harris classification (Figure 34-3)

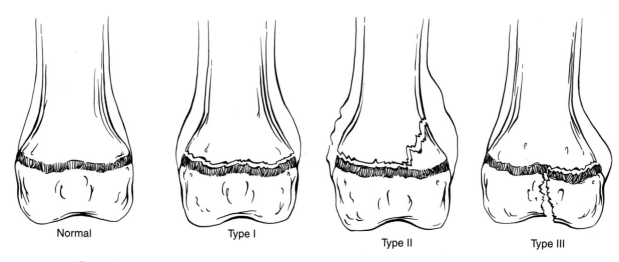

Figure 34-3 The Salter-Harris classification. *(From Eiff MP, Calmbach WL, Hatch R, Higgins MK. Fracture Management for Primary Care. Philadelphia: WB Saunders, 1998:254.)*

Table 34-4   Definitions of Fractures—cont'd

Fracture	Fractures involving the epiphyseal plate at the end of the long bone of a growing child
Salter Type	**Description**
I	The growth plate is fractured
II	The growth plate and the metaphysis are fractured
III	The growth plate and the epiphysis are fractured
IV	The metaphysis, growth plate, and epiphysis are fractured
V	Nothing "broken off," compression injury of the epiphyseal plate

Type IV   Type V

Figure 34-3—cont'd For legend see opposite page

Table 34-5   Types of Fractures

Bone/Joint	Fracture Description	Mechanism of Injury	Complication(s)
Clavicle	Most common location is middle third of the clavicle, common in children and young adults	Indirect through a fall on the lateral shoulder or an outstretched hand or a direct blow to the clavicle	Uncommon, rarely subclavian vessels trapped
Humerus	Proximal humerus fracture, common in elderly patients	Young adults high-energy trauma, fall onto arm or elbow	Loss of motion, nonunion, nerve and vascular damage
Elbow	Supracondylar fractures most common in children and elderly patients	Fall on extended or flexed elbow	Loss of motion, ulnar nerve palsy, varus or valgus deformity
Wrist	Colles' fracture, fracture of the distal radius, common in elderly patients, related to osteoporosis in this age group	Fall on the outstretched hand with wrist in extension	Stiffness of the finger joints and shoulders, carpal tunnel syndrome, rupture of tendons (Figure 34-4)
	Scaphoid fracture	Fall on the outstretched hand or direct blow to hand	Delayed union, nonunion, avascular necrosis

Continued

Table 34-5	Types of Fractures—cont'd		
Bone/Joint	**Fracture Description**	**Mechanism of Injury**	**Complication(s)**

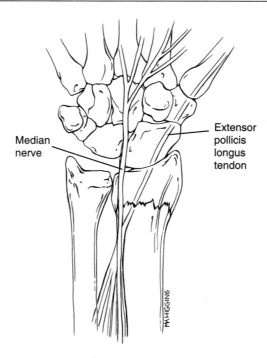

Figure 34-4 The median nerve may be associated with a distal radius fracture. *(From Eiff MP, Calmbach WL, Hatch R, Higgins MK. Fracture Management for Primary Care. Philadelphia: WB Saunders, 1998:80.)*

Bone/Joint	Fracture Description	Mechanism of Injury	Complication(s)
Fingers	Boxer fracture of the 5th metacarpal neck (Figure 34-5, *A* and *B*)	Direct impact on metacarpal head with hand in clenched position	Prominent metacarpal head in palm, rotational malunion
	Mallet finger, avulsion fracture of the distal phalanx	Forced flexion of fingertip actively extended	Mallet finger deformity
Rib	Nondisplaced rib fractures most common	Blunt trauma or severe paroxysms of coughing	Pneumothorax, trauma to internal organs and vessels
Pelvis	Pelvic fracture	Automobile passenger, pedestrian accidents or minor fall in older patients	Hemorrhage, rectal injuries, ruptured diaphragm, nerve root injury
Hip	Femoral neck fracture	Minor trauma secondary to a fall, common among older adults owing to osteoporosis, women > men	Avascular necrosis

Table 34-5	Types of Fractures—cont'd		
Bone/Joint	**Fracture Description**	**Mechanism of Injury**	**Complication(s)**

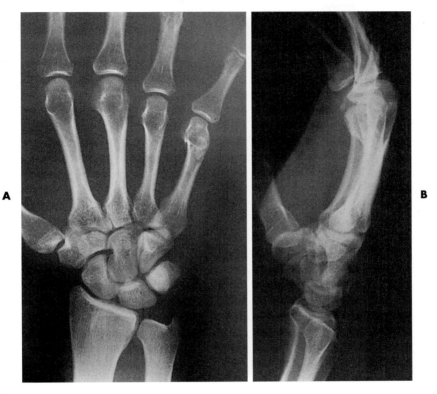

Figure 34-5 A, Anteroposterior views. **B,** Lateral view of a boxer's fracture. *(From Eiff MP, Calmbach WL, Hatch R, Higgins MK. Fracture Management for Primary Care. Philadelphia: WB Saunders, 1998:50.)*

Knee	Tibial plateau	Direct blow or twisting injury	Loss of range of motion, early degenerative joint changes, infection, nerve and vascular injuries
Ankle	Ankle fractures are intra-articular injuries	Plantar flexion and inversion injury—"twisted ankle"	Associated 5th metatarsal fracture
Foot	Calcaneal fracture	Fall from a height and lands on the heels	Associated compression fractures of lumbar spine, compartment syndrome

Continued

Table 34-5	Types of Fractures—cont'd		
Bone/Joint	**Fracture Description**	**Mechanism of Injury**	**Complication(s)**
Toes	Phalangeal fractures	Blunt trauma *Type I:* Fracture of growth plate *Type II:* Fracture of growth plate with fracture of metaphysis *Type III:* Fracture of growth plate and portion of epiphysis *Type IV:* Single fracture through growth plate, metaphysis, and epiphysis *Type V:* Nothing fractured, crushing injury to growth plate	Maceration secondary to taping Potential for growth disturbances

Developmental Dysplasia of the Hip (DDH)

Developmental dysplasia of the hip encompasses all dysplastic hip disorders. DDH is associated with ligamentous laxity and is detectable at birth. DDH is more common among females and is more likely to be noted in the left hip in breech presentation. There is an increased incidence in North American Indians and whites of northern European ancestry. Most afflicted neonates are detectable at birth and are asymptomatic. Parents may notice a limp, a waddling gait pattern, or a limb-length discrepancy when the infant begins to walk. Physical examination reveals a positive Ortolani's click test. In older children, secondary adaptive changes may be evident, including waddling gait and symmetry of the gluteal thigh and labial folds. The goal of treatment is to contain the femoral head within the acetabulum while the acetabulum develops and the hip stabilizes. An abduction brace is usually sufficient for newborns and infants. The brace should be continued until acetabular development and joint stability have occurred.[13]

Pes Planus (Flatfoot)

Flatfoot is an abnormally low or absent longitudinal arch. It may be congenital or may result from trauma or tendon degeneration. Flexible flatfoot is more common and involves a normal foot shape in infants. Flexible flatfoot is usually painless. Physical examination reveals the heel in valgus alignment and the forefoot abducted and a loss of longitudinal arch on weight bearing. The range of motion is normal, but secondary contracture of the Achilles tendon may develop in older children. Management is usually not required. Modifications to shoe and orthotic devices have not been proved to alter the natural development of a longitudinal arch. If fatigue symptoms or activity-related discomfort persists, shoe modification provides support.[11,13]

Osgood-Schlatter Disease

Osgood-Schlatter disease results from repetitive injury or small avulsion injuries at the bone-tendon junction where the patellar tendon inserts into the secondary ossification center of the tibial tuberosity. The typical history includes pain exacerbated by running, jumping, and kneeling activities. Physical examination reveals tenderness and swelling at the insertion of the patellar tendon into the tibial tubercle. Radiographs during the acute phase reveal soft tissue swelling. In chronic patients, heterotopic ossification may be noted anterior to the tibial tuberosity. Management involves activity modification to permit healing of the microscopic avulsion fractures. Athletes may return to full training in 6 to 7 months.[13]

CHALLENGES AND REWARDS FOR PAs IN ORTHOPEDICS

PAs working in orthopedic surgery encounter a number of challenges. Although some patients demonstrate improvement and/or cure of their problems, other orthopedic patients have chronic disabling conditions that do not improve. PAs may find it difficult to help patients make the behavioral changes needed to improve their musculoskeletal status. For example, obesity exacerbates most orthopedic problems, but losing weight constitutes one of the more difficult challenges for patients and clinicians.

As with any subspecialty practice, PAs in orthopedic surgery may find limited opportunities to use the full range of their primary care skills.

Rewards for orthopedic PAs include the satisfaction of helping patients regain function and improve their quality of life. Many PAs find it particularly satisfying to see athletes resume their training and succeed in their sports (often the PAs who choose this field enjoy participating in athletic activities themselves).

CONCLUSION

PAs in orthopedics must develop a thorough knowledge of anatomy and must sharpen their history and physical examination skills because most diagnoses are based on this foundation. In addition to helping patients and exercising their clinical skills, orthopedic PAs enjoy participating in outpatient, inpatient, and surgical care. As the U.S. population ages, this surgical subspecialty is likely to continue to offer a wide range of opportunities for PAs.

CLINICAL APPLICATIONS

1. Practice the orthopedic special tests listed in Table 34-3.
2. If you accepted a position in an orthopedic surgery practice, what knowledge and skills would you need to update?

3. Interview a patient who has recovered from an orthopedic injury. What rehabilitation approaches were successful for this patient? Why?

REFERENCES

1. American Academy of Physician Assistants. 2001 PA Census. Available at www.aapa.org. Accessed 1 August, 2002.
2. American Academy of Physician Assistants. 1998 PA Census. Available at www.aapa.org. Accessed 1 August, 2002.
3. Magee DJ. Orthopedic Physical Assessment, ed 2. Philadelphia: WB Saunders, 1992.
4. Greene WB. Essentials of Musculoskeletal Care, ed 2. Rosemont, Illinois: American Academy of Orthopaedic Surgeons, 2001.
5. Bickley LS. Bates Guide to Physical Examination and History Taking, ed 7. Philadelphia: JB Lippincott, 1999.
6. Cipriano JJ. Photographic Manual of Orthopaedic Tests. Baltimore JB: Williams & Wilkins, 1985.
7. Anderson BC. Office Orthopedics for Primary Care Diagnosis and Treatment, ed 2. Philadelphia: WB Saunders, 1999.
8. Matsui M. The painful shoulder: Is it impingement syndrome? Journal of the American Academy of Physician Assistants 2000:13.
9. Slolane PD, Slatt LM, Ebell MH, Jacques LB. Essentials of Family Medicine. Baltimore: Lippincott, Williams & Wilkins, 2002.
10. O'Neil DM. Understanding inflammatory disorders of the upper extremity. Journal of the American Academy of Physician Assistants 2001:14.
11. Swiontkowki MF (ed). Manual of Orthopaedics, ed 5. Philadelphia: Lippincott, Williams & Wilkins, 2001.
12. Puffer JC. 20 Common Problems in Sports Medicine, ed 1. New York: McGraw-Hill, 2001.
13. Bergaman AB. 20 Common Problems in Pediatrics, ed 1. New York: McGraw-Hill, 2001.

RESOURCES

PAs in Orthopedic Surgery. *This specialty organization of the American Academy of Physician Assistants (AAPA) was organized to address the needs and interests of PAs working in orthopedics. Contact information is available at the AAPA web page at www.aapa.org.*

Anderson BC. Office Orthopedics for Primary Care Diagnosis and Treatment, ed 2. Philadelphia, PA: WB Saunders, 1999. This comprehensive text addresses the evaluation and treatment of common orthopedic problems from a primary care perspective.

CHAPTER 35

Dermatology

P. Eugene Jones

INTRODUCTION

This chapter presents an overview of dermatology for physician assistants (PAs) in training as well as for new or experienced graduates who may be contemplating dermatology as a clinical specialty. Dermatology is a visually oriented specialty that offers a unique perspective on health care and includes patients from every age and demographic group. Dermatology can be a deceivingly complex specialty, and the breadth and depth of dermatologic diagnoses can be daunting. By middle age, the number of dermatologic conditions experienced tends to increase to the point that many people intermittently seek care for differing types of skin, hair, and nail disorders. Dermatology is a rewarding specialty that enables the clinician to become adept in a number of surgical procedures while establishing long-standing clinician/patient relationships because of the chronicity of many dermatologic disorders that may require decades of follow-up care.

HISTORY OF DERMATOLOGY

Since the beginning of recorded history, physical and written reference is made to the adornment and ailments of the skin, hair, and nails. Mummified bodies from Egypt and ancient papyrus documents reflect the presence of assorted lesions, tattoos, and piercings. The Hebrew Bible of 2700 years ago describes dermatologic diseases and therapies, suggesting that disorders were of divine infliction. Centuries later, the ancient Greek and Roman civilizations attempted to distinguish dermatologic diseases by external and internal causes. More than 200 years ago, modern dermatology evolved among groups of Austrian, English, French, and German dermatologists, who developed the origins of the modern-day nosography of dermatologic disorders.[1] As the specialty evolved, dermatology was combined with syphilology owing to the variable cutaneous manifestations of syphilis. Before the formation of the American Board of Dermatology in 1932, dermatologists were recognized by The Section on Dermatology and Syphilology of the American Medical Association.[2]

WHAT IS DERMATOLOGY?

Dermatology includes the diagnosis and treatment of pediatric and adult patients with benign and malignant disorders of the skin, mouth, external genitalia, hair, and nails, as well as a number of sexually transmitted diseases. To be certified as a dermatologist, a physician must have had at least 4 years of postgraduate residency training accredited by the Accreditation Council for Graduate Medical Education. The first broad-based general clinical (internship) year is followed by 3 years of intensive training in dermatology, including dermatopathology and dermatologic surgery.

A certified specialist in dermatology may subspecialize and become certified for Special Qualification as follows:

➤ **Dermatopathology** (Special Qualification in Dermatopathology)—Although all dermatologists have training and experience in dermatopathology, Special Qualification in Dermatopathology, signifying advanced competence, can be obtained by either a board certified dermatologist or a pathologist. Special Qualification involves additional extensive training and experience in the evaluation of tissue specimens submitted from dermatologic patients.

➤ **Immunodermatology** (Special Qualification in Dermatological Immunology/Diagnostic and Laboratory Immunology)—An immunodermatologist is a dermatologist who, through additional specialty training, has developed expertise in the study of the cause, diagnosis, treatment, and outcome of skin diseases involving the immune system. These physicians have a basic understanding of such diseases from the perspective of anatomic and clinical pathology, as well as from the interpretation of immunologic analyses of tissue cells and body fluids.[3]

DERMATOLOGY ORGANIZATIONS
Society for Dermatology Physician Assistants

The Society for Dermatology Physician Assistants (SDPA), founded in 1993 by Joe Monroe, PA-C, represents both part-time and full-time dermatology PAs. Listing the large number of U.S. and international dermatologic societies and their purposes is beyond the scope of this chapter. However, a link to most of these organizations can be found at the SDPA website—http://home.pacifier.com/~jomonroe/. This site provides a wealth of current and useful information for the PA who may be interested in dermatology. The site includes many helpful links to hundreds of other relevant sites; major topics of these include academies and organizations, international sites, journals and publications, commercial sites, e-mail lists, disease-specific information, searchable sites/search engines, skin cancer–related sites, dermatology practice/dermatology PA web sites, and information on universities, colleges, and schools.

Dermatology Demographics

According to the National Center for Health Statistics, as of 1999, 33 million office visits were made to approximately 13,700 U.S. dermatologists annually, and approximately 10.4 million visits to office-based physicians occurred because of skin rash.[4] According to the American Academy of Dermatology, nearly 8.2 million cases of dermatitis and 4.9 million cases of acne were reported in 1996.[3]

The 2001 Census Report from the American Academy of Physician Assistants[4] reports that 1.8% of PAs practice in dermatology. However, the demand for dermatology PAs currently exceeds the supply, particularly for PAs with dermatology experience.

The range of services provided by dermatology PAs is extensive and includes general dermatology with a concentration on common skin, hair, and nail disorders; skin cancer surgery, including shave, punch, and excisional biopsies; cryosurgery; electrodessication and curettage; lesion excision; and Mohs micrographic surgery. LASER (Light Amplification by Stimulated Emission of Radiation) use by dermatology PAs is commonplace; carbon dioxide, ruby, alexandrite, neodymium:yttrium-aluminum-garnet (Nd:YAG), argon, tunable dye, pulsed tunable dye, KTP, NLite, and erbium LASERs are used for treatment of a variety of cutaneous conditions.

Dermatology PA Residency Training

Currently, three postgraduate residency training programs in dermatology are available for PAs. The University of Texas Southwestern Medical Center at Dallas offers a comprehensive 12-month program that includes a range of dermatologic surgical and clinical experiences directed by staff attending board certified dermatologists—weekly didactic sessions to include grand rounds at an academic medical center dermatology department, journal club, case studies, dermatopathology instruction, and basic science lectures.

The Northeast Missouri Regional Medical Center/Kirksville College of Osteopathic Medicine (NMRMC/KCOM) Physician Assistant Dermatology Residency in Kirksville, Missouri, is an intensive 12-month program of clinical and didactic instruction. It is modeled after the American Osteopathic College of Dermatology's first year Dermatology Residency at NMRMC/KCOM. Graduates are well equipped with the knowledge and surgical skills necessary to care for the dermatologic patient.

The Dermatology Associates of Tallahassee & Nova Southeastern University offers a 12-month postgraduate residency program in Tallahassee, Florida. The program is designed to continue the training of physician assistants in dermatology and dermatologic surgery and includes a complete didactic program leading to a master's degree in medical sciences (MMS) and a certificate of completion in dermatologic surgery.

CLINICAL DERMATOLOGY
The Dermatologic Interview

In addition to the standard medical history elements of chief complaint, present problem or illness, past medical history, family history, personal and social history, and review of systems, the dermatologic interview often requires the clinician to concentrate on detailed occupational and medication use histories, drug and other allergies, aggravating and alleviating factors, and indicators of atopy. Atopy indicators may include a past or current history of hay fever, allergic rhinitis, asthma, sinusitis, keratosis pilaris, ichthyosis vulgaris, dry skin, wool insensitivity, removal of collar labels from clothing due to irritation, Dennie-Morgan folds, and palmar hyperlinearity. Another example of the need for an extensive medical history is the patient with chronic urticaria, the cause of which may be difficult to determine.

The Dermatologic Examination

A proper dermatologic examination consists of several elements. Following a thorough history and review of systems, sectional draping and exposure with appropriate chaperone presence as needed allows the clinician to visualize the entire body without compromising patient modesty. One of the most important elements of the examination is the distribution of lesions. A fully clothed patient who rolls up one sleeve or one pant leg to reveal a "rash that is all over my body" is getting an inadequate examination. Patients typically do not examine their scalp, back, buttocks, or posterior legs, and the presence and distribution of lesions in these areas may provide substantial clues to the correct diagnosis. Dispensing medication requires complete visualization of the lesion distribution so that sufficient medicinal quantities can be estimated and prescribed.

Skin Examination Tools

A centimeter ruler is necessary to measure lesions for documentation and to track changes in size, shape, and configuration. A Wood's lamp is useful in examining patients suspected of having conditions that may fluoresce in different colors, including *Microsporum*-related tinea capitis (green) and erythrasma (coral red). A handlight or penlight is necessary to inspect orifices, particularly the oral mucosa, for associated findings such as Wickham's striae in lichen planus. A magnifying lens enhances subtle lesion features, and skilled dermatologic clinicians are adept at using epiluminescence microscopy for differentiating pigmented lesions.

Skin Lesion Distribution

Lesion distribution is one of the most important elements in correctly diagnosing a patient's condition. Many diseases have similar clinical appearances, but their distribution influences the differential diagnoses.

➤ **Generalized**—covering much of the body surface in a regular arrangement pattern.
➤ **Localized**—restricted to one particular body area.
➤ **Symmetrical**—lesions appear to be distributed in a similar arrangement on differing sides of the body.
➤ **Asymmetrical**—lesions are not distributed in a symmetrical pattern.
➤ **Discrete**—lesions are distinctly separate from each other with identifiable borders.
➤ **Grouped**—lesions appear in clusters or groups.
➤ **Confluent**—lesions are coalesced together from smaller into larger areas where the borders may become ill-defined.
➤ **Sun-exposed**—lesions appear on areas of the body that are more sun-exposed than others.
➤ **Intertriginous**—appearing within the skin folds.

Skin Lesion Configuration

➤ **Annular**—round or circular with areas of central clearing.
➤ **Arciform**—a partial circle.
➤ **Circinate**—round, circular.
➤ **Iris or targetoid**—targetlike (bull's eye) lesions of annular configuration with central color contrast.
➤ **Linear**—straight.

➤ **Margination**—defining lesion borders by degree of sharpness and definition.
➤ **Serpiginous**—wandering, uneven borders.
➤ **Zosteriform**—in a dermatomal distribution.

Primary Lesions

A primary skin lesion is a cutaneous change caused directly by the presenting disease process. The key to accurate description and interpretation of cutaneous disease is identification of the primary lesion. The following presentations constitute primary skin lesions (Table 35-1).

Secondary Lesions

Secondary skin changes result from external factors such as infection, trauma, scratching or friction, and changes caused by healing (Table 35-2).

COMMON PROCEDURES IN DERMATOLOGY
Skin Biopsy

Skin biopsy requires the PA to choose the best surgical technique that will gain the most useful information with the least amount of tissue, resulting in the best cosmetic outcome. The three common categories of skin biopsy are shave, punch, and excisional. For an excellent discussion on skin biopsy procedures for physician assistants, see DiBaise M. Dermatologic procedures. In: Asprey DP, Dehn RW (eds). Clinical Procedures for Physician Assistants. Philadelphia, 2001, WB Saunders, 2001, p. 333.

Shave   The shave biopsy technique can serve the dual purpose of either a biopsy or an excision, depending on the size and depth of the lesion. The shave technique is primarily indicated for epidermal and superficial lesions when a portion of the tissue is sufficient for dermatopathologic examination. If dermal depth is required, or if the lesion extends to subdermal tissue, then a punch, excision, or incisional biopsy is recommended.

Punch   For full-thickness specimens or larger surface area lesions requiring only a small amount of tissue for diagnostic purposes, the punch biopsy technique is preferred. Additionally, if special studies such as light or

Text continued on p. 773

Table 35-1   Primary Skin Lesions

Description	Examples	
Macule A flat, circumscribed area that is a change in the color of the skin; less than 1 cm in diameter	Freckles, flat moles (nevi), petechiae, measles, scarlet fever	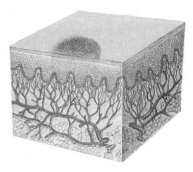
Papule An elevated, firm, circumscribed area less than 1 cm in diameter	Wart (verruca), elevated moles, lichen planus	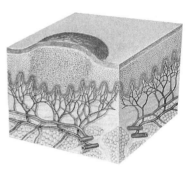
Patch A flat, nonpalpable, irregularly shaped macule larger than 1 cm in diameter	Vitiligo, port-wine stains, mongolian spots, café au lait spot	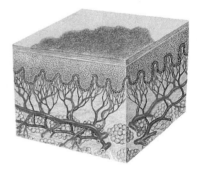
Plaque Elevated, firm, and rough lesion with flat-top surface greater than 1 cm in diameter	Psoriasis, seborrheic and actinic keratoses	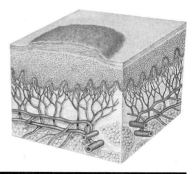

Modified from Thompson JM, Wilson SF. Health assessment for nursing practice. St. Louis: Mosby, 1996.

Table 35-1 Primary Skin Lesions—cont'd

Description	**Examples**	
Wheal Elevated, irregularly shaped area of cutaneous edema; solid, transient; variable diameter	Insect bites, urticaria, allergic reaction	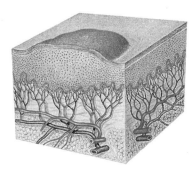
Nodule Elevated, firm, circumscribed lesion; deeper in dermis than a papule; 1 to 2 cm in diameter	Erythema nodosum, lipomas	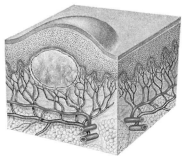
Tumor Elevated and solid lesion; may or may not be clearly demarcated; deeper in dermis; greater than 2 cm in diameter	Neoplasms, benign tumor, lipoma, hemagioma	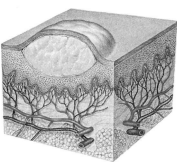
Vesicle Elevated, circumscribed, superficial, not into dermis; filled with serous fluid; less than 1 cm in diameter	Varicella (chickenpox), herpes zoster (shingles)	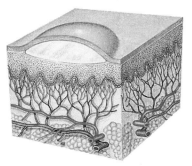

Continued

Table 35-1 Primary Skin Lesions—cont'd

Description	Examples	
Bulla Vesicle greater than 1 cm in diameter	Blister, pemphigus vulgaris	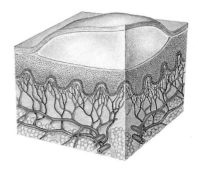
Pustule Elevated, superficial lesion; similar to a vesicle but filled with purulent fluid	Impetigo, acne	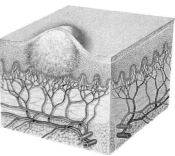
Cyst Elevated, circumscribed, encapsulated lesion; in dermis or subcutaneous layer; filled with liquid or semisolid material	Sebaceous cyst, cystic acne	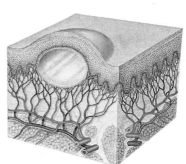
Telangiectasia Fine, irregular red lines produced by capillary dilation	Telangiectasia in rosacea	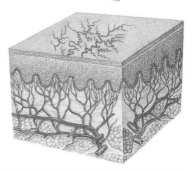

Table 35-2   Secondary Skin Lesions

Description	Examples	
Scale Heaped-up keratinized cells; flaky skin; irregular; thick or thin; dry or oily; variation in size	Flaking of skin with seborrheic dermatitis following scarlet fever, or flaking of skin following a drug reaction; dry skin	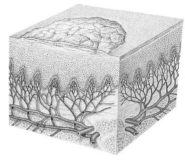
Lichenification Rough, thickened epidermis secondary to persistent rubbing, itching, or skin irritation; often involves flexor surface of extremity	Chronic dermatitis	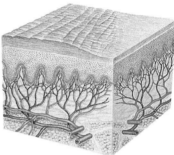
Keloid Irregularly shaped, elevated, progressively enlarging scar; grows beyond the boundaries of the wound; caused by excessive collagen formation during healing	Keloid formation following surgery	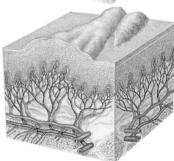
Scar Thin to thick fibrous tissue that replaces normal skin following injury or laceration to the dermis	Healed wound or surgical incision	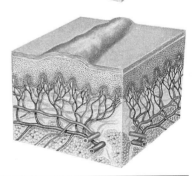

Modified from Thompson JM, Wilson SF. Health assessment for nursing practice. St. Louis: Mosby, 1996.

Continued

Table 35-2   Secondary Skin Lesions—cont'd

Description	Examples	
Excoriation Loss of the epidermis; linear, hollowed-out, crusted area	Abrasion or scratch, scabies	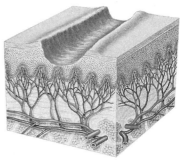
Fissure Linear crack or break from the epidermis to the dermis; may be moist or dry	Athlete's foot, cracks at the corner of the mouth	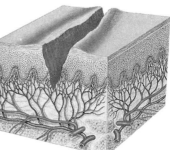
Erosion Loss of part of the epidermis; depressed, moist, glistening; follows rupture of a vesicle or bulla	Varicella, variola after rupture	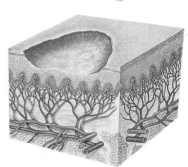
Ulcer Loss of epidermis and dermis; concave; varies in size	Decubiti, stasis ulcers	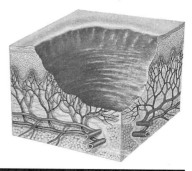

Table 35-2   Secondary Skin Lesions—cont'd

Description	Examples Excoriation	
Crust Dried serum, blood, or purulent exudate; slightly elevated; size varies; brown, red, black, tan, or straw. Scab on abrasion; eczema	Scab on abrasion, eczema	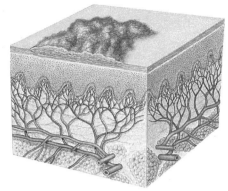
Atrophy Thinning of skin surface and loss of skin markings; skin translucent and paperlike	Striae; aged skin	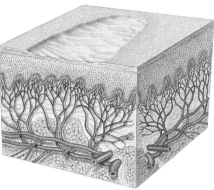

electron microscopy, immunofluorescence, or cell cultures are required, the punch technique is usually employed.[5]

Excisional   Excisional biopsies are indicated when complete removal of the lesion is desired, for a suspicious lesion of relatively small size, or for pigmented lesions with atypical features.[6]

Electrosurgery

The most common form of electrosurgery used in dermatology is electrodessication, which is typically accompanied by curettage of electrodessicated lesions. Diagnostic certainty must be a factor because there is no residual tissue for dermatopathologic evaluation following electrosurgery. With the lowest possible power setting that results in tissue destruction, electrodessication is frequently used for elimination of spider and vascular (cherry) hemangiomas, verrucae, superficial nonmelanoma skin cancer, and actinic keratoses.[1]

Cryosurgery

Cryosurgery has several indications and advantages over other surgical modalities in selected dermatologic patients with appropriate lesions.

The portability and ease of cryosurgical application render it advantageous for most body areas. Cutaneous lesions with more sharply demarcated borders are typically more responsive to cryosurgery, and the rapid healing is an additional advantage.[6] Although cryosurgery is contraindicated in patients with cryoglobulinemia, cold intolerance, or cold urticaria, it is especially useful in elderly, high-risk surgical patients, and patients with coagulopathies and pacemakers because of its ease of application and the relatively minimal associated risks (Table 35-3).[7]

Potassium Hydroxide Test

All patients who present with a scaly rash deserve a potassium hydroxide (K^+OH^-) test to rule out the presence of dermatophyte (fungal and yeast) infections. The K^+OH^- test is performed by gently scraping across the advancing edge of a scaly rash with a glass slide or a No. 15 surgical blade and collecting the cellular debris and scale on a glass slide. One to three drops of 20% K^+OH^- solution is applied to the scale to dissolve the cell walls, and a glass coverslip is applied. Using K^+OH^- with dimethyl sulfoxide (DMSO), gently heating the

Table 35-3 Cryogens and the Centigrade Temperature	
Cryogen	**Temperature° (C)**
Ice	0
Salt ice	−20
CO_2 slush	−20
CO_2 snow	−70
CO_2 solid	−78.5
Liquid nitrous oxide	−89.5
Liquid nitrogen	−20 (swab)
Liquid nitrogen	−195.8 (spray/probe)

From Jones PE. Cryosurgery. In: Asprey DP, Dehn RW (eds). Clinical Procedures for Physician Assistants. Philadelphia: WB Saunders, 2001:385.

slide, or waiting 10 to 15 minutes will hasten the dissolution of the keratin and make it easier to see the fungal elements. Begin by examining the slide under low microscope power with the condenser lowered. In a dermatophyte (tinea) infection, look for branching hyphae. In candidiasis, look for budding yeast.

Scabies Prep Test

All patients presenting with intractable nocturnal pruritus and a typical burrowlike rash or papules in the interdigital web spaces between the fingers or in the waist, axillae, buttocks, or external genitalia warrant a skin scraping examination to rule out scabies. Burrows or unexcoriated papules are vigorously scraped with a No. 15 blade coated with mineral oil, and the cellular debris is transferred to a glass microscope slide. A glass coverslip is applied and the findings are examined under low power to detect the diagnostic presence of mites, eggs, or fecal pellets (scybala).[1]

Tzanck Smear

The Tzanck smear is helpful in the diagnosis of herpetic lesions such as herpes simplex, varicella zoster virus, and herpes zoster. The procedure involves gently unroofing an intact vesicle with a No. 15 blade and scraping the underside of the vesicle in a perpendicular fashion with the edge of the blade. The material is smeared onto a glass microscope slide and is allowed to air-dry, or is rapidly fixed with alcohol (ETOH). After it has dried, the slide is stained with either Wright's or Geimsa stain and is gently rinsed. When it has been air-dried again, the slide is examined under low power for multinucleated giant cells.[1]

Acetowhitening

To facilitate the diagnosis of condyloma acuminata lesions, moisten a gauze pad with 3% to 5% acetic acid (vinegar is 5%), and apply the pad to suspected genital warts for 5 to 10 minutes. Condyloma lesions will whiten and appear as circumscribed macular/papular lesions with a granular surface and a punctate vascular pattern.[8]

Mohs Micrographic Surgery

Developed by Frederic E. Mohs, MD, in the 1930s, the Mohs micrographic surgical procedure has been refined and perfected for more than half a century. Dr. Mohs developed a unique technique of color-coding excised specimens and created a mapping process to accurately identify the location of remaining cancerous cells. Clinical studies have shown that Mohs micrographic surgery has a 5-year cure rate of up to 99% in the treatment of basal cell and squamous cell carcinomas. Mohs micrographic surgery is primarily used to treat basal and squamous cell carcinomas, but it can be used to treat less common tumors, including melanoma.[9]

CASE STUDY 35-1

A 40-year-old man presents with a scalp lesion that has been present for approximately 20 years, according to the patient. A maternal aunt died from malignant melanoma 5 years earlier. He reports having a "mole in his scalp" that his barber thought had been changing over the past 8 months. The patient is a nurse who had heard that "moles with hair growing from them" were always benign. Examination of the scalp reveals a 2-cm asymmetrical multicolored nevus with an irregular border and papular elevation on one side. An excisional biopsy reveals a malignant melanoma.

Patients with a positive family history of melanoma, one or more blistering sunburns, excess cumulative lifetime sun exposure, and lighter hair, eye, and skin coloration are more susceptible to developing malignant melanoma. Complete skin examinations (to include hair-bearing areas) are necessary for the evaluation of changing or suspicious lesions. Any lesion that changes in size, shape, or color, or becomes symptomatic, should be evaluated as soon as possible, even if the lesion has been present for many years. Melanomas arising from previously benign-appearing nevi are not uncommon. In this Case Study, the patient suffered from inoperable metastatic disease and died 11 months after diagnosis.

CASE STUDY 35-2

A 44-year-old woman with a long-standing history of psoriasis reports for follow-up care. She had developed "new lesions" on her thighs and self-treated twice daily with Psorcon® (diflorasone) ointment, a group I topical steroid previously prescribed for plaque psoriasis of the elbows and knees. She asks about the presence of "stretch marks" and bleeding near the new lesions.

Although the patient thought she was doing the right thing by applying Psorcon® to the lesions she assumed were psoriatic, she had not been told to avoid using superpotent steroidal preparations in areas of thinner skin, such as the groin, intertriginal spaces, and face. A complete evaluation of the new lesions, including a punch biopsy, revealed a new diagnosis of erythema annulare centrifigum, a condition unrelated to the previously established diagnosis of psoriasis. The patient developed striae with scattered shallow ulcerations because of the thinness of the intertriginal skin on the proximal thighs and the occlusive effect of the thighs rubbing together. The shallow ulcerations healed with topical antibiotic therapy, but the striae remain a permanent reminder of the potential adverse effects of misused topical steroids.

CONCLUSION

Dermatology is a medical subspecialty that attracts the visually oriented clinician who is interested in a variety of patient conditions and age ranges. The growing interest in LASER therapy, cosmetic dermatology, and extended surgical opportunities makes the specialty particularly attractive to clinicians having or desiring advanced psychomotor skills. The patient evaluation element requires advanced skills in gathering a detailed and often elusive history to determine allergic or occupational origins of skin lesions. Dermatology is a rewarding specialty that challenges the mind while simultaneously honing cutaneous surgical skills.

REFERENCES

1. Freedberg IM, Eisen AZ, Wolff K, Austen KF, Goldsmith LA, Katz SI, Fitzpatrick TB. Fitzpatrick's Dermatology in General Medicine, ed 5. New York: McGraw-Hill, 1999.
2. http://www.dermato.med.br/hds/. Accessed 28 November, 2001.
3. http://www.aad.org/. Accessed 26 November, 2001.
4. http://www.cdc.gov/nchs/fastats/skin.htm. Accessed 30 November, 2001.
5. 2001 AAPA Physician Assistant Census Report. Alexandria, VA: American Academy of Physician Assistants, October 6, 2001.
6. O'Sullivan RB, Padilla RS. Excision. In: Ratz JL (ed). Textbook of Dermatologic Surgery. Philadelphia: Lippincott-Raven Publishers, 1998.
7. Jones PE. Cryosurgery. In: Asprey DP, Dehn RW (eds). Clinical Procedures for Physician Assistants. Philadelphia: WB Saunders, 2001.
8. Habif TP. Clinical Dermatology: A Color Guide to Diagnosis and Therapy, ed 3. St. Louis: Mosby, 1996.
9. http://www.mohs.net/about.html. Accessed 26 November, 2001.

C H A P T E R 3 6

Oncology

Susan Blackwell and Lee A. Daly

INTRODUCTION

Cancer has been an affliction of mankind throughout history. The Chinese physician Huang Ti gave the first description of tumors in *Nei Ching,* the oldest written treatise of internal medicine. He included five forms of therapeutic care in his treatise—spiritual cure, pharmacology, diet, acupuncture, and treatment of respiratory diseases. Later, Hippocrates included the treatment of tumors within his *Corpus Hippocraticum,* one of the documents that established him as the father of medicine.[1] Over past centuries and still today, the diagnosis of cancer is accompanied by fear, helplessness, and uncertainty, which affects not only the patient but the family and community as well. Cancer is understood as a group of diseases characterized by unchecked development and proliferation of abnormal cells. The treatment of cancer combines disease-specific scientific knowledge, public health awareness, and sensitivity. The challenge of oncology is to successfully combine compassion and medical acumen at this delicate time in a patient's life.

It is for these reasons that the practice of oncology can be an intellectually and personally rewarding subspecialty for physician assistants (PAs). The oncology PA has the opportunity to apply medical knowledge and physical diagnosis skills developed during PA education, as well as to hone excellent interpersonal skills in caring for patients during what might be the most difficult experience of their lives. Cancer occurs with increasing incidence throughout the middle years of life and later. Therefore, as our population continues to age, the need for PAs in oncology subspecialties is growing.

DEMOGRAPHICS

The American Cancer Society has estimated that in the year 2003, 1,334,100 new cases of cancer will be diagnosed, and 556,500 will die from their disease.[2] In this country, at the turn of the century, cancer was the eighth leading cause of death. However, at the beginning of the 21st century, cancer has become the second leading cause of death following heart disease.[3] Currently, an estimated one in four deaths in the United States is caused by cancer. However, cancer death rates declined in men and women from 1992 to 1998, and cancer incidence rates decreased among men and slightly increased among women during this same period. Although cancer death rates continue to decline, the total number of recorded cancer deaths in the United States continues to increase owing to the aging and growing U.S. population.

In the year 2002, the three most commonly diagnosed cancers in women were expected to be cancers of the breast, lung and bronchus, and colon and rectum. Prostate, lung and bronchus, and colon and rectum were expected to be the most commonly diagnosed cancers in men. The most common cause of cancer death among men and women is cancer of the lung and bronchus (Figure 36-1).[2]

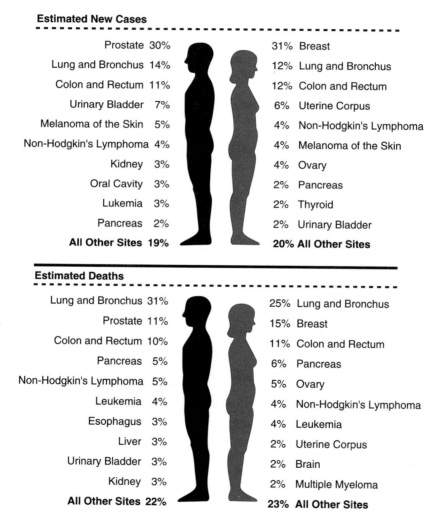

Estimated New Cases

Prostate	30%		31%	Breast
Lung and Bronchus	14%		12%	Lung and Bronchus
Colon and Rectum	11%		12%	Colon and Rectum
Urinary Bladder	7%		6%	Uterine Corpus
Melanoma of the Skin	5%		4%	Non-Hodgkin's Lymphoma
Non-Hodgkin's Lymphoma	4%		4%	Melanoma of the Skin
Kidney	3%		4%	Ovary
Oral Cavity	3%		2%	Pancreas
Lukemia	3%		2%	Thyroid
Pancreas	2%		2%	Urinary Bladder
All Other Sites	**19%**		**20%**	**All Other Sites**

Estimated Deaths

Lung and Bronchus	31%		25%	Lung and Bronchus
Prostate	11%		15%	Breast
Colon and Rectum	10%		11%	Colon and Rectum
Pancreas	5%		6%	Pancreas
Non-Hodgkin's Lymphoma	5%		5%	Ovary
Leukemia	4%		4%	Non-Hodgkin's Lymphoma
Esophagus	3%		4%	Leukemia
Liver	3%		2%	Uterine Corpus
Urinary Bladder	3%		2%	Brain
Kidney	3%		2%	Multiple Myeloma
All Other Sites	**22%**		**23%**	**All Other Sites**

*Excludes basal and squamous cell skin cancers and in situ carcinomas except urinary bladder.
Percentages may not total 100% due to rounding.

Figure 36-1 Ten leading cancer sites for estimated new cancer cases and deaths by sex, United States, 2002.*

Not only does cancer have an impact on individuals and their families, it also impacts our society as a whole. Estimates indicate that two of every three families in America are affected by cancer. The annual cost of cancer exceeds $100 billion, which includes direct medical costs, indirect morbidity costs, and indirect mortality costs. In addition, millions of cancer survivors are alive in the United States today. The American Cancer Society estimates that two thirds of patients with cancer survive for 5 years or longer. Many have undergone curative treatment and have returned to normal lifestyles; however, many others live with permanent disabilities and pain.[3]

PATIENT CARE

The care of the oncology patient begins with a detailed history and physical examination. Although cancer patients may present with vague complaints, they often reveal at least one symptom that can be directly relayed to the underlying disease. Some of the most common nonspecific symptoms are fatigue, pain, anorexia, insomnia, and nausea. Often patients present with a palpable mass; some may present with symptoms indicative of their particular type of cancer. For example, lung cancer patients may present with dyspnea on exertion or hemoptysis. Anemia from occult bleeding is common in the GI cancer patient. Debilitating back pain in an elderly patient is suspicious for myeloma. Eliciting a complete review of systems aids in identifying a significant symptom that the patient may discount or fail to mention.

Information from the past medical history may reveal risk factors for a specific diagnosis or may indicate co-morbidity such as renal disease or cardiac impairment that could affect subsequent treatment options for cancer. The social history may uncover smoking, alcohol consumption, and environmental or occupational exposures related to the cancer diagnosis. In addition, the social history should provide the health care team with an understanding of the patient's social support and special needs. The family history becomes increasingly more informative and important as counseling and prevention strategies for unaffected family members in higher-risk groups are identified. Refer to Chapter 49 for detailed information on family pedigrees.

A thorough history accompanied by a complete physical examination and basic laboratory tests may prevent an oncologic emergency. The PA should begin with a basic screening examination followed by more organ-specific and symptom-specific examinations. A thorough examination may lead to identification of lymphadenopathy, hepatomegaly or other physical findings that suggest advanced disease. The presence of a superficial enlarged lymph node may allow for tissue sampling of this node and diagnosis, obviating the need for other, more invasive procedures.[4]

CASE STUDY 36-1

Mr. G is a 46-year-old man who presented with complaints of tenesmus and rectal bleeding over 3 months. He had no complaints of anorexia, weight loss, fatigue, constipation, or change in stool caliber. On physical examination, a firm mass was palpated in the rectum with moderate discomfort and slight bleeding. The lungs were clear and no organomegaly, abdominal tenderness, or hyperactive bowel sounds were noted.

Colonoscopy was performed, which revealed a 1.8 cm × 5.6 cm mass in the anterior wall of the distal rectum near the anal verge. A biopsy of the mass was positive for moderately differentiated adenocarcinoma. Transrectal ultrasound revealed the mass to be nearly circumferential with involvement of the muscularis propria near the level of the prostate. This mass was noted on magnetic resonance imaging (MRI) of the abdomen and pelvis, with no involvement of the seminal vesicles or the prostate gland. There was no evidence of metastatic disease in the lungs, liver, or abdomen. Chest x-ray was negative and blood counts, chemistries, and carcinoembryonic antigen (CEA) were all within normal limits. This cancer was staged as T2N0M0.

Family history was negative for cancer in parents, siblings, grandparents, or other members. Multimodality therapy using preoperative chemoradiation and surgical resection was discussed with the patient and his wife, and they were provided information for both standard therapy and research protocol options. The probability of cure with surgery alone is approximately 50%; the addition of chemoradiation increases this to 65% for patients with resectable disease.

The patient opted for standard therapy and received daily continuous-infusion fluorouracil by portable pump with radiation therapy for 5 to 6 weeks. Four weeks after completion of chemoradiation, he underwent an abdominal perineal resection with surgical closure of the anus and formation of a colostomy. He then received 4 months of adjuvant chemotherapy with daily continuous-infusion fluorouracil alone. This therapy was generally well tolerated with mild to moderate fatigue, anorexia, diarrhea, neutropenia, and skin irritation in the radiation field. The only major long-term complication was severe erectile dysfunction.

Submitted by Michael E. Poole, PA-C, MPH

MULTIDISCIPLINARY APPROACH TO CANCER TREATMENT

Over the past few years, the value of a multidisciplinary approach to the care and treatment of a cancer patient has been increasingly recognized. In many institutions, disease-specific multidisciplinary cancer clinics offer patients the opportunity to be evaluated by the medical oncologist, surgical oncologist, radiation oncologist, nutritionist, physical therapist, and social worker at the time of their first or second clinic visit. Whether the PA is employed in medical oncology, surgical oncology, or radiation oncology, the opportunity to take care of patients and to coordinate care in this setting is challenging, intellectually stimulating, and personally satisfying. Certainly for the patient, the family and the referring physician, the possibility of an entire team of cancer specialists working together to meet the individual needs of the patient in a timely manner is optimal. In the multidisciplinary approach to patient management, each discipline performs a complementary function.

Historically, surgery is the oldest treatment for cancer, and until recent years, it was considered the only treatment that offered potential cure for cancer patients. Surgery has become a very popular career choice for physician assistants. Subspecialties such as thoracic oncology are growing areas in which the surgical PA may find a niche. The primary care physician most often refers to a surgeon for biopsy and pathological diagnosis; therefore, the surgical oncology team is often the first to see a patient with a newly diagnosed or suspected cancer. The surgeon not only provides the pathological diagnosis but is instrumental in the extensive staging needed for the cancer patient. The surgical oncology team is responsible for keeping up with advances in surgical techniques and the expanding knowledge of cancer biology.[5]

After Roentegen's discovery of x-rays in 1895 and the Curies' discovery of radium several years later, the biological effects of ionizing radiation were recognized and soon were used to treat a variety of malignant and nonmalignant conditions.[6] Radiotherapy has both curative and palliative indications in the treatment of patients with cancer. Radiation is often given in conjunction with surgery, as well as chemotherapy. Patients undergoing radiation experience varied symptoms, most often related to the organs that are within the direct radiation field, such as esophagitis and dysphagia from the treatment of oral cavity cancers, esophageal cancers or lung cancers. Radiation dermatitis and skin breakdown can occur, and patients often have associated fatigue and nausea. Patients receiving brain radiation, whether for a primary central nervous system (CNS) tumor or a metastatic lesion, can experience a myriad of symptoms, including severe fatigue, disequilibrium, nausea, vomiting, confusion or short-term memory loss, and hair loss. Radiotherapy prior to surgery is often employed to decrease the amount of normal tissue removed for resection of the tumor. Radiotherapy is an integral and indispensable modality for pain relief and palliation of other symptoms such as metastatic disease to bone or obstructing bronchial lesions.[5]

Medical oncology specializes in the use of systemic forms of treatment for cancer, such as chemotherapy, biological modulators, and immunotherapy. However, the role of the medical oncologist extends far beyond the delivery of these agents. Traditionally, the medical oncologist serves as the internist in the multidisciplinary management of cancer. For the most part, the surgical oncologist and the radiation oncologist provide specialized care of short duration. However, the medical oncology team is responsible for the continued and long-term follow-up of the cancer patient. From the time of diagnosis to the long-term follow-up of survivors or to the end-of-life care for patients with incurable disease, the medical oncology team provides treatment, symptom management, and supportive care.[5]

CASE STUDY 36-2

Mr. P is a 49-year-old married father of three, who works as an electrician. He was referred to the multidisciplinary lung cancer clinic by his primary care provider. Mr. P had been in good health all of his life. Approximately 4 months before presentation, Mr. P developed right shoulder pain. Treatment with nonsteroidal anti-inflammatory drugs (NSAIDs) brought a brief period of relief, but the pain returned and continued to worsen. He then developed pain in his right forearm and fourth and fifth fingers with associated numbness. He presented to his primary care physician (PCP) who noted a right Horner's syndrome. Chest x-ray revealed a mass in the right superior sulcus. Chest computed tomography (CT) confirmed a 6 cm × 6 cm superior sulcus tumor. There was no evidence of mediastinal node enlargement.

Mr. P had noted increased fatigue and decreased stamina but had continued to try to work. His appetite was good, although he had a 5-pound weight loss in the past month. He denied shortness of breath, dyspnea on exertion, cough, sputum production, or hemoptysis. Past medical history was remarkable for hypertension diagnosed 3 years prior. He denied any drug allergies. He had smoked one pack of cigarettes a day for 25 years and stopped 3 years ago. Review of systems was negative for headaches, fever, chills, and night sweats. He denied chest pain, abdominal pain, constipation, diarrhea, nausea, or vomiting. He denied numbness or tingling in his extremities, other than the numbness and pain in his right fourth and fifth fingers.

On physical examination, he appeared well, and vital signs were stable. Karnofsky performance status was 80%. His skin was without rashes, and there was no cervical, supraclavicular, axillary, or inguinal adenopathy. He had a right-sided Horner's syndrome. There were no oral lesions. No abnormalities in the lungs, heart, and abdomen were found. Extremities showed no clubbing, edema, or cyanosis. Neurological examination revealed the cranial nerves to be grossly intact, the reflexes symmetrical and 2+, and the strength 5+/5. He had decreased sensation in an ulnar distribution of the right forearm and hand.

Mr. P was scheduled for a brain CT and bone scan to complete his staging workup. Both of these were negative for distant disease. A whole body positron emission tomography (PET) scan showed a large area of hypermetabolic activity in the right upper lobe, but no other focal abnormalities were seen, and there was no evidence of mediastinal, hilar, or axillary abnormalities. Mr. P was referred to thoracic surgery and underwent bronchoscopy and cervical mediastinoscopy. The bronchoscopy revealed no endobronchial lesions. The mediastinoscopy was negative for evidence of malignancy at 2R, 4R, 4L, and level 7 lymph nodes. Mr. P underwent pulmonary function tests, which were adequate for surgery. He returned to the multidisciplinary thoracic oncology clinic a week following his mediastinoscopy. He was seen in conjunction with the radiation oncology department and in follow-up by surgical oncology team members.

Mr. P was thought to be a good candidate for neoadjuvant treatment prior to resection of the superior sulcus tumor. He was also a good candidate for treatment in a clinical trial and met with the research nurse to discuss the current neoadjuvant trial of concurrent chemotherapy and radiation. Mr. P agreed to treatment on this protocol, and informed consent was obtained. He received 6 weeks of concurrent radiation and chemotherapy. During this treatment, he experienced mild nausea, which was treated with antiemetics, moderate esophagitis treated with narcotics and viscous lidocaine, mild radiation dermatitis, and moderate fatigue, but only a 5-pound weight loss. Erythropoietin injections were given to maintain his hemoglobin above 12 gm/dL.

At the completion of his adjuvant chemotherapy and radiation, he underwent repeat staging with chest CT, which showed that the right upper lobe mass had decreased in size, measuring approximately 4.5 cm in largest dimension. A repeat brain CT was negative for metastatic disease.

Mr. P was taken to the operating room approximately 4 weeks after completing his neoadjuvant therapy. He underwent right thoracotomy, right upper lobectomy with chest wall resection, and removal of ribs 1 to 3. Final pathology showed a residual poorly differentiated adenocarcinoma as dispersed mild clusters of cells within a 2.5 cm × 2 cm × 2 cm mass containing fibrosis and necrosis, typical of treated tumor. There was no lymphatic or vascular invasion. There was extension to the parietal pleura, but the chest wall margin was free of tumor. The posterior rib margins were free of tumor, and the anterior rib margins were negative for tumor following decalcification. Additional lymph node dissection, including level 11 and level 7, was negative for malignancy.

Mr. P had an uneventful postsurgical hospital course and was discharged without incident. He returned to the multidisciplinary clinic 2 weeks after surgery, at which time he was doing well, although he was experiencing post-thoracotomy pain and continued shoulder and right arm pain. He noted some slight weakness in his right hand and was referred for physical therapy and occupational therapy. He continued to require narcotics for pain control. The management plan for Mr. P included follow-up in the multidisciplinary thoracic oncology clinic monthly for 4 months, where he would be evaluated by the surgical and medical oncology teams. After that, he would be seen in the medical oncology department every 3 months for the first year, every 6 months for 5 years, and yearly thereafter.

GOALS OF TREATMENT

Most patients with cancer receive some type of therapy once a histologic diagnosis has been made and the extent of disease is known by appropriate staging. Accurate staging provides a basis for both the provider and the patient to weigh individual benefits and risks associated with a treatment. If the intent of therapy is curative, both the oncology team and the patient are more apt to accept toxicities to achieve that goal. However, in the setting of palliative treatment for advanced disease, the goals are to enhance quality of life and, when possible, to extend life. The balance of risk to benefit is different. A discussion of benefits in relationship to risks in clear layperson terms is vital for shared decision making.

Whether therapy has a curative or a palliative intent, its success depends on a sound understanding of the patient's disease and performance status, and acceptance of the treatment plan. Most cancer therapies have associated toxicities; therefore, one of the PA roles in oncology is to address complications of both the disease and its treatment.[4] A comprehensive patient assessment before, during, and after therapy is essential to determine the efficacy of treatment and to manage its adverse effects. Prompt recognition and appropriate intervention for complications of cancer therapies, as outlined in Table 36-1, may prevent more serious problems.[7]

In many ways, supportive care becomes essential to the success of cancer treatment. Failure to treat the symptoms of cancer and of cancer therapy may lead to a patient's withdrawal from treatment and, possibly, to a lost opportunity for cure. Inclusion of the patient's family and support network whenever possible aids in treatment planning. However, a patient's confidentiality must be consistently respected. It is important to discuss in detail the diagnosis, treatment implications, and survival so that the patient and his family may make plans, have a better understanding of the clinical situation, and cope with potential risks and financial costs.[4]

CASE STUDY 36-3

Ms. J is a 43-year-old premenopausal woman who presented with a self-detected right breast mass of 2 weeks' duration. Previous mammograms 9 months earlier were unremarkable. Repeat mammogram revealed new architectural change in the right upper outer quadrant. Ultrasound demonstrated a solid mass. Initially, fine-needle biopsy was nondiagnostic. She underwent excisional biopsy for a 2.5-cm invasive ductal carcinoma with negative surgical margins. Estrogen and progesterone receptors were positive. She opted for

Table 36-1   Complications of Cancer Therapies

Chemotherapy	Surgery	Radiation Therapy	Biotherapy
Fatigue	Fatigue	Fatigue	Flulike symptoms
Changes in hematological values	Pain	Changes in hematological values	Fatigue
Low white blood cells	Change in mobility	Low white blood cells	Loss of appetite
Low red blood cells	Changes in nutrition	Low red blood cells	Altered taste sensation
Low platelets	Potential for postoperative infection	Skin changes	Slowed thinking
Nausea and vomiting	Skin changes	Dry desquamation	
		Moist desquamation	Reversible changes in liver enzymes and hematological values
Mucositis: oral, rectal, and vaginal			Inflammatory reactions at injection sites
Skin changes		Site-specific adverse effects	
Alopecia			
Darkened nail beds			
Changes in sexuality			

breast-conserving surgery and had an axillary node dissection with 3 of 17 lymph nodes involved with cancer. Radiological evaluation, including bone scan and chest/abdomen CT, was within normal limits, ruling out distant disease.

Ms. J was otherwise healthy, except for an active 20-pack-year smoking history. Family history was remarkable for a maternal grandmother alive at 87 years old after mastectomy for breast cancer at age 57, and two maternal great aunts who had breast cancer late in life. Her mother and two sisters are alive and well. She was nulliparous. She lived alone, with supportive family nearby.

Her tumor size, three involved lymph nodes, and premenopausal status placed her in an intermediate to high risk category for recurrence. An estimated 40% risk of systemic recurrence within 10 years was discussed. Chemotherapy and the use of tamoxifen are shown to increase disease-free and overall survival in women with similar histories. The chemotherapy and tamoxifen benefit was estimated at a relative 50% reduction of her risk, or an absolute 20% reduction. The short-term and long-term risks of chemotherapy were reviewed with Ms. J, and chemotherapy options were presented.

She decided to enroll in a multicenter treatment trial and was randomly assigned to the standard treatment arm of four cycles of doxorubicin and cyclophosphamide over 12 weeks. She tolerated her chemotherapy with only minimal nausea. She received radiation to her breast and lower axilla over 6 weeks. Ms. J completed 5 years of oral tamoxifen this year and is without evidence of disease.

ISSUES IN ONCOLOGY

When people are given the diagnosis of cancer, profound changes occur not only in their life, but also in the lives of their families. In years past, the word *cancer* was equated with death. Perhaps one of the most disturbing aspects of cancer is the fear of the unknown. In the past, physicians often tried to downplay the extent of the illness, attempting to protect patients from what they viewed as a devastating diagnosis. Patients and their families often felt shame and sought to keep the diagnosis a secret. This fear and secrecy compounded the emotional burden felt by patients and their families. The American Cancer Society was founded in 1913 to try to counteract public fears and to teach that there was the possibility of cure with early diagnosis and treatment. Advances have enhanced detection, improved treatments, and increased cure rates.

Pioneering work that focused on psychosocial issues of cancer patients has revealed that patients do better when fully informed of their illness, treatment options, and prognosis. The more information patients and families are given, the more likely they are to cope successfully with the adverse effects associated with treatment. In addition to fear of the unknown and possible death, cancer patients are faced with numerous other psychological and social stresses, such as dependence on others, disability, disfigurement, strain on relationships, sexual issues, spiritual distress, job discrimination, and financial issues. Returning to school, the workplace, and society after treatment adds additional stress. The oncology PA may need flexibility in scheduling extra time with the patient to address these psychosocial issues. Patients' psychosocial needs vary. The ability to comfortably discuss all these issues and to make appropriate referrals is vital for optimal care of the oncology patient.

Repeated and continued counseling prior to treatment, during treatment, and after completion of treatment is necessary and has been shown to be reassuring, not frightening, to the patient. A hopeful, compassionate attitude may succeed even when a treatment is not effective. During this time, the patient and family gain confidence and trust in the PA. They become more effective participants in their care when they feel their concerns and needs are recognized. Ultimately, it is the patient's decision as to what treatment to undergo, and the oncology team must be prepared to accept the possibility that the patient may not follow the advice of the team. Reassurance that care will be provided no matter what the patient chooses is paramount.[4,7,8,9]

When it becomes inevitable that a patient will die from cancer, the appropriate discussion of end-of-life issues with the patient and his or her family becomes a matter of great importance. Studies have shown that terminally ill patients benefit significantly from being able to discuss their feelings and fears about death. The most common cause of death in patients with cancer is infection, followed by respiratory failure, hepatic failure, and renal failure. Usually, many months pass between the diagnosis of metastatic cancer and the development of these complications. Timely information about the narrowing effective treatment options provides a framework for patients to determine the level and extent of medical intervention that they desire. Hospice provides an extraordinary service for cancer patients and their families and usually results in a positive and satisfying experience for the medical team, as well as the patients' families. The PA will most likely have an integral involvement with hospice team members, communicating with them sometimes on a daily basis up until the death of the patient.[4,10,11] Refer to Chapter 28 for details about hospice care and to Chapter 46 for further discussion of issues related to dying and death.

REWARDS AND CHALLENGES IN ONCOLOGY

Oncology is an exciting field with advances occurring at a rapid rate. Who would have thought that someone like Lance Armstrong who suffered from brain metastases could come back to win the Tour de France multiple times? The 5-year survival rate for all cancer is now estimated at 50%.[7] Oncology not only is academically challenging, but it offers the PA the opportunity to profoundly affect patients' lives and future practice patterns. In addition, the clinical trials in cancer diagnosis and treatment, with their far-reaching scale and scope, are perhaps the largest such efforts undertaken in modern medicine. PAs have the opportunity to enroll patients in these trials, thus impacting the standard of care for years to come.

The demands and stresses of patient care are heightened in oncology. Patients are often ill and debilitated. What may seem like a small thing, such as touching a patient's shoulder, may signal compassion and hope when the patient feels despair. The uncertainty of the effectiveness of a particular treatment for an individual patient is a persistent reality. Unique toxicities are inherent to oncology therapies; some of these predispose patients to life-threatening complications. The PA has the opportunity to become well acquainted with the patient and his immediate and extended family, and in certain cases, may become personally and emotionally attached. Being involved in decisions about withholding or stopping treatment, dealing with the impact of unrealistic expectations from some patients and families, and the repeated impact of patient deaths can lead to depression and burnout. Monitoring oneself for symptoms of increased stress and emotional fatigue, setting up a support system, and taking time off are important coping strategies. In the practice of oncology, one must be able to accept the inadequacies of medicine, recognize one's limitations, try to maintain a healthy diet and exercise program, and allow time for relaxation and recreation.[8]

CONCLUSION

Whether the physician assistant decides to enter the field of oncology in a community private practice setting or in a university academic setting, the opportunity for personal, educational, and professional success is unlimited. The potential to be involved in clinical trials and in the development of new therapies to try to improve survival with exciting research and new surgical techniques, new drugs, and new advances in supportive therapies makes oncology a fascinating and ever-changing field of medicine. To provide hopeful and compassionate patient care that includes education, counseling, and support to patients and their families during one of the most devastating and difficult times of their lives is, above all, the greatest reward.

CLINICAL APPLICATIONS

1. If you were involved in the care of the three patients presented in the cases in this chapter, what psychosocial issues, including family issues, would you anticipate? Develop a plan for counseling and patient education to address these issues.
2. Why is the patient's input important when deciding on a treatment plan?
3. If you secured employment as a PA in oncology, what would you find challenging and rewarding?

REFERENCES

1. Lee HSJ (ed). Dates in Oncology. New York: The Parthenon Publishing Group, 2000.
2. Jemal A, Thomas A, Murray T, Thun M. Cancer Statistics, 2000. A Cancer Journal for Clinicians 2002;52:23.
3. Wingo PA, Parkin DM, Eyre HJ. Measuring the occurrence of cancer: impact and statistics. In: Lenhard RE Jr, Osteen RT, Gansler T (eds). The American Cancer Society's Clinical Oncology. Atlanta, GA: American Cancer Society, 2001.
4. Longo DL. Neoplastic disorders. In: Braunwald E, Fauci AS, Kasper DL, Hauser SL, Long DL, James JL (eds). Harrison's Principles of Internal Medicine, ed 15. New York: McGraw-Hill, 2001.
5. Holland JF, Frei E, Kufe DW, Bast RC Jr, Pollock RE, Weichselbaum RR. Principles of multidisciplinary management. In: Bast RC Jr, Kufe DW, Pollock RE, Weichselbaum RR, Holland JF, Frei E (eds). Cancer Medicine. Hamilton, Ontario, Canada: BC Decker, 2000.
6. Mieszkalski GB, Brady LW, Yaeger TE, Class R. Radiotherapy: basis for current major therapies for cancer. In: Lenhard RE Jr, Osteen RT, Gansler T (eds). The American Cancer Society's Clinical Oncology. Atlanta: American Cancer Society, 2001.
7. Rieger PT, Escalante CP Complications of cancer treatment. In: Boyer KL, Ford MB, Judkins AF, Levin B (eds). Primary Care Oncology. Philadelphia: WB Saunders, 1999.
8. Lederberg MS, Massie MJ. Psychosocial and ethical issues in the care of cancer patients. In: Devita VT Jr, Hellman S, Rosenberg SA (eds). Cancer Principles and Practice of Oncology. Philadelphia: JB Lippincott, 1993.
9. Lenhard RE Jr, Osteen RT. General approach to cancer patients. In: Lenhard RE Jr, Osteen RT, Gansler T (eds). The American Cancer Society's Clinical Oncology. Atlanta: American Cancer Society, 2001.
10. Gerber LH, Levinson S, Hicks JE, Gallelli P, Whitehurst J, Scheib D, Sonies BC. Evaluation and management of disability: rehabilitation aspects of cancer. In: Devita VT Jr, Hellman S, Rosenberg SA (eds). Cancer Principles and Practice of Oncology. Philadelphia: JB Lippincott, 1993.
11. Hughes MK, Weinstein S. Medical decision making at the end of life: hospice care and care of the terminally ill. In: Boyer KL, Ford MB, Judkins AF, Levin B (eds). Primary Care Oncology. Philadelphia: WB Saunders, 1999.

RESOURCES

Boyer KL, Ford MB, Judkins AF, Levin B (eds). *Primary Care Oncology*. Philadelphia: WB Saunders, 1999. *A useful, comprehensive text for the primary care practitioner.*

The American Cancer Society's Clinical Oncology. Atlanta, GA: American Cancer Society, 2001. *The American Cancer Society's journal provides the latest research and recommendations on cancer diagnosis and treatment.*

www3.cancer.org. The American Cancer Society's web site features a wealth of information for patients and their families and for health care professionals.

CHAPTER 37

Infectious Disease Medicine

Venetia L. Orcutt and Durward A. Watson

INTRODUCTION

Just as the physician assistant (PA) concept emerged during the 1960s in response to demands for more available, accessible, and affordable health care,[1] it is likely that the selection of the infectious disease practice by physician assistants reflects the response of these individuals to the demands emerging from the advent of the human immunodeficiency virus (HIV)/ acquired immunodeficiency syndrome (AIDS) epidemic in the 1980s. The 1990s demonstrated small yet steady increases in the absolute numbers of physician assistants in this internal medicine subspecialty that offers a variety of roles and rewards. Because no studies have been done to date on the utilization of physician assistants in the infectious disease subspecialty, this chapter provides anecdotal information concerning the scope of practice of physician assistants who select infectious disease as their practice. Additional goals of this chapter are to discuss the following:

➤ The historical development of infectious disease as a specialty.
➤ The most common roles of PAs within the specialty.

➤ The roles and rewards of working in this arena.
➤ Representative case studies of those most often encountered by health care professionals involved in the care of infectious disease patients.

HISTORY OF INFECTIOUS DISEASE

Infectious disease as a specialty arose only after significant advances had been made in the field of medicine. Especially during the years after World War II, the industrialized world benefited from the development of chemotherapeutic agents, the expansion of public health practices, and profound discoveries in the fields of microbiology and immunology, all of which led to significant decreases in the incidence of mortality and morbidity due to infectious processes. It was in this exciting and changing environment that the infectious disease specialty, as it is recognized today, had its beginnings.

Kass,[2] in providing a historical perspective, suggested three distinct phases of the emergence of infectious disease as a specialty area of medicine. In the first and earliest phase, all clinicians were by default infectious disease specialists in that a large proportion of problems addressed in an ordinary practice setting involved infectious processes. There was little to provide in terms of effective preventive measures or treatments for infectious disease during this phase, and the medical research community's focus was on the description of clinical syndromes and the natural history of processes rather than on treatments. The advances in public health measures and the prosperity that characterized the early 19th century heralded the second phase in the history of infectious disease. Microbes were recognized as a cause of disease and specific vaccines were developed. These advances began the trend toward decreasing mortality and morbidity secondary to infectious disease. It wasn't until the understanding among members of the scientific community was enhanced regarding the recognition, prevention, and treatment of these diseases that a shift in the focus of the general practitioner could occur. It was no longer necessary for every clinician to be a specialist because many diseases were now more easily controlled through prevention or treatment. This further allowed those practitioners who were specifically drawn to infectious disease to focus their attention on new approaches to these diseases and the efficacy of older approaches, and to become the storehouse of knowledge about previously common diseases that were becoming more and more rare occurrences. Thus, this third phase saw the differentiation of the infectious disease specialist from other types of clinicians. As a result, the average infectious disease specialist today serves as a consultant to other clinicians in the treatment of patients affected by a myriad of infectious diseases.

PHYSICIAN ASSISTANTS IN INFECTIOUS DISEASE PRACTICE

Census data from the American Academy of Physician Assistants (AAPA) suggest that less than 1% of responding physician assistants indicated involvement in the infectious disease subspecialty in 1991, the first year that data were collected. Over the past decade, more have chosen this area as their primary practice focus (Table 37-1), yet the percentage of physician assistants in an infectious disease practice has remained steady at less than 1%.[3] However, these numbers do not reflect the vast number of primary care physician assistants who treat patients affected by the problems generally seen in an infectious disease practice.[4]

Physician assistants may assume a variety of different roles in the infectious disease specialty arena. They provide outpatient and inpatient care in public and private settings, and they may provide clinical, research, consultation, or educational services.

Table 37-1   PAs in Infectious Disease, by Region, Sex, and Year

	Northeast		Southeast		North Central		South Central		West		
	Male	**Female**	**Male**	**Female**	**Male**	**Female**	**Male**	**Female**	**Male**	**Female**	
											TOTALS
1992	9	9	6	15	1	4	2	6	5	4	61
1993	2	12	5	12	1	3	4	8	5	7	59
1994	8	10	5	9	2	4	4	6	6	4	58
1995	9	11	7	15	5	4	7	11	5	8	82
1996	10	15	7	11	1	3	6	6	8	8	75
1997	11	17	10	17	2	2	8	5	6	8	86
1998	8	16	14	15	1	4	6	7	9	7	87
1999	11	13	12	19	3	4	5	10	11	15	103
2000	15	16	12	16	2	6	3	12	8	16	106
2001	16	20	11	18	2	5	5	8	6	13	104

AAPA Census data, 1992-2001.

In the outpatient setting, PAs are typically involved in the routine management of patients, which includes the initial evaluation of presenting patients with elicitation of historical information, performance of the physical examination, ordering of appropriate diagnostic tests, interpretation of test results, and the development and implementation of management plans. Often PAs are involved in the interdisciplinary team approach to patient management and find themselves interfacing with infusion pharmacists and nurses, home health care providers, dietitians, and social workers.

Many infectious disease practices are engaged in clinical research. In this setting, PAs, in conjunction with other study staff members, assume the investigator functions of protocol management. These functions may include determination of patient inclusion and exclusion criteria, performance of entry and interim history and physical examinations, and oversight of clinical events occurring during the study period. Of particular importance are the identification and management of serious adverse outcomes, and the submission of appropriate documentation to the sponsoring organization. Opportunities abound for physician assistants to contribute to the growing knowledge of this specialty and to participate in publications. Inpatient settings provide physician assistants a means of participating in the management of the hospitalized patient. Although many of the roles in this setting mirror those in the outpatient arena, often PAs serve as consultants to admitting primary care clinicians. Additionally, PAs are involved as educators as they participate in teaching rounds conducted at the hospitals or serve as preceptors for students who are completing an infectious disease elective course.

This variety of roles provides PAs with opportunities for significant personal satisfaction and continued career growth. The infectious disease specialty is an evolving area of medicine. Ongoing advances in the areas of virology, immunology, bacteriology, and chemotherapeutic agents provide the opportunity for involvement in cutting edge medicine that lends itself to continued intellectual stimulation. The immense personal satisfaction of assisting patients in moving from feelings of overwhelming loss of function due to an infectious disease process to a place of empowerment and control is one of the many rewards of working in this specialty. The ability to share this dynamic field with future physician assistants adds to the overall feeling of satisfaction experienced by PAs in infectious disease medicine

CLINICAL ASSESSMENT IN THE INFECTIOUS DISEASE SPECIALTY OUTPATIENT SETTING

Physician assistants working in an infectious disease setting need to have a basic understanding of the pathophysiology, clinical presentation, and treatment of viral, bacterial, fungal, and parasitic infections. Although dramatic progress has been made over the past several decades in the treatment and prevention of these infections, infectious diseases continue to be responsible for significant morbidity and mortality in both the developed and the developing regions of the world. In the United States, infections frequently encountered in clinic and hospital settings include *viral infections* caused by such agents as HIV, herpes simplex virus, hepatitis B (HBV), hepatitis C (HCV), influenza virus, and cytomegalovirus (CMV); *bacterial infections* responsible for various sexual transmitted diseases (STDs), pneumonias, tuberculosis, colitis, necrotizing skin infections of the diabetic, and osteomyelitis; *fungal infections* such as cryptococcus and histoplasmosis affecting the pulmonary tree, the skin, and/or the cerebrospinal fluid; and *parasitic infections* of the skin and gastrointestinal system.

Clinical evaluation of the patient referred to an infectious disease practice is based on the established principles of obtaining a medical history, performing a thorough examination, and ordering pertinent laboratory, radiographic, and skin antigen/antibody testing to support a working clinical assessment. Concern about the immune status of a patient is usually raised on the basis of the frequency or severity of infections, or, as is often the case in a specialty setting, the finding of an unusual, opportunistic infectious agent. One screening approach to a patient with suspected infectious disease is provided in Table 37-2.[7]

History

Initial evaluation of the patient includes an extensive history, which should draw out the patient's general

Table 37-2 Screening Evaluations for Infectious Disease Patients

History	Medications and treatments
	Frequency, severity, distribution, type of infections
	Vaccination history, especially live vaccines
	Causative infectious agents
Physical examination	Weight, height, vital signs
	Hair: sheen, pigmentation
	Oropharynx: thrush, oral hairy leukoplakia, ulcers, gingivitis, dentition
	Lymphatics: assess cervical, supraclavicular, axillary, inguinal
	Chest: adventitious breath sounds, diaphragmatic excursion, anteroposterior diameter
	Cardiovascular: rhythm, rate, heart sounds, gallops
	Abdomen: organomegaly, presence of tenderness, mass, ascites
	Musculoskeletal: fractures, stature, strength
	Neurological: central nervous system examination, sensory discrimination
	Skin: wounds, abscesses, lesions, rash, cellulitis, edema, telangiectases, eczema
	Extremities: edema, dorsalis pedis/posterior tibialis pulses, edema
Routine laboratory tests	Complete blood count
	Differential: lymphopenia, neutropenia, eosinophilia
	Peripheral smear
	Platelets
	Chemistries
	Creatinine/blood urea nitrogen
	Liver function tests
	Lipid panel
	Thyroid panel
	Serologies
	HIV-1 ELISA ab test with reflexive Western blot
	Hepatitis antibody panel for A, B, C
	RPR and MHA-TP
	Toxoplasmosis immunoglobulin G (IgG)
	Serum cryptococcal ag
	Urine histology ag
	CMV antigenemia
	EBV-ab
	Immunoglobulins
	IgA, IgM, IgG, IgE
	Inflammatory markers
	Erythrocyte sedimentation rate, C-reactive protein
	Cultures: wound, blood, cerebrospinal fluid, sputum for routine bacterial C/S, fungus
	Stool assays for routine C/S, cryptosporidia, ova and parasites, *Clostridium difficile*, white blood cell count

Modified from Mandell G, Bennett J, Dolin R. Principles and Practice of Infectious Disease, 5th ed. Philadelphia: Churchill Livingstone, 2000:149.

health status, drug history, sexual history and current sexual behaviors, history of previous hepatitis infections, previous vaccinations, and risk assessment for opportunistic infections. The history should delineate the patient's general well-being, the presence of any constitutional symptoms, history of infectious disease (both childhood and adult), previous hospitalizations, and immunization history. Drug history should include allergic reactions and history of prescribed and over-the-counter medications. Frank discussion of past and present illicit drug history, tattooing, and piercings should be documented. Sexual history includes previous sexually transmitted diseases, current sexual activity, obstetrical and gynecological history, contraceptive use, and encounters with partners at risk for HIV, HBV, HCV, and STD infections (i.e., gonorrhea, syphilis, and herpes simplex virus). Background information should be elicited with respect to foreign travel and current and previous residences; occupation and hobbies should also be noted. Any history of past transfusion should be elicited.

Physical Examination

A comprehensive physical examination should be completed, with emphasis on documentation of weight, height, and temperature; careful funduscopic and oral examination should be performed, along with dermatological evaluation of the sensory dermatomes, hands, feet and nail beds; complete lymphatic evaluation; and rectal and genital assessments. Pelvic examinations and Papanicolaou smears should be performed on any postmenarchal HIV infected woman every 6 months for the first year and annually thereafter.

Laboratory Evaluation

An initial baseline hematology and chemistry panel should be obtained, along with a urinalysis and thyroid panel. The chemistry panel should include renal function tests (blood urea nitrogen, creatinine), liver function tests (serum bilirubin, transaminase enzymes, alkaline phosphatase, lactate dehydrogenase), serum amylase, lipase levels, and a lipid profile that fractionates the patient's serum cholesterol and fasting triglycerides. Baseline HIV antibody testing by enzyme-linked immunosorbent assay (ELISA) and

reflexive Western blot should be obtained when the patient's permission has been received (document in chart). Baseline serologies for syphilis (rapid plasma reagin [RPR] and microhemagglutination–*Treponema pallidum* [MHA-TP]); toxoplasmosis; hepatitis A, B, and C; and Epstein-Barr virus are routinely drawn. In addition, baseline purified protein derivative (PPD) with controls and chest x-ray should be ordered.

A majority of physician assistants working in the infectious disease specialty setting are primarily involved with the evaluation and management of patients impacted by HIV and common co-morbid infections such as HBV and HCV. Therefore, a working knowledge of specific laboratory evaluation of the patient believed to be impacted by these infections is warranted.

➤ If HIV is confirmed by antibody testing, a baseline measurement of absolute CD4+ T cells and percentages allows the clinician to assess the patient's risk for developing specific opportunistic infections. Baseline plasma HIV RNA by polymerase chain reaction (PCR), or viral load, taken on two occasions 2 to 4 weeks apart[5] at least 6 to 12 months following exposure to HIV, identifies the patient's "set point" and permits assessment of the patient's relative risk for disease progression.[6]

➤ If hepatitis B is confirmed on serology, a hepatitis B DNA assay is performed to assess viral load; hepatitis B antibody/antigen testing is obtained to assess the patient's relative infectivity status.

➤ If hepatitis C is confirmed, hepatitis C RNA will provide a baseline viral load; genotyping is performed to help the clinician predict the relative success ratio for treatment intervention, and a liver biopsy is performed to assess degree of fibrosis and to rule out hepatic carcinoma.

In some cases, the patient's history and physical findings may lead to consideration of some other specific infections or conditions. When cytomegalovirus infection is suspected or confirmed, a serum CMV antigenemia assay is obtained and followed to remission. Likewise, if cerebrospinal fluid cryptococcal disease is known or suspected, serum cryptococcal antigen is obtained and followed. Urine histoplasma antigen testing can help confirm a diagnosis of histoplasmosis.

When congenital immune deficiency is suspected, immunoglobulins and serum electrophoresis are obtained. For deep skin structure (cellulitis) and bone infections (osteomyelitis), tissue cultures are obtained for identification of aerobic and anaerobic organisms with sensitivities to direct antimicrobial therapy. For these patients, baseline inflammatory markers (C-reactive protein and erythrocyte sedimentation rate) are drawn and followed.

An excellent reference for descriptions of the commonly used laboratory tests mentioned previously and in Table 37-2 is Harrison's Principles of Internal Medicine, 15th ed, Part 7 (entitled "Infectious Diseases" [New York: McGraw-Hill, 2001].

CASE STUDY 37-1

Trouble with adherence

Mr. A, a 29-year-old gay, Hispanic male, presented in May of 2001 as a clinically stable, HIV-infected male who had not seen a physician for longer than 6 months. He reported having gotten "tired of going to the doctor all the time for my HIV." Mr. A is an accountant by profession, plays soccer in a community league, and was not involved in a long-term relationship as of this initial office visit. The patient was first diagnosed in 1992 at an anonymous testing center operated by a local service agency. The patient reported no history of serious opportunistic infections and had no clinical complaints at his first visit. He did recall an episode of urethral gonorrhea in his early 20s and reported having had hepatitis A in the past. The patient also reported that he had undergone surgical excision of penile and rectal condylomata in the past.

Mr. A had begun his last regimen of antiviral medications (efavirenz 600 mg at bedtime, didanosine 200 mg chewable tablets on an empty stomach twice daily, and stavudine 40 mg every 12 hours) in 1998 but had not taken his medicines over the past "3 or 4" months. Furthermore, the patient indicated that he had had trouble adhering to his three medications; his previous physician had told him that he should not skip doses but that if he did, he should discontinue his medications. Aside from his most recent regimen, the patient

knew that he had been on "a lot of medications" in the past, including "Crixivan (indinavir) and Viracept (nelfinavir)."

Available medical records showed that he had a "see-saw" pattern of viral loads since January of 2000. At that time, his viral load was 117,931 copies/mL; 2 months later, his viral load dropped to 2500 copies/mL, but it rose back to 45,600 copies/mL before nadiring at fewer than 400 copies/mL in May of 2000. Over the subsequent 12 months, the patient's viral load had steadily risen and was recorded at 26,459 copies/mL at the time of his initial visit in the office. No prior CD4 cells were available; his CD4 cell count in May of 2001 was low, at 159 cells/mm^3.

Discussion

Here, the clinician is faced with two familiar problems with HIV-infected patients who are seen for an initial office visit—lack of complete medical records (complete records from 1992 would be helpful) and a pattern of nonadherence.

Knowledge of the patient's previous regimen(s) would be helpful so the clinician could avoid prescribing a regimen that is likely to fail for the patient. However, prudent use of resistance testing[8] up front with this patient fills in some important gaps. Indeed, a viral genotype in this patient revealed that he was completely resistant to efavirenz and other members of the non-nucleoside reverse transcriptase inhibitor (NNRTI) class of antiretrovirals. The patient was also found to have acquired a number of other resistant mutations among the nucleoside reverse transcriptase class, including those conferring likely resistance to zidovudine, lamivudine, and stavudine. Armed with these findings and surrogate markers (viral loads, CD4 cell counts) that suggested the patient was at risk in the foreseeable future for developing opportunistic infections such as *Pneumocystis carinii* pneumonia,[9,10] the clinician had acquired sufficient information to develop clinical interventions.

But first, it is imperative that the patient's tendency to disrupt therapy is addressed. If Mr. A is not to repeatedly fail subsequent regimens and thus, ultimately succumb to his underlying infection, adherence counseling is necessary. Depending on the available clinical personnel, some measure of adherence counseling is bound to be addressed by the physician assistant. Questions to be addressed are summarized in Table 37-3. Investing time up front to address the patient's concerns will go a long way to ensure future successful management of the patient's HIV infection.

In the end, simple key messages of relevance to a patient's situation need to be presented in a straightforward and inviting manner. The importance of adherence to both medications and appointments, the basics of resistance and cross-resistance, and the need for communication between patient and clinician are universal in all adherence counseling. Without sounding pessimistic, it would be wise to convey the limited number of available regimens and the danger that Mr. A may eventually "run out of options." The challenge in these sessions is to strike a balance between being positive, so that the patient feels motivated, and being honest and direct, so that he or she understands the consequences of nonadherence.

Mr. A was eventually placed on a regimen of zidovudine, lamivudine, and abacavir, which has recently been combined into one single tablet to be taken every 12 hours. The patient missed his initial 6-week follow-up to check surrogate markers but returned at the 8-week interval after being prompted by phone contact. At that time, his viral load had dropped to 2000 copies/mL, with a corresponding rise in his CD4 cell count to 240 cells/mm^3. At 12 weeks after initiation of the new regimen, the patient's viral load had dropped to 228 cells/mL and his CD4 cell count was more than 400 cells/mm^3. It is notable that despite objective evidence of partial resistance to zidovudine and lamivudine on his baseline viral genotype, when these were provided in combination with a third powerful agent as a single tablet that the patient can take when brushing his teeth in the morning and evening, the patient's viral surrogate markers dramatically improved, thus enhancing the possibility that the patient may eventually attain remission of his infection.

CASE STUDY 37-2

Co-morbidity: to wait or not to wait

Ms. S is a pleasant 51-year-old African-American single mother employed as a detective in a large metropolitan police department, who transferred to the practice for management of her co-morbid HIV and HCV infections in May of 1999, after her previous physician had retired. Her husband died of complications of AIDS in 1995, and she feels that he was the most likely source of her infection. In May of 1999, her HIV viral load was 122 copies/mL and her CD4 count was higher than 900 cells/mm^3; her hepatitis C viral load was more than

Table 37-3	An Adherence Primer
Questions	Does the patient drop into and out of therapy? Why?
	Does the patient self-interrupt therapy? Why?
	What beliefs does the patient hold about his/her HIV medications?
	Is he/she concerned about the number or the size of his/her pills?
	What is the patient's greatest difficulty in taking his/her medications?
	Concomitant clinical problems such as depression? Drug addiction?
	What additional challenges does the patient confront: Financial? Children? Language barriers? Job stress? Transportation?
Support	Is there anyone that the patient can identify (and perhaps bring into the office) who can commit to supporting him or her in the adherence program?
	Does the patient have access to you by phone to ask questions regarding medications?
	Is there an additional clinical staff member (adherence nurse, social worker) who can meet with the patient at regular intervals to monitor adherence?

850,000 copies with a high normal serum glutamate pyruvate transaminase (SGPT) of 49. She had no hepatic stigmata and her liver span was not appreciated on percussion. She was naïve to antiretroviral medications for HIV and in the past was unable to tolerate therapy for hepatitis C because of adverse effects (Table 37-4).

She has a past medical history of hypertension. She has had one tubal pregnancy and a subsequent tubal ligation. Her 7-year-old daughter is HIV-infected, clinically stable, and under physician management at a regional children's health care center that has a large, well-funded treatment clinic for pediatric HIV.

Discussion

Ms. S represents a sizable number of patients encountered in an HIV-oriented practice who are co-morbidly infected with hepatitis C. Approximately one third of the 800,000 people living with HIV in the United States are infected with hepatitis C.[11] With respect to her HIV infection, Ms. S has been fortunate; she has maintained stable low viral loads and high CD4 cell counts over the subsequent 3 years since her initial evaluation in the clinic. The Department of Health and Human Services guidelines, published in April of 2001, support delaying treatment regimens in clinically stable HIV-infected individuals who demonstrate CD4 cell counts above 350 cells/mm^3 and viral loads lower than 55,000 copies/mL.[12,13] Thus, Ms. S has remained naïve to antiretroviral therapies. Of note, she experienced a community-acquired pneumonia in January of 2001, which she believes she caught from her daughter. She was treated successfully with intravenous quinolone antibiotic therapy as an outpatient.

On the other hand, the same "wait and see" approach cannot be taken with Ms. S's hepatitis C

Table 37-4 Adverse Effects of Interferon and Ribavirin

INTERFERON

Constitutional adverse effects	Nausea
	Myalgias
	Flulike symptoms, low-grade fever, lethargy
Myelosuppression	Thrombocytopenia
	Leukopenia
Autoimmune diseases	Hypothyroidism or hyperthyroidism
	Hyperglycemia, overt diabetes
Psychiatric adverse effects	Depression, occasionally suicidal ideation
	Emotional lability, short temper
	Psychosis

RIBAVIRIN

Hemolysis	High-risk patients include those with coronary artery disease, pulmonary disease, preexisting hemolytic disorders, and retinopathy (diabetes, hypertensive)
Teratogenesis	Pregnancy must be avoided if either partner is taking ribavirin
Mouth ulcers	
Hypersensitivity skin rashes	
Psychiatric and some constitutional symptoms associated with interferon may be exacerbated by ribavirin	

Modified from Massachusetts Medical Society. AIDS Clinical Care, vol 12, p 73 (Table 1—Side Effects of Interferon and Ribavirin).

infection. Hepatitis C virus (HCV) is a "flavivirus" that was discovered in the mid-1980s.[14] HCV is usually contracted by percutaneous exposure, but rates of sexual and perinatal transmission of HCV are significantly higher among HIV-positive patients. Approximately 20% to 30% of HCV-infected patients spontaneously clear the virus, usually within a few months of infection. The remaining 70% to 80% become chronically infected in the absence of treatment, which ultimately results in cirrhosis, hepatic failure, and hepatocellular carcinoma.[14]

Ms. S was staged in preparation for a new attempt at therapeutic intervention for HCV. Her serum transaminases remained normal, which occurs in approximately 20% to 30% of chronically infected patients. Her liver biopsy revealed fibrosis of moderate grade, without histological evidence of cirrhosis. Predictably, Ms. S had a genotype of 1. Approximately 75% of U.S. patients with HCV have a genotype of 1, and studies demonstrate that these patients have significantly poorer initial and sustained response to traditional interferon-α injections and oral ribavirin.[15]

We elected to wait until the availability of the "pegylated" interferon-α formulation before initiating new therapy for Ms. S. The new formulation, made available in the United States in October of 2001, allows for a slower release of interferon-α and the possibility of maintaining sustained plasma levels of the drug with more effective viral suppression.[16] Reducing the number of times per week that she had to self-inject her medications (from 3 times to once weekly) was attractive to this working mother; the possibility of improved tolerance was also a factor in our decision to wait. Nevertheless, within 2 weeks of initiation of therapy, her hemoglobin dropped to 10.5 g, and weekly subcutaneous erythropoietin was initiated to counteract hemolysis due to oral ribavirin. The patient's hemoglobin has subsequently been maintained between 10 and 11 g on maintenance erythropoietin. Her 6-week follow-up hepatitis C viral load by PCR is pending; a significant drop would be predictive of a good response. Given her genotype, if she is continuing

to respond at 6 months, we intend to treat for a total of 48 weeks.

CASE STUDY 37-3

Things are not always as they seem

Mr. H is a 52-year-old white male dockworker with a history of nicotine abuse and remote intravenous drug use who developed fever and cough 5 days before hospitalization. His primary care physician had initially obtained a clear chest x-ray and had treated him empirically with antibiotics for "bronchitis." The patient temporarily defervesced, but his fever rebounded and was accompanied by new dyspnea and weakness. Upon admission, the patient appeared acutely ill with a temperature of 102.5° F and a respiratory rate of 28. His examination demonstrated conjunctival petechiae, a midsystolic click, and a holosystolic murmur. Echocardiogram demonstrated severe mitral regurgitation and "vegetation" off the septal leaf of the mitral valve. The patient's admission blood cultures revealed Gram-positive cocci in chains that were then identified as group viridans streptococci out of two bottles. Mr. H responded to an 8-week course of intravenous penicillin G therapy, and a repeat echocardiogram obtained late in the course of therapy demonstrated 70% ejection fraction, persistent mitral regurgitation, and "tiny" vegetation off the mitral valve septal leaf. The patient was released to his primary care physician at the end of 8 weeks of intravenous antibiotic therapy, with instructions to pre-medicate with oral penicillin before dental procedures. Shortly after returning to work, the patient was "showing off" to his fellow workers by performing a backflip off the loading dock. Posterior neck pain developed, that worsened over the next couple of weeks despite rest and nonsteroidal anti-inflammatories. In addition, the patient began running a low-grade fever. Magnetic resonance imaging (MRI) demonstrated possible osteomyelitis at C6-C7 with phlegmon. Mr. H was placed back on continuous intravenous penicillin therapy and is waiting surgical evacuation of phlegmon and rod placement to stabilize his cervical spine.

Discussion

Infective endocarditis (IE) results from various bacteria, including streptococci, staphylococci, enterococci, gonococci, and Gram-negative bacilli. Heart valves are commonly affected, with "vegetation" consisting of bacterial mass, fibrin, and platelet aggregation, appreciated on the surfaces of the valvular leaflets by echocardiogram. Although Mr. H initially reported that he had stopped abusing intravenous cocaine more than a year before his hospitalization for endocarditis, it is more likely that an event producing high-grade bacteremia (e.g., dental extraction, bronchoscopy with rigid scope, GI scoping, shooting drugs) occurred within a 2-week "incubation period" before the diagnosis of endocarditis was established.[17] Streptococci account for 60% to 80% of bacterial agents in infective endocarditis. Phlegmon refers to a diffuse inflammatory reaction to streptococcal infection that forms a suppurative mass that may extend into deep subcutaneous tissues, muscles,[18] and in this case, vertebral bodies. The patient was resumed presumptively on continuous intravenous penicillin therapy and, in the opinion of the orthopedic surgeon, required removal of infected cervical vertebrae and rod insertion at the time of evacuation of phlegmon.

Following his recovery from infective endocarditis with an adequate prolonged course of intravenous antibiotics, the patient's relapse with a second serious infection raises the probability of ongoing drug addiction. Following surgery, the patient will require an additional 6 weeks of intravenous antibiotic therapy. The patient is at high risk for abusing his intravenous line for extracurricular drugs, and enrollment in a drug treatment facility is planned following acute recovery from surgery.

CONCLUSION

Selecting infectious disease as a specialty area of practice will provide the physician assistant with opportunities in outpatient and inpatient settings and public and private settings, as well as in the educational and research arenas. It is a growing practice area for the utilization of physician assistants and offers rewards that include continued intellectual stimulation, clinician/patient satisfaction, and the knowledge of working in cutting edge medicine while assisting the growth and recovery of patients. The case histories within this chapter represent just a few of the various clinical problems encountered within infectious disease practice; they are provided to stimulate in the reader further consideration of this remarkable field of practice.

CLINICAL APPLICATIONS

1. Contact and visit the local or regional health department in your area. Health departments are excellent resources for rates of antibiotic resistance to various pathogens, STD services, and much more. List the available services and contact numbers for future use in your practice. What infectious diseases are most prevalent in your area? What is the prevalence of hepatitis C in your area?

2. Contact the local social services organizations in your area. What specific services are available for patients affected by HIV/AIDS? By hepatitis C?

3. Familiarize yourself with the current standard of care for community-acquired pneumonia. What nosocomial infections are most prevalent in the major hospital settings in your area?

REFERENCES

1. Carter RD. Sociocultural origins of the PA profession. J Am Acad Phys Assist 1992;5:655.
2. Kass EH. History of the specialty of infectious diseases in the United States. Ann Intern Med 1987;106:745.
3. Census report. Alexandria, VA: American Academy of Physician Assistants, 1991-2001.
4. Zmigrodski JA. The lonely road. Primary care providers coping with AIDS. Physician Assist 1995;19:21.
5. Carpenter C, Feinberg M, Aubry W. Report of the NIH panel to define principles of therapy of HIV infection (draft). Bethesda, MD: National Institutes of Health, 1997.
6. Mellors J, Kingsley L, Rinaldo C. Quantitation of HIV-1 RNA in plasma predicts outcome after seroconversion. Ann Intern Med 1995;122:573.
7. Mandell G, Bennett J, Dolin R. Principles and Practice of Infectious Disease, 5th ed. Philadelphia: Churchill Livingstone, 2000.
8. Saag M. HIV resistance testing in clinical practice. Ann Intern Med 2001;134:475.

9. Mellors J, Kingsley L, Rinaldo C. Quantitation of HIV-1 RNA in plasma predicts outcome after seroconversion. Ann Intern Med 1995;122:573.

10. Report of the NIH panel to define principles of therapy of HIV. Washington, DC: National Institutes of Health, April 2001.

11. Chung A, Kim A, Polsky B. HIV/hepatitis B and C co-infection: pathogenic interactions, natural history and therapy. Antivir Chem Chemother 2001;12(suppl 1):73.

12. Guidelines for the use of antiretroviral agents in HIV-infected adults and adolescents. Washington, DC: U.S. Dept of Health and Human Services, April 2001.

13. Pomerantz R. Initiating antiretroviral therapy during HIV infection: confusion and clarity. JAMA 2001;286.

14. Craven D, Nunes D. Managing hepatitis C infection in HIV-positive patients. AIDS Clin Care 2000;12:71.

15. Landau A, et al. Efficacy and safety of combination therapy with interferon-alpha2b and ribavirin for chronic hepatitis C in HIV-infected patients. AIDS 2000;14:839.

16. Heathcote E, Shiffman M, Cooksley W, et al. Peginterferon alfa-2a in patients with chronic hepatitis C and cirrhosis. N Engl J Med 2000:343:1673.

17. Mandell G, Bennett J, Dolin R. Principals and Practice of Infectious Diseases, 5th ed. Philadelphia: Churchill Livingstone, 2000.

18. Dorland's Illustrated Medical Dictionary. Philadelphia: WB Saunders, 1988.

RESOURCES

AIDS Education Global Information System. Available at http://www.aegis.com. *This web site may be the largest HIV/AIDS database in the world. Filled with multiple fact sheets, daily briefings, and links to various additional resources, this site can be a valuable asset to the busy clinician seeking more information for practice or to provide to patients.*

Bartlett J, Gallant J. Medical Management of HIV Infection. Baltimore: Johns Hopkins University Press. *Annually updated authoritative clinical management pocket text reflecting the author's efforts to keep abreast of and gather news of new developments from more than 40 journals. Treatment recommendations presented are based largely on federal guidelines when they exist—antiretroviral therapy for adults, pregnancy management, opportunistic infection prophylaxis, management of occupational exposure, and management of tuberculosis co-infection.*

Braunwald E, Fauci A, Kasper D, et al. Harrison's Principles of Internal Medicine, 15th ed. New York: McGraw-Hill, 2001. *Definitive medicine text with the chapter on human retroviruses co-authored by Anthony Fauci, MD. Dr. Fauci is the foremost authority on HIV in all its social, economic, and clinical dimensions. A current edition of* Harrison's *should be handy in the clinician's office for quick reference and review.*

Centers for Disease Control and Prevention. Available at http://www.cdc.gov. *This web site provides entry to the leading federal agency whose mission is to promote health and quality of life by preventing and controlling disease, injury, and disability. A must bookmark for clinicians involved in the infectious disease specialty. A list of available list serves is also maintained on the National AIDS Clearinghouse web site at* http://www.cdcnac.org.

Dolin R, Masur H, Saag MS. AIDS Therapy. New York: Churchill Livingstone, 1999. *A comprehensive text on the management of patients affected by HIV. This edition also provides a thorough resource appendix of professional web resources, research resources, clinical trial information, and more.*

Federal Drug Administration, Good Clinical Practices (21CFR). Available at http://www.fda.gov. *Code of Ethics published by the FDA that governs the conduct of clinical trials that use human subjects conducted by FDA-approved clinicians. This manual provides guidelines for physician assistants and other professionals who participate as clinical investigators in clinical research.*

Infectious Diseases Society of America. Available at http://www.idsociety.org. *Representing physicians, scientists, and other health care providers who specialize in infectious disease practice, the IDSA's mission is to promote and recognize excellence in patient care, education, research, public health, and prevention of infectious disease. This web site is a rich resource complete with practice guidelines, education and research opportunities, policy statements, and links to other helpful infectious disease–related sites.*

Physician Assistant AIDS Network. Available at http://www.paan.org. *The Physician Assistant AIDS Network (PAAN) is a nonprofit organization devoted to promoting the networking of physician assistants engaged in HIV/AIDS practice. This web site includes a newsletter, information about jobs in the field, and much more.*

Sande MA, Volberding PA. The Medical Management of AIDS, 6th ed. Philadelphia: WB Saunders, 1999. *Sande and Volberding were two of the first physicians to publish a comprehensive text devoted to the management of AIDS. This sixth edition continues to provide detailed information for clinicians involved in the evaluation and treatment of patients affected by HIV.*

U.S. Department of Health and Human Services Health Resources and Services Administration (HRSA). Available at http://hab.hrsa.gov/D/4web/news.htm. *The HRSA's HIV/AIDS Bureau's monthly newsletter featuring current clinical issues. A sampling of recent in-depth articles includes the topics of HIV and homelessness, HIV in women of color, palliative and supportive care, pediatric HIV/AIDS, and a new decade of AIDS in the United States. The annual HIV/AIDS Treatment Update is available with every January issue; it provides the most recent standard of care guidelines for treating practitioners written by a panel of leading HIV/AIDS experts in the United States.*

CHAPTER 38

Geriatric Medicine

Vyjeyanthi S. Periyakoil, Steven Johnson, and Gwen Yeo

INTRODUCTION

This chapter provides an overview of geriatric medicine oriented to the beginning clinician; included here are basic information and clinical perspectives that are useful to the clinician in approaching the social and medical complexities associated with care of the older person. For further reference, a number of excellent textbooks and other materials are described in the resource section at the end of the chapter.

The health care of elders in the United States presents the clinician with social, medical, spiritual, and political challenges that cut across the full spectrum of race, religion, and social standing. When these challenges are successfully met, however, physician assistants (PAs) in geriatric practice can experience enormous satisfaction and a sense of important contribution to the well-being of both patients and society.

Our society is growing older just as our medical care has become more sophisticated at an ever-increasing cost. By the year 2030, mid-range projections indicate that approximately 22% of the U.S. population will be 65 years of age or older. In the 1990s, approximately 30% of our health care dollars are spent on the 13% of the population in that age range. Each medical practice is now experiencing the effects of this increase in the older population and decrease in resources and compensation. The publication of this chapter coincides with dramatic changes in the compensation of primary care providers and a growing political movement to provide access to health care for every American. The challenge to all PAs is to provide competent, cost-effective, functionally oriented, ethnically competent health care to each older person in their practices.

Beyond the social challenge is the real medical challenge of elder care. As the body ages, the wear and tear of poor health habits and disease takes an increasing toll. Effectively diagnosing and managing health concerns that span multiple organ systems in a sensitive and humane manner is a challenge to any clinician. Because PAs are now compensated by Medicare for hospital and nursing home care of elders and are actively recruited for practices that include a large segment of elders, most PAs will at some time in their careers face the complex challenges of caring for the elderly patient.

In addition to the medical concerns, the care of older persons touches on the personal and spiritual. PAs will be called on not only to manage health care but also to help patients, spouses, and families cope with and adjust to the emotional and financial burdens of disability, loss of independence, and death. These issues call on the personal strength, philosophy, and, at times, spiritual perspective of the health care provider to address the difficult realities of disability and death facing families and patients from diverse social and ethnic backgrounds with various levels of social support and financial resources.

The complexity of the medical concerns of older persons is most often not amenable to the 15-minute "quick" visit and offers poor financial compensation for the time spent. (See the helpful tool, "10 Minute Screener for Geriatric Conditions"[1] [Table 38-1].) The same complexity makes many people unable to care for the most dependent parent or relative at home, given the economic and cultural realities of the United States in the 21st century. The alternative is an expensive placement in an all too often impersonal nursing facility. Geriatric providers numb themselves to the pain and despair because there seems to be no other solution. It is important to recognize, however, that PAs are in an excellent position to provide desperately needed continuity of care.

In accepting the challenge of the profession, PAs will find themselves on the cutting edge of the medical, social, and economic changes that are affecting our entire society. By being involved, they can help shape the ways in which elders are approached and their care and well-being are managed. Each student and PA in practice looking at elder care might ask, "Do I want this system of care to be my future and my children's future?" As members of a profession that is evolving to meet the rapidly changing demands of a complex health care system, PAs will be part of the solution to provide competent, compassionate, cost-effective elder care.

GERIATRIC CARE

Although protocols were being written in the 1970s for PAs to manage chronic diseases such as diabetes and hypertension, the importance of PAs in providing competent and compassionate geriatric care was increasingly recognized and documented during the 1980s. In the mid-1980s, two large-scale national studies of practicing PAs, most of whom were in primary care, found that approximately 40% of the respondents' patient contact time was spent with patients age 55 and older.[2,3] Major activities that occupied the time of PAs in the care of these older patients were health education and counseling, taking histories, and performing physical examinations. Patients were most often coming in for follow-up of chronic conditions or uncomplicated acute conditions, such as constipation and urinary tract infection. With

Table 38-1   10-Minute Screener for Geriatric Conditions

Problem	Screening Measure	Positive Screen
Vision	Two parts: 1. Ask: "Do you have difficulty driving or watching television or reading or doing any of your daily activities because of your eyesight?" 2. If yes, then: Test each eye with the Snellen chart while the patient wears corrective lenses (if applicable)	Yes to question and inability to read >20/40 on Snellen chart
Hearing	Use audioscope set at 40 dB; test hearing using 1000 and 2000 Hz	Inability to hear 1000 and 2000 Hz in both ears, or inability to hear frequencies in either ear
Leg mobility	Time the pt after asking: "Rise from the chair. Walk 20 feet briskly, turn, walk back to the chair, and sit down."	Unable to complete task in 15 sec
Urinary incontinence	Two parts: Ask: "In the past year, have you ever lost your urine and gotten wet?" If yes, then ask: "Have you lost your urine at least on 7 separate days?"	Yes to both questions
Nutrition, weight loss	Two parts: Ask: "Have you lost 10 lb over the past 6 months without trying to do so?" Weigh the patient	Yes to the question or weight <100 lbs
Memory	Three-item recall	Unable to recall all items after 1 minute
Depression	Ask: "Do you often feel sad or depressed?"	Yes to the question
Physical disability	Six questions "Are you able to do strenuous activities like fast walking or bicycling?" "...do heavy work around the house, like washing windows, walls, or floors?" "...go shopping for groceries or clothes?" "...get to places out of walking distance?" "...bathe, either a sponge bath, a tub bath, or a shower?" "...dress, including putting on a shirt, buttoning and zipping, and putting on shoes?"	No to any of the questions

From Mopore AA, Su AL. Screening for common problems in ambulatory elderly: clinical confirmation of a screen instrument. Am J Med 1998;100:440.

the recognition that PAs were playing such important roles in the care of older patients, emphasis on geriatrics increased in PA training programs in the late 1980s, with encouragement from federal grants and contracts. Recently, some PAs are being employed in practices that are totally geriatric, especially in outpatient geriatric clinics, in senior apartment complexes, in some Veterans Affairs (VA) Medical Centers, and in private practices that follow large numbers of frail older patients in nursing homes and at home.

The contribution of these PAs to providing excellent, well-accepted, cost-effective geriatric care is being increasingly recognized in the ongoing national debate concerning the best model for American health care.

The role of the PA in geriatric care is similar to the role of the PA in providing any health care—that is, to provide thorough, cost-effective, safe health care within current state legislation that regulates the scope of PA practice. Geriatric practice differs, however, in several significant ways.

Medicare Regulations

Medicare is the federal health insurance program for Americans age 65 years and older. Until 1998, Medicare regulations were burdened with an "incident to provision ratio" that limited the care provided by the PA. The Balanced Budget Act of 1997 (Public Law 105-217), effective January 1, 1998, gave PAs explicit statutory Medicare coverage and increased the rate of reimbursement for some services. The bill passed in no small part because of input and lobbying by the American Academy of Physician Assistants.

PAs may be reimbursed for health care provided in outpatient offices or clinics without the requirement of "direct physician supervision" (interpreted as the supervising physician being on-site). PAs are also reimbursed in the hospital, surgical, and skilled nursing home settings. The rate of reimbursement in outpatient settings, first-assist in surgery, hospital care, and skilled nursing care is 85% of the rate of reimbursement for a physician.

An excellent resource for the details of the latest legislation and interpretation is the American Academy of Physician Assistants, Department of Government and Professional Affairs, 950 North Washington Street, Alexandria, VA, 22314-1552; telephone, 703-836-2272.

Time and Perspective

Geriatric practice also often differs in time and perspective, in that geriatric PAs frequently need to spend time learning and understanding their patient's medical status over the course of time compared with their counterparts in other types of practice. Time is often the critical factor in eliciting a thoughtful and comprehensive history, especially in cases with multiple chronic conditions. Many older patients need more time to disrobe and dress again. The geriatric PA may have to schedule driving time to visit a nursing home patient whose condition has changed or for a routine continuity-of-care visit. Another extremely important factor is knowledge of the context: geriatric patients often have multiple chronic medical problems as their baseline, which are often managed by multiple medications. When the elderly patient who is chronically ill develops an acute condition, a prior therapeutic relationship with the patient and a clear sense of the patient's baseline are extremely important because these enable the provider to identify the subtle signs (e.g., confusion, decreased appetite, listlessness) that may often be the only clues for an underlying infection. Thus, although initially the PA may need to spend more time getting to know an elderly patient, he or she will then more easily be able to spot acute or chronic changes and, in many cases, to preempt problems before they arise. It is important for PAs to recognize the larger time element required, especially during the initial phase of the care relationship with the older person, and to schedule appropriately, allowing physicians to spend their time in a more cost-effective manner in the office. Once such a meaningful therapeutic patient/PA relationship has been established, the PA will be of enormous help to the physicians in that he or she will be able to establish the contextual framework for the patient's illness, thereby significantly increasing the overall efficacy of the practice.

APPROACH TO THE ELDERLY PATIENT

"Geriatric" patients do not easily lend themselves to generalizations, either medical or scientific. Gerontology is still a "young" field, and there remains a great deal to learn about the aging process. Many previous assumptions about aging have been found to be untrue owing to the interaction of disease and disuse.[4] Aging is commonly viewed as *usual* (the gradual loss of function and independence with increasing years) or *successful* (remaining active and functional in the physical, cognitive, and emotional realms until death).[4]

There are vast differences between people within all age groups in terms of strength, endurance, cognition, and general health, but more dramatically so among elders. For example, people in their 70s, 80s, and even 90s regularly complete the 26-mile, 385-yard Boston Marathon. The aging process depends on the complex interaction of genetics, disease, health habits (e.g., smoking and alcohol consumption), diet, and exercise. Generalization about physiological and anatomical changes with age would not be helpful to the new clinician. Each patient in the "elderly" category (65 years or older) needs to be approached only on the basis of health status and without the expectation of disability.

With that caveat, some important age-related changes seem to occur in spite of an active and healthy lifestyle. These changes are summarized by system in the sections that follow.

Sensory Changes

With older age, there is an increased incidence of cataracts and a consequent decrease in visual acuity, resulting in, among other risks, an increased incidence of falls. There is an age-related reduction in the ability to hear higher frequencies (presbycusis), resulting in communication difficulties. On the whole, when one is communicating with an elderly person who is known to have sensory impairment, it is important to speak slowly and clearly, sit close to the person, and make sure one's face is in the light. These simple measures can reduce confusion and anxiety and make for a more successful clinical encounter.

There also appears to be a decrease in acuity of taste in advanced age, so that food tends to be perceived as bland. The clinical consequence can be a decreased appreciation for food and a loss of appetite, which can lead to significant weight loss and nutritional deficiency. The aging skin is more porous and therefore tends to lose increased body water by direct evaporation through the skin, thus resulting in increased insensible fluid losses.

Cardiovascular Changes

The resting cardiac output does not change with age. There is a slight decrease in the heart rate and a compensatory increase in stroke volume. Heart rate response to exercise is decreased in elders secondary to a decrease in the beta-adrenergic response. Also diastolic dysfunction is seen during both rest and exercise in older adults.

Coronary artery disease is the most common cause of death among those 65 years and older. A well-balanced healthy diet and regular exercise have a tremendous positive impact on the cardiovascular changes associated with aging. A *reasonable* diet and exercise program should be strongly encouraged for everyone because even persons in advanced years have been able to increase their stamina and aerobic fitness if they exercise regularly.

Endocrine Changes

Aging is associated with deteriorating glucose tolerance changes, and peripheral glucose utilization is thought to be the major factor in this phenomenon.[5] Thyroid function is generally normal in physiological aging, although older patients tend to have low triiodothyronine (T_3) levels. There is an increase of 2% to 5% in the prevalence of hypothyroidism in those over age 65, and the prevalence continues to rise with age. The clinical implication for the clinician is to consider hypothyroidism when confronted with complaints of fatigue, depression, loss of initiative, confusion, dry skin, and constipation. Serum parathyroid hormone (PTH) increases in the elderly and this increase correlates with a decline in vitamin D levels; treatment with $1,25\text{-}(OH)_2\text{-}D_3$ results in a decrease in PTH levels. Age-related increases in PTH are thought to be a major factor accounting for age-related bone loss.

Immunological Changes

There is an overall decrease in immunity with age, resulting in a greater prevalence of infections (e.g., pneumonia and urinary tract infections), shingles, Gram-negative bacteremia, and severe episodes of influenza. Aging is accompanied by changes in both cellular and humoral immunity. The function of lymphocytes is altered with decreased proliferative capacity of T lymphocytes in aging. Macrophage function is altered and delayed-type skin hypersensitivity (DTH) declines. Also, elders often present an atypical clinical picture, with absence of fevers, presence of hypothermia, altered eating patterns, delirium, and agitation in response to infection. They may also fail to mount a leukocytosis in response to infections. The clinical implication is that even simple illnesses in the elderly should be monitored closely and treated aggressively as indicated.

Renal Function

There is an overall decrease in kidney mass and loss of parenchymal mass. The total number of glomeruli decreases with age and the renal vasculature undergoes sclerotic changes. All of these changes result in a progressively decreasing glomerular filtration rate (GFR). Concomitantly, with increasing age, there is a reduction in lean body mass, which results in decreased creatinine production. Therefore, the creatinine can continue to remain falsely low or "normal," even in the face of decreasing GFR and compromised renal function. Even the commonly used Cockcroft and Gault equation (Creatinine Clearance = [140 − age] × Body Weight in kilograms/[72 × Serum Creatinine]) can lead to a mean underestimation of the measured creatinine clearance of 12.1 mL/minute in a group of healthy patients.[6] Therefore, calculated creatinine clearances should be avoided in the elderly in favor of short-duration, timed urine collections to measure the actual creatinine clearance. To avoid overmedication, any medicine excreted by the kidneys should be carefully considered and monitored.

Functional Status

The essential perspective in caring for the older patient is one of function. Can a diabetic patient see well enough to be able to self-administer insulin? Can a patient easily swallow antibiotic tablets for bronchitis, or would a liquid be easier and promote compliance? Can a patient (limited by arthritis) remove the cap from the medication bottle or easily remove the tablets from the office samples the PA has given him or her? The question that should always underlie any change of condition or new diagnosis is, "How does this affect this person's ability to manage the activities of daily living?"

The activities of daily living (ADLs) are, in essence, a survey of the degree of independence in basic personal self-care. Instrumental activities of daily living (IADLs) survey an individual's ability to manage household and business affairs in the context of the society at large. ADLs and IADLs (Table 38-2) are typically assessed by self-report. It is not unusual for the clinician to receive conflicting assessments of an individual's self-care abilities, depending on who is offering the assessment—patient, spouse, caregiver, or friend. At times, the only accurate method of assessment is to observe the patient in the home or a structured environment.

It is important in treating older or infirm persons not to assume functional competence or to expect them to achieve perfect compliance with the usual off-hand and complex instructions health professionals routinely give out. To diagnose and treat is the usual goal of the clinical encounter. With older patients who have medically complex problems, the goal extends to assessing their ability to perform or

---

Table 38-2 ADLs and IADLs

ACTIVITIES OF DAILY LIVING
Feeding
Dressing
Ambulation
Toileting
Bathing
Transfer (bed, chair, toilet)
Continence
Grooming
Communication
INSTRUMENTAL ACTIVITIES OF DAILY LIVING
Writing
Reading
Cooking
Cleaning
Shopping
Laundry
Climbing stairs
Using telephone
Managing medication
Ability to be employed or to perform outside work (gardening)
Ability to travel

Modified from Kane RW, Ouslander JG, Abrass IB. Essentials of Clinical Geriatrics, ed 3. New York: McGraw-Hill, 1994.

comply with the treatment and, if necessary, arranging for the resources to assist a patient whose function is impaired in any way.

Ethnic Differences

In addition to adapting to the age-related changes listed so far that affect the provider/patient encounter, PAs need to learn skills that enable them to be culturally competent. It is important to recognize that within the exploding population of older American adults, the numbers of elders in the four major ethnic minority categories (American Indian/Alaska Native, African American, Asian/Pacific Islander, and Hispanic) are growing even more rapidly than the total group number; these groups are expected to account for one third of all Americans age 65 and older by the year 2050.[7]

Within each of these government-designated categories, there are extremely heterogeneous cultural groups. Elders from each group are more likely than younger members to maintain their culturally based expectations of health care and health beliefs, which may conflict with Western health care providers' traditional methods of assessing and managing chronic diseases and caring for dying patients. Although it is beyond the scope of this chapter to address ethnogeriatric issues in detail, readers are encouraged to consider carefully the application of the material presented in Chapter 8 regarding interactions with elders from ethnic populations other than their own.

ISSUES IN GERIATRIC CARE

One of the ways geriatrics differs from general adult medical practice is the relative frequency of some common problems that are infrequently found in middle-aged patients. For example, older patients often present with confusion or falls, both of which can be symptoms of a wide variety of underlying acute or chronic conditions that affect one or more of a number of organ systems. The atypical or vague presentation of disease, including myocardial infarctions without perceived pain, is legendary in geriatrics. It is not uncommon for older patients to come in with nonspecific complaints of malaise and be found to have a serious disease process or organ failure. On the other hand, there are also serious functional impairments, such as incontinence, that patients commonly fail to

mention at all to their providers, so that unless specific questions are asked, such impairments go undiagnosed and untreated. The detective work needed to solve the mysteries involved in geriatric care presents its own unique challenges. Some of the keys that assist in that detective process are described in the sections that follow.

Complications of Pharmacotherapy

CASE STUDY 38-1

Mrs. S is a 72-year-old widow who lives alone in an apartment complex. Her two sons live nearby. During World War II, she was in a German concentration camp, and since then, she has had intermittent psychiatric disturbances. At one time, she was diagnosed as having schizophrenia, but she is currently diagnosed as having paranoia. During the past 10 years, Mrs. S has also been diagnosed as having congestive heart failure, hyperparathyroidism, hypertension, and chronic obstructive pulmonary disease.

One day, she is brought into the office by her older son, who reports that her landlady found Mrs. S wandering in the snow, talking incessantly, disoriented, tearful, and apparently hallucinating. She had fallen several times on the ice. Her face is flushed and she is lightly clad, even though it is cold outside. Her temperature is 102° F, pulse and respirations are rapid, and pupils are dilated. She is apparently very agitated but cannot speak above a whisper. She appears very frightened but recognizes and embraces the doctor. Her lips and mucous membranes are bone-dry. Examination reveals the following: bruises over the arms and legs and on the forehead; lung fields clear, heart-sinus tachycardia, no murmur, moderate cardiomegaly; abdomen—no organomegaly, no tenderness or decreased bowel sounds, hard stools in rectum.

Mrs. S's son has brought all her current medications, as he was instructed to do when he phoned for the appointment. The following medication bottles are pulled from the bag: digoxin, 0.125 mg daily; potassium (Slow-K); furosemide (Lasix), 20 mg bid; Fleet Phospho-Soda, 1 tsp tid; flavoxate (Urispas), one twice a day; propantheline bromide (Pro-Banthine), 15 mg ac; thioridazine (Mellaril), 50 mg tid; amitriptyline (Elavil), 75 mg hs; ibuprofen (Motrin), 400 mg tid; propoxyphene compound (Darvon Compound-65), 1 q4hr, prn; flurazepam (Dalmane), 15 mg hs, prn; and benztropine mesylate (Cogentin), 2 mg bid.

Mrs. S is hospitalized and all medications are stopped; infection, injury, and thyroid, diabetic, and metabolic/electrolyte imbalances are ruled out. Over the course of a week, she returns to normal. The diagnosis of anticholinergic psychosis is confirmed.

In later discussions with Mrs. S and with the psychiatrists and other physicians who treated her, the PA pieces the following history together: different doctors had seen her at different times, and each had given her medications for the current complaint without looking at the entire set of medications. When she began showing symptoms that could have been adverse effects of previous medications, such as depression or agitation, new drugs were added for those symptoms. Primary care physicians had been hesitant to change her psychiatric medications, and psychiatrists left her somatic drugs to her general physicians.

How could this happen? Unfortunately, similar cases are not uncommon. Some of the causes include the following: many elders are taking a large number of medications from different providers; confusion is a common reaction to toxic medication levels or drug interactions in elders; family members and others can attribute confusion to "just getting old" or "senility." For appropriate prescription practices and avoidance of polypharmacy, the following recommendations have been made to health care providers by the American Geriatrics Society[8]:

1. *Obtain a complete drug history.* Be sure to ask about previous treatments and responses, as well as about other prescribers. Ask about allergies, over-the-counter (OTC) drugs, nutritional supplements, alternative medications, alcohol, tobacco, caffeine, and recreational drugs.

2. *Avoid prescribing before a diagnosis is made.* Consider nondrug therapy. Eliminate drugs for which no diagnosis can be identified.

3. *Review medications regularly and before prescribing a new medication.* Discontinue medications that have not had the intended response or are no longer needed. Monitor the use of prn and OTC drugs.

4. *Know the actions, adverse effects, and toxicity profiles of the medications you prescribe.* Consider how these might interact with or complement existing drug therapy.

5. *Start long-term drug therapy at a low dose, and titrate dose on basis of tolerability and response.* Use drug levels when available.

6. *Attempt to maximize dose before switching or adding another drug.* Encourage compliance with therapy. Educate patients and/or caregivers about each medication regimen, the therapeutic goal, its cost, and potential adverse effects or drug interactions. Provide written instructions.

7. *Avoid using one drug to treat the adverse effects of another.* Attempt to use one drug to treat two or more conditions.

8. *Avoid combination products.*

9. *Communicate with other prescribers.* Don't assume patients will—they assume you do!

10. *Avoid using drugs from the same class or with similar actions (e.g., alprazolam and solpidem).*

GERIATRIC SYNDROMES
Dementia

Dementia is the most common cause of mental decline in old age. Dementia can be defined as an acquired syndrome of decline in memory and other cognitive functions sufficient to affect daily life in an alert patient. Dementia takes an immense toll on the physical, psychosocial, and economic well-being of patients and their families and also the society at large.

Alzheimer's dementia accounts for approximately two thirds of all dementia cases, and vascular dementia (multiple infarcts in the cortical and subcortical gray matter and the internal capsule, or white matter demyelination in the frontotemporal cortex resulting in dementia) causes an estimated 15% to 25%. In recent years, dementia associated with Lewy bodies (DLB—dementia plus parkinsonian signs/detailed visual hallucinations leading to secondary delusions and alterations of alertness or attention) and frontotemporal dementia have received increased attention. As people age, they usually experience such memory changes as slowing in information processing, but these kinds of changes are benign. In contrast, dementia is a progressive and disabling pathological condition that is not an inherent aspect of normal aging.

Alzheimer's disease (AD), the most common and well-known form of dementia, is estimated to affect about 4 million people in the United States. It is expected that an estimated 14 million Americans will suffer from AD by the year 2040. The prevalence of AD increases with age, with an estimated 6% to 8% occurring in patients 65 years of age or older, and an estimated 30% noted among those age 85 or older.

Both caregivers and patients may misinterpret initial symptoms of AD (e.g., memory loss) as normal age-related changes, and physicians may not recognize early signs or may misdiagnose them. The two greatest risk factors for AD are age and family history. Genetic mutations on chromosomes 1, 14, and 21 are responsible for the rare forms of familial AD that begin before age 60. The apolipoprotein E gene (*APOE*) on chromosome 19 is a risk factor for the commonly occurring late-onset AD.

Gradual onset and progressive decline in cognitive functioning characterize AD; motor and sensory functions are usually spared until late stages. Memory impairment is a core symptom of any dementia, and this is seen even in the earliest stages of AD. Difficulty learning and retaining, aphasia, disorientation, visuospatial dysfunction, and impaired judgment and executive functioning are typical symptoms of AD.

The cognitive impairment of dementia profoundly affects the patient's IADLs and eventually the ADLs so that eventually the patient becomes completely dependent on the caregiver. Recognition of dementia may be further complicated by the presence of depression. Patients with primary dementia commonly experience symptoms of depression, and depressed patients present with cognitive complaints that exceed objectively measured deficits.

Dementia Workup Patient and family member interviews and office-based clinical assessment are the most important diagnostic tools for dementia. A comprehensive history and physical examination with special attention to the onset and rate of progress of cognitive problems; the use of quantified screening tests of cognitive function, such as Folstein's Mini-Mental State Examination (for copies of this examination, please call 617-587-4215); and laboratory evaluations to rule out hypothyroidism (thyroid-stimulating hormone [TSH]), syphilis (Veneral Disease Research Laboratory [VDRL]), and B_{12} deficiency are recommended. Brain imaging studies should be considered in patients if:

➤ Dementia onset occurs at an age younger than 65 years.
➤ The condition is post acute (symptoms have occurred for less than 2 years).
➤ Focal neurologic deficits are present.
➤ The clinical picture suggests normal-pressure hydrocephalus (triad of onset within 1 year, gait disorder, and unexplained incontinence).

Management of Dementia Primary treatment goals for patients with dementia are to enhance and preserve quality of life and to optimize functional performance by improving cognition, mood, and behavior. Both pharmacologic (donepezil, galantamine, and rivastigmine) and nonpharmacological treatments (e.g., stimulation therapy, reminiscence therapy) are available, and the latter should be emphasized. Working closely with the patient and caregivers to establish a trusting relationship and a therapeutic alliance facilitates management. It is of critical importance that care providers make long-term health and financial care plans while the patient is still in the early stages of dementia when they are able to participate in these crucial decisions. Caregivers are often subject to enormous stresses and should be referred to caregiver support groups because these have been shown to effectively alleviate stress. Respite care and other community resources like dementia adult day care offer caregivers relief and help postpone patient institutionalization.

Delirium

CASE STUDY 38-2

Mr. S is an 88-year-old white male veteran with a past medical history of Alzheimer's disease (AD), mild hypertension, and gallbladder disease status post cholecystectomy (35 years ago). The VA geriatric clinic interdisciplinary team was very familiar with Mr. S, having cared for him for the past 3 years. His AD had been diagnosed 5 to 6 years ago. He had initially lived by himself, but as his AD progressed, his daughter Sandy, who is his surrogate decision maker, moved him to a residential care facility. Over the past year, Mr. S seemed to be deteriorating with increased memory problems and difficulty recognizing acquaintances, and needing some help with ADLs. His recent Mini-Mental State Examination (MMSE) was 17/30 (his education level was high with a master's in aeronautic engineering).

One morning, Sandy brought Mr. S to clinic and requested to see only the geropsychologist, saying, "Today, Daddy's issues are not medical problems; it is purely psychiatric." The residential facility staff had also noted that the patient had become very confused and agitated over the past week. His confused mood was noted to wax and wane over time. The agitation had not been related to any particular events; nor had there been any new employees or any other changes in residential care routines. On two notable occasions, Mr. S was heard screaming out, "Fire! Fire!" and one night, he actually dialed 911 and reported a fire in the facility (which had led to a police investigation of the facility premises). Further history revealed that the residential facility staff had in fact noticed that he had been eating poorly but was afebrile and otherwise asymptomatic.

Patient's medications:

Lisinopril 10 mg per day

Multivitamin 1 tablet per day

Tylenol 500 mg tid for arthritis

No history of other over-the-counter medications or herbal medications

Allergies: No known drug allergies.

Physical examination: Mr. S was able to recognize his primary care physician (PCP) but seemed very listless. When asked about the fire episode, he became agitated and repeatedly said, "Fire! Fire," and was clutching his groin region while saying this. His daughter Sandy was very embarrassed at this and admonished her dad for this behavior.

Vitals: Temp of 97.6° F, BP 134/82, RR 12, and HR 76

HEENT: Normocephalic, atraumatic. Pupils reacting equally to light and accommodation.

Neck: Supple with trachea in the midline.

Chest: CTAB

Heart: RRR with no murmur, rub, or gallop.

Abd: Soft, positive for bowel sounds, mild diffuse tenderness to percussion (especially in the suprapubic region) with voluntary guarding to palpation.

Extr: No cyanosis, clubbing, or edema.

Rectal exam: Significantly enlarged hard, nodular prostate with guaiac-negative stool.

Discussion: At this point, the physician believed that Mr. S's enlarged prostate had probably caused urine retention with a secondary urine infection, which was clinically confirmed by suprapubic tenderness. His delirium was thought to have been secondary to his urine infection. The clinic nurse did a bladder scan and determined that Mr. S's postvoidal residue was 280 mL. A stat UA was consistent with a urinary tract infection, and Mr. S was given a course of antibiotics and was started on tamsulosin and pyridium.

The bigger concern was the newly diagnosed prostate enlargement. Because a malignancy was suspected, a prostate-specific antigen was ordered and a follow-up appointment was scheduled in 2 weeks. Over the next several days, Mr. S's confusion lessened, but he continued to remain weak and listless and also developed severe back pain (thought to be due to bony metastasis and later palliated with opioids). His PSA came back as significantly elevated at 125 units. A clinical diagnosis of prostate cancer was made and the geriatrician offered to refer Mr. S to a urologist for further workup. Because the patient was deemed incompetent to make any medical decisions, further discussions were held with his daughter who was his durable power of health care attorney. After several discussions with Sandy, the physician ordered a bone scan, which was consistent with extensive bony metastasis. Sandy refused further workup of the presumed prostate cancer because her father had previously specifically expressed the wish not to have any invasive medical procedures; a prostate biopsy was therefore not an option. Mr. S continued to deteriorate rapidly and was admitted to the VA Inpatient Hospice Unit for comfort care. He died peacefully 2 weeks later, and an autopsy confirmed the diagnosis of metastatic prostate cancer.

Delirium or an "acute confusional sate" is a very common geriatric syndrome that is underdiagnosed. As many as one third of all hospitalized elderly patients may have delirium. Delirium is an independent risk factor for poor medical outcomes in the elderly. An advanced age, history of dementia, poor functional status, and sensory impairment are some of the predisposing factors for delirium. Acute infection, postoperative state, acute myocardial infarction, and alcohol withdrawal are common precipitating factors. Iatrogenic delirium is extremely common among the elderly, with drugs with anticholinergic effects being one of the most common culprits. Other causative drugs include antihistamines, antiparkinsonism drugs, benzodiazepines, and H_2-blockers. Management of delirium includes withdrawing the offending drug (if any); treating the underlying cause; providing supportive care, including a well-lit, safe, and familiar environment; and reassuring both the patient and the family.

Urinary Incontinence

Unfortunately, incontinence frequently is not mentioned by patients and often is not asked about by providers. It is all too often mistakenly assumed by patients to be a normal function of aging. In reality, it certainly is not inevitable and is usually treatable.

Urinary incontinence of one or more episodes in the past month affects about 20% of people over age 60 in the community, 50% of those in institutions, and twice as many women as men. One third to one half of affected patients have never sought medical attention for it.

The adverse effects of incontinence can be extremely troubling, resulting in skin breakdown, frequent urinary tract infection, and falls (from rushing to the toilet or slipping in urine). The psychological impact of incontinence can lead to social isolation and depression. There can be tremendous stress on the family or caregivers, and the resulting dependency often results in institutionalization of an incontinent patient. The economic costs can be considerable when supplies, laundry, labor, and the medical cost of managing complications are totaled. The total direct costs alone have been estimated at more than $10 billion per year in the United States.

Incontinence can be classified as acute or chronic. Acute incontinence in an otherwise healthy person is usually secondary to infection or inflammation (e.g., atrophic vaginitis or urethritis). A mnemonic that covers the primary differential diagnosis is shown in Table 38-3. It is important to note that the differential diagnosis for acute incontinence covers a wide range of possibilities, including restricted mobility.

The principal types of chronic urinary incontinence can be categorized as stress, urge, overflow, or functional; many patients have more than one type.

Table 38-3 A Mnemonic for the Treatable Causes of Dementia

D	Drugs
E	Emotional disorders
M	Metabolic or endocrine disorders
E	Eye and ear dysfunctions
N	Nutritional deficiencies
T	Tumor and trauma
I	Infection
A	Arteriosclerotic complications (myocardial infarction, congestive heart failure) and use of alcohol

Modified from Kane RW, Ouslander JG, Abrass IB. Essentials of Clinical Geriatrics, ed 3. New York: McGraw-Hill, 1994.

Stress Incontinence Involuntary loss of urine, usually a small amount, secondary to increased intra-abdominal pressure (as from a cough or laugh). Common causes are weakness and laxity of the pelvic floor musculature and weakness of the bladder outlet or urethral sphincter.

Urge Incontinence Leakage of urine, usually a large amount, because of the inability to delay voiding after the sensation of bladder fullness is perceived. Common causes are detrusor muscle instability, either alone or associated with a local genitourinary condition (urinary tract infection, urethritis, tumor, stones), and central nervous system disorder (parkinsonism, cerebrovascular accident, dementia).

Overflow Incontinence Leakage of urine resulting from mechanical forces on an overdistended bladder. Common causes are anatomical obstruction, such as urethral stricture secondary to benign prostatic hypertrophy or cystocele; acontractile bladder associated with diabetes or a spinal cord injury; and neurogenic bladder, which results from a detrusor-sphincter dyssynergia associated with multiple sclerosis and other suprasacral cord lesions.

Functional Incontinence Inability to toilet due to impaired cognitive or physical function, environmental barriers, or psychological unwillingness (depression, anger, or hostility).

The PA's approach to incontinence should include the following measures:

➤ A thorough history to quantify the amount of urine lost and circumstances of the incontinent episodes.

➤ A physical examination, including abdomen, genital, rectal, and neurological screening and mobility/joint examination.

➤ Laboratory assessment of urine with culture and sensitivity testing.

➤ Other laboratory tests, depending on history and physical findings.

On the basis of findings, the type of incontinence can be classified. For the most common types affecting older women—stress and urge—the nonpharmacological, noninvasive behavioral intervention known as *pelvic muscle* or *Kegel exercises* has been found in a majority of cases to substantially reduce or eliminate incontinence problems. PAs can improve the quality of life of many of their older patients who have lost control of their urination by giving them the instructions described in the Box and then scheduling regular follow-up visits to monitor and reinforce their progress. Pharmacological interventions are also available for urge incontinence if the behavioral interventions are unsuccessful.

Instability and Falls

Falls account for a significant number of cases of injury and death among the elderly. Accidents are the sixth leading cause of death among the elderly, and falls account for two thirds of accidental deaths.[9] Besides the acute trauma noted in patients who present in the emergency department or office, a significant number of unreported falls with resulting soft tissue injury and psychological stress occur, leading to decreased independence and a reduced sense of autonomy.

Falls are a multifactorial problem in the elderly. The intrinsic factors affecting stability and predisposing an older person to falls include the following:

1. Changes in vision, including depth perception and acuity.
2. Decreased proprioception.
3. Decreased lower extremity muscle strength.
4. Increased postural sway.
5. Changes in gait, both speed and height of step.
6. Almost any disease process that exacerbates the expected aging changes, especially dementia, depression, cardiovascular disease, arthritis, podiatric problems, diabetes, peripheral neuropathy, and stroke.

Extrinsic factors play an important role in falls and include the following:

1. Poor lighting.
2. Irregular surfaces (cracks in the sidewalk, short or irregular steps).
3. Slick surfaces (throw rugs).
4. Furniture too high or too low.
5. Bathroom fixtures without support bars or at an inappropriate height.

Falls require a careful medical evaluation, including assessment of orthostatic blood pressure changes,

INSTRUCTIONS FOR PATIENTS FOR PELVIC MUSCLE (KEGEL) EXERCISES

Identifying and Contracting (Tightening) Your Pelvic Muscle: The pelvic muscle is the muscle you tighten to stop your urine flow and to keep from passing gas or, if you are a woman, to "pull up" your vagina. Women can easily feel if they are tightening this muscle by placing one or two fingers in their vagina and contracting around their fingers.

It is important to be able to contract your pelvic muscle without contracting your abdominal muscles, which could cause you to leak urine. To determine if you are tightening your abdominal muscles, place a hand on your abdomen while you tighten your pelvic muscles. If you feel your abdomen tighten, you need to practice relaxing your abdomen while continuing to contract your pelvic muscles.

Practicing Pelvic Muscle Exercises: First, empty your bladder. Sit or lie in a comfortable place and relax for a minute. Then, tighten your pelvic muscle (without tightening your abdomen). Keep it tight for 10 seconds. Then, relax for 10 seconds. Repeat for a total of 15 contractions. Do these 15 contractions three times each day. If you are not able to hold the muscle tight for 10 seconds or are unable to repeat 15 times, just do it as many times as you can. Your ability to perform the exercise will improve with time.

What to Expect: The benefit increases the longer you practice the exercises. Most women notice a decrease in their frequency of incontinence within 4 to 6 weeks. Studies have shown that this exercise program is effective in reducing incontinence by an average of 70% and completely eliminates incontinence in about one third of women after 6 weeks. As the exercises become familiar, you can practice them anytime, such as when you are watching television, driving, or in bed.

If Incontinence Persists: If incontinence persists, there are additional treatment options of medication or surgery that you may want to discuss with your doctor.

cardiovascular status, neurological deficits such as mentation, musculoskeletal conditions, foot disorders, and sensory deficits (especially visual) (see box). A careful review of medications, particularly psychotropic agents, is especially important for those elderly patients who report a history of falls.

Fall prevention strategy requires attention to those factors that can be medically or surgically corrected, for example, cataract surgery or medication adjustment. Physical disabilities can be addressed with physical therapy and, if appropriate, assistive devices like walkers and canes. A home health nursing evaluation or a home visit by the PA may help address the extrinsic factors. Community resources like the senior center often provide information on low-cost installation of bathroom and hallway bars.

The Frailty and Injuries Cooperative Studies of Intervention Techniques (FICSIT) addressed the following eight factors that influence falls[10]:

1. Postural hypotension.
2. Use of sedative/hypnotic medication.
3. Use of more than four medications.
4. Toilet and bathtub safety.
5. Environmental hazards.
6. Abnormal gait, transfers, and balance.
7. Lower and upper extremity strength and range of motion.
8. Foot problems.

The intervention group experienced a 30% reduction in falls. This study clearly demonstrates the value of a careful approach and intervention to prevent further falls. An important note needs to be made of exercise in the prevention of falls. Studies demonstrate that even the very old can benefit from exercise and weight training. The practice of Tai Chi has been shown to reduce the incidence of falls.[11]

Dizziness and Syncope

Dizziness can be classified as vertigo (rotational sensation), presyncope (impending faint), disequilibrium (loss of balance without head sensation), or lightheadedness.[12] Benign positional vertigo (BPV) is a common cause of dizziness among elders and manifests as episodic dizzy spells that are usually precipitated by changes in position, such as turning, rolling over, getting into and out of bed, or bending over. These spells are often brief (5 to 15 seconds) and usually relatively mild. Presyncope is the sensation of near-fainting caused by diminished cerebral perfusion; it occurs secondary to cardiac causes (arrhythmias) or vascular causes (orthostatic hypotension) or vagal stimulation, which in some cases can result in syncope (micturition syncope). Syncope is defined as a sudden, transient loss of postural tone and consciousness not due to trauma and with spontaneous full recovery. Like presyncope, syncope is generally caused by a reduction in cerebral perfusion. The clinical history, physical examination, and electrocardiogram have been found to be the most useful steps in evaluating syncope,[13] and they should be used in most patients to determine whether further testing is needed.

Sleep Problems

Difficulty falling asleep, nighttime awakening, early morning awakening, and daytime sleepiness are common sleep problems experienced by elders. Risk factors for sleep disturbance include chronic illness, mood disturbance, lack of physical activity, and increased physical disability. Older people report an earlier bedtime and an early awakening. They also report decreased total sleep time with fragmented sleep patterns characterized by frequent arousals during the night and diminished deep sleep (stages III and IV of sleep). Consequently, older patients may report dissatisfaction with the quantity and quality of their sleep and often attribute their low energy, easy fatigability, and excessive daytime sleepiness to poor nighttime sleep.

Screening Older Patients for Sleep Problems

The National Institutes of Health Consensus Statement on the Treatment of Sleep Disorders of Older People recommends that the following three questions be asked:

1. Is the person satisfied with his or her sleep?
2. Does sleep or fatigue interfere with daytime activities?
3. Does the bed partner or others complain of unusual behavior during sleep, such as snoring, interrupted breathing, or leg movements?

Although a detailed account of the diagnosis and management of sleep problems is beyond the scope of

this chapter, the authors wish to emphasize that the clinician should review medications and other medical conditions and should try to avoid long-term usage of sedative/hypnotics in older patients because these are associated with many adverse effects, including secondary depression and increased incidence of hip fractures.

DEPRESSION

Depression is underdiagnosed and undertreated in the elderly.[14] Late-life depression has been found to be associated with higher than expected mortality rates and persistent impairment.[15]

Older patients tend to be more preoccupied with somatic symptoms (e.g., constipation, insomnia, and pain) and report depressed mood and guilty preoccupations less frequently, so depression may often be masked. The gateway symptoms of depression, including persistent feelings of a sad mood (in the absence of normal causes like recent bereavement) and anhedonia or loss of pleasure, are hallmarks of depression and are helpful in the identification of depression in most medically ill patients. Furthermore, the gateway symptoms are less likely to overlap with those of a medical illness.

The diagnosis of major depression in older persons is complicated by the overlap of symptoms of major depression with those of physical illness (e.g., weight loss, insomnia, loss of libido, changes in bowel habits). Debilitated patients and those with serious illness may be preoccupied by thoughts of death or worthlessness. The elderly also are often taking numerous medications (e.g., beta-blockers, steroids, H_2-blockers), which can complicate the picture even further. Certain medical conditions (e.g., hypothyroidism) that commonly occur in the older adult also predispose to depression. As individuals grow older, they often experience a loss of friends, family, personal function, economic resources, and social position. Any such loss (especially the loss of a spouse) can precipitate a reactive depression that should be addressed by the health care provider. To simply regard depression as a natural component of aging and to thereby dismiss it disregards the possible serious consequences.

Clearly, the identification of depression in the elderly is a diagnostic challenge. Untreated depression can significantly reduce the patient's quality of life and can cause immense suffering. Depression can result in increased morbidity and mortality in patients who have co-existent medical illnesses. Development of depression in patients following a myocardial infarction, congestive heart failure, or cardiac bypass surgery has been shown to increase mortality from cardiovascular events.

Depression can impair judgment, leading to risks not usually taken and ultimately to an accident or fall. Lack of appetite and loss of sleep can seriously affect the frail elderly and exacerbate underlying disease. The withdrawal and apathy that may be the first signs of depression can result in severe social isolation and lack of self-care. Depression can precipitate a downward spiral of biological and social events, ultimately leading to morbidity and death.

Depressed older patients with co-morbid physical illness, who live alone, who are male, and/or who are alcoholic are at high risk for suicide. Persons age 65 and older represent less than 13% of the population but account for 25% of suicides. The older depressed patient is more likely to attempt suicide, more likely to commit suicide violently (firearms and hanging), and more like to succeed compared with younger counter-

parts. "Psychological autopsy" studies have shown that older adults who commit suicide were often suffering from a major depression. The vast majority had seen a primary care physician within 1 month of the act. Therefore, the need for frequent screening of the elderly patient for depression cannot be overemphasized. The short form of the Geriatric Depression Scale (Figure 38-1) is a rapid and effective tool for screening the elderly patient for depression.

Steps in the diagnosis of depression in the older adult include the following:

1. A quick review of medications for possible depressive adverse effects (e.g., steroids, beta-blockers, benzodiazepines).
2. A social history focusing on recent changes in finances, living circumstance, new diagnosis of disease, and loss of friends or family.
3. Screening with the short form of the GDS (see Figure 38-1).
4. Focused history and physical examination for the early manifestations of disease or a change in existing disease.
5. Screening of TSH to rule out hypothyroidism as appropriate.

Choose the best answer for how you felt over the past week.

1. Are you basically satisfied with your life?	yes/**no**
2. Have you dropped many of your activities and interests?	**yes**/no
3. Do you feel that your life is empty?	**yes**/no
4. Do you often get bored?	**yes**/no
5. Are you in good spirits most of the time?	yes/**no**
6. Are you afraid that something bad is going to happen to you?	**yes**/no
7. Do you feel happy most of the time?	yes/**no**
8. Do you often feel helpless?	**yes**/no
9. Do you prefer to stay at home, rather than going out and doing new things?	**yes**/no
10. Do you feel you have more problems with memory than most?	**yes**/no
11. Do you think it is wonderful to be alive now?	yes/**no**
12. Do you feel pretty worthless the way you are now?	**yes**/no
13. Do you feel full of energy?	yes/**no**
14. Do you feel that your situation is hopeless?	**yes**/no
15. Do you think that most people are better off than you are?	**yes**/no

NOTE: Score bolded answers. One point for each of these answers. Cut-off: Normal = 0-5; above 5 suggests depression. For additional information on administration and scoring, refer to the following sources: Sheikh JI, Yesavage JA: Geriatric Depression Scale: recent evidence and development of a shorter version, *Clin Gerontol* 1986;5:165-172. Yesavage JA, Brink TL, Rose TL, et al: Development and validation of a geriatric depression rating scale: a preliminary report, *J Psych Res* 1983;17:27.

Figure 38-1 The Geriatric Depression Scale (short form, GDS). *(Courtesy Jerome A. Yesavage, MD.)*

It is important to note that elders who emigrate to the United States from other countries are at special risk for depression. This is especially true if they come to live with younger family members and find themselves isolated at home most of the time while the others in their household are at work, or if they come as refugees after having experienced traumatic events in their homeland. One difficulty in diagnosing depression among these immigrant elders (in addition to lack of a common language for communication, which is often the case) is that the symptom complex may not be the same as those described in American psychiatric literature. Depressed Asian elders, for example, especially those from China or Southeast Asia, have been found to be much more likely to present with somatic symptoms such as loss of appetite, sleep disturbances, and even headaches or stomachaches and to not reveal feelings of sadness or dysphoria.

Once the cause of the depression has been diagnosed, appropriate treatment should be pursued. If necessary, referral to a psychiatrist or other therapist who specializes in the treatment of older adults should be considered. Depression is usually a treatable disease and should not be regarded as a hopeless circumstance to be endured and hidden.

GERIATRIC WOMEN'S HEALTH

Today, U.S. women can expect to live into their 80s and beyond. Many of the health risks that characterize these later years of life for women can be attributed to postmenopausal changes. Physiological aging of the woman accelerates after menopause, especially in the genital tract. The ovarian follicular estrogen (estradiol) diminishes dramatically in the postmenopausal woman, and estrone—a low-potency estrogen derived from androstenedione—takes over as the major estrogen. Progesterone, derived mainly from the adrenals, also diminishes. The genital organs undergo atrophy, resulting in sclerotic ovaries, a smaller atrophied uterus, a pale foreshortened narrow vaginal canal (sometimes causing dyspareunia), and the loss of acidic vaginal pH, causing increased vulnerability to infection. The hormonal changes caused by menopause also result in accelerated osteoporosis, so that by age 70 years, 50% of bone mass is lost in

women, compared with men, who lose 25% of bone mass by age 80 years.[16] Increased levels of cholesterol, triglycerides, and low-density lipoprotein (LDL) and decreased levels of high-density lipoprotein(HDL) secondary to ovarian failure increase the older women's predisposition to heart disease.

Hormonal Replacement Therapy

Data regarding postmenopausal hormonal replacement therapy (HRT) continue to evolve. At the time of the writing of this chapter, HRT is an appropriate option for postmenopausal women who are not at high risk for breast or endometrial cancer. Women with intact uteruses should be taking a combination of estrogen and progesterone, and women who have undergone hysterectomy can take estrogen alone. There is no age limit for HRT; it can be given to women in their 70s and 80s. HRT helps in the prevention of osteoporosis; has a positive effect on hot flashes, vaginal dryness, and the lipid profile, and possibly on heart disease; but may increase the risk of thromboembolic disease and possibly the risk of breast cancer. Currently, researchers are looking at selective estrogen receptor modulators (SERMs) as a possible alternative to standard HRT in women at risk for breast cancer because SERMs help decrease postmenopausal osteoporosis without increasing the risk for breast cancer.

SEXUALITY AND AGING

CASE STUDY 38-3

Mrs. C is 75 years of age and has been happily married for 10 years. Her husband, who is in the end stages of Parkinson's disease, has recently developed an inappropriate and hostile fixation on sex that is part of a progressive dementia. In reviewing her circumstances with the PA, Mrs. C relates a history of physical closeness that she has cherished. When she and her husband retired to bed each night, they would hold each other, kiss, and touch. They would talk and share the day's activities, as well as their hopes, dreams, and troubles. Now that her husband is unable to participate in that closeness, she says with sorrow, "When you grow old, you become withered and ugly. No one wants to touch you anymore."

As life expectancy increases, it is important to recognize that continued sexual activity is an essential component of old age in promoting satisfactory relationships and good quality of life. Many older patients maintain sexual interest and capacity as long as they have their health, a healthy partner, and a good relationship with that partner. Normal change in sexual function in men is manifested in the following ways:

1. The need for more time for arousal.
2. The need for more time for reaching orgasm.
3. Less-rigid erections.
4. Orgasms that last for a shorter time than when they were younger.
5. Less force of ejaculation and less volume of ejaculate.

Older women are often more concerned about their appearance and their desirability. Although women's multiorgasmic capacity remains throughout life, postmenopausal hormonal changes result in physical and psychological changes. In addition, older women are often primary caregivers for their aging partners and are often greatly burdened by caregiver stress syndrome. Because women tend to outlive their male counterparts, they may have difficulty finding good partners and meaningful relationships.

Often, there is a generational difference between the health care provider and the elderly patient that can cause some discomfort for both parties. The provider should approach the issue with an open-ended question that allows the patient to choose to participate and voice concerns or questions. For example, during the review of systems, the PA could ask, "Are there any sexual or relationship issues or questions you would like to discuss this visit?" A sensitively elicited sexual history, a focused physical examination as directed by the history, diagnosis and treatment of sexually transmitted diseases when present, offering HRT to women as appropriate, and offering overall guidance and support continue to remain important components of care of the aging patient.

PROSTATE DISEASE

Benign prostatic hypertrophy is one of the most common conditions among aging men, accounting for more than 1.5 million office visits and about 250,000 surgical procedures annually in the United States. A nonmalignant enlargement of the epithelial and fibromuscular components of the prostate gland that may result in irritative (frequency, urgency, nocturia) and/or obstructive (hesitancy, intermittency, weak stream, incomplete emptying) urinary symptoms is almost universal among older men. If left untreated, it can result in significantly diminished quality of life in the older man. Treatment options include lifestyle modification (avoidance of caffeine, decrease in late evening fluid intake), avoidance of problematic medications (e.g., anticholinergic drugs), and treatment with appropriate medications like alpha-adrenergic antagonists (e.g., doxazosin, terazosin, tamsulosin) and 5α-reductase inhibitors (finasteride). Surgery is reserved for patients who have severe symptoms that are refractory to medical treatment, or for patients who are unable to tolerate the adverse effects of medication.

Prostate cancer is a cancer of old age. Its incidence increases with age and it is rare in men younger than 40 years of age. Autopsy studies in which the entire prostate was examined have revealed histological evidence of prostate cancer in 30% of men over age 50 and 80% of men over age 80. Prostate cancer usually arises in the peripheral zone of the prostate and remains asymptomatic in most patients, especially in the early stages. At present, there is no direct evidence that early detection decreases mortality rates due to prostate cancer. Most men with prostate cancer die with the disease, not from it. Serum prostate-specific antigen (PSA) is a nonspecific test, with elevations in PSA occurring in BPH and prostatitis, and transiently in response to conditions such as ejaculation and prostatic massage, or even a digital rectal examination. The U.S. Preventive Services Task Force, the American College of Physicians, and the Canadian Task Force on the Periodic Health Examination have recommended *against* routine PSA screening for prostate cancer.

Acute bacterial prostatitis is characterized by fever, chills, dysuria, and a tense or tender prostate as seen in older men with indwelling urinary catheters; an infectious agent is not identified in 80% of cases. Treatment includes antibiotics, and hospitalization may be required in severe cases.

Chronic bacterial prostatitis presents classically as recurrent bacteriuria, and continuous low-dose antibiotic suppressive therapy can be considered for patients with frequent symptomatic relapse.

COMPLEMENTARY AND ALTERNATIVE MEDICINE

The National Center for Complementary and Alternative Medicine of the National Institutes of Health defines complementary and alternative medicine (CAM) as "an unrelated group of non-orthodox therapeutic practices often with explanatory systems that do not follow conventional biomedical explanations." Herbal products have become increasingly popular, in part because patients may feel that these products are "natural" and therefore safe, and because they are available without a prescription. The Food and Drug Administration (FDA) does not regulate herbal products. Thus herbal therapies can be promoted for health conditions without proof that they work or that they are safe for people to use. CAMs of particular interest to older patients because of the conditions they are alleged to help alleviate are St. John's wort (depression), kava (anxiety), valerian (sleep problems), ginkgo (memory loss), saw palmetto (prostate symptoms), and glucosamine with chondroitin (arthritic pain).

Although many elders use CAM, many will not voluntarily or willingly divulge this. The PA who spends time establishing a trusting relationship with patients will be able to elicit information about CAM usage by using sensitive and gentle questioning. Once the information has been elicited, the PA should strive to be nonjudgmental and should provide evidence-based information about the safety and efficacy of the CAM that the patient is using.

ELDER ABUSE

Evaluation of the geriatric patient cannot be considered complete unless the issue of elder abuse/mistreatment has been addressed. The term *elder mistreatment* denote acts of omission or commission that result in harm or threatened harm to the health or welfare of an older adult. The national incidence of elder abuse is approximately 450,000 cases annually; with a prevalence range of 700,000 to 1.2 million older adults, elder abuse occurs in approximately 4% of those age 65 years or older.[17] Abuse can be physical abuse

(including sexual abuse), emotional abuse, intentional or unintentional neglect of the debilitated or demented patient, financial exploitation, or abandonment, or it may be a combination of these.

Poverty, dependency of the elderly person for caregiving needs, functional disability, frailty, and cognitive impairment are some of the risk factors for elder abuse. Clues to elder abuse include patients who look ill-dressed with poor personal hygiene; are malnourished, listless, or apathetic; are brought to clinic or the emergency department by someone other than the caregiver; present with fractures or bruises in various stages of healing, unexplained bruises, or unusual bruises (e.g., bruises in inner arms or thighs); have cigarette, rope, or chemical burns; or have facial lacerations and abrasions or marks occurring only in areas of the body usually covered by clothes. Evidence that material goods are being taken in exchange for care or that personal belongings (house, jewelry, car) are being taken over without consent or approval, as well as reports of being left in unsafe situations or of inability to get needed medication, can be indicators of underlying abuse. Astute PAs who maintain a heightened suspicion for potential elder abuse can identify cases by a careful history and a discerning physical examination, and by watching for subtle changes in the physical and psychosocial status of the patient over time.

Social Support

Older persons who are involved with, and supported by, their families or members of another important social network are generally healthier and happier than those in isolation. Loss of social support can signal real risk for frail elders. Referral to social services or an outreach community program can help provide a safety net of social support for those at risk. In some cases, a "buddy system" of daily phone calls to check in can alert care providers to a sudden change in a patient's condition or, if there is no answer, to the possibility of a fall.

Screening

Cancer is the second major cause of death in people over 65 years of age, following cardiovascular disease. Leukemia, as well as cancer of the digestive tract, breast, prostate, skin, and urinary tract, increases in incidence at least up to the age of 84. During the annual visit by an older patient for evaluation and health care maintenance, the examiner needs to take the increased risk for cancer into account and screen appropriately.

Table 38-4 lists comprehensive recommendations for screening and health promotion strategies for older adults.

UTILIZING HEALTH RESOURCES IN THE COMMUNITY

A major part of geriatric primary care is knowing the important health-related support services available for older adults in the community, knowing when they are indicated to support the maintenance of older patients' functional status and quality of life, and then helping elders access the services they need. Because a truism in geriatrics is that it is by nature a multidisciplinary enterprise, to be a successful provider is to be a team player. Unfortunately, in many medical settings, the other members of the geriatric team—the social worker, the psychologist, the chaplain, the home care nurse, and the therapists, for example—are employed by other organizations and are less accessible for coordination of care than the medical provider might prefer.

This section describes some of the major types of services primary care providers should be familiar with in their local communities. Keeping current phone numbers of such resources in the office directory can be a useful means of dealing with common geriatric situations, such as the need for posthospitalization care for an older widow who lives alone, the mild depression and growing isolation of a retiree, or the increasing stress and fatigue of an older woman trying to care for her mildly demented husband. In addition to the resources discussed here, there are hundreds of others that would be valuable in helping older patients improve or maintain their health and quality of life.

Information and Referral Services

A logical place to start for most community resources is one of the agencies organized (1) to maintain current listings of services older adults need and (2) to provide the appropriate information to elders or their advocates. To find the local equivalents of the services listed in this section, the PA could consult an Information and Referral (I&R) service in one of two agencies.

Area Agencies on Aging (AAAs) are available to plan and coordinate services for older adults in every corner of the United States. One of the requirements imposed by the Older Americans Act, which created the AAAs, is that they maintain I&R services for the region they cover, usually including one or more counties. Unfortunately, AAAs frequently have some other official designation, such as "Department on Aging" or "Senior Services Council," and they may be associated with a governmental or a private nonprofit agency, but one can usually find the phone number for the local AAA or its I&R through the listings in the front of the telephone directory under "Senior" or "Aging" services.

Another excellent source of I&R services is the local *multipurpose senior center,* which is available in almost every town or suburb of any size. Most senior centers offer among their services a comprehensive I&R department that has up-to-date information on services elders need, such as housing, home health care, transportation, home-delivered meals, and nursing homes, for the particular area they serve.

Case Management or Care Coordination

An important role within the geriatric team is for a person to coordinate the myriad of fragmented health and social services and agencies a frail elder with multiple problems might need. A *case manager* (or care coordinators, as they are called in some communities) not only deals with medical services but also assesses need and helps to arrange for transportation, in-home assistance (such as home-delivered meals and homemaker services), assistance with business affairs, and, if needed, more supportive housing such as assisted living. They also follow up to see that the services are delivered and are satisfactory. Unfortunately, case managers are not yet available in all communities and to all older residents, but they are increasingly part of community-based long-term care services designed to provide alternatives to institutional care for frail elders. Private case management programs are also growing in many areas.

Table 38-4   Summary of Preventive Medicine and Screening Recommendations for Older Adults*

Maneuver	Evidence†	Recommendation (Source)	Grade†
SCREENING‡			
Blood pressure	1	Every examination at least every 1-2 years (USPSTF)	A
Physician breast examination	1	Annually >40 (ACS, USPSTF)	A
Mammogram	1	Annually >50 (ACS) or every 1-2 years, ages 50-69 (USPSTF, ACP); continue every 1-3 years, ages 70-85 in willing and appropriate patients (AGS, USPSTF)	A;C>69
Pelvic examination/ Pap smear	II	Every 2-3 years after three negative annual examinations can the or discontinue after age 65-69 (ACS, USPSTF, CTF, AGS)	A;C >65
Cholesterol	I-III	Adults every 5 years (NCEP); less certain for elderly	B;C >65
Rectal examination	II	Annually >40 (ACS)	C
Fecal occult blood test	II	Annually >50 (ACS)	B
Sigmoidoscopy	II	Every 3-5 years >50 (ACS)	B
Visual acuity test	III	Periodically in older adults (various)	B
Test/inquire for hearing impaired	III	Periodically in older adults (various)	B
Mouth, nodes, testes, skin, heart, lung examinations	III	Annually (ACS, AHA)	C
Glucose	III	Periodic in high-risk groups (USPSTF)	C
Thyroid function	III	Clinically prudent for elderly, especially women (USPSTF)	C
Electrocardiogram	III	Periodically >40-50 (AHA)	C
Glaucoma screening	III	Periodically by eye specialist >65 (USPSTF)	C
Mental/functional status	III	As needed; be alert for decline (USPSTF)	C
Osteoporosis (bone densitometry)	III	NR/as needed (USPSTF)	C
Prostate examination/ prostate-specific antigen	III	Annually >50 (ACS); NR (USPSTF)	C-D
Chest x-ray	III	If needed for treatment decision (USPSTF)	D
PROPHYLAXIS/COUNSELING			
Exercise	I-II	Encourage aerobic and resistance exercise as tolerated (USPSTF, AHA)	A
Tetanus-diphtheria vaccine	I-II	1 series then booster every 10 years (ACP, USPSTF)	A
Influenza vaccine	I-II	Annually >65 or chronically ill (ACP, USPSTF)	B
Pneumovas	II	23-valent at least once >65 (ACP, USPSTF)	B
Calcium	II	800-1500 mg/d (various)	B

Table 38-4 Summary of Preventive Medicine and Screening Recommendations for Older Adults*—cont'd

Maneuver	Evidence†	Recommendation (Source)	Grade†
PROPHYLAXIS COUNSELING			
Estrogen	II	Postmenopausal women (various)	B
Aspirin	I-II	Men >50 80-325 mg qd-qod (various) (USPSTF)	C

Modified from Goldberg TH, Chavin SI. Preventive medicine and screening in older adults. J Am Geriatr Soc 1997;45:351.

NR, Not recommended for routine screening in asymptomatic individuals, although it may be useful when clinically indicated.

*Recommendations on prevention and screening in older adults, summarized from this paper and other literature.

†Grades of evidence and recommendations adapted primarily from U.S. Preventive Services Task Force. Grades are those given by the Task Force except when none are available and grades are assigned by authors.

‡Screening recommendations apply only to asymptomatic individuals; specific clinical circumstances may necessitate different testing and treatment schedules. Where no upper age limits are listed, screening should continue until approximately age 85 or when the patient is not a treatment candidate because of limited active life expectancy/quality.

Sources include the following: American College of Physicians (ACP), American Cancer Society (ACS), American Geriatrics Society (AGS), American Heart Association (AHA), Canadian Task Force (CTF) of the periodic Health Examination, National Cholesterol Education Program (NCEP), U.S. Preventive Services Task Force (USPSTF), and authors' interpretation of the literature.

Multipurpose Senior Centers

It is safe to say that the lives of millions of elders across the nation are enhanced by participation in their local senior centers, which typically offer a wide range of programs at no or low cost for healthy independent elders. Day programs provided in a center for older adults who live in the community enable elders to do the following:

➤ Take classes in subjects such as fitness (frequently ranging from armchair exercises through yoga to aerobics), music of various types, languages, financial management, and self-management for chronic disease.

➤ Eat a nutritious low-cost lunch subsidized with Older Americans Act funds.

➤ Learn about and take advantage of special services or programs for senior citizens, such as travel and tours, hypertension screening, and assistance with tax forms.

➤ Visit with friends in an attractive, upbeat environment that encourages older adults to be active and stay involved with the world.

PAs would do well to become acquainted with the staff and activities in the local senior center, so that they can refer patients there for a wide range of health-related support services, including nutrition, fitness, health screenings, health education, health insurance assistance and counseling, and antidotes to depression for elders who are isolated and lonely.

Day Care/Day Health Care Programs

Just as multipurpose senior centers are important health centers for generally healthy, independent elders, day care (sometimes called "social day care") and day health care programs serve a similar function for frail elders. Both usually offer programs for movement impaired or cognitively impaired older adults who need assistance, and the programs are typically offered 5 days a week. Both are designed to provide respite for the family caregivers of frail elders, frequently enabling adult children to keep frail elders in their homes when both children and spouse work outside the home. Some day centers also accept elders who are incontinent. Both models typically offer transportation, and the cost is usually figured on a sliding scale. Programs commonly include music, arts and crafts, current events, and a nutritious lunch. In addition, the day health care programs provide nursing, social work, and physical and occupational therapy services on the basis of assessed need. For the elder at risk of institutionalization, these centers are extremely important resources that can help maintain the elder at home for much longer than would otherwise be the case, because the staff can monitor changes in the patient's health and functional status on a daily or weekly basis and can keep the PA informed about problems, such as reactions to medications or acute confusion that might signal an infection.

In-Home Care

Many patients prefer to remain at home as long as possible, and because that desire often represents the option that both supports the patient's highest quality of life and is the most cost-effective, the goal of geriatric care is often to keep a patient at home. There is great comfort in being in familiar surroundings and, if possible, being cared for by family and friends. To that end, the PA should know about a variety of resources available to assist patients who prefer to be at home but need professional and other types of support that cannot be provided by the informal support system.

The *home health care* industry has become extremely sophisticated and offers a wide range of services to the homebound elderly person. In-home care through home health agencies should be considered as a possible resource to prevent nonacute hospitalization or placement in a skilled nursing facility. The services provided vary, depending on the agency, and can include physical therapy; occupational therapy; social work to evaluate and coordinate assistance with financial, social support, and mental health resources; hospice care for dying patients and their family members; and skilled nursing support. Skilled nursing care can include intravenous (IV) hydration, IV antibiotics, wound care, management of medication, follow-up of office assessment, fecal disimpaction, placement of urinary catheters, drawing of blood for laboratory assessment, pain control, and a nursing assessment of the patient's condition. The skilled nursing care and affiliated services provided by home health agencies can be extremely important in maintaining continuity of posthospitalization care for older patients.

The role of the PA in home health care includes the following:

➤ Evaluate the patient medically, and recommend a course of treatment.

➤ Document the need for the services provided by the home care agency.

➤ Act as liaison for the agency to monitor care and outcomes and provide support for the staff if medical questions arise.

➤ Understand the resources and financial constraints involved in recommending home care, and ensure that all parties understand the scope of needed services and the cost.

Although most PAs in practice know and work with home health agencies, older patients can often profit from less skilled and more varied support at home. In many cases, the prevention of institutionalization depends on the availability of someone to assist the elder with ADLs and IADLs at home. This assistance, referred to as *homemaker or chore services,* can often be provided by the same home health agencies that furnish skilled professional care. The advantages of going through the agency are that workers are screened and bonded for security and may have some training, and that substitutes can be provided if a worker is absent. The disadvantage is that the services obtained through a home health care agency may be more expensive than those arranged privately. Some communities maintain registries of names of possible assistants.

Home-delivered meals are provided in most communities on a sliding fee scale for elders medically certified as homebound through Older Americans Act funds, but there may be a waiting list to receive such services. Other in-home services, such as *home repairs and renovations* for wheelchairs, are frequently also available; the best source of information is a case manager or an I&R service.

An especially important service for very frail or at-risk elders who are living alone is an *alert system.* These are electronic monitors that can be attached to clothing or worn around the neck so that an elder who has fallen or otherwise has an emergency can easily contact a central switchboard, which then summons assistance as needed. The private systems that are widely advertised on TV tend to be much more expensive than those run in many communities through a local hospital or other health care agency. Communities also frequently have volunteer programs to provide *friendly visiting or telephone reassurance* on a regular basis for homebound elders at risk for isolation.

Senior Housing

Many choices of housing are especially designed for older adults and provide all degrees of support needed. When PAs are included in the process of recommending or deciding on residential options, it is imperative that they know the differences between levels of care so that the support available in the living environment can be matched to the level of care needed. The most important principle to use in those decisions is that of *the least restrictive environment,* meaning that elders need to be given the option of living in the type of environment that allows them the most freedom possible while giving them the support they need. The major options available in most communities are described here.

Independent Living
Many attractive choices are commonly available for healthy independent elders who would like to move from their current homes for reasons such as security, level of maintenance needed, and change of location. Of course, those who can pay market prices can buy or rent in elegant retirement communities with many added amenities and services operated by for-profit corporations, but many areas also have very attractive senior apartment complexes subsidized by the U.S. Department of Housing and Urban Development (HUD) for low- and moderate-income elders. The latter are owned and operated by private nonprofit agencies; if an elder's income and assets are low enough to qualify, the rent is one third of income, no matter how small the income. The major disadvantage of the HUD-subsidized senior housing is that these complexes are in such demand that they have long waiting lists. Some areas also have other models of senior housing for middle-income elders, with many agencies now moving to monthly rent and options of additional services in the apartments if needed. Senior housing for independent elders usually has an on-site manager and often has an activity director or social worker. This housing always includes kitchen facilities, but many facilities serve at least one meal a day in an attractive dining room.

Assisted Living
Assisted living housing facilities may also go by a variety of other names—residential care, board and care, personal care, and community care. They are distinguished by the level of assistance they provide without license to provide health care. They all provide three meals a day, assistance with some ADLs such as bathing, supervision of medications, and transportation; other services are frequently added. In larger facilities, a variety of activities are commonly planned and offered through an activities director. In most states, assisted living facilities are not required to have nurses on staff, but many do.

Nursing Homes
The distinguishing feature of nursing homes, which offer the most intensive level of care on a continuous basis, is that they provide skilled nursing care. Some nursing homes are not licensed. However, if they are reimbursed for services by either Medicaid or Medicare, they must meet basic minimum standards of staffing, sanitation, nutrition, and nursing care and are licensed through the state. Facilities that are technically classified as nursing facilities frequently call themselves "convalescent hospitals," or they use a variety of other terms, such as "manor" or "home," that do not really distinguish them from assisted living facilities. A very important growing role for PAs in geriatrics is to provide a level of continuous medical care for nursing home patients, which has been very rare to date, by spending longer and more comprehensive visits and being more available to the nursing home staff to respond to their concerns.

Continuing Care Communities
Some facilities have two or more of the levels of care previously described and generally offer very comfortable and pleasant lifestyles for a variety of needs. The older models often are associated with religious communities, and many newer models have been developed by for-profit corporations that require a large "buy-in" down payment on admission. Some newer multiple-level facilities require only monthly payments, which increase with more intensive levels of care. The advantages of these continuing care communities is that they offer security for the future for elders with progressive chronic illness, and they are convenient

for couples with one member in need of more intensive care. The disadvantage is that they are frequently too expensive for low- or middle-income elders.

CONCLUSION

Caring for the elderly is intense but very rewarding work. Geriatrics offers the PA student a unique opportunity to provide holistic care. The nature of PA training is intense and clinically oriented. There is tremendous value in seeing what is "normal" and contrasting that with the physical manifestation of disease. The geriatric population often offers the student the opportunity to observe the "abnormal" findings associated with aging and the disease processes that sharpen the clinical learning process.

Students may struggle with the fundamentals of the history, physical examination, and diagnosis, as well as the options for treatment. However, medical care is more than ascertaining the correct diagnosis and treatment. Working with elders enables the PA student to struggle with the social, emotional, and cultural challenges inherent in working with the medically complex person. Also, patients benefit tremendously by being in the care of a provider who takes the time to get to know the person behind the disease and to provide care that takes into account the physical, psychological, social, functional, and spiritual components of need. For the student to avoid the challenge of treating older patients because they are too complex, too hard to talk with, or simply too difficult is to lose an essential learning experience that cuts across all medical disciplines to the core of the health care experience, which is to make a difference and help patients find meaning in their lives amid the challenges generated by their illnesses.

CLINICAL APPLICATIONS

1. Summarize age-related changes for each body system that are common in elderly patients.
2. Identify four steps in assessing the medication status of elderly patients.
3. List eight common causes of reversible dementia in the elderly. Which cause is the most common?
4. Describe how you would teach pelvic muscle exercises to a patient with incontinence.

5. List eight components of a safety assessment of the home environment of an elderly patient.
6. Discuss your perceptions of the challenges and satisfactions of caring for elderly patients.

Acknowledgments

The authors would like to express their appreciation to Dr. David Thom, who has extensively researched and taught medical students about urinary incontinence, for his contribution to this section.

REFERENCES

1. Moore AA, Su AL. Screening for common problems in ambulatory elderly: clinical confirmation of a screen instrument. Am J Med 1998;100:440.
2. Yturri-Byrd K, Glazer-Waldman H. The physician assistant and care of the geriatric patient. Gerontol Geriatr Ed 1984;5:33.
3. Schafft G, Fasser CE, Cyr AB. Final Report: The Assessment and Improvement of Knowledge and Skills in Geriatrics. Arlington, VA: American Academy of Physician Assistants, 1985.
4. Rowe JW, Kahn RL. Successful Aging: The MacArthur Foundation Study. New York: Pantheon, 1998.
5. Fink RI, Kolterman OG, Koa M, et al. The role of glucose transport system in the post receptor defect in insulin action associated with human aging. J Clin Endocrinol Metab 1984;58:721.
6. Malmrose LC, Gray SL, Pieper CF, et al. Measured versus estimated creatinine clearance in a high functioning elderly sample: MacArthur foundation study of successful aging. J Am Geriatr Soc 1993;41:715.
7. Racial and Ethnic Diversity of America's Elderly Population. Washington, DC: U.S. Bureau of the Census and National Institute on Aging, 1993.
8. Reuben DB, Herr K, Pacala JT, et al. Geriatrics at Your Fingertips. New York: American Geriatric Society, 2000.
9. Steinweg K. The changing approach to falls in the elderly. Am Fam Physician 1997;7:1815.
10. Tinetti ME, Baker DI, McAvay G, et al. A multifactorial intervention to reduce the risk of falling among elderly people living in the community. N Engl J Med 1994;331:821.
11. Wolf SL, Barnhart HX, Kutner NG, et al. Reducing frailty and falls in older persons: an investigation of Tai Chi and computerized balance training. J Am Geriatr Soc 1996;44:489.
12. Drachman DA. A 69-year-old man with chronic dizziness. JAMA 1998;280:2111.
13. Linzer MD, Yang EH, Estes M, et al. Diagnosing syncope: part 1: value of history, physical examination and electrocardiography. Ann Intern Med. 1997;126:989.
14. NIH Consensus Conference. Diagnosis and treatment of depression in late life. JAMA 1992;268:1018.

15. Denihan A, Kirby M, Bruce I, et al. Three-year prognosis of depression in the community-dwelling elderly. Br J Psychiatry. 2000;176:453.

16. Grimley Evans J. The significance of osteoporosis. In Smith R (ed). Osteoporosis. London, England: Royal College of Physicians, 1990.

17. The National Elder Abuse Incidence Study: Final Report. The National Center on Elder Abuse at The American Public Human Services Association in Collaboration with Westat, Inc. Washington, DC: National Aging Information Center, 1998.

RESOURCES

AGS Panel on Chronic Pain in Older Persons. The management of chronic pain in older persons. J Am Geriatr Soc 1998;46:635. *These clinical practice guidelines were developed and written by a multidisciplinary expert panel under the auspices of the Panel on Chronic Pain in Older Persons of the American Geriatrics Society.*

Jacox A, Carr DB, Payne R, et al. Management of Cancer Pain. Clinical Practice Guideline No. 9. Rockville, MD: U.S. Department of Health and Human Services, Public Health Service, Agency for Health Care Policy and Research, March 1994. AHCPR Pub. No. 94–0592/3. *The AHCPR guidelines provide an evidence-based approach to the assessment and management of pain in cancer patients.*

Small GW, Rabins PV, Barry PP, et al. Diagnosis and treatment of Alzheimer disease and related disorders: consensus statement of the American Association for Geriatric Psychiatry, the Alzheimer's Association, and the American Geriatrics Society. JAMA 1997;278:1363. *This is a consensus statement addressing a variety of dementia issues, including diagnosis, treatment, management, and public policy. Clinicians may find some of the management topics helpful for their clinical practices.*

Health Care Financing Administration. Medicare and You 2000. Rockville, MD: U.S. Government Printing Office, 2000. Pub. No. HCFA-10050. *This user friendly, well-written booklet is intended to help older people use the Medicare program. It describes Medicare's structure, function, and covered services, and also describes the supplemental (medigap) insurance.*

Health Care Financing Administration. 2000 Guide to Health Insurance for People with Medicare. Rockville, MD: U.S. Government Printing Office, 2000. Pub. No. HCFA-02110. *This handbook provides detailed information about the Medicare supplemental medigap insurance policies.*

http://www.medicare.gov. *This web site is an excellent resource that supplies patients and providers with information about the Medicare program. It also provides information about the nursing homes available in each community in the United States.*

The National Center on Elder Abuse at The American Public Human Services Association. The National Elder Abuse Incidence Study. Final Report: September 1998. Washington, DC: National Aging Information Center, 1998. *The National Elder Abuse Incidence Study research provides a national incidence estimate*

of elder abuse, which can serve as a baseline for future research and service interventions about elder abuse.

O'Hara M, Kiefer D, Farrell K, et al. A review of 12 commonly used medicinal herbs. Arch Fam Med. 1998;7:523. *This excellent review article provides useful and practical clinical information.*

Astin JA. Why patients use alternative medicine: results of a national study. JAMA 1998;279:1548. *This paper provides information about what motivates people to use alternative therapies. The following factors were found to be associated with CAM usage: having more education, poorer health status, a transformational experience that changes the person's worldview, an interest in spirituality and personal growth psychology, anxiety; suffering chronic pain or urinary tract problems; and belonging to a cultural group identified by a commitment to environmentalism or feminism.*

Abrams WB, Berkow R, Fletcher AJ (eds). The Merck Manual of Geriatrics. New York: Merck Sharp & Dohme Research Laboratories, 1990. *In the format of the original Merck Manual, this comprehensive reference was designed to be a practical handbook for clinicians dealing with older patients. One- to five-page descriptions of hundreds of acute and chronic conditions are arranged in thumb-tabbed chapters by organ system.*

Bortz WM. We Live Too Short and Die Too Long: How to Achieve and Enjoy Your Natural 100-Year-Plus Life Span. New York: Bantam, 1991. *An optimistic view of aging for the layperson of any age written by a prominent geriatric clinician. Reviews the research on fitness and function in old age, with emphasis on Bortz's theory that disuse accounts for much of the loss of function in many domains and organ systems that is traditionally ascribed to aging.*

Ham RJ, Sloane PD (eds). Primary Care Geriatrics: A Case-Based Approach, ed 2. St Louis: Mosby, 1992. *A valuable educational resource using case-based chapters designed for individual study. The sections cover general principles and practice issues in geriatrics, the major syndromes, common and acute problems, common problems in the hospital, and common problems in the nursing home. Each chapter within the sections (e.g., ethics; rehabilitation; confusion, dementia, and delirium; vision; hearing; estrogen therapy; hypothermia) is written by a geriatric specialist and is built around case histories. Each chapter also includes learning objectives, study questions, and post-tests.*

Kane RW, Ouslander JG, Abrass IB. Essentials of Clinical Geriatrics, ed 4. New York: McGraw-Hill, 1997. *The most popular and usable reference and educational tool for clinical medicine practice with older adults, written by leading geriatricians. Highly recommended for clinicians who prefer to have one comprehensive guide.*

Mace NL, Rabins PV. The 36-Hour Day: A Family Guide to Caring for Persons with Alzheimer's Disease, Related Dementing Illnesses, and Memory Loss in Later Life. Baltimore: Johns Hopkins Press, 1982. *A classical guide for family caregivers to help them cope with the overwhelming problems encountered as a family member goes through the various stages of dementia. Continues to be published by numerous sources a decade after its first printing, is available in Spanish and other languages, and can be obtained through local Alzheimer's Associations.*

Tideiksaar R. The Role of Physician Extenders in the Care of the Elderly Patient. In: Ham RJ (ed). Geriatric Medicine Annual. Oradell, NJ: Medical Economics, 1986. *Written by one of the nation's leading geriatric PAs, this chapter presents a strong argument for the need for PAs and other physician extenders in geriatric care. Specific suggestions are made for roles that PAs can play to provide more effective and less costly care for elders, including initial assessments, home visits, telephone contact for follow-up, health screening and education, and inservice education in geriatrics to other health care providers.*

Yeo G, Tully D. Model Geriatric Clerkship for Physician Assistant Students: The Continuum of Elder Care. Stanford, CA: Stanford University School of Medicine, Division of Family Medicine, 1987. *This manual includes curriculum outlines for six curriculum units, descriptive materials, detailed suggestions for implementation, and clinical resource material for the establishment of a geriatric clinical rotation for PAs based on roles PAs are likely to have in clinical practice. Units deal with communication skills, evaluation of health status, management of common health problems in noninstitutionalized elders, health promotion and disease prevention, family and elder counseling, and long-term care issues. Assessment forms and an extensive bibliography are included. The manual was developed with support from the Bureau of Health Professions of the U.S. Health Resources and Services Administration and is available in PA training programs.*

American Geriatrics Society, British Geriatrics Society, and American Academy of Orthopaedic Surgeons Panel on Falls Prevention. Guidelines for the prevention of falls in older persons. J Am Geriatr Soc 2001;49:664. *This publication aims to guide clinicians in assessing fall risk and managing older patients at risk of falling or who have fallen. The following areas are addressed: assessing older persons who have had one or more falls, or those who report recurrent falls or abnormalities of gait or balance. Interventions for the management of falls by older persons in various settings are also addressed.*

CHAPTER 39

Correctional Medicine

R. Scott Chavez

INTRODUCTION

Although physician assistants (PAs) working in correctional medicine have a demanding and difficult role, the rewards they receive are unlike those received from any other health care discipline. There are advantages and disadvantages to working in correctional medicine, and this field of health care holds an interest and challenge with which few can compare. This chapter describes the past, present, and future of correctional medicine and the contribution that PAs can make.

To help the reader fully appreciate correctional medicine, its definition, history, case law, and standards are presented first. The second section of the chapter describes the role of the PA in correctional settings. A discussion of incarcerated patients' health problems and their management is also presented. The third section forecasts the future for PAs in correctional medicine. The chapter concludes with a discussion of why PAs should consider correctional medicine as a career selection.

WHAT IS CORRECTIONAL MEDICINE?

Correctional medicine is the art and practice of delivering health care to incarcerated men, women, and children. As a specialty, correctional medicine is a rather new development in the history of medicine. The delivery of health care in correctional settings is founded on case law. It was not until the early 1970s that state and federal courts examined and defined health care in correctional facilities.

The defining of standards of care, the structuring of health care systems in jails and prisons by professional health providers, and the establishment of medical autonomy in correctional settings were forces that shaped correctional medicine as a specialty.

A *prison* is a state or federal facility that confines individuals to serve a sentence of longer than 1 year; however, in most jurisdictions, the length of sentence is longer. A *jail* is an institution in a local municipality (city, county, or town) where one awaits trial, sentencing, and transfer to other facilities after conviction, or is serving a sentence that is usually less than 1 year. A *juvenile detention center* is a facility that holds individuals who have protected legal status as minors. *Parole* is defined as community supervision after a period of incarceration; *probation* means that an offender is still serving a criminal sentence but is living in the community.[1]

WHAT ARE THE ADVANTAGES OF WORKING IN CORRECTIONS?

Working in corrections has several advantages. PAs in this public health arena can practice their clinical skills, and health providers working in corrections are challenged daily to provide a high level of care to a disadvantaged class. The PA's education, training, and skills are put to the test daily.

The health care needs of the incarcerated population are complex. The PA also has the opportunity to provide public health care to a specific group. For many of the incarcerated, health care in jail or prison is the only health care that they have received in their lives. Some practitioners regard corrections as a dynamic field that is at the forefront of the public health care delivery system in the United States.

Correctional health care offers practitioners a group of patients in whom compliance, assessment, and efficacy of treatment can be monitored. Correctional health is at the forefront of health access issues. As the United States struggles with questions of health care access, financing, and minimal standards of care, correctional health care is the field in which these issues are examined by the courts. Correctional health care may turn out to be the model for minimal levels of accessible care in the United States.

Correctional medicine gives the PA an opportunity to practice medicine. The PA sees health care problems that often go unattended in the "free world" (i.e., outside correctional institutions) because of poor access or lack of purchasing power. The health status of the incarcerated ranges from healthy to walking sick. It has been estimated that 95% of arriving inmates require medical attention, and that in 66% of cases, this contact is the first with a health professional. In addition, every inmate has a 50% likelihood of being a drug abuser, a 5% possibility of being severely mentally disturbed, and a 15% chance of having a serious emotional problem.[2] In 1976, there were 6425 sentenced drug offenders in U.S. federal prisons, accounting for 26.6% of the total federal prisoner population. Ten years later, the sentenced drug offenders incarcerated in U.S. federal prisons rose to 12,119, accounting for 38.1% of this total population. In 1996, there were 50,754 sentenced drug offenders, who accounted for 60.8% of the total federal prisoner population.[3] Because of long-term multiple-drug use and alcohol abuse, resulting in concomitant diseases and disorders, the correctional PA sees a myriad of health care problems in his or her medical career.

Correctional medicine also allows the PA to administer health care. The correctional mission is to confine and restrain individuals from society. The health care mission is to provide care and cure. At times, these missions collide, and it becomes the responsibility of health staff to work out solutions administratively; thus correctional medicine provides PAs opportunities to develop administrative skills. The field needs individuals who have the capacity to resolve conflict and integrate two opposing philosophies.

Because many correctional facilities are located in rural areas and the salaries are set by government pay scales, correctional health salaries are not as competitive as those in other employment settings. However, defining a competitive salary is not always easy.

Aside from the base rate, other factors that should be considered are raises, bonuses, promotional opportunities, and overtime pay. For part-time coverage, PAs can consider a professional service contract with the correctional institution.

Some correctional institutions provide differential pay for "hazardous" or "shift" work to compensate for less attractive working conditions. Salary is just one component of a compensation package, however. Other benefits to consider are health and life insurance, vacation, holiday and sick pay, pregnancy leave, disability pay, pension plans, tuition reimbursement, continuing professional education stipends or allowance, reimbursement for job interviews and moving expenses, housing allotments, free meals or other emoluments, job placement assistance for spouses, family leave, child care subsidy or allowance, employee health care programs (such as stress management courses and smoking cessation clinics), and employee assistance programs that provide short-term counseling or referral when personal problems have begun to affect an employee's job performance.

Another "compensation" often overlooked by PAs is the working conditions, which include the workplace and environment, the hours, and the number of days worked. The ambience of clinics and offices is certainly important to a positive working experience. Correctional institutions have a public image of oppressive, crowded, and unpleasant surroundings. The truth of the matter is that many correctional institutions' health services clinics look like any "free world" medical office or clinic. Owing to litigation, court consent decrees, or standards of care, many prisons and jails have been required to maintain health clinics that are clean, spacious, and well equipped. In fact, many correctional health clinics are so well controlled that they are often safer, cleaner, and more pleasant places in which to work than are some "free world" clinics. However, some correctional institutions do not have modern facilities for health services, which may hamper recruitment efforts.

Safety is a major concern for security. In this regard, all employment applicants must be cleared by security personnel. Security clearance for an employee may include any of the following actions: job-related age or physical ability requirements and screening, photograph and/or fingerprinting, credit or character reference checks, and a check of arrest or court records. Some correctional systems have lengthy security clearance procedures, whereas others (e.g., trusty camps or work release units) may have none at all. In either case, however, the prospective applicant should be aware that a security clearance may delay the beginning of employment for 2 weeks to 3 months.

WHAT ARE THE RISKS OF WORKING IN A CORRECTIONAL FACILITY?

The question most frequently asked by health professionals who are thinking about employment in corrections is, "How safe is it?" Research on prisoner/staff violence is underdeveloped and exact rates of inmate-to-staff assaults are not available. It is difficult to answer the question of how safe it is to work in a correctional facility because of the lack of definitions, classifications, and perceptions.

First, there is no standardized definition or classification of inmate assaults. An inmate can assault a staff member in nonphysical and physical ways. Inmates can be hostile or menacing in their responses by verbal or nonverbal cues. Physical assaults can take the form of spitting, pushing, slapping, scratching, punching, biting, kicking, and the more serious, stabbing, shooting, or choking. As a result of this wide variance, there is no consistency in reporting prevalence and rates of inmate assaults on staff.

Second, there is a wide variance in the data that are collected. The Bureau of Justice Statistics has collected some data on state and federal prisoner assaults, reporting .5% assaults on almost 350,000 correctional workers; however, there is no information collected for jail settings, and the data are not classified into custody or health staff, nor are they classified according to type of assault[4]. This makes any inference to staff "safety" of limited value.

Third, the perception of threat influences the perception of risk. Some health staff members are threatened and feel unsafe by nonphysical assaults (e.g., shouting); others may feel threatened by the overwhelming numbers and presence of inmates. Health staff working in corrections must be able to accept a wide range of human behavior so as not to feel threatened, or at least to minimize the risks of working in these institutions.

Given the previous discussion, we do not know the complete risk for those working in correctional environments. Anecdotally, most correctional health care workers report few incidences of inmate assaults. Jaye Anno, a leading correctional health care authority, observes that, "the proportion of health professionals that have been physically assaulted annually is probably even lower than the overall rate."[4] Bottoms explains that the reason why there are so few inmate assaults on staff is that there is a very rigid social order that controls and represses such behavior.[5] This social order and control are not present in other institutions such as hospitals, nursing homes, or mental hospitals. It is for this reason that health staff members are more likely to suffer an occupational injury inflicted by a patient in the emergency department or other noncorrectional setting.

WHAT ARE THE DISADVANTAGES OF WORKING IN CORRECTIONS?

There are several disadvantages to working in corrections. They include challenges to medical autonomy, overcrowded conditions, recruitment and retention of qualified health care workers, and cost containment.

The challenge to medical autonomy arises from the conflict between corrections and medicine. Corrections is based on the military model, which is founded on ranks or levels of authority, tradition, and direct supervision. Health care is based on the "team approach" model, which fosters collaborative action, sharing of power and authority, and independent thought. Correctional staff members derive their power from government and the institution itself, whereas health staff members derive power from outside the institution, such as a board of medical examiners' authority or court-ordered health care. In some ways, health staff work in the prison or jail at the discretion or permission of corrections personnel. As a result of inmate litigation, the state or federal courts may order or impose specific actions on correctional administrators; health care is just one such action. In these situations, corrections authorities have admitted health care staff to the institution under duress. This,

at times, results in tension between corrections and health care.

The custody needs of security and order invariably collide with medical needs for access and therapy; it is this challenge to medical authority and autonomy that adds to the pressures and frustrations that "free world" PAs do not encounter.

Another disadvantage to working in corrections relates to financial factors and cost containment. Correctional systems have undergone tremendous change over the past decade. The push for mandatory sentencing and the criminalization of narcotic and drug abuse and mental illness have resulted in overcrowding of our nation's jails and prisons. The Bureau of Justice Statistics reports that at mid-year of 2001, there were 631,240 jail inmates and 1,334,255 prisoners in the 50 states, the District of Columbia, and the Federal Government.[6]

The explosion in the number of new prisons and jails to house this population has had a profound effect on the fiscal management of correctional systems. In a climate of tight state and county budgets, there are constant challenges to cut and contain costs in providing health care to the incarcerated.

The difficulty in recruiting qualified and competent health care professionals is another problem adding to the frustration of working in corrections. Burnout and stigma are recruitment impediments experienced in corrections. Partly owing to the location of prisons (i.e., away from metropolitan areas), the stigma of the working environment, and noncompetitive salaries, it is extremely difficult to recruit health personnel. The professional burnout of health staff in corrections experience reflects the difficulties in dealing with the issues. The social stigma of working in corrections is another factor influencing recruitment.

Owing to the difficulty in recruiting health professionals, many departments of corrections and jail systems have improved working conditions by offering such temptations as higher salaries, guaranteed shifts, shift differential pay, increased fringe benefits, hazardous duty pay, and continuing medical education for professional staff.

On the other hand, it has become much easier today than in the past to attract and retain qualified correctional health professionals. Corrections officials have learned that they must be competitive with the "free world" to attract all types of professionals, including health care workers. In addition, there is an increase in the respectability of correctional medicine. Many practitioners are willing to consider correctional health care as a career because "free world" practice settings offer many impediments to the practice of medicine. PA employment opportunities in corrections are increasing.

Still, why would anyone want to work in corrections? What attracts providers to the field? As one leading author in the correctional health care field has pointed out:

> Prison and jail inmates are overwhelmingly poor, are disproportionately minorities, and have the added stigma of having been charged with transgressing society's laws. They do not vote, are essentially without power, and there are few special interest groups concerned with their welfare. Why should anyone care whether the health services provided to these individuals are adequate? Perhaps because ... the care and treatment provided to the incarcerated is a reflection of the degree of professionalism attained by the field of correctional medicine and a hallmark of a civilized society.[4]

To help the reader understand why correctional medicine remains an attraction and why this specialty is at the forefront of the major issues facing the United States, a discussion of the history and legal foundations follows.

HISTORY OF CORRECTIONAL MEDICINE

A society is judged by how it accepts responsibility for those entrusted to it. Hubert Humphrey once observed that a society that cannot educate its infirm, sick, poor, or disabled is a government without compassion and a soul.[7]

Our society is based on laws, and government has a responsibility to incarcerate those who violate its laws or rules; however, the needs of the violators do not cease the moment they become wards of the state. Society's obligation to provide the basic needs of food, shelter, clothing, and health care to those it is punishing by incarceration must be met.

In the early 1970s, federal district courts framed judicial opinion that recognized government's constitutional duty to provide health care to inmates. Today, judicial review has established that an organized system of professional medical, dental, and psychiatric care must be guaranteed to each inmate. In fact, the incarcerated are the only class with a protected right to health care access. However, this has not always been the case. The United States has had gulag conditions in its jails and prisons. Abuses have been well documented.

The literature is filled with illustrations of generally unsanitary living conditions and practices in correctional facilities. Studies performed in the early 1970s described inadequate lighting, heating, and ventilation.[8,9] One study in Pennsylvania described cockroaches in the dining room and rat droppings in the kitchen.[10] Other literature describes lice and vermin infestations and mouse bites. Personal space was nonexistent, and bathroom facilities were often unsanitary. One survey in the late 1970s found that "46 percent of federal inmates and 44 percent of state inmates lived in high-density, multiple occupancy units."[11] In a landmark case, it was demonstrated that a quadriplegic who spent many months in a state corrections' medical and diagnostic center's hospital developed bed sores that eventually became infected with maggots. His bandages were not changed for days, and the stench permeated the entire ward. Medical and court records demonstrated that in the month before his death, his dressings were changed and he was bathed only once.[12]

A businesswoman who had been sentenced to a week in the Cook County Jail for contempt of court in 1969 filed suit for atrocities inflicted on her by staff and inmates. In her complaint, she stated that she was subjected to an examination in a search for concealed narcotics with unsterilized vaginal instruments. Her complaint further stated that the attending physician took away her cardiac prescription medicine and never returned it.[13]

In another case, a geriatric stroke patient, rendered partially incontinent, was forced to sit on a wooden bench beside his bed every day because the staff did not want to frequently change his bed linen or attend to him. On one occasion, he fell from the bench and one of his legs became edematous and cyanotic. The circulatory compromise was never attended to, and he subsequently had the leg amputated. He died 1 day after the amputation.

Factors Impeding Change

There were many reasons why penal conditions were allowed to deteriorate to this level. Prior to the 1970s, a judicial doctrine of "hands off" was applied to correctional institutions, based on a belief that specific constitutional provisions did not exist for the courts to interpret correctional environments. Aside from the Eighth Amendment's general prohibition against cruel and unusual punishment, the courts believed that there was no judicial precedent to interfere with prison administration.

Public officials, citing limited resources and low public priority, were reluctant to change prison conditions. Correctional administrators, referring to public concern for security and order, maintained that health care was a low priority that did not contribute to the goal of custody.

Prison administrators' indifference to inmates' conditions also contributed to the deterioration of prison life. There was a widespread belief that deprivation is *the* role of corrections and that it is justified. Many correctional staff members still believe that inmates do not deserve basic human considerations.

Also contributing to the inhumane conditions in the penal system is an environment that is predicated on control. Correctional staff members control an inmate's life. Corrections determines when, where, how, and why an inmate is allowed to move about the prison or jail confines. In an environment where power over inmates is important, control over access to medical care becomes equally important, and abuses occur too easily.

There is little incentive to change conditions because the relationship between staff and inmates fosters hostile interactions. Staff members often stereotype the inmates as secretive and untrustworthy, and inmates often regard staff as vindictive, unfair, and controlling.

Finally, the medical profession had little motivation to change the inhumane conditions. As has been stated previously, the courts did not interpret prisoner health care as a constitutionally protected right, so the medical community had no legal basis for change. The prison doctor, after all, lacked legal authority, social status, or regulatory standards of care to argue his or her case for reform; nor did the community acknowledge the public health ramifications of local jail or prison conditions.

Factors for Change

Indifference to the inhumane conditions in the American penal system began to lessen in the 1970s. Society's obligation to improve correctional facilities and provide adequate living conditions became recognized. Change was supported on ethical, humanitarian, public policy, and legal grounds. In this context, correctional health became a part of the public health agenda.

In the 1970s, there was a growing belief that good health care should be a right extended to everyone and not a privilege available only to those who could afford it. The courts began to interpret government's role as providing basic necessities of life to its charges, including prisoners, and decided that access to health care was a necessity.

The establishment of standards of care became an issue for change. When services are provided in a two-tiered system, one for "paying" patients and one for "nonpaying" patients, good medical care cannot be promoted. The establishment of minimal standards of care acceptable for everyone, including the incarcerated, was another step toward reform.

Correctional authorities themselves began to support improvement to correctional health.[14] It became increasingly clear that the duty of the jailer was not simply to keep secure those entrusted to custody, but to care for them as well. In fact, the belief that the effort to maintain security would be assisted if health care conditions improved in the correctional facility began to emerge. Order and security would be better achieved if improving inmates' health services reduced prison violence.

Humanitarian and public health concerns also fostered change in correctional health. The humanitarian argument hinged on the belief that society had an even greater responsibility to provide health care to the incarcerated because prisoners were not free to choose their care. The social agenda in the 1970s was to champion international human rights, yet human rights in our own penal system were an embarrassment. Improving the inmate conditions for humanitarian reasons became the socially right thing to do.

Public health authorities began to review the community health problem inside prisons and jails as well. Providing adequate health care to inmates was just as important for the community because the added costs and consequences to the public health budget would become evident after the prisoner was released. Released prisoners who failed to receive adequate health care while in prison would invariably require help (and perhaps more costly support) from a variety of government-sponsored welfare programs. In one way or another, the cost of correctional health care is shouldered by society.

Finally, a legal mandate to change the deplorable conditions in prisons and jails came during the early 1970s. Any resistance to change was met by a growing body of case law that propelled correctional administrators to improve conditions and meet minimum standards of care.

> The case that signaled the beginning of the reversal of the "hands-off" doctrine with respect to prisoners' rights to medical care was *Newman v. Alabama*. In this October 1972 decision, a United States district court found the whole state correctional system of Alabama to be in violation of the Eighth and Fourteenth Amendment rights of the inmates, by failing to provide them with *adequate and sufficient* medical care. The court placed the state's correction agency under injunction and demanded immediate remedies for all existing deficiencies. Cost considerations were held not to be sufficient defense for failing to provide care. Subsequent review at the circuit court level upheld this landmark decision.[4]

Since 1972, many class action suits have alleged unconstitutional conditions and inadequate health care services. The American Civil Liberties Union noted, in its 1990 "Status Report," that 45 states had some litigation against the prison system for unconstitutional conditions.[15] Between 1972 and 1974, many state and local correctional systems were brought before the courts in suits relating to specific inmates' rights, health, and well-being. The cases were often nonbinding to all jurisdictions, however, or were not equally applied to all classes of incarcerated people (e.g., some applied only to detainees or to civil commitments). Furthermore, court decrees are binding only to those participating in a suit. The lack of federal legislation or Supreme Court opinion on prisoners' right to health care was problematic to any continued and real reform in the correctional system.

The U.S. Supreme Court finally addressed the constitutional issue of prisoners' medical care in the case *Estelle v. Gamble*. The Court reflected lower court decisions by stating that the "denial of medical care may result in pain and suffering which no one suggests would serve any penological purpose."[16] Further, the Court stated that the infliction of unnecessary suffering is inconsistent with contemporary standards of decency, and concluded that "deliberate indifference to serious medical needs of prisoners constitutes the 'unnecessary and wanton infliction of pain' proscribed by the Eighth Amendment. This is true whether the indifference is manifested by prison doctors in their response to the prisoner's needs or by prison guards in intentionally denying or delaying access to medical care or intentionally interfering with the treatment once prescribed. Regardless of how evidenced, deliberate indifference to a prisoner's serious illness or injury states a cause of action."[17] The *Estelle v. Gamble* case set the national standard for what was to become modern-day correctional health care.

THE DEVELOPMENT OF STANDARDS

It is important for PAs working in correctional medicine to understand the fundamental principles and minimal standards of care of this specialty. In 1976, the American Public Health Association (APHA) published the first national health care standards written specifically for correctional institutions. These standards were comprehensive in their approach to the issue of correctional health care, with the exception of enforcement. APHA provided no mechanism to implement, monitor, or maintain its standards.

A second set of standards, although not as detailed as the APHA's, was published in 1977 by the American Medical Association (AMA). These standards were specific to health care delivery in a jail setting. In 1979, the AMA published its standards for health care in prisons. A major difference from the APHA's correctional health standards was that the

AMA standards were tied to an accreditation program. In 1983, the AMA program for jail and prison accreditation came under the authority of the National Commission on Correctional Health Care (NCCHC). The NCCHC is a not-for-profit 501(c)3 organization whose board of directors comprises individuals named in the Box of professional associations.

The representatives to NCCHC guide the accreditation program and the maintenance of standards. The NCCHC's accreditation program demonstrates an institution's efforts at compliance and has become accepted by the courts as proof of attaining a minimum level of care. The NCCHC is constantly monitoring its accreditation program to provide additional detail and direction to the field through subsequent revisions to the standards. The most recent jail and prison revisions occurred in 2002. The juvenile detention standards will be revised in 2003.

A third set of standards used in the field of correctional health is promulgated by the American Correctional Association (ACA), a membership organization for correctional workers such as wardens and custody staff. The ACA performance-based standards have been based on input from medical personnel; however, representation from PAs has been limited and disorganized, unlike NCCHC's standards.

Other sets of correctional standards have been issued by the American Nurses Association and the American Psychiatric Association; however, no accreditation service has been associated with these standards. Their focus is to primarily guide nursing or psychiatric practice in correctional institutions.

Essentially, the standards address three basic inmate rights that have emerged from case law: the right of access to care, the right to care that is ordered, and the right to a professional medical judgment. Over the years, the courts have enumerated the essential elements of a health care program in corrections (see the Box).

Establishment of standards of care was a critical step toward prison and jail health care reform. Standardizing health services in corrections meant that health care providers were expected to perform comparably with their free world counterparts. This led to the employment of licensed, qualified, and professional health care providers. The past 20 years has

---

PROFESSIONAL ASSOCIATIONS NAMED BY THE NCCHC BOARD OF DIRECTORS

American Academy of Child & Adolescent Psychiatry
American Academy of Pediatrics
American Academy of Physician Assistants
American Academy of Psychiatry & the Law
American Association of Physician Specialists
American Association of Public Health Physicians
American Bar Association
American College of Emergency Physicians
American College of Health Care Executives
American College of Neuropsychiatrists
American College of Physicians–American Society of Internal Medicine
American Correctional Health Services Association
American Counseling Association
American Dental Association
American Diabetes Association
American Dietetic Association
American Health Information Management Association
American Jail Association
American Medical Association
American Nurses' Association
American Osteopathic Association
American Pharmaceutical Association
American Psychiatric Association
American Psychological Association
American Public Health Association
American Society of Addiction Medicine
John Howard Association
National Association of Counties
National Association of County and City Health Officials
National District Attorneys Association
National Juvenile Detention Association
National Medical Association
National Sheriffs' Association
Society of Correctional Physicians
The Society for Adolescent Medicine

seen tremendous changes in correctional medicine. The control of health services by health care providers has led to professionalization of the field, which illustrates ways that correctional medicine can be rewarding and stimulating. The remainder of the chapter is devoted to these two concepts.

PROFESSIONALIZATION OF CORRECTIONAL MEDICINE

The professionalism of correctional medicine has, in recent years, become most evident in the development of academic degree programs, national conferences on correctional health, and a national certification program. Academic degree programs with correc-

tional health emphasis are offered at several universities, providing advanced education to PAs, physicians, and nurses.

Since 1976, a national conference on health care in corrections has been held annually. Currently, three national meetings are held on correctional health care. An annual meeting of the American Correctional Health Care Services Association (ACHSA) is held in the spring of each year, and the NCCHC holds national meetings in the spring and fall. These meetings attract health care professionals from a variety of disciplines and correctional administrators for the purpose of discussing the major administrative and health issues in corrections.

ESSENTIAL ELEMENTS OF A HEALTH CARE PROGRAM IN CORRECTIONS

Medical Services
- A health administrator should be selected and should have responsibility for budgeting, planning, staffing, and supervising health services.
- The health care system should be based on policies and written procedures and protocols.
- Inmates are entitled to a prompt medical history.
- There should be sufficient staff who are appropriately trained to perform health care services.
- Staff should be trained in administration of medication.
- There should be a procedure that allows inmates' health complaints to be triaged by persons appropriately trained.
- Inmates should receive examinations by staff who are trained in physical diagnosis.
- Pharmaceuticals should be used under medical supervision.
- Inmates should be allowed to have access to adequate laboratory and x-ray services.
- Inmates should have complete and adequate medical records.
- Emergency medical care should be available 24 hours a day, 7 days a week.
- Correctional and health staff should have effective and comprehensive in-service training programs.
- The health staff should schedule regular clinic visits.
- The health staff should have a system for monitoring inpatients.
- Medical records should undergo periodic review to determine patient compliance.
- Health care should be performed by qualified, trained workers and not by inmate assistants.
- Health services should undergo internal and external audits for determination of compliance with acceptable professional standards.

Dental Services
- Inmates are entitled to same-day evaluation and treatment of dental emergencies.
- Inmates should have been seen for nonemergency dental treatment within 1 week of a request.
- Dental staff should have a priority system for the orderly treatment of dental patients.
- Health staff should develop a system to track how care is ordered and provided without delay.
- A dental care quality assurance and audit plan should be adopted.

Continued

ESSENTIAL ELEMENTS OF A HEALTH CARE PROGRAM IN CORRECTIONS—cont'd

Mental Health Services
- Inmates are entitled to an evaluation process that adequately screens for mental health treatment needs.
- Mental health treatment is more than segregation and monitoring.
- There should be sufficient mental health staff who are appropriately trained to provide mental health care.
- Correctional officers should be trained in preventive suicide precautions.
- There should be a clearly written policy and an ongoing training program on suicide prevention.

Special Diets
- Inmates are entitled to prescribed therapeutic diets for serious medical problems.
- Confidentiality of Personal Medical Information.
- Inmates are entitled to protected information and nondisclosure of medical records.
- Inmates have a clear protected right, under the Fourteenth Amendment of the United States Constitution, to informed consent for medical treatment and the right to refuse medical care.

Due Process
The Supreme Court also has affirmed the lower court's finding that the following minimum procedures were required before transfer of a prisoner to a mental hospital:
- A prisoner should receive written notice that a transfer to a mental hospital is being considered.
- Prisoners are entitled to a hearing, and after sufficient notice, they should be permitted to prepare and respond to the transfer.
- Prisoners are entitled to an opportunity to be heard in person, to present documentary evidence, to present testimony of witnesses by the defense, and to cross-examine witnesses called by the state.
- Inmates are entitled to an independent decision maker who may act on their behalf.
- Prisoners should receive a written statement as evidence and reasons for transfer.
- Prisoners should have a competent and independent advisor who is free to act solely in the inmate's best interests.
- The process should be effective and timely.[18]

The American Public Health Association has a committee on jail and prison health, which is a part of the medical care section of the APHA national conference. Papers and presentations are offered at all three annual meetings.

A third way that correctional medicine has become further professionalized is through the Certified Correctional Health Professional (CCHP) program offered by NCCHC. This program was initiated in 1990 and is administered by a Board of Trustees that ensures the validity and reliability of the certification program. Peter Ober, PA-C, JD—the AAPA representative to the NCCHC Board of Directors—is the 2002-2003 chairman of the CCHP Board of Trustees.

He observes that the certification program is "an outstanding process that has come to include some of the finest and most professional individuals in correctional health. Their effort to maintain a professional level of care in difficult work environs is always amazing."[18]

The CCHP program provides two levels of certification. The first is a basic certification, which is based on minimal requirements of 3 years of correctional health care experience, three referenced recommendations, and a valid credential or license in one's professional discipline. Upon meeting these requirements, the correctional health professional is sent a self-assessment examination to earn basic certification. The basic certification must be maintained by demonstrating annual participation in continuing education related to correctional health care.

DEVELOPMENT OF THE CODE OF ETHICS

The American Correctional Health Services Association (ACHSA) had its origins in 1975 as an organization of prison health administrators. Today, ACHSA has a multidisciplinary membership of about 1000 correctional health professionals. ACHSA participates on the NCCHC board and is an affiliate of the American Correctional Association (ACA), an organization that primarily represents department of correction officials.

The NCCHC publishes two major publications for correctional health care providers: *CorrectCare* is a quarterly newspaper that deals with timely and important issues in the field. *The Journal of Correctional Health Care* is a peer-reviewed journal that publishes research and scholarly work in the field. This journal is available through subscription, but *CorrectCare* is distributed free upon request. Another publication, *Corhealth,* is ACHSA's bimonthly membership newsletter, which is available only to members.

Because correctional health professionals have addressed issues pertaining to their standards of practice, attention has been drawn to developing a code of ethics for practitioners. Health professionals with

---

AMERICAN CORRECTIONAL HEALTH SERVICES ASSOCIATION CODE OF ETHICS

Preamble
Correctional health professionals are obligated to respect human dignity and act in ways that merit trust and prevent harm. They must ensure autonomy in decisions about their inmate-patients and promote a safe environment.

Principles
Correctional health professionals should:
- Evaluate the inmate as a patient or client in each and every health care encounter.
- Render medical treatment only when it is justified by an accepted medical diagnosis. Treatment and invasive procedures shall be rendered after informed consent.
- Afford inmates the right to refuse care and treatment. Involuntary treatment shall be reserved for emergency situations in which there is grave disability and immediate threat of danger to the inmate or others.
- Provide sound privacy during health services in all cases and sight privacy whenever possible.
- Provide health care to all inmates regardless of custody status.
- Identify themselves to their patients and not represent themselves as other than their professional license or certification permits.
- Collect and analyze specimens only for diagnostic testing based on sound medical principles.
- Perform body cavity searches only after training in proper techniques and when they are not in a patient/provider relationship with the inmate.
- Not be involved in any aspect of execution of the death penalty.
- Ensure that all medical information is confidential and that health care records are maintained and transported in a confidential manner.
- Honor custody functions but not participate in such activities as escorting inmates, forced transfers, security supervision, strip searches, or witnessing use of force.
- Undertake biomedical research on prisoners only when the research methods meet all requirements for experimentation on human subjects and individual prisoners or prison populations are expected to derive benefits from the results of the research.

From American Correctional Health Services Association. http://www.corrections.com/achsa/.

careers in correctional medicine are becoming more aware of their ethical responsibilities to the inmate-patient, to the correctional institution, to the field of correctional health, and to society. In early 1990, ACHSA began work on drafting a code of ethics for health professionals working in corrections. See the Box for the ACHSA Code of Ethics.

The Academy of Correctional Health Professionals (ACHP) is another membership organization that has recently been created, with the mission of creating a professional community for the advancement of correctional health care. The organization promotes professional development through education and information exchange within the correctional health care community, in order to advance the science and ethical practice of correctional health care. The ACHP advocates for improvement in correctional health care by keeping policymakers, the public, and other interested parties informed about health care to the incarcerated.

WHAT ARE THE ETHICAL ISSUES INVOLVED IN CORRECTIONAL HEALTH?

Biomedical ethics for physician assistants has been discussed elsewhere in this text (see Chapter 6). This discussion is focused on the ethical dilemmas in correctional health care. These ethical issues, although not new to correctional health professionals, are new to ethical research and the body of medical-ethical literature. Three tenets are central to all medical-ethical literature:

➤ The provider has an ethical and moral edict to "do no harm."

➤ The provider must be an advocate for the patient's "best interests."

➤ The patient has a right to self-determination in which the patient's preference will prevail.

The unique dilemmas that correctional health care providers face stem from situations in which confidentiality of patient information must be violated because custody staff must be informed of an inmate's specific medical information in order to protect the patient, the staff, or other inmates. Correctional health staff must confront ethical dilemmas when they are asked by security to perform body cavity searches, to collect forensic information, and to assist or pronounce death

at an execution. The unique role of the correctional health care provider is to be the primary care provider for the inmate-patient and not to use this privileged relationship for disciplinary purposes. Ethical dilemmas stem from the fact that the correctional health care provider is a state employee, and the state expects the provider to do what is necessary to maintain the mission of corrections.

Another unique ethical dilemma that the correctional health care provider faces is hunger strikes. Correctional health care providers have a moral and ethical responsibility not to interfere with striking inmates—particularly when the intent of strike is to improve conditions in the prison. Yet the provider also has a responsibility to ensure that no harm comes to his or her patients.

Patient/Provider Relationships

A correctional facility operates on the principle of rank, not equality, and the hierarchy is clear. Correctional staff have status, rights, and privileges over prisoners. The military operational structure, uniforms, and other symbols of authority all serve to control inmates. Choices and decisions are limited and controlled. How, where, and when a prisoner will get medical care are choices that are not made by the prisoner. The ethical dilemma for the correctional health care provider in encouraging patient self-determination, maintaining autonomy, and promoting the patient's "best interest" is that it runs counter to the correctional goal of coercing inmates into obeying the rules and regulations.

In the "free world," the provider/patient relationship is based on mutual trust and respect. The "free world" patient chooses a physician on the basis that the physician will do only what is in the best interest of the patient. In corrections, however, the inmate-patient does not choose the health care provider. The provider is often viewed by patients as a correctional employee, someone who traditionally does not act in the patients' best interest. It is the challenge, and perhaps the distinction, of correctional medicine that the health professional must persuade the inmate-patient that trust, advocacy, and the inmate-patient's best interest will come before corrections. The correctional health care provider is under a greater ethical burden to ensure access to health care for all patients and is faced with a greater challenge not to become co-opted by a hardened "security" attitude.

Privileged Communication

The legal concept of privileged communication protects the patient/doctor relationship. Confidentiality is a cornerstone of the concept of privileged communication. Both are necessary to foster open and honest relationships and are paramount to effective health care delivery. However, the correctional health care provider's duty to public health (e.g., tuberculosis or the acquired immunodeficiency syndrome [AIDS]) and the responsibility to protect staff and inmates from contraband (e.g., drugs or weapons) often conflict with the duty of confidentiality. If the provider acquires information that indicates that a patient may be an immediate danger to self or others, the provider has a greater responsibility to inform the institution's officials.

Preserving confidential communication is difficult in any circumstance, and it is extremely difficult in jails and prisons. After all, an inmate's movement within the institution cannot be kept secret, and any trip to the medical clinic becomes public knowledge. The gossip mill is very active in prisons and has the potential to erode confidence and trust in the institution's health care providers and health care system.

Confidentiality is important not only to the privacy of an inmate, but also as an underpinning for the truthtelling necessary for an adequate history and physical assessment. Histories of drug and alcohol abuse, as well as incidents related to trauma or to sexual attack or behavior, are far more likely to be explained accurately to a provider if the inmate is sure of the privacy of the communication. Inmates' secrets should be protected and guarded.

Informed Choice

Informed consent and the right to refuse care take on different nuances in a correctional setting. The patient's right to an informed choice ensures that particular values and preferences will direct the health care provided. Informed consent is predicated on the fact that the health care provider has given the patient sufficient information about the probable diagnosis; the prognosis for recovery; the risks, benefits, and outcomes of alternative available treatments; and the possible outcome of refusing medical care.

Informed consent and refusal practices inside prisons are more complicated than free world practices. Legally, inmates have a right to consent to medical treatment; however, they do not have an equal right to refuse care.

In one case, the court concluded that an inmate who was refusing dialysis could have his right to refuse care overruled if the administration of the prison would be adversely affected by the inmate's refusal and subsequent death.[19] In another case, inmates refused care on the basis of an allegation that the physician was brutal and sadistic.[20] The inmates claimed to prefer to suffer from their medical conditions rather than endure the physician's deliberately painful care. The court ruled that when an inmate does not appear for scheduled treatment or care, the facility administrators must determine whether the reason is that the symptoms abated, that there was a schedule conflict with another program or a family visit, that the prisoner was prevented from coming, or that some other disincentive to meet medical appointments was operative.

This ruling now applies to correctional medicine in all institutions. The correctional clinic, like its free world counterpart, should record a "no show" in the medical record. Prison officials must, however, determine the exact cause when an inmate fails to appear for treatment, as was described previously. Failure to do so may constitute a denial of care.

Medical Autonomy

The correctional environment presents another dilemma for the health provider—medical autonomy. Medical autonomy is defined as the primacy of professional and medical judgment, without interference from nonmedical personnel. This concept is particularly difficult to uphold in correctional systems, in which the administrative authority controls the budget. Medical autonomy as it relates to patient care, however, is a principle specifically recognized in the standards of both the NCCHC and the ACA. The observance of this ethical tenet is the basis for the delivery of all health care in correctional facilities.

Body Cavity Searches

Correctional health personnel face another ethical dilemma when they are asked to search body orifices for contraband. Because body cavity searches are done solely for custodial purposes, correctional health staff should absolutely refuse to perform them. Some individuals, within and outside of correctional settings, advance the belief that body cavity searches should be conducted by correctional health staff because these staff members:

1. Are more likely to be adept.
2. Are probably more considerate of the inmate's feelings.
3. As correctional employees, have a responsibility to protect the institution from contraband.

However, PAs and other correctional health staff should refuse to perform a body cavity search because to perform one would compromise their neutral role and endanger the patient/provider relationship.

This ethical dilemma is addressed in standards of both the NCCHC and the APHA. The standards state that it is inappropriate and unethical for correctional health staff to perform body cavity searches. It is not unethical for community health care providers, who do not have a direct provider/patient relationship with inmates, to perform a body cavity search. The best approach, however, is to have trained correctional officers perform a body cavity search when it is justified to protect either the inmate or others. For a warranted body cavity search on a prisoner, the AMA has provided very clear guidelines:

➤ The (nonmedical) persons conducting these searches should receive training from a physician or other qualified health care provider regarding how to probe body cavities so that neither injuries to the tissue nor infections from unsanitary conditions result.

➤ Searches of body orifices should not be performed with the use of instruments.

➤ Searches should be conducted in privacy by a person of the same sex as the inmate.[21]

In the final analysis, the question of when such searches are to be conducted is a correctional decision, and determining who should conduct them is a professional decision. Owing to the fact that having medical personnel conduct body searches adversely affects and compromises the ethics of the provider/patient relationship, such correctional health staff should refrain from body cavity searches.

Forensic Information

Health staff face other ethical dilemmas that are unique to the correctional setting. They may be asked to collect forensic information to be used for adversarial or disciplinary proceedings, such as evaluating mental health status for prosecution or execution, drawing blood to determine chemical use or for DNA analysis, and using radiological equipment to discover contraband. Because only medical professionals should carry out these procedures, such requests present a special problem for correctional health staff.

The ethical model requires consistency, and to that end, correctional health staff should refuse to collect forensic information. It would be preferable for security to obtain medical and psychiatric services outside the prison walls for the purpose of gathering biomedical information for legal proceedings. The NCCHC standard on forensic information supports this position. NCCHC recognizes, however, that maintaining such a position is not always practical nor is it always possible, and it does permit correctional health staff to perform "court ordered laboratory tests or radiology procedures . . . with the consent of the inmate."[22] Additionally, NCCHC permits correctional health staff to gather forensic evidence in sexual assault cases if requested to do so by the victim.

Related to the issue of forensic information is DNA blood specimens. DNA is drawn for genetic "fingerprinting," and as such has become admissible evidence. Several states have passed laws requiring convicted sex offenders or felons to be "fingerprinted" via DNA analysis. Correctional health staff are more often being asked to draw these specimens. The NCCHC standard allows correctional health staff to obtain DNA specimens with the consent of the inmate. If an inmate refuses, the collection of blood specimens for DNA analysis should be performed by community health care providers and not by correctional health staff. Protecting the patient/provider relationship is very important for maintaining mutual trust and advancing good clinical care. Correctional health workers must take extra steps to guard their relationship with inmate-patients.

PAs IN CORRECTIONS

PAs will continue to play an integral role in delivering health care to prisoners. PA education will need to address the role that PAs have in corrections, and should consider correctional facilities as sites for student clinical rotations. In fact, many PA programs already have clinical rotations in correctional sites.

The following case studies illustrate the roles of PAs in correctional medicine.

CASE STUDY 39-1

Jim K, PA-C, works at the federal Corrections Institution and federal Prison Camp at Oxford, Wisconsin. The correctional institution is a medium security facility with about 1100 male prisoners, and the minimum security camp has about 150 prisoners. Jim began working at the federal prison as a National Health Service Corps scholarship recipient. The most difficult aspect of his job, he observes, is dealing with the manipulative behavior and secondary gain that inmates attempt. Some of the administrative and security-related duties were also a surprise to him when he first started.

Although a majority of the patients he sees have viral illnesses and musculoskeletal problems, Jim notes that inmates do have serious health problems such as asthma, cardiac failure, and trauma. Jim states that the hardest thing he has to do is to treat trauma patients during evening shifts. For example, when a fight recently broke out between two rival gangs, one prisoner was so severely injured that 31 injury assessments were necessary. Jim recommends working in corrections, but only if the PA has some experience.

CASE STUDY 39-2

Kelly S, PA-C, has been working at the U.S. Penitentiary, Terre Haute, Indiana, for the past 18 months. The facility is a maximum security institution with 1300 male prisoners, 300 of whom are in lock-down status. Kelly's primary duties are to see the daily acute care sick-call patients, see clinic patients returning from consulting doctors, and be available for emergencies. Her typical workweek is 40 hours in length with rotating call once every 2 months. On average, she sees 30 patients a day. She believes that she has seen clinical pathology that she would not have seen in the civilian community, and that she could not have asked for better training. She notes the disadvantages as being that she does not provide pediatric or female care.

Because the patient population is controlled, it is easy to spend the time necessary to research reference textbooks to determine the best course of treatment, and it is easy to follow patients for continuity of care. For this reason, Kelly believes, inmates get some of the very best health care possible.

Initially, she was frightened about working in a prison; however, after receiving "excellent" training in which she learned how to appropriately respond to a variety of difficult situations, her trepidation about working in corrections began to ease. Now, after 18 months on the job, Kelly feels very safe in the correctional environment. In fact, she notes, inmates generally respect and protect health providers and do them no harm because it is the health care workers who provide support, comfort, and dignity to their lives.

CASE STUDY 39-3

Why would a PA want to work in a correctional facility? Ed F, PA-C, has worked at Cermak Health Services at the Cook County Jail in Chicago, Illinois, for 6 years. The jail admits more than 100,000 detainees annually, with about 60% being released within 90 days, and 10,000 inmates in permanent housing. One third of the housing is maximum security. Twelve physicians and nine PAs provide health care services.

Ed observes that his job involves a managed care system, only with very specialized patients. His average day consists of seeing individuals with a lot of pathology, who have not sought medical care or taken care of themselves. His patients are some of the most violent gang members in Chicago. What keeps him there is his interest in providing high quality of care to a difficult patient population and the health care challenges that this presents. Cermak sees one third of the city's syphilis cases and provides service to the largest psychiatric hospital in the Midwest. His patients present with a wide range of problems, such as abuse, chronic illness, trauma, gunshot wounds, and even leprosy.

Cermak Health Services is accredited by the NCCHC and must adhere to standards of care and quality assurance activities. Ed notes that providers must maintain a high level of medical documentation and record keeping to maintain their accredited status.

What is the most difficult part of his job? Because corrections is always the last on the list for funding and bureaucratic attention, Ed finds it difficult to get things done. Dealing with the county bureaucracy makes it difficult sometimes to administer and provide clinical services.

How Many PAs Are Employed in Correctional Medicine?

The American Academy of Physician Assistants Census of 2001 identified approximately 52,000 PAs (28,000 who are non-AAPA members and 24,000 who are AAPA members). It is estimated that approximately 1076 PAs work in correctional institutions (2.9% of nonmembers and 1.1% of members).[23]

This figure does not, however, reflect the number of PAs who provide services to the incarcerated in a local physician's office or hospital emergency department. Such PAs are not counted as correctional PAs because they are not employed directly by a correctional facility. However, many community primary care physicians and PAs have contracts with local jails or prisons to provide health care to inmates. These PAs and physicians often do not see themselves as working in correctional medicine. Nonetheless, the courts have ruled that these providers have no lessening of obligation or responsibility in meeting the standards of care to inmates.

The U.S. Supreme Court settled the issue of liability in 1988.[24] An inmate sued a physician, who was under contract with the state of North Carolina to provide orthopedic services at a state prison hospital, for failing to schedule surgery for an acknowledged and

recommended procedure. The inmate was discharged while his ankle was still swollen and painful. The Supreme Court determined that the private physician's delivery of medical treatment was state action and that he "acted under color of state law" and thus was directly accountable to the state. The Court concluded the liability as follows:

> The fact that the State employed [the doctor] pursuant to a contractual arrangement that did not generate the same benefits or obligations applicable to other state employees does not alter the analysis. It is the physician's function within the state system, not the precise terms of his employment, that determines whether his actions can fairly be attributed to the State. Whether a physician is on the state payroll or is paid by contract, the dispositive issue concerns the relationship among the State, the physician, and the prisoner. Contracting out prison medical care does not relieve the State of its constitutional duty to provide adequate medical treatment to those in its custody, and it does not deprive the State's prisoners of the means to vindicate their Eighth Amendment rights. The State bore an affirmative obligation to provide adequate medical care to [the prisoner]; the State delegated that function to [the private doctor]; and [the private doctor] voluntarily assumed that obligation by contract.[24]

Private practice PAs who treat offenders in their office may not see themselves as correctional health care workers, but their responsibilities to uphold the Eighth Amendment rights of prisoners are not abated.

At one time, PAs interested in correctional medicine organized themselves into the Correctional Health Care Caucus (CHCC) of the American Academy of Physician Assistants (AAPA). Recognized as a caucus in 1997, CHCC serves to "provide a forum for correctional health care PAs to meet, network, and reduce the feeling of isolation due to the high stress, intense environments in which they work (e.g., managing pathological patients and security) and the need to uphold high ethical standards." However, the CHCC has suffered from a lack of leadership and has been placed on inactive status by the AAPA.

There is potential for PAs in correctional health administration, health delivery, and policymaking. Growth is also seen in city and state facilities as more managed care organizations get into this billion dollar industry. Although the CHCC is inactive today, it may be resurrected when more PAs become involved in correctional medicine.

What Are the Public Health Issues?

Correctional medicine is at the vanguard of many of the public health threats and has great potential for PAs who want to specialize in public health medicine. Many people believe that the only public health care being delivered in the United States is in correctional settings. The reduction of public health care funding and community resources, coupled with the fact that corrections is federally mandated to provide health care, makes jail or prison the only place that many of the indigent get health care. As was previously mentioned, it is widely recognized that correctional medicine is the first—and perhaps only—contact with health care for many patients.

A recent report on the "Health Status of Soon-to-Be-Released Inmates" demonstrates that improving the health care of inmates can also benefit public health in two important ways.[25] First, the community's health is improved when the transmission of communicable diseases from inmates who are released with untreated conditions is reduced. The implementation of disease prevention programs in jails and prisons is an important step toward diminishing the rate of communicable disease in the non-incarcerated community. Second, the public financial burden is reduced when jails treat inmates before their release. Inmates who return to the community with undiagnosed or untreated communicable disease, chronic disease, and mental illness continue to drain on public health resources. Treating them in a closed environment and releasing them into the community healthier than before is a better use of public health dollars.

There is another important advantage to reaching this population while it is still incarcerated. It has been consistently demonstrated in the literature that inmates have high rates of co-infection with multiple diseases.[25] Because the incarcerated have a high rate of drug abuse, and because substance abusers are at very high risk for human immunodeficiency virus (HIV)/acquired immunodeficiency syndrome (AIDS),

sexually transmitted diseases, hepatitis B and C, tuberculosis (TB), and chronic diseases, the rate of co-infection among prisoners is extremely high. It only makes sense, from a clinical perspective, that treating existing conditions can prevent other diseases from developing.

AIDS, TB, hepatitis B and C, substance abuse, and mental illness are a few of the major health threats that a PA will encounter in correctional medicine. This section briefly presents the status and issues of these public health threats in corrections.

AIDS   AIDS in prisons, jails, and juvenile confinement centers is a major health concern. Of the estimated 229,000 persons living with AIDS in the United States in 1996, 17% passed through a correctional facility that year.[25] The prevalence of AIDS among inmates is six times higher than the prevalence among the total population in the United States.[26] The AIDS epidemic has produced many perplexing legal, ethical, and medical controversies. Decisions over AIDS testing, as well as treatment, housing, and therapeutic clinical trials for HIV-positive prisoners, have generated recent case law.

The courts have sent confusing messages by upholding the practice of mandatory HIV testing and the refusal to conduct mandatory HIV testing.[27-30] The NCCHC position protects the rights of the individual patient and suggests that correctional institutions should avoid mandatory testing and encourage inmates with risk factors to agree to be tested.[31] NCCHC also supports the concepts of providing educational programming to help inmates avoid acquiring and transmitting HIV/AIDS, and offering appropriate standard of care treatment to all inmates with HIV infection.[32]

A recent development in the field of correctional health care has been the creation of clinical guidelines for correctional health care providers.[32] Using existing evidence-based medicine to ensure that the latest developments in clinical care were incorporated, the NCCHC developed guidelines that "encourage total disease management, which requires clear indicators of the severity of the patient's condition and whether the condition is stable, improving or deteriorating."[32] As of July of 2002, the NCCHC had written clinical guidelines for asthma, diabetes mellitus, epilepsy, high blood cholesterol, high blood pressure, and HIV. These guidelines are unique because they alert the health clinician to commonly found barriers in correctional facilities that hinder appropriate treatment and care. The guidelines can be extremely helpful to PAs and other clinicians who are new to correctional medicine.

A petition for services by a hypertensive inmate denied enrollment in a prison boot camp was heard by the Court in *Pennsylvania Department of Corrections v. Yeskey* (1998).[33] The Court ruled that correctional institutions are not exempt from the provisions of the Americans with Disabilities Act (ADA) and must make reasonable accommodations for disabled inmates. Moreover, in other rulings, the Court has stated that HIV-related discrimination is prohibited under the ADA. As a result of these rulings, coupled with improved highly active antiretroviral treatment (HAART), treatment and care of HIV cases in prisons and jails have improved and the number of prison deaths related to AIDS has steadily declined every year since 1995.[34]

Research in correctional settings has had an onerous past. Abuses have been documented in which prisoners were tested for new vaccines, chemotherapeutic agents, or cosmetics without consent or with consent that was obtained under coercion. In 1976, the problem of research on prisoners was addressed by the National Commission for the Protection of Human Subjects of Biomedical and Behavioral Research. The Commission concluded that strict and prohibitive conditions should be applied to research in prisons and jails. In 1981, a federal law was passed stipulating that research in prisons and jails is restricted to behavioral (e.g., study of the cause and effect of criminal behavior and incarceration) or organizational (e.g., study of the correctional system and its effect on the incarcerated), conditions affecting prisoners as a class (e.g., hepatitis, alcoholism, drug addiction, and sexual perversions), and practices that could improve the health or well-being of the subject (e.g., AIDS clinical trials). Research protocols approved by an institutional review board may proceed only after the Secretary of the U.S. Department of Health and Human Services has approved the research.

Increasingly, HIV-infected inmates are asking to participate in therapeutic clinical trials. Many state departments of corrections preclude inmates from participating in clinical trials because of the restrictive federal regulations or because correctional administrators are reacting to the past abuses of prisoner research and wish to avoid negative publicity. Many professionals in correctional health argue that the opportunity for inmates to access AIDS therapeutic clinical trials should be allowed; it is only a matter of time before there is litigation over this issue.

One final note on AIDS in corrections. There is a general perception that people are contracting AIDS in prison. In reality, the transmission of HIV in correctional institutions has not been corroborated by the literature,[25] and there have been no recorded incidents of a health care worker contracting AIDS while employed in a correctional facility.

Tuberculosis TB is a health problem in correctional institutions. Prisons and jails are environments that are conducive to the spread of air-borne infection among inmates, staff, and visitors. In 1997, more than 130,000 inmates tested positive for latent TB infection; because the jail population includes repeat offenders, an estimated 566,000 inmates with latent TB infection entered and were released from jails in 1996.[25] In 1996, an estimated 35% (12,200) of all people with active TB served time in a correctional facility. The NCCHC estimates that the prevalence of active TB among inmates is between 4 and 17 times greater than the rate among the total U.S. TB population.[25] TB outbreaks in California and South Carolina prisons have been reported and further illustrate how serious the problem is. For example, in 1999, a cohort of 323 men who had been in one South Carolina prison dormitory building from 1 to 152 days during 1999-2000 were followed and given tuberculin skin testing (TST) throughout the year. As of November of 2000, 31 current or former inmates, and one medical student, had contracted TB.

What can correctional institutions do to halt the spread of TB? The single most important step is to contain or isolate TB-positive inmates in order to reduce the spread of TB.[35] Jails and prisons can implement comprehensive quality improvement activities that monitor the screening and containment efforts of jail and prison personnel, which is an important component of TB reduction. Correctional institutions can collaborate with public health departments to ensure that prevention and control measures are instituted and can improve upon their TB information systems and process of assessment.

Hepatitis Hepatitis B and C are evolving to become major health issues in corrections. "Based on the estimated 155,000 inmates released with current or chronic hepatitis B infection in 1996, between 12% and 15% of all individuals in the country with chronic or current hepatitis B infection in 1996 spent time in a correctional facility that year."[25] The prevalence of hepatitis C in prisons and jails is even more alarming. The NCCHC estimates that, "1.3 to 1.4 million releasees infected with hepatitis C infection in 1997 suggests that an extremely high 29% to 32% of the estimated 4.5 million people infected with hepatitis C in the United States served time in a correctional facility that year. The 17.0% to 18.6% prevalence range of hepatitis C among inmates—probably an underestimate—is 9 to 10 times higher than the estimated hepatitis C prevalence in the nation's population as whole."[25]

Corrections provides an opportunity for PAs to be directly involved in the public health of the country. By supporting policies that routinely vaccinate all inmates, or susceptible inmates, against hepatitis B; by offering educational sessions to correctional officers and inmates; and by promoting and presenting strategies to avoid the transmission of disease, correctional PAs make a valuable contribution to public health initiatives in this country.

Other Areas Other areas of major concern and opportunity in corrections are substance abuse, health care for youth, and mental illness. PAs wanting to concentrate their clinical experience in these areas could find opportunities in corrections.

There is significant alcohol and drug abuse in this country. "It is estimated that 1 out of 7 people in the U.S. abuse or are dependent on alcohol and that an additional 1 out of 20 individuals abuse or are dependent on other drugs."[36] In fact, substance abuse

accounts for a good portion of the crime-related activity in the United States. The Bureau of Justice Statistics reports reveal that more than "75% of jail inmates had used illegal drugs at some time and that 13% had committed their crimes to get money for drugs."[37]

In 1989, the average daily population of all youth incarcerated in the United States was 1891, and in 1990, it was 2140—a 13.2% increase in this custody class.[38] In 1997, 2.8 million U.S. juveniles were arrested by law enforcement agencies; however, only a small percentage (4.4) of these arrests were for violent crime such as murder, forcible rape, robbery, or aggravated assault.[39] This means that many nonviolent youth are being processed into the juvenile and criminal justice systems who require appropriate adolescent care. The medical and mental health needs of the incarcerated juvenile are great. First contact with a health care provider, for many detained juveniles, comes when they are initially incarcerated.

Mental illness, once treated in psychiatric hospitals and community health centers, is now being treated in our jails and prisons. "Researchers have documented that the prevalence of severe mental disorders is significantly higher in jails than in the general population."[25,40] Future opportunities for PAs in corrections are abundant.

CONCLUSION

The United States continues to incarcerate offenders at unprecedented rates. Owing to mandatory, fixed, and longer sentencing, and to the wars on crime and drugs, overcrowding in our nation's jails and prisons has become the major issue confronting the future of corrections.

With the development of standards, case law, professional organizations, codes of ethics, and national certification, one would expect improvement in the correctional health care system. Although there has been vast improvement since the 1970s, there are still considerable problems with prisons, jails, and juvenile detention centers in terms of how they are funded and managed.[41] Unfortunately, competition for the corrections budget is extremely tight and, because health care programs are supportive of the custody mission, many program dollars are redirected to custodial operations.

The poor health habits of the incarcerated, such as substance abuse, smoking, and sedentary lifestyles, have put them at high risk for AIDS, TB, diabetes, heart disease, hypertension, and sexually transmitted diseases. Inmates also have a high incidence of mental illness or mental retardation as well. As a result, prisoners are staying longer, getting older, and becoming sicker. The correctional health profession will have to confront and help solve the issue of long-term care and the terminally ill. B. J. Anno observes, "As we move toward the twenty-first century, it is appropriate for those of us in the field of correctional medicine to embrace the challenge and goals of *Healthy People 2000*. We need to advocate for the inclusion of 'the least of us' in the nation's broad health care mission to increase the span of healthy life for Americans, reduce health disparities among Americans, and achieve access to preventive services for all Americans. Other groups may be more deserving of adequate health care than inmates, but few are more needy."[4]

The future of correctional medicine depends on how well its professionals can focus on preventive health care, reduce costs, demonstrate high quality, and gather information that may influence change for their patients. With these goals, the PA can have an important and rewarding public health career in correctional medicine.

CLINICAL APPLICATIONS

1. If you were considering a position in correctional medicine, how would you determine whether you would prefer to work in a local, state, or federal facility? What clinical skills would you need to acquire or review for a position in correctional medicine?

2. If you worked in correctional medicine, what do you think you would find rewarding and challenging?

3. Describe how the role of PAs in correctional medicine involves the public health arena.

REFERENCES

1. U.S. Department of Justice, Bureau of Justice Statistics. Available at http://www.ojp.usdoj.gov/bjs/abstract/pp99pr.htm.

2. Medicine behind bars: hostility, horror and the Hippocratic oath. Med World News 1971;12:26.

3. Bureau of Prisons. Available at http://www.bop.gov/fact1297.html. Accessed 3 March, 1998.

4. Anno BJ. Correctional Health Care: Guidelines for the Management of an Adequate Delivery System. Washington, DC: U.S. Department of Justice, 2001.

5. Bottoms AE. Interpersonal violence and social order in prisons. In: Tonry M, Petersilia J (eds). Prisons. Chicago: The University of Chicago Press, 1999.

6. Beck AJ, Karberg JC, Harrison PM. Prison and Jail Inmates at Midyear 2001. Washington, DC: U.S. Department of Justice, April 2002 (NCJ 191702).

7. Litman TJ, Robins LS (eds). Health Politics and Policy. New York: Wiley, 1984.

8. Law Enforcement Assistance Administration. Local Jails: A Report Presenting Data for Individual County and City Jails from the 1970 National Jail Census. Washington, DC: U.S. Government Printing Office, 1974.

9. Law Enforcement Assistance Administration. Survey of Inmates of Local Jails 1972: Advance Report. Washington, DC: U.S. Government Printing Office, 1974.

10. Law Enforcement Assistance Administration: The Nation's Jails, Washington, DC: U.S. Government Printing Office, 1975.

11. Mullen J, Smith B. In: American Prisons and Jails, Volume I: Summary of Findings and Policy Implications of a National Survey. Washington, DC: National Institute of Justice, 1980:61.

12. *Newman v. Alabama*, 349 F. Supp. 285 (MD Ala 1972); *aff'd*, 503 F.2d 1320 (5th Cir. 1974); *cert. denied*, 421 U.S. 948 (1975).

13. Menninger K. The Crime of Punishment. New York: Viking, 1969.

14. Inmates' Legal Rights. Washington, DC: National Sheriffs' Association, 1974.

15. National Prison Project. Status Report: State Prisons and the Courts. J Natl Prison Proj 1990;22:7.

16. *Estelle v. Gamble*, 429 U.S. 103, 97 S. Ct. at 290 (1976).

17. *Estelle v. Gamble*, 429 U.S. 104-105, 97 S. Ct. at 291 (1976).

18. Peter Ober, personal communication, July 11, 2002.

19. *Vitek v. Jones*, 445 U.S. 494-500, 100 S. Ct. at 1264-1268 (1980).

20. *Commissioner of Correction v. Myers*, 399 NE 2d 452 (Mass 1979).

21. *White v. Napoleon*, 897 F2d 103 (3d Cir 1990).

22. American Medical Association. Report E.E. of the Board of Trustees. Searches of Body Orifices. Chicago: AMA, 1980.

23. AAPA 2001 Physician Assistant Census, personal communication with Kevin Marvel, Vice President of Data Services and Analysis. AAPA, July 11, 2002.

24. *West v. Atkins*, 487 U.S. 42, 108 S. Ct. 2250 (1989).

25. National Commission on Correctional Health Care, Report to Congress. The Health Status of Soon-to-Be-Released Inmates. Chicago: Author, 2002.

26. Centers for Disease Control and Prevention. HIV/AIDS Surveillance Report, 1997. Atlanta, GA: U.S. Department of Health and Human Services, 1997.

27. Dean-Gaitor HD, Fleming PL. Epidemiology of AIDS in incarcerated persons in the United States, 1994-1996. AIDS 1999;13:2429.

28. *Dunn v. White,* 880 F2d 1188 (10th Cir 1989).

29. *Glick v. Henderson,* 855 F2d 536 (8th Cir 1988).

30. *Harris v. Thigpen,* 727 F. Supp. 1564 (M.D. Ala. 1990).

31. National Commission on Correctional Health Care. Position Statement on the Administrative Management of HIV in Corrections. Available at http://www.ncchc.org/links/hiv.html. Accessed 2002.

32. NCCHC's Clinical Guidelines. Available at http://www.ncchc.org/.

33. *Pennsylvania Department of Corrections v. Yeskey,* 524 U.S. 206 (1998).

34. Maruschak, LM. HIV in Prisons and Jails, 1999. Bureau of Justice Statistics Bulletin, July 2000. Available at www.ojp.usdoj.gov/bjs/pub.

35. Abt Associates. An Evaluation of TB Prevention and Control Measures in Large City and County Jails. Draft Report Prepared for the National Center for HIV, STD, and TB prevention. CDC Draft Report Contract Number 282-98-0006, April 23, 2002.

36. Group for the Advancement of Psychiatry, Committee on Alcoholism and the Addictions. Substance abuse disorders: a psychiatric priority. Am J Psychiatry 1991;148:10, 1291.

37. Drugs and Jail Inmates. Washington, DC: Bureau of Jail Statistics Special Report, 1989.

38. Jail Inmates, 1990. Washington, DC: Bureau of Jail Statistics Bulletin, 1990.

39. U.S. Department of Justice, Federal Bureau of Investigation. Crime in the United States, 1997. Uniform Crime Reports. Washington, DC: U.S. Department of Justice, 1998.

40. Abram T. Co-occurring disorders among mentally ill jail detainees. Am J Psychol 1991;104:1036.

41. U.S. Department of Justice, Civil Rights Division, Special Litigation Section. Jails and Prisons Investigations. Available at http://www.usdoj.gov/crt/split/findsettle.htm.

RESOURCES

Anno BJ. Correctional Health Care: Guidelines for the Management of an Adequate Delivery System. Washington, DC: U.S. Department of Justice, 2001. *Anno provides a comprehensive review of the history of correctional health care, as well as the current medical and legal issues related to the delivery of health care in correctional facilities.*

Journal of Correctional Health Care. Published by the National Commission on Correctional Health Care, Chicago. *This peer-reviewed journal, published semiannually, contains articles related to research and analysis in correctional health care.*

CorrectCare. Published by the National Commission on Correctional Health Care, Chicago. *This quarterly newspaper includes articles on timely topics and newsworthy developments in correctional health care. It also includes conference listings and employment opportunities.*

Academy of Correctional Health Care Professionals, P.O. Box 11117, Chicago, IL 60611, 877-549-2247. Web site: http://www.correctionalhealth.org. *The Academy of Correctional Health Care Professionals is an organization for correctional health care professionals. Through publications, educational activities, and special events, the Academy provides professional leadership in the field.*

American Correctional Health Services Association, P.O. Box 10, Glenn Dale, MD 20769, 877-918-1842 (Voice—Toll-free), 301-918-1842 (Voice). Web site: http://www.corrections.com/achsa. *ACHSA provides support, skill development, and educational programs for health care personnel, organizations, and decision makers involved in correctional health care.*

Certified Correctional Health Professional, 1300 W. Belmont Ave., Chicago, IL 60657, 773-880-1460. *This organization certifies individuals for their knowledge of the minimum standards of care in prisons, jails, and juvenile detention centers. Individuals successfully completing the examination become CCHPs. Regional workshops and conferences are held for CCHPs to maintain their knowledge base. CCHPs meet annually at the NCCHC's conference.*

C H A P T E R   4 0

*Occupational and Environmental Medicine**

Maryann Ramos

INTRODUCTION

Occupational and environmental medicine is a clinical specialty that addresses worksite and environmental concerns and such community health and policy issues as atmospheric pollution, product safety, health promotion, and benefits values management. Environmental medicine has been defined as the branch of medical science that addresses the impact of chemical and physical stressors on individuals and groups. Both occupational and environmental medicine use

similar skills and focus on the recognition and prevention of hazardous exposures.[1]

Physician assistants (PAs) deliver health services in the workplace by extending the occupational and environmental physician, just as is done with other medical specialties. One occupational medicine reference states that PAs are "well trained to do general physical examinations and because of this are excellent for doing preplacement examinations for any type of job in which such an examination is not restricted to a physician by government mandate."[2] Another reference states, "Physician assistants can provide many clinical and non-clinical services at significantly lower cost. The quality of care has repeatedly been demonstrated to be comparable to

---

*The views expressed in this chapter are the personal views of the author, not necessarily those of the Department of Defense, the DiLorenzo Tricare Health Clinic, or the Pentagon Civilian Employees' Health Service.

traditional services and often with evidence of better patient empathy on the part of the allied health providers."[3]

Occupational and environmental medicine is a combination of disciplines that encompass hazard exposure prevention from chemical, physical, biological, or psychological threats in the workplace community. Occupational medicine clinicians treat and help prevent maladies caused by chemical exposure. Examples of work-related illnesses from toxic chemicals include lethargy, forgetfulness, and upper extremity tremors caused by lead poisoning in battery makers, as well as bladder cancer in benzidine dye workers. Biologically induced exposures include hepatitis B in those exposed to blood, byssinosis in cotton workers, and poison ivy (*Rhus*) contact dermatitis in utility workers. Examples of physically induced illnesses are carpal tunnel syndrome in typists and occupational hearing loss in factory workers. Post-traumatic stress syndrome incurred during military service is an example of a psychologically induced workplace illness.[4]

Settings in which occupational and environmental health is practiced may include the employee health service of a hospital, a clinic in a production plant or mine, or the corporate medical director's office. PAs administer services in occupational health settings by performing annual physical examinations required by the Occupational Safety and Health Act, screening employees for environmental exposures such as lead or mercury, or giving medical advice to employees preparing for business travel to other countries.

HISTORY OF OCCUPATIONAL MEDICINE

Medical care in the workplace dates back to ancient history. The Egyptian, Imhotep, made the connection between work and illness in 2980 BC. In about 350 BC, Hippocrates, the father of medicine, admonished followers to observe the environment of their patients. Luke, an apostle of Christ, later noted the same connection. Agricola and Paracelsus studied the effects of gold and mercury on certain workers in the 1500s.

Bernardino Ramazzini is considered the father of occupational medicine. His book *Diseases of Tradesmen* was published in 1713. This work gave us profound insight into occupation-related illnesses.

Dr. Ramazzini was a physician who stressed the importance of a person's ability to work without the hindrance of a disease that makes labor a curse rather than a pleasure. He described the diseases of metal diggers, painters, midwives, glass makers, potters, sewer workers, those who inhaled noxious gas, and those who held their bodies in improper postures while they worked. He amended Hippocrates' list of medical history questions by adding one about the patient's occupation.

The following is taken from *Diseases of Tradesmen:*

> The arts that men practice are various and diverse and from them may arise various diseases. Accordingly, I have tried to unearth in the shops of craftsmen, for these shops are schools whence one can depart with more precise knowledge, whatever may appeal to the taste of investigators, and, which is the main thing, to suggest medical precautions for the prevention and treatment of such diseases as usually affect the workers...a doctor...should...question ...carefully, What occupation does he follow?[5]

It became clear to London physicians John Hill and Percival Pott that illness was related to habits or work exposure, especially occupationally or environmentally caused cancer. In 1761, Dr. Hill described the elevated prevalence of cancer of the nasal passages among tobacco snuff abusers. In 1775, Dr. Pott perceptively reported the first occupational cancer—an increased prevalence of scrotal cancer among chimney sweeps heavily exposed to soot in their work. Dr. Pott also described tuberculosis of the bone, a condition that bears his name.

Other types of skin cancer were noted in the 1800s to be linked to occupational exposure to inorganic arsenic and to tar and paraffin oils containing polycyclic aromatic hydrocarbons. In the same era, an association between bladder cancer and occupational exposure to certain dyes was made. Not until 1935 was the first case report of bronchogenic carcinoma in a patient with asbestos exposure published. Some types of cancer occurring in the 1930s, such as that among radium watch dial painters, who routinely licked their radium-tipped brushes to obtain a fine point, had not yet reached the public eye.[6]

LABOR ORGANIZATIONS' CONTRIBUTION

In the United States, during the Industrial Revolution, labor organizations' concerns brought safety problems to the forefront. Massachusetts created the first factory inspection department in the country in 1867, and enacted the first job safety law, requiring metal guards on textile spinning machinery. In the 1870s and 1880s, the Knights of Labor, the leading labor organization, demanded "the adoption of measures providing for the health and safety of those engaged in mining and manufacturing, building industries, and for indemnification . . . for injuries." The U.S. Bureau of Labor was created in 1888. In 1910, the Labor Commissioner led an investigation of the match industry in the first major public act to control occupational disease.

In Great Britain, during the same period, a centralized system of factory inspection was established in 1878. Sir Thomas Morison Legge became the first Medical Inspector of Factories in 1898. Legge wrote *Lead Poisoning and Lead Absorption* with K.W. Goadby in 1912, and also described the entities of anthrax, glassblowers' cataract, work-related skin cancer, toxic jaundice, and poisoning by phosphorus, arsenic, and mercury. He lectured extensively in many hospitals where he stressed the need to educate medical students about occupational diseases. Legge was knighted for his work in 1925.

Alice Hamilton was the first American physician to devote a lifetime to occupational medicine. She was the first woman professor at Harvard Medical School, and she made great contributions to the cause of preventing workplace injury and illness. She wrote her first article concerning workplace safety in 1907, urging Americans to join "every civilized country" in making workers immune from the "sacrifice of life and health."[4] Hamilton went on to write *Industrial Poisons in the United States* in 1925, *Industrial Toxicology* in 1934 (5th edition 1998, edited by R.D. Harbison), and *Exploring the Dangerous Trades* in 1943. She studied the problems of lead poisoning and, working with the American Association for Labor Legislation, helped reduce that disease among bathtub enamellers in 1906. Her recommendations concerning matchmakers' phossy jaw, which led to jaw bone breakdown, led to substitution

of dangerous white phosphorus with safer phosphorous sesquisulfide in "strike-anywhere" matches. The U.S. Bureau of Labor published a document based on her work, prompting passage of the White Phosphorus Match Act, which prohibited the export and import of matches made of white phosphorus. This was one of the most effective reforms and is an excellent example of substitution of a safe component for one that caused unnecessary disease and death. Hamilton later studied the effects of carbon monoxide in steelworkers, carbon disulfide–causing neurological disease in the viscose rayon industry, and mercury in hat makers.[7]

LEGISLATION

The real burst of activity and concern for occupational health and safety as well as accompanying legislation began after 1900, once the modern industrial economy gained full steam and labor became more of a political force.[7]

By 1900, most states had enacted minimal legislation dealing with employment hazards. More than 200 publications concerning occupational disease appeared before that year.

Implementation of the Workers' Compensation system was a very important step in the health care of workers. Workers' Compensation is a government-driven no-fault system that enables employees to receive benefits for medical care and lost wages incurred through work-related injury and illness. Before enactment of Workers' Compensation, common law governed. An employee who was injured had to prove negligence on the part of his or her employee to recover damages. In addition, three common law defenses known as contributory negligence, assumption of risk, and the fellow servant rule had to be overcome as well. The result was a time-consuming, uncertain process that was expensive to worker and employer. The no-fault system eliminated the need to prove negligence and permitted the employee to receive benefits more easily, but it set limits on the benefits granted.[8]

Workers' Compensation was first enacted in Germany in the late 1800s. Around 1900, Great Britain adopted its own Workers' Compensation laws. In 1911, Wisconsin enacted the first U.S. Workers'

Compensation law based on the British concept of a no-fault system of benefits provided to most workers who had incurred work-related injury. Then, other American states began to enact Workers' Compensation laws. New York's law was at first declared unconstitutional and then was passed. By 1948, all states had Workers' Compensation legislation.

In 1913, the National Safety Council was organized and began its "safety first" educational program. In 1914, the U.S. Public Health Service established the Office of Industrial Hygiene and Sanitation for research in occupational health. This agency was the forerunner of the National Institute for Occupational Safety and Health (NIOSH).[5]

In 1936, the Walsh-Healey Public Contracts Act was passed requiring compliance with health and safety standards by employers receiving federal contracts over $10,000. Shortly thereafter, the federal government provided funds to states for industrial health and safety programs, and the Bureau of Mines was authorized to inspect and investigate mine hazards. The Atomic Energy Act was passed in 1954, establishing radiation safety standards. The Nuclear Regulatory Commission currently provides oversight of these standards.

Enforcement of these laws was sketchy, and those with occupational disease rarely received compensation for work-related disabilities because of the difficulty in proving causal effect and the lack of exposure data. In addition, the role of toxins ingested, inhaled, or absorbed through a person's skin, and those that may accumulate outside a workplace, may confuse the picture of workplace exposures. This is sometimes called a confounding variable. These confounders also make the diagnosis of occupational cancer for a cigarette-smoking worker exposed to a workplace lung toxin quite difficult. In addition, increased pollution of the working environment and a concurrent 29% increase in industrial accident rates raised more doubts about the reliability of workplace exposure data.

The death of 78 miners in a 1968 coal mine explosion in Farmington, West Virginia, paved the way for the 1969 Coal Mine Health and Safety Act. In 1970, the Federal Occupational Safety and Health Act was passed. In 1972, the Black Lung Benefits Act was passed. The Toxic Substances Control Act (TOSCA) became law in 1976. TOSCA provided for extensive restriction of the hazards of the chemical industry.

The Occupational Safety and Health Act, commonly called OSHA, has as its core the general duty clause, which holds that businesses, with the exception of railroads, mining, and weapons manufacturing industries, must promote a safe and healthy workplace. All but the smallest workplaces such as domestic sites are covered under this overarching piece of legislation. The intent of the legislation is to control risk by setting specific safety and hygiene standards, enforceable by inspectors who respond to complaints from workers (whistleblowers) or after a major disaster such as workplace death.[8]

OSHA introduced a new Cooperative Compliance Program in 1996, a strategic, "data-driven" initiative specifically aimed at reducing workplace injuries and illnesses. The first and foremost requirement for an on-site inspection is that the motivation for an investigation be driven by site-specific data. This gives OSHA the ability to target establishments with high rates of injury or illnesses based on actual data from that worksite. There is an emphasis on cooperation between company management and OSHA to bring a preventable workplace problem to its swiftest conclusion.[9]

An addition to OSHA, the Occupational Exposure to Bloodborne Pathogens Act was passed in 1992. This initiative was aimed at preventing transmission of hepatitis B virus and human immunodeficiency virus (HIV) in the workplace, and at preventing more than 200 deaths per year from hepatitis alone. Those with potential exposure to blood or body fluids must receive training, and employers must make provisions for environmental controls such as hand washing facilities, hepatitis B vaccine, and protective equipment for the health care worker.[10]

DELIVERY OF OCCUPATIONAL HEALTH SERVICES

The national rate of nonfatal occupational injuries and illnesses in private industry in 1996 was 6.2 million, according to the U.S. Bureau of Labor Statistics. The resulting rate is 7.4 cases for every 100 full-time workers. Although the number of injuries and illnesses requiring recuperation away from work declined for all occupations by about 20% from 1992 to 1996, injuries and illnesses for truck drivers increased by nearly 5%. Between 1992 and 1996, fatal occupational injuries decreased from 6217 to 6112 fatalities. Highway traffic accidents and homicides led the job-related fatalities in 1996. These two causes amounted to 37% of worker fatalities. Highway accidents are increasing, with 22% of fatal occupational injuries due to motor vehicle accidents, the majority occurring while victims were driving or riding in a truck.[11-13] Homicide continues to be a leading cause of job-related deaths, accounting for 912 deaths or 15% of fatal work injuries in 1996, with robbery the primary motive for deaths. Falls accounted for 11% of fatal work injuries, 20% of those due to falling from or through roofs.[14]

Comprehensive knowledge is required to act on these statistics, provide preventive strategies and worker education, and treat the worker. However, primary care practitioners deliver most of the care to patients who are injured or become ill at work. Performing job preplacement or return-to-work examinations, deciding whether a toxic exposure at work is causing an illness, and filing Workers' Compensation forms are all common duties of occupational and environmental medicine. Knowledge of work processes and the work environment, harm related to toxic exposures, and the OSHA Act all help the practitioner deliver the best care. The work-relatedness of disease may be missed in the absence of a suspicion linking the health problem to the workplace. In addition to workplace hazards, specific maladies such as occupational asthma, cumulative trauma disorder, and the depression of "downsized or surplus" workers are of concern.[15] Other concerns for health delivery to employees include patient/physician confidentiality, the Americans with Disabilities Act, and screening for substances of abuse. Safeguarding patient confidentiality involving how issues of safety and management are served is a fine line that may easily be overlooked without oversight by an experienced practitioner. Since the advent of the Americans with Disabilities Act in 1992, pre-employment examination before a job offer is no longer performed. Instead, a preplacement examination is done without

relationship to the initial hiring decision; it focuses on a specific set of essential job tasks, including advocating for reasonable accommodations. Employment decisions remain in the sphere of the personnel manager, medical recommendation nothwithstanding.[16] Another important medical legal concern involves testing for substances of abuse. Some 7 million interstate truckers and commercial drivers must be tested biannually for general health fitness to operate a vehicle and to ensure they are free from substances of abuse. Collection agents must be trained to conform to legal standards for evidence gathering. Collection must follow strict standards that include specimen labeling, donor signature, tamper-proof packaging, and special handling.[15]

In addition to caring for a work-related wound, referring for specialty evaluation may be warranted. Two examples include a metal-containing foreign body in the eye and tendon lacerations. A foreign body containing iron might prudently be referred to an ophthalmologist because of possible complications. Hand surgeons might best be consulted if a tendon laceration is suspected.

In general, follow-up and interaction with managers should be done following an occupational injury, with discussion that may center on fitness for return to work, as well as the availability of a light duty assignment. Other uniquely employee-related problems that may need intervention include work hardening or help in tracking Workers' Compensation benefits.

An entry must be made in the OSHA log whenever a death occurs on the job. In addition, entries are made when an illness or an injury is job-related and results in a specified amount of lost time, or when the patient receives prescription medication. This log is a tracking device used by OSHA to evaluate the safety of the industrial workplace. It should be notated in the case of a minor work-related injury that requires only first aid treatment; no entry on an OSHA log is necessary.

Confidentiality must be maintained between the patient-worker and the manager. The employer needs to know only whether the employee is medically able to return to work. If there is a period of recuperation, an estimate of the length of that period is made, with a clinical follow-up date, if necessary. Unless there is danger to the employee or others, the employer need not be told the exact nature of the illness. Information management at times may demand information that would violate patient confidentiality. However, the practitioner must refrain from divulging confidential medical information when that information is not needed to make an administrative decision. To maintain the employee's confidence as well as to uphold the law, worker privacy must not be compromised.[17]

DUTIES IN OCCUPATIONAL MEDICINE

PA involvement in occupational medicine escalated in 1978, when noted business and union leaders, responding to cost containment in industry, recommended the use of PAs in the workplace as extenders of physician services.[18] Duties that were assigned to PAs consisted of annual employee physical examinations, some form of exercise stress testing, occupational health education, and treatment of work-related injuries.[19] Many worker injuries involve common strains and sprains and extremity injuries such as uncomplicated lacerations. The primary care training of PAs makes them well suited for entry-level delivery of workplace care.[2,3]

Traditionally, the physician assistant has provided general care in underserved areas. The same holds true in occupational and environmental medicine. It has been the practice to use PAs at dangerous workplaces that need medical care delivery on-site. These sites may be industrial and may employ fewer than 400 people; they may be in remote locations, such as on oil drilling rigs in the ocean. Similarly, PAs have successfully provided health care during construction of the Alaskan pipeline. In most cases, the PA was the only health care professional on-site, with a supervising physician accessible only by telephone and helicopter.[20] In 1973, some 150 PAs were stationed along the 800-mile pipeline at 37 sites and provided most of the hands-on medical coverage with backup telephone supervision supplied by physicians. Many times, the cold climate prevented emergency evacuation via planes and helicopters.[21]

Besides histories and physical examinations, the duties of the PA may include health promotion, emergency care, counseling, safety assessments, environ-mental hazards identification, record keeping, and evaluation of worker rehabilitation, disability leave, and ability to return to work. Responsibilities may also include referring employees to community health resources, performing OSHA medical surveillance for specialized monitoring (hearing conservation, asbestos exposure tracking, respirator medical clearance), and implementing strategies directed to employer needs and organizational goals.[22]

The job descriptions in Tables 40-1 to 40-3 provide specific job duties for occupational medicine PAs. Table 34-1 describes an administrative, policy-making position; Table 40-2 describes a hospital-based employee health care position; Table 40-3 outlines a supervisor's tasks.

PROFILING THE PHYSICIAN ASSISTANT PRACTICING OCCUPATIONAL MEDICINE

A questionnaire sent to 124 physician assistants known to be working in occupational medicine demonstrated how the PA's role in occupational medicine had grown in 20 years. Respondents were at plant sites, in private industrial medicine clinics, and on corporate medical staffs.

The average survey respondent was a 36-year-old white man with a bachelor's degree in a natural science and with formal education as a PA. The typical work setting was a large corporation of 3500 or more employees. The PA saw about 26 patients daily, caring mainly for sick or injured workers. Those in private industrial medicine clinics spent most of their time in direct patient care and had minimal interaction with safety officials or plant management.[23]

Corporate medical staff PAs were described as those who reported directly to the corporate medical director. They saw patients and participated in health evaluations, ran health education classes, performed administrative tasks, and maintained contact with medical departments of other company divisions around the country.

Thirty-eight percent of 47,280 physician assistants responded. Six hundred thirteen PAs worked in occupational medicine. That figure represents 3.6% of individuals eligible for PA practice in the United States.[24]

Table 40-1 Job Description: Occupational Medical Program Specialist, Human Resources Department

Objective: Plans, directs, and coordinates medical services, including medical service contracts, cost accounts, and preventive medicine services; offers expert opinions concerning exposures to hazards; and provides and evaluates medical services for the company.

Dimensions: Supervises the company's contracts for employee physical examinations and consulting medical director services. Interfaces with the consulting medical director in matters concerning occupational medicine. Provides the company with technical and administrative expertise for compliance with legal standards (i.e., applicable Nuclear Regulatory Commission, State Department of Labor, and federal safety and health regulations and standards).

Principal Accountabilities: Develops contract specifications and policies and procedures to execute medical programs on a company-wide basis.

Supervises the execution of the company's physical examination program to maintain compliance with the Nuclear Regulatory Commission and the State Department of Labor regulations and commitments.

Advises and educates workers and managers about hazards in the workplace and their health effects by searching the literature and compiling data relating to workplace exposures. Initiates literature searches of toxic hazards by supervising literature searches, then synthesizes a position paper with input from the consulting medical director.

Personally provides clinical support to employees in monitoring chronic health problems; offers medical counseling and referral to medical or surgical services; and coordinates clinical screening services such as those for cholesterol and blood pressure.

Promotes healthy habits and activities by introducing wellness education, describing risks for workplace, while traveling, and at home.

Works in conjunction with the Consulting Medical Director to expedite Workers' Compensation and lost-time injury issues.

USING PHYSICIAN ASSISTANTS IN OCCUPATIONAL MEDICINE

Just as PA utilization is expanding in other segments of health care, the trend in occupational medicine is to employ a growing number of PAs. One area in which PAs are playing a rapidly increasing role is in a workplace health and safety program. A graduate of a PA program needs little additional training to be qualified to conduct biological monitoring for work exposures, perform preplacement examinations, provide education and counseling, perform comprehensive health maintenance activities, assume some administrative responsibility, and treat occupational injuries and diseases.[6]

The National Commission on Certification of Physician Assistants conducted a practice analysis that identified physician assistant knowledge and skills in 1998. These parameters included the follow-

ing knowledge and skills relative to occupational and environmental medicine: preventive health maintenance, for example, screening and immunizations; monitoring of occupational or environmental exposures and follow-up; and maintenance of databases in poison control, correlating toxins and target organs.

Areas as diverse as health promotion, training, and research all provide avenues in which the PA is welcome. Health promotion in the workplace has been found to be effective in bringing down the cost of health benefits by preventing lost time and unnecessary illness or injury. PAs have taken over this training role admirably, based on their own training as health educators.

The concept of health promotion is that of *primary prevention*. In primary prevention of back injury, for instance, the new worker is taught to lift correctly, using concepts such as assessment of the load (Can I

Table 40-2 Job Description: Physician Assistant in Employee Health

Summary: This position is accountable for ensuring quality medical care for employees.

Nature and Scope: Reports to the Medical Director of Employee Health Service. The PA is responsible for giving complete, comprehensive pre-employment examinations to establish a health survey and database for every employee candidate, including all employees and full-time students.

Functions as a health care provider for employees with minor emergencies. Maintains medical records using a problem-oriented approach and ensures confidentiality for all patients seen.

Provides instruction in safety and good health practices and is responsible for immunizations as approved and recommended by the Centers for Disease Control and the hospital's Infection Control Committee. The incumbent will be actively involved in the wellness program endorsed by the hospital and any other projects under the supervision of the Medical Director.

Works directly or indirectly with the emergency department physician, as indicated by privileges. He or she is expected to recognize and interpret signs and symptoms and initiate appropriate diagnostic and therapeutic measures.

This position requires a minimum of a bachelor's degree and a certificate from an accredited PA program, as well as certification by the National Commission on Certification of Physician Assistants, plus appropriate state licensure as required.

Principal Accountabilities: The PA will work cooperatively with the employee health physician in the identification, treatment, and management of epidemiological problems. Initiates requests for consultations for problems out of the scope of the employee health service.

Provides urgent care for conditions that would not reasonably require the PA to seek immediate management by the physician, including but not limited to suturing superficial lacerations, immobilizing trauma victims before x-rays are taken, and removing a foreign body superficially embedded in the cornea. Initiation of emergency treatment for cardiopulmonary arrest is started by the PA as the physician is being called.

Other duties may be delegated by the physician, depending on experience and training and as hospital or clinic privileges allow.

Table 40-3 Employee Health Coordinator: Occupational Health

Position Summary: This position is accountable for ensuring quality medical care for employees.

Nature and Scope: Reports to the Director of Employee Health. This incumbent oversees all phases of the occupational health clinical program. Implements program goals and policies that have been established by the medical and administrative directors. Works in coordination with the business manager in matters concerning budget, marketing, and personnel management.

Facilitates the coordination of occupational health clinic services with the other services offered in the entire occupational health program.

Maintains liaison with client companies to provide a continuum of interest and credibility through personal communication efforts.

Continued

Table 40-3 Employee Health Coordinator: Occupational Health—cont'd

Is responsible for the quality assurance program of the employee health service, such as monthly statistics on exposure and screening for tuberculosis (TB), hepatitis, rubella, and AIDS of employees seen in the employee health clinic. He or she is an active participant in the hospital safety and infection control committees and must interface with the personnel responsible for those committees.

Is responsible for developing and implementing a wellness program for the employees of the hospital and other organizations as appropriate and for coordinating the activities of such programs.

Coordinates the daily activities of the employee health clinic to allow for routine physical examinations; treatment of acutely ill employees; epidemiological follow-ups; routine screenings for tuberculosis, hepatitis, rubella, and AIDS; employee education; and wellness-related activities.

Is responsible for giving complete and comprehensive pre-employment physical examinations and for documenting findings in a systematic manner on a problem-oriented medical record. The incumbent shall maintain the privacy of the patient and the confidentiality of the medical record. He or she is responsible for immunizations as recommended by the Centers for Disease Control (CDC) and the Infection Control Committee. The incumbent must also be able to accurately assess those employees who present for treatment and must initiate appropriate diagnostic and therapeutic measures according to protocol. In addition to the previously listed responsibilities, the incumbent is responsible for any other duties as deemed appropriate.

Directs and assigns work to clinicians and secretaries, and provides managerial support, such as personnel counseling, recruitment and/or dismissal, and general performance reviews for these workers, including day-to-day disciplinary needs.

Endeavors to provide state-of-the-art expertise and counsel to client companies in matters of occupational health and safety, Workers' Compensation, and any other relevant areas of occupational medicine.

Facilitates the whole health care rendering process for the client's employees, from entry to return-to-duty.

With the assistance of the program's Business Manager or Marketer, obtains new clients and develops new services for clients.

The Code of Ethical Conduct for Physicians Providing Occupational Medical Services, published by the American College of Occupational and Environmental Medicine, will be followed in carrying out all previously listed duties and responsibilities.*

Principal Accountabilities: The incumbent is a permanent member of the Safety Committee and the Infection Control Committee. He or she will work cooperatively with the Physician Director and Infection Control Nurse/Epidemiologist.

Generates monthly statistical reports on TB, rubella, hepatitis, and AIDS, as well as other epidemiological investigative reports to be presented to the Director of Emergency Services and the Infection Control Committee.

Is responsible for treatment and/or referrals for problems of employees presenting to the employee health clinic.

Coordinates a wellness program for employees and other organizations as appropriate.

Initiates a weekly meeting with the emergency department Medical Director to discuss medical care rendered and other timely issues.

Reviews and revises policies and procedures on at least an annual basis.

The Employee Health Coordinator must possess a bachelor's degree in health care (master's preferred) and must have a background in public health, industrial, or ambulatory care settings. He or she must possess management skills as demonstrated by education and/or experience. He or she must possess appropriate licensure as required.

---

*Code of Ethical Conduct, Board of Directors of the American College of Occupational and Environmental Medicine. Adopted October 25, 1993.

lift this material alone or does this job need more than one person?), correct lifting techniques of holding the object close enough to control the load and using the legs and abdominal muscles in addition to the muscles of the back, and maintaining lordosis in the cervical and lumbar spine. *Secondary prevention,* or taking corrective measures after the fact, is a useful strategy. In secondary prevention, those who have experienced back strain or sprain should be performing exercises to strengthen musculature and help discourage advanced back injury.

Another aspect of prevention is that *a PA can efficiently administer worksite health promotion, sometimes called wellness.* Worksite health promotion, a rapidly growing form of preventive health service, may include health risk appraisal with communication of findings to the individuals tested. It may also assist in helping individuals achieve and maintain physical and mental fitness, control alcohol use, avoid or quit using tobacco and other drugs, wear seat belts, and otherwise maintain health protective habits.

These programs provide opportunities to control high blood pressure, reduce elevated blood cholesterol, prevent obesity, and address other health hazards. Wellness and health promotion programs correlate with lower medical costs by decreasing hospital days and admissions, reducing sick leave, and increasing productivity.[25]

Research studies address the cost of compensable low back pain, the costliest occupational injury. The total compensable cost for all low back pain in the United States was estimated to be $11.7 billion in the 1995 claims year.[26] A PA who has spent much of her life's work in the ergonomics research section of an insurance company found that the prevalence of low back disability has increased dramatically. This conclusion was based on numbers of disability claims filed, the disability duration, or both. Of interest is that over the time of the study period, 1988 through 1996, the average cost of a claim decreased by 41.4% and the median cost increased by 19.7%.[27]

OTHER ROLES

The successful utilization of PAs at one major corporation provided an example of a career ladder for the PA in occupational medicine. Positions for PAs were divided into four levels: level I PAs performed basic assessment and screening tests with supervision, and participated in established programs. Level II PAs had limited input into policymaking; independently performed health risk assessment, health education, and counseling; independently implemented care in accordance with set objectives as well as personal expertise; and monitored occupational health programs.

Level III PAs had significant input into policymaking. They possessed a broad knowledge of occupational health, including ergonomics, epidemiology (dealing with interrelationships of host, agent, and environment), and toxicology (dealing with poison detection, chemistry, and pharmacological actions), as well as a broad knowledge of company policy and objectives. This PA supervised others and had full responsibility for a medical facility, while complying with PA clinical supervision requirements. A level III PA had a baccalaureate and 7 years' experience that had to include 5 years in occupational health.

Level IV PAs had extensive input into policymaking. Their expertise was in occupational health; they had a broad knowledge of company policy and objectives, as well as exercising administration and management authority. They coordinated activities, including advising others, independently or under administrative supervision. There was extensive PA participation in developing, implementing, monitoring, and evaluating programs, including involvement in budgetary needs and cost containment. Educational requirements for level IV PAs were a master's degree in the appropriate health field and 10 years of occupational health experience.[20]

Most occupational health PAs working in hospitals practice in employee health departments. These job functions are frequently within the purview of the emergency department or an employee health section. See Tables 40-1 and 40-2 for specifics in position descriptions of PAs in employee health.

The counterpart of the PA in Europe is the feldsher. These workers have been used extensively in occupational medicine in Russia. In this Russian innovation, mid-level practitioners are trained to deliver clinical services to the population, especially in satellite agricultural clinics. The full-time training course for feldshers consists of ongoing instruction 6 days a week for 6 classes a day in groups of 10 to 15 students for a period of 3 years. The Russian journal, *Feldsher Akush,* publishes articles on the role of the feldsher in the workplace. One title concerns prevention and treatment of trauma among agricultural workers; the other concerns encouraging workers to develop a healthy lifestyle.[28,29] Countries as far flung as Great Britain and Liberia, The Netherlands, and New Zealand utilize PAs in general medical practice and, although numbers are few, they may be used in the workplace as well. Other physician assistants work in Canada, especially in the military, where medical care is delivered to the fighting and training force. In developing countries in which manual labor dominates, it seems inevitable that PAs will be utilized for occupational treatment and prevention.

OCCUPATIONAL MEDICINE TOOLS

Two tools of the occupational practitioner are screening and surveillance. *Screening* is the search for previously unrecognized diseases caused or influenced by work-associated factors. A typical screening method is a questionnaire seeking suggestive symptoms or exposures, such as the asbestos questionnaire used for workers with asbestos exposure shown in Figure 40-1 and the respiratory questionnaire shown in Figure 40-2. Further diagnostic tests are usually necessary to confirm the diagnosis and evaluate the severity of the condition.

Surveillance is a system of monitoring the occurrence of disease among workers on the basis of reports of cases. This strategy helps in identification of clusters of work-related medical problems so they may be controlled before reaching epidemic proportions. The following case studies exemplify the use of surveillance.

CASE STUDY 40-1

Chief complaint

A 25-year-old black male laborer comes in for his first visit. "I get tired, I feel nervous, food doesn't taste right, and I can't sleep. I have stomach pain and I've taken Tums but they don't help. I've felt so jittery that I've been snapping at everyone. I can't even stand being around myself! This has been going on for about 4 months."

Past medical and family history

A review of his medical history form reveals that he has received vaccinations for diphtheria, tetanus, and polio, and has not been exposed to tuberculosis. He has been in good general health all his life. There is no history of surgery or accidents. There is no family history of neurological or cardiac disease. His father died in an auto accident 10 years ago.

Social history

He denies cigarette smoking or other tobacco use. He admits drinking two beers a day. He denies psychological pressures. He denies illegal drug use. He is a heterosexual, practices safe sex, and reports no sexual problems. He lives with his mother and brothers.

Work history

He has worked for 4 years for a construction firm as a laborer. Until 6 months ago, his jobs had been limited to working on new building construction. For most of that time, he was a hod carrier, using a wheelbarrow to transport wet cement from the large cement truck to areas of a building site inaccessible to a truck with an automatic cement chute. He says he was reassigned to general labor division, helping with gutting and reconstruction of old buildings, 6 months ago. He goes down to the building basement and retrieves parts of the wooden framing removed by carpenters who bang it down and saw up partitions to make way for the new framing. He says conditions are dusty, that his clothes get covered with white powder, and that he sometimes coughs at work. He says his cough is much better on weekends. He denies a chronic cough or shortness of breath.

Physical examination

Vital signs: blood pressure, 120/80; pulse, 80; respirations, 16. An unplanned weight loss of 10 lb is noted.

Notable physical findings include anxious and fidgety demeanor, fingernail pallor, increased deep tendon reflexes, and tremor of outstretched hands.

Laboratory tests

Complete blood count: serum lead level of 120 g/m³; normal is less than 50 g/m³.

Text continued on p. 862

ASBESTOS MEDICAL QUESTIONNAIRE

1. Name _____

2. Social Security Number _____

3. Present Occupation _____ Company _____

4. Address _____

   _____

5. Telephone Number _____

6. Interviewer _____

7. Date _____

8. Date of Birth _____

9. Place of Birth _____

10. Sex: Male _____   Female _____

11. Marital Status: Single _____ Married _____ Widowed _____ Separated/Divorced _____

12. Race: White _____ Black _____ Asian _____ Hispanic _____ Indian _____ Other _____

13. What is the highest grade completed in school? _____

    (For example, 12 years is completion of High School)

OCCUPATIONAL HISTORY

14. a. Have you ever worked full-time (30 hours per week or more)?   Yes _____ No _____

    b. Have you ever worked for a year or more in any dusty job?   Yes _____ No _____ Does not apply _____

       Specify job/industry _____ Total years worked _____

       Was dust exposure: Mild _____ Moderate _____ Severe _____

    c. Have you ever been exposed to gas or chemical fumes in your work?   Yes _____ No _____

       Specify job/industry _____ Total years worked _____

       Was exposure: Mild _____ Moderate _____ Severe _____

    d. What has been your usual occupation or job (the one you worked longest at)?

        1. Job occupation _____

        2. Number of years employed in this occupation _____

        3. Position/job title _____

Figure 40-1 Sample of an asbestos exposure questionnaire. *(Courtesy Medicus, P.C., 1245 Route 9, Wappingers Falls, NY 12590.)*

4. Business, field or industry _____

5. State the years worked (e.g., 1960-1969) _____

Have you ever worked:

e. In a mine?   Yes _____   No _____

f. In a quarry?   Yes _____   No _____

g. In a foundry?   Yes _____   No _____

h. In a pottery?   Yes _____   No _____

i. In a cotton, flax or hemp mill?   Yes _____   No _____

j. With asbestos?   Yes _____   No _____

PAST MEDICAL HISTORY

15.   a. Do you consider yourself to be in good health?   Yes____ No____ If no, state reason _____

_____

b. Have you any defect of vision?   Yes ____ No____ If yes, state nature of defect _____

c. Have you any hearing defect?   Yes____ No____ If yes, state nature of defect _____

d. Are you suffering from or have you suffered from:

1. Epilepsy (fits, seizures, convulsions)?   Yes _____   No _____

2. Rheumatic fever?   Yes _____   No _____

3. Kidney disease?   Yes _____   No _____

4. Bladder disease?   Yes _____   No _____

5. Diabetes?   Yes _____   No _____

6. Jaundice?   Yes _____   No _____

CHEST COLDS AND CHEST ILLNESSES

16.   If you get a cold, does it usually go to your chest? (*Usually* means more than half the time.)   Yes ____ No ____

Don't get colds   ____

17.   a. During the past three (3) years, have you had any chest illnesses that kept you off work,   Yes ____ No ____

indoors at home, or in bed?

IF YES TO PART a:

b. Did you produce phlegm with any of these chest illnesses?   Yes ____ No ____

Figure 40-1, cont'd For legend see p. 855.

c. In the past three (3) years, how many such illnesses with increased phlegm did

   you have?   # of illnesses   _____

18.   Did you have any lung trouble before the age of 18?   Yes _____ No _____

19.   Have you ever had any of the following?

   a. Bronchitis attacks?   Yes _____ No _____

      IF YES TO PART a:

   b. Was it confirmed by a doctor?   Yes _____ No _____

   c. At what age was your first attack?   Age _____

20.   a. Have you ever had pneumonia or bronchopneumonia?   Yes _____ No _____

   b. Was it confirmed by a doctor?   Yes _____ No _____

   c. At what age did you first have it?   Age _____

21.   a. Have you ever had hay fever?   Yes _____ No _____

      IF YES TO PART a:

   b. Was it confirmed by a doctor?   Yes _____ No _____

   c. At what age did it start?   Age _____

22.   a. Have you ever had chronic bronchitis?   Yes _____ No _____

      IF YES TO PART a:

   b. Do you still have it?   Yes _____ No _____

   c. At what age did it start?   Age _____

23.   a. Have you ever had emphysema?   Yes _____ No _____

      IF YES TO PART a:

   b. Do you still have it?   Yes _____ No _____

   c. Was it confirmed by a doctor?   Yes _____ No _____

   d. At what age did it start?   Age _____

24.   a. Have you ever had asthma?   Yes _____ No _____

      IF YES TO PART a:

   b. Do you still have it?   Yes _____ No _____

   c. Was it confirmed by a doctor?   Yes _____ No _____

Figure 40-1, cont'd For legend see p. 855.

d. At what age did it start? Age _____

e. If it stopped, state at what age. Age _____

25. Have you ever had:

a. Any other chest illnesses? Yes ____ No ____

If yes, please specify

_____

_____

b. Any chest operations? Yes ____ No ____

If yes, please specify

_____

_____

c. Any chest injuries? Yes ____ No ____

If yes, please specify

_____

26. a. Has a doctor told you that you had heart trouble? Yes ____ No ____

IF YES TO PART a:

b. Have you ever had treatment for heart trouble in the past ten (10) years? Yes ____ No ____

c. Has a doctor told you that you had high blood pressure? Yes ____ No ____

IF YES TO PART a:

d. Have you had any treatment for high blood pressure (hypertension) in the past

ten (10) years? Yes ____ No ____

27. a. When was your last chest x-ray? _____

b. Where was the x-ray taken? _____

FAMILY HISTORY

28. Was either of your natural parents ever told by a doctor that he or she had a chronic lung condition such as:

	FATHER			MOTHER		
a. Chronic bronchitis?	Yes ____	No ____	Don't know ____	Yes ____	No ____	Don't know ____
b. Emphysema?	Yes ____	No ____	Don't know ____	Yes ____	No ____	Don't know ____

Figure 40-1, cont'd For legend see p. 855.

c. Asthma?   Yes ___ No ___ Don't know ___   Yes ___ No ___ Don't know ___

d. Lung cancer?   Yes ___ No ___ Don't know ___   Yes ___ No ___ Don't know ___

e. Other chest conditions?   Yes ___ No ___ Don't know ___   Yes ___ No ___ Don't know ___

29. Are your parents currently alive?

a. Father   Yes ___ No ___ Don't know ___

b. Mother   Yes ___ No ___ Don't know ___

30. Please specify:

Father   _____ Age if living   Mother   _____ Age if living

_____ Age at death   _____ Age at death

_____ Don't know   _____ Don't know

_____ Cause of death   _____ Cause of death

31. a. Do you usually have a cough? (Count a cough with the first smoke or first going

   out of doors. Exclude clearing of throat.) If no, skip to question 31c.   Yes ___ No ___

   b. Do you usually cough as much as 4 to 6 times a days four or more days out of the week?   Yes ___ No ___

   c. Do you usually cough at all on getting up or first thing in the morning?   Yes ___ No ___

   d. Do you usually cough at all during the rest of the day or night?   Yes ___ No ___

   IF YES TO QUESTION 31a, b, c, or d, ANSWER THE FOLLOWING. IF NO, CHECK "Does not apply."

   e. Do you usually cough like this on most days for 3 or more

   consecutive months during the year?   Yes ___ No ___ Does not apply ___

   f. For how many years have you had the cough?   # of years _____

32. a. Do you usually bring up phlegm from your chest? (Count phlegm with the first

   smoke or on first going out of doors. Exclude phlegm from the nose. Count swallowed

   phlegm.) If no, skip to 32c.   Yes ___ No ___

   b. Do you usually bring up phlegm like this as much as twice a day four (4) or more

   days out of the week?   Yes ___ No ___

   c. Do you usually bring up phlegm at all on getting up or first thing in the morning?   Yes ___ No ___

   d. Do you usually bring up phlegm at all during the rest of the day or night?   Yes ___ No ___

   IF YES TO QUESTIONS 32a, b, c , or d, PLEASE ANSWER QUESTIONS 32e and 32f. IF NO, SKIP TO 33a.

Figure 40-1, cont'd For legend see p. 855.

e. Do you bring up phlegm like this on most days for 3 consecutive months or more

during the year?   Yes ___ No___

f. For how many years have you had trouble with phlegm?   # of years ___

33. a. Have you had periods or episodes of (increased) cough and phlegm lasting for 3 weeks

or more each day? (For those who usually have cough and/or phlegm.)   Yes ___ No___

IF YES TO PART a:

b. For how long have you had at least one such episode per year?   # of years ___

34. Does your chest ever sound wheezy or whistling:

a. When you have a cold?   Yes ___ No___

b. Occasionally apart from colds?   Yes ___ No___

c. Most days or nights?   Yes ___ No___

IF YES TO 34a, b, or c:

For how many years has this been present?   # of years ___

35. a. Have you ever had an attack of wheezing that has made you feel short of breath? Yes ___ No___

IF YES TO PART a:

b. How old were you with your first attack?   Age in years ___

c. Have you had two or more such episodes?   Yes ___ No___

d. Have you ever required medicine or treatment for the(se) attack(s)?   Yes ___ No___

36. If disabled from walking by any condition other than heart or lung disease, please describe and proceed to

question 38a.

Nature of condition(s) _____

37. a. Are you troubled by shortness of breath when hurrying on the level or walking

up a slight hill?   Yes ___ No___

IF YES TO PART a:

b. Do you walk slower than people of your age on the level due to breathlessness?   Yes ___ No___

c. Do you ever have to stop for breath when walking at your own pace on the level?   Yes ___ No___

d. Do you ever have to stop for breath after walking about 100 yards or after a few

minutes on the level?   Yes ___ No___

Figure 40-1, cont'd For legend see p. 855.

    e. Are you too breathless to leave the house or breathless on dressing or climbing

       one flight of stairs?   Yes ____ No____

38.   a. Have you ever smoked cigarettes? (*No* means less than 20 packs of cigarettes or 12 oz.

       of tobacco in a lifetime or less than 1 cigarette a day for 1 year.)   Yes ____ No____

       IF YES TO PART a:

    b. Do you still smoke cigarettes? (As of 1 month ago.)   Yes ____ No____

    c. How old were you when you first started regular cigarette smoking?   Age _____

    d. If you have stopped smoking cigarettes completely, how old were you when you stopped?   Age _____

    e. How many cigarettes do you smoke per day?   packs/day_____

    f. On the average of the entire time you smoked, how many cigarettes did you smoke per day?   packs/day_____

    g. Do or did you inhale the cigarette smoke?   Yes ____ No____

    h. If yes, how much? _____ Slightly _____ Moderately _____ Deeply

39.   a. Have you ever smoked a pipe regularly? (*Yes* means more than 12 oz. of tobacco

       in a lifetime.)   Yes ____ No____

       IF YES TO PART a:

    b. How old were you when you started to smoke a pipe regularly?   Age _____

    c. If you have stopped smoking a pipe completely, how old were you when you stopped?   Age _____

                                        Still smoking   _____

    d. On the average over the entire time you smoked a pipe, how much tobacco

       did you smoke per week? (Average pouch contains 1 1/2 oz.)   Oz. per wk. ____

                                      Does not apply   _____

    e. How much pipe tobacco are you smoking now?   Oz. per wk. ____

                                       None _____

    f. Do you or did you inhale the pipe smoke?   Yes ____ No____

    g. If yes, how much? _____ Slightly _____ Moderately _____ Deeply

Figure 40-1, cont'd For legend see p. 855.

40. a. Have you ever smoked cigars regularly? (*Yes* means more than 1 cigar a week for 1 year)   Yes ___ No ___

   IF YES TO PART a:

   b. How old were you when you started smoking cigars?   Age ___

   c. If you have stopped smoking cigars completely, how old were you when you stopped?   Age ___

   Still smoking   ___

   d. How many cigars did you smoke per week over the entire time you smoked? (Average)   # per wk. ___

   e. How many cigars are you smoking now?   # per wk. ___

   None ___

   f. Do you or did you inhale the cigar smoke?   Yes ___ No ___

   g. If yes, how much? ___ Slightly ___ Moderately ___ Deeply

SIGNATURE _____   DATE _____

Figure 40-1, cont'd For legend see p. 855.

Diagnosis
Work-related lead exposure.

Lead
Typical early signs of exposure in adults include abdominal colic, headache, and fatigue. At high levels or in later stages, one may see peripheral motor neuropathy with wristdrop or footdrop and anemia.

Chronic exposure
Consistent with interstitial fibrosis and renal failure. Reproductive problems include association with spontaneous abortion, premature delivery, and membrane rupture; fetal brain development and cognitive development are affected.

   Construction Standard. OSHA lead standard is 40 g/m^3 over an 8-hour day (known as time-weighted average, or TWA). With a routine exposure at 50 g/m^3, one can expect about 40 g/m^3 as a laboratory result.

Treatment
➤ Recommend that safety and health officer and manager immediately remove worker from any job site where lead may be a factor.
➤ Begin chelation therapy.
➤ Recommend that worker refrain from home and recreation lead exposure (e.g., soldering with lead and making bullets).
➤ Request that worker return for an appointment in 4 weeks for follow-up of lead level.
➤ Notify safety and health officer for addition to OSHA log as required by law.
➤ Recommend that safety and health officer and manager immediately screen co-workers for lead levels.
➤ Recommend an industrial hygiene consultation to begin an environmental exposure survey and to make heating, ventilation, and air conditioning (HVAC) recommendations if air contains toxic levels or wipe samples are above permissible levels.

Text continued on p. 868

..1910.134 Appendix C
Appendix C to Sec. 1910.134: OSHA Respirator Medical Evaluation Questionnaire (Mandatory)

To the employer: Answers to questions in Section 1, and to question 9 in Section 2 of Part A, do not require a medical examination.

To the employee:

Can you read (circle one): Yes/No

Your employer must allow you to answer this questionnaire during normal working hours, or at a time and place that is convenient to you. To maintain your confidentiality, your employer or supervisor must not look at or review your answers, and your employer must tell you how to deliver or send this questionnaire to the health care professional who will review it.

Part A. Section 1. (Mandatory) The following information must be provided by every employee who has been selected to use any type of respirator (please print).

1. Today's date:_____

2. Your name:_____

3. Your age (to nearest year):_____

4. Sex (circle one): Male/Female

5. Your height: _____ ft. _____ in.

6. Your weight: _____ lbs.

7. Your job title:_____

8. A phone number where you can be reached by the health care professional who reviews this
   questionnaire (include the Area Code): _____

9. The best time to phone you at this number: _____
10. Has your employer told you how to contact the health care professional who will review this
    questionnaire (circle one): Yes/No
11. Check the type of respirator you will use (you can check more than one category):
    a. _____ N, R, or P disposable respirator (filter-mask, non-cartridge type only).
    b. _____ Other type (for example, half- or full-facepiece type, powered-air purifying, supplied-air,
       self-contained breathing apparatus).

12. Have you worn a respirator (circle one): Yes/No

If "yes," what type(s):_____
_____

Part A. Section 2. (Mandatory) Questions 1 through 9 below must be answered by every employee who has been selected to use any type of respirator (please circle "yes" or "no").

1. Do you *currently* smoke tobacco, or have you smoked tobacco in the last month: Yes/No

Figure 40-2 Respirator Medical Evaluation Questionnaire (Mandatory). *(From U.S. Department of Labor, Occupational Safety and Health Administration, 1910.134 Appendix C. Available at http://www.osha. gov/SLTC/respiratory_advisor/oshafiles/medicalrequirements1.html#Appendix%20C. Accessed 22 April 2002.)*

2. Have you *ever had* any of the following conditions?
   a. Seizures (fits): Yes/No
   b. Diabetes (sugar disease): Yes/No
   c. Allergic reactions that interfere with your breathing: Yes/No
   d. Claustrophobia (fear of closed-in places): Yes/No
   e. Trouble smelling odors: Yes/No

3. Have you *ever had* any of the following pulmonary or lung problems?
   a. Asbestosis: Yes/No
   b. Asthma: Yes/No
   c. Chronic bronchitis: Yes/No
   d. Emphysema: Yes/No
   e. Pneumonia: Yes/No
   f. Tuberculosis: Yes/No
   g. Silicosis: Yes/No
   h. Pneumothorax (collapsed lung): Yes/No
   i. Lung cancer: Yes/No
   j. Broken ribs: Yes/No
   k. Any chest injuries or surgeries: Yes/No
   l. Any other lung problem that you've been told about: Yes/No

4. Do you *currently* have any of the following symptoms of pulmonary or lung illness?
   a. Shortness of breath: Yes/No
   b. Shortness of breath when walking fast on level ground or walking up a slight hill or incline: Yes/No
   c. Shortness of breath when walking with other people at an ordinary pace on level ground: Yes/No
   d. Have to stop for breath when walking at your own pace on level ground: Yes/No
   e. Shortness of breath when washing or dressing yourself: Yes/No
   f. Shortness of breath that interferes with your job: Yes/No
   g. Coughing that produces phlegm (thick sputum): Yes/No
   h. Coughing that wakes you early in the morning: Yes/No
   i. Coughing that occurs mostly when you are lying down: Yes/No
   j. Coughing up blood in the last month: Yes/No
   k. Wheezing: Yes/No
   l. Wheezing that interferes with your job: Yes/No
   m. Chest pain when you breathe deeply: Yes/No
   n. Any other symptoms that you think may be related to lung problems: Yes/No

5. Have you *ever had* any of the following cardiovascular or heart problems?
   a. Heart attack: Yes/No
   b. Stroke: Yes/No
   c. Angina: Yes/No
   d. Heart failure: Yes/No
   e. Swelling in your legs or feet (not caused by walking): Yes/No
   f. Heart arrhythmia (heart beating irregularly): Yes/No
   g. High blood pressure: Yes/No
   h. Any other heart problem that you've been told about: Yes/No

6. Have you *ever had* any of the following cardiovascular or heart symptoms?
   a. Frequent pain or tightness in your chest: Yes/No
   b. Pain or tightness in your chest during physical activity: Yes/No
   c. Pain or tightness in your chest that interferes with your job: Yes/No
   d. In the past two years, have you noticed your heart skipping or missing a beat: Yes/No
   e. Heartburn or indigestion that is not related to eating: Yes/ No
   f. Any other symptoms that you think may be related to heart or circulation problems: Yes/No

Figure 40-2, cont'd For legend see p. 863.

7. Do you *currently* take medication for any of the following problems?
   a. Breathing or lung problems: Yes/No
   b. Heart trouble: Yes/No
   c. Blood pressure: Yes/No
   d. Seizures (fits): Yes/No

8. If you've used a respirator, have you *ever had* any of the following problems? (If you've never used a respirator, check the following space and go to question 9)
   a. Eye irritation: Yes/No
   b. Skin allergies or rashes: Yes/No
   c. Anxiety: Yes/No
   d. General weakness or fatigue: Yes/No
   e. Any other problem that interferes with your use of a respirator: Yes/No

9. Would you like to talk to the health care professional who will review this questionnaire about your answers to this questionnaire: Yes/No
   Questions 10 to 15 below must be answered by every employee who has been selected to use either a full-facepiece respirator or a self-contained breathing apparatus (SCBA). For employees who have been selected to use other types of respirators, answering these questions is voluntary.

10. Have you *ever lost* vision in either eye (temporarily or permanently): Yes/No

11. Do you *currently* have any of the following vision problems?
    a. Wear contact lenses: Yes/No
    b. Wear glasses: Yes/No
    c. Color blind: Yes/No
    d. Any other eye or vision problem: Yes/No

12. Have you *ever had* an injury to your ears, including a broken ear drum: Yes/No

13. Do you *currently* have any of the following hearing problems?
    a. Difficulty hearing: Yes/No
    b. Wear a hearing aid: Yes/No
    c. Any other hearing or ear problem: Yes/No

14. Have you *ever had* a back injury: Yes/No

15. Do you *currently* have any of the following musculoskeletal problems?
    a. Weakness in any of your arms, hands, legs, or feet: Yes/No
    b. Back pain: Yes/No
    c. Difficulty fully moving your arms and legs: Yes/No
    d. Pain or stiffness when you lean forward or backward at the waist: Yes/No
    e. Difficulty fully moving your head up or down: Yes/No
    f. Difficulty fully moving your head side to side: Yes/No
    g. Difficulty bending at your knees: Yes/No
    h. Difficulty squatting to the ground: Yes/No
    i. Climbing a flight of stairs or a ladder carrying more than 25 lbs: Yes/No
    j. Any other muscle or skeletal problem that interferes with using a respirator: Yes/No

Part B Any of the following questions, and other questions not listed, may be added to the questionnaire at the discretion of the health care professional who will review the questionnaire.

1. In your present job, are you working at high altitudes (over 5,000 feet) or in a place that has lower than normal amounts of oxygen: Yes/No
   If "yes," do you have feelings of dizziness, shortness of breath, pounding in your chest, or other symptoms when you're working under these conditions: Yes/No

Figure 40-2, cont'd For legend see p. 863.

2. At work or at home, have you ever been exposed to hazardous solvents, hazardous airborne chemicals (e.g., gases, fumes, or dust), or have you come into skin contact with hazardous chemicals: Yes/No
If "yes," name the chemicals if you know them:_____
_____
_____

3. Have you ever worked with any of the materials, or under any of the conditions, listed below:
a. Asbestos: Yes/No
b. Silica (e.g., in sandblasting): Yes/No
c. Tungsten/cobalt (e.g., grinding or welding this material): Yes/No
d. Beryllium: Yes/No
e. Aluminum: Yes/No
 f. Coal (for example, mining): Yes/No
g. Iron: Yes/No
h. Tin: Yes/No
 i. Dusty environments: Yes/No
 j. Any other hazardous exposures: Yes/No
If "yes," describe these exposures:_____
_____
_____

4. List any second jobs or side businesses you have:_____
_____

5. List your previous occupations:_____
_____

6. List your current and previous hobbies:_____
_____

7. Have you been in the military services? Yes/No
If "yes," were you exposed to biological or chemical agents (either in training or combat): Yes/No

8. Have you ever worked on a HAZMAT team? Yes/No

9. Other than medications for breathing and lung problems, heart trouble, blood pressure, and seizures mentioned earlier in this questionnaire, are you taking any other medications for any reason (including over-the-counter medications): Yes/No
If "yes," name the medications if you know them:_____

10. Will you be using any of the following items with your respirator(s)?
a. HEPA Filters: Yes/No
b. Canisters (for example, gas masks): Yes/No
c. Cartridges: Yes/No

11. How often are you expected to use the respirator(s) (circle "yes" or "no" for all answers that apply to you)?:
a. Escape only (no rescue): Yes/No
b. Emergency rescue only: Yes/No
c. Less than 5 hours per week: Yes/No
d. Less than 2 hours per day: Yes/No
e. 2 to 4 hours per day: Yes/No
 f. Over 4 hours per day: Yes/No

12. During the period you are using the respirator(s), is your work effort:
a. *Light* (less than 200 kcal per hour): Yes/No
If "yes," how long does this period last during the average
shift:_____hrs._____mins.

Figure 40-2, cont'd For legend see p. 863.

Examples of a light work effort are *sitting* while writing, typing, drafting, or performing light assembly work; or *standing* while operating a drill press (1-3 lbs.) or controlling machines.

b. *Moderate* (200 to 350 kcal per hour): Yes/No
If "yes," how long does this period last during the average
shift:_____hrs._____mins.
Examples of moderate work effort are *sitting* while nailing or filing; *driving* a truck or bus in urban traffic; *standing* while drilling, nailing, performing assembly work, or transferring a moderate load (about 35 lbs.) at trunk level; *walking* on a level surface about 2 mph or down a 5-degree grade about 3 mph; or *pushing* a wheelbarrow with a heavy load (about 100 lbs.) on a level surface.

c. *Heavy* (above 350 kcal per hour): Yes/No
If "yes," how long does this period last during the average
shift:_____hrs._____mins.
Examples of heavy work are *lifting* a heavy load (about 50 lbs.) from the floor to your waist or shoulder; working on a loading dock; *shoveling; standing* while bricklaying or chipping castings; *walking* up an 8-degree grade about 2 mph; climbing stairs with a heavy load (about 50 lbs.).

13. Will you be wearing protective clothing and/or equipment (other than the respirator) when you're using your respirator: Yes/No
If "yes," describe this protective clothing and/or equipment:_____
_____

14. Will you be working under hot conditions (temperature exceeding 77 deg. F): Yes/No

15. Will you be working under humid conditions: Yes/No

16. Describe the work you'll be doing while you're using your respirator(s):
_____
_____

17. Describe any special or hazardous conditions you might encounter when you're using your respirator(s) (for example, confined spaces, life-threatening gases):
_____
_____

18. Provide the following information, if you know it, for each toxic substance that you'll be exposed to when you're using your respirator(s):
Name of the first toxic substance:_____
Estimated maximum exposure level per shift:_____
Duration of exposure per shift:_____
Name of the second toxic substance:_____
Estimated maximum exposure level per shift:_____
Duration of exposure per shift:_____
Name of the third toxic substance:_____
Estimated maximum exposure level per shift:_____
Duration of exposure per shift:_____
The name of any other toxic substances that you'll be exposed to while using your respirator:
_____
_____
_____

19. Describe any special responsibilities you'll have while using your respirator(s) that may affect the safety and well-being of others (for example, rescue, security):
_____

Figure 40-2, cont'd For legend see p. 863.

CASE STUDY 40-2

Chief complaint

A 45-year-old white woman has pain in her wrists and hands, sometimes radiating into the forearm. It sometimes wakens her at night.

History of present illness

This woman has been working at an automobile parts plant for 3 years. Over the past 4 months, there were layoffs at the plant, and her quota of parts was increased. She denies any hobbies or home activities that involve twisting pressure on her wrists.

Social and family history

She works on an assembly line and has a daily quota. Her work involves pressing an "o" ring onto a rod with pliers to make a part for an auto window mechanism. She has been a two-pack-a-day cigarette smoker for 20 years and is a social drinker (takes two drinks at an occasional party). She states that she had the usual childhood diseases and complete vaccinations. She is married with no children.

Past medical history

She has been in good health all her life with the exception of lumbosacral strain that required a 1-week convalescence 2 years ago. She complains of occasional back pain when she overworks or doesn't lift using the appropriate muscles. She denies diabetes mellitus, rheumatoid arthritis, or thyroid problems.

Physical examination

Positive findings included decreased sensation in the median nerve distribution tested by sharp-dull discrimination. Pain is noted on direct pressure of the carpal tunnel bilaterally. (The carpal compression test, performed by applying direct pressure on the carpal tunnel, is probably the most sensitive test.) Pain is exacerbated by dorsiflexion of the wrist. Tinel's sign is positive (tingling or shocklike pain is elicited on volar wrist percussion). Phalen's sign is positive (pain or paresthesia in the distribution of the median nerve when the patient flexes both wrists to 90 degrees, with the dorsal aspect of the hands held in apposition for 60 seconds).

Diagnosis

Tendonitis of wrists; carpal tunnel syndrome to be ruled out.

Treatment

Removal of the worker from the assembly line. Splinting of the hand and forearm at night. Referral to an orthopedic surgeon to seek alleviation of symptoms, which may require the injection of corticosteroids into the carpal tunnel for some patients.

PROFESSIONAL DEVELOPMENT AND FUTURE ROLES

The undergraduate training of the PA does not usually include specifics about occupational health. Ambulatory and emergency medicine concepts are certainly taught, but specialty areas such as hearing conservation, prevention tactics against dust diseases, and Occupational Safety and Health Administration (OSHA) examinations are usually not covered.

Master's degree programs in preventive medicine and occupational health are available at schools of public health and other graduate schools throughout the country that address prevention. Applicants must possess a baccalaureate degree and meet specific admission requirements for the institution in question. Many programs offer part-time schedules for working professionals.[30]

One such graduate program at the University of Oklahoma, Oklahoma City, exists solely for PAs. It is offered as part of the existing occupational health curriculum conducted by the Department of Environmental Health in the College of Public Health, and is cooperatively sponsored by the Physician Associate Program of the College of Medicine.[31]

SHORTAGE OF PHYSICIANS AND PHYSICIAN ASSISTANTS IN OCCUPATIONAL AND ENVIRONMENTAL MEDICINE

According to a study sponsored by the Institute of Medicine's Subcommittee on Physician Shortage in Occupational and Environmental Medicine, there is a shortage of 3100 to 5500 physicians in occupational medicine. This includes a shortage of 1600 to 3500 fully trained specialists and 1500 to 2000 clinicians. Clinicians specializing in occupational and environmental medicine (OEM) are primary care physicians with special competence in the field who can serve as consultants and educators when specialists are not needed or are unavailable.

Other authors call for expanding the availability of master's programs in public health so that established physicians can complete the degree and receive practical experience on a part-time basis.[32]

Demands for patient service in a setting where an OEM physician delegates tasks to an OEM PA may help alleviate this shortage. Both the desire to contain costs and the wish to ensure quality of service delivery might increase PA utilization in this specialty.

The total number of physician assistants practicing by the year 2015 is expected to grow to 79,000. Approximately 3.7% of PAs are currently practicing in OEM. If this prediction proves accurate, and the current percentage of PAs choosing to practice in occupational and environmental medicine holds steady, there will be approximately 2900 PAs practicing in OEM in 13 years.[33] Well-trained PAs supervised by occupational physicians may well provide the answer to the manpower shortage.

THE PHYSICIAN/PA TEAM

A group of physicians looked critically at America's health care needs and envisioned the health professional who became the physician assistant. The physician could more effectively care for patients when working as part of a physician/PA team.[34] The efficiency of this team model has led to its utilization in all medical and surgical specialties. The physician/PA team may be so effective because the education of the PA follows the medical school model. PA students may share classes, facilities, and clinical rotations with medical students. The similarity of training sites, faculties, and medical education parameters leads to homogeneity of thought in the clinical workplace.[35] The Pew foundation wrote, "The traditional relationship between PAs and physicians, the hallmarks of which are frequent consultation, referral, and review of PA practice by the supervising physician, is one of the strengths of the PA profession. The characteristics of this relationship are also considered to be the elements of professional relationships in any well-designed health system."[36]

The AAPA Policy Manual states that the physician/PA team relationship is fundamental to the PA profession and enhances the delivery of high-quality health care. As the structure of the health care system changes, it is critical that this essential relationship be preserved and strengthened.[34]

There is a shortage of physicians as well as PAs in occupational medicine.[37,38] In a year 2000 practice analysis survey done by a national testing group to refine the clinical context of the physician assistant certifying examination, 1% of the 2716 respondents identified themselves with industrial medicine. However, many of the PAs in general practice prize the knowledge of preventive health maintenance such as screening and occupational or environmental exposures and follow up.[39] It is interesting to note that numbers of PAs in the OEM practice setting are expected to rise to help physicians bridge the gap that the National Institute for Occupational Safety and Health (NIOSH) projects in the early years of the 21st century.[40]

Although one of the bases on which PAs were based was cost containment, current health care costs in business make the profession even more attractive. Workplace application of PAs has been shown to be cost-effective. To ensure the future growth of PAs working in the occupational and environmental medicine field, there must be an attempt to increase mainstream exposure to the field during PA training.

The physician assistant in occupational medicine can care for the healthy worker, focus on preventive medicine, deliver emergency care to injured workers, perform preplacement examinations, provide screening and monitoring, handle administrative tasks, and assist the corporate medical director. These delegated tasks are accomplished with the same cost-effectiveness that has made the physician assistant an integral part of the physician/PA team for America's health care delivery system for years. As industry looks for ways to provide quality care to its employees, the demand for PAs in occupational and environmental medicine will continue to grow. The challenge for PAs will be to fill this demand, helping to minimize the dangers that people face from various environmental exposures in the workplace.

PROFESSIONAL OCCUPATIONAL MEDICINE ORGANIZATIONS

The American Academy of Physician Assistants in Occupational Medicine (AAPA-OM) was founded in 1981 as the professional association for PAs in the field. The main functions of the AAPA-OM are to render services to the medical profession and the public and to develop and enforce continuing medical education (CME) programs for PAs involved in the practice of occupational medicine. The AAPA-OM is also pledged to promote high-quality care delivered by PAs involved in occupational medicine. Educating occupational medicine professionals and employee consumers, as well as recruiting PA students to the specialty, will help achieve this goal.

In 2001, the AAPA-OM had almost 200 members. The organization has held CME sessions in conjunction with the American Academy of Physician Assistants (AAPA) and the American College of Occupational and Environmental Medicine. Future conferences are anticipated with both PA and physician groups.

The mission statement of AAPA-OM is as follows:

The American Academy of Physician Assistants in Occupational Medicine serves its members by providing a forum for exchange of information and ideas to ensure delivery of the highest quality, state-of-the-art preventive services. In order to maintain safe and healthy workers and work environments, we strive to form mutually beneficial relationships with other occupational health and safety professionals. We endorse and support the code of ethical conduct as established by the American College of Occupational Medicine.[41]

AAPA-OM has promoted specialty training at the annual conference of the AAPA for many years. At least one full day of occupational or environmental course offerings is provided during the conference. The courses offer both new concepts and reviews aimed at the PA already working in the area of occupational medicine, and are also of interest to the generalist who cares for the ill and injured worker.

The American College of Occupational and Environmental Medicine (ACOEM) is the organization to which most occupational physicians belong. The directions of modern occupational medicine in the United States took shape with the formation of the then-named American Occupational Medical Association (AOMA) in 1916. Since that time, the name has been changed to include the concept of environmental medicine; the final change became effective January 1, 1992 when the association became the American College of Occupational and Environmental Medicine. Stating that occupational and environmental medicine disciplines are clearly intertwined, the ACOEM reflects the issues encountered by the occupational-environmental physician.[42]

ACOEM is known as the world's largest society dedicated to promoting the health of workers through clinical practice, research, and teaching. Its membership includes specialists in all branches of medicine because the concerns of occupational and environmental medicine touch virtually every physician's practice. Educational activities take place in the form of two national conferences annually—the American Occupational Health Conference each spring, and the State of the Art Conference each fall. Scientific sessions are conducted on a variety of occupational and environmental medicine issues, as are in-depth postgraduate seminars at each conference.

Physician assistants have delivered lectures as part of the Occupational Physician/Occupational Physician Assistant Team Section of ACOEM. This Section exists to strengthen the team concept via educational pursuits and interactive communication. Affiliate membership for physician assistants was established by membership vote during the American Occupational Health Conference in April of 2002. This affiliation promises global opportunities with membership benefits of education, access to colleagues, employment opportunities, and valuable expertise. Publications available to members include the *ACOEM Report* (newsletter), the monthly peer-reviewed *Journal of Occupational and Environmental Medicine* (JOEM), the ACOEM Membership Directory, a recommended Library Listing, position papers, and practice guidelines (personal observation).

Regional ACOEM component societies offer continuing medical education on the local level. The component societies elect delegates to the policymaking body of the ACOEM. In 1948, the American Board of Preventive Medicine (ABPM) was formed and joined AOMA in encouraging research in occupational medicine and fostering training of physicians. Since then, significant growth has taken place in this field. Today, ABPM certifies physicians in general preventive medicine, public health, and aerospace medicine, including more than 6100 member physicians.[41]

There is room for growth for primary care PA providers to learn and use occupational and environmental medicine concepts in their practice. There is a growing trend among family practice physicians and emergency physicians, along with their PA counterparts, to deliver care to workers. Many cities and towns have few occupational and environmental medicine specialists and PAs who provide the first line of care to workers. For the benefit of public safety, health care providers should know how to perform Department of Transportation commercial drivers' license examinations, manage nurse and day care workers' inoculation schedules, and recommend that managers employ workers under light duty restrictions as part of a return to work schedule.

FUTURE ROLES

There is room for growth in occupational and environmental medicine among primary care providers, especially for the physician assistant. The PA in occupational medicine can care for the healthy worker, focusing on preventive medicine; deliver emergency care to those who are injured on the job; perform preplacement examinations; carry out screening and monitoring; handle administrative tasks; and assist the corporate medical director, all with the same cost-effectiveness that made the PA an integral part of America's health care delivery system.

Providing care in the workplace offers great satisfaction to a PA. Starting a wellness program or running a health fair to encourage healthy behaviors, knowing that he or she is intervening between an employee and early illness, is a positive accomplishment. Seeing those who have responded to rapid emergency care return to the workplace is especially rewarding. It is gratifying to have an employee with a strong family history or early, nonfatal myocardial infarction embrace the offer of a company-sponsored exercise program and the recommendation of a healthy diet.

CONCLUSION

As industry looks for ways to provide quality care for its employees in the most cost-efficient manner possible, the demand for PAs in occupational medicine will continue to grow globally. The challenge for PAs will be to fill this demand, helping to minimize the dangers that people face from various environmental exposures in the workplace, satisfied that they have contributed to an area of medicine that has been underpopulated all too long.

REFERENCES

1. American College of Occupational and Environmental Medicine home page. Available at http://www.acoem.org. Accessed 20 April, 2002.
2. Silver RR. Basic Occupational Medicine: A Guide to Developing Delivery Systems. Boca Raton, FL: CRC Press, 1991.
3. McCunney RS. A Practical Approach to Occupational and Environmental Medicine. Boston: Little, Brown & Co, 1994.
4. Key MM, Henschel AF, Butler J, et al (eds). Occupational Diseases: A Guide to Their Recognition. NIOSH Publication No. 77-181. Washington, DC: Department of Health, Education, and Welfare, September 1978.
5. Rom WN. The discipline of environmental and occupational medicine. In: Rom WN (ed). Environmental and Occupational Medicine. Boston: Little, Brown & Co, 1983.
6. Storm AH. Occupational health and safety programs in the workplace. In: Levy BS, Wegman DH (eds). Recognizing and Preventing Work-Related Disease, ed 1. Boston: Little, Brown & Co, 1983.
7. Sicherman B. Alice Hamilton: A Life in Letters. Cambridge, MA: Harvard University Press, 1984.
8. Welter ES. The role of the primary care physician in occupational health. In: Zenz C (ed). Occupational Medicine, ed 3. Chicago: Year Book Publishers, 1994.
9. Widess E. Toxic tort litigation and United States occupational and environmental legislation. In: Rosenstock L, Cullen MR (eds). Textbook of Clinical Occupational and Environmental Medicine. Philadelphia: WB Saunders, 1994.
10. Occupational Safety and Health Administration, U.S. Department of Labor. OSHA High Injury/Illness Rate Targeting and Cooperative Compliance Programs, CPL2-0.119. Washington, DC: OSHA, November 25, 1997.
11. Bureau of Labor Statistics. Workplace Injury and Illnesses in 1996. Washington, DC: U.S. Department of Labor, December 17, 1997.
12. Bureau of Labor Statistics. National Census of Fatal Occupational Injuries, 1996. Washington, DC: U.S. Department of Labor, August 7, 1997.
13. Bureau of Labor Statistics. Lost-Worktime Injuries and Illnesses: Characteristics and Resulting Time Away From Work, 1996. Washington, DC: U.S. Department of Labor, April 23, 1998.

14. Bureau of Labor Statistics. Fatal Occupational Injuries by Incident or Exposure, 1992–1996. Washington, DC: U.S. Department of Labor, September 15, 1998.

15. Greaves WW, Pearson JK. Occupational medicine—a primary care perspective. Patient Care 1996;30:28.

16. Himmelstein JS, Pransky GS. The ADA and you: implications for the occupational health professional. J Occup Med 1992;34:501.

17. Person JK, Rosenstock L, Salvaggio JE, Weida TJ. We're all practicing occupational medicine. Patient Care 1996; 30:42.

18. Cawley J. The physician assistant profession: current status and future trends. J Public Health Policy 1985;6:78.

19. Elliott CH. The physician assistant in occupational medicine. PA Drug Update 1984;September:42.

20. Lang RH, O'Braint CR, Good J, et al. The ARCO Medical Department Job Family Matrix. Paper presented at The American Occupational Health Conference, Kansas City, MO, April 1985.

21. Randall G. Physician assistants on the trans-Alaska pipeline project. Newsline for Physician Assistants 1997; September:4-7.

22. Ramos M. Occupational medicine: how PAs keep the workplace safe. Physician Assistant 1989;13:79.

23. Sharp G. AAPA-OM Survey. American Academy of Physician Assistants in Occupational Medicine Newsletter, 1992;January:2.

24. 2001 AAPA Physician Assistant Census Report, 1998-2002. Volume 1, page 10.

25. Breslow L, Fielding J, Herrman AA, Wilbur CS. Worksite health promotion: its evolution and the Johnson and Johnson experience. Prev Med 1990;19:13.

26. Murphy PL, Volinn E. Is occupational low back pain on the rise? Spine 1999;7:691.

27. Hashemi L, Webster BS, Clancy EA. Trends in disability duration and cost for workers' compensation LBP claims (1988-1996). J Occup Environ Med 1998;40:1110.

28. Voronin NI, Shtarberg AI. The role of the feldsher in the prevention and treatment of trauma among agricultural workers. Feldsher Akush 1989;54:12.

29. Afonina EV. Work organization of the occupational pathology department of a provincial hospital. Feldsher Akush 1989; 54:10.

30. Graduate Education for Public Health. Association of Schools of Public Health, Washington DC, 1984.

31. The Graduate Program in Occupational Health for Physician Assistants. University of Oklahoma Health Sciences Center, Oklahoma City, OK 73190. Association of Physician Assistant Programs, 1997, ed 15:120.

32. Rosenstock L, Rest KM, Benson JA Jr, et al. Occupational and environmental medicine: meeting the growing need for clinical services. N Engl J Med 1991;325:924.

33. Fair S, Kohlhepp WC, Amato PE. Occupational medicine: physician assistants can meet the need. J Am Acad Physician Assistants, February 2002.

34. The American Academy of Physician Assistants. Issue Brief: The Physician-PA Team, April 4, 2001.

35. White GL, et al. Physician assistants and Mississippi. J Miss State Med Assoc 1994;25:353.

36. The Pew Health Professions Commission. Charting a Course for the Twenty-First Century: Physician Assistants and Managed Care. San Francisco, CA: UCSF Center for the Health Professions, 1998.

37. Teichman RF, Goldstein MD. Filling the void of well-trained occupational medicine physicians: a challenge for the 1990s. J Occup Med 1990;32:124.

38. Brandt LB, Beinfield MS, Laffaye HA, Baue AE. The training and utilization of surgical physician assistants: a retrospective study. Arch Surg 1989;124:348.

39. Hooker RS, Freeborn DK. Use of physician assistants in a managed health care system. Public Health Rep 1991;106:90.

40. Cawley, JF, Andrews MD, Barnhill G, Webb L, Hill IK. What makes the day: an analysis of the content of physician assistants' practice. J Am Acad Physician Assistants 2001;5:41.

41. AAPA-OM Board of Directors. AAPA-OM Newsletter, 1997.

42. Shaptini LA. J Occup Med 1991;33:907.

RESOURCES

Zenz C. Occupational Medicine: Principles and Practical Applications, ed 3. Chicago: Year Book Medical Publishers, 1994. *The reference book for occupational medicine. It is arranged into major sections consisting of important administrative factors, clinical occupational medicine, the physical occupational environment, the chemical occupational environment, and behavioral or psychosocial considerations. Its major goal is to acquaint practitioners with the basic operations of various occupational medicine departments, including employee health services in hospitals and community practice–related medicine; and to give an outline of certain administrative functions and some fundamentals of Workers' Compensation.*

Levy BS, Wegman DH. Occupational Health: Recognizing and Preventing Work-Related Disease, ed 1. Boston: Little, Brown & Co, 1983. *The fourth edition, published in 1999, has 864 pages but omits references to PAs. These soft-covered books are very readable. The first edition gives a good description of the role of the PA in occupational medicine. The third edition gives an explanation of causative contributions based on risk analysis. Both editions highlight recognition and prevention of occupational diseases, cover hazardous workplace exposures well, and describe occupational disorders by system. The latest edition includes useful appendices on researching toxic effects of chemical substances and professional educational opportunities.*

Harbison RD (ed). Hamilton and Hardy's Industrial Toxicology, ed 5. St. Louis: Mosby, 1998. *This is an excellent reference for hazardous substance toxicity, occupational exposure, and occupational health as well as risk assessment. It is based on the* books originated by Hamilton in 1934, which he later collaborated on with Harriet L. Hardy, another Harvard Medical School professor. Hamilton's pioneer wisdom is a compilation of current industrial hygiene practice combined with the authors' clinical experience as internists especially interested in industrial disease.

Silver RR. Basic Occupational Medicine: A Guide to Developing Delivery Systems. Boca Raton, FL: CRC Press, 1991. *This thin book is devoted to the special skills and knowledge necessary for the development of the industrial medical practitioner and an industrial medical practice within a hospital group or as a solo practitioner. It describes the usefulness of PAs in the occupational sphere; however, the description of the interaction between the PA and consultants exhibits scant knowledge of interprofessional cooperation or sensitivity.*

Rom WN (ed). Environmental and Occupational Medicine, ed 2. Boston: Little, Brown & Co, 1992. *This is a highly respected reference book that emphasizes the connection between the larger environment and an occupational exposure. It is well structured with excellent illustrations of occupational diseases.*

LaDou J (ed). Occupational Medicine, ed 2. Norwalk, CT: Appleton & Lange, 1997. *This book is a favorite soft-cover reference. The sections on occupational exposures by substance and the chapters on toxicology of specific chemical agents and target organ damage make this an affordable alternative for those in general medicine practice. Although relatively short, chapters devoted to environmental health, building-associated illnesses, and biostatistics and epidemiology offer a compact resource.*

Newsletter, American Academy of Physician Assistants in Occupational Medicine. Published quarterly by the AAPA, 950 N. Washington St., Alexandria, VA 22314-1552; (800) 596-4398; fax (703) 684-1924. Web site: http://www.aapa.org/paom.htm.

Journal of Occupational and Environmental Medicine. *The official publication of the American College of Occupational and Environmental Medicine is published monthly by Williams & Wilkins, 428 E. Preston Street, Baltimore, MD 21202-3993.*

Occupational Medicine: State of the Art Reviews (quarterly publication of Hanley & Belfus, Inc., 210 South 13th Street, Philadelphia, PA 19107). *The reviews, each about 190 pages, concentrate on one aspect of occupational medicine. Examples are back to school programs, pulmonary disease prevention, the nuclear energy industry, health hazards of farming, and the management perspective.*

Amdur MO, Doull J, Klassen CD (eds). Casarett and Doull's Toxicology: The Basic Science of Poisons, 5th ed. New York: McGraw-Hill, 1995. *This excellent book is the authoritative source book for toxicity of substances and their ability to poison or injure. Besides its readable and comprehensive information on basic toxicology, the chapter on occupational toxicology describes threshold limit values and time-weighted averages, describes clinical workplace survey techniques, and provides other practical information for the occupational clinician.*

Acute Low Back Problems in Adults: Assessment and Treatment. AHCPR Publication No. 95-0643. Rockville, MD: U.S. Department of Health and Human Services, Public Health Service, Agency for Health Care Policy and Research, December 1994. *Quick reference guide for clinicians.*

Ramos M. Guidelines on the role of physician assistants in occupational and environmental medicine. Available at http://www.aapa.org/ominfo.html. Accessed 22 April 2002.

CHAPTER 41

Behavioral Science: Essentials in Practice

F. J. Gino Gianola and H. James Lurie

INTRODUCTION

The physician assistant (PA) is one of the front-line providers who identifies and addresses the mental health needs of patients in the majority of clinical practices. Observations over the past 30 years by the authors indicate that this is the case regardless of practice location (inner city, suburban, or rural) or type (family practice, internal medicine, women's health, pediatrics, surgery, or transplant medicine). In this chapter, we describe common psychiatric problems confronting the PA today. We then provide some basic building blocks and resources for treatment of those problems.

As health practitioners work each day with the sick and the worried well, they strive for the mental as well as physical health of their patients. Before attempting to evaluate the mental health of a patient, clinicians should review their personal coping mechanisms in order to avoid projecting their own value systems onto the patient. The task for the PA who is

considering a psychiatric diagnosis is to gather data, evaluate, reflect, and formulate and implement therapies directed toward the needs of specific individuals.

We have included the *Diagnostic and Statistical Manual of Mental Disorders,* 4th edition (DSM-IV), criteria to familiarize the student with the classification system used for mental disorders.[1] This is also a valuable resource for practicing PAs who must use this system when completing insurance forms. The Resources section at the end of the chapter provides suggestions for further reading, including several Internet sites that can offer day-to-day assistance with questions on mental health.

MENTAL HEALTH

Improving mental health in the United States has been seen as a desirable goal. However, in recent years, restrictive guidelines for reimbursement by managed care services public and private insurance providers have imposed serious limitations on the ability of clinicians to assess and treat emotional problems that present in a clinical setting. Often, it is difficult for a PA to offer the in-depth services needed. At the same time, the patient who has been referred to a mental health practitioner or clinic is usually limited to a set number of reimbursed outpatient visits per year.

Compounding the problem are underserved populations who often have little access to mental health professionals. For better or worse, in remote and rural areas, the major source of mental health services is the primary care practitioner.[2] The American Academy of Family Practice in its mental health discussion paper, "Provision of Mental Health Care Services by Family Physicians," addressed the necessity of including basic mental health care services in a uniform benefits package. This discussion paper estimates that depression, anxiety disorders, and somatization occur in 20% to 30% of the primary care population.[3]

It has long been recognized that depression, anxiety, and somatization are disorders that commonly present in primary care settings. At the same time, the stigma attached to seeking help for emotional problems (including acknowledging the problem to oneself) often delays recognition and treatment of these disorders, sometimes for decades. Stoic feelings (e.g., "...if I'm a little blue or nervous, I have to deal with it myself...," or "...if I tell my doctor I'm depressed or nervous and receive treatment, do I have to mark it on my job application or insurance forms that ask, 'Have you ever been treated for a mental illness?' Will this jeopardize my job or my insurance coverage?") hinder a person from seeking mental health care. An additional complication is that mental health issues are seen very differently in the context of different racial and ethnic cultures. A problem that might be referred for psychiatric evaluation in one culture may be referred to a priest in another, and a family elder in a third. It seems clear, however, that PAs should be able to make accurate assessments of the most common emotional problems that present in primary care settings, establish at least a tentative diagnosis, have definite ideas about treatment (possibly in consultation with their preceptor physician or with a mental health professional), and be aware of community

resources for referral, patient education, support, and additional treatment.

Emotional problems that greatly impact the lives of patients have always been a major part of medicine. As was noted earlier, research suggests that between 40% and 70% of patients who present in an outpatient primary care setting have a primary emotional problem either as the major reason for their visit or as a major component of their physical complaint.[4] With the recent information explosion in neuroscience, as well as the increasing availability of pharmacological agents to treat specific psychiatric syndromes, the armamentarium of both psychiatric specialists and primary care practitioners has been increased enormously. Despite this hopeful state, many psychiatric disorders in primary care are underdiagnosed or misdiagnosed.[5] Unless the correct questions are asked, anxiety disorders and depressive disorders—two of the most common conditions seen in primary care settings—are often missed. The patient then returns with a myriad of puzzling somatic complaints.

Over the past 20 years, increasing emphasis has been placed on accurate classification of mental disorders for purposes of both research and reimbursement. The major classification system used in the United States is published in the *Diagnostic and Statistical Manual of Mental Disorders* (DSM), developed by the American Psychiatric Association, which is now in its fourth edition; hence the criteria are from the "DSM-IV" classification.[1] Wherever possible in this chapter, reference to this classification system is made because health care practitioners are expected to use this classification system when completing patient reimbursement forms for both private and public insurance providers (e.g., managed care, health maintenance organization, Medicare, Medicaid, and Social Security reimbursement forms).

The purpose of this chapter is to describe, with case examples, many of the major psychiatric syndromes likely to be seen by PAs, especially in primary care settings. We also provide some suggestions about brief psychotherapy (counseling). Because mental health issues pervade all aspects of medicine, this chapter obviously cannot be complete. However, the authors' hope is that it may serve as an introduction to psychiatric conditions, which are inseparable from those of "physical medicine," even if their descriptions appear to polarize the differences between "mind and body."

PSYCHOTHERAPY

People come to a primary care provider because they are anxious and worried. They miss work because they are experiencing a new or chronic pain. Often, they are concerned about issues that are more vague—not feeling "right" or wondering about a new pain or physical symptom. They may be having trouble sleeping, or they may be feeling anxious about some ill-defined sense of malaise. The "conventional" separation of mind and body simply does not apply to most patients. People develop symptoms after experiencing stress, and any physical symptom in turn induces stress and worry. The internal dialogue may go: "Is this the first symptom of a fatal disease? Am I developing heart trouble like what my father had when he was my age? Does this lump mean I have breast cancer? Is my PA going to suggest that my breast needs to be removed?"

The PA's role is to give information, identify issues, and educate, but most of all to give comfort to the patient who often has no other place to raise fears and worries with, and to receive reassurance and comfort from, a concerned yet objective provider.

For the PA who is willing, psychotherapy in a medical context is a natural, very helpful intervention, and it often takes much less time than expected. Psychotherapy in a medical context does not mean psychoanalysis. It does not mean an hour of counseling provided on a weekly basis. It does mean a focused intervention relevant to the specific patient and his or her concerns, often around a medical diagnosis. Following are eight suggestions about how to provide brief psychotherapy in the context of a medical encounter.

1. Listen for and inquire about the patient's concerns, both medical and psychological. Prioritize your patient's appointment time to listen to, clarify, and identify the concerns of the patient. The first 5 minutes of every scheduled encounter should be spent in assisting the patient to articulate his or her genuine concerns.

"...so, since you developed that pain, you wonder if you have the same heart disease that your Dad had at your age..."

Part of clarifying the patient's concerns involves finding out if an event (e.g., a change at home or at work, an anniversary, a birthday) might be a contributing factor. Clarifying a patient's statement often means repeating it in your own words, asking, "Do you mean...?", and restating the concerns (which may be multiple) in as simple and straightforward a manner as possible.

2. Empathize with the patient's apprehension and anxiety.

"...it must be very wearing on you to have that pain and not know whether it's serious or not ..."

3. Help the patient identify how the medical/psychological concern is affecting how he or she feels.

"...I'm always keyed up, worrying, about what might happen to my family. I can't sleep at night, and I'm having trouble concentrating at my job. My wife noticed I'm keyed up, but I haven't wanted to worry her, too... And sometimes, I've been feeling really down..."

"...so, you've been feeling anxious, fearful, and sometimes really down, too..."

4. In a sensitive and empathetic manner, develop a plan with the patient to help clarify the reality of the patient's concerns.

"What I think we should do first, is to get a more detailed history of all your symptoms—anything leading up to them; any stress contributing to them. We should then do a good physical exam and get some lab work and an ECG, and maybe a stress test (depending on what the ECG reveals). We need to make some time to go over the results. It is also crucial that we talk about how we can deal with your anxiety, which is really making your life so uneasy."

5. Educate the patient in an empathic manner about heart disease and anxiety. Affirm that feeling anxious is normal and is not a sign of weakness. Reassure the patient that depression often follows anxiety about a real or feared loss. Although this is "normal," both depression and anxiety must be monitored so they do not turn into serious, disabling conditions.

6. Offer your opinion about what would be helpful, but remember that the patient is the one who ultimately decides what is to be done. Arguing with or confronting the patient is rarely productive: Patients will "talk with their feet" and take neither your advice nor your medication. They are unlikely to return for the next appointment. Ultimately, by supporting the patient's choice, you can maintain an open dialogue and educate so as to be available to the patient even if you disagree with his or her current choice.

7. When you meet with a patient with a severe mental illness or who appears to be disregarding your opinions and "medical facts," it is important to explore his or her attitudes about having a particular diagnosis, taking medications, and having to "change behavior" for treatment to be beneficial. Try questions such as these:

   "...Do you feel that taking medication for depression is a sign of weakness?" or "...Does it seem that cutting down on fats and sugars is just too much of a sacrifice?"

8. A regular appointment schedule for follow-up is important in many cases. You and the patient will be able to evaluate how the patient's various concerns are resolving or whether the patient may need a referral to a mental health specialist.

REFERRAL: HOW AND WHEN

When a PA makes a referral to a specialist for liver disease, the reason is that the issues of the disorder are beyond the scope of the practice, knowledge, and skill of the PA. The referral seems straightforward, and both the PA and the patient tend to accept the need for more "expert" opinion for management and treatment.

PAs and patients have a tendency to be much more ambivalent about referral to a counselor, a psychiatrist (a doctor of medicine trained in psychological issues and also able to prescribe medications), or a psychologist (a person with expert training in the diagnosis and treatment of psychological problems with the use of behavioral and other therapies). Patients often do not understand that a referral to someone accustomed to dealing with complex psychological situations is like any other medical referral. Rather than being an admission of failure or weakness, this referral is simply a procedure to help the patient resolve symptoms as expeditiously as possible. The PA needs to remain positive about the referral, negotiating with the patient about keeping in touch and continuing to care for the patient's other medical problems.

   "...Gordon, you have what's called technically 'a major depression,' which is a biochemical disorder of the nervous system. Although it was set off by your divorce, we've talked about how it runs in your family, and you have mentioned that in the past you had a bad setback when you were in college. We've tried a couple of medications but you're still feeling pretty teary and sad. I'm worried about you. I'd like you to see a colleague that I've worked with, who is much more familiar with a wide variety of other treatments and medications that might be helpful for you. I want to keep seeing you here in the office and, with the help of my colleague, I'm sure this situation will improve. I need your agreement before I make the referral..."

MENTAL STATUS EXAMINATION

As with other types of referrals, before you refer your patient to a mental health specialist, it is imperative that you gather data. Information on the mental status examination (MSE) can be found in the box on p. 878. This formal mental status examination is used when needed, especially in cases in which you are concerned about a psychotic disorder.

The Mini-Mental Status Examination (MMSE) (see box on p. 878) is most often used for determination of dementia or delirium. This test takes about 10 minutes. It includes fewer categories than the complete MSE, and the MMSE is scored. The problem with using the MMSE is that it is insensitive to patients with a low educational level, poor language skills, or impaired vision. Scores for patients with lower educational levels or poor language skills tend to be lower. The primary care provider should be aware of the cultural insensitivity of the MMSE when incorporating the tool into an examination. The provider should be careful not to misinterpret the cultural insensitivity of the test by presuming that the results reflect a lower educational level.

MENTAL STATUS EXAMINATION (MSE)

Appearance	Level of consciousness: alert, hypervigilant, drowsy, stuporous
	Dress, grooming, idiosyncrasies
Behavior	Cooperative, aggressive, ambiguous, hostile
Speech	Rate: rapid, forced, slowed
	Volume: loud, soft monotone, dramatic
	Quality: flowing, peculiar
Affect/Mood	Silly, anxious, labile, controlled, unreserved, blunted, flat
Thought process	Tangential, disorganized, loose associations, flight of ideas
Thought content	Delusions, grandiose, paranoid, bizarre
	Document precisely what the patient appears to believe
	Thought broadcasting, thought insertion
	Suicidal or homicidal ideations, including plan and intent
Perception	Hallucinations, illusions (auditory, visual, somatic, tactile)
	Belief in hallucinations that originate inside or outside, how many voices
Cognition	Level of awareness: aware of situation
Level of alertness	Orientation to person, place, and time
Memory	Immediate, short-term, and long-term
Attention	Digital span serial 7s; spell *world* backward
Calculation	Ability to calculate change from a transaction, addition, subtraction
Fund of knowledge	
Abstractions	Proverb interpretation, similarities
Insight	Knows something is wrong, understands illness is present and is psychiatric
Judgment	Does the behavior match stated goals; response to standard questions (What would you do if you smelled smoke in a crowded theater?); Is patient behaving appropriately for the situation?

MINI-MENTAL STATUS EXAMINATION

The MMSE includes the following tasks:

Orientation (10 points)	What is the date: (year, season, date, day, month)—5 points
	Where are we: (state, country, town, hospital, floor)—5 points
Registration (3 points)	Name three objects: Each one spoken distinctly with a brief pause. Patient repeats all three with one point for each. Score is determined by first repetition. Record number of trials needed to learn all three objects.
Attention and calculation (5 points)	Either serial 7s counting backward from 100, or spell *world* backward. Points are awarded for each correct answer up to the first miscalculation or misspelled letter.
Recall (3 points)	Recite the 3 objects memorized in the Registration Section.
Language (9 points)	Patient names two objects that he or she is shown (watch, pencil) (1 point each)
	Repeat a sentence: "No if's, and's, or but's." (1 point)
	Follow a three-stage command: Take a piece of paper in your right hand, fold it in half, and put in on the floor. (3 points)
	Read and obey the following: Write on a blank piece of paper, "Close your eyes." Ask the patient to read and do what it says. (1 point)
	Ask the patient to copy a design (intersecting pentagons). All 10 angles must be present, and 2 must intersect. (1 point)

Total maximum score is 30 points. Commonly, a score of less than 24 is indicative of dementia or delirium.

DEPRESSIVE DISORDERS

CASE STUDY 41-1

A 70-year-old widower whose wife died 2 years ago presents to a primary care office because of weight loss, fatigue, a persistent cough, and "feeling run down." At one time a heavy smoker, the patient now smokes only half a pack of cigarettes a day. The patient has always prided himself on his independence and athletic stamina but began to lose interest in his usual daily walks about a year after his wife died. Clinically, the patient is alert, but he looks slightly sad and anxious. He states that he doesn't enjoy much of anything anymore, except for watching sports on TV. His sleep is restless. His speech is slightly slowed. His memory and concentration are slightly decreased. Physical examination reveals some bilateral rhonchi. An extensive workup was done for medical problems that might explain his symptoms. All laboratory tests, including chest x-ray, are relatively normal. On the second visit for these complaints, he begins to discuss his sorrow after his wife's death and the fact that he sometimes wishes he were dead so he could "join her." In response to specific questions about suicidal ideation, he says he has considered suicide and has a loaded gun but "wouldn't have the guts to use it." After intensive treatment for a depressive disorder, most of the patient's symptoms disappear. Within 2 months, he says that, although he still greatly misses his wife, he now feels "more his old self" (see Clinical Applications at end of chapter).

Depression is one of the most common conditions seen in medicine, affecting 10% to 20% of the population at any given time, with 4% to 8% of the population having full-blown clinical depression. Women have twice the incidence of depression as men.[6] (In depression, as in several other disorders such as schizophrenia, Alzheimer's disease, anxiety disorders, and alcoholism, neuroendocrine differences between men and women produce different incidence ratios and different clinical courses.[7]) For unclear reasons, the incidence of depression has gradually increased throughout this century. More people are becoming depressed and at an earlier age.[6,8] According to experts, only one quarter of depressed individuals receive treatment.[9] As was mentioned previously, some of this occurs because many people with depression feel that seeking help is a sign of moral weakness. In other cases, health practitioners either minimize depressive symptoms as "normal," or do not ask the right questions to establish a diagnosis.

Although everyone has depressed feelings or a depressed mood from time to time in response to disappointment or loss, such feelings usually go away after a short time and respond to reassurance and affection. Depression as a disorder is more pervasive and disabling and does not rapidly remit. Current clinical research suggests that signs and symptoms of a depressive disorder are related to biochemical changes in the brain. Once established, such symptoms left untreated usually do not disappear in less than a year. Depression is also associated with a worse outcome when it occurs with physical illness, such as coronary artery disease.[9,10]

It has been the authors' experience and observation that primary care providers tend to treat depressed patients for too brief a time and at too low a dose of medication.

Major Depression (DSM-IV 296.2)

Signs and Symptoms Five or more of the following symptoms during the same 2-week period are needed for this diagnosis. At least one of the symptoms is either a depressed mood or a loss of interest or pleasure in usual activities. These (single episode) symptoms cause significant distress, are not due to substance use, and are not caused primarily by bereavement.

1. Depressed mood most of the day, nearly every day.
2. Diminished interest or pleasure in most activities.
3. Significant weight loss (>5% body weight loss in a month) or decrease or increase in appetite.
4. Insomnia or hypersomnia nearly every day.
5. Motor agitation or retardation nearly every day.
6. Fatigue or loss of energy.
7. Feelings of worthlessness or excessive guilt.
8. Decreased ability to think or concentrate.

9. Recurrent thoughts of death, suicidal ideation, or a suicide attempt or specific plan.

In Case Study 41-1, although it was possibly triggered by the death of his spouse, this man's depression fit the criteria for a major depression and required medication, supportive individual counseling, referral to a support group, and mobilization of his support network to achieve remission of his symptoms. The sleep disturbance and depressed mood responded fairly rapidly. His energy level and appetite took a longer time to readjust.

Differential Diagnosis   A number of common illnesses, nonprescription drugs, and prescribed medications can produce depression. Illnesses include cancer, viral disease, endocrine abnormalities, anemia, stroke, and liver disease. Medications, including oral contraceptives, steroids, some β-blockers, L-dopa, and methyldopa, can cause depression. Drugs that can trigger depression include alcohol and narcotics; withdrawal from amphetamines or cocaine can do the same. Depressive symptoms can also exist in schizophrenia, dementia, and anxiety disorders. Depression is found in manic-depressive illness in which an individual has elevated mood, increased energy, decreased need for sleep, and poor judgment alternating with the more classical symptoms of major depression.

Treatment   Treatment measures include medications, focused psychotherapy, and emotional support. Many medications are available and effective in treating depression. However, in primary care settings, patients often do not receive medications long enough and in adequate dosages for them to be effective. Prescribing a "mild" (subtherapeutic) dose of an antidepressant is often useless. If a patient's depression requires medication, the patient requires a full, therapeutic dose.

Support can come from family, friends, and primary care providers. Support represents the mainstay of treatment for depression. Experts in the treatment of depressive disorders also advise clinicians who treat depressed patients to do the following[11]:

➤ Establish a supportive and positive relationship.
➤ Have regular appointments with the patient.

➤ Maintain a hopeful attitude with the patient.
➤ Set realistic goals.
➤ Explore and confront negative thinking through diaries and discussion with the primary care clinician.
➤ Involve the family and/or other supportive individuals.

Focused counseling usually requires referral to a mental health professional and is often useful if depression persists despite adequate medication and support, or if the patient has more than two episodes of major depression.

Anxiety Disorders

CASE STUDY 41-2

A 16-year-old girl with spina bifida dropped out of high school after she had several panic attacks at school. These were triggered initially by the fact that she was being teased by other students for occasional episodes of urinary incontinence at school. She became increasingly fearful of leaving her house, and over several months became fearful of being alone at home in the absence of family members. She became anxious and tremulous at the thought of going outside. During her occasional episodes of panic, she experienced rapid heartbeat, a sense of doom, a feeling that she might be choking to death, trouble catching her breath, sweating, and numbness of her hands. On several occasions, her worried parents brought her to an emergency department because she thought from her symptoms that she was having a heart attack. Eventually, she consented to come to a primary care clinic to rule out medical causes for her condition. She had told her parents after her last panic attack (which lasted 3 hours) that she would rather be dead than continue to experience "these terrible episodes." After treatment was begun with both medication from her PA and behavioral techniques administered by a psychologist, her symptoms of both panic attacks and generalized anxiety were sufficiently alleviated that she could gradually return to school on a limited basis. Stabilization of her symptoms took a number of months and involved a number of different medication trials, but eventually was moderately successful (see Clinical Applications at the end of the chapter).

Anxiety disorders are very common in the general population and in primary care practice. About a third of otherwise normal individuals have sporadic panic attacks, and about 1% to 2% of the population have severe enough symptoms to be diagnosed as having a panic disorder. Severe fearfulness of leaving the home environment and severe specific phobias occur in 2% to 5% of the general population, and about one fifth of people have milder phobias. About 5% of the general population have symptoms of generalized anxiety. Anxiety symptoms are often misdiagnosed and undertreated.[9,10]

In many cases, anxiety is accompanied by depression. Although the primary care provider often treats the symptoms of anxiety adequately, the depression is frequently not treated appropriately. If medication is prescribed, it may be at too low a dose or for too short a time.

Several different conditions are included under the general heading "anxiety disorders." These include post-traumatic stress disorder (PTSD), obsessive-compulsive disorder (OCD), panic disorder with or without agoraphobia, social phobia (social anxiety disorder), and specific phobia.

Generalized Anxiety Disorder (DSM-IV 300-02)

In this disorder, there is excessive anxiety and worry more days than not about a number of events or activities. The person finds it difficult to control the worry, and anxiety and worry are associated with three or more of the following six symptoms:

1. Restlessness.
2. Being easily fatigued.
3. Difficulty concentrating.
4. Irritability.
5. Muscle tension.
6. Sleep disturbance (difficulty falling or staying asleep, or restless, unsatisfying sleep).

Anxiety, worry, or physical symptoms cause significant distress or impairment in social, occupational, or other important areas of functioning.

Pharmacological Treatment of Anxiety Disorders It is well beyond the scope of this chapter to describe in detail the specific treatments available for the different forms of anxiety disorder. However, pharmacological treatments are generally used to treat each type of anxiety disorder. The difficulty in generalizing about treatment in large part results from research that increasingly indicates that different areas of the brain are involved in the different disorders, and that different neurochemical mechanisms mediate their clinical expression. In general, however, antianxiety agents, such as buspirone and the benzodiazepines, are used for generalized anxiety disorders, whereas disorders involving panic often respond to the newer antidepressants, especially the selective serotonin reuptake inhibitors (SSRIs). Older antidepressants such as the monoamine oxidase inhibitors (MAOIs) are very effective but tricky to use because of their dangerous interactions with certain foods and medications.

Phobias and social avoidance problems are treated with a combination of antianxiety medications, along with behavioral treatments such as relaxation training and desensitization to the feared stimulus.[4,6] Certain kinds of social anxiety, such as performance anxiety, respond to β-blockers, a type of antihypertensive agent.

Obsessive-compulsive disorder requires both treatment with SSRIs (often in high doses) and training that enables the patient to stop and interrupt obsessive thinking or compulsive rituals. "Cognitive restructuring" is often useful for this disorder. The patient learns to "correct" his or her obsessional thinking (e.g., "I know that even if I feel I must wash my hands, nothing bad will happen if I stop myself from doing it").[11]

The treatment of PTSD is highly complex and often involves specialized group and individual therapy, as well as antidepressants and antianxiety medications.

In patients with each of these conditions, the PA who is interested can often play a major role in identifying the disorder; in less complex cases, the PA can also be instrumental in providing treatment. The PA can serve as a "case manager" and triage person for patients with those disorders that often fluctuate in intensity throughout the life span.

Situation-Specific Anxiety in Medically Ill Patients

According to Dubovsky,[6] certain types of anxiety arise in response to specific situations, especially in the medically ill. These include the following:

1. *Separation anxiety.* Anxiety occurs when the patient is separated from an important caregiver. This may express itself in fearfulness, disruptive behavior, physical complaints, or increased demands for attention.

2. *Stranger anxiety.* Although normal in childhood, this is manifested by distress or increased complaints when the patient is confronted by unfamiliar health care providers.

3. *Anxiety about dependency.* These individuals are threatened by any situation that makes them feel dependent. They may devalue those who offer help or may refuse to comply with treatment.

4. *Anxiety about loss of control.* This type of anxiety occurs when important decisions are taken out of the hands of patients, such as when they require hospitalization. These patients argue about diagnosis, are noncompliant, may fail to keep appointments, and may remain oppositional to regain a sense of control.

5. *Anxiety about the meaning of an illness.* Such patients may, for example, engage in inappropriately seductive behavior if they are worried about no longer being attractive.

6. *Signal anxiety.* Patients may overreact to medical situations if such situations evoke "bad" thoughts or emotions that the patient has previously tried to suppress.

Differential Diagnosis

A variety of medical conditions can produce symptoms that mimic anxiety disorders. These include cardiovascular disease such as paroxysmal tachycardia; endocrine or metabolic disorders, such as hypoglycemia or thyroid disease; multiple sclerosis; acute organic brain syndromes of any cause; tumors such as pheochromocytoma or carcinoid; pulmonary disorders, including hypoxemia and pulmonary embolism; and infectious agents such as tuberculosis. Medications and nonprescription drugs that may cause anxiety include central nervous system stimulants such as amphetamines, cocaine, caffeine, monosodium glutamate, theophylline, and neuroleptics (which produce akathisia, a kind of motor restlessness).

Nonpharmacological Treatment Approaches

In addition to medication, a variety of other treatments are often effective for these disorders. These include reassurance, explanations, and patient education about treatments (especially if the patient has specific concerns about the treatment), systematic exposure to feared situations, and relaxation and visualization techniques to assist in immediate reduction of anxiety. For treating phobias, systematic desensitization is often used together with medication. In the office, the patient initially uses a relaxation technique and then progressively visualizes scenes of increasing anxiety, signaling the clinician as the anxiety appears and relaxing again until the anxiety disappears. Outside of the office, the patient actually enters the scenes that were visualized, transferring the habit of relaxation to the actual phobic setting. Other techniques include providing support, encouraging the patient to use mechanisms such as exercise that have previously been helpful in stressful situations, and encouraging denial for those patients who tend to dwell too much on the danger they are in. Family counseling is sometimes useful to help individuals maintain progress, so that the family does not inadvertently encourage dependence or regression.

Panic Disorder with Agoraphobia (DSM-IV 300.2)

Signs and Symptoms   Recurrent, unexpected panic attacks. A discrete period of intense fear or discomfort occurs, in which four or more of the following symptoms develop abruptly and reach a peak within 10 minutes:

➤ Palpitations, pounding, or accelerated heart rate.
➤ Sweating, trembling, or shaking.
➤ Sensation of shortness of breath or smothering.
➤ Feeling of choking, chest pain, or discomfort.
➤ Nausea or abdominal distress.
➤ Feeling of dizziness or lightheadedness; fainting.
➤ Feeling of unreality or of being detached from oneself.
➤ Fear of losing control or going crazy.
➤ Fear of dying.

At least one of the attacks must have been followed by fear of having additional attacks, worry about the consequences of the attack (e.g., going crazy), or a significant change in behavior related to the attacks.

Agoraphobia is diagnosed when the following two symptoms occur:

1. Anxiety about being in places or situations from which escape might be difficult or embarrassing, or where help may not be available in case of another panic attack. (Agoraphobia often involves being outside the home alone, being in a crowd or standing in a line, being on a bridge, or traveling by car, train, or bus.)
2. Situations are avoided or endured with marked distress.

Panic Disorder Without Agoraphobia (DSM-IV 300.01)

Although panic attacks (see earlier) occur in this situation, accompanied by concern about additional attacks, the patient is not immobilized to the point of avoiding such situations.

Agoraphobia Without History of Panic Disorder (DSM-IV 300.22)

The patient has a fear of developing paniclike symptoms without having experienced the symptoms that meet the criteria for panic disorder.

Specific Phobia (DSM-IV 300.29)

An excessive or unreasonable fear in the presence or in anticipation of a specific situation or object (e.g., insects, flying, heights). Exposure to the phobic stimulus almost invariably provokes an immediate anxiety response.

Social Phobia (DSM-IV 300.23A)

Marked and persistent fear of one or more social or performance situations in which the person is exposed to unfamiliar people or to possible scrutiny by others. The individual fears that he or she will act in a way that will be humiliating or embarrassing. Exposure to the feared situation almost invariably provokes anxiety or a panic attack. Individuals avoid such situations or endure them with intense anxiety; this avoidance interferes with their normal routine, occupational functioning, or social activities or relationships.

Obsessive-Compulsive Disorder (OCD) (DSM-IV 300.3)

The person has either obsessions or compulsions. Obsessions are recurrent intrusive and inappropriate thoughts, impulses, or images that cause marked anxiety or distress that the individual attempts to ignore or suppress. Compulsions are repetitive behaviors (e.g., hand washing, checking) or mental acts (e.g., praying, counting, repeating words) that the person feels driven to perform in response to an obsession. With both obsessions and compulsions, the individual recognizes that the obsessions or compulsions are excessive or unreasonable.

Post-traumatic Stress Disorder (PTSD) (DSM-IV 309.81)

The individual has experienced, witnessed, or been confronted by events that involved threatened death or serious injury, or a threat to the physical integrity of self or others. The person's response involved intense fear, helplessness, or horror. The traumatic event is persistently re-experienced in one or more of the following ways:

1. Recurrent and distressing recollections of the event, including images, thoughts, or perceptions (e.g., "flashbacks").
2. Recurrent distressing dreams of the events.
3. Acting or feeling that the event is recurring.

This includes a sense of reliving the experience, illusions, hallucinations, or dissociative flashback episodes, including those that occur on awakening or when intoxicated. Symptoms are accompanied by intense psychological distress, including persistent symptoms of increased arousal (e.g., difficulty falling asleep, irritability, difficulty concentrating, hypervigilance, and exaggerated startle response). There is persistent avoidance of stimuli associated with the trauma, as well as numbing of general responsiveness by reactions such as avoiding thoughts or conversations associated with the trauma and avoiding activities that arouse recollection of the trauma, inability to recall aspects of the trauma, diminished interest in significant activities, feelings of detachment or estrangement from others, restricted range of affect (e.g., unable to have loving feelings), and the sense of a foreshortened future (doesn't expect to have a career or a normal life span).

PSYCHOTIC DISORDERS

Beginning in the 1960s, motivated by the success of new antipsychotic medications, a humanitarian effort was undertaken to discharge patients from mental hospitals and place them back into their communities. For financial reasons, many individuals with chronic psychosis who previously had lived for years inside a protected hospital setting were released precipitously into the community. Although some of these efforts were successful, many patients were unable to mediate the demands of community living. They ended up homeless, incarcerated in prison, or rehospitalized. In recent years, younger patients who develop severe mental illness, especially schizophrenia, may never be hospitalized but may still have great difficulty coping in the community. They run afoul of the law because of poor judgment and often use alcohol and drugs as a way of coping with their psychotic symptoms. Although many of these individuals have their mental illness supervised by mental health professionals, such individuals usually have their health care needs met by primary care providers, including PAs. It is important, therefore, for PAs to be aware of signs and symptoms of psychotic disorders and to work collaboratively with mental health professionals in identifying early symptoms of decompensation.

Schizophrenia

Signs and Symptoms Schizophrenia usually arises during the late teens and early 20s. It is often preceded by a "prodromal phase" in which a person whose previous functioning was reasonably good becomes disorganized, withdrawn, and suspicious. The person shows increasingly impaired reality testing. To meet DSM-IV criteria for schizophrenia, an individual must show, during the "active" phase of the disorder, continuous signs of a disturbance for at least 6 months. Two or more of the following symptoms must be present during a 1-month period:

1. *Delusions.* The patient exhibits fixed, false ideas that are inconsistent with his or her culture or religion and cannot be corrected by rational argument. They may be poorly organized or complex and somaticized. They may be bizarre and sometimes are associated with a depressed or elevated mood.

2. *Hallucinations.* These are perceptual experiences that occur in the absence of an actual stimulus. Auditory and visual hallucinations are most common. Olfactory, tactile, and complex visual hallucinations are more common with other organic mental syndromes, such as intoxication, seizure disorders, and tumors.

3. *Disorganized speech.* This symptom is often a reflection of both the individual's difficulty in concentration and the bizarre content of the individual's thoughts. It may also show the unusual form of the individual's thinking (e.g., a patient's conversation is "derailed" when he says a word that reminds him of a word with a similar sound, even though there is no other connection between the words). A patient may also have "loose associations" in which he or she interprets abstract sayings in a highly idiosyncratic fashion, for example, "a table and a chair are alike because they sit together to pray."

4. *Gross disorganization or catatonic behavior.* In this situation, the patient may become severely withdrawn, mute, and unresponsive to questions or requests and may even be incontinent.

5. *Negative symptoms.* The patient shows affective flattening (no emotional expression), may display limited or absent speech, and reveals the absence of interest in any activities or participation.

The person with schizophrenia also shows a marked deterioration in areas of work, interpersonal relations, and self-care compared with previous levels of functioning.

Antipsychotic medications have become increasingly refined so that newer medications produce fewer adverse effects than do the older medications used for the treatment of psychosis. Many individuals who had some remission of hallucinations and delusions were very troubled by motor stiffness, involuntary motor restlessness, and at times, acute motor spasms. In addition, negative symptoms were usually not helped by the older medications. Now, many patients using the newer antipsychotic medications are able to live independently, can be employed, and have a much brighter affect and a higher energy level. Despite these improvements, many individuals with residual schizophrenia continue to display poor judgment, exhibit intermittent drug or alcohol abuse or dependence, have difficulty managing money, and receive marginal health care. This is often so because of poor compliance, confusion about the need for medical follow-up, poor coping and problem-solving skills, and problems in trusting authority figures. During assessment of an individual with schizophrenia who presents to a primary care setting, the following questions are crucial:

➤ Is the patient currently taking antipsychotic medications regularly; does he or she know how much and how often?

➤ What is the patient's source of financial security? Can he or she buy and take medications that the PA might prescribe?

➤ How impaired is the patient currently? Is the patient oriented? How intact are memory and judgment? Is the need to continue on medication and to have follow-up acknowledged by the patient? Does the patient understand the medical conditions you are assessing and treating? Can the patient be relied on to take medications? Does the patient need supervision for medication compliance?

➤ Is the patient currently using/abusing recreational drugs or alcohol? Are these a major impediment to compliance with the medical regimen?

➤ Who else in the patient's support system can be contacted for assistance to help with compliance (e.g., a case manager, mental health personnel, family members)?

Differential Diagnosis   Psychotic thinking may sometimes be associated with other disorders besides schizophrenia. These include delirium, dementia, toxic states, and mood disorders. Also included is psychosis associated with severe depressive illness or with manic-depressive illness, especially during the manic phase when grandiose delusions are very common.

Treatment   Although mental health professionals usually undertake the treatment of schizophrenia, a treatment team is often necessary for an individual with schizophrenia to remain stable. This team often includes a case manager (to "keep track" of the afflicted individual and often manage his or her money), family members (who need education about

the disorder to help provide appropriate support and structure), a primary care team to keep track of the medical aspects of the patient's condition, and, whenever possible, a community advocacy component (such as the National Alliance for the Mentally Ill) to keep track of resources in the community, educate health and mental health providers, and serve as a source of legal and financial advocacy if necessary.

Delirium and Dementia

Because the population of the United States is growing older and is living longer, an important component of primary care practices involves (and will increasingly involve) assessment and management of individuals who, as they become older, develop increasing memory problems. Major diagnostic categories of particular concern are delirium and dementia.

Delirium (DSM-IV 293.0)   Delirium is a syndrome that involves a disturbance in consciousness, which shows the following characteristics:

1. Disturbance of consciousness, with reduced clarity of awareness of the environment and with reduced ability to focus, sustain, or shift attention.
2. A change in cognitive abilities, such as memory deficit, disorientation, language disturbance, or the development of a perceptual disturbance.
3. The disturbance develops over a short period and tends to fluctuate over the course of the day.

Delirium can be secondary to medication or drug intoxication (e.g., minor tranquilizers), metabolic conditions (e.g., diabetic ketoacidosis), medication or substance withdrawal (e.g., abrupt withdrawal of benzodiazepines), or acute physical illness (e.g., a febrile illness). Because in an elderly person delirium often occurs in tandem with a more fixed and permanent memory problem (i.e., dementia), it is crucial that a primary care provider take a careful history and do a thorough mental status and physical examination to differentiate how much the memory problem is related to an irreversible process and how much is related to an acute medical problem.

Dementia (DSM-IV 290.1)   Dementia is a chronic disturbance of memory, judgment, and intellectual functioning, without prominent clouding of consciousness. Onset is often insidious. Two of the most common forms of dementia are dementia of the Alzheimer's type and vascular dementia (related to cerebral anoxia or small brain infarcts).

Dementia of Alzheimer's Type
Criteria for dementia of the Alzheimer's type include multiple cognitive deficits manifested by both of the following:
1. Memory impairment (impaired ability to learn new information or to recall previously learned information).
2. One or more of the following cognitive disturbances:
   a. Aphasia (language disturbance).
   b. Apraxia (impaired ability to carry out motor activities despite intact motor function).
   c. Agnosia (failure to recognize or identify objects despite intact sensory function).
   d. Disturbance in executing functioning (i.e., planning, organizing, sequencing, abstracting).
3. Cognitive deficits that cause significant impairment in social or occupational functioning and that represent a significant decline from a previous level of functioning.
4. Course that is characterized by gradual onset and continuing cognitive decline.[12]

Vascular Dementia (DSM-IV 290.4)
Vascular dementia has similar criteria, except that focal neurological signs and symptoms or laboratory evidence of cerebrovascular disease is present, and the clinical course usually shows episodic rather than gradual decline (as in Alzheimer's-type dementia).

A number of diagnostic tests, such as the Mini-Mental Status Examination, are useful for documenting the degree and type of impairment, especially when a patient is followed over an extended time.[13] Because elderly patients are especially sensitive and embarrassed about memory or other cognitive losses, an evaluation for dementia and delirium must be done with great tact, sensitivity, and reassurance.

CONCLUSION

The primary care practitioner should be familiar with common emotional problems that present in clinical settings, be able to make an assessment (sometimes with consultation from a mental health specialist), and have sufficient knowledge, compassion, empathy, and skills to be able to develop a subsequent effective course of action, ranging from pharmacological intervention to referral for counseling, support, additional education, or, if necessary, hospitalization. The outcome of medical treatment in primary care settings (for instance, with diabetes or hypertension) depends as much on awareness of the interaction or co-morbidity between medical and psychological factors or conditions as on knowing the dosage of the appropriate medication. The mind and body have never been separate domains; research increasingly is documenting their interdependence for homeostasis and health.[14] However, as Faber observes, "In the final analysis, the goal of neuropsychiatric assessment is to understand the patient and explain his or her predicament, leading to maximally effective treatment. Mainly through empathy and pertinent observation, clinicians can understand psychologically the patient's pain, distress, and dysphoria."[15]

CLINICAL APPLICATIONS

1. What is the most common mental health coverage provided by Medicare, Medicaid, and private insurers? For your patients, are inpatient or outpatient therapies reimbursed better? What is the average number of outpatient visits covered? What is the ceiling coverage for inpatient care, and is there a limit to the number of times a patient can be admitted for inpatient treatment? For the provider, does inpatient or outpatient care lead to better reimbursement?
2. What type of training do religious leaders (e.g., ministers, priests, rabbis) receive for counseling their members?
3. Would you access members of the religious community for counseling patients in your practice who are members of their congregations? If yes, how would you access them? What about patient confidentiality?
4. What are some of the economic effects of untreated depression and anxiety? On the patient, on the local community, nationally?

5. In Case Study 41-1 of the 70-year-old widower, what are your specific treatment options, and what specific medications would you use and why? What are your follow-up strategies?

6. This patient states that he feels like his "old self" after 2 months of receiving your therapies. What are your major concerns? What are your follow-up plans at this point?

7. What is the estimated number of cases of depression in your community? Why? What are the percentages by age?

8. In Case Study 41-2, the 16-year-old has returned to school on a limited basis. In your community, what types of social service and school support exist for children reentering school after mental health treatment, including medications? Is there a systematic way of teaching children without disabilities about their classmate with physical and mental challenges, especially for children who are preteens and teens?

9. This teenager is presently stabilized. What is your follow-up plan for her at this point in her therapy? What is your major concern? Why?

10. Specifically, how do you involve the family in her continued therapy?

11. Let us assume she is now visiting colleges to make a choice of where to go. She and her family ask what they should look for to ensure her continued successful therapy. How would you approach this question? What would you do now?

REFERENCES

1. Diagnostic and Statistical Manual of Mental Disorders, ed 4 (DSM-IV). Washington, DC: American Psychiatric Press, 1994.

2. Hartley D. Rural primary care practitioners are a major source of mental health services. Rural Health Quarterly 1997;7:1.

3. AAFP Position Paper on the Provision of Mental Health Care Services by Family Physicians, 1996. Available at http://www.aafp.org/practice/mentalhe.html.

4. Marmor J. In: Lurie HJ (ed). Practical Management of Emotional Problems in Medicine. New York: Raven, 1982.

5. Sheikh JI. Anxiety disorders. In: Coffey CE, Cummings JL (eds). Textbook of Geriatric Neuropsychiatry. Washington, DC: American Psychiatric Press, 1994.

6. Dubovsky SL. Clinical Psychiatry. Washington, DC: American Psychiatric Press, 1988.

7. Seeman MV. Psychopathology in women and men: focus on female hormones. Am J Psychiatry 1997;154:1641.

8. Weller EB, Weller RA. Mood disorders. In: Lewis M (ed). Child and Adolescent Psychiatry. Baltimore: Williams & Wilkins, 1991.

9. Glassman GH, Stoll AL. Depression and the course of coronary artery disease. Am J Psychiatry 1998;155:4.

10. Salzman C, Lebowitz BD (eds). Anxiety and the Elderly. New York: Springer, 1991.

11. Towbin K, Riddle MA. Obsessive-compulsive disorder. In: Lewis M (ed). Child and Adolescent Psychiatry. Baltimore: Williams & Wilkins; 1991.

12. Diagnostic Criteria from DSM-IV. Washington, DC: American Psychiatric Association, 1994.

13. Folstein M, Folstein S, McHugh P. Mini-Mental State: a practical method for grading the cognitive state of patients for the clinician. J Psychiatr Res 1975;12:189.

14. Andreason N. Editorial: What shape are we in? Gender, psychopathology, and the brain. Am J Psychiatry 1997;154:1637.

15. Faber R. Neuropsychiatric assessment. In: Coffey CE, Cummings JL (eds). Textbook of Geriatric Neuropsychiatry. Washington DC: American Psychiatric Press, 1994.

RESOURCES

Diagnostic and Statistical Manual of Mental Disorders: Primary Care Version. Washington, DC: American Psychiatric Association, 1995. The basic manual for DSM-IV categories. *This edition is especially for the primary care provider and should be on your bookshelf for billing for your services and clarification of the diagnostic categories.*

Herman R, Kaplan M, LeMelle S. Psychoeducational debriefings after the September 11 disaster. Psychiatric Services 2002;53:479. *A useful article about the preventive effects of psychoeducational debriefings after a major disaster, and the beneficial impact this practice has on patients.*

Fishkind A. Calming agitation with words, NOT DRUGS. Current Psychiatry 2002;1:33. *Suggestions for primary care practitioners on how to calm down agitated and potentially violent patients, including what to say and how to say it. The article also outlines "rules" for how to approach agitated patients in general, especially those with a major mental disorder.*

Practice guidelines for the treatment of patients with bipolar disorder [revision]. Am J Psychiatry 2002;159:32. *Among the suggestions for dealing with a patient who is manic-depressive, these guidelines include specific ideas about how to discuss the illness with patients, as well as the kinds of psychological treatments and medications that are likely to be helpful.*

Amador X. I Am Not Sick. I Don't Need Your Help. Books for Life, Vida Press, 1150 Smith Road, Peconic, NY 11958 (pp 52-108). *This book is excellent in providing practical advice for both health practitioners and family members for dealing with the denial and resistance to accepting medications and therapy often displayed by patients with a mental illness. This book has been highly endorsed by the National Alliance for the Mentally Ill as a "bible" for family members in effectively dealing with a family member who has a mental illness.*

Hilliard JR. Manual of Clinical Emergencies in Psychiatry. Washington, DC: American Psychiatric Press, 1990. *A concise monograph regarding psychiatric emergencies and how they should be approached. Designed for psychiatric specialists and primary care providers.*

Knesper DJ, Riba MB, Swenk TL. Primary Care Psychiatry. Philadelphia: WB Saunders, 1997. *A comprehensive, lucid book that covers most topics the primary care provider will encounter in practice. Includes very good tables for reference.*

Maxwell J, Ward N. Essential Psychopathology and Its Treatment. New York: WW Norton & Co, 1995. *This is a well-written effective text of psychiatric diagnoses, which includes DSM-IV categories and case studies. It is a great read and provides essential information on diagnosis and treatment.*

Miller WR, Rollnick S. Motivational Interviewing. New York: Guilford, 1991. *A useful "how to do it" book that discusses therapeutic interviewing as it may apply to a primary care setting.*

http://healthlinks.washington. edu/clinical/psychiatry.html. *A good web site that points to resources and patient information, as well as some guidelines. Also includes three web guides, a medical matrix, a medical world search, and mental health net multiple links with these guides.*

http://www.psychlink.com. *A site that provides new professional resources and a database for mental health providers, as well as information for patients. Worth a visit.*

CHAPTER 42

Military Medicine

John L. Chitwood

INTRODUCTION

Shortages in U.S. health care systems (civilian and military) during the 1960s resulted in needs not being fulfilled by physicians. Shortfalls in military physician recruiting were made more serious by the unpopular war in Vietnam. The decrease in availability of health care providers to U.S. Department of Defense (DOD) beneficiaries became a reality, and physician scholarship programs were initiated to bring more physicians into the military services. This shortage was not helped by the length of time in the "training pipeline" it took for a physician to be educated. Even after a medical student had been selected to receive a scholarship that obligated him/her to military service, it took 5 years for a general medical officer (GMO, who has no residency training) to be educated, and up to 9 years for a board eligible physician to be trained. Physician assistants (PAs) and other physician extenders, such as nurse practitioners, were seen as the short-term answer to a potentially long-term problem.[1]

PA training programs were established in the U.S. Army, the U.S. Navy, and the U.S. Air Force in 1971. Enlisted military members with broad military and medical backgrounds were selected for advanced training as new health care professionals. Each curriculum consisted of 1 year of didactic training at various military educational facilities, and a 1-year rotational clinical practicum in a military hospital. After completion of the 2-year program, all new graduates were credentialed by either the military hospital to which they were assigned or the military hospital that had medical supervision over their clinical practice. These graduates were credentialed to provide routine and emergency primary care under the direct or indirect supervision of a physician. Secondary to manpower ceilings, these military training programs have been activated, deactivated, and then reactivated since 1977. When PAs had been initially trained in the military, they were used in the enlisted and warrant officer ranks. The Air Force began commissioning PAs as officers in 1978, the Navy in 1989, and the Army in 1992.

Originally, the military training programs awarded only certificates of completion because PA programs were viewed as advanced coursework for highly trained technicians that utilized the experience of existing military corpsmen. Military PA graduates now receive a certificate that enables them to sit for the National Commission for Certification of

Physician Assistants (NCCPA) certifying examination, along with a Bachelor of Science degree from a sponsoring university. A competitive bid process determines the sponsoring university. Military programs continue to grant a certificate so that, should there ever be a problem with the degree-granting institution's Accreditation and Review Committee for PA Programs (ARC-PA) status, graduates of a military program would still be eligible to sit for the NCCPA examination.

Before 1996, the Navy PA program trained students in one class annually in San Diego, California. The Air Force PA program educated 75 students in three matriculated classes annually, and the Army had 50 students enrolled in two classes each year. The U.S. Coast Guard relied on recruiting civilian PAs or sending enlisted personnel to a variety of civilian PA educational programs. In 1990, the U.S. Air Force School of Health Care Sciences began training Coast Guard PA students who received officer commissions upon graduation. The Navy also enrolled students in the Air Force program in the early days of military PA training. In 1996, all military PA training programs were consolidated into a single program located within the U.S. Army Medical Department Center and School at Fort Sam Houston, San Antonio, Texas. In the Interservice Physician Assistant Program (IPAP), there is a mixed faculty for didactic and clinical instruction that comprises PAs, science officers, and physicians, who represent each uniformed service and all contract civilian personnel. IPAP educates up to 200 students per year. This leads to a total yearly enrollment of up to 400 (200 in phase 1 and 200 in phase 2), making IPAP the largest PA program in existence. The IPAP curriculum confers 95 semester hours in the didactic phase at Fort Sam Houston and 50 hours during the clinical phase. Two thirds of the didactic phase hours are coded at the graduate level by the University of Nebraska (the affiliated university). All of the clinical phase hours have been coded as graduate level. This means that graduates of IPAP have a minimum of 91 semester hours of undergraduate work (60 are from prerequisite course work) and 113 graduate level hours. After the didactic phase, the students return to their host services' medical treatment facilities for clinical preceptorships.

Nonmilitary students from other federal agencies also attend IPAP.

The military services continue to rely heavily on IPAP to meet their respective PA inventory shortfalls. The recruitment of civilian PAs into active duty or into the National Guard or Reserve components is problematic for several reasons:

➤ Overall disparity in pay between the military services and the civilian sector.

➤ The maximum base pay of an O1E (second lieutenant with more than 4 years of enlisted service) is $31,662.00.[2] The average starting salary of a PA in 2001 was $59,839.00.[3] The military began offering the Thrift Savings Plan in January of 2002, and more than 30% of officers elected to participate during the first month.[4] It is too early to evaluate if this 401K-type plan will affect recruiting and retention.

➤ Some civilian-trained PAs may be overwhelmed by military productivity standards. The productivity expected (25+ patients per day) is not excessive; however, the support infrastructure (physical, fiscal, and personnel) is not as flexible and efficient as in civilian health care models.

➤ Adaptation to the role of a professional military officer first, and to the role of medical provider second, may appear to be too demanding and stressful. The application of these two standards can be disconcerting.

➤ The scope and demands of military practice may be broader than some PA roles in civilian practice. Military PAs often practice fairly autonomously in remote and austere situations. It is expected that they function by providing quality care with minimal support and consultation. It is not uncommon for the PA to rarely see the preceptor and to have only telephonic/radio contact on an as-needed basis.

Because the attrition of PAs continues in each branch of the uniformed services, service recruitment goals are not being met. However, it has become increasingly apparent that the granting of commissioned officer status to military PAs was a significant step in the right direction toward helping to solve PA manpower shortfalls. Incentives such as bonuses and educational scholarships, which have been used to recruit other medical professionals, should be used to recruit/retain PAs in the various components of the armed services.

The credentials committees of the various medical treatment facilities (MTFs) recommend to the MTF commander the individual clinical privileges of student and graduate military PAs, who are assigned to or provide care within the medical support areas of the MTF. Hospital commanders define in writing the scope and limits of the clinical practice for each PA and designate the supervising physician(s). Clinical privileges for PAs are determined on initial assignment, are reevaluated after any change of assignment, and are reviewed annually, unless more frequent evaluation is necessary.[5]

At present, there are approximately 1100 active duty PAs in the uniformed services. A majority of these PAs are working in primary care, family practice, emergency departments, troop medical clinics, or dispensaries. PAs are considered to be the "gatekeepers" of the DOD health care system. Having repeatedly been proven cost-effective, PAs are providing quality medical care while increasing accessibility to medical care for all types of DOD beneficiaries.

SCOPE OF PRACTICE

Military PAs principally work in primary care and family practice. They can also be found in acute care ("fast track") and emergency services. Military PAs may specialize in aviation medicine, bone marrow transplant, cardiovascular perfusion, education, emergency medicine, occupational medicine, orthopedics, otolaryngology, oncology, public health, and general surgery. However, procedures performed by a PA must not exceed his/her authorized competency level.

The military PA must keep abreast of innovations in primary patient care and combat. Eighty percent of Army PAs are assigned to combat or field maneuver units, the remainder being assigned to outpatient care at installation hospitals or to administrative positions. A majority of Air Force and Navy PAs are assigned to family practice clinics, but more combat operational roles are opening up to them at remote air bases and aboard ships because of their participation in Operations Desert Shield and Desert Storm. Specialty-trained PAs must keep their skills current in the ever-changing technologies of their respective specialties and in family practice to maintain their NCCPA certification.

PAs in the U.S. Coast Guard must also be included in any discussion of military PAs. The Coast Guard is more than 200 years old and is a part of the U.S. Department of Transportation during peacetime and the DOD during war. PAs in the Coast Guard have the same rank structure as PAs in the Navy. During wartime, they are federalized under the operational direction of the Department of the Navy. Coast Guard PAs are assigned to each Polar Class or Wind Class Icebreaker ship as the sole health care provider. They are also utilized as general medical officers in shore assignments. In addition, Coast Guard PAs perform medical administrative duties (such as serving as consultant to the U.S. Coast Guard Health and Safety Directorate) and are assigned as senior medical officers to post security units for worldwide deployment (e.g., in Korea, Turkey, and the Desert Storm operations area). Coast Guard PAs, similar to other military PAs, attend the Army flight surgeon training course and are designated as aviation medical officers. They attend the Tri-Service Combat Casualty Care Course, and are certified in advanced cardiac life support (ACLS) and advanced trauma life support (ATLS). They can also attend graduate specialty training and can earn graduate degrees. For this purpose, a Coast Guard PA instructor is permanently assigned to the IPAP school in San Antonio.[6]

ROLE OF PAs IN THE MILITARY

Peacetime   Like their civilian counterparts, PAs in military service improve the productivity of a physician's practice, reduce patient waiting time, manage emergencies effectively, reduce pressure on the physician, improve patient access to professional care, and lower the costs of that care. It must be noted that when PAs see patients, not only are they personally productive but this also allows the physicians in their practice setting to see the more difficult to treat patients. It has been hypothesized that PAs can see 80+% of the patients in a given practice.[6] This figure can be further defined by stating that PAs can effectively manage 80% of the disease/injury processes of their physician colleagues. Moreover, these 80+% of disease processes may account for well over 90% of the patients seen.

Wartime   Military PAs provide routine and resuscitative unit level medical care and evacuation to sick, wounded, and injured personnel from forward combat locations. The proper place for a PA in any wartime scenario is in the second echelon of care—aid stations, medical treatment platoons, air-transportable hospitals, naval ships, convalescent centers, outpatient care positions at evacuation and surgical hospitals, and Special Forces operations. Specialty-trained PAs, especially those trained in orthopedics and emergency medicine, may be used in nearly every echelon of care. In war, PAs perform the following functions:

1. Conduct and/or supervise training of unit personnel in first aid, sanitation, personal hygiene, medical evacuation procedures, and the medical aspects of injury prevention.
2. Arrange for a unit preventive psychiatry program that includes unit leader training in methods of preventing psychiatric disorders and combat stress casualties.
3. Perform triage on and treat sick, wounded, or injured persons.
4. Refer patients who require additional treatment to a higher echelon of care.[5]

With the battlefield of the future being more fluid, it has been proposed that the PA should be the commander of "roving" medical units stationed along the transitory forward line of battle. This means that PAs will be the senior medical providers of those injured or ill on the front lines. These units will hold patients for longer periods before evacuation, in theory making them second and third echelon facilities. This will result in only the more unstable patients being transported to support facilities for definitive treatment. Delayed transport will be further complicated by evacuation of patients to facilities that are intertheater rather than intratheater. Examples of these types of patients are those whose battle injuries may require surgery and/or prolonged hospitalization, and combat stress casualties in need of definitive care and rest away from the battlefield environment. Referrals such as these represent approximately 5% to 20% of the patients seen by a PA under combat conditions.

Therefore, PAs may be solely responsible for 80+% of disease/injury treatment in or near the battlefield.

The Service Impact

Although PAs in uniformed services have been largely used in primary care and for troop care in maneuver units, they are also educated in the care of every type of DOD beneficiary. The additional use of specialty-trained PAs is cost-beneficial and represents an optimal utilization of a health care resource to extend the capabilities not only of the primary care physician but also of the highly trained specialist physician. Although the military has been in the forefront of creating formalized residency training programs for PAs, the DOD has been severely lagging in the utilization of PAs in specialty areas. If the civilian model were followed, 74% of military PAs would be utilized in non–family practice/general medicine areas.[3] Because of the high shortages of all health care providers in military medical specialties, civilian market–driven patterns are worth considering.

The daily working relationships of physician/PA partnerships foster unity of thought and medical logic that permit relative autonomy of practice by PAs when the military situation so dictates. PAs may be independently assigned to units that are deployed to remote areas of the world. In such instances, the medical decisions made by PAs follow accepted guidance and standards in that they are the senior medical officers on-site.

Military PAs are in a relatively new health care profession that provides an innovative level of medical care previously unavailable. No other health care provider can be substituted for a PA, just as a PA cannot substitute for any other health care provider. PAs are the only mid-level providers who are educated according to the medical model to extend the capabilities of physician services in all treatment settings. Any discussion of the substitution of health care that PAs provide can be addressed only at the level of health care delivered—either increased, as with a physician, or decreased, as with a corpsman. Proper utilization of health care extenders such as PAs, along with nurses and corpsmen, creates a health care team capable of delivering routine and emergency primary care under the direct or indirect supervision of a physician. Each team works toward the common goal of improving the quality, accessibility, and cost effectiveness of health care. The utilization of PAs with corpsmen in such health care teams enhances the availability of care and provides an excellent role model for enlisted personnel who might be considering health care careers.[7]

A Typical Day

Although the organization and delivery of PA services differ somewhat among the various branches of the military, many of the basic functions of PAs are similar. For illustration purposes, the following section describes a typical Army PA.[7]

PAs in the Army are primarily assigned to a combat or combat support maneuver unit (e.g., an infantry or artillery battalion). Each infantry battalion has approximately 800 soldiers and each artillery battalion has about 400 soldiers. The PA is the primary care provider. He/she begins the day between 0530 and 0600 hours, conducting "sick call" in the battalion aid station. There, the PA may see 15 to 35 soldiers with varying illnesses, complaints, and injuries. Most conditions evaluated by the PA are upper respiratory infections, skin diseases, gastrointestinal problems, and musculoskeletal injuries. The PA is assisted by medical corpsmen, who obtain histories, measure vital signs, and may perform minor treatments or dressing changes. The PA in the aid station can manage many of the patients' complaints and dispositions, but 5% to 20% of patients presenting for sick call are referred to a troop medical clinic (TMC) for further laboratory workup or further referral to a physician. The TMC serves the population of at least three battalions as well as soldiers in other units within the brigade-sized element, that is, 3000 to 5000 soldiers.

After sick call, the PA then moves to the TMC to continue to provide primary care to the soldiers and to others presenting to the TMC for that sick call. The PA is joined by other PAs from like battalions within the brigade, as well as by one or two physicians specifically assigned to the TMC; all provide primary care. One of the physicians, designated as the "brigade surgeon," is the primary supervising physician for all the PAs assigned to units within the brigade. Official sick call closes at mid-day.

In the afternoons, Army PAs may spend their time performing routine annual physical examinations on active duty soldiers, or they may remain in a TMC or move to a hospital-based clinic located on the installation (post) to see family members or retired personnel by appointment. In this manner, the Army PA could see up to 40 patients on an average day. Patients may present with diabetes, hypertension, or thyroid disease, all of which are managed by the PA. The PA may also refer to or consult with a supervising physician or a specialist physician on any patient regarding treatment.

This scenario does not address the PA's other duties as a platoon leader, trainer, planner, and manager of medical assets. This scenario does not take into account the PA's extra duties and "call" performed in emergency rooms, nor does it consider the duties performed when a PA is deployed to a field or combat location anywhere in the world.

COST-BENEFIT ANALYSIS

Patient care provided by PAs cannot be distinguished from physician care in the primary care setting. Although most studies suggest that PAs can perform 80% of the services performed by doctors, the percentages vary with the location of the PA's practice, the practice setting, and the specialty. Because of this equality of outcome, when cost-benefit comparisons are made for PA services, the benefit is the same, regardless of whether a physician or a PA cares for the patient.

In a valid cost-benefit analysis, a reliable method for determining the costs (salary and benefits) and benefits (costs of patient care elsewhere if purchased) must be used. Currently, the DOD does not determine actual medical manpower costs for individuals or identifiable groups of providers. The actual cost per provider should be readily available based on the medical officer's Social Security Administration Number (SSAN). For a valid cost-benefit comparison between different providers (by groups or as individuals), a ratio must be computed. Because ratios are the purest form of analytical comparison, it would be useful if the DOD used them in making health care manpower decisions. If the actual cost of a PA were used (actual salary and benefit costs), the cost portion of the formula would be substantially lower than that of other providers who receive their salary based on a higher pay grade and with more extensive monetary benefits, such as professional pay and bonuses. The number of patient visits, categorized by beneficiary type and diagnosis, would accurately determine the benefit figure used in the ratio and would determine the value of the services represented.

Because access to valid information as outlined earlier (by SSAN or provider group) is not available secondary to privacy act restrictions, a simpler method for determining value will be used: value of services rendered less the most common military salary/benefits figure.

REASONS FOR COMMISSIONING

Today, PAs are commissioned officers in all the uniformed services. Reasons for commissioning include the following:

➤ Recognizes PA professional duties and responsibilities.
➤ Confirms the professional comparability of PAs with other nonphysician health care providers.
➤ Promotes the attractiveness of the position as a career.
➤ Enhances retention of current PAs in military service.
➤ Increases the ability of the military to recruit PAs from civilian sources and PA programs.

COST-BENEFIT ANALYSIS OF PAs IN THE MILITARY

Benefit

Military PAs see an estimated (conservatively) average of 25 patients per day.
Military PAs earn 30 days (i.e., 4 weeks, including weekends) of leave (vacation) a year.
Military PAs usually travel on temporary duty (TDY or TAD) orders for an average of 2 weeks a year.
A workweek is defined as 5 days.
Therefore, military PAs see 5750 patients per year (52 weeks per year − 4 weeks leave − 2 weeks TDY) = 46 (weeks worked in patient care per year) × 25 (patients per day) × 5 (days per week).

Determining the value of each patient visit is somewhat more complicated secondary to conflicting data. Because of the conflicts, the lowest figure available–$105 per outpatient visit purchased[8]–was used as the monetary value of an outpatient visit. This does not take into account the systems that the military and their contractors have established for determining costing. There are many confounding factors–overhead, fixed and variable costs, and so forth; however, this type of "productivity"-based calculation is widely accepted in the medical community.

Therefore, the economic impact of a military PA is: 5750 (patient visits per year) × $105 (cost of purchasing an outpatient visit) = *$603,750.00.*

This needs to be offset by the direct cost of employing the military PA. DOD PAs range in rank from O1E ($2638.50/mo = $31,662.00 direct taxable compensation per annum[2]) to O6 ($7675.20/mo = $92,102.40 direct taxable compensation per annum[2]). More PAs hold the rank of O3 than any other ($4549.50/mo = $54,594.00 direct taxable compensation per annum[2]). This does not take into account nontaxable housing allowances and subsistence allowances for which the DOD PA may be eligible. It also does not factor in board certification pay for which many PAs are eligible (requires a graduate degree relevant to PA practice and NCCPA board certification). It is conceded that the most accurate way to determine the costing of a PA is by having access to the actual cost accounting numbers based on all DOD PAs' SSANs. Given this concession, the comparison salary used here for DOD PAs is for an O3 with maximum time in grade = *$54,594.00.*

NET value of a military PA to DOD = $603,750.00 - 54,594.00 = *$549,156.00.*
This leads to an enviable cost/benefit ratio of 0.090.

➤ Encourages patient acceptance of the health care provided by PAs, whose rank is now comparable to that of other health care providers.

➤ Lends a structure to PA forces to help define career progression.

CONCLUSION

Since the draft ended in 1973, the military services have demonstrated that the utilization of PAs provides high-quality, cost-effective medical care. This care is accepted by all categories of patients treated by military PAs and has received exceptionally favorable reactions from commanders and management personnel. Utilizing PAs has dramatically improved access to care within the military health care system, leading to a lower cost of care per beneficiary. The PA is now viewed by the military as an integral part of the health care system.

PAs are expected to be used in the future in their present specialties, but the required numbers will probably fluctuate as the population of the military rises and falls. Primary care utilization and specialty training for PAs will be driven by demand, by the availability of other medical personnel, and by the funding of PAs within the uniformed services.

It is expected that the Army will continue to use PAs largely in field maneuver units as well as in fixed medical treatment facilities. The Air Force will continue to use PAs in fixed base clinics and hospitals. Navy PAs will provide similar primary and specialty care on board ships and at fixed base clinics and hospitals. Finally, Coast Guard PA utilization will parallel that of their counterparts in the Navy.

The military PA works and practices in unique settings and with unique demands. Schafft and Cawley[9] have stated that the medical provider is standing in the middle of the struggle among increases in demand for health services, quality of care, and cost containment. These demands are, and will continue to be, placed on all PAs, both civilian and military. Military PAs have committed to their challenges historically and will continue to meet the demands of patient care and operational readiness now and in the future. Their job satisfaction and superb morale come with their commitment to doing the best job possible under any conditions.

CLINICAL APPLICATIONS

1. Describe the changes in the training of military PAs since 1996.
2. Describe the "typical" day for a military PA. Compare that day with a "typical" day for a civilian PA in primary care.
3. List eight reasons for the commissioning of PAs in the military.
4. Discuss the contribution of active duty and reserve PAs to Operation Desert Storm and military operations in Bosnia and Afghanistan.

Acknowledgments

Many thanks to David H. Gwinn and Jimmie E. Keller, authors of previous versions of this chapter. Their tutelage, as always, was greatly appreciated.

Disclaimer

The author is solely responsible for the contents of this chapter. It is not a position paper representing the Department of Defense or any governmental entity.

REFERENCES

1. A Study for Special Pay for Allied Health Professionals: The Military Physician. A Draft Report to the U.S. Congress. Washington, DC: U.S. Dept of Defense, Office of the Assistant Secretary of Defense for Health Affairs, 1989.
2. FY2002 Pay Chart. Available online at www.dtic.mil.
3. 2001 American Academy of Physician Assistant (AAPA) Census Report. Alexandria, VA: AAPA, 6 October 2001.
4. Air Force Times, Military Times Media Group. Springfield, VA: U.S. Air Force, 18 February 2002.
5. Army Field Manual 8-15, Medical Support in the Theater of Operations. Washington, DC: U.S. Department of Defense, 1972.
6. Correspondence from Col. (ret.) Jerrold L. Wheaton, MD, MPH.
7. Army Regulation 40-48, Nonphysician Health Care Providers. Washington, DC: U.S. Department of Defense, 7 November 2000.
8. Evaluation of the TRICARE Program, FY2000 Report to Congress.
9. Schafft GE, Cawley JF. The Physician Assistant in the Changing Health Care Environment. Rockville, MD: Aspen Publishers, 1987.

CHAPTER 43

Alternative Roles

Sarah F. Zarbock

INTRODUCTION

The physician assistant (PA) profession has achieved several important milestones in approaching its 35th anniversary. It has evolved from a small group of graduates of the Duke University program in 1965 to approximately 35,000 PAs today. The impetus for the development of the PA profession came from a physician shortage in the 1960s. PAs were intended to fill this gap in access, predominantly in family practice and primary care settings. They were trained as generalists, with PA program curricula geared to providing the information, skills, and experience needed to be a real assistant to the physician. It was projected not only that PAs would improve overall access to primary care in this country but also that they would appreciate the demand for and have the motivation to accomplish a geographical distribution to medically underserved areas of the country. In fact, "primary

care," "underserved," and "rural areas" were the buzzwords of the admission process into PA programs. Nationally, the need had been defined, and the concept of the PA had been specifically developed to match that need.

Census Data

Understandably, data about the PA profession have focused more on what PAs do than on what they do not do. In other words, the tracking, collection, and analysis of information have emphasized the roles that PAs play in clinical practice rather than alternative roles or opportunities that some have pursued outside clinical medicine. Therefore, one can only speculate indirectly about those who have chosen other roles.

Most practice data have been collected by the American Academy of Physician Assistants (AAPA) as part of its membership census and survey process. In 1984, approximately two thirds of PA members of the Academy were employed in primary care settings, including family medicine, general practice, emergency medicine, pediatrics, and occupational health.[1] Census data obtained by the AAPA in 1991 show that the numbers shifted slightly. Approximately 56% of those PAs surveyed in 1991 indicated that they practiced in a primary care setting, and 7.1% stated that they were no longer in clinical practice. Of this latter group, 11% had left the profession entirely, 22.6% were unemployed by choice, and 26.2% were in teaching or in research and administration, most likely still in a health care–related field.[1]

In 1996, the census survey was expanded to include those PAs who were not members of the AAPA during 1996, with a similar sampling for the 1997 census. In that year, of the 32,782 individuals surveyed, 19,860 were AAPA members and 12,922 were not. Completed surveys were received from 12,400 members (62.4% participation rate) and 2806 nonmembers (21.7%).[2] Of the total respondents, 11.4% (n = 1730) stated that they were not in clinical practice—a significant increase from the 1991 data. As in earlier years, more than half of the 1997 respondents (52.6%) reported that their primary specialty is one of the primary care fields. Also as in previous census reports, information was not available on the types of employment of those PAs who are no longer practicing clinically.

Another census was completed by the AAPA in 2001.[3] In that year, more than 47,280 surveys were mailed, representing 90% of the 52,716 PAs eligible to practice. Of the 28,417 surveys sent to AAPA members, 15,012 (53%) were returned; 24,299 nonmembers were sent surveys, and 20% (n = 4930) were returned. Of 19,942 respondents, 12.2% (n = 2423) stated that they were not in clinical practice—slightly more than 11.4% of respondents to the 1997 survey. Overall, 48.5% reported that their primary specialty was one of the primary care fields (compared with 52.6% reported in 1997).

Development of Alternatives

The initial primary care role of the PA was well established and fulfilled by the first graduates and remained relatively stable for the first 10 years of the profession. Anecdotal evidence, however, indicates that some PAs had begun to select alternative professional pathways, including employment in specialty areas of clinical medicine as well as nonclinical positions. There has been no formal evaluation or data collection on the specific elements of the evolutionary process away from clinical roles, nor any tabulation on exactly what alternative roles had been established. In addition to the PAs who went into medical or surgical subspecialties, it appeared that PAs were filling professional roles customarily occupied by other medical professionals, most notably nurses and house staff physicians, or were choosing health care–related positions such as hospital administrators and pharmaceutical company representatives. Some became educators, predominantly with PA programs, whereas others created entirely new roles, particularly entrepreneurial PAs who formed their own companies.

There are several reasons for the increase of PAs in alternative roles. Some PAs want jobs that provide greater financial remuneration than is available in traditional clinical practice. With their background in medicine, they are familiar with the vocabulary within the medical field and can knowledgeably participate with other medical professionals. They also have both formal education in PA programs and experience within clinical practice that enable them to understand the medical "system"—who the players are, how the different professionals fit together to provide care, and the mechanics of health care provision.

Initially, a majority of PAs went directly from PA school into clinical practice. It was apparently not possible or at least not common for them to consider alternative employment settings during the nascent stages of the profession. In those first years, PAs filled the traditional positions envisioned for them. PAs who have been in clinical practice for longer periods, however, may be more susceptible to burnout, an often-mentioned reason for choice of another professional path.

Employment patterns for PAs are extremely variable. Certainly, PAs leave clinical practice for a wide variety of reasons and, as the PA profession "ages," PAs are reaching—or have reached—retirement. Anecdotal evidence also supports that there are some

PAs, usually women, who are reentering the profession after completing their child-rearing activities. As one long-time observer has noted, "In any profession, a number of people would be expected to explore new and expanding areas of opportunity, and the PA profession seems like a reasonable springboard for this. Because a large number of PAs sought this profession after making one or more career changes, it seems only natural that they be afforded this view as well if they seek career latitude or an alternative role."[4]

According to AAPA data, although the mean age of students entering PA programs has stayed relatively stable at about 26 years, there is a wide range of ages.[1] Older PA students therefore have previous employment experience. Some PAs would identify themselves as beginning a second or third career. Some may want a career that offers an opportunity for advancement, in conjunction with wanting more control over their future than previous jobs gave them.

Some factors involved in the choices of alternative roles probably also relate to the original motivators for PAs in choosing the medical field. PAs say that they want to work closely with patients and that they value their special niche because they are able, in general, to spend more time with patients than their physician colleagues. PAs are interested in patient education, which they regard as one of their most important professional tasks.

Probably the major influence on PAs, both those who stay in clinical practice as well as those who seek alternative roles, is the advent of managed care, with its substantial influence on the economics of medicine. It is certainly not clear at this time how managed care will affect PA practice.[5] There is also disagreement about whether, with the expanding number of PA programs, there will be too many or too few PAs.[6,7]

The interesting aspect of PAs in alternative roles is that they remain very committed to their profession, especially to the importance of the unique place they occupy in relationship to their patients. In fact, most of the PAs interviewed either still maintain some form of clinical contact or clearly value their clinical experience and intermittently desire to return to clinical practice. In spite of choosing alternative opportunities, they all remain PAs, first and foremost, and all express a loyalty to and pride in being part of the PA profession.

EXAMPLES OF ALTERNATIVE ROLES

There are certainly a variety of ways to interpret the newer data from the 2001 AAPA Census Report. What are the reasons why more PAs are not in clinical practice? Retirement? More who are choosing alternative paths? Why are a smaller percentage of PAs practicing in primary care fields? Increasing specialization? Changing demographics of patients and providers? However, the goal of this chapter is not to interpret data but, rather, to show how others do it. The best way to learn about alternative roles is to hear the personal stories of people who have gone in new directions. This section of the chapter summarizes interviews with PAs in alternative roles, including updates on several PAs 4 years after the initial interview, and then again 4 years later. These stories reflect their personal evolution, as well as the evolution of the health care system.

Those who have made alternative choices value and often miss their clinical involvement with patients. None of the PAs interviewed for this chapter explored alternative roles because they did not enjoy or did not feel rewarded by spending time with patients. In fact, the opposite is true. Of the PAs interviewed, none made the move as a negative reaction to what they had been doing. Rather, their clinical experience was the foundation for their next career steps.

The following case studies illustrate a variety of alternative roles for PAs in service.

Entrepreneurial Spirit

Frank R. is president of his own company, which specializes in scientific communications and the development of clinical symposia and in-hospital training programs. He remembers vividly the day he left clinical practice.

"I was working in an HMO family practice in the town where I grew up. On this particular day, I was doing urgent clinic—seeing one patient with asthma, another with a hot abdomen, a third with paroxysmal atrial tachycardia, and the last with a finger laceration. As I was practically running from room to room, I realized that the physician was taking blood

pressures as part of a routine follow-up appointment for hypertension. Somehow, the roles had become reversed."

That was in 1983, and Frank had been in clinical practice since his 1977 graduation from PA training. His concerns about the limitations of being a PA are not unique. He was struck by the irony that one of his patients, a city sanitation worker whose job did not require specialized education, was making almost twice Frank's salary. In addition to the frustration of his day-to-day professional life and the relatively low financial reward, he realized that there was little opportunity for advancement. He had substantial responsibility but scant authority, and he believed that as a PA in clinical practice, he had very little if any say about his future.

To make any changes in his professional status, Frank decided that he needed more education. He therefore returned to graduate school to earn a master's degree in hospital administration. Although he later had jobs in health care marketing and advertising, he felt he still did not have the professional autonomy he sought. While working for the scientific division of another company, he realized he could do it better. He founded his own company in 1989 with three pharmacists and a pharmacist attorney. The company now employs 19 people and has billings in excess of $3 million annually.

Over the years, Frank has watched the PA profession evolve, and now he observes that more and more PAs are making alternative choices. In recognition of the growing numbers of nonclinical PAs and in an effort to bring them together, he co-founded the Caucus of Executive and Administrative Physician Assistants. With membership in excess of 150 PAs, the Caucus provides an opportunity for those not in clinical practice to meet, network, share experiences, and have a special camaraderie.

"We need to be in positions of influence and authority," Frank says. "I see it happening all around me in the other medical professions, such as physicians, nurses, and pharmacists." These people are policymakers, who have the power to change the health care delivery system in which PAs function. Frank feels strongly that PAs need to be much more a part of this change. Yet he is also ambivalent about having

left clinical medicine altogether and gone into business. Although his PA background has enabled him to better understand both the end-consumer's and client's needs in a business that clearly has been quite successful, Frank still believes that he is not always taken seriously by those in the business of medicine. In fact, a physician executive friend suggested that he keep two business cards: one with the "PA-C" after his name and one without it.

"I see enormous opportunities within the health care field, and I see the other professions taking advantage of what's out there. I think it's a serious mistake for clinical PAs not to consider how nonclinical PAs fit into the scheme of things. We should avail ourselves of the opportunity to play a role in influencing how major health care decisions are made."

A Better Mousetrap

As a director of research and development for a continuing medical education (CME) consulting firm, Nancy S. knew not only what was a good idea but also how she could make it better.

"My sister-in-law worked for an organization that marketed enduring materials for CME to nurses. They had developed a very good product in their audio and video professional education cassettes on cardiology and emergency medicine. However, in all humility, I felt that I could do it better and could also market it to my PA colleagues."

After working in clinical practice for a while and then having two children, Nancy was already looking for something else to do. Therefore, she rewrote the Advanced Cardiac Life Support preparatory course for audiocassette and accompanying workbook, and first marketed it at the 1988 PA professional conference. On the basis of a very positive response to her new product, she went on to develop a video, which won an award at a prestigious film festival for technical and educational films. The recognition by the media and other professionals was especially satisfying and provided the impetus to refine the product for distribution to other sources.

"I was able to combine my clinical experience, my background in education, and my love for writing. My being a PA bears a direct relationship to this type

of work and enables me to feel that I am making my own special contribution to our profession. I would really love to do this full time. However, there are several other priorities in my life these days."

Nancy acknowledges that the amount of time required to run her own business is substantial, despite the fact that there are advantages to being her own boss, working on her own schedule, and being able to work at home.

"I want always to be clinically involved," Nancy comments. "It's what being a PA is all about. I would love to spend more time developing the videos because there is a need for this type of CME. However, I realize there just isn't time to do everything, and I may have to postpone that choice for a while."

Answering the Call

Salt Lake City is a long way from their home in rural Pennsylvania, a relocation that Nancy, her husband, and their two girls made 2 years ago to expand the family business. It was also quite a distance from the suburban family practice where she worked the 1-day-a-week time that she volunteers now at a community health center for the homeless. She is absolutely clear, though, that the path she has taken is the correct one and that it is in keeping with her spiritual life.

"I've always wanted to work in a medical mission, and believe that all that has come to pass is the result of prayer. My life is incredibly enriched by being obedient to the call."

She acknowledges that it has been a big adjustment for everyone in her family. She was concerned, at first, that she might be putting her own health at risk because of the high incidence of infectious illnesses she sees in the clinic patients and because she has a chronic illness herself. Her husband was also anxious about her choice of volunteer work. But their faith is strong and she just knew that this is what she had been asked to do.

"Of course, I took appropriate infection control precautions and my fears have gradually subsided. I know that burnout here is high and, because it is so emotionally draining, no one works more than 3 days in a row."

Nancy remarks that she does not see her volunteer work as a PA as a way to "combine" her professional life and her faith because one is not separate from another. Instead, she comments that everything she *does* is her faith and it's what she has been called on to do.

"My work at the clinic has been an incredible blessing, and I am now entering my second year of service. I prayed for outreach and this was the answer."

Something Different

Kathy S. initially left her job as a PA on the Neuro-oncology Service at a metropolitan children's hospital because she wanted to learn something new. Aware that there is considerable advancement opportunity in the field of pharmaceutical sales, she responded to an advertisement in the newspaper, and was hired by a major pharmaceutical firm as an "Oncology Specialty Representative."

"I didn't realize that I had an edge on the competition when I interviewed for the job. Pharmaceutical sales have become quite technical, so they were actually looking for someone with a clinical background," who was able to understand the technical information about the product without just memorizing the package inserts. Although most of her colleagues were nurses and pharmacists, and they all functioned on the same level, having a PA on the team was unique.

Kathy's hospital experience proved to be an advantage because she felt comfortable in the hospital setting, whereas some of her colleagues found it somewhat intimidating. She better understood and was more sensitive to the time constraints on potential customers, and had a special appreciation for the work done by the nurses.

In her new job, however, she was also less active, no longer a member of the team providing direct patient care—a prior source of considerable professional stimulation and reward. In addition, as a pharmaceutical representative, she had changed from being a real ally of the physician to a potential enemy, a pain in the neck, or someone from whom to obtain money.

"It was a bit hard to get accustomed to this change in my professional relationship to my medical colleagues. I think it relates far more to preconceptions

about the reps than to the reality of what we can offer."

After the birth of her first child, Kathy began working part time in an administrative position at a local community hospital, but she still speaks highly of the benefits of her pharmaceutical rep job.

"Had I not become pregnant," she notes, "I would have stayed, doing what I was doing. I had a great deal of schedule flexibility, the opportunity to work with some very interesting professionals, and a good salary and benefit package. I believe that it's one of the more challenging and definitely appropriate alternative roles for PAs."

New Directions

Laurie L., a surgical PA for 13 years at a hospital in Chicago, had become tired of the rigors of the job and the unpredictability of her day. She liked the hospital and the people with whom she worked, but she was at the peak of her salary range and had no upward mobility. She learned that there was a position available as quality assurance (QA) coordinator. Although she had heard about risk management (RM) at the annual AAPA conference and appreciated the need for good follow-up and appropriate documentation, her preconceived notion of QA work related mostly to being responsible for reporting to medical records and reviewing charts, which did not seem particularly challenging or stimulating.

Despite her ambivalent feelings, however, she pursued the issue. On meeting with the vice president in charge of hiring, she learned that in addition to overseeing both QA and RM, the position involved creating a whole new department for quality management, safety, and infection control. She indicated her enthusiasm for this expanded role, continued with the application and interview process, and got the job.

"I was thrilled to have the opportunity to organize an entire department, from creating job descriptions, hiring, preparing a budget, overseeing QA activities, and providing infection control to having responsibility for clinical risk management."

A major advantage of her new role was that she was in the same hospital, working with people who already trusted and respected her. She had the clinical background and experience to know the practical aspects of her new position but also to understand the realities of clinical practice—the system was not perfect. This blend reinforced her appreciation of how her PA colleagues contributed to maintaining high-quality care. Perhaps because PAs did not have the same credentials as physicians, were in dependent positions, and consequently were under closer scrutiny, they were more diligent and meticulous.

Fortunately, her knowledge and experience are portable. Laurie's career path has changed recently because her marriage has required relocation to another metropolitan area. She remains optimistic about pursuing her options of either returning to surgical care or, more likely, advancing her career in quality assurance and risk management. "I now have the credentials and experience to have a wider employment choice. It's as if I have two careers, a very comforting duality in these health care delivery times."

Distance Traveler

Tom C. is a 1970 graduate of the first MEDEX program, at a major university's school of public health and community medicine. Before attending the program, however, he had been a Green Beret, Army Special Forces, medic in Vietnam. While there, he had trained members of the Montagnards, a non-Vietnamese ethnic minority group, to be medics. Tom fully anticipated that as a PA, he would be in a stateside urban practice. It was not until he heard that a physician who ran a mission hospital in Vietnam was back in town on a recruiting trip that "something clicked."

"I proposed to her setting up a village health worker training program in the central highlands of Vietnam. She agreed, so I went back to Vietnam for 2 years, and founded and directed the program in two provinces that covered 500,000 people. It was an incredibly challenging and rewarding experience, heightened even more by, as a single parent, my adopting a Montagnard child."

On his return in 1973, Tom joined a MEDEX group of a school of medicine at another university. In 1986, he was appointed that program's Human Resource Development Director. He has trained students, trainers, and supervisors in many countries in

Asia, the Pacific, Latin America, the eastern Caribbean, and Africa. He has helped create a competency-based curriculum, and has also served as both resource person and consultant. Teaching in international primary health care (PHC) provides a wonderful opportunity to learn about different cultures and their health care problems and how to deal with limited resources. He was selected to receive his alma mater's "1981 Distinguished Alumnus Award" for his leadership in the PHC system development and his contributions to international health.

Tom travels about 60% to 80% of the time. Although at this point in his life, he would like to work specifically with only one overseas program, the demand for his services is understandably high.

"I think I've always been a lifelong learner, and the cross-cultural perspective has also helped me learn about myself. Even though I guess I'm not a 'typical' PA, being a physician assistant has allowed me to have a special experience. I've seen that we all have the same basic human needs, and there truly are more similarities than differences between cultures. For example, all parents want their kids to have it better than they did." He laughingly concludes, "I see that frequently as I now watch my 30-year-old adopted son taking care of my two grandchildren."

Advance Planning

Susan W. knew before she went to PA school that she wanted also to go to law school in order to combine medicine and law in her career. After 2 years of clinical practice, she returned to school to get her JD degree.

"The shortcoming of today's lawyers is that they are deciding issues involving medical professionals without truly understanding what it is like to be in clinical practice," she says.

Although she began her new career as a medical malpractice trial attorney, she found the work too adversarial and combative—a search for peoples' weaknesses and how to exploit them. Consequently, she switched her legal specialty and became involved in risk management, first as a consultant and then as part of the risk management team at a metropolitan children's hospital. The new job was ideal because it enabled her to use her legal expertise to assist health care providers in making themselves risk-proof and helping them to prevent injury.

Her PA background enhanced her credibility with other medical professionals; they believed they could talk to her in their own language about the realities of practicing medicine. Most of her legal colleagues were impressed by her dual background, and in the process of working with her, they learned a great deal about the PA profession. They respected Susan for her unique qualifications of combined medical knowledge and clinical experience.

Unfortunately, some of her co-workers, especially physicians, believed that she had gone into "the enemy camp,"—the perception many people in clinical medicine have about lawyers. Her PA peers, however, were more supportive and understanding about her career decision.

Susan has now become the Assistant Vice President for Medical Affairs at another children's hospital. In her new job, she is responsible for physician relations, contract negotiations, quality assurance, risk management, medical staff, and the residency program. She acknowledges that her new job is both an incredible professional opportunity and a challenge for her to expand her career.

"PAs tend to think of themselves only in a clinical perspective, but really there are numerous other ways for them to use their knowledge base and experience. Medicine plus law was a good combination for me. If PAs are interested in nonclinical experiences, I strongly urge them to pursue opportunities beyond the clinical realm."

Health Care Consultant

"I have always loved working with patients," notes Ron R., a managing partner in a health care consulting firm. *"As a matter of fact, from time to time, I toy with the idea of going back to clinical medicine, but I feel that I am making an even larger contribution to health care by what I am doing now."*

Ron had been in clinical practice for well over 10 years when he was first exposed to the business side of medicine. His first foray into a nonclinical role was in 1982, when he took over as the director of a health promotion institute. From there, he took a job in a company specializing in market research for the pharmaceutical industry, and then became involved in the field of medical practice management, his company's specialty.

His knowledge of and experience in clinical practice are the cornerstones of the organization, enabling them to more effectively compete with others in practice management. This advantage is especially noticeable when the company is working with physicians, who seem to listen differently to someone who can speak their language and who knows what it is like to practice medicine. The credibility of the company is enhanced because in its special projects, there is always the involvement of a clinical person.

> *"There is a particular mind set of those in clinical medicine," Ron says. "They need to know that you really understand their problems, that you have been where they are. An MBA is fine, but our ability to fully understand and appreciate what goes on in the clinical setting really gives us the competitive edge."*

Ron feels that he is making an important contribution to improving the quality of the health care delivery system, and he continues to wholeheartedly agree that PAs play an important part in the health care field. He remembers his previous clinical experience as very rewarding and believes that he gave both his employers and his patients good service.

> *"I have no regrets. I feel particularly fortunate that my background as a PA is such an important resource for the company."*

Five years later in 1998, the health care landscape had gotten far more complex than it was when Ron was last interviewed. He took his consulting business of assisting academic practices with reimbursement issues and expanded into capitation analysis, managed care contract negotiations, refined tools for practices' financial performance, and strategic management.

> *"It is both challenging and rewarding to help medical practices run themselves like real businesses, showing physicians how they can turn their clinical work into income," in which the right questions get asked and the best solutions are created. He continually finds examples of how his clinical*

background as a PA gives him the competitive edge.

> *"The largest source of lost revenue for physician practices is that services are provided but appropriate and documented charges are not applied. It would be highly unlikely, if not impossible, to be able to identify which services went 'uncaptured,' that is, were not charged, without knowing about clinical practice."*

Because of his clinical expertise as a PA, Ron believes that he is able to give better service to his clients. "I just don't think that you can learn the clinical side of medicine without going through it." He remarks that when he looks for consultants to work for him, he wouldn't think of hiring anyone without a clinical background. Even after having been away from clinical practice for more than 15 years and now with an MPH under his belt, he continues to think of himself, to some extent, as a PA.

> *"Next to practicing as a physician, it offers the best clinical background in terms of the breadth of knowledge," he says. "I still use my clinical experience almost everyday."*

Fortuitous Circumstances

Karl K. has come a long way from his 5 years of clinical practice. His neighbor, a nurse with systemic lupus erythematosus, had a severe pulmonary infection related to the SLE. She needed information about morphine administration and turned to him for advice. Karl quickly realized that a good teaching film was needed. At about the same time, he was introduced to an employee of a small company that produced films, videos, and teleconferences. What began as a coincidental introduction became a full-time involvement when he went to work for the company. Now a vice president of the company, Karl is involved in marketing its services as well as producing and directing many of its productions.

> *"Everything that I did when I was in clinical practice has helped me in this job, including understanding what goes on in the clinical setting and the relationships among health care providers."*

Karl's transition into an alternative role is typical, in that he was not actively searching for a way out of clinical practice. In retrospect, however, he realizes that as a clinician, he had very little control over his life in terms of what decisions were made and by whom. Now, although he is not necessarily making more money, he has more control over his future and the direction it will take. As the unofficial medical director within his company, he also has a special relationship with his colleagues. He does not compete with them, but rather they work together in a synergistic partnership.

He especially enjoys producing something tangible that he can see, touch, and feel, and experiences immense satisfaction when a project has been completed and he can hold the finished product in his hand.

Yet despite his own career choice, Karl voices what many others feel about their concern for the future of the PA profession. As more and more PAs become more clinically specialized or seek nonclinical career opportunities, fewer PAs will be working in the way the profession was initially intended—as front-line primary care practitioners. Perhaps because the profession is still relatively small in comparison with other health care professions (e.g., physician and nursing), the loss of a single member is more noticeable. Karl muses on this observation.

> *"I see many of my PA colleagues get stuck in positions without room for advancement. Frustrated, they go into a specialty practice or choose nonclinical alternatives. I worry that perhaps as a profession we are setting ourselves up for criticism by moving too far away from our primary care roots."*

Five years later in 1998, nothing was as sure as change, and Karl's professional track was a perfect example.

> *"After I left my previous job in electronic medical media, I became chief operating officer of a national foundation focusing on research and education in cardiology. From there, I went on to start my own company. Working for myself has been—and still is—one of the most satisfying experiences in my career. Not only am I able to do work that I enjoy, I now have the time to work with some foundations who have asked me to sit on their Board of Directors."*

Karl's area of expertise is pharmaceutical marketing and medical communications. His clients include pharmaceutical companies, publishers, and medical device manufacturers for whom he produces symposia, video programs, video teleconferences, and specialized publications. He has worked with many of his clients for over a decade.

Karl remarks that because he is a PA, although not currently in practice, he has an extra degree of credibility that puts him a step ahead of the competition. His clients know that he has been in the "clinical trenches," so to speak. The major change he sees is that his clients must now adapt to a different set of decision makers. Again, the influence of managed care is felt even in the field of medical marketing and communication.

> *"My clients, especially the pharmaceutical companies, want to reach the managed care plans as well as individual physicians. In the past, physicians had the latitude of writing for any medication they wanted,"* he says, and adds that *"those days are coming to an end. Now, many physicians are beginning to have to limit their prescription choices to what is in a given formulary. So, basically, they are being pushed out of the driver's seat. Pharmaceutical companies have to shift their emphasis if they are to stay ahead of their competitors."*

One piece of good news, however, is that pharmaceutical companies are more informed about the roles played by PAs, and they are including them more in their educational outreach. These companies are also realizing that PAs can make an impact on the bottom line. Therefore, both parties benefit when pharmaceutical companies want to reach the PA audience.

> *"Even though I occasionally get a tug to return to patient care, I thoroughly enjoy my work and will be doing it for the foreseeable future,"* but Karl concludes, *"who would have guessed I would see my retirement activity as seeing patients again."*

Opportunity Knocks

Leslie K. contracted hepatitis B three quarters of the way through her postgraduate surgical training. At the end of the PA residency program, she was physically drained and began looking for a job in surgery that was less demanding than the rigorous schedule of a house medical officer. She accepted a temporary assignment at a small medical publishing company that wanted to start a publication focusing on the teaching rounds in a large metropolitan hospital's emergency department. Although this new concept never sold, she was brought in-house as a medical editor and eventually helped launch a journal for PAs. Several years later, when she learned that a professional PA organization wanted to start its own clinical, peer-reviewed journal and needed a managing editor, she applied and got the job.

> *"It was a challenge to create the journal. I felt I could be quite creative in identifying the needs of the PA reader and in selecting topics, finding authors, and soliciting manuscripts," she notes. "It is very gratifying to know that my PA colleagues benefit from reading the articles in the official organization journal."*

An especially satisfying aspect of her work is helping PAs who want to write to learn about the article development process, from the idea stage, through the outline, to actual writing and revising, and then to the final product.

At times, Leslie finds the job frustrating, especially because it is not always easy to work with authors, some of whom take editorial commentary personally. On the other hand, she has the opportunity to work with her PA colleagues, many of whom are just beginning to submit their written work and who she believes benefit from her encouragement and practical assistance.

There is an explosion of technology in medical publishing and in the amount of information the clinician needs to know. These trends provide an excellent opportunity for PAs who are interested in writing for pharmaceutical companies, developing patient education materials, and reporting on the results of clinical trials. Both professionals and the lay public need more and more information explained to them, and Leslie appreciates how very important it is that PAs become more involved and proficient in written communication.

Leslie's job as editorial director requires that she remain familiar with PA practice and the clinical informational needs of PAs, but she feels quite removed from the day-to-day realm. She comments on this distance.

> *"I have been away from the clinical world for quite some time now, and I worry that it would be difficult to reenter as a practicing PA. In truth, that makes me uneasy, and I suppose it is the major downside for me in choosing to do what I do."*

This concern is often voiced by PAs who have chosen alternative nonclinical employment options. Leslie's suggestion for meeting the needs of many nonclinical PAs who may want to return to clinical work is to develop some form of reentry courses.

In the meantime, she is sufficiently occupied by the challenges of producing a high-quality medical journal for PAs, and she believes that by continuing to encourage her colleagues to contribute to the journal, she is giving something back to her profession.

Five years later in 1998, Leslie's career path had brought her back to clinical medicine when she volunteered one shift a week at a county health department clinic that provided care for Medicaid and the working-poor populations. This family practice setting seems a far cry from when she was a surgical PA at an inner city hospital. In the interim, she has worked exclusively as editor of the *Journal of the American Academy of Physician Assistants,* which included a 10-year period when she was not active clinically at all.

> *"People always ask me what it's like to reenter clinical practice," she remarks, "and I must admit that I had a certain amount of trepidation. To help me make the transition, I developed my own reentry curriculum of studying journals and textbooks and spending time with clinic practitioners." She adds that having a mentoring relationship with the supervising physician is a very important ingredient in successful reentry.*

Now with four children, the logistics—not to mention the financial aspects—of her life are complicated. Although she intends to continue to volunteer for another year, she is wondering about whether or not to go back to work full time, and in what type of setting. Although what she is doing now will certainly enhance her chances in finding satisfying employment, she believes that attending a formal reentry program would be especially helpful. But what's the chance of having that type of educational opportunity available in a health care environment that may soon have enough PAs?

Leslie asks, "Will PA programs or other institutions be motivated to help PAs return to clinical practice if jobs are being filled by new graduates or current graduate PAs?" She adds that the nursing profession has developed refresher courses for nurses who have been out of the clinical realm for a while, so there is definitely a precedent. However, the future for PAs who want to come back is still unclear.

For the meantime, she says that in her current role, there is a need for PAs to become better writers and to increase their understanding of research and the medical literature. She concludes, "Being an editor of *JAAPA* has been a challenging and satisfying professional experience, and I see the job market expanding for medical writers and editors."

Clinical Research

Rick K. was employed at a university medical center and was involved in both clinical practice and research when he was approached by a pharmaceutical company to provide an outside referral in order to conduct clinical drug studies. Because such requests were made repeatedly and the in-hospital physicians had neither the staff available nor the expertise to participate in studies, Rick formed his own consulting company to secure, place, and conduct clinical trials in private practice settings. On the basis of his initial success and proven track record in this field, he was offered his current opportunity—to start a research center at a private clinic.

> *"This was a classic example of opportunity knocking,"* he notes. *"And I answered."*

Rick likes the competitive environment of clinical research studies, especially working with cutting-edge pharmaceutical products that are not being used by anyone else. He is currently involved in investigating pharmaceutical products for the treatment of breast cancer, acute respiratory tract infection, arthritis, hypertension, and pediatric infection. He has already helped develop an antianginal, an antihypertensive, and an anti-HIV agent.

He finds it rewarding to work with new products that offer significant advances in treatment as well as therapies with fewer adverse effects and other properties that enhance patient compliance. In addition, Rick has complete autonomy, both administratively in running the center and clinically in following the protocol.

However, he misses the patient contact and taking care of people—his primary reasons for entering the PA profession. From time to time, he becomes tired of the administrative problems and longs for the relative simplicity of patient care. Yet he also acknowledges that the benefits of his current role are the diversity of responsibility, control over his own future, a potentially higher salary, and job security he would never achieve as a clinical PA. He also believes that PAs in clinical practice have been limited in terms of career opportunities and upward mobility. He encourages PAs to consider expanded roles within the health care system.

> *"I feel that I am very fortunate because every day I go to work and do exactly what I want to do, and am well regarded by other professionals in the field. In all honesty, I have never been happier."*

Five years later in 1998, Rick's professional life continued to expand in his niche in clinical research from being Director of Clinical Research as well as Director of Clinical Laboratory and Health Screening Departments for his previous employer to becoming the Executive Director and CEO of one of the subsidiaries of a site management company for clinical research.

"The direction of my career would have totally surprised me 5 or 10 years ago, before the advent of managed care," he says. "Because of the changes in health care in this country, physicians are seeing their incomes crunched, and they are looking for additional sources of revenue." Rick's employer manages research in physicians' offices, which is being funded by the pharmaceutical companies, and all three parties are served. He remarks, "Patients participate in clinical trials that may be beneficial; pharmaceutical companies are able to test new agents and devices; and physician practices get added income for their involvement. I see it, basically, as a win-win-win situation."

Rick oversees nine research centers that manage research in 25 physician offices, involving a total of

155 physicians. He describes his role as multifunctional. As a PA and as a clinical coordinator certified by the Association of Clinical Research Professionals, he is able to participate in the research itself by performing histories and physical examinations, and by overseeing the administration of new drugs. "I am also a full-time administrator," he adds, "supervising the support and nursing staff, as well as establishing new research centers."

He was concerned about managed care and that, with budget cuts, PAs might be one of the casualties. He now sees that there is so much opportunity for PAs and that there are niches, such as the one he has made for himself, within the practice of medicine. "I feel that I am established in a decision-making seat, a location where major differences can be made."

Rick took another step up the corporate ladder in 2000, when he became the President, CEO, and Chairman of the Board of Clinical Research Consultants, Inc., a private pharmaceutical research company funded by 11 individuals. As one of the major stockholders, Rick has an opportunity to provide input into the strategic direction of the company. By entering the private sector, he has gained an autonomy that suits him well.

> "My recent career change has positioned me to play a more proactive role in the health care marketplace. I have eliminated as much as possible the negative impact of being required to have physician supervision and oversight, as well as contending with insurance payment requirements and being restricted by working for someone else. I now have a greater opportunity to control my destiny."

Rick now employs other PAs, nurse practitioners, and nurses, and he contracts with the physicians who are employees of his company. He acknowledges that he has the best of both worlds. He still sees patients, but he is no longer at the mercy of a physician or medical practice in terms of his income, his benefits, and the direction of his career. The physicians and other staff are now dependent on Rick to determine salary and benefits and to set the company's direction. He admitted that it is a totally different equation when one is in charge and is not working for someone else.

Rick's PA roots continue to go deep.

> "I would not have the opportunities to achieve what I have accomplished today had I not been a PA," he admitted. "I still meet many PAs who are frustrated with salary caps, required time commitments, and limitations on their ability to practice by physicians, hospitals, medical boards, and insurance companies." He has been fortunate to find another niche in his career and to not have his goals defined by someone else. "I am not held back by what others want me to do. I now have the freedom to soar as high as I can go."

Best of Both Worlds

It has been 10 years since Steve N. was contacted by a hospital administrator with a request to find PAs to staff a clinic in a community near Phoenix, Arizona. Steve realized that there was a business opportunity to fill this need, formed a simple partnership with a PA colleague, and contracted with the administrator to provide what was wanted. Although his first partner went his own way, Steve is now president of his own company, and together with his second PA partner, he still has that original contract. For liability reasons, they changed the partnership to a corporation. From their success and word-of-mouth advertising through the hospital, they now have 18 PAs working for them.

> "It's basically a supply and demand situation," Steve comments. "There are more physicians than PAs in this area, and the service we provide is a low risk for all concerned."

The physician is "leasing" the PA, not hiring the PA as an employee. If the arrangement does not work out, another PA is found to do the job. It is a similar low-risk situation for the PAs. They have flexibility in hours and place of employment. Some of the PAs even work at more than one facility on a rotating schedule.

Steve finds that there are advantages and disadvantages to owning his own company. On the one hand, he has considerable autonomy and control over his career, as well as the opportunity to promote the PA concept at every encounter. However, the job takes away from leisure time with his wife and children. PAs and physicians call him at any time of the day or night, so he feels that he is "on call" almost all the time. He is also somewhat cautious about working with some physicians.

Steve has also stayed in clinical practice all along because he still believes in the importance of being involved with patient care. Although he originally decided on continuing clinical work for the income, that reason is less true now that his company has become so successful.

"Maybe I'm just too altruistic about caring for patients. That's what our training and experience prepares us to do. I'll probably continue having both jobs because both are so important to how I view myself as a professional."

Five years later in 1998: "The managed care landscape has had a dramatic impact on the company that I have with another PA. Whereas we used to have contracts for providing PAs to private physicians or hospitals, our major contract is with the Indian Health Service in Phoenix," Steve notes. Although he continues to work clinically in the same infertility and gynecology practice as he has for the past 16 years, his PA leasing service has changed considerably. At least half of the PAs had been employees, but now all the PAs who work for them are independent subcontractors.

"Small companies such as ours just cannot get the price breaks, for instance, on health insurance for employees, or setting up 401Ks—we have no economy of scale." He goes on to add that the Indian Health Service (IHS), which uses PAs in the emergency department of the Phoenix Indian Medical Center, has not been able to find sufficient coverage. *Although they could contract with individual PAs, it is more convenient and efficient for them to work directly with Steve's company—the IHS gets the PAs, Steve gets the paperwork.*

Another reason that Steve believes they still retain a competitive edge is that they are working with PA colleagues. In fact, Randy, Steve's business partner, occasionally works alongside his employees. Steve wonders, however, about the future of his business.

"With two PA programs in town, many PA jobs in the area are being directly filled with new graduates. It also means that we have two valuable resources from which to find PAs to work for us at IHS. Unfortunately, I think our days are numbered in this community because there are more jobs than PAs." He is philosophical when he concludes, *"The government is our*

major client now and, honestly, if these federal contracts go away, we might be out of business."

Steve added one more entry to his resume, when, in July of 2000, he became director of an Internet-based master of science program for practicing PAs at the local school of health sciences. He somehow still manages to continue practicing as a PA in gynecology. However, he is now an independent contractor for his own company because his supervising physician retired. He still subcontracts with several PAs, maintains the contract with the Indian Health Service, and participates in clinical research studies.

"I looked for other employment opportunities when my supervising physician retired. However, I was at a disadvantage by being a male practitioner in gynecology in a county with an abundance of nurse practitioners in the same specialty. Moving into academia provided more job security and a chance to further my own education by getting my master's degree."

Steve now has greater financial opportunity than when he was paid a salary from the private practice. Although he continues to be frustrated by paperwork and insurance requirements, he still tries to spend as much time as possible with his patients.

"I find that I spend more time these days trying to find ways to work the system—getting managed care organizations to provide services, requesting more free samples to give to patients, or finding a way for patients getting a consult or service at a discount."

As with a growing number of PAs, Steve sees that retirement door is getting closer, but he also sees himself as an aging dinosaur who is trying to keep up with the rapid changes in medicine—from both clinical and management points of view. Although he doubts that he will continue his clinical practice after retirement, he still sees a role for himself in administration or education, or as an employer.

Volunteerism Pays Off

Ann E. thoroughly enjoyed her experience as a state PA chapter president, especially the time she spent developing prescriptive practice legislation. She liked organizing and pulling people together and became quite interested in political issues. She was also troubled by the fact that legislators had the authority to make policy decisions without real knowledge of what was happening in the field. In 1988, the state senator who had been a sponsor for a PA bill and chairman of the senate's health care committee offered her a job as a legislative analyst researching health care bills. At the same time, she joined the community board of a health center for the elderly. When the new mayor in her city took office, a member of the transition team also was on the board and recommended Ann for the job of director of the city's health department.

"This is an incredible opportunity," Ann says. "I oversee the health care of 76,000 people in a densely populated working-class city in the metropolitan area."

She has many responsibilities as director, including overseeing the board of health; community sanitation; restaurant, food, and housing inspection; hazardous waste contamination cleanups; and enforcement of laws dealing with environmental crimes. Ann also administers school and environmental health services, the city's AIDS commission, lead paint poisoning prevention, and tuberculosis monitoring. Her clinical experience has helped her to identify and appreciate the priorities in public health planning, and to combine public and private efforts to meet the needs of the community.

"Our city needs as much as you can give it," she comments. Ann believes that PAs can find similar challenges and satisfactions within the political system by becoming a part of policymaking and programs that address the health care needs of a community. She believes that her clinical background is a significant asset.

Ann did not plan to go in the direction that she has, but as she learned more about health policy and what needed to be done within the system, her goals became much clearer. Although she is subject to the winds of political change because she is a mayoral appointee, she knows where she will be working at least for the next 2 years because the mayor has just won reelection.

Ann's new (as of October 1997) job as Director, Division of Public Health, City of Portland (Maine) is no less busy than her previous employment as

Director, City of Somerville (Massachusetts) Health Department. Under her former "umbrella," she worked on two initiatives of which she is justifiably proud:
1. Passage of comprehensive tobacco control regulation in the city in 1992.
2. The Community Health Agenda, a community health assessment and improvement initiative that led to the merger of the Somerville Hospital and the Cambridge Hospital.

For both achievements, she won, in 1995, the prestigious Dr. Nathan Davis Award granted by the American Medical Association for Outstanding Career Public Servant at the Local Level.

But that was then, and this is now. "I have a new and exciting opportunity to work within a larger and more influential—in terms of numbers of individuals served—public health department because Portland covers many of the health needs of about 250,000 when the surrounding towns are included." She adds that her perspective as a PA, together with her legislative and public health experience since when she was in clinical practice, has provided her with an important vantage point within the health care scene.

"My eyes have been opened to see the needs within the community, both in Somerville and in Portland, that are not met by the traditional system of health care. In contrast with Somerville, in which the emphasis was on enforcement of regulations, in Portland it is on prevention and health promotion as well as the provision of primary care service."

Although she has a larger department to direct, she has an in-place infrastructure with capable program managers to do what needs to be done. That includes a homeless health program; a clinic, staffed by volunteer providers, for people without insurance; two school-based health centers; a sexually transmitted diseases and HIV testing clinic; five child health clinics; and outreach programs for intravenous drug users for HIV prevention.

"As my career advanced," she acknowledges, "I became increasingly in a position to look at and effect change among major providers of care and, to a certain extent, influence how things progressed. I feel that my move to Portland is the next important

step I can take to make a difference in the delivery of health care."

In 1997, Ann had just begun her new job as Director, Division of Public Health, city of Portland. Her department had 80 employees, and she was responsible for overseeing a $3 million budget and more than 30 federal, state, and privately funded grants. Ann played a leadership role in securing the City Council's passage of an ordinance to ban smoking in restaurants, an effort that led to a statewide ban the following year. Her career path took another turn when she served as a Senior Health Policy Fellow in the Office of the Surgeon General. The 1-year fellowship was supported by the PA Foundation, and its purpose was to promote close collaboration between the government and providers on prevention initiatives.

> *"I was presented with a wonderful opportunity to learn more about the inside workings of the federal government and to make a difference in improving the health of the nation. At the end of this fellowship, I was hired as a consultant to work until the end of the Surgeon General's term in February 2002 on several of the Surgeon General's initiatives. I also had the pleasure to frequently introduce myself as 'the first PA in the Office of the Surgeon General.'"*

Ann's early experience in practicing as a PA sensitized her to the critical importance of access to health care. She provided care for too many uninsured patients whose illnesses could have been more effectively treated or prevented sooner had they been insured and had access to good health care. Obtaining health insurance coverage for high-quality health care services for all people continues to be an important challenge for the nation, as well as for the PA profession.

> *"I have always found that my PA background keeps me focused on what is best for the care of patients. My goals have been to identify what can be done to improve their care and the systems that care for them, and what can be done to prevent illness and premature death at the individual, community, and system levels."*
>
> *"I am currently in the process of exploring new employment opportunities for the future,"* she said, *"both in government and in the private sector. I project that I will continue to work on efforts to improve*

health care, especially through prevention. As it has so much already, my background as a PA will continue to provide me with an invaluable perspective."

Educating New PAs

Don P., director of a state university's PA program, believes that he has achieved the perfect blend in his professional choice. In addition to his program responsibilities, he teaches students, and, until being called up for military service during Operation Desert Storm, he spent a third of his time in clinical practice. He worked for 1 year in rural Idaho in family practice after graduation, but when he was asked to return as academic coordinator of the program, he jumped at the chance.

> *"I suppose I was flattered to be asked to return to the program as a faculty member, but I think I always knew at some level that I wanted to be part of the educational process for PAs and would probably have gotten into that aspect eventually. It was just a matter of time."*

There is no doubt in Don's mind that he will always want to have some clinical involvement with patients. Temporarily away from clinical practice now, he is certain that it won't be long until he returns. Equally important for him is contact with PA students. He is continually amazed by the diversity of their backgrounds as well as their dedication and enthusiasm; he strongly believes that the PA profession is unique in this regard.

Don notes that it is sometimes difficult to have to work within the bureaucracy of a large university medical school. Although the inherent game of politics is not a major detractor, he finds it difficult to have to "work the system" in order to get what he needs, particularly because PAs are so much in demand on the open medical market and it seems that they cannot be educated fast enough.

> *"I feel fortunate to be able to blend my administrative, teaching, and clinical roles. But I must admit that it's the students who really make the difference. Hopefully, by participating in their education, I am making my own important contribution to my profession."*

"Although I continue to be a PA program director, I have had to relinquish my clinic time over the last year and a half because of the 'busy-ness' related to the changes in health care," Don comments. He says that he finds himself "at the table" more often lately, especially because he is at an academic health center. "We've had to look at things quite differently in terms of getting more into the primary care area and away from highly specialized medicine. I'm pleased to say that 75% of our 500 graduates are working in primary care." However, the spending of medical education dollars has also changed, and a legislatively mandated council will have the authority to decide how—and for whom—the money will be spent.

"I get farther away from my clinical role, as I get more involved in both teaching and program management." As president of the Association of Physician Assistant Programs, Don also enjoys working with his faculty colleagues. The organization is developing a peer-reviewed journal and a research institute, as well as an endowed fund, the interest income from which will be earmarked for research conducted by PA program faculty.

> "I certainly never envisioned the PA role diversification that we see today—whether in clinical practice, PA program development, or faculty professional activities. But I believe that part of what PAs learn is to be flexible and adaptable, both talents that are needed in today's changing health care scene."

Five years later, Don continued as the director of the PA program and was still involved in teaching, research, and clinical care. He also continued to be frustrated by more to do and less time to do it.

"I am trying to be more adept at managing my time, using different strategies to increase my output without sacrificing quality. Of course, there are always limits to what can be done," he admits. He has found that one of the best ways to both reduce the number of tasks and shelter the time he already has is by simply saying, "No."

With the graying of PAs, retirement is now on the horizon. How will that major change influence how time is spent? "I am amazed that I will be reaching retirement within the next 5 years," Don says. "I often feel like I just graduated from school and taken my first job as a PA in a professional world where practically no one had heard of us."

But retirement does not mean that Don will slow down. He would like to become more involved in humanitarian projects by teaching and providing care, perhaps on the international level. "Retirement will also provide me with that precious commodity—time. Finally, I will be able to spend all day, if I want to, on oil painting."

One Final Story

I was asked to write this chapter because of my own professional road, a somewhat "scenic" tour through a variety of careers, culminating with the best one—being a PA. As an English education major, I developed an interest in writing. Then, as the owner of a needlework mail order company, I realized the personal importance of working for myself. It was not until a great deal later, however, when I heard about the PA concept, that I finally settled into the career that I knew I would have for life. This certainty of professional choice is frequently voiced by PAs, especially those who have had previous occupations.

After graduation, I gained clinical experience, predominantly in the field of adult and pediatric hospice care, in both private practice and community and tertiary care hospital settings. Yet, interspersed throughout my clinical years were opportunities for medical writing, in the forms of health education for patients, grantsmanship for the development of new clinical programs, and marketing and public relations for my specialized background in hospice care. My clinical practice always seemed ultimately to steer me in another direction. Perhaps it just provided me with the opportunity to write or, in fact, enabled me to see that my most important and satisfying professional contribution was not patient care but what I could do with my writing to enhance it.

Today, what at one time was just an avocation has become my vocation. Without a doubt, my life as a freelance medical writer and editor has been possible only because I became a PA. As is true of many choices we all make, I am not sure that the direction of my professional life was always consciously made. It may have merely been a case of being in the right place at the right time. With hindsight, however, I am confident that the tour was worth it, because the destination provides that "best fit" feeling we all hope to achieve.

As I have gotten older, I have begun to look more closely at my professional career path, and not just at what I need to do now to ensure that I can have some satisfying existence after I retire. Unfortunately, when you work for yourself, there doesn't really seem that there is *any* age at which you can afford to retire.

But, assuming for the time being that I have made appropriate financial arrangements, I turn my mind to what I actually want to be doing for the next 15 years. And I find myself feeling a tug at my heart because I am thinking that I might not ever be a practicing PA again. I am well suited to the freelance life, being able to create my own schedule, juggle different projects, and be my own boss, and never planning or attending my own meetings—with myself.

I was looking through a drawer the other day when I came upon my stethoscope, curled up and nestled next to my reflex hammer. I paused and allowed myself to remember my clinical days—visiting hospice patients at home, fine-tuning fluids and electrolytes on bone marrow transplant kids, and taking care of garden-variety admissions in a community hospital. Those days seemed so long ago and, yet, they didn't. I can't remember many names but I do remember many faces, many stories, many happy endings, and, yes, quite a few sad ones.

I believe that life is just a series of choices. Certainly, one of my more important ones was to become a freelance medical writer and editor. Another choice was to move to a very rural area to be nearer my family but also in which PA employment opportunities were scant. I had chosen to become very involved in my community and was able to participate as much as I wanted because my schedule was my own to bend and flex. Throughout this time, I had intermittently thought about going back to clinical work but never really went any farther than thinking about it. And now it had been 7 years since I had listened through my stethoscope or elicited a reflex with my hammer.

I had been making choices all along—some active and some passive, but choices nonetheless. A correlate of this is that people do what they want to do and leave behind what they don't want to do. In other words, there is always a reason, although it is not always a conscious one, for the directions that we take in our lives. Had I, in fact, at some level, made a choice not to return to clinical practice? Was I doing what I really wanted to do?

I had just completed the writeups of the eight individuals whom I had re-contacted, and I realized that there is a common thread that connects all of us. We are all PAs—maybe not still in clinical practice—but all individuals who had dramatically changed our lives by selecting this particular professional path. I suspect it is safe to say that not one of us knew, when we were new graduates, that we would be doing what we are doing today. We, in fact, may not even be sure of what we will be doing tomorrow. I know I am not. But I feel reasonably comfortable saying for all of us, that becoming a PA was one of the most important and valuable decisions that we ever made. That decision has opened so many wonderful and surprising doors. Although I do not know which will be my next door to open, I can assure you that it will be connected in some way to being a PA. I'll keep you posted.

Just when I thought I had probably done it all, another opportunity came into view and, again, my career path took an abrupt turn. It all began on a sunny August afternoon as I was returning from yoga with a friend, who is a teacher at the local junior boarding school. I accidentally stepped on a book on the floor of the passenger side and, when I went to retrieve it, saw that it was about how teaching Latin could be used to teach English. "Hmmmm," I thought, and innocently remarked, "I took 5 years of Latin in high school, and I actually got my undergraduate degree in secondary school English education." My friend's surprised reply was, "You did?" The rest, as they say, is history. Since then, I have taught English to 7th and 8th graders and am now both a yoga *and* a teaching colleague with my friend.

So where does that leave my life as a PA? Although I still work as a freelance medical writer and editor, it's been about 12 years since I provided patient care. I love to watch "E.R." (I made a complicated diagnosis while Dr. Green was still going through the differential) and perk up when I hear a discussion about just any medical topic. I have even taught a class on Bone Marrow Transplantation, my previous clinical specialty, to both 5th and 9th graders at my school.

Throughout all of this, I have maintained my certification and, 2 years ago, dragged my way through the Pathway II requirements. My 6-year stretch is up soon, and I will need to become re-certified. I dread the moment when I have to admit to myself, "You haven't seen patients in years. You don't have any reason to stay certified as a PA."

I have mixed emotions about closing the PA professional door. When I tracked down and interviewed five of the PAs whose stories are in this chapter, I realized that they, too, had taken major steps away from clinical practice but were still PAs in their hearts. I have now reached a point in life where I don't want any more turns in my career path. Retirement is becoming more of a reality and less of a dream. Upon reflection, I can't imagine my life without being a PA. I have a feeling that most PAs, whether still providing patient care or exploring new opportunities, could say the same for their lives, too.

CONCLUSION

As PAs, we are well positioned in the medical health care system. We combine the strong background of education and experience with both a belief in our unique professional role and contribution to patient care and a high level of enthusiasm and dedication. Clearly, PAs are choosing interesting, challenging, diverse, and rewarding alternative career options, for both personal and professional reasons. Despite the variety of motivations for going in another direction, PAs continue to support the important contributions made by their colleagues in clinical practice. Some continue in practice themselves, even as they have changed their professional choices. They all seem to have a strong sense of loyalty and connection to the profession. Although sounding trite, the phrase "Once a PA, always a PA" has a familiar ring of truth.

In any profession, some practitioners take new and different paths. As PAs celebrate another anniversary of the profession and beyond, it is important that we continually recognize and appreciate our roots. Perhaps learning about PA colleagues who have taken different roads will give the reader a stimulus for change. It is a distinct pleasure to be able to salute both those PAs who continue to provide exceptionally valuable care to patients and those who have chosen to travel an alternative road.

CLINICAL APPLICATIONS

1. If you wanted to expand your role as a PA into related areas, such as research, public health, business, publishing, consulting, or PA education, how would you find out what additional preparation you might need? How would you decide which alternative roles might interest you?

2. You overhear two colleagues talking about a PA who works full time in PA education and has not been in clinical practice for 5 years. They refer to the faculty member as "not a real PA." How would you respond? How would you respond if the same statement were made about a PA who works in research, consulting, or public health?

3. You are a PA in a primary care practice. A colleague PA who has not been in clinical practice for 10 years, but has maintained certification, asks you to design a program to help her return to clinical practice. What would you include in a "reentry program"?

REFERENCES

1. Conversation with Judith B. Willis, MA, PA-C. Director of Research, AAPA (Sept., 1992).
2. 1997 AAPA Physician Assistant Census Report. Alexandria, VA: AAPA, 1997.
3. 2001 AAPA Physician Assistant Census Report. Alexandria, VA: AAPA, 2001.
4. Hooker RS, Cawley JF. Physician Assistants in American Medicine. New York: Churchill Livingstone, 1997.
5. Davis A, Griffin D, Kahwaty B, et al. Managed care: What issues do clinicians face in an evolving system? J Am Acad Physician Assist 1997;10:18.
6. Cawley JF, Jones PE. Are there (a) too many, (b) too few, or (c) just enough PAs? The possibility of an impending health professions glut. J Am Acad Physician Assist 1997;10:80.
7. Hooker RS. Are there (a) too many, (b) too few, or (c) just enough PAs? Is there an undersupply of PAs? J Am Acad Physician Assist 1997;10:81.

RESOURCES

Baker JA, Oliver D, Donahue W, et al. Predicting role satisfaction among practicing physician assistants. J Am Acad Physician Assist 1989;2:461. *Addresses the more traditional clinical practice roles and highlights areas of professional satisfaction for PAs: independence, responsibility for patient care, and acceptance by patients. Also underscores the issues of promotions, salary increases, and career advancement.*

Carter R, Perry H (eds). Alternatives in Health Care Delivery: Emerging Roles for Physician Assistants. St. Louis: Warren H Green, 1984. *The first comprehensive text about the PA profession, which provides a wealth of information about the development of the PA concept, the contribution of PAs to health care, PA program curricula, and the certification and licensure processes. Numerous clinical roles are discussed, as well as issues related to job satisfaction, reimbursement, and hospital privileges.*

Hooker RS, Cawley JF. Physician Assistants in American Medicine. New York: Churchill Livingstone, 1997. *An in-depth look at the development and current status of the profession, including PA education, specialization, and roles in primary care inpatient settings. Describes nonclinical roles and opportunities for PAs as well as their relationship with other professionals. Interesting information included on the economic and legal aspects of PA practice and speculation on the future direction of the profession. Appendices provide model state legislation, the Code of Ethics, and a list of PA programs.*

Sadler A, Sadler B, Bliss A. The Physician's Assistant: Today and Tomorrow. Cambridge, MA: Ballinger, 1975. *A landmark book on the PA profession that defines the clinical role of PAs in the landscape of health care in the 1970s. Includes discussions of legal, organizational, and competency concerns for the profession, and is an intriguing review of the origins of PAs.*

Schafft G, Cawley J. The Physician Assistants in a Changing Health Care Environment. Rockville, MD: Aspen Publishers, 1987. *Provides an important bridge between the earlier works on traditional role definition and the part PAs play in an evolving medical marketplace. Includes a discussion of how current PA roles have been defined and speculates on the development of alternative roles, including a thought-provoking chapter on the future of PAs in a "multi-tiered" health care system.*

Zarbock S, Harbert K. Physician Assistants: Present and Future Models of Utilization. New York: Praeger, 1986. *Based on a conference, this book contains descriptions of PAs in geriatric, HMO, surgical, and tertiary care hospital settings. Also has practical information about nurse/PA relationships and a chapter on the use of PAs in strategic planning and marketing.*

CHAPTER 44

Critical Incident Stress Management: Managing Traumatic Stress With Group Crisis Intervention

Kenneth R. Harbert

INTRODUCTION

On September 11, 2001, the largest act of terrorism that Americans have ever witnessed occurred, killing more than 3000 people in New York City alone.[1] That day was a defining moment in the history of traumatic events in the United States. Since the beginning of recorded time, history has been full of traumatic events of both natural and human origin, which have left physical and mental scars on the victims and survivors. Traumatic events are unexpected and uncontrollable. Traumatic events affect the psychological functioning and adaptation of victims to everyday life thereafter.

Victor Frankl, who survived the concentration camps during World War II and went on to study traumatic stress, referred to a sense of self-actualization that occurred as the result of his experience. He stated, "It did not really matter what we expected from life but rather what life expected from us. We needed to stop asking about the meaning of life and instead to think of ourselves as those who were being questioned by life. Life ultimately means taking the responsibility to find the right answer to its problems and to fulfill the tasks it constantly sets for each individual. The meaning of suffering is not to change others: its meaning is that it changes you."[2]

915

STRESS

Hans Selye defined stress as the state manifested by a specific syndrome, which consists of all the non-specifically induced changes within a biological system. Later, he wrote that the nonspecific response of the body to any demand made on it is stress.[3]

Simply put, stress is the tension, strain, or pressure felt by a person. The stress or crisis in our daily lives offers the opportunity to advance from one level of maturity to another. Maslow focused on the self-actualized individual, noting that people are capable of virtually limitless growth and development when they are in the midst of the pain and turmoil of events such as divorce and physical illness.[4] Crisis may be defined as a serious occasion or turning point that presents both danger and opportunity.

A predicament is not crisis; a predicament is a condition or situation that is unpleasant, dangerous, or embarrassing. An emergency may or may not be a crisis because an emergency is the result of an unforeseen combination of circumstances that call for immediate action. A crisis does not necessarily follow a traumatic event. Nor does crisis lead to emotional or mental breakdown. Crisis does not occur in isolation, and often there is a dynamic interplay with stress and sometimes trauma. Yet trauma is not a stress, a crisis, or a predicament, nor is it an emergency. Traumatic stress is an extreme event out of the normal range of daily life.

TRAUMA

Freud defined trauma as "what occurs when the organism's protective barrier which modulates incoming stimuli is overwhelmed by the intensity of the organism's reaction."[5] Mitchell and Bray define traumatic stress as the "stress response produced when a person is exposed to a disturbing traumatic event." The reaction to such a traumatic event may be immediate or delayed.[6] Traumatic stress occurs when our interpretation of traumatic events, our coping ability, and the limitations of our individual or group resources lead to stress so severe that we cannot find relief.

Traumatic stress has had many names over the past 50 years, including yet not limited to, shell shock, traumatic neurosis, combat fatigue, operational exhaustion, and other names; yet even today, researchers and clinicians are still trying to define it.

Traumatic stress is elusive because as our society changes, so does society's view of the true definition of trauma. History has a way of repeating itself, but it also has a way of being forgotten. Today, there are those who incorrectly deny the existence of the Holocaust during World War II. Most of us have forgotten the great flood of 4000 BC in the Tigris and Euphrates valley in which thousands drowned, as well as the Coconut Grove Melody Lounge fire in Boston in 1942 that killed 492 people. Charles Dickens, Florence Nightingale, Sigfried Sassoon, and many other famous authors have written about their traumatic symptoms after experiencing traumatic events in their lives. These were not events of distress but rather traumatic events outside the realm of normal everyday life that had lifetime effects on these survivors, their rescuers, their caregivers, and even their families.

Traumatic stress differs from general stress, cumulative stress, or even distress. Traumatic events affect the psychological functioning and adaptation of victims to the sequelae of the event. Although history has documented a great deal about how traumatic stress affects individuals, researchers still are trying to understand the interactions of individuals and the stressor event, including such variables as the individual or group personalities, the coping processes involved, and the psychobiological mechanisms affected by trauma. The differences between disasters of natural origin and traumatic events of human origin are striking simply because the uncontrolled, violent forces of nature (e.g., fire, water, and wind) are minuscule in comparison to disasters from human sources. A good example of this is the horrific outcome of September 11, 2001. The cities of New York and Arlington and the entire world were affected by the events of that day, as was the entire world, as CNN broadcasted the event over and over again for viewers to share in this immense traumatic event. One day, the twin towers were there; the next, they were gone, and the worldview of many in the United States had changed. The images of the firemen raising the American flag at Ground Zero and the American flags on cars and businesses throughout the United

States are symbols of people trying to deal with a traumatic event that was not a natural disaster but a trauma inflicted on humans by humans.

In 1991, Donovan defined traumatology as "the study of natural and man-made trauma, the social and psychobiological effects thereof, and the predictive-preventive-interventionist pragmatics which evolve from that study."[7] He later reported that traumatology recognizes that experience, the most elemental of human phenomena, is mediated physiologically and thus has physiological consequences. The physiological response experience is interpretative, which is one of the reasons why different individuals respond differently to potentially traumatic events. If experience can be formative and de-formative, it can also be re-formative. In 1993, Figley used the term *traumatology* to describe the investigation and applications of knowledge related to the immediate and long-term psychosocial consequences of highly stressful events and the factors that affect those consequences.[8]

Several authors have suggested that there is a natural reaction to a traumatic event in both behavior and emotion, physiologically and psychologically.[8-10] Figley defined this traumatic stress reaction as a collection of conscious and unconscious actions and emotions that occur as an individual attempts to deal with the stressors of a traumatic event and the period immediately afterward.[11] Traumatic stressors may include not only exposure to a traumatic event itself, but also the degree of perceived risk of exposure to traumatic events; this has been reported very clearly after the event of September 11, 2001 in New York City.[12]

A traumatic stress reaction begins with the response to the event or the patient encounter and continues as long as symptoms are present. Symptoms may be swift in onset, as in an acute reaction, which follows minutes after a critical incident. This response is a normal grief response, as would be expected after a tragedy. If intense symptoms persist, or if the symptoms appear sometime after the tragedy and continue, a cumulative or delayed stress reaction is present. A post-traumatic syndrome of symptoms may last months or decades. Avoidance behavior may occur, and the emotional response may impair the person's ability to function and relate to other people.

Many factors determine how and whether persons will be affected by traumatic stress, including age, experience, expectations, interpretations, and perceptions of the traumatic event. Adaptation to a traumatic life event may be affected by personality, nature of the stressors experienced, coping resources, support resources, history of co-morbidity, and the nature of the recovery, which may involve a positive change in character.

Health care professionals can use basic coping mechanisms to manage acute or delayed stress reactions that do not cause life-disrupting changes, such as recurring nightmares or intrusive thoughts. Ochberg suggests four categories to focus on for improving coping skills in victims of acute or delayed stress reactions: education, holistic health, social support, and social integration. If primary assessment reveals severe symptoms, counseling or other supportive therapy is needed.[13] Prevention programs that stress awareness and education may circumvent the onset of symptoms. Flannery and Everly have stated that acute care should focus on "stabilization of escalating distress, mitigation of acute signs and symptoms of distress, and restoration of adaptive independent functioning or facilitation of access to higher levels of care."[13]

UNDERSTANDING TRAUMATIC STRESS

Although we have learned a great deal about how traumatic stress affects people, we are still trying to understand the interactions of individuals and the stressor event, the personalities attributed and coping processes involved, and the psychobiological mechanisms affected by trauma.

Pierre Janet in 1889 is credited as the first psychologist to study and treat traumatic stress, including hysterical and dissociate symptoms.[14] He studied the recognition of the brain and its inability to integrate traumatic memories as the core issue in post-traumatic stress disorder (PTSD) and then discovered the importance of the fundamental biphasic nature of traumatic stress.[14] Janet thought that the physiological response to trauma accounted for the continued emergency responses to subsequent stresses. Experiences that overwhelm coping mechanisms set the stage for a person to react automatically with excessive emotional reactions to subsequent stressors. He thought that fear needed to be tamed for proper cognitive appraisal and appropriate action to occur.

Freud stated also that the fixation of the trauma is biologically based.[15] The traumatic neurosis is the result of an "extensive rupture in the barrier against stimuli."[16] In 1911, Oppenheim was credited with coining the term *traumatic neurosis.*

Little was known about the underlying physiological mechanisms of this traumatic response until Selye described the pituitary-adrenalin cortical response to experimental stressors in 1936. In 1950, he went on to describe a general adaptation syndrome, which detailed characteristic responses to major personal threats as the following: alarm, resistance, and ultimately, sheer exhaustion. He separated stress into *eustress,* or good stress, such as that caused by marriage, and *distress,* such as that caused by divorce.[17]

Psychiatrists often used the terms *shell shock* and *effort syndrome* in World War I to describe the traumatic stress of that period. The term *shell shock* was coined because of the artillery blasts that left men deaf, emotionally numb, and wandering aimlessly through the trenches. Later, in World War II, this traumatic stress was called "battle stress or combat stress reaction" because of the environment in which this phenomenon occurred. This term applied to soldiers who appeared fatigued and had shortness of breath, palpitations, headache, excessive sweating, and inability to function, and who were withdrawn and/or depressed during or after battles.[18]

As a result of experience with traumatic stress disorders, the term *gross stress reaction* was included in the first edition of the *Diagnostic and Statistical Manual of Mental Disorders,* in 1952.[19] *Gross stress reaction* was defined as a reversible and transient response to stress. This diagnosis was removed in the second edition, only to return after significant modification in the third and fourth editions. The new interpretation states that acute stress disorders are human responses to a traumatic event that the person experienced, witnessed, or was confronted with, such as an event that involved actual or threatened death or serious injury, or a threat to the physical integrity of self or others.[20]

The early concepts of traumatic stress disorder focused on emotional reactions to environmental stimuli, such as earthquakes, fires, and occupational burnout. In the 1970s, traumatic stress disorders were viewed as the results of psychosocial stress, such as that observed in Holocaust victims, Vietnam veterans, and rape and abuse victims, and even as the results of occupationally induced stress, such as that seen in police officers, nurses, paramedics, fire fighters, and physicians. As a result of the psychiatric morbidity associated with Vietnam veterans, the phrase *posttraumatic stress disorder (PTSD)* was finally coined.

Psychobiology of Traumatic Stress

The limbic system plays an important role in guiding the emotions that stimulate the behavior necessary for self-preservation and survival of the species. It is responsible for such complex behaviors as feeding, fighting, fleeing, and reproducing, and it also assigns to experience free-floating feelings of significance, truth, and meaning.[21] The limbic system is also the primary area of the central nervous system (CNS) wherein memories are processed and is the most likely location of an explanation for the memory disturbances that follow trauma.

The hippocampus, which records the spatial and temporal dimensions of experiences in memory, does not fully mature until the third or fourth year of life. The hippocampal localization system remains vulnerable to disruption, and severe or prolonged stress can suppress hippocampal functioning.[22] The limbic system is involved in "kindling," or repeated stimulation, and oversees sensitization of limbic neuronal circuits and neuronal firing at lower thresholds. Trauma can cause long-term alterations in neuronal excitability, which may lead to lasting neurobiological and behavioral changes mediated by alterations in the temporal lobe.[23]

Lowered serotonin activity in traumatic stress is at the core of the diminished efficacy of the behavioral inhibition system, which in turn is responsible for the continuation of emergency responses to minor stresses long after the actual trauma has ceased.

The body responds to increased physical or psychological demands by releasing norepinephrine from the locus ceruleus and adrenocorticotropin (ACTH) from the anterior pituitary. Peripherally, the body's stress response consists of the secretion of norepinephrine by the sympathetic nerves and of epinephrine by the adrenal medulla. Stimulated by ACTH, the adrenal cortex secretes glucocorticoids. These hormones help mobilize the energy necessary to deal with stressors ranging from increased glucose release to enhanced immune function. In a well-functioning organism, stress produces rapid and pronounced hormonal responses. However, chronic persistent stress blunts this effective stress response and induces sensitization. After prolonged stress, corticotropin-releasing hormone (CRH) secretion leads to less cyclic adenosine monophosphate (cAMP) formation and ACTH release because of downregulation of corticotropin-releasing factor (CRF) receptors. Thus, the release of the stress hormone ACTH is controlled by complex regulatory mechanisms. Multiple factors such as CRH, vasopressin, catecholamines, and other hormones stimulate ACTH release by acting on the anterior pituitary. The simultaneous release of these catecholamines (exciters), corticosteroids and serotonin (moderators), and endogenous opioids (providing pain analgesia, emotional blunting, and memory shortening) allows our nervous system to deal with life-threatening events. Balance is the key to this psychobiological cascade. When overarousal occurs, rage, panic, and agitated behavior are present.

Rapidly expanding knowledge of the effects of trauma on the CNS provides the awareness that memory and ongoing functions of memory are at the core of the psychological disruptions seen with chronic traumatic stress disorders and with PTSD. A variety of psychopharmacological agents that affect the physiological arousal system, including clonidine, benzodiazepines, monoamine oxidase (MAO) inhibitors, and tricyclic antidepressants, reduce the long-term effects of inescapable shock and seem to have some use in the pharmacotherapy of PTSD. Medications can be used to relieve depression and to improve sleep, suppress intrusive images, and calm explosive anger.

In 2001, Roger Pitman, a Harvard Medical School psychiatrist, proposed that the amygdala is more relevant than the hippocampus to the development of PTSD because the amygdala is involved in the acquisition of a conditioned fear response. With the use of magnetic resonance imaging (MRI) studies, he found that the amygdala does not change during PTSD, and by administering the antiadrenaline drug propanolol within 6 hours of a traumatic event, he reduced PTSD by blocking the effects of noradrenaline in the amygdala.[24]

Traumatic and untreated stress can cause physical illness, the loss of self-realization, and/or loss of self-growth and can disrupt our life-course trajectory.[25]

CAREGIVERS AND TRAUMATIC STRESS

Trauma affects both victims and caregivers. The role of caregivers during traumatic events is physically and emotionally demanding. Caregivers are expected, by society and by peers, to provide treatment to the victims of traumatic events regardless of how extensive. They are also expected to cope with these events without having serious emotional problems themselves. Patients and peers often expect superhuman outcomes with unreal expectations. Often, caregivers encounter a traumatic event to which they react with severe inner turmoil. The response of the caregiver varies. Many recover fully within days or weeks of the event. A few may be so overwhelmed that their ability to function at work and in relationships with family members and friends is jeopardized. The ultimate goals of therapy and recovery are to restore dignity and self-worth, promote emotional stability and expressiveness, and offer peace to the affected caregiver. Both traditional and nontraditional therapies are of value. State, national, and international organizations offer referral and counseling assistance.[26]

The Shock Trauma Center in Baltimore, Maryland, was one of the first major medical trauma facilities to offer support services to its trauma staff. Marge Epperson-Sebour, a social worker in the family services section, was concerned with the turnover of experienced staff nurses. She developed a series of educational stress management programs in the mid-1970s.[27] In Australia, Robinson worked with fire, emergency workers, and hospital staffs to reduce the negative impact of stress on staff members.[28] Mitchell addressed the issues of emergency medical personnel, which he described as "critical incident stress," using a term borrowed from the field of organizational behavior that identified powerful predictors of success or failure on the job. He defined "a critical incident" as a crisis or traumatic event that can exert such a stressful impact that it overwhelms an individual's usual coping mechanisms.[29]

In 1990, the Geisinger Medical Center in Danville, Pennsylvania, established one of the first interdisciplinary critical incident stress management (CISM) teams within a rural tertiary medical center that served more than 34 rural counties within central Pennsylvania. The team was formed with the support of the nursing department, and included physicians, physician assistants (PAs), nurses, social workers, emergency medical personnel, mental health specialists, pastoral counselors, and an assigned administrator. All team members received basic and advanced training from the International Critical Incident Stress Foundation. The nursing and PA members of the team were all active members of a regional CISM team and had participated in a number of CISM interventions. The team was established to respond to any issues, concerns, and/or critical events on a 24-hour, 7-day-a-week basis. This interdisciplinary model was presented in 1990 at an annual research conference sponsored by the Agency for Health Policy and Research and later was used as a model for a number of regional and national hospital CISM teams.[30]

The PA, nurse, or physician who has dealt with the mass casualties resulting from a fire, a train derailment, a plane crash, or a combat situation may continue to have difficulty on the anniversary of that event or when confronted by a similar event or incident. Sometimes, these difficulties may include intrusive thoughts or sleep disorders.

Caregivers who provide life-saving skills for seriously ill or dying patients often find it difficult, if not impossible, to share their feelings and fears with family and friends who did not share in the experience. It is difficult or even impossible for their family and friends to understand the realities of emergency departments even after they have seen many of these traumatic events on television shows such as "E.R." The role and perception of the caregiver about the event and his or her sense of guilt or responsibility for a negative outcome have enormous consequences for putting the event or incident into the proper healthy perspective. One positive outcome of the tragic events

of September 11, 2001, in New York City and in Virginia was the outpouring of caring for the emergency medical rescuers who died in both of these tragic events and a renewed respect for caregivers throughout the world.

The bottom line for most troubled caregivers is the question, "What can I do about the situation?" versus "What is wrong with me?" If the symptoms of trauma are viewed as a situational problem that affects others in similar circumstances and not as a problem resulting from their own failure to cope, individuals will strive to make the situation more tolerable. Caregivers expect superhuman effort from themselves, but often they are the first to counsel their patients not to expect perfection from themselves or from life. Yet when faced with having traumatic stress symptoms, caregivers may exhibit guilt, shame, fear of stigmatization, and concerns about personal confidentiality.[31] Healing can begin at a very basic level by allowing caregivers to express meaningful appreciation for what each has done and suggestions for how they can help each other after the event has ended. People have a need for appreciation, support, respect, and approval from their co-workers, during and after the time of crisis.[32]

A traumatic stress disorder is often triggered by a particular event in the near or distant past that has caused stress to the caregiver. It is not uncommon, for example, for a caregiver who has responded without emotion to dozens of adults injured in motor vehicle accidents to suddenly crumple emotionally at the sight of a disfigured child or infant. The trauma may be relived over time simply by discussing the event or by being near where the event occurred. Also, the caregiver may have confused emotions when faced with his or her children when returning home after the event.

The lifetime prevalence of post-traumatic stress disorder is estimated to be from 1% to 3% of the general population. It is also known that another 5% to 15% may experience other forms of this disorder. Among high-risk groups such as police, fire personnel, physicians, nurses, and emergency medical personnel, the lifetime prevalence is estimated to be 16% to 20%. Post-traumatic stress can be a normal survival mechanism. Post-traumatic stress disorder is a pathogenic version of that mechanism.

Not everyone develops post-traumatic stress disorder after a traumatic event. The variables include the individual preexisting biological and psychosocial factors and the individual perceptions of the events that follow. Recent research has shown that this disorder has a great deal to do with the stressor's subjective meaning to a person. Other key factors include the victim's understanding of the event, accepting the perceptions of self and others, focusing on the situation and stressors, feeling a sense of guilt after the event, and/or inability to share the event with others.

The immediate interventions that are provided for the individual or group after a traumatic event deliver emotional first aid, offer stabilization, mitigate stress, offer a sense of normalization, and offer the opportunity for restoration of daily living. Crisis intervention at the right time, for the right reasons, and for the right people provided by trained individuals can help make a difference in mitigating the effects of traumatic stress.

Wilson suggests that therapeutic goals for traumatic stress should include the following[33]:

➤ Providing therapeutic support.
➤ Developing the ability to express emotions.
➤ Promoting interest in meaningful activities.
➤ Exploring feelings of helplessness.
➤ Placing feelings in perspective.
➤ Evoking positive emotions.
➤ Reducing the cycle of numbing, intrusive thoughts, distortion, and dissociation.

INTERVENTIONS FOR TRAUMATIC STRESS
Crisis Intervention

Flannery and Everly have defined crisis intervention as "the provision of emergency psychological care to victims so as to assist those victims in returning to an adaptive level of functioning and to prevent or mitigate the potential negative impact of psychological trauma."[34]

Crisis intervention is also crisis management, a short-term helping process that focuses on resolution of the immediate problem through the use of personal, social, and environmental resources. It is related to but differs from psychotherapy. Crisis intervention offers assistance for those dealing with psychological crisis, especially when it is sudden, unexpected, and life threatening.

The Coconut Grove Melody Lounge fire in 1942 that killed 492 people resulted in a classical study of bereavement and defined the grieving process that people go through after the sudden death of a relative.[35] Lindemann found that survivors of this disaster who developed serious psychopathologies had failed to go through the normal process of grieving.[28] Processing grief consists of mourning one's loss, experiencing the pain of such loss, and eventually accepting the loss while adjusting to life without the loved one or object.[36]

In 1964, Caplan developed the conceptual framework for understanding crisis, including the process of crisis development.[37] His framework of crisis intervention focused on five hallmarks: early intervention (immediacy); intervention with close physical proximity to the acute crisis manifestation (proximity); acute problem-focused intervention (expectancy); short intervention consisting of one to three contacts (brevity); and simple, direct interventions to prevent confrontation (simplicity).[38] He also emphasized a community-wide approach to crisis intervention. His later studies focused on crisis prevention—that is, the mastery of stress as well as the importance of social, cultural, and material "supplies" necessary to avoid crisis.[39]

These studies were extremely valuable to mental health professionals in explaining the development and resolution of crisis. Caplan's focus on prevention rather than simply on the treatment of disease encouraged Mitchell in the development of his concept of CISM.

Interpretation of the crisis experience implies that people in crisis are unable to take charge of their lives. People who accept this view when in crisis will be less likely to participate actively in the crisis resolution process and thereby will diminish their potential for growth.[40] Individuals and groups in crisis need an opportunity to do the following[41]:

➤ Experience and express their feelings of fear, panic, loss, and pain within a safe environment.
➤ Become fully aware and accepting of what has happened to them.
➤ Resume activity and begin reconstructing their lives with the social, physical, and emotional resources available.

➤ Be listened to with concern and sympathy.

➤ Understand the reality of what has happened, a bit at a time.

➤ Make contact with relatives, friends, and other resources needed to begin the process of social and physical reconstruction.

Emotional recovery requires that a traumatized person be able to incorporate events into his or her own system of meaning and to maintain at least some perception of self-control. If a situation seems beyond one's control, self-blame may be used as a way of coping with the event. It is important that victims attribute responsibility to its true sources rather than to themselves. Interpreting a person's anger and demand for compensation as dependency conflict is a form of blaming the victim. Traumatized people should be linked to self-help and advocacy groups through which they might channel their anger into constructive action for necessary change.[42] Individuals have different perceptions of traumatic events, the understanding of which is central to coming to terms with and resolving a crisis.

Without communication, we cannot understand another's interpretation of an event or issue, and we may become a hindrance to constructive crisis resolution. CISM, as one model of group crisis intervention, offers the uniqueness of others' perceptions and the satisfaction of people helping others and helping themselves.[43] As people are brought together to discuss the traumatic event, they discover that the interpretations of the event are as diverse as the group members themselves. Communication helps persons tell their traumatic experience through emotional display, behavior, and verbal communication. Often, victims find that friends or counselors may not listen because the event or incident is too overwhelming, but that those who participated in the event or incident are willing to discuss it in the hope of resolving their feelings, thoughts, and memories of the event.

The basic principles of crisis intervention are to intervene immediately, stabilize the victim or the community, facilitate understanding about what has happened, focus on problem solving within what is possible for the victim, and encourage self-reliance to restore a sense of independent functioning.[13]

The comprehensive, integrated, multi-component CISM system offers a full range of services that span the crisis spectrum from the pre-crisis phase, through the acute crisis phase, and into the post-crisis phase, as well as referral for formal mental health assessment and treatment.[35] CISM is considered comprehensive in that it consists of interventions that may be applied to individuals, small functional groups, large groups, families, organizations, and even entire communities.[13]

The right type of intervention is essential, as too are the proper timing and choice of people who need assistance. Different interventions exist. At times, individual support is needed; at other times, team or group support is needed. As a system consisting of multiple crisis intervention components, CISM offers interventions that begin in the pre-crisis phase and continue until the crisis is over.[44]

CRITICAL INCIDENTS—WHAT ARE THEY?

A critical incident involves a situation that causes individual health care providers, or a group, to experience unusually strong emotional reactions. Critical incidents have the potential to interfere with caregivers' ability to function during or after the event. A major disaster with multiple casualties or multiple deaths, the sudden death of a faculty member, or the violent death of a peer are all types of critical incidents, but an event or situation does not have to be of this magnitude to classify it as a critical incident.

A critical incident is defined as any event with sufficient impact to produce significant emotional reactions in people at the time of occurrence or later.[43] These events are considered to be outside the range of ordinary human experience. The incident may lead to development of post-traumatic stress disorder if the issues caused by the incident or event are not resolved by the person effectively and quickly. The following are examples of critical incidents that may involve PAs:

➤ Verbally or physically abusive patients, visitors, and/or family members.

➤ Suicide attempts by patients, staff members, faculty, or students while in the hospital or clinic, or in a patient familiar to staff over a long period.

➤ Death of a child or infant as the result of abusive behavior.

➤ Sexual abuse of a child or infant that results in morbidity or mortality.

➤ Prolonged resuscitation efforts involving trauma, emergency department (ED), Life Flight (aeromedical evacuation), and neonatal intensive care unit teams or individuals.

➤ Sudden accidental death of a peer, faculty member, or student.

➤ Violent death of a professional peer, faculty member, or student while at work or at home.

➤ Sudden dramatic rise in morbidity or mortality over a long period (longer than 10 working days) within a close-knit inpatient unit (e.g., ED or intensive care unit),

➤ Suicide of a co-worker, team member, faculty member, or student.

➤ Caring for a seriously ill co-worker, family member, relative, or close friend.

➤ Caring for a seriously ill prisoner with guards and weapons present over a long period (longer than 10 working days).

➤ Hostage situations in the hospital, clinic, or unit.

➤ Staff or team member hostility toward each other that appears abusive and unresolved.

➤ Multiple-casualty situations or natural or human-made disasters.

➤ Impairment of a co-worker that affects patient care and team interaction and cohesiveness.

➤ Intense work or training sessions that cause sleep deprivation, or hazardous environments that are potentially harmful to staff or students.

➤ Any other significant event within the health care or academic institution.

To assist health care workers, Flannery has developed a CISM approach for health care providers of child and adult services in emergency departments; inpatient, outpatient, or day programs; homeless shelters; and community-based residences. The model includes individual crisis counseling, group debriefings, staff/victim support, staff/victim family counseling, and professional referral when needed.[49]

CRITICAL INCIDENT STRESS MANAGEMENT—HOW AND WHY IT WORKS

Crisis intervention has evolved, as has the conceptual framework of how and when to use the right model of intervention. The concept that crisis intervention should offer more than one intervention is not new. Bordow and Porritt demonstrated that multi-component crisis intervention was more effective than one single intervention.[46]

Raphael suggested the use of a broader spectrum approach to crisis intervention, especially for emergency medical personnel.[47]

Critical incident stress management (CISM) was developed and is currently utilized by Dr. Jeffrey Mitchell. Mitchell is a former fire fighter and paramedic who teaches stress management, crisis intervention, and the psychological effects of disasters. In the late 1970s and after the Air Florida crash in Washington, D.C. in 1982, Mitchell started conceptualizing his "Mitchell model" for CISM. More than 400 CISM teams use this model today worldwide. These teams have assisted with disasters and critical incidents all over the globe over the past 10 years.

CISM is one model of traumatic stress management services for groups and individuals that is a comprehensive, integrated multi-component crisis intervention system.[45] The core components of CISM include the following:

1. Pre-crisis planning/education.
2. Individual crisis intervention (one-on-one).
3. Small group crisis intervention—defusing.
4. Small group crisis intervention—critical incident stress debriefings (CISDs).
5. Large group crisis intervention—demobilizations (for public safety, rescue, disaster personnel).
6. Large group crisis intervention—crisis management briefing (CMB) for civilian populations, schools, businesses, communities, and so forth.
7. Organizational consultation.
8. Family crisis intervention.
9. Pastoral crisis intervention.
10. Mechanisms for follow-up and referral.

CISM offers a comprehensive approach for the victims of natural and man-made disasters, as well as for emergency mental health personnel, that provide support to victims and rescuers during traumatic events. It also provides a method of screening individuals who may need further assistance or referral.

It was never designed with routine in mind. CISM should be applied only to those events that are extraordinary.[45] The best way to assess the need for this type of comprehensive CISM model is to determine whether the event or incident has generated strong feelings among individuals or groups of caregivers. Basic criteria for use of the CISM model include the following:

➤ Many individuals of a common group appear distressed after an event or incident.
➤ Personnel make significant errors after an event or incident.
➤ Personnel request help.
➤ The event or incident is extraordinary, unlike any other.
➤ Staff members die, are injured, or are abused.
➤ Individuals involved in the event or incident are not able to continue at their normal level of professional functioning.
➤ Personnel involved in the event or incident demonstrate numerous behavioral changes.
➤ Distress among staff or individuals continues beyond 3 weeks.

CISM is an early intervention strategy, a means of mitigating traumatic stress that provides a safe, supportive opportunity for individuals to express, self-disclose, and understand their emotions. CISM focuses on helping participants explore their perceptions of the event, allowing for confirmation of the incident and the roles of individuals or a group during the event. CISM also offers the opportunity for members of the group to express fears, concerns, and regrets within a group of peers, with the value of the added support of a professional and/or peer who was not at the incident or involved with the group.

Only individuals who have been specifically trained in the concepts of CISM should use this technique. Having a background in medicine, psychiatry, psychology, nursing, or any other professional discipline does not automatically ensure that individuals understand or can use these methods. CISM was developed specifically for emergency personnel, but it has had great success when used with other professionals and groups. The key to successful use of this technique is that the CISM team leader and other CISM team members must have been appropriately trained in these components through specific courses offered through the International Critical Incident Stress Foundation (ICISF).

CISM is a group-focused team approach to mitigating the harmful effects of stress. This team approach comprises a mental health professional and several peer support personnel (not involved in the incident or event or not well known by those who need CISM). CISM is a group process, with a meeting or discussion designed to reduce stress and enhance recovery from stress, based on the hallmark principles of crisis intervention and health education. It has been designed to stabilize cognitive and affective processes and to further mitigate the impact of a traumatic event. It is not a critique of the incident or event.

CISM provides support services for a group or team that has experienced something out of the ordinary. CISM is not psychotherapy, nor is it a substitute for psychotherapy. CISM accelerates the rate of normal recovery, in normal people who are having normal reactions to abnormal events. These techniques may not solve all of the problems that arise during the CISM intervention. The core elements of CISM allow for the basic mental health screening of individuals who may require further mental health assistance. Use of these basic interventions may lead to the introduction of mental health personnel, offering an essential bridge for further follow-up with appropriate mental health professionals.

Adaptation and accommodation of specific interventions to fit the circumstances are essential if the best help is to be delivered to those who need it. Standardized training and CISM team experiences are crucial elements in the use of the right group of response personnel, including appropriate mental health personnel.

Pre-crisis Planning/Education The first intervention in the CISM system is labeled "pre-crisis planning and education" and occurs in the pre-crisis phase. This intervention is designed to set the appropriate expectation for the potential event while enhancing behavioral responses to the event. It is appropriate for high-risk personnel, such as health care workers in a high-risk area, or health care students who will face trauma situations.

The goals of pre-crisis planning and education include setting appropriate expectations for actual experiences, increasing cognitive resources relevant to a crisis, and/or teaching behavioral stress management and personal coping techniques with the goal of preventing psychological dysfunction and disorder.

Stress management education begins before the traumatic event occurs. Education is one of the most important components of a systematic, comprehensive, multi-component approach to the management of traumatic stress. An informational discussion about traumatic stress and types of interventions would benefit PA students and graduates. PA programs could offer this in concert with their discussions regarding eustress and distress.

PA programs might consider the importance of providing this type of training before having students enter their clinical preceptorships, and then should evaluate the need for this type of training within their region for practicing PAs.[24]

Demobilization   Another CISM intervention is demobilization. This intervention can be used at mass disaster sites to assist disaster response personnel to decompress and transition from the incident site to home or work. This quick informational and rest session is applied when operational units have been released from service at a major incident that requires more than 100 personnel. The demobilization consists of a process whereby teams or groups receive 10 minutes of information from a CISM team member about stress, trauma, and coping techniques, followed by 20 minutes of refreshments and comfort within a safe environment. Ideally, demobilization is provided by a trained CISM team member experienced in dealing with mental health issues.

Crisis Management Briefing   Crisis management briefing (CMB) is a large group, crisis intervention technique that can be used to mitigate the levels of crisis and traumatic stress in the wake of terrorism, mass disasters, violence, and other "large-scale" crises involving up to 300 people. CMB is a practical four-phase group crisis intervention technique that is designed to be highly efficient in that it requires only 45 to 75 minutes to conduct and may be used for large groups consisting of 10 to 300 individuals.[48] Phase One consists of bringing together individuals who have experienced a common crisis event. Phase Two involves providing the most credible facts of the crisis event delivered by a highly credible spokesperson. This phase is focused on controlling rumors, reducing anticipatory anxiety, and offering a sense of control to victims of the event. This phase also offers the opportunity to provide factual information and explain what is not known about the event. Phase Three involves having credible health care professionals discuss the most common reactions to traumatic stress and, if terrorism is involved, discussing the implications of the event. Because terrorism is an action undertaken to achieve a political or theological goal that creates terror or horror among victims, a credible expert should be utilized. Phase Four involves addressing personal coping and self-care strategies that may be of value in mitigating distressing reactions to the crisis event. Simple and practical stress management concepts and strategies are offered. Reference information is provided to participants, along with contact information for additional future CISM interventions.

Defusing   A technique called *defusing* is a shortened version of the debriefing. This intervention may take 25 to 45 minutes; it involves group discussions of the event or incident and is designed to mitigate the impact of the event, accelerate the recovery process, and assess the need for future interventions and/or other services. Defusing is also designed to reduce cognitive, emotional, and physiological symptoms. Defusing is made up of three components. These include the introduction phase used to describe the process, motivate participants, stress confidentiality, and clarify that it is not a critique but rather a process for helping participants to help themselves. The exploration phase focuses on what happened to the personnel involved; the experience is clarified, reactions and experiences are shared, facts are separated from fiction, and the need for further intervention is assessed. The final phase provides stress management information, offers a summary of the exploration, and focuses on normalizing the experience and reactions to the event. Educational information is given out, as is information about opportunities for future follow-up interventions. The defusing should take place within 8 hours after the incident has ended.

Critical Incident Stress Debriefing

Critical incident stress debriefing (CISD) is the most complex of all the CISM interventions. CISD was originally designed to reduce stress in emergency personnel, but over the past 10 years, it has been applied to diverse groups, including college students, educational systems, law enforcement, health care systems, nursing personnel, military personnel, PAs, and physicians.[49] CISD is one specific model of psychological debriefing, developed by Mitchell, and is a group process that employs both crisis intervention and educational processes.

CISD focuses on mitigating or resolving the harmful effects of work-related trauma and psychological distress associated with a critical incident or traumatic event. The CISD team is a partnership between mental health professionals and peers who are interested in preventing and mitigating the negative impact of acute stress on themselves and others. Mental health professionals who serve on CISM teams should have at least a master's degree in psychology, social work, psychiatric nursing, or mental health counseling. Peer support members should have received specific training in the basic and/or advanced concepts of CISM from the International Critical Incident Stress Foundation (ICISF) and also should have completed the ICISF course on assisting individuals in crisis.

The CISD and defusing processes are group meetings or discussions about a traumatic event, or a series of traumatic events. The CISD and defusing processes are solidly based in crisis intervention and educational intervention theory. CISDs and defusings are designed to mitigate the psychological impact of a traumatic event and prevent the subsequent development of a post-traumatic syndrome; they serve as an early identification mechanism for individuals who will require professional mental health follow-up after experiencing a traumatic event.

CISD is used with a homogeneous group of individuals who have experienced a traumatic event or crisis. The technique should be used at least 24 hours after the traumatic event has ended, or at least 24 hours after individuals have been operationally disengaged from the event with the clear expectation of not returning to the event. Timing is essential if CISD is to be effective in mitigating the adverse psychological impact of a traumatic event. CISD's goals include the following:

➤ Offer early intervention.
➤ Provide an opportunity for catharsis.
➤ Offer a safe, secure venue in which participants can verbalize trauma.
➤ Begin in the cognitive domain and move to the affective domain.
➤ Provide group support.
➤ Enhance peer support.
➤ Offer an opportunity for assessment of individual and group responses to traumatic stress.

CISD comprises a seven-stage group intervention. The CISD team–led process starts at the point that is easiest to discuss, and then moves gradually into more emotionally intense group discussions. The group is gradually brought back out of the intense discussions to the less intense discussions. The seven phases of CISD include the introduction phase, the fact phase, the thought phase, the reaction phase, the symptom phase, the teaching phase, and the reentry phase.

CISD provides a finite behavioral structure. The process starts by engagement of the cognitive domain. This structure is ideal for those persons engaged in cognitive analysis or denial mechanisms. It aligns with their psychological posture rather than contradicting or opposing it, thus avoiding the risk of initiating group conflict. As the CISD process continues, affective ventilation or self-disclosure may be achieved.[47]

Introduction Phase

The introduction sets the stage for the other phases of the debriefing. The objectives to achieve during this phase include the introduction of CISD team members, the introduction of the team leader (establishing the leadership of the team), an explanation of the purpose of the meeting, and an explanation of the process, rules, and guidelines of CISD, which include the following:

➤ No one in the group has rank over another.
➤ All participants speak for themselves only.
➤ Recorders and note taking are not allowed.

➤ CISD is not a critique or an investigation.

➤ Participants are instructed not to disclose any information that would jeopardize an investigation or would constitute an admission of criminal activity or deliberate violations of policies and/or procedures.

➤ No one is allowed to leave the room and not return. Everyone is important to the complete process, and everyone is there to help themselves and each other.

➤ Whatever is stated in the room is confidential and stays in the room. This applies to the team as well as to participants.

➤ Participants are asked to turn off pagers, radios, and other distracting devices.

Other objectives of the debriefing include gaining the cooperation of participants, answering any questions or concerns from the group, and encouraging mutual help and understanding. Often, the key elements to healing are talking about the event, having time to deal with it, and allowing tears to flow among those who understand the pain.

Fact Phase   The first phase, which is the fact phase, allows participants to describe the traumatic event from their own perspective. Facts are a collection of items outside of oneself. Facts are impersonal. A discussion of facts is not as distressing as attempting to talk about how one feels, which involves more personal material. The following Case Study illustrates the fact phase.

CASE STUDY 44-1

The team leader starts by stating:

"We realize that some of you do not want to be here. You may not need help, but staying here now may help someone else who needs your help to get through this event. You have all shared a bad experience. It's sad that bad things happen to good people; that's why we are here. We were not present during the event. We only know bits and pieces of the incident. It would be very helpful to hear from each of you about what your role was during the incident, and what you saw and heard. If you choose not to speak, that is okay. Just shake your head and we will pass right over you to the next person in the circle."

This should be repeated by the team leader, who says that what we need to know is:

➤ Who you are (first name and profession, e.g., Harriet—physician assistant).

➤ What your job or role was during the incident (trauma team—PA).

➤ What happened during this event from your point of view and only your point of view.

Often, during the answers to these questions, participants spontaneously begin to show emotions. Mitchell has stated, "When participants in a debriefing are asked to describe the facts of the situation and they begin to express their emotions, it is generally a sign of how badly they have been affected by the event."[45]

Thought Phase   The next phase is the thought phase. This phase begins with the team leader asking the participants to state what their first or most prominent thought was once they got off an auto pilot mode of operating or functioning. This phase allows the participants to describe their cognitive reactions to the event and to begin to transition to the affective domain. The thought phase is the transitional phase between the factual world and the world that is close and personal. Facts are often outside of a person, but thoughts are internal and are part of the inner person. This is the phase in which participants may express anger at team members or at others regarding the event. The CISD team must always be alert to participant reactions during this phase.

Reaction Phase   The most emotional phase of CISD is the reaction phase, which follows the thought phase. This phase identifies the most traumatic aspect of the event for participants who wish to speak and allows for cathartic ventilation. This phase is entirely in the affective domain. The key question, raised by the team leader, for this phase is, "What was the worst thing about this incident, event, or situation for you personally?"

Other questions that follow for the group may include the following: "What bothered you the most?" "If you could erase one part of this event, what would it be?" "What aspect caused you the most pain?" The discussion at this point is free flowing. Until this phase, the team leader has directed each of the questions to each member of the group in a round-robin fashion, usually from right to left, from the team leader to the last person in the circle. During this phase, anyone who wishes to speak may do so. This is the toughest point for the participants. They are now wrestling with the emotions they have begun to connect with the event. Some comments will trigger strong verbal group responses.

Emotions often pour out. Sometimes, these emotions are held back, but the body language of the participant is screaming in anger, grief, or sorrow. This phase may last anywhere from 10 to 40 minutes total. When the discussion drops off or questions asked by the team members end with little or no response, it is a signal to move on to the next phase—the symptom phase.[45]

Symptom Phase   The symptom phase is another transition phase. Mitchell describes that the objective in this phase is to begin to move the group back from the emotionally laden content of the reaction phase toward the more cognitively oriented material. The symptom phase is a natural part of the overall process from the cognitive domain to the emotional and then back to the cognitive domain. Mitchell states, "The debriefing is always continued to the end to complete the process and to restore people to the cognitive level they began with during the debriefing, so that they can resume the normal responsibilities of their lives, armed with their customary set of psychological defenses intact."[45]

The symptom phase is initiated when the team asks the participants to describe any cognitive, physical, emotional, or behavioral experiences they may have encountered while they were working or since the event occurred. Mitchell states that on occasion, "The participants are reluctant to bring up their symptoms because they fear that they are the only ones with these feelings or symptoms and that their symptoms may be abnormal."[49] This phase identifies any symptoms of distress that the group wishes to share and potentiates the initial transition from the affective domain back to the cognitive domain.[24] The symptom phase typically lasts 15 to 20 minutes. Once the

number of responses has decreased dramatically, the team makes a decision to move into the next phase of the debriefing—the teaching phase.

Teaching Phase   The teaching phase facilitates a return to the cognitive domain by normalizing and demystifying the event and the reactions of the participants. The CISD team empowers the participants with stress management and coping techniques that can be used to reduce current and potential future stress. A natural transition is to describe the symptoms mentioned in the symptom phase as being normal for someone who has experienced a traumatic event. Team members are active in describing typical symptoms of distress and forewarn the group about other symptoms they might encounter. Instructions are given regarding diet, exercise, rest, talking to significant others, talking to each other, supporting each other, and avoiding alcohol and caffeine. This phase allows team members to direct specific information to individual participants with concerns or issues of discomfort. While the whole group gets the message, the individual receives the information important to himself or herself. This is also the time to ask, "Did anything happen during the event to make it a little less painful or chaotic?" It is a great time to point out the successes, and the fact that everyone did what was expected of them and what they were trained for, and they did it well. With this closing comes the final phase—the reentry phase.

Reentry Phase   The last phase of the debriefing is the time to clarify issues, answer questions, make summary statements to the group, and return the group to their normal functions. This phase effects closure of the discussions that have just occurred in the debriefing.

The team leader may end the debriefing by saying, "Let us try to summarize what we have covered here during this process together." The entire CISD team should be included in this final discussion and should offer thoughts from their hearts and minds. This is the time for respect, encouragement, appreciation, support, and final direction. Team members may wish to end this session with personal contact, thanking each participant verbally, shaking hands, offering positive eye contact, and congratulating each member for participating.

Individual Crisis Intervention (One-on-One)

Another intervention is individual one-on-one crisis support, which can be applied on-scene during a crisis event or at any time after such an event. The key factor here is that this intervention is provided one-on-one. The CISM model is known as the SAFER model. The SAFER model represents a specific protocol that peer counselors or mental health professionals can use for conducting individual crisis response interventions. The SAFER protocol includes *s*tabilization of the situation, *a*cknowledgment of the crisis, *f*acilitation of understanding, *e*ncouragement of adaptive coping, *r*estoration of independent functioning, and *r*eferral for continued care. It may be used on-site or on-scene, or anywhere at any time after the initial crisis or event has occurred. Only trained personnel should use this model of intervention.[45]

HOW PAs CAN BENEFIT FROM LEARNING ABOUT AND USING CRITICAL INCIDENT STRESS MANAGEMENT

PAs are academically and clinically prepared to provide health care services. They offer these services to diverse patient populations from crowded urban areas to remote rural environments. It is not uncommon for the PA to offer psychosocial services to patients while helping patients cope with illness and/or injuries. The standards and guidelines for an accredited educational program call for "PAs to have a functional understanding of personality development, child development, normative responses to stress, psychosomatic manifestations of illness and injury, responses to death and dying, and behavioral patterns related to the maintenance and restoration of health."[50]

Many PA educational programs offer courses in behavioral aspects of medicine that instruct students in the concepts of patient counseling. PA programs could explore the addition of a course that addresses the issues of traumatic stress and its impact on both patients and providers. A course of this type would be valuable for students in terms of both their own future mental health as caregivers and the mental health of their patients. The concepts and theories involved in

dealing with compassion fatigue, professional burnout, distress, and traumatic stress have changed dramatically, and, as lifelong learners, PAs need to know how to care for their patients and how to care for themselves. A basic course might address the nature of stress, the types of stress encountered by caregivers, and particular types of provider/patient conflict and stress. In addition, students should learn basic crisis interventions that they can use for both patients and themselves.

Many courses of this type are offered by the International Critical Incident Stress Foundation (ICISF) located in Ellicott City, Maryland. The ICISF offers courses throughout the world, including basic CISM, advanced CISM, psychotraumatology, CISM and children, peer support/crisis intervention, and many others. Information regarding courses and locations of worldwide teams can be found on the web at www.icisf.org, or by calling 410-750-9600 for routine information (the emergency number is 410-313-CISD). The ICISF has teams all over the world. If an event occurs and a PA or patients need help, this phone number connects the caller with a local or regional CISM team that will assist. Other organizations that offer similar courses include the Association of Traumatic Stress Specialists (www.atts-hq.com), the American Academy of Experts in Traumatic Stress (www.aaets.org/), the Florida State University Traumatology Institute (www.fsu.edu/~trauma/), and the International Society for Traumatic Stress Studies (www.istss.org).

State and regional continuing medical education coordinators should consider offering to their state members lectures on compassion fatigue and dealing with traumatic stress. Continuing education is the key to surviving traumatic stress as a caregiver. Traumatic stress is a relatively common event in the lives of health care providers today, especially those who deal with emergency, occupational, trauma, and psychiatric medicine.[51] Health care professionals who work in disaster management, emergency departments, Life Flight operations, critical care units, remote sites, and/or with other agencies such as ski patrols, dive clubs, parachute clubs, or military units should consider exploring these type of courses as part of their lifelong learning to help themselves and to help others.

CONCLUSION

As Frankl has stated, "It does not really matter what we expect from life but rather what life expects from us that matters."[2] Traumatic stress will not disappear from our lives, but our conceptual approach to dealing with traumatic events and victims of traumatic events must be grounded in interventions that make a difference in our patients' lives and our own. The health care professional who cannot care for himself or herself cannot provide humanistic quality care for others.

The goals of crisis intervention for traumatic stress include restoring hope, offering dignity, focusing on self-worth, promoting emotional stability, and finally, offering peace with oneself without a sense of guilt. The primary goal of CISM and other crisis intervention techniques is to help others help themselves.

CLINICAL APPLICATIONS

1. Distinguish between stress and trauma. Discuss the psychobiology of traumatic stress.
2. Identify factors that contribute to caregivers' experiences of traumatic stress. Why are caregivers more likely than members of the general population to develop post-traumatic stress disorder?
3. Discuss examples of critical incidents that might be encountered in clinical settings by a PA student or a PA.
4. List the seven components of CISM, and explain how to assess the need for CISM.
5. List the seven phases of the CISD protocol.
6. If you or your team needed CISM interventions, how would you access these services?
7. If you were interested in training to become a CISM leader, what steps would you take?

REFERENCES

1. Dead and missing. New York Times. December 26, 2001:B2.
2. Frankl VE. Man's Search for Meaning. New York: Pocket Books, 1959.
3. Selye H. The Stress of Life. New York: McGraw-Hill, 1956.
4. Maslow A. Motivation and Personality. New York: Harper & Row, 1970.
5. Strachey J. The Complete Psychological Works of Sigmund Freud. London: Hogarth Press, 1920.
6. Mitchell J, Bray G. Emergency Services Stress: Guidelines for Preserving the Health and Careers of Emergency Services Personnel. Englewood Cliffs, NJ: Brady Publishing, 1990.
7. Donovan D. Traumatology: a field whose time has come. J Trauma Stress 1991;4:433.
8. Figley C. Forward. In: Wilson J, Raphael B (eds). International Handbook of Traumatic Stress Syndromes. New York: Plenum, 1993.
9. Figley C, Horowitz M. Stress Response Syndrome. New York: Jason Aronson, 1976.
10. Selye H. Handbook of Stress. New York: The Free Press, 1976.
11. Figley CR. Trauma and Its Wake. New York: Brunner/Mazel, 1985.
12. Galea S, et al. Psychological sequelae of the September 11 terrorist attacks in New York City. N Engl J Med 2002;346:982.
13. Flannery R, Everly G. Crisis intervention: a review. Int J Emerg Mental Health 2001;2:119.
14. Janet PL. Automatisme psychologique: essai de psychologie experimentale sur les formes inferieures de l'activité humaine. Paris: Felix Alcan, 1889.
15. Wilson JP, Raphael B. International Handbook of Traumatic Stress Syndromes. New York: Plenum, 1993.
16. Freud S. Introduction to Psychoanalysis and War Neuroses. London: Hogarth Press, 1919.
17. Selye H. The Stress Without Distress. Philadelphia: JB Lippincott, 1974.
18. Hymans KC, Wignall FS, Roswell R. War, syndromes and their evaluation: From the U.S. Civil War to the Persian Gulf. Ann Intern Med 1996;125:1822.
19. Diagnostic and Statistical Manual of Mental Disorders, ed 1. Washington, DC: American Psychiatric Association, 1952.
20. Diagnostic and Statistical Manual of Mental Disorders, ed 4. Washington, DC: American Psychiatric Association, 1994.
21. MacLean PO. Brain evolution relating to family, play, and the separation call. Arch Gen Psych 1985;42:505.
22. Squire LR. Memory and the Brain. New York: Oxford University Press, 1987.
23. Post RM, Pickar D, Ballenger JC, Naber D. Endogenous opioids in cerebrospinal fluid: relationship to mood and anxiety. In: Post RM, Ballenger JC (eds). Neurobiology of Mood Disorders. Baltimore: Williams & Wilkins, 1984.
24. Pitman RK, et al. Special section. Hippocampus 2001;11:73.
25. Wilson J, Friedman M, Lindy J. Treating Psychological Trauma and PTSD. New York: Guilford Press, 2001.
26. Harbert K, Hunsinger M. Traumatic stress for health care workers. J Am Acad Physician Assistants 1991;4:384.
27. Epperson M. Families in Sudden Crisis. Social Work Health Care. New York: Plenum Press, 1977.
28. Robinson R. Stress reactions in emergency medical crews. J Trauma Stress 1983;5:1.
29. Everly GS, Mitchell JT. Innovations in Disaster and Trauma Psychology: Critical Incident Stress Management. Ellicott City, MD: Chevron, 1997.

30. Harbert K, Hunsinger M. The development of an interdisciplinary CISM team within a rural tertiary care center. Agency for Health Policy and Research, Primary Care Research Conference, Atlanta, Georgia, 1990.

31. Luce A, Firth-Cozens J, Midgley S, Burges C. After the Omagh bomb: posttraumatic stress disorder in health service staff. J Traumatic Stress 2002;15:27.

32. Pines A, Aronson E. Career Burnout. New York: Free Press, 1986.

33. Wilson J. Identity, Trauma, Transformation, and Healing. New York: Brunner/Mazel, 1989.

34. Flannery R, Everly G. Crisis intervention: a review. Int J Emerg Mental Health 2001;2:119.

35. Cobb S, Lindemann E. Neuropsychiatric observation after the Coconut Grove fire. Ann Surg 1943;117:814.

36. Lindemann E. Symptomatology and management of acute grief. Am J Psychiatry 1994;101:329.

37. Caplan G. Principles of Preventive Psychiatry. New York: Basic Books, 1964.

38. Caplan G. Support Systems and Community Mental Health. New York: Behavioral Publications, 1991.

39. Caplan G. Mastery of stress. Am J Psychiatry 1981;138:413.

40. McGee RK. Crisis in the Community. Baltimore: University Park Press, 1974.

41. Wilson JP. Trauma, Transformation, and Healing: An Integrative Approach to Theory, Research, and Post-traumatic Therapy. New York: Brunner/Mazel, 1989.

42. Everly G. Critical incident stress management: proposed international standard of care for crisis intervention. Paper presented at the 9th Montreux Congress on Stress, Montreux, Switzerland, 1991.

43. Mitchell JT. When disaster strikes: the critical incident stress debriefing process. J Emerg Med Serv 1983;36.

44. Everly GS. CISM: A New Standard of Care in Crisis Intervention: LIFENET. Ellicott City, MD: Newsletter International Critical Incident Stress Foundation, 1997.

45. Mitchell J, Everly G. Critical Incident Stress Debriefing, An Operations Manual for CISD, Defusing and Other Group Crisis Intervention Services, ed 3. Ellicott City, MD: Chevron, 2001.

46. Bordow S, Porritt D. An experimental evaluation of crisis intervention. Soc Sci Med 1979;13:251.

47. Raphael B. When Disaster Strikes. New York: Basic Books, 1986.

48. Everly G. Crisis management briefings (CMBs): large group crisis intervention in response to terrorism, disasters, and violence. Int J Emerg Mental Health 2002;2:53.

49. Flannery R. The Assaulted Staff Action Program: Coping with the Psychological Aftermath of Violence, Innovations in Disaster and Trauma Psychology. Ellicott City, MD: Chevron, 1998.

50. Accreditation Standards for Physician Assistant Education. Accreditation Review Commission on Education for the Physician Assistant, Marshfield, Wis, 2001.

51. Sorenson S. Preventing traumatic stress: public health approaches. J Traumatic Stress 2002;15:3.

RESOURCES

Baldwin D. Trauma Information Page. Available at www.traumapages.com/. *This site offers the latest information concerning concepts, research, and definitions of traumatic stress. An excellent resource for those needing articles, other links, and current definitions of treatment and management of traumatic stress.*

Mitchell J, Everly G. Critical Incident Stress Debriefing, An Operations Manual for CISD, Defusing and Other Group Crisis Intervention Services, ed 3. Ellicott City, MD: Chevron, 2001. *This text deals with the integrated, multi-component intervention system that spans the entire crisis spectrum from pre-crisis phase and on-scene support to final follow-up. In fewer than 400 pages, the authors (world leaders in the field of critical incident stress management) focus on the foundations of crisis intervention and CISM stress management. (International Critical Incident Stress Foundation, Inc. Available at www.icisf.org. This site provides information concerning ICISF and offers a 24-hour hotline for emergencies, with immediate answers regarding local, state, or international trained teams available for response to any emergency or disaster. Also, the site offers training information, course descriptions, signs and symptoms of traumatic stress, and information on faculty members available to provide training.)*

Wilson JP (ed). Trauma, Transformation, and Healing: An Integrative Approach to Theory, Research, and Post-Traumatic Therapy. New York: Brunner/Mazel, 1989. *This text offers valuable insight into the psychobiology of trauma. Wilson offers more than 20 years of experience in studying everything from the combined effects of neurophysiology to the vulnerabilities and responses to traumatic events. The more interesting chapters explore the use of "sweat lodges" as focused therapeutic modalities for victims and discuss the research that demonstrates how trauma can cause abnormal reactions in the brain, resulting in a change in affect and emotional reactions. This is an excellent source for the practitioner seeking an understanding of the theory of post-traumatic therapy for victims of trauma.*

Flannery R. The Assaulted Staff Action Program: Coping with the Psychological Aftermath of Violence, Innovations in Disaster and Trauma Psychology. Ellicott City, MD: Chevron, 1998. *This book focuses on a CISM approach to crisis intervention for coping with the aftermath of violence. It is a very helpful text for health care professionals and health care institutions.*

Raphael B, Wilson J. Psychological Debriefing: Theory, Practice and Evidence. New York: Cambridge, 2000. *This excellent text explores both theory and practice concerning the use of psychological debriefing. It offers a broad range of discussion regarding the use of and evidence for psychological debriefing.*

Wilson J, Friedman M, Lindy J. Treating Psychological Trauma and PTSD. New York: Guilford, 2001. *A holistic model for treating PTSD. This book offers an in-depth look at the symptomatology and treatment options for traumatic stress and PTSD. The editors are all internationally known experts in the field of traumatic stress and PTSD. Excellent resource for practitioners treating PTSD.*

CHAPTER 45

Health Care for the Homeless

Peggy A. Valentine and Dawn Morton-Rias

INTRODUCTION

The physician assistant (PA) profession was established to address the unmet health needs of the medically underserved and disenfranchised in America. Graduate PAs and PA students continue the tradition of service for those in need by providing much needed health care for the underserved in rural, urban, suburban, and frontier communities throughout the United States. One population increasingly in need of health care services includes those who experience homelessness.

Individuals and families may experience homelessness as a result of a wide range of personal, social, and economic challenges and situations. Regardless of the genesis, homeless adults, children, and families constitute a growing population of medically underserved. Through national health care for the homeless projects, community-based practices and clinics, emergency service centers, correctional facilities, and community hospitals, PAs positively impact the health status of America's homeless. Similarly, through preceptorships and clinical training affiliations, PA students may be introduced to the clinical opportunities and professional rewards experienced through service to this richly diverse patient population.

HOMELESSNESS IN THE UNITED STATES

A generally accepted definition of *homeless* is "living on the streets" or in homeless shelters.[1] According to the Stewart B. McKinney Act, 42 U.S. C, a person is considered homeless who lacks fixed, regular, and adequate night-time residence and whose primary residence is a facility designed to provide temporary living accommodations. Some researchers argue that these definitions are too narrow and should include persons who have lost their residence and live with friends or relatives on a temporary basis.[2]

How many homeless persons are there? The actual number of homeless individuals or those who experience homelessness is difficult to determine. Data may be collected by counting the number of individuals, over a specific period, who access temporary housing facilities, shelters, and service organizations designed to help meet the needs of the homeless. Other methods include counting the numbers of those actually seen living on the street, over a specific period, in selected locations nationwide and extrapolating the findings. The National Coalition for the Homeless acknowledges the challenge in counting the numbers in its Fact Sheet, "How Many People Experience Homelessness," and describes several methods used to estimate the numbers.[1] Similarly, Burt (1996) outlines methods for counting the number of homeless individuals in the United States, and acknowledges that exact figures are difficult to ascertain.[2]

Challenges with methodology notwithstanding, it is conservatively estimated that 760,000 people are homeless on any given night, and 1 to 2 million people experience homelessness over a 1-year period. Approximately 12 million U.S. adults have been homeless at some point in their lives.[3,4] As has been illustrated, determining the "actual number" of homeless individuals remains difficult and probably results in an underestimation of the actual size of the population and the extent of the challenges they face. In effect, the number of homeless patients and clients actually encountered by health and social service agents or counted may represent only the "tip of the iceberg."[5]

Homelessness in the United States is not a new phenomenon. It has been seen at various points in U.S. history in association with difficult economic times. During the depression of 1870 and the Great Depression of the 1930s, for example, the number of homeless was reported to "increase markedly at once." The homeless population of the Great Depression were described as "transients" and included hobos, migrant workers, and tramps. The estimated number of transients by the late 1930s ranged from 300,000 to 3,000,000.[6]

From the 1950s to the early 1970s, the homeless population was often described as mostly male, "skid row" alcoholics.[7] Various reasons were sought to explain why alcoholics became homeless. In the late 1960s, Bahr[7] tried to establish a relationship between the size and stability of parental families, extent of drinking, and homelessness, but found none. Others have suggested that alcohol abuse, conditions of the job market, and a shrinking housing market for people with alcoholism contribute to homelessness.[8] The National Alliance to End Homelessness estimates that 25% or more of homeless individuals abuse alcohol

or other drugs as a way to avoid boredom and loneliness and to lift spirits.[9]

Another commonly referenced event that contributed to contemporary homelessness was the deinstitutionalization of the mentally ill. The 1999 Fact Sheet, Why Are People Homeless, published by The National Coalition for the Homeless, asserts that "while the exact relationship between addition and homelessness remains complex and controversial, rates of alcohol and drug abuse are disproportionately high among the homeless population". Many people who are addicted to alcohol and drugs never become homeless, but people who are poor and addicted are clearly at increased risk of homelessness.[10] During the 1960s, a movement to establish comprehensive community-based psychiatric centers resulted in the release of many persons who had been housed in overcrowded and underfunded state hospitals. Unfortunately, many of those released to the community were unable to work because of their disabilities and had limited resources with which to care for themselves. Many were unable to adjust to the stresses of community living. In addition, the quality of community resources and availability of care for the newly released individuals varied. This change is thought to have contributed to the numbers of homeless. In 1955, approximately 560,000 persons were housed in psychiatric institutions.[11-14] By 1984, 132,000 persons resided in these institutions. Recent studies suggest little change. Koegel and associates (1996), in their compilation of research and essays on homelessness, estimate that 20% to 25% of the single adult homeless population suffer from some form of severe or persistent mental illness. Currently, a new wave of deinstitutionalization of the mentally ill, denial of services, poor or absent discharge planning, and other changes related to managed care arrangements continue to contribute to homelessness among the mentally ill. For these reasons, many mentally ill persons are homeless.[15]

Other events in recent history that have affected homelessness include the economic recessions of the past 2 decades. Many factories and businesses have closed, and many companies have merged or downsized to reduce costs. As a result, thousands of workers have lost jobs and homes.[13] A new subgroup, the *situationally distressed,* has joined the homeless population. Current economic conditions, including changes in the stock market and in employment rates, suggest that the trend may continue.[15]

In 1985 Fischer and Breakey asserted that the homeless were a very diverse group consisting of four groups commonly identified as follows[16]:

1. *Chronically mentally ill.* The people in this group have a history of being mentally disabled, and may be recently deinstitutionalized. They may or may not use an ambulatory mental health clinic. The U.S. Conference of Mayors Reports of 1991 and 1998[14] indicated that approximately 25% to 29% of the homeless population were mentally ill. It is estimated, however, that only 5% to 7% of homeless persons with mental illness require institutionalization. In 2000 they reported that an average of 22% of homeless people are considered mentality ill. This does not include suburban and rural populations.[17,18]

2. *Street people.* The people in this group are often described as "bag ladies and grate men." They usually isolate themselves from others and do not use shelters. In choosing their own place to eat and sleep, they tend to set up in parks, doorways, vacant buildings, and subways or under bridges. The prevalence of mental illness and alcohol abuse may be high in this subgroup.

3. *Chronic alcoholics and substance abusers.* For the people in this group, lifestyle revolves around acquiring and consuming drugs. The chronic alcoholics comprise mostly males over the age of 45 years. In a study conducted at a Boston shelter, 9% of women and 36% of men used drugs. In the same study of a street sample, 25% of women and 39% of men used drugs.[19] A 1991 survey of the homeless in 28 U.S. cities cited substance abuse as a characteristic in 40% of the homeless. Even today, following poverty and lack of affordable housing, substance abuse is considered a major contributing factor in the experience of homelessness. Furthermore, the nation lacks enough drug treatment programs to meet the needs of the homeless.[20]

4. *Situationally distressed.* This group consists of those who may have a recent history of being unemployed and having been evicted from their residence, or they may be traveling in search of jobs. This subgroup frequently includes single persons and families.

Other important elements of the homeless population must be considered. The 1998 Conference of Mayors survey of 30 cities also found that the nationwide homeless population comprises 49% African Americans, 32% Caucasians, 12% Hispanics, and 3% Native Americans, and as with the domiciled population, the exact demographic breakdown varies according to geographic location. The National Coalition for the Homeless reports that in 1998, the U.S. Conference of Mayors' survey of homelessness in 30 cities found that 25% of the urban homeless population comprised children under the age of 18, 3% were unaccompanied minors, 45% were single men, 14% were single women, and families accounted for 38% of the homeless population. A typical homeless family consists of a woman with two or three children who became homeless for one of a number of reasons: poverty, lack of affordable or subsidized housing, domestic violence or abuse, personal crisis (eviction) or loss of support, unemployment, underemployment, and/or lack of marketable skills.[9]

Many homeless families have experienced difficulty in acquiring support.[21,22] Some have been turned away from emergency shelters that were designed to provide short-term housing for the homeless. A recent survey of 18 U.S. cities indicated that 70% of these cities must turn away homeless families owing to lack of resources. As a result, some families have resorted to living in cars and using public restrooms as changing and bathing facilities.[15,21,22]

Poverty, unemployment, and underemployment are inextricably linked to homelessness and "the experience of homelessness or situational homelessness." According to the U.S. Bureau of the Census Population Survey 2000, although the poverty rate declined from 11.8% in 1999 to 11.3% in 2000, the number of poor people continues to exceed 31 million and the average household income in 2000 remained unchanged from 1999. Approximately 40% of all persons living in poverty are children, and many are African American.[23] The 1996 welfare reform legislation may further increase the risk of homelessness for certain families. The Aid to Families with Dependent Children (AFDC) program was repealed and replaced with a block grant program called Temporary Assistance to Needy Families (TANF). The benefits provided are below the poverty line. Further, denial of Supplemental Security Income (SSI) to legal and non-legal immigrants increases the risk of homelessness for this group.[24]

Another group of homeless includes runaway and throwaway youth. Every year, approximately 1 million people younger than 18 years of age run away from home or are forced out of their homes (thrown away). Precipitating events indicate a high incidence of physical, emotional, and sexual abuse. Many are traumatized from these experiences. Some may use drugs or resort to prostitution. As young people leave home and enter the world of homelessness, they find that their resources are limited. They generally cannot stay in adult shelters, and few cities offer teen shelter.[9]

The last but certainly not least group worthy of discussion includes the homeless military veterans. It is estimated that veterans make up 23% of the homeless population. Various reasons have been cited for their inclusion among the homeless, such as a high incidence of alcoholism, major psychiatric disorders, impaired cognitive functioning, and social and economic deprivation.[15,17]

WHY IS THERE HOMELESSNESS?

Why do we have homelessness in this wealthy and progressive nation? Hopper and Hamberg[25] offer insight from two perspectives:

1. The individual is unable to acquire housing owing to a particular circumstance.
2. Society has failed to provide suitable mechanisms that will enable all citizens to be housed.

The following discussion explains the major factors accounting for homelessness.

Housing Shortage

Lack of affordable rental housing for low-income persons is often cited as an important cause of homelessness. With each passing decade, fewer Americans can afford to purchase a home; by the 1970s, the proportion had dropped to one half of families, and by 1976, only one quarter of families could afford new homes. During the recession of the 1980s, the demand for rental units increased, and one half of poor families paid more than 72% of their income for rent. This trend has continued into the 21st century. Poor families are therefore at greater risk of becoming homeless.[12] It is estimated that the United States has a shortage of 4.7 million affordable housing units. The greatest unmet housing needs occur among families with children, the elderly, and disabled individuals with low income.[26]

Unemployment

Economic opportunities have shifted over the past 15 to 20 years, to include a declining number of manufacturing jobs, expansion of lower-paying service jobs, and an increased demand for a highly skilled or professional workforce. Industrial plant closings, the collapse of many Internet-based companies, mergers and downsizing, and a shift to part-time jobs all have contributed to rising unemployment. The number of weeks that one can receive unemployment benefits is limited. When a person's benefits run out, the risk of becoming homeless increases.[27]

Unemployed and homeless people continue to experience great difficulty in acquiring a job owing to lack of a permanent address and/or telephone number, and limited means of transportation. Further, they may not be able to make a "good impression" when being interviewed because of difficulty in maintaining personal hygiene.[9]

Level of Education

One's level of education may affect one's chances of becoming homeless. For example, persons with lower levels of education have difficulty in acquiring anything other than low-paying, service-type positions. The income from these positions is often insufficient to meet the rising costs of housing, thus contributing to homelessness. Higher educational and technical training requirements for jobs over the past 10 years, arising from technological advances, such as computerization of the workplace, have precipitated changes in the workforce opportunities for the undereducated. There is a decline in jobs available to persons who do not have high school diplomas.[1,15] It is estimated that 27 million Americans are functionally illiterate; illiterate adults earn 42% less than high school graduates.[9,15]

Unfortunately, many of today's young people are not attaining the educational foundation to ensure their future employability. More than a quarter of American high school students drop out, and in some inner city settings, more than half of high school students leave school before graduation. Many of these dropouts have great difficulty entering the workforce and are at risk for becoming homeless in the future.

RESOURCES FOR THE HOMELESS

Religious organizations and missions have historically attempted to assist the homeless by providing shelter facilities. In many U.S. cities during the 1980s, municipal and voluntary agencies began to focus on the multifaceted needs of the homeless. Military facilities such as large armories were converted to shelters to house single adults. Municipal buildings and hotels were renovated to provide shelter.

Shelters are in great demand, even though they were not originally intended to provide broad-based human services. Shelters were established to provide services for only a few days, on the assumption that homelessness resulted from an acute crisis that would be resolved in a short time.

Shelter facilities are not all alike. Operational guidelines include entry requirements, duration of stay, and types of eligible clients. The atmosphere may vary from small cozy havens where guests can receive the best in social services to large congregational centers that offer few services. For example, in New York City, approximately 4500 single adults are housed every night.[1,9] Tier I facilities (shelter for single adults) may range from 800-bed armories to church and school basements that each sleep only a few. Other facilities may offer residence for battered women and their children, where a 24-hour hotline is available and residents can receive counseling and support services.

The type and quality of shelter services vary greatly from one facility to another. Some provide access to shower facilities, clothing, toiletries, and food services. Food services may range from coffee and sandwiches to one or two hot meals a day.

HEALTH ISSUES

People experiencing homelessness generally suffer from chronic health challenges related to their homeless status. The incidences of frostbite, trauma, tuberculosis, and skin infection are understandably higher among the homeless. Homelessness interferes with maintenance of adequate nutrition, hygienic practices, and other health promotion activities. In addition to the health challenges associated with living conditions, homeless patients experience higher rates and poorer outcome from chronic illnesses such as hypertension and diabetes.

Access to health care for homeless individuals differs greatly from that for the general or domiciled population. For example, the average person with resources usually requests evaluation of health status by a practitioner at the onset of signs and symptoms suggestive of a disorder or as follow-up to a chronic disorder to maintain his or her state of health. Ideally, this evaluation occurs in an outpatient setting. The management plan may include the use of diagnostic and therapeutic modalities, home care, and dietary modifications. Emergency services are reserved for acute conditions.

In contrast, homeless individuals do not access services until signs, symptoms, or the disease process impedes their mobility and interferes with their ability to acquire food, clothing, shelter, or other substances. They rarely make routine office visits for health screening, immunizations, or follow-up of chronic disorders. Therefore, many homeless individuals are seen by the health care provider late in the course of illness and require extensive treatment. Complications are common, recovery is problematic, and there is a high incidence of relapse.

Recovery from seemingly benign conditions is often complicated by the unavailability of supportive care. For example, bedrest, nutritious meals, a warm environment, and the use of over-the-counter medications are the normal measures most people use for flu symptoms. The homeless way of life does not provide such niceties, and recovery from the flu is difficult if one sleeps in an abandoned car or boarded-up building in the winter.

HEALTH CARE NEEDS

Many of the health care needs of homeless individuals can be managed by PAs. As primary health care providers, PAs are capable of serving this population because many of the medical conditions treated are similar to those of domiciled patients or those not homeless. Table 45-1 lists the types of medical problems commonly encountered in the homeless. There are high incidences of infectious diseases and trauma, in association with poor living conditions. For example, in crowded shelters, homeless persons are more apt to acquire upper respiratory infections and skin infestations. Those who have limited access to clean clothing, bathroom facilities, and toiletries may suffer from skin infections, dental cavities, toothache, and athlete's foot. Traumatic disorders include injuries associated with fighting to protect possessions or falling down from drunkenness, thermal skin burns from sleeping on grates to stay warm in winter, and frostbite from sleeping outdoors in freezing temperatures and having improper or unprotective footwear.

Table 45-1   Common Acute and Chronic Ailments of 23,745 Homeless in 16 U.S. Cities

Ailments	Percentage (%)
ACUTE DISORDERS	
Upper respiratory infections	33
Traumas	23
Minor skin ailments	14
Infestational disorders	4-5
CHRONIC DISORDERS	
Hypertension	14
Gastrointestinal ailments	14
Peripheral vascular diseases	13
Problems with dentition	9
Neurological disorders	8
Eye disorders	8
Cardiac disease	7
Genitourinary problems	7
Musculoskeletal ailments	6
Ear disorders	5
Chronic obstructive pulmonary disease	5

Data from Wright JD, Weber E. Homelessness and Health. New York: McGraw-Hill, 1987:104; reprinted with permission from Valentine P. PA students reach out to the homeless. J Am Acad Physician Assistants 1990;3:504.

The health status of the homeless is further affected by dietary patterns. Most do not get enough food to eat and have irregular patterns of eating. Many homeless persons have no money to purchase food, and they frequent charity organizations such as soup kitchens and shelters. The food served is fairly nutritious and offers some variety, but most resources are unable to serve more than one meal per day.[28]

Some homeless individuals do not go to shelters or soup kitchens, but eat instead from garbage bins. As a result, this group is more likely to suffer gastritis and other gastrointestinal ailments than those who do go to soup kitchens and shelters.[28]

PAs can treat many health disorders of the homeless "on the spot" and can arrange hospital transport for more acute illnesses. In the process of treatment, the PA must remember that follow-up is difficult. For example, it may be difficult to find a homeless individual living on the streets. Therefore, treatment must be realistic for the setting.

UNIQUE CHALLENGES TO PROVIDING HEALTH CARE TO THE HOMELESS

In selecting employment, PAs often acquire jobs that meet their personal interests. PAs who choose to work with the homeless are most likely concerned about social and health issues of an underserved population, and feel that they can "make a difference."

There are many challenges to providing health care to the homeless, which some PAs find exciting. First, it is difficult to elicit a medical history. Historical information may be limited owing to lack of privacy in a nontraditional provider setting, and the patient may be guarded about disclosing sensitive information. The patient may omit key elements of the history of present illness out of fear of rejection and reprimand. Further, if the PA records historical information in the presence of the patient, the patient may stop talking. In order to acquire candid and explicit information, the PA may have to defer recording until after the encounter.

Another challenge may be completing a comprehensive physical examination. Because not all homeless individuals go to clinics or shelters, health assessment may occur in nontraditional settings, such as on the street or in mobile vans. Facilities to ensure privacy may not be available. Patients may not be physically able to disrobe, or they may be embarrassed about their condition or about body odor and uncleanliness. The PA will need to demonstrate compassion, flexibility, and creativity to complete the health assessment.

The PA will be further challenged in conducting and interpreting diagnostic studies. For example, placement and timely interpretation of a purified protein derivative (PPD) tuberculin test may be difficult because the patient may not return for follow-up. Further, diagnostic radiographs may not be obtained owing to lack of funds, lack of medical insurance, poor patient compliance with referral, difficulties in patient transport to appropriate facilities, and patient reluctance.

Other challenges include treatment and management of infections, injuries, and chronic ailments. Homeless individuals are prone to acquiring upper respiratory infections because of crowded living conditions in shelters, or environmental exposure from sleeping outdoors. Many suffer minor trauma and secondary infections from falls, cuts, and bruises. Seemingly minor injuries of the extremities can progress to cellulitis and ulceration. Chronic conditions such as venous stasis ulcers are exacerbated by prolonged standing, improper footwear, exposure to the elements, and poor hygiene. PAs rely on their clinical skills and knowledge of epidemiology in this population. PAs can reduce the morbidity and mortality associated with these illnesses through early intervention and "on the spot" treatment with appropriate medication or other resources. The PA should be able to arrange referral or immediate transport to the appropriate facility for follow-up care.

Working with homeless individuals also yields rewards and satisfaction. PAs feel a sense of satisfaction through patient feedback. Homeless patients are often very appreciative of health services rendered and openly express their feelings of gratitude.

By working in the homeless environment, PAs are in a position to manage acute conditions and arrange emergency transport. It is not uncommon for them to manage drug overdose, heatstroke, thermal injuries, and pneumonia. Saving a life or immediately improving the health status of a person is personally satisfying.

PAs who work in the homeless setting need never question their value as health care providers. Because of the many medical and social needs of the homeless, the demand for PA services will continue. In working with this special population, PAs have an opportunity to be creative in their treatment approaches and to provide care to the truly needy.

WAYS STUDENTS CAN LEARN ABOUT HOMELESSNESS

The educational curriculum of most PA programs is designed to produce primary health care practitioners to work in a variety of settings, including those of the medically underserved. Historically, provision of services to the medically underserved has included the homeless, and PAs have established a role in providing care to this population.[26] It therefore behooves students to acquire experience in working with the homeless through PA educational training.

Students can gain hands-on working experience with the homeless during the clinical training year. This can be accomplished through establishing linkages with shelters or street outreach teams that provide medical services to the homeless. Students can work with primary care providers at these settings.

The benefits of this learning experience include the following:

➤ Opportunity to dispel preconceived notions about causes and effects of homelessness.
➤ Making firsthand observations of the psychosocial and economic issues that affect health maintenance and provision of health services.
➤ Participation in the team approach to providing comprehensive health services.
➤ Participation in the management of a variety of medical and psychiatric disorders.
➤ Gaining a sense of helping those in need and who feel overlooked by society.

In preparing for this clinical experience, students can work with the homeless during their didactic year of training. As volunteers, students can assist with preparation and serving of meals at a soup kitchen, offer tutorial assistance to children living in shelters, or work on a hotline for battered women.

Like graduate PAs, students can make a valuable contribution to the health care of homeless people.

CLINICAL APPLICATIONS

1. Ms. D is a 26-year-old mother of three young children, who presents to the free clinic complaining of diarrhea and fever for the past 5 days. She recently left her husband, who physically abused her, for the second time and has been living for 2 weeks in a boarded-up vacant apartment building without running water or electricity. She wants to find a more suitable residence for herself and her children, but she is unemployed and unskilled.

   ➤ What factors have contributed to Ms. D's homelessness?

   ➤ What are the health issues for Ms. D?

   ➤ What are the potential risks for her children?

   ➤ What can you do to assist the family?

2. Mr. J is a 64-year-old unemployed truck driver with a history of alcoholism for many years. He has lived on the streets for the past 5 years. A typical day is spent walking continuously within a 10-block radius. Occasionally, he becomes hostile, yelling profanity and throwing stones at abandoned buildings. He has stuffed pieces of newspaper in his ears to muffle "the voices."

   ➤ What factors have contributed to Mr. J's homelessness?

   ➤ What are the health issues for Mr. J?

   ➤ What can you do to assist Mr. J?

REFERENCES

1. National Coalition for the Homeless Fact Sheet #2, How Many People Experience Homelessness," and Fact Sheet #3, "Who is Homeless." February 1999. Available at nch.ari.net/numbers.html.

2. Burt M. Practical Methods for Counting Homeless People: A Manual; for States and Local Jurisdictions, ed 2. Washington, DC: The Urban Institute, 1996.

3. National Law Center on Homelessness and Poverty. Mean Sweeps: A Report on Anti-Homeless Laws, Litigation and Alternatives in 50 U.S. cities, 1996. Washington, DC: National Law Center on Homelessness and Poverty, 1996.

4. Link B, Phelan J, Bresnahan M, et al. Life-time and five-year prevalence of homelessness in the U.S.: new evidence on an old debate. Am J Orthopsychiatry 1995;65:347.

5. Applebaum RP. Counting the homeless. In: Momeni JA (ed). Homelessness in the United States: Data and Issues. New York: Greenwood Press, 1990.

6. Caplow T. Transiency as a cultural pattern. Am Sociolog Rev 1940;5:731.

7. Bahr HM. Family size and stability as antecedents of homelessness and excessive drinking. J Marriage Family 1969; 31:477.

8. Benda BB, Hutchinson ED. Homelessness and alcohol. In: Belcher JR, DiBlasio FA (eds). Helping the Homeless: Where Do We Go From Here? Lexington, MA: Lexington Books, 1990.

9. The National Alliance to End Homelessness. What You Can Do to Help the Homeless. New York: Simon and Schuster, 1991.

10. National Coalition for the Homeless Fact Sheet Number 1, Why Are People Homeless, June 1999 http://nationalhomeless.org/causes/html.

11. Linn MW, Caffey EM, Klett J, et al. Day treatment and psychotrophic drugs in aftercare. Arch Gen Psychiatry 1979;36:1055.

12. Momeni JA. No place to go: a national picture of homelessness in America. In: Momeni JA (ed). Homelessness in the United States. New York: Greenwood Press, 1989.

13. Blackwell B, Breakey W, Hammersly D, et al. Psychiatric and mental health services. In: Brickner PW, Scharer LK, Conanan BA, et al (eds). Under the Safety Net. New York: WW Norton, 1990.

14. Butra R. The Great Depression of 1990. New York: Dell, 1990.

15. Baumohl J. Homeless in America: A compilation of research and essays. New York: Oryx Press, 1996.

16. Fischer PJ, Breakey. Homelessness and mental health: an overview. Int J. Mental Health 1985–86;14: 6–11.

17. U.S. Conference of Mayors Reports. Homelessness and Hunger, 1991, 1998 and 2000.

18. Federal Task Force on Homelessness and Severe Mental Illness. Outcasts on Main Street: A Report of the Federal Task Force on Homelessness and Severe Mental Illness, 1992. Delmar, NY: National Resource on Homelessness and Mental Illness, 1992.

19. Milburn NG. Drug abuse among homeless people. In: Momeni JA (ed). Homelessness in the United States. New York: Greenwood Press, 1989.

20. Williams L. Addiction on the Streets: Substance Abuse and Homelessness in America, 1992. Washington, DC: National Coalition for the Homeless, 1992.

21. Lee MA, Haught K, Redlener I, et al. Health care for children in homeless families. In: Brickner PW, Scharer LK, Conanan BA, et al (eds). Under the Safety Net. New York: WW Norton, 1990.

22. Huttman ED. Homelessness as a long-term housing problem in America. In: Momeni JA (ed). Homelessness in the United States. New York: Greenwood Press, 1989.

23. U.S. Bureau of the Census. Poverty in the United States: 1996 Current Population Reports. Series P60-198. Washington,

DC: U.S. Bureau of the Census, 1997 and 2000. Current Population Reports. Series P60-214. Washington, DC: U.S. Bureau of the Census, 2001.

24. Greenberg M, Baumohl J. Income maintenance: little help now, less on the way. In: Homelessness in America. Washington, DC: Oryx Press, 1996.

25. Hopper K, Hamberg J. The making of America's homeless: from skid row to new poor, 1945-1984. In: Bratt RG, Hartman CW, Meyerson A (eds). Critical Perspectives on Housing. Philadelphia: Temple University, 1986.

26. U.S. Department of Housing and Urban Development. Rental Housing Assistance at a Crossroads: A Report to Congress on Worst Case Housing Needs. Washington, DC: HUD, 1996.

27. Thorne RA, Zandler C, Waller JB Jr, et al. Entitlements. In: Brickner PW, Scharer LK, Conanan BA, et al (eds). Under the Safety Net. New York: WW Norton, 1990.

28. Cohen BE, Burt MR. Food sources and intake of homeless persons. In: Momeni JA (ed). Homelessness in the United States. New York: Greenwood Press, 1989.

RESOURCES

National Coalition for the Homeless: Online Directory of Local Homeless Service Organizations. Available at www.national-homeless.org. *National clearinghouse on causes, cases, needs, and special issues related to homelessness.*

Brickner PW, Scharer LK, Conanan BA, et al (eds). Under the Safety Net. New York: WW Norton, 1990. *An edited book written by participants in the Health Care for the Homeless program, which is funded by the Robert Wood Johnson and Pew Foundations. Provides a comprehensive view of the specific health issues affecting this population and draws attention to the need for society to address major social problems such as homelessness.*

Lezak A, Edgar E. Preventing Homelessness Among People with Serious Mental Illness: A Guide for States. Delmar, NY: National Resources Center on Homelessness and Mental Illness, 1998.

The National Alliance to End Homelessness. What You Can Do to Help the Homeless. New York: Simon & Schuster, 1991. *A small paperback that provides many suggestions for addressing homelessness. Contains a variety of practical approaches and a listing of national organizations that provide services to the homeless.*

Valentine P. PA students reach out to the homeless. J Am Acad Physician Assistants 1990;3:504. *Describes how students in the Howard University PA Program gained hands-on experience working with homeless people in Washington, DC. Contains information about client characteristics, health problems seen, and desirable characteristics of PAs who care for the homeless.*

CHAPTER 46

Dying and Death

Nanci Cortright Rice

INTRODUCTION

One of the most challenging aspects of the physician assistant's practice is caring for dying patients and their families. Few PAs are prepared to handle the emotional stress they experience while dealing with a patient they cannot cure. This is in part due to the training that physician assistants and other health professionals receive. Most of their medical education focuses on diagnosing and treating patients. Clinical medicine courses provide information on identifying diseases and selecting the appropriate treatment regimen. Little of the curriculum is devoted to helping physician assistants cope with the death of their patients, and even less of the curriculum addresses the knowledge and skills necessary to care for the families of patients who have died. As a result, many PAs feel that they have failed when a patient dies. It is sometimes difficult for them to view death as a natural occurrence, especially if the patient who is dying is young. In order to reduce these feelings of inadequacy, PAs and other health professionals sometimes avoid patients who are dying, or they curtail the amount of time spent with them during hospital stays or office visits.

Additionally, when PAs are caring for a patient who is dying, they are forced to examine their own mortality. Questions concerning their personal views of life and death may enter the minds of PAs caring for dying patients. Feelings of confusion and apprehension about their own mortality may unconsciously inhibit the amount of time PAs spend with their patients. Other health professionals, who share similar feelings, also avoid or limit the contact that they have with dying patients and their families. Thus, dying patients, who often need additional support from health care providers, may find a void in their care. One of the most important roles for PAs is to fill this void by providing comprehensive care for patients and their families throughout the dying process and after death. In order to provide such care, it is important for PAs to understand the attitudes and feelings of patients facing death in today's society.

CHANGES IN DYING AND DEATH IN THE UNITED STATES

Circumstances surrounding death have changed drastically over the past 50 years. Before the second half of this century, most people died at home. Unless people had an illness that required immediate hospitalization, it was unusual for them to be seen by medical professionals at the time of death. Their families and friends would stay by the bedside providing comfort and care for them. As a result, people usually died at home, in their own beds, with loved ones around them. Funeral services were often held at the home of the deceased, and the body was prepared for

burial by family members. In many cases, especially in rural areas, the burial site was somewhere on the person's property or in a nearby cemetery. Subsequently, the extent of most health care professionals' involvement in the dying process of their patients was less than it is today, and the extent of the families' and friends' involvement was much greater. Both of these transitions have led to the changes that have occurred in dying and death in the United States.

Other changes have also occurred in the type and extent of medical care patients received during the dying process. In the early 1900s, the leading cause of death was infectious disease (Figure 46-1); medical

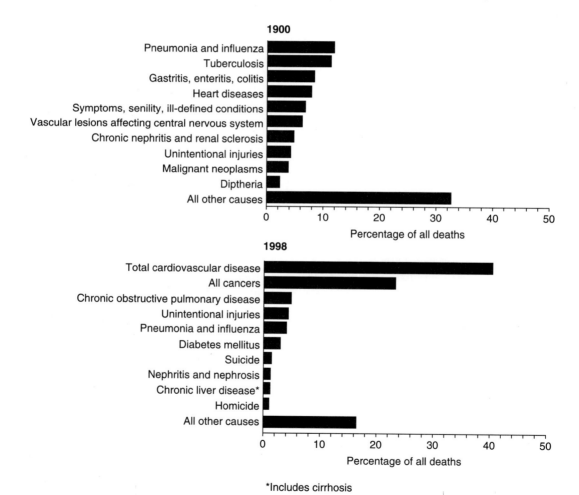

Figure 46-1 Causes of death in the United States, 1900 and 1998. *(From 1990: U.S. Bureau of the Census; 1998: National Center for Health Statistics, CDC.)*

care was limited to treating symptoms and being unable to effect a cure. With the advent of antibiotics, the leading causes of mortality changed from communicable diseases to lifestyle-related causes. In addition, the life expectancy of Americans increased significantly over the past century. In 1900, people had an average life expectancy of 47.3 years. Presently, the average life expectancy at birth is approximately 77 years.[1]

As the population started to lived longer, the types of illnesses encountered in later life varied, and the chances of developing a number of different life-threatening diseases increased. In addition, technological advances in medicine have rapidly escalated since the 1960s. The practice of cardiopulmonary resuscitation (CPR) has enabled many patients who previously would have died to be revitalized and maintained. With the development of mechanical respirators (later referred to as *ventilators*), health care practitioners have been able to keep people breathing almost indefinitely. Artificial hydration and nutrition have allowed basic functions to be maintained, and prophylactic administration of antibiotics has curtailed secondary infections. These changes in the ways in which people die, the increases in life expectancy, and the advances in technology have influenced almost every aspect of health care, including ethical, legal, and financial ones. The changes have altered the type and the amount of care patients who are dying receive during the last months and weeks of their lives. It is important that PAs are cognizant of these changes and the impact that they may have on their practice.

In response to these changes, laws such as the Patient Self-Determination Act have been enacted that relate to the rights of the dying patient to determine what type, if any, of life-prolonging and life-sustaining treatment they will receive. Living wills and durable power of attorney for health care laws continue to be reviewed and expanded within most states to reflect the changing legal needs of patients who are dying. Legislation regarding organ donation and transplantation has been developed to protect the rights of dying patients while providing adequate opportunities for the living to procure needed organs. It is a responsibility of all PAs to be aware of the state

and federal laws governing these death-related matters and to provide the necessary resources to enable patients and families to comply with them. Further discussion of death-related legislation may be found in Chapter 6 of this text.

UNDERSTANDING THE PATIENT WHO IS DYING

It is well recognized that most Americans have been poorly socialized about dying and death. Although death is portrayed daily in the media, it is often addressed in a cavalier manner, with dead people being shown on the evening news telecasts between the weather and sports reports. Young people in U.S. society are first exposed to death through cartoons in which the characters killed in one scene appear instantly in the next scene alive and well. It is common practice not to allow children to view the body of a dead person, even if it was a close relative of the child, and to discourage children from attending the funeral services of the deceased. Children's concepts of death, unless otherwise explained, are formed by the perceptions that derive from what they see on television, read in the newspaper, view at the movies (many of which are horror films), or overhear by listening to adults. Death education is rarely incorporated into the curricula of elementary or secondary school programs and is infrequently introduced in the home environment. Thus, unless adults have made specific efforts to discuss dying and death with young people during childhood or adolescence, children develop strong fears and premonitions regarding death that they carry into adulthood.

For physician assistants, the importance of being aware of how death is addressed in society and is introduced to children is twofold. As professionals, PAs need to be aware that patients may not have fully developed their own meaning of life and death and, in some cases, may not have experienced the death of a loved one. It is important to understand that the fear of the unknown, combined with the lack of opportunity to explore their feelings on death, will intensify their apprehension. On a personal level, PAs must also be aware of how their own early exposure to the topic of death may influence their approach to dying patients. Patients and their families often feel that health care providers "avoid" or "abandon" them during the dying process. If this perception is correct, it may reflect the response of health care professionals to fears and anxieties about their own mortality. Physician assistants have an obligation to their patients and to themselves to carefully examine their attitudes and feelings about dying and death before caring for patients who are dying.

STAGES OF DEATH AND DYING

As has previously been noted, changes in dying and death in this country have forced health care professionals to review more closely how they relate to patients who are dying and their families. In an attempt to better understand the feelings of these patients, Elisabeth Kübler-Ross interviewed patients with terminal illnesses over 2½ years and described her experiences in a book entitled *On Death and Dying,* which was published in 1969.[2] This work proved to be important for many reasons. It was the first publication that specifically addressed the need to talk with dying patients in order to learn more about their feelings, setting the stage for additional work in the area of *thanatology* (the study of dying and death), which Kübler-Ross and others explored. The book also identified specific emotional phases, or "stages," that the patients she interviewed experienced during the dying process.

As Kübler-Ross explains, the commonality of these stages does not negate the uniqueness of death for an individual; rather, it enhances appreciation of the range of emotions patients may encounter. Patients do not necessarily experience each stage, nor do they necessarily proceed in the order presented here. The physician assistant's role is to be attentive to patients' needs and allow them the opportunity to discuss their thoughts and feelings about life and death.

Denial and Isolation

To understand this first stage, one need only remember a personal loss of someone or something of great import. Perhaps it was a loved one who died, or a pet that was accidentally hit by a car, or a significant possession that was stolen. Often, the first reaction to this situation is one of disbelief. As Kübler-Ross notes, when people discover that they have a terminal illness, they first greet the news with a statement of denial, "It can't be true." The lack of realization that this could be happening to them may be so intense that they deny treatment suggestions and, in fact, seek other health care providers to support their denial. It is a difficult time for PAs, who recognize the importance of beginning a therapeutic regimen for these patients to possibly extend their time left to live. For patients, however, it is a time of adjustment. They are not ready to discuss treatment when they have not yet acknowledged their condition as terminal. Over time, patients begin to realize that the diagnosis is accurate and may seek to retreat from the world. They are uncertain with whom they want to share the information, and sometimes they try to protect their loved ones by sheltering them from knowing about their terminal illness. The extent of isolation varies from patient to patient, as does its duration.

Anger

As patients begin to realize that their illness is terminal and that they have a limited amount of time to live, they often express anger and resentment. They may question why *they* are dying, rather than someone who is older or has been ill for a long time. A frequently asked question is "Why me?" The anger is directed at many different targets. Patients are angry with their health care providers about the lack of medical treatment to cure their disease. They express feelings of frustration and even jealousy toward their friends and family, who will go on living after they have died. Patients may also have angry feelings toward God for "allowing" them to die. Family members and health care providers find it difficult to be with a dying patient in this stage, who may be aggressive or defiant. It is also frustrating for patients, who feel a loss of control over their lives. The challenge for PAs is to provide continued care without taking personal offense at the patient's anger.

CASE STUDY 46-1

PA student B is on a surgery rotation and is involved with the team who is caring for Ms. R, a 56-year-old woman who was admitted for evaluation of a mass on her chest x-ray. The student knows that during Ms. R's surgery 2 days ago, a large malignant tumor was found and Ms. R has a poor prognosis.

The student sees the patient before morning rounds to check on her postoperative progress. Ms. R is upset and angry and says to student B, "What's wrong with me? Why won't you people tell me anything? I want to know what you found!" The student feels very uncomfortable trying to respond to Ms. R and says, "I don't know but I'll try to find out."

The student approaches the staff PA on the service and repeats Ms. R's questions. Student B is upset that Ms. R has not been informed about her disease or prognosis and asks the PA if that is deceitful.

The PA responds that Ms. R has been told that she has lung cancer, both by the attending physician and by the PA herself. The PA points out that Ms. R is in a state of shock and denial about her disease and that it takes time to assimilate such bad news.

The PA and student visit Ms. R together. The PA says, "Student B tells me that you have some questions. I want you to know that I'll try to answer any question you have." Ms. R asks what the surgery showed, and the PA describes the cancer and the extent of the disease. Ms. R bursts into tears and says, "I guess you told me, I just couldn't believe this was happening to me." Over the next few days, Ms. R seeks more information and seems to be coming to terms with her situation.

Bargaining

As Kübler-Ross explains, this stage is less definable but very helpful to the patient. Bargaining occurs when patients realize that the condition they have is terminal and that the hope for cure is not a viable one. Therefore, what they hope for is more time. This stage is an attempt to prolong the inevitable death and to eliminate or reduce the pain and physical suffering they may be experiencing. An aspect of bargaining that most patients exhibit during this stage is the promise of good behavior for a reward of more time. Patients often express the wish for more time for a specific reason, such as to attend a special event (e.g., a child's graduation) or experience an important

milestone (e.g., their 40th birthday). It is not always clear with whom they are bargaining. Sometimes, patients bargain with their health care providers and other times with God. Physician assistants can be helpful during this time by allowing patients to experience this stage but being cautious not to provide false expectations. The wish to make things "all better" for patients and their families must not be confused with promises of unrealistic outcomes.

Depression

As the disease progresses, patients become more acutely aware that their condition is terminal. It seems obvious that at this time, patients experience depression. They are no longer able to deny that their illness is life threatening and that life, as they have known it, will change. Their physical discomfort becomes more pronounced, and the fatigue and weakness limit their daily activities. In addition, patients receiving selected treatments may encounter debilitating adverse effects, such as nausea and vomiting. They also may feel uncomfortable with their physical appearance. They may have lost weight and hair and may have undergone skin changes. As a result, patients are aware that people recognize there is something different about their appearance, and they are asked questions like "What's wrong?" A combination of the physical and mental stresses the illness has placed on them leaves patients feeling tired and depressed.

Patients also become depressed about losing or "leaving behind" people they love. They and their loved ones experience anticipatory grief (grieving for someone who has not yet been lost) as they begin to acknowledge that death is approaching. Often, patients begin to detach themselves from their significant others as part of this process. It is difficult for friends and families to understand this separation, which may therefore contribute to the intensity of the situation.

In addition, patients are depressed about what they have not yet accomplished or experienced in their lives. The realization that they no longer have unlimited time forces them to reflect on what they wish they had done in their lives, "but never got around to." Although everyone acknowledges cognitively that death is inevitable, most people believe they have plenty of time to do what they desire. Depression stems from the realization that their time to die is approaching and they have yet to live their lives.

Physician assistants can be especially helpful during this time by recognizing the possible sources of the patients' depression and by being respectful of their feelings of loss. When appropriate, it is beneficial to explain to family members that part of the dying process often includes a separation phase. Patients may carefully select with whom they spend time and what they discuss. Physician assistants can advise families that supporting patients during this time may simply mean holding their hand or staying by the bedside.

Acceptance

In the final stage, as described by Kübler-Ross, patients come to accept that they are dying. Although it is not a happy time for patients, they often have a sense of peace and contentment. They also feel a need to organize their personal affairs. They attend to financial concerns, especially those related to beneficiaries and to funeral arrangements. Often, there is a shift of energy from seeking curative medical treatments to making plans for their family's future security.

It is also a time for patients to complete "unfinished business." Reflections about their lives may take place with their loved ones as they recall events they shared together. Goodbyes, spoken and unspoken, occur among close friends and family at this time. With uncertainty as to when death may actually occur, patients become focused on daily living and spend their time selectively. Physician assistants can help patients at this time by providing resources when requested, such as counseling services, and by continuing to provide supportive care to patients and their families.

HOSPICE CARE

The concept of *hospice care* (derived from the Latin word *hospitium,* meaning "hospitality or lodging") originated years ago when dogs were sent to rescue people lost in the mountains and bring them to a place to rest and renew. Recently, the term came to be associated with caring for the sick, specifically the terminally ill. A model many modern hospices have emulated is the St. Christopher's Hospice in London, England, founded by Dame Cicely Saunders in the late 1960s. Following closely the philosophies and structure of the St. Christopher's Hospice, the first hospice program in the United States was started in 1974 in New Haven, Connecticut. The Connecticut Hospice began as a home care program, but by the latter part of that decade, it also included an inpatient facility. The "hospice movement" rapidly grew in this country, resulting in the establishment of hospices in every state and the formation of the National Hospice Organization. Although the reasons for the overwhelming acceptance of the hospice concept vary, recognition of the need for an alternative to dying in an institution was at the forefront of the movement.

The hospice concept represents an overall philosophy that dying is a normal occurrence in the life cycle and should be addressed as openly and comfortably as possible by patients and their families. Hospice programs recognize that hospitals and nursing homes have not adequately cared for patients who are dying, especially from the psychosocial perspective. In traditional care settings, medical intervention has often been initiated or continued when patients may not have preferred it. The hospice seeks to determine the wishes of dying patients and then adheres to those wishes as closely as possible, including patients' desires to die at home. *Hospice,* used in the general sense, refers to providing supportive care to patients who are dying and to their families. Programs are provided through various settings, such as hospital-based units, home care agencies, complete inpatient facilities, and continuum care units. Although the settings differ, all hospice programs have specific characteristics and objectives (Table 46-1).

Hospice care focuses on providing palliative care (i.e., treating symptoms and making patients comfortable), which involves a variety of pain-reducing and pain-alleviating strategies, such as the use of medication and relaxation techniques. An important aspect of the medication administration in hospice programs is providing patients with regularly scheduled or self-administered pain medicine, rather than requiring patients to repeatedly request medication. This allows

Table 46-1   Objectives of Hospice Care

- Define the terminally ill person and his or her family as the unit of care.
- Involve the terminally ill person and his or her family as part of the care planning team, allowing them to retain final say in decision making concerning care.
- Provide a professional interdisciplinary care planning team that plans care in cooperation with the terminally ill person and his or her family.
- Make services available 7 days a week, 24 hours a day.
- Make available specially trained volunteers, as well as physical therapy, occupational therapy, speech therapy, and other services as needed.
- Maintain central administration and record keeping.
- Focus on care in the home when this is feasible and desired by the terminally ill person and his or her family. Coordinate inpatient care when necessary.
- Maintain continuity of services wherever the terminally ill person is cared for (at home, in an institution, or in a special residential facility).
- Maintain appropriately high staff-to-patient ratio whether home care or inpatient service is provided.
- Provide symptomatic relief of the terminally ill person's physical distress and symptoms.
- Make counseling available.
- Maintain open, direct, and honest communication with the terminally ill person and his or her family.

From Sendor VR, O'Connor PM. Hospice and Palliative Care. Lanham, MD: Scarecrow Press, 1997.

for relief of distress while also helping patients feel less dependent on staff members.

Another important aspect of hospice care is the inclusion of a multidisciplinary team. Patients who are in hospice programs receive care and support from many allied health care professionals, such as PAs, physical therapists, and occupational therapists. The teams also include nurses, physicians, social workers, and members of the clergy. Trained volunteers are a major part of many hospice programs. When patients are in the home, volunteers support the families by providing basic care (e.g., feeding and bathing) and by offering other helpful services, such as reading to the patients. Through the use of a variety of caregivers, hospice programs are able to provide for patients' physical, mental, emotional, and spiritual needs.

A unique aspect of hospice care is the provision of support to families throughout the patients' lives and after their death. The patients' loved ones are considered part of the overall care unit whose needs are considered and addressed by the hospice team. In addition to providing support to families of patients who are dying at home, many hospices include an inpatient facility where patients can be admitted when

families can no longer provide care or simply need a rest themselves. Unlike acute care centers, where patients are admitted, treated, cured, and discharged, hospice inpatient facilities provide care to patients who know they are dying and who need palliative treatment in a supportive environment. Additionally, patients' families and friends are encouraged to communicate with the team so that their needs are known and addressed. An essential part of hospice care is the promotion of this communication, even after the patient has died. Support throughout the bereavement period has proved to be an effective means of assisting families and friends in the healing process and of preventing related problems.

Physician assistants will become increasingly important to the hospice movement as they provide referral services to dying patients and as they continue to function as members of hospice teams.

RESPONSIBILITIES TO DYING PATIENTS

Providing care for dying patients and their families' demands involvement by physician assistants in various ways. First, there must be ongoing, honest communication between patients and PAs. Repeatedly, dying patients express their need to trust their practitioners and to be adequately informed about their conditions. Second, patients may sometimes find it difficult to speak openly about their emotions. Physician assistants may facilitate the process by asking questions such as, "Is there anything you want to talk about that we have not discussed?" Third, when appropriate, PAs may arrange for family conferences to offer support and information. In order to meet the psychosocial needs of patients and their families, PAs may provide resources, including information on support groups, counseling services, and hospice programs. Finally and most important, PAs must help patients learn to cope with their condition, physically and mentally. Through palliative care and support services, patients may find hope and learn to live life as fully as possible, despite the terminal nature of their illness.

CASE STUDY 46-2

Mrs. F is a 48-year-old medical technologist with terminal breast cancer. Mrs. F has told the primary care PA that she does not want to talk to her husband about her death. Although Mr. F has been supportive and involved in each step of her treatment, Mrs. F reports that he seems unable to recognize that she has little time left. The PA asks Mrs. F how she feels about talking about her death with Mr. F. She replies, "I'm afraid. I'm not afraid of dying. I'm worried for him, and I'm afraid that I'll start crying and I won't be able to stop."

The PA asks an open-ended question about Mrs. F's relationship with her husband. Mrs. F responds, "We've been so close. He's my best friend. I guess I feel lonely." The PA suggests that Mr. F may feel lonely as well and that sharing their feelings might be good for both of them. The PA also points out that crying is a natural human reaction at this time.

At the next visit, Mrs. F appears physically weaker but more peaceful than in previous weeks. She reports that she and her husband spent the entire weekend talking and crying. She says, "I feel like I have my husband back. I was so lonely and now I have my friend to talk to again. I know he's sad, but I know he'll be OK."

CARE FOR THE DYING CHILD

One of the most difficult experiences in the physician assistant's practice is caring for a child who is dying. The psychological needs of the child and his or her family are complex and varied. Many times, the child is "protected" from hearing the truth about the illness because the family is not prepared to accept the possibility of losing a child. Although the situation is challenging, the PA may be instrumental in encouraging truthful, language-appropriate communication with the child. This may be accomplished through open discussions with the family and with assistance from child-related support groups that specialize in helping children with terminal illnesses. Regional children's hospices, state and national cancer associations, and local Ronald McDonald Houses provide education, support, and resource materials for health care professionals and dying children and their families.

Recently, other new resources have been developed to assist parents, teachers, and health care professionals who are caring for children with a terminal illness. A number of on-line support groups have been established that allow caregivers to share their thoughts, feelings, and advice with others. These groups are particularly helpful to parents who are homebound with their child and are unable to get to regional support groups at hospitals. Caregivers utilizing these sites have indicated that they find useful information regarding the dying and grieving processes, as well as feeling a connection with others who are experiencing similar suffering. The physician assistant may refer parents and teachers to these resources and encourage on-line networking as another way of communicating. The Resources section of this chapter provides a selection of these web sites.

As with adult patients, children need to have support and encouragement throughout their care, especially when they are dying. The challenge for the PA is to assist the child to live as fully as possible, despite the terminal illness.

CLINICAL APPLICATIONS

1. You are caring for a 43-year-old woman with terminal acquired immunodeficiency syndrome (AIDS), who has two teenage children. She tells

you tearfully that she knows she does not have much time, but she is afraid to talk to her children about her sadness at separating from them. She feels that she needs to be "strong for them" and does not want to burden them with her sorrow. What do you say?

2. Your patient is a 62-year-old man who was diagnosed with colon cancer and had a partial colectomy 2 days ago. You participated in the surgery and have been following his progress postoperatively. When you see him early this morning, he angrily complains about the nursing staff, the constant noise outside his room, and his inability to sleep, and that "nobody tells me what's going on here." He has previously been calm and cooperative in all of your interactions. How do you feel and how do you respond?

3. Your patient is an 11-year-old girl with terminal leukemia. You have been involved in her care over the past month as her condition has deteriorated. Today, on morning rounds, she seems happier and confides in you that, "I'm going away today." You are aware that her parents have been unable to talk with their daughter about her impending death and have focused their attention on all available treatment options. You are sure that the child will die very shortly. How do you handle this situation?

REFERENCES

1. Healthy People 2010: Understanding and Improving Health. Washington, DC: U.S. Department of Health and Human Services, Public Health Service, 2000.
2. Kübler-Ross E. On Death and Dying. New York: Macmillan, 1969.

RESOURCES

Barton D (ed). Dying and Death: A Clinical Guide for Caregivers. Baltimore, MD: Williams & Wilkins, 1977. *Presented in this guide is a two-part overview (approaches and perspectives) on caring for patients who are dying. An important contribution to this publication is the inclusion of chapters written by patients living with life-threatening illnesses.*

Buckingham RW. Care of the Dying Child. New York: Continuum Publishing Corp, 1989. *An overview of several aspects of caring for children who are dying. Specific chapters address parental guilt and grief, truth telling, teachers, and adolescents who are dying. In addition, the author includes appendices with related information on hospice care for children and bereavement support.*

Davidson GW (ed). The Hospice: Development and Administration, ed 2. Washington, DC: Hemisphere, 1985. *A comprehensive text on organizing and maintaining hospices that includes examples of model programs, a framework for training interdisciplinary teams, and a discussion of related ethical and legal issues.*

Gonda TA, Ruark JE. Dying Dignified: The Health Professional's Guide to Care. Menlo Park, CA: Addison-Wesley, 1984. *Guidebook utilizing case studies and practical models to assist health care professionals who are providing care for dying patients. A specific discussion is included on the facts and patterns surrounding death in the United States.*

Healthy People 2010: Understanding and Improving Health. Washington, DC: U. S. Department of Health and Human Services, Public Health Service, 2000. *Provides national priorities for improving the health status of the U.S. population.*

Kübler-Ross E. On Death and Dying. New York: Macmillan, 1969. *After interviewing patients who are dying, the author describes specific stages persons may experience throughout the dying process.*

Kübler-Ross E. Questions and Answers on Death and Dying. New York: Macmillan, 1974. *Presents frequently asked questions about death and dying and offers answers designed to assist health care professionals and lay people.*

Leming MR, Dickinson GE (eds). Understanding Dying, Death, and Bereavement. New York: Holt, Rinehart and Winston, 1985. *A college level textbook that provides a psychosocial perspective on dying and death for students from various fields. A valuable resource for professionals caring for patients and for individuals seeking a greater understanding of death.*

Sendor VF, O'Connor PM. Hospice and Palliative Care: Questions and Answers. Lanham, MD: Scarecrow Press, Inc, 1997. *An excellent resource guide for health care professionals interested in all aspects of hospice care. Using a question and answer format, the authors address specific issues related to hospice care, including criteria for admission, payment structures, palliative care, advance directives, and bereavement care. Although the book is intended for patients and their families, it is an important work about the progressive hospice movement that should be read by all health care providers. The final chapter and the appendix contain important resources and documents related to hospice and caring for the dying.*

Torchia DM. Advance directives. Physician Assist 1992;16:79. *An overview of the legislation regarding patients' rights to determine life-sustaining treatment, including the Patient Self-Determination Act, living wills, and durable power of attorney laws. Emphasis is placed on the role of physician assistants as it relates to the legislation.*

www.nhpco.org. *This web site of the National Hospice and Palliative Care Organization includes information about hospice programs, third party support for hospice services, and research resources.*

www.cancer.org. *This American Cancer Society web site provides message boards for discussion, information for patients and family members, and access to support groups.*

www.dying.about.com. *This web site provides access to a large menu of topics related to dying, death, and grieving, including legal and funeral information.*

www.GriefNet.org. *GriefNet.org is an Internet resource for people dealing with grief, death, and major loss and provides access to e-mail support groups.*

CHAPTER 47

International Health Care

David H. Kuhns

INTRODUCTION

Physician assistants have actively participated in the delivery of international health care since the inception of the PA profession. PAs work with many international organizations, both private and governmental. PAs have served, and continue to serve, with international relief organizations in Cambodia, Brazil, Tonga, Peru, Guatemala, Nicaragua, Afghanistan, Djibouti, and Somalia, to name just a few. Other PAs are employed by private multinational corporations, supporting the oil-drilling crews above the Arctic Circle in Siberia or providing primary care to expatriates and their families living in China and Saudi Arabia. Many more PAs serve with U.S. Armed Forces throughout the world in a variety of environments. PAs work with other branches of the U.S.

government as well. Some serve as Peace Corps workers, and more experienced PAs serve as Peace Corp Medical Officers (PCMOs). As PCMOs, PAs provide the medical support for Peace Corps volunteers in a given country. Recent developments have brought the PA concept to the U.S. Foreign Service. Also of note is the fact that PAs are now being recruited for service with the Central Intelligence Agency for deployment overseas. Suffice it to say that PAs who want to practice in other countries now have many more options than they did just a few years ago. Overall, the number of PAs who work internationally remains quite small. Of the estimated 29,000 practicing PAs, only about 200 list themselves with international (or Armed Forces) addresses in the 1997-1998 *AAPA Directory of Members and Information*

Resources. This does not reflect the number of PAs who work overseas for short periods.

The actual clinical roles and responsibilities of international PAs are as varied and diverse as the many countries and cultures in which they work. Thus, for the same reasons that it is difficult to describe the role of a "typical" PA practicing anywhere in the United States, it is equally difficult to identify the "typical" PA role in foreign countries.

Although the Russian "feldsher" and the Chinese "barefoot doctor" are often cited as examples of analogous mid-level practitioners in foreign settings, the idea of the physician assistant was developed and, for all practical purposes, remains based in North America. Although the American model grew out of the Vietnam experience, Canadian PAs have served in the military since World War II, and they are currently exploring models for civilian employment in Canada.

Meanwhile, the export of the model of a mid-level practitioner has begun, with many nurse practitioners already working in the British Isles. U.S.-based PA consultants are working with the British government to develop a new provider level that ultimately may look like a PA as we know it or may take a somewhat different direction. At the same time, there are initiatives to develop PA analogs in the Netherlands and Italy. Although the spread of the PA model to Europe has occurred relatively recently, it is not the first. PA models can be found in the African countries of Liberia and Lesotho, and on the Asian subcontinent of Pakistan and Afghanistan.

Physician assistants who choose to work in an international environment have many options. These options depend on the PAs, who must first determine whether they will seek employment or serve on a volunteer basis. PAs then need to identify the target population (expatriates or indigenous) they are interested in serving. Once they have decided where, how, and with whom they want to work, PAs can begin an often lengthy application process. Passports, application forms and references, security clearances and background checks, screening health examinations, necessary vaccines, language skills and other pertinent training, and interviews are just some of the many steps that are likely to be required.

Working for the U.S. government, either in the capacity of the military PA or with other governmental organizations (e.g., Foreign Service), usually entails providing care to a generally young and healthy expatriate staff. The "standards of care" are expected to be similar to treatment for the same problem in a typical medical facility in the United States. Diagnostic equipment and supplies, although perhaps rudimentary, are likely to be familiar to even the inexperienced provider. Advanced care may sometimes be available by transporting the patient back to the continental United States by air ambulance or other similar service.

At the other end of the health care spectrum is work in developing countries. Providing health care to indigenous populations through nongovernmental organizations (NGOs) can offer PAs a far greater challenge on many levels. Novice PAs (in terms of international experience) will likely face a rather unsettling experience when they realize that many of their preconceptions about what constitutes a "norm" in medical standards of care in the United States cannot, and for a variety of reasons must not, apply to the delivery of health care in a developing country. PAs may face medical conditions that they never imagined, disease states of which they know little or nothing, and an overwhelming lack of resources, such as hospitals without running water or an oxygen delivery system. Frequently, the medical and diagnostic equipment, if available, is very basic. Laboratory studies might be limited to determination of a hemoglobin value and microscopic examinations of urine and blood (for cell count and differential, as well as thick and thin prep slides for malaria), as well as stool for ova and parasites. Diagnostic and "hands-on" physical evaluations frequently are performed through the use of interpreters, thus increasing the time required for even a simple examination. The organizations listed in the Box can provide additional information.

The PA who chooses to work with an indigenous population will have to decide if he or she wants shorter terms—3 to 6 months, for example, doing emergency relief where conditions are likely to be stressful. The generally safer alternative is to work in developmental projects for longer terms, for example,

9 to 12 months. These developmental projects typically have more infrastructure.

The PA serving indigenous populations will likely confront many other hurdles beyond language differences. There may be significant cultural, societal, and religious issues to address. Despite these factors, and perhaps because of them, the rewards of investing oneself in such a venture are often immeasurable.

PRACTICAL CONSIDERATIONS
General Issues

The experience of many internationally experienced PAs demonstrates the need for a well-conceived plan. PAs who hope to practice internationally would be well advised to research all aspects of such a commitment. This section addresses a number of major hurdles that PAs have encountered. Although the list of topics below is comprehensive, it is by no means complete.

The Box presents a set of guidelines for PAs considering international work, which were adopted by the American Academy of Physician Assistants (AAPA) in 2001. All PAs working internationally need to adhere to these guidelines, as well as to the *Guidelines for Ethical Conduct for the Physician Assistant Profession.*

ORGANIZATIONS FOR INTERNATIONAL HEALTH CARE

American Academy of Physician Assistants
www.aapa.org/international.html
Ellen Butler, Assistant Director, International Affairs
703/836-2272, ext. 3307
ellenb@aapa.org

Canadian Academy of Physician Assistants
www.caopa.ca
Canadian Academy of Physician Assistants
Canadian Forces Medical Services School
Canadian Forces Base Borden
Borden, Ontario L0M 1C0 CANAD

Physician Assistants for Cross-Cultural Involvement
www.paxi.org
PAXI
146 West 200 South
Bountiful, UT USA 84010-6218

Fellowship of Christian PAs
www.fcpa.net
Fellowship of Christian Physician Assistants
4 Grieb Court
Wallingford, CT 06492-2637

American Society of Tropical Medicine and Hygiene
www.astmh.org
60 Revere Drive, Suite 500
Northbrook, IL 60062 USA
Phone: 847/480-9592
astmh@astmh.org
For information on tropical medicine training programs:
www.astmh.org/certification/courslst.rtf

GUIDELINES FOR PAS WORKING INTERNATIONALLY

Policy of the American Academy of Physician Assistants
1. PAs should establish and maintain the appropriate physician/PA team.
2. PAs should accurately represent their skills, training, professional credentials, identity, or service, both directly and indirectly.
3. PAs should provide only those services for which they are qualified via their education and/or experiences, and in accordance with all pertinent legal and regulatory processes.
4. PAs should respect the culture, values, beliefs, and expectations of the patients, local health care providers, and local health care systems.
5. PAs should take responsibility for being familiar with, and adhering to, the customs, laws, and regulations of the country in which they will be providing services.
6. When applicable, PAs should identify and train local personnel who can assume the roles of providing care and continuing the education process.

Licensure/Registration

There is no universal means by which PAs are permitted to receive authorization to work in a foreign country. In some cases in which expatriate PAs are serving an expatriate patient population, official approval from foreign governments is obtained through a series of clinical competency examinations. In some countries, PAs will be breaking new ground as they explore the ways by which they can perform the tasks and deliver the level of care for which they are trained. One such "ground breaker," Donald Prater, worked in Nanjing, China, for a U.S.-based company, providing health care to hundreds of expatriates and their families who live in that region. Even though he was not providing medical services to the local residents, Chinese authorities required that he take the Chinese medical examination (in English) so that he could see his expatriate patients on a fee-for-service basis.

More commonly, governmental approval is awarded to the agency with which the PA is working (e.g., American Refugee Committee). Thus, the PA is allowed to work under the umbrella of that organization. Consequently, that agency will typically require that credentials and letters of recommendation be submitted as the first step in going "to the field." Experience indicates that PAs, as fully licensed, certified, and registered providers in the United States, can usually practice their clinical skills to the full scope of their training. However, the actual scope of practice for the international PA can, and often does, vary widely.

Physician/Physician Assistant Relationship

The physician/PA relationship in international settings can be informal or it can be very tightly structured. The supervising physician can be in immediate proximity, working alongside the PA in a refugee camp, or in the capital city of the country where the PA is working. Another option is that the supervising physician in the United States may be available by satellite communications. This is the model that many private multinational companies follow. It is important to remember that because there are no distinct or universal rules that govern international PA practice (except those constraints of the state wherein the PA is duly licensed or registered), practice standards for PAs in international settings unfortunately remain vague and ill defined.

Malpractice

Although the myriad aspects of U.S.-based medical practice differ from those of international practice, and malpractice is not usually an issue in international practice, PAs must always provide the same high level of care for which they have trained, regardless of where in the world they find themselves. PAs should check with their insurance carriers before departing because insurance carriers rarely provide coverage outside the United States.

PAs must never represent themselves as physicians, either at home or abroad. The problems that could occur as a result of such misrepresentation may be devastating for an individual PA, and may even have long-reaching effects on the PA profession.

When the PA is working overseas, it remains his or her responsibility to account for absences from clinical practice at home. This may require that adequate documentation be provided for any extended absences, including formal verification from the international employer or the organization.

Continuing Education

Continuing medical education (CME), although not usually an issue for the countries in which the PA may work, is nonetheless a requirement for maintaining licensure and certification. Maintaining certification by the National Commission on Certification of Physician Assistants (NCCPA) becomes an issue only if the PA is outside of the United States for a year or longer. From a practical perspective, Category 1 CME credits are best obtained either by "stockpiling" before leaving the United States, or by using multimedia presentations available in compact disk (CD) format. Recent developments allow the globetrotting PA to access various Category 1 CME programs online from Internet cafes around the world.

QUALIFICATIONS
Medical Skills

The ability to improvise with limited resources is an essential skill. Of particular value is a reliance on a basic "hands-on" approach to medicine. To highlight this issue, Cameron McCauley, an experienced international PA, tells of a time during his PA training when he was learning to evaluate heart murmurs. Like most of his peers, he scoffed at the need for physical assessment skills when technology such as echocardiograms would confirm the diagnosis. Cameron was humbled many years later, when he found himself working in a remote village without any hope of accessing such technology. Instead, he used those basic physical diagnostic skills he had learned years before to determine that a young patient had a ventricular septal defect. The child was then referred to the distant capital city where his diagnosis was confirmed and the defect was surgically corrected.

It is important to remember that there are usually few advanced resources available. The PA will seldom find advanced diagnostic options, such as ultrasound or computed tomography (CT), or even the basics of plain radiography. As an example of the paucity of resources that can be faced, when the author worked in Somaliland (northwestern Somalia) in 1994, there was only one electrocardiogram (ECG) machine in the entire country. The nearest x-ray unit was 2 hours away and could be reached only by driving over rough roads, with the patient bouncing along in the back end of a beat-up Land Rover.

Tropical Medicine

Patients in developing countries do not have the same causes of morbidity and mortality as those in the United States. Instead of cancers and cardiovascular diseases, patients in developing countries typically succumb to the ravages of infectious diseases. Even such relatively straightforward illnesses as gastroenteritis, acute respiratory infections like pneumonia, and measles are the leading causes of death. Treatment is usually simple, that is, *if* the patient can access the proper medication in time. Clinicians can spend years learning to specialize in infectious tropical disease; however, there are several short courses in American universities that can provide excellent training over a couple of weeks to a few months.

Public Health

Because infectious diseases are so commonplace throughout the rest of the world, a strong emphasis must be placed on prevention of these problems. Therefore, it is essential that PAs, especially those working in infrastructure development and capacity building, develop an understanding of the basic principles of public health. Many accredited schools of public health are available in the United States, but only a relative few offer specialty training in international health.

Management and Teaching Expertise

Frequently, PAs are sought not just as clinical providers, but as trainers or supervisors of local staff. In Jalalabad, Afghanistan, the author served as the Project Medical Coordinator for New Hadda, an emergency refugee camp of more than 80,000 people who had fled the fighting in Kabul, the capital, but were then unable to escape to neighboring Pakistan. Health care provided in the camp was the responsibility of the international humanitarian aid agency, Doctors Without Borders, which provided primary care through a series of clinics staffed by Afghan doctors and nurses. As the project medical coordinator, I was responsible for the overall delivery of medical care in the camp clinics, some limited clinical practice, the provision of supplies and drugs to the clinics, and some limited clinical teaching, as well as all aspects of public health in the camp. To accomplish this, I regularly collaborated with representatives from other local and international NGOs, the local Ministry of Health, the United Nations International Children's Emergency Fund (UNICEF), and the World Health Organization.

Language Skills

A second language (e.g., French, Spanish, Russian, Persian, or Arabic) can open many doors and allow for an ease of communication with patients and professional counterparts. The alternative—total reliance on interpreters—can result in frustration for all parties involved. Nuances of the medical history can be missed, and the interpreter can sometimes act as a screen, perhaps keeping details vague or even misleading the PA.

OTHER CONSIDERATIONS
Stress

Living in harsh environments is stressful. The sound of gunfire can fill the air throughout the night. Insects, crawling and flying, can plague the living space. Accommodations are typically Spartan. Adequate rest becomes a precious commodity. The days are often long and demanding. In addition, working and living with the same group of people, day in and day out, provides additional challenges. There must be some opportunity for rest and recuperation to avoid what many see as inevitable burnout. It is very common for expatriates working in large refugee camp environments to work 7 days a week, 12 or more hours each day. Workers share a common feeling that there is so much work that needs to be done and so little time in which to do it. Therefore, many NGOs insist that workers take time away, to the extent that this can be done without affecting the operations of the project.

Medications and Standards of Treatment

Medications, if they are available, may not be familiar to the PA because they are sometimes antiquated by most Western standards. Usually, no multi-generational cephalosporins are available, not just because of the cost, but because resistance has not yet been a significant issue in the area. As a result, inexpensive but nonetheless effective drugs such as chloramphenicol or penicillin G are still used extensively.

Another common observation is that patients from the local population often expect that when they come to a clinic or a hospital, they will be treated and will *always* receive some sort of medication. A patient encounter in which the patient does not walk out with medications can be felt to be unsatisfactory from the patient's perspective, even though the PA may have otherwise given appropriate treatment and provided proper patient education. A visit without medications can be viewed by the patient as substandard care.

Traditional Health Care

Maintaining an open mind is important when one is confronted with traditional and folk medicines. These methods, although usually unfamiliar to U.S.-born PAs, often play a significant role for patients. We must remember that after the PA and other international expatriate staff members leave, the responsibility for ongoing health care usually falls back onto the traditional health care worker.

In Afghanistan, the author learned of the traditional resuscitation technique used by traditional birth attendants (TBAs) for stillborn infants. The TBA places the placenta on the face of the infant, with the thought that the placenta had provided life to the child in the womb and it should do similarly after birth. To attempt to change this misconception would involve much work and more than a simple message that the TBA "is wrong." It is essential that changes be introduced according to a well-conceived approach. Undermining a community's confidence in a local provider would have long-term ramifications.

An awareness of how a community relies on traditional healers is important if one is to understand what the community expects of the PA. Expatriates must realize that their presence, however long, is still seen as transient by the indigenous populations. It is therefore important to remember that, especially in emergency relief settings, when the expatriate leaves, there will be little left but footprints in the sand.

Personal Health and Safety

Although working in war-ravaged and developing countries represents its own challenge, typically the greatest risk to expatriates occurs while they are traveling by car or truck. Injuries from motor vehicle accidents remain the primary reason for expatriates with Doctors Without Borders to return from the field for medical reasons. Other common medical problems are due to tropical diseases such as malaria, as well as to gastroenteritis.

Land Mines

More than 60 countries are still littered with more than 60 to 80 million land mines; therefore, these indiscriminate killers represent a significant threat not just to the local population but to expatriate relief workers as well. It is imperative that a mine awareness training program be completed by expatriate PAs before they go to work in a land mine–infested country. PAs must always maintain a keen sense of safety when working in such an environment. Elizabeth Sheehan, a PA with vast international experience, tells of an incident when she was traveling through a heavily mined area of Cambodia. In front of her car, a cow was wandering down the dirt road. Suddenly, the cow exploded as it stepped onto a mine, showering Liz's car with cow parts.

Security

Expatriate PAs can sometimes find themselves in dangerous environments. Although they may be volunteers, the stipend of a few hundred dollars a month that they may receive is still significantly more than the average annual income for many locals. As a result, volunteer relief workers have been held hostage, and others have been threatened at gunpoint. There have been robberies, kidnappings, assaults, and even deaths among field workers of most major international relief organizations. Although the economic motivation for these acts seems clear, perhaps less obvious are the political overtones common in some developing countries. One such tragedy occurred on December 17, 1996, when six workers with the International Committee of the Red Cross in Chechnya were murdered as they slept. The reason for the attack was believed to be political. The murderers were never identified.

Reentry

Returning home from an overseas experience often proves difficult, and returning PAs should not count on a smooth transition. Family members, other loved ones, and co-workers can seldom understand fully what the returned PA may have seen or experienced. Common experiences have been identified among returning relief workers. An example of such an experience is the "supermarket event." Kate Herlihy, who spent 2 years working for the American Refugee Committee in a Cambodian refugee camp, speaks of the disdain and shock that she felt when she entered a supermarket at home. She was overwhelmed by the variety of pet food, after she had cared for starving people just a few days earlier.

More serious symptoms of post-traumatic stress disorder can also occur. Depression and even suicide have been reported in returned volunteers. It is therefore important to provide a mechanism for adequate debriefing on return and a means to follow up in a timely manner. Many international organizations offer psychological debriefings as part of ongoing support for their workers, paid and volunteer. It can be helpful to speak with a psychologist, psychiatrist, or other mental health expert if the PA has a difficult time with the reentry process.

Topics for Preparation

When a PA is considering taking the time to work overseas, it is important that he or she learn about all the possible aspects of such a commitment. The list below includes a selection of topics to be researched:

➤ What is the overall mission of the organization?
➤ What is the organizational approach to the problems—individual and curative, or more utilitarian public health focused, or perhaps a blend of both?
➤ What happens if you get to the post and you discover it is not what you had expected?
➤ What security parameters will be followed?
➤ Will the PA be self-sufficient, functioning outside the established health care system, or will he or she work along side local counterparts in existing health support structures?
➤ Will there be a salary or a stipend for you as a volunteer?
➤ What will happen if you have a needlestick or some other human immunodeficiency virus (HIV) risk exposure?
➤ Who will pay the necessary expenses of your travel, room, and board?
➤ What provisions are made for your medical and/or psychological care both during and after a mission?
➤ Will you have time off while in the field? If so, what are the options for that time?
➤ What about repatriation to the United States in case of medical or family emergencies?
➤ What about life insurance?
➤ Will medical supplies and equipment be provided, or will you have to bring everything yourself?
➤ Is there a training or orientation program available, or will you be expected to go directly to the field?
➤ Is the situation stable enough for the PA to be accompanied by a spouse or other family member?
➤ How do you relax when you are under stress?
➤ How do you function in a team? How do you feel about living and working, day in and day out, in a cramped living space, surrounded by smokers?

➤ What about the job that you will be leaving behind? Is there any chance that the job, and any promises regarding the security of that job, will not be maintained? If not, what is your fall-back plan?

Case Study 47-1, written from the author's personal experience, illustrates the challenges and satisfactions of work in international health care.

CASE STUDY 47-1

For my first mission with Doctors Without Borders, or *Médecins Sans Frontières (MSF)*, I had asked for a "stable" situation on which to cut my teeth. The reply from headquarters was that I had the opportunity to go to Somaliland (northwestern Somalia), where MSF had been working for almost a decade. The area was considered quite stable, by MSF standards. It had been a couple of years since fighting had dominated the area. It was also hundreds of miles, and a separate and distinct country, from Mogadishu, where the scene was much more volatile. Our project, based in the city of Burao, was to continue to strengthen the existing health structures through a collaborative effort with the Ministry of Public Health (MOPH). As the Country Medical Coordinator, I was the leader of the small team of two other expatriates, a Dutch nurse, and an English logistician, as well as about 40 local staff, consisting of doctors, nurses, and various nonmedical support staff

Because MSF was in the process of scaling back operational involvement, my job was supposed to be primarily nonclinical. However, I was also told that I could probably integrate my clinical background into my daily work. Between negotiations with my counterpart, the hospital director, I would make ward rounds and discuss management of patients with the Somali doctors and nurses. Overall, it was proving a rather interesting departure from my experience in emergency medicine. My focus was no longer centered on a single patient at a time; instead, I now looked at improving the quality of medical care for a whole city and the regions beyond.

My first couple of weeks in Burao was overwhelming. I tried to establish some sense of order

in my life. I had just left a tertiary care center in Portland, Maine, and I was now working in a hospital that lacked such amenities as running water or even continuous electricity for 24 hours a day. Goats and sheep wandered about the grounds of the hospital compound, leaving behind a different sort of "land mine" to discover. I could literally walk through a pile of sheep dung and then step into the operating theater. There, the patient could be found situated on a table with a large fan turning directly overhead. On the wards, patients lay on the bare springs of decrepit beds. If patients were fortunate enough to have a mattress or bed linens, the patient's family had provided them. Hospital windows had no intact glass or screens. The ceilings of the wards were stained from rain that had leaked through the countless bullet and shrapnel holes in the roof. During the rainy season, I saw the staff madly shuffling children in cribs around the room in a futile effort to avoid the many leaks that plagued the entire hospital. I developed an overwhelming sense of seeing that there was so much work that needed to be done and so little time or money to do what was really needed. Eventually, that sense of frustration grew less when, on several occasions, community elders would approach me and thank me for the "help that MSF was providing to this impoverished and forgotten country."

I eventually shifted my focus from trying to reproduce what I knew to be a standard of health care and turned to a more pragmatic approach. It would not matter if we could provide drugs, supplies, and diagnostic equipment like x-ray machines, if they would then be lost to damage from the rains. We turned our focus to rehabilitating the infrastructure of the hospital—repairing the roof, replacing windows, and other simple efforts. Our efforts were starting to pay off. A sense of accomplishment was shared by the whole team. Unfortunately, our joy was short-lived. The political climate was changing acutely, and tensions were rising. The night air became quieter as people started to hoard their precious ammunition.

One particularly quiet night was suddenly disrupted by the sound of tanks rolling through the city streets. The next morning, the expatriate team was evacuated back to our base of operations in the adjacent country of Djibouti, a postage stamp–sized country located about 2 hours flying time to the West. There we could relax over a beer and contemplate our next actions. Our downtime was limited to a short few hours. A freak storm had struck the area, resulting in a tremendous flash flood that hit the city of Djiboutiville. Walls of water spilled out of the rugged mountain areas and dumped into the flood plains from which the city arises. Shanty towns in the city's periphery suffered the most, with thousands of homes destroyed. More than a hundred people were swept away by the rapidly rising waters, while hundreds of others escaped to safety when they were eventually plucked from roofs and treetops by helicopters sent by the local detachment of the French military. While the fetid waters also struck the MSF office and forced my colleagues to flee to the roof, I was out of danger.

The flood was only the first blow. Another killer was stalking the population and awaiting the chance to pounce. With the flood came the opportunity for that culprit—cholera. Cholera is endemic in the area. These simple bacteria thrive in the milieu of a hot, humid environment and in the poor sanitation found in such a developing country. Untreated, cholera can result in a 50% mortality rate. Like so many other infectious diseases, the highest mortality is among the elderly, children, and those with significant medical problems. Within a few hours of exposure, the body responds to the infection with gastrointestinal symptoms. Abdominal cramps, nausea, vomiting, and profound diarrhea, often described as "rice water" in appearance, are the classical presentation.

The city was trying to recover from the flooding, dealing with the displacement from the floods, and planning for the inevitable cholera outbreak. MSF responded by offering our assistance. Within the world of emergency medical relief, MSF is well known as an authority on managing cholera epidemics. With huge stores of prepackaged supplies available in European warehouses, MSF can respond to an emergency in a matter of days. The

logistical support network is well organized and quite efficient, the product of many similar responses during the past decades. In just 3 days, two additional expatriate staff, an experienced nurse and a logistician, joined our team. The tents, intravenous fluids, chlorine for water treatment and disinfections, and the remainder of our cholera treatment center (CTC) supplies arrived the next day from Amsterdam. Our job was to establish a CTC near the hardest hit area of the city. The residents were already poor, with limited resources. Many were Somalis who had fled the fighting in their homeland and settled in Djibouti, awaiting peace in their homeland. In Djibouti, they lived in shanties—simple wood frame structures covered with corrugated sheets of metal and plastic sheeting. Drinking water supplies had been contaminated. Children suffered from malnutrition and were subject to malabsorption diarrheas.

As a novice to the ravages of cholera, I soon found myself in the uncomfortable role of being the senior medical person in charge of the CTC. The good news was that the treatment for cholera is simple: Replace fluids at a greater rate than they are being lost. If patients can tolerate oral fluids, they receive oral rehydration salts (ORS). If unable to keep that down, patients receive nasogastric (NG) feedings of ORS. If patients were profoundly dehydrated, as so many were, intravenous (IV) replacement of fluids is the only option left. The local staff that made up the backbone of our CTC was, as a rule, excellent in assessing and treating patients. My job was to ensure that we treated patients according to the protocols of the World Health Organization (WHO). As the senior medical person on the scene, I was also the one to whom the staff turned if they were unable to place an NG tube or find an IV site.

I still recall treating a child about 2 years old, weighing only 6 or 7 kilograms (the result of chronic malnutrition). He was floppy and unresponsive, with poor skin turgor and sunken eyes, and in shock from the profound fluid loss of his vomiting and diarrhea. The child was held suspended by his feet, while I waited for his neck veins to distend. I placed an external jugular line and started the process of rehydrating the child. Accustomed as I was to working in a level I trauma center, I was initially taken aback by the WHO protocol for the aggressive IV rate of 30 ml/kg/hr that is recommended in volume replacement for cholera. My skepticism ended when I saw the tremendous volume of liquid stools that just poured out of these children. To hold a child, floppy and lethargic, in shock from this dramatic gastroenteritis was eye-opening. Suddenly it became clear why cholera claims so many victims around the world each year. The days in the CTC were long and demanding, but my reward was seeing the child who had been at death's door a few hours earlier, now bright-eyed and alert in the arms of his grateful mother.

We soon handed over the day-to-day supervision of the CTC to the Djiboutian Ministry of Health. Meanwhile, our team made preparations to return to Somaliland. We learned that tens of thousands of civilians had fled the fighting in the cities and had returned to their traditional home in the Somali "bush" country. Because this displaced population had no provisions for medical care, MSF volunteered to help. My team was soon traveling back into Burao. There, we planned for a series of assessment missions to determine the extent of the problem we were facing.

It was on such a mission on December 23, 1994, that I found myself in the settlement of Hor Fadda, normally just a stopover in the desert for bands of nomadic shepherds. The "village" was little more than hundreds of simple huts surrounding a muddy watering hole the size of a tennis court. Countless goats, sheep, camels, and humans muddied the water as they all sought to quench their thirst. Surrounding the water hole were thousands of people who had fled the fighting in the capital city of Hargeisa. These refugees, mostly women, elderly men, and children (the young men were back in the city as fighters), were living in makeshift shelters constructed of branches and covered with plastic sheeting, while the men slept outside on the ground, wrapped from head to toe, shroudlike, with thin wool blankets. The only permanent structure in the village was a small, mud-walled hut that we converted to a temporary clinic where we initially treated patients. We then set up a large canvas tent that we had brought with us. That night, the tent would serve as our shelter. The following day, the tent served as the base for a clinic that provided health care to the 15,000 people in the camp.

Later that evening, we shared a meal of boiled mutton and rice. I sat back, enjoyed a cup of chai, relished the warmth from the fire, and took the time to relax a bit and to reflect on the events of the day. It had been a very long day that started at dawn with a 6-hour trip in an elderly Land Rover, bouncing over dirt roads, at times feeling like I was in the midst of a National Geographic special. The one thing that kept me from enjoying much of the journey was that the Somali countryside had been littered with land mines, the result of many years of civil war. We were now traveling roads that normally we would have avoided because of that threat from land mines. However, now the stakes were different: Thousands of people were in need of assistance and, if we did not go, no one else was available. We traveled the well-worn roads and kept our fingers crossed. As we sat around the campfire, it was quiet—much quieter than I had yet experienced during my time on the horn of Africa. My thoughts turned to my loved ones, safe at home on the other side of the world. Christmas was less than a day away and here I was, in the desert, sitting around a campfire.

The silence was broken when Mohammed, one of the staff, asked me if I watched Western movies. I turned to see his toothy smile as he told me that the scene we were in was "just like in the movies." I chuckled and wondered what this man's image of America really was. I was surprised as he then described the typical cowboy scenario portrayed by John Wayne or Gary Cooper. He continued, "We could make a movie and call it 'Night in Hor Fadda,'" which caused us to laugh as we both continued to build the image upon the foundation that he had so accurately depicted.

It was during that evening that I realized how much I had experienced in a little over 2 weeks. I had been through the start of a civil war, a flash flood, a cholera outbreak, and a journey into the bush, where I had witnessed the devastating effects of war on civilians. Although physically and emotionally exhausted, I had survived. More important, at least to me, I felt good about what I had done. I started to lose some of my self-pity and instead started to feel that I was here for a purpose, and that I had, in some small way, made a difference. On some clear nights as I look skyward, Mohammed's voice and handsome face echo in my mind. I smile when I see him.

CONCLUSION

Working in an international environment can be a rich and rewarding experience. Although sometimes dangerous, and clinically challenging, it can also be very demanding, both physically and emotionally. Uniformly, PAs with such international expertise have had valuable experiences that continue to influence and enrich their lives in many ways. Jean Carpenter, who worked as a lay missionary with Maryknoll in Guatemala and Nicaragua, tells of her wonderful experience working and living with the native people, "seeing another way of life, another way of practicing medicine, and a chance to live as few other Americans have."

Acknowledgments

I want to thank the following individuals who worked with me on the AAPA's former International Affairs Committee for their contributions to this chapter: Richard Rohrs, Ellen Kuo, Kathy Pederson, Rebekah Halpern, Janet-Ditto Boswell, James White, and David Guinn. A special thanks to Ellen Butler, Assistant Director, International Affairs and Leadership, at the AAPA.

CLINICAL APPLICATIONS

1. If you were interested in a position in international health care, how would you research the opportunities for PAs? How would you match your skills to the health care needs and practice settings of international communities?
2. If you secured an international position as a PA, how would you obtain information about the language, culture, politics, infrastructure, and health care system of the area? What else would you want to know before going to an international setting?

RESOURCES

Cahill M. A Framework for Survival: Health, Human Rights, and Humanitarian Assistance in Conflicts and Disasters. New York: Routledge, 1999. *Provides the reader an appreciation of the breadth and depth of effort required to address the many recent international humanitarian crises.*

DuFour D, Kromann Jensen S, Owen-Smith M, et al. Surgery for Victims of War. Geneva, Switzerland: International Committee of the Red Cross, 1990. *A primer on the management of war-related injuries. This practical book belongs on the shelf of anyone working with such devastating trauma, either in the actual war environment or as the trauma specialist of a major emergency department. Don't expect photos or drawings as it works from the assumption that the basics are covered.*

Leaning J, Briggs S, Chen L (eds). Humanitarian Crises: The Medical and Public Health Response. Cambridge: Harvard University Press, 1999. *An excellent text that addresses the various health related interventions in the setting of humanitarian emergencies.*

Levy B, Victor S (eds). War and Public Health. New York: American Public Health Association, 2000. *The editors have assembled an impressive array of experts in the field from whom they draw valuable insight into the horrors of war and the variety of impact that results.*

Maren M. The Road to Hell: The Ravaging Effects of Foreign Aid and International Charity. New York: The Free Press, 1997. Médecins Sans Frontières. Refugee Health: An Approach to Emergency Situations. MSF, 1997. *This compact book, written by the leading international humanitarian relief agency, Doctors Without Borders, provides both the depth and breadth of information on how to best deliver medical care to refugee populations. This is a "must read" for anyone who has worked in the field or dreams of doing so. Maren has done both, and he writes of the impact that relief work can have, both good and bad.*

Werner D. Where There Is No Doctor. Palo Alto, CA: The Hesperian Foundation, 1992. *This text has served as the bible for primary health care to indigent populations all over the world. Although directed to a lay audience, the book also provides insight to health professionals on how they can teach concepts and techniques in simple, effective terms.*

CHAPTER 48

Residency Programs

David P. Asprey

INTRODUCTION

In the early 1970s, formal educational programs were developed to provide physician assistants (PAs) with a postgraduate specialty education experience utilizing the physician internship or residency training model of education. These residency programs provided the graduate PA with an opportunity to gain additional didactic and clinical experience in a specialty area of medicine that would build on the primary care PA or surgical assistant (SA) training acquired from the entry-level PA program. Most of the residency programs are located within larger teaching hospitals or clinics throughout the United States. Many of these PA residency programs were developed in response to the call to reduce the number of physician residents in training. As the number of physician residents available to hospitals decreased, PAs were viewed as a desirable substitute for the traditional house staff. Consequently, PA residencies

developed to respond to the need for additional house staff in the hospitals.

PA residency programs vary in length, area of specialty training, amount of didactic education, credential awarded upon completion, and number of residents admitted each year. In response to the wide degree of variety in the residency programs, some individuals have proposed a need for accreditation[1] and standardization.[1,2] Although the residency programs can generally be viewed as successful, they have struggled to mature and stabilize owing in part to lack of an accreditation mechanism and the tenuous nature of PA residency program funding.

HISTORY OF POSTGRADUATE RESIDENCY EDUCATION

The first postgraduate PA program was initiated in 1971 by Montefiore Medical Center in affiliation with the Albert Einstein School of Medicine in New York.

Montefiore Medical Center began employing and educating PAs to replace surgical house officers. These PA residents were employed and trained alongside physician surgery house officers and were substituted in the place of surgical physician residents.

In 1975, Norwalk Hospital and the Department of Surgery at the Yale School of Medicine established a 1-year surgical residency program exclusively structured for PAs, which combined didactic and clinical instruction. By 1980, six postgraduate residency programs existed. The number of programs has increased and decreased in recent years, reaching a peak of approximately 25 programs in recent years. Currently, 25 programs are members of the Association of Postgraduate Physician Assistant Programs (APPAP), offering residencies in 10 different specialty areas. The 1996 census was the last time that the American Academy of Physician Assistants (AAPA) reported data on residency programs attended by its responders. At that time, the data indicated that of 13,256 respondents, 708 (5.3%) PAs reported having attended a PA postgraduate residency program.

Relatively little has been published in the literature regarding PA residency programs. A few of the individual programs have reported their experiences.[3-5] In 1982, Cawley and Katterjohn[6] completed a survey of available postgraduate residency training programs regarding their program activities from 1979 to 1981. Although this study was not published, the findings from the study are available as part of the Proceedings of the Paper Presentation Session from the 10th Annual PA Conference.[6]

In 1987, Keith and Doerr[3] completed a study and published data regarding their experience in surgical PA postgraduate residencies. They conducted a survey of the graduates of the Montefiore Medical Center Surgical Residency Program. The results of this survey from the 110 respondents showed that 86% remained employed as PAs. Information on the specialties of these PAs is presented in Table 48-1. Of the 110 respondents, 86 (78.2%) were employed by institutions and 24 (21.8%) were employed by physicians in private practice. This survey also included a salary analysis, which indicated that graduates of postgraduate residency programs earned significantly higher pay than PAs practicing in the same specialty

Table 48-1 Specialty Practice of the Montefiore Surgical Residency Gradiates Employed as PAs

	Number	Percent
Surgery	66	69.5%
Primary care	16	16.8%
Emergency medicine	8	8.4%
Educational administration	5	5.3%
Total	95	100%

who had not completed a postgraduate residency program. The average salary of the respondents was 21% greater than the national average salary of PAs.

The graduate residents were asked to comment on their perceptions about the degree to which their training prepared them for their jobs. About 72% indicated satisfaction with the preparation they had received, 20% believed they were overprepared, and 8% felt inadequately prepared for the positions they held.

Two additional studies were conducted in 1998 by Asprey and Helms, who obtained and reported data from PA residency program directors and from currently enrolled PA residents.[7,8]

ASSOCIATION OF POSTGRADUATE PROGRAMS

At the American Academy of Physician Assistants Annual Meeting in Los Angeles in May of 1988, a group of representatives of postgraduate PA residency programs met to formalize a national postgraduate PA program organization. Bylaws were written and approved by the eight founding programs, and subsequently, the Association of Postgraduate Physician Assistant Programs (APPAP) was formed to further the specialty education of PAs.[9]

The stated purposes and goals of the APPAP include the following:

➤ Assisting in the development and organization of postgraduate educational curricula and programs for PAs.

➤ Assisting in defining the role of the PA (with emphasis on the specialties).

➤ Assisting in the development of evaluation methodologies for postgraduate educational curricula and programs.

➤ Serving as an information center to PAs, with programs training PAs at the entry level, as well as professionals in other medical and health care disciplines and the public, with respect to postgraduate educational curricula and programs for PAs.[9]

The APPAP maintains a formal liaison with the American Academy of Physician Assistants and the Association of Physician Assistant Programs (APAP) and works with these organizations on mutual goals to further the PA profession and postgraduate PA education. Additional information regarding current member residency programs, bylaws, and general information can be viewed at the web site (http://www.appap.org).

APPAP MEMBER PROGRAMS

The member programs of APPAP are formal postgraduate PA programs that offer structured curricula, including didactic and clinical components, to educate PAs who are eligible or certified by the National Commission on Certification of Physician Assistants (NCCPA) for a defined period (usually 12 months) in a medical specialty. Currently, 10 areas of specialization are available at APPAP member programs, including dermatology, emergency medicine, family medicine, oncology, orthopedic surgery, pediatrics, psychiatry, rural primary care, surgery, and urology. The current APPAP member programs and their areas of specialty training may be reviewed at the Association's web site.

PA postgraduate residency programs may be categorized as two basic types.[7] The first type is the traditional physician residency model or apprenticeship model. These programs possess a modest amount of practically oriented didactic curriculum combined with an intense clinical rotations experience that leads to a certificate of completion. The second type is an academic model program. These programs combine a highly structured and formalized didactic education (through courses taken for academic credit) with an intense clinical rotations experience that typically leads to a master's degree (or credit towards a master's degree) upon completion. APPAP member programs follow several models of training with varying titles, including fellowships, master's degree programs, and residencies. All APPAP member programs must award a certificate or a degree or provide graduate academic credit.

RESIDENCY PROGRAM ACCREDITATION AND ESSENTIALS

Currently, there is no accreditation agency or mechanism for PA residencies. However, in published articles, members of the profession have called for greater standardization and accreditation of PA residency programs.[1,2] In addition, APPAP has expressed interest in developing a means of accreditation for PA residency programs. Although there is ongoing interest by the APPAP in developing an accreditation process, the membership has felt that it is financially prohibitive to the currently small number of member programs.

In an attempt to accomplish the goal of PA residency accreditation, APPAP has met with several organizations in the profession to discuss the feasibility of developing a collaborative mechanism for PA residency program accreditation.[10] Specifically, APPAP has discussed this issue with AAPA, APAP, and the Accreditation Review Committee on Education for the Physician Assistant (ARC-PA). Recently, two organizations within the profession have proposed the development of specific taskforces charged with investigating the feasibility of developing and implementing an accreditation system for PA postgraduate residency programs. The residency programs have not yet developed an accreditation system; however, APPAP has taken an initial step in developing its own set of program essentials, which are intended to identify the desirable elements of a PA residency program. These essentials were developed and approved in 1991 by the member programs. Compliance with the essentials is voluntary and is not reviewed or enforced by any external entity. However, APPAP member programs must agree to adhere to the essentials as a condition of membership. The PA residency program essentials for postgraduate physician assistant programs may be viewed at the APPAP web site.

RESIDENCY GRADUATE EMPLOYMENT OPPORTUNITIES

Employment opportunities and roles for PAs are rapidly expanding to include a high proportion of specialty areas. Because of this diversity and specialization, formal postgraduate training is assuming a greater importance as an adjunct to PA primary care education. Postgraduate curricula are designed to build on the knowledge and experience acquired in PA school, enabling the PA to competently assume a role as physician assistant on a specialty health care team. Many postgraduate programs have pioneered the role of the PA in these specialty areas and offer experienced role models as well as formalized instruction.

Very little objective information has been published comparing the number of employment opportunities and the salaries commanded between residency-prepared and non–residency prepared PAs. However, there is anecdotal information and a general belief that the residency-prepared PA has a competitive edge when applying for PA positions and commands additional salary.

GENERAL CHARACTERISTICS OF EXISTING PROGRAMS

Admission Requirements

Residency programs vary considerably in their specific requirements for eligibility for the programs. All require graduation from an accredited PA program. In addition, a majority of programs require NCCPA certification or eligibility for the NCCPA examination for admission. Some programs also require state licensure or eligibility or advanced cardiac life support certification; in other cases, a specific degree is required.

Application Process

PA residency programs are competitive and admission requires the completion of an application package. This includes items such as an application form, a copy of the certificate of completion from the PA program, a copy of the NCCPA certification (if applicable), transcripts, educational and work history or resume, letters of recommendation, and a narrative describing the candidate's interest in the residency and the specialty area. In addition, nearly all residency programs require a personal interview. Residency directors have reported using many different criteria in making admissions decisions for their programs. Commonly used measures include interest in the specialty, the interview, letters of recommendation, level of motivation, academic performance, interpersonal skills, desire to continue education, and possession of a degree.

Class sizes vary from as few as 1 student to as many as 18. Competition for admission to these residency programs is generally quite high. Programs may experience applicant-to-enrollee ratios in excess of 10:1.[6,11] Demographically, a 1998 study of enrolled residents revealed a balanced sex distribution, with 14% of residents representing a minority; the average age was 34.4 years. Most residents (61%) have not worked as PAs at the time of enrollment in the program.[7,8]

Selecting a Residency Program

Residents have often indicated that the way they learned about the residency program was either through information provided by the PA program they attended or from a fellow student or colleague. Residents identify improved ability to compete for a job in their specialty, interest in acquiring additional knowledge and skills before entering practice, improved future earning potential, and the desire for increased competence in the specialty area as the items that had the greatest influence on their decision to attend residency. The majority of enrolled residents reported that they had applied to a single residency program.[8]

Curriculum

PA residency programs vary in length from 12 to 22 months. Internship model programs typically are 12 months in length (a few are 15 months in length), and the academic model programs are 20 to 22 months long.

Curriculum content varies based on whether the program is an internship model or an academic model, and according to the specialty of the clinical training received in the residency. All residencies have a didactic component, either at the beginning of the residency or incorporated throughout the residency. The didactic element may constitute formal courses or a series of lectures, conferences, grand rounds, and other programs. Residency directors have reported the average number of hours of didactic curriculum in their program to be 249 hours for internship model programs and 531 for academic model programs.[7] Enrolled residents have estimated their total number of hours of didactic education associated with the residency program they attended to be 350.4 hours for residents in internship model programs and 413.4 hours for residents enrolled in an academic model program.[8]

Clinical Hours Worked

A concern that has been voiced by residents regarding their training is the number of clinical hours they are required to work per week. The number varies dramatically from specialty to specialty and from program to program, but residents tend to work considerably more than a traditional 40-hour workweek. Residents in academic model programs reported working 44.1 clinical hours per week. Residents enrolled in internship model programs reported working an average of 72.3 clinical hour per week.[8]

Stipend/Fringe Benefits

Compensation is dependent on the nature of the residency (internship versus academic model) and the total benefits package. Data from a study of program directors in 1998 identified that stipends varied from $25,000 to $42,000 per year. The mean salary for all residents was $34,902. Benefits packages vary considerably but generally include such items as health insurance, malpractice insurance, paid vacation time, and life insurance.[7]

Credential Awarded

The most commonly awarded credential is the certificate of completion or training. In some instances, the residency program is also linked to an academic institution that grants a master's degree. Other residency programs offer an opportunity to earn credit for courses toward a master's degree.

RESIDENT PERCEPTIONS OF TRAINING

Residents' perceptions of their training in general are very positive. Table 48-2 presents findings about residents' levels of satisfaction with various aspects of their training.[8] It also categorizes the data on

Table 48-2   Summary of Residents' Satisfaction Levels[8]

Educational Experience	Very High	High	Low	Very Low
Clinical supervision received	15 = 32.6%	24 = 52.2%	6 = 13%	1 = 2.2%
• High vs. low satisfaction	High = 84.8%		Low = 15.2%	
Degree of responsibility	19 = 43.2%	24 = 54.5%	1 = 2.3%	0 = 0%
• High vs. low satisfaction	High = 97.7%		Low = 2.3%	
Degree of autonomy	14 = 31.8%	22 = 50.0%	8 = 18.2%	0 = 0%
• High vs. low satisfaction	High = 81.8%		Low = 18.2%	
Salary or stipend	3 = 7.3%	20 = 48.8%	14 = 34.1%	4 = 9.8%
• High vs. low satisfaction	High = 56.1%		Low = 43.9%	
Benefits package	10 = 24.4%	17 = 44.7%	7 = 18.4%	4 = 10.5%
• High vs. low satisfaction	High = 69.1%		Low = 28.9%	
Didactic education	15 = 32.6%	25 = 54.4%	3 = 6.5%	3 = 6.5%
• High vs. low satisfaction	High = 87.0%		Low = 13.0%	
Clinical education	16 = 35.6%	23 = 51.1%	3 = 6.7%	3 = 6.7%
• High vs. low satisfaction	High = 86.7%		Low = 13.4%	
Overall residency training	16 = 34.8%	30 = 65.2%	0 = 0%	0 = 0%
• High vs. low satisfaction	High = 100%		Low = 0.0%	

satisfaction into high and low categories for broader comparisons. All residents reported satisfaction in the summary evaluations of their residency training experiences and substantial satisfaction in the areas of degree of responsibility and didactic and clinical education. Residents were least satisfied with the salary and benefits packages. When asked if they would recommend their residency program to other PAs interested in their specialty, 71.7% (n = 33) answered "definitely," and 28.3% (n = 13) said "probably." None replied that they would not recommend their training program.

Included in this chapter is an interview of a PA who attended a residency. This interview explores the PA's perceptions of her residency experience and her reasons for electing to attend a residency program.

CASE STUDY 48-1

This 28-year-old female PA attended the Illinois Bone and Joint Institute Postgraduate PA Orthopedic Residency and graduated in July of 2000. She did not practice as a PA before entering the residency program. Currently, she works in an orthopedic practice with two physicians who specialize in sports medicine and total joint replacements.

Q: Why did you elect to attend an orthopedic residency program rather than taking a position in an orthopedics practice after graduating from PA school?

A: I knew that I wanted to work in a surgery specialty and after considering my options, I believed that orthopedics would provide me with the greatest level of satisfaction and flexibility in the future. I wanted to feel confident in my ability to take care of orthopedic patients when I took my first job and knew the residency would do that for me. I believed that I would get a better, more systematic educational experience in the residency program than I would in a regular practice position. I also felt that the residency would significantly expand my opportunities for finding a job in the specialty.

Q: What exposure to the specialty of orthopedics did you receive in your entry-level PA program education?

A: I completed a 4-week elective orthopedics rotation.

Q: Describe the curriculum in your residency program.

A: There was no formal separate orientation; however, the first 2 weeks served as a practical orientation to the hospital system and the paperwork. A regular lecture series occurs weekly that provides the residents with specific knowledge of how to diagnose, treat, and manage various orthopedic conditions. The rotations are preset as 3-month blocks assigned to different surgical teams. The teams are separated into a joint and spine team and a sports medicine and hand, foot, and ankle team. Although there is no elective rotation, there is opportunity to seek out specific experiences if you have interest in a particular area.

Q: With what types of procedural activities did you gain experience?

A: I developed skills in suturing and surgical assisting, casting and fracture reduction, reduction of dislocations, and management of patients with major trauma, as well as preoperative and postoperative care skills.

Q: Was there a research element in your residency program?

A: Yes, we were expected to identify a research topic or project and work with a physician mentor in producing a research paper.

Q: How was your performance in the residency program evaluated?

A: We received regular feedback from the physicians that we worked with closely. They would give us suggestions on a regular basis about how to improve our technique and our management of patients. We also received a summary evaluation from the residency program at the middle and near the end of the program. We did not complete an objective examination to assess our knowledge of orthopedics.

Q: What unique knowledge and skills do you feel you acquired that were beyond what you received in your PA program education?

A: I expanded my knowledge and skills in almost every area related to orthopedics. My procedural and surgical skills have showed the greatest improvement; my ability to manage patients preoperatively and postoperatively has also been enhanced.

Q: Who served as your teacher in the residency?

A: Primarily, it was the staff physicians, but it's a team approach and physician-residents and PAs also contributed to my overall education.

Q: What compensation did you receive during the residency?

A: We received a stipend of $40,000 during the year and have a traditional benefits package with things such as malpractice insurance, health insurance, life insurance, vacation, and sick leave.

Q: How long is the residency?

A: It was 12 months in length.

Q: How many hours did you work during an average week?

A: I would guess it averaged around 70 to 80 hours per week.

Q: How many residents were enrolled in your program?

A: Five PA residents were enrolled in my program.

Q: What job opportunities did you find were available when you had completed the residency?

A: I believe I had 7 offers. Many of them came from the physicians with whom I was working during the residency. Others came from groups that would contact the residency program to express an interest in one of the graduates. I really felt that the residency created a lot of job opportunities for me that wouldn't have been there if I had not been through the residency.

Q: What were the negative aspects of being a PA resident?

A: I really thought the residency program was great, and my experience has been that all of the negative aspects or sacrifices involved were short-term ones. You do work a lot of hours and you have less autonomy over your schedule than someone in a traditional job, but I think the benefits far exceeded the short-term costs. Certainly you have fewer opportunities for a robust social life or leisure time to spend with your family, but that limitation was restricted to a single 12-month period.

Q: Any final comments?

A: I thought that my residency training experience was excellent and I would highly recommend it to anyone who is interested in orthopedics.

CONCLUSION

PA residency education continues to evolve. These programs can generally be considered successful in preparing graduate PAs to practice effectively in a specialty area of medicine. Considerable interest has been demonstrated by applicants to the residency programs and by institutions interested in developing new PA residency programs. The PA profession is unique in that it has both academic model–type residencies and more commonly, the internship model residency. It seems reasonable to conclude that at some point in the future, as more PA programs offer a master's degree upon completion, level of interest in the residency programs granting a master's degree (academic model programs) may decline. PA residents in general are very satisfied with their educational experiences and would recommend the residency program to others.

APPAP plans to continue working to achieve a mechanism for program accreditation. If PA residency programs are able to achieve their goal of developing an accreditation mechanism, this may also serve to address issues related to the financial stability of the programs. Until PA residency programs have an accreditation mechanism, it seems unlikely that they will be recognized by other agencies for loan deferment or in competing for training funds.

CLINICAL APPLICATIONS

1. If you were interested in PA residency education, how would you find out about the distinctive features of each program?
2. What are some of the pros and cons associated with attending residency programs?
3. Would you choose a residency program with a certificate or a master's degree? Why?
4. Interview two PAs working in specialty areas—one who attended a residency program and one who did not. Ask them to describe their PA careers and how they acquired the knowledge and skills related to their specialties.

REFERENCES

1. Katterjohn KR. Legislation: the increasing interest by hospitals in substituting PAs for housestaff. Physician Assist Health Practitioner 1979;3:8.
2. Timmer S. Call for uniform guidelines for postgraduate surgical residency programs. J Am Acad Physician Assist 1991;4:453.
3. Keith DE, Doerr RJ. Survey of a physician assistant internship concerning practice characteristics and adequacy of training. J Med Educ 1987;62:517.
4. McGill F, Kleiner GJ, Vanderbilt C, et al. Postgraduate internship in gynecology and obstetrics for physician assistants: a 4-year experience. Obstet Gynecol 1990;76:1135.
5. Brandt LB, Beinfeld MS, Laffaye HA, et al. The training and utilization of surgical assistants: a retrospective study. Arch Surg 1989;124:348.
6. Cawley JP, Katterjohn KR. A survey of postgraduate residency training programs for physician assistants. Association of Physician Assistant Programs. In: Proceedings of the Paper Presentation Session, Tenth Annual Physician Assistant Conference. Washington DC: 1982.
7. Asprey D, Helms L. Description of physician assistant postgraduate residency training: The director's perspective. Perspectives on Physician Assistant Education 1999.
8. Asprey D, Helms L. A description of physician assistant postgraduate residency training: The resident's perspective. Perspectives on Physician Assistant Education 2000.
9. Association of Postgraduate Physician Assistant Programs (1997-1998), National Membership Directory. Philippi, WV: National Directory of Postgraduate PA Programs, 1997.
10. Association of Postgraduate Physician Assistant Programs. Recognition of Postgraduate Physician Assistants. Report to the AAPA Education Council and the APAP Board of Directors. Albuquerque, NM: APPAP, October 23, 1994.
11. Cornell PA. Surgical residencies. Adv Physician Assist 1997;5:48.

RESOURCE

Association of Postgraduate Physician Assistant Programs web site (http://www.appap.org). *This APPAP web site provides a wealth of information about PA residencies, including a listing of programs.*

CHAPTER 49

Genetics in Primary Care

Chantelle Wolpert and Michael Rackover

Introduction	**Current and Future Issues/Trends in Genetics**
Identification of At-Risk Patients	**Genetic Counseling**
Analyzing a Family History	**Current and Future Roles of PAs in Genetics**
Many Genetic "Paths," One Disease	• **Case Study 49-1**
"Destination"	• **Case Study 49-2**

INTRODUCTION

Physician assistants (PAs) and other health care providers believe they rarely see a patient with an inherited disorder, leading many to think that learning medical genetics has limited value.[1] However, this is an outdated belief. In the past, medical genetics was confined to the identification and treatment of rare diseases. This time period is sometimes referred to as the "old genetics." Today, knowledge from genetic research has ushered in the era of "the new genetics." Many researchers now consider, "Genetics [as] the central science of medicine and health care..."[2] because all disease has a genetic component. Recognizing and addressing this facet of health is becoming a critical aspect of patient care.

Several advances have led to this era of "new genetics":

1. It has been shown that most adult-onset, chronic diseases have a genetic component, be it an increased genetic susceptibility or a single, disease-causing gene.[3] Among the chronic diseases recently proven to have a genetic component are coronary heart disease, diabetes mellitus, asthma, mental health disorders, Alzheimer's disease, osteoporosis, glaucoma, and breast and colon cancer.[4]

2. Clinical applications of genetic research are now starting to reach the primary care setting. GENETests™, a web site sponsored by the University of Washington that catalogs genetics clinics and laboratories around the world, has nearly 50,000 registered users.[5] This resource lists more than 1000 clinics and more than 500 laboratories that test for nearly 1000 diseases. Genetic testing and counseling are now standard components of prenatal and oncological care in this country. Pediatric and neonatal care providers frequently use the services of clinical geneticists and genetic counselors.

3. Medical genetic research breakthroughs are frequently featured in the popular press, both in print and on the Internet. Additionally, many Americans use the Internet to search for information pertaining to their health. A recent survey by the Pew Internet and American Life Project found that 62% of U.S. adult Internet users (73 million people) have gone on-line to look for health information.[6] As a result of this increased

media attention, a growing number of patients now ask about their risk for developing disorders that "run in their family." In order to make the most of the clinical applications brought about by new medical genetic technology and patient requests for genetic information, PAs will need to cultivate a better understanding of genetics, including terminology and concepts.[7]

IDENTIFICATION OF AT-RISK PATIENTS

As more is learned about genetic factors that contribute to commonly occurring diseases, as well as to less commonly occurring diseases, it becomes possible to identify patients who are at increased risk for developing, or having a child with, a genetic disease or a disease with a significant genetic component. At-risk patients can be offered specific medical monitoring, education about lifestyle, and medical prevention practices, and in some instances, genetic testing, with the ultimate goal of reducing the morbidity and mortality associated with the disease. Accurate understanding of health risks is often of significant psychosocial benefit because people frequently overestimate their risk for developing a disorder that "runs in the family." This information can be important in life planning.

Education regarding the genetic factors affecting a patient's health may be pertinent to other family members, and patients can be advised to convey such information to their families. In some instances, it may even be possible to offer treatment in order to prevent or delay the onset of a chronic disease. For example, individuals with a family history of coronary artery disease can be offered preventive treatment such as dietary changes and exercise or folic acid supplementation to reduce homocysteine levels.[8]

In order to practice preventive medicine, PAs need to incorporate "genetic thinking" into their daily clinical encounters. An improved understanding of genetics will help PAs to identify at-risk patients. The key method for identifying these at-risk patients is through a family history. By eliciting a *comprehensive* family history, the PA acquires a powerful data source from which to begin analyzing the patient's familial risk factors for the development of disease.[9-11]

However, too often, the typical written record of family history information is not comprehensive enough to capture the significance of familial risk factors. For instance, documenting that a patient has a parent with a history of hypertension and coronary artery disease would not be as comprehensive as drawing a pedigree. The pedigree documents all relatives with hypertension and coronary artery disease, along with age of onset and an inquiry into other risk factors for heart disease. (See Case Studies 49-1 and 49-2 at the end of this chapter.)

A comprehensive family history includes the following components:

➤ A multi-generational family history (usually at least three generations), including ethnicity, drawn in pedigree form using standardized pedigree symbols.

➤ Pertinent health information about each closely related relative (parents, grandparents, siblings, aunts, uncles, cousins, children), including age of onset for adult-onset diseases such as hypertension and breast cancer.[12]

Recently, the Core Competency Working Group of the National Coalition for Health Professional Education in Genetics (NCHPEG) recommended that, "all health professionals possess the core competencies in genetics...to enable them to integrate genetics effectively and responsibly into their current practice."[13] Included in the core competencies are two items related to the family history. The first states that, "all health professionals should understand the importance of family history (minimum of three generations) in assessing predisposition to disease." The working group also recommended that, "all health care professionals should be able to gather family history information, including an appropriate multigenerational family history." Family medical histories are dynamic and should be updated periodically.

ANALYZING A FAMILY HISTORY

The family history can be used to assess which patients are at risk for specific diseases. Family histories may reveal a known genetic disorder in the family, or they may sometimes show a disorder with a clear-cut inheritance pattern (e.g., autosomal dominant, autosomal recessive, or X-linked inheritance).[9]

In these instances, the PA and the patient may agree that genetic counseling and possibly genetic testing may be useful. However, a family history will typically show one or more chronic, adult-onset disorders such as hypertension, glaucoma, or diabetes mellitus. This seemingly vague information is just as important clinically as the family histories that demonstrate a clear-cut inheritance pattern because it may indicate an increased risk for the disorder.

Many Genetic "Paths," One Disease "Destination"

Advances in genetic research, including research through the Human Genome Project (HGP), show that some diseases once thought to be a single clinical entity are actually a group of disorders with a similar clinical presentation but different etiologies. For instance, there are more than four Alzheimer's disease genes, and these different forms of Alzheimer's disease are not distinguishable based on the clinical presentation, except for the age of onset of the disease.[14] All types of Alzheimer's disease are characterized by progressive dementia and would meet current clinical diagnostic guidelines. All share the telltale senile plaques and neurofibrillary tangles found in the brains of Alzheimer's patients, as well as other clinical similarities. Similarly, there are more than three genes associated with diabetes mellitus, and also more than three genes associated with breast cancer. This knowledge leads clinicians to stop thinking of disorders as distinct clinical entities and instead to recognize that they are simply "clinical descriptions."

Genetic health professionals call the clinical presentation of a disorder a *phenotype*. The names of diseases are often just "phenotypic" descriptions of clinical findings.[4] For example, retinitis pigmentosa, once considered a unique disease entity in itself, is now recognized as one physical finding in many disorders. Another more familiar example is the "diagnostic" term *hypertension*. Hypertension describes a phenotype that can be caused by conditions ranging from polycystic kidney disease to "essential" or idiopathic hypertension. Successful treatment of hypertension depends in large part on the underlying cause. Over time, clinicians will be able to treat disorders according to their genetic etiology.

CURRENT AND FUTURE ISSUES/TRENDS IN GENETICS

Medications are currently prescribed according to certain guidelines such as a patient's weight, allergies, and other medications that the patient is taking. However, even after these considerations, patients with similar symptomatology may have widely differing responses to the medication. As biological differences caused by genetic profiles that result in differing responses are uncovered, prescriptive practice will change. Pharmaceutical companies will be able to recommend which patients should receive specific medications based on their genetic profiles.[15] Clinicians will have more information to consider in determining which medications to prescribe.

In the future, patient management will be based on an individual's metabolism. This will allow health care providers to write the best prescription the first time around, thus bypassing severe adverse reactions or ineffective treatments. The pharmacotherapeutic industry, with potentially the most to gain financially from these developments, may become a driving force for the application of primary care medical genomics.

GENETIC COUNSELING

Receiving a diagnosis of a genetic disorder can have a profound impact for both the patient and the family members. It is clear that aside from the need for medical and genetic information, families affected by genetic disorders have educational, social, and psychological needs that require attention.[16-18] For instance, certain predictable reactions have been observed in families. Often, parents of a child with an inherited disorder feel profound guilt at having transmitted the gene to their child. In other families, the family member who does not have the inherited disorder or outlives the affected family member may feel guilty. Sometimes, this phenomenon is termed "survivor guilt." In other instances, family members at risk for developing a late-onset disorder live with intense anxiety about the future. Another very common occurrence is that other family members may incorrectly infer that they are at risk for having a child with a genetic disorder. Attempts to help families cope with these varied needs have resulted in the emergence of a model of genetic education and counseling called genetic counseling.

Genetic counseling has evolved into a profession. For more than 30 years, genetic counselors have been members of the health care team providing comprehensive and consistent medical genetic services, while also tending to the social and emotional welfare of the patient and his or her family.[19,20] In the United States, the first master's degree training program for genetic counseling was established in 1971. Since then, the profession has grown tremendously. There are now more than 2500 genetic counselors in the United States and 25 genetic counseling training programs. Many industrialized countries have adopted the U.S. model of training for genetic counselors, and master's-level training programs now exist in Canada, Australia, Great Britain, and South Africa.

As the profession grows, the definition of genetic counseling continues to evolve. Genetic counseling is currently defined as "a communication process that helps an individual and/or family"[21] to:

1. Comprehend the medical facts, including the diagnosis, probable course of the disorder, and available management approaches.
2. Appreciate the way heredity contributes to the disorder and the risk of recurrence in relatives.
3. Understand the alternatives for dealing with the risk of recurrence and the medical facts relating to a disorder.
4. Make informed, independent decisions, free of coercion, by utilizing the necessary facts and information about available genetic testing and medical treatment.
5. Access local and national support resources.

Because the diagnosis of a genetic disorder in an individual often leads to identification of other family members who may be at risk for having or passing on a genetic disorder, genetic counselors often work with entire families. Even when genetic testing is not available, early identification of at risk patients and their family members can be valuable and quite possibly life-saving.

The demand for genetic education and counseling will likely increase as knowledge accumulates about the genetic components of commonly occurring disorders like breast cancer, Alzheimer's disease, heart disease, diabetes mellitus, and osteoporosis. As a result, many professionals, including genetic educators, physicians, PAs, nurses, social workers, medical geneticists, and genetic counselors, will provide genetic education and counseling.

As they provide beneficial genetic counseling to patients and their families, professionals must have a full understanding of the dangers of eugenics. The abuse of genetic information has led to many atrocities in the past. In Germany, the Nazis murdered nearly 7 million "genetically defective" people during World War II and forced sterilization of nearly half a million others.[22] The United States also has a checkered past with respect to eugenics. In the early 20th century, the United States passed laws allowing sterilization of the mentally handicapped and limiting the number of "genetically inferior" ethnic groups that were allowed to immigrate.

To prevent such abuses from occurring again, the genetic counseling profession has followed in the footsteps of other health care professions to establish a code of ethics to guide professional behavior. Policies such as *nondirectiveness*, prevention of genetic discrimination, respect for patients' beliefs, complete disclosure, and informed consent are components of these ethical principles.[23] Nondirectiveness, one of the major tenets of genetic counseling, is described as enabling "clients to make informed independent decisions, free of coercion, by providing or illuminating the necessary facts and clarifying the alternatives and anticipated consequences."[24]

Genetic counseling has become a vital part of medical genetics. With the knowledge gained from the past and the tools to help patients choose their paths, genetic counseling will continue to be invaluable in the rapidly growing field of human genetics.

CURRENT AND FUTURE ROLES OF PAs IN GENETICS

As the "new genetics" takes hold, there will be a sharper focus on family histories to identify individuals at risk for different disorders. Identifying patients at risk may ultimately result in PAs playing a main role in recognizing risk factors, offering screening or treatment for disorders, recommending tests, and referring at-risk or inquisitive patients to genetic health care providers.[25]

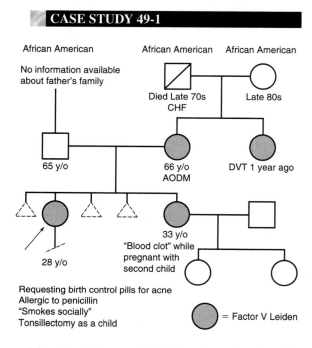

African American   African American African American

No information available about father's family

Died Late 70s CHF   Late 80s

65 y/o   66 y/o AODM   DVT 1 year ago

28 y/o   33 y/o "Blood clot" while pregnant with second child

Requesting birth control pills for acne
Allergic to penicillin
"Smokes socially"
Tonsillectomy as a child

◯ = Factor V Leiden

Diane is a 28-year-old African American female, who presents for a first appointment and inquires about a prescription for oral contraceptives. She states that she read an advertisement about a birth control pill that helps "control acne."

The patient's past medical history is remarkable for an allergy to penicillin and a tonsillectomy at age 5. The patient smokes "socially," and has a 5-pack-year history.

The patient's past medical history is remarkable for a sister who had a "blood clot" while she was pregnant and a maternal aunt who had a "DVT." Additionally, the patient's mother has adult-onset diabetes mellitus and has had three miscarriages, but medical information about these occurrences is not available. The patient's maternal grandmother is alive and well and in her late 80s. The patient's maternal grandfather died in his late 70s of congestive heart failure. The patient's father is 65 years old and in good health. Medical information about his family is not available.

The patient was advised that she was not a candidate for oral contraceptives because of her family history of "blood clots." Further evaluation revealed that the patient carried one factor V Leiden gene. This family history is an example of an inherited thrombophilia that follows an autosomal dominant pattern of inheritance.

Discussion

Forty percent of individuals under the age of 50 who are admitted for a thrombotic episode have an identifiable, inherited thrombophilia. Factor V Leiden is one of several inherited thrombophilias. An individual who carries one copy of the factor V Leiden gene (heterozygote) has a 7-fold greater increase of having a thrombotic episode than an individual in the general population. If an individual carries two copies of the factor V Leiden gene (homozygote), then he or she has an 80 times greater chance of having a thrombotic episode. Factor V Leiden disorder exhibits a *gene dosage* effect, which means that one copy of the gene may cause clinical problems, and two copies of the gene is even more likely to cause clinical problems.

Knowing that an individual has a genetic risk or predisposition means that environmental factors can be modified. In this instance, the patient can be advised not to use oral contraceptives, not to smoke, and to seek medical advice before becoming pregnant.[26]

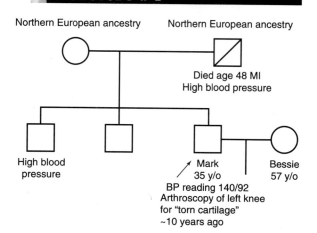

Northern European ancestry   Northern European ancestry

Died age 48 MI
High blood pressure

High blood pressure   Mark 35 y/o   Bessie 57 y/o

BP reading 140/92
Arthroscopy of left knee
for "torn cartilage"
~10 years ago

Mark is a 32-year-old Caucasian male whom you have seen for several urgent care visits over the past 2 years. He presents at this visit for a routine history and physical. He has no current complaints, and his personal medical history is significant for an arthroscopy of his left knee at age 25 for "torn cartilage." Physical examination is remarkable for a blood pressure of 140/92. Upon reviewing the chart, you notice that on two other occasions, Mark had similar blood pressure readings.

A family history reveals that Mark has two older siblings, one with high blood pressure. His father had hypertension, and Mark states that his father passed away at age 48 from a myocardial infarction (MI).

Discussion

This case demonstrates a significant family history of hypertension. Most notable is the fact that the patient's father had hypertension and had a fatal MI in his late 40s. The patient's brother also has hypertension. It is unclear what actually caused the father's MI. The pedigree in this family is consistent with an autosomal dominant pattern of hypertension, but it is known that environmental factors can affect blood pressure.

A search of the Online Mendelian Inheritance in Man (OMIM) and GENETests™ databases does not reveal any identified genes associated with an autosomal dominant essential hypertension.[27,28] However, given the "strong" family history of hypertension, Mark is worked up and treated according to current guidelines. The patient is counseled that because of his family history, he should pay close attention to this condition and work with the health care team to control his blood pressure. Mark is asked to find out the exact cause, if possible, of his father's MI because this information may affect his treatment.[28]

This case shows that even when genetic testing is not available, family medical history can be useful in determining the threshold for medical treatment.

CLINICAL APPLICATIONS

1. Research and write your family pedigree. Would analysis of your pedigree result in changes in your own health risk behaviors?

2. If you were the PA in Case Study 49-1, how would you counsel Diane about the risks of oral contraceptives? What alternatives could be offered?

3. If you were the PA in Case Study 49-2, how would you counsel Mark about his risk of cardiovascular disease? What modifications in his life style would be recommended?

REFERENCES

1. Wolpert CM. Genetic history: a key to diagnosis. Physician Assistant 1994;18:23.
2. National Coalition for Health Professions Education in Genetics. Available at http://www.nchpeg.org/.
3. http://www.pbs.org/faithandreason/transcript/coll-frame.html.
4. Wolpert CM, Melvin E, Speer MC. Complex genetic disorders: evaluating when genetic research findings are applicable for genetic counseling practice. Journal of Genetic Counseling 1999;8:73.
5. GENETests™: Genetic Testing Resource. Directory of Medical Genetics Laboratories. Available at www.genetests.org.
6. Pew Internet and American Life Project. Vital decisions. Available at http://www.pewinternet.org/reports/toc.asp?Report=59.
7. Rackover MA, Peay HL, Wolpert CM. The need for genetic literacy among physician assistants. Perspectives on Physician Assistant Education 2001;12:113.
8. Clark R, Stansbie D. Assessment of homocysteine as a cardiovascular risk factor in clinical practice. Annals of Clinical Biochemistry 2001;38:624.
9. Wolpert CM. Genetic history: a key to diagnosis. Physician Assistant 1994;18:23.
10. Pharoah PDP, Stratton JF, Mackay J. Screening for breast and ovarian cancer: the relevance of family history. Br Med Bull 1998;54:823.
11. Rose P, Humm E, Hey K, Jones L, Huson SM. Family history taking and genetic counseling in primary care. *Fam Pract* 1999;16:78.
12. Bennet R. The Practical Guide to the Genetic Family History. New York: Wiley-Liss, Inc, 1999.
13. Core Competency Working Group of the National Coalition for Health Professional Education in Genetics. Recommendations of core competencies in genetics essential for all health professionals. Genetics in Medicine 2001;3:155.
14. St. George-Hyslop PH. Molecular genetics of Alzheimer disease. Biological Psychiatry 2000; 47:183.
15. Roses AD. Pharmacogenetics place in modern medical science and practice. Life Sciences 2002;70:1471.
16. Epstein CJ. Who should do genetic counseling, and under what circumstances? Birth Defects: Original Article Series. 1973;9:39.

17. Kessler S. Psychological aspects of genetic counseling VI. A critical review of the literature dealing with education and reproduction. Am J Med Genet 1989;34:340.

18. Kessler S. Process issues in genetic counselling. Birth Defects Original Article Series 1992;28:1.

19. National Society of Genetic Counselors. Genetic counseling as a profession. In: National Society of Genetic Counselors. Wallingford, PA: National Society of Genetic Counselors, Inc, 1983.

20. Reed S. A short history of genetic counseling. Social Biology 1974;21:332.

21. Fine B, Koblenz M. Conducting pre-test patient Education. In: Humanizing Genetic Testing: Clinical Applications of New DNA Technologies. Chicago, IL: Northwestern University, 1994.

22. http://fcit.coedu.usf.edu/Holocaust/people/victims.htm.

23. National Society of Genetic Counseling. Code of Ethics, Section II, No. 3. Adopted in 1992.

24. http://www.nsgc.org/about_code.asp.

25. Wolpert CM. Human genomics in clinical practice: bridging the gap. Clinicians Review 2000;10:67.

26. American College of Medical Genetics consensus statement on factor V Leiden mutation testing. Genetics in Medicine 2001;3:139.

27. Online Mendelian Inheritance in Man (OMIM). Available at http://www.ncbi.nlm.nih.gov/omim/. Accessed 29 May 2002.

28. GENETests™: Genetic Testing Resource. Directory of Medical Genetics Laboratories. Available at www.genetests.org. Accessed 29 May 2002.

RESOURCES

GENETests™ at www.genetests.org. *This web site, sponsored by the University of Washington, catalogs genetic clinics and laboratories around the world. It lists more than 500 laboratories that test for almost 1000 diseases.*

CHAPTER 50

Complementary and Alternative Medicine

Emily WhiteHorse

INTRODUCTION

Complementary and alternative medicine (CAM) refers to the use of approaches, therapies, and treatments that are not considered part of the biomedical (conventional) model of medicine. CAM also encompasses a broad range of philosophies and beliefs regarding the nature of health, healing, illness, and disease different from those on which our health care system is based. Other terms such as *integrated* or *holistic* medicine have also been used.

By definition, *complementary* refers to those approaches or therapies that are used in addition to conventional medicine treatments, such as the use of acupuncture with physical therapy and medications in patients with chronic pain syndromes. *Alternative* refers to those approaches or therapies that are used instead of or in place of conventional medicine, for example, the use of homeopathy and homeopathic remedies instead of pharmaceutical medications. In everyday use, this clear distinction is lost.

The biomedical model is based on clearly defined philosophies and approaches to health and illness that are based on the beliefs and values of Western scientific culture. Many complementary and alternative approaches represent philosophies, beliefs, values, and approaches of health care systems from other cultures and other countries, such as the use of the meridian system and the concept of *Qi* in the diagnosis and treatment of illness in traditional Chinese medicine. In addition, some CAM approaches emerge from visionary ideas initiated by individuals within a given culture, for example, craniosacral therapy.

Every health care system in the world is based on the dominant beliefs, values, and expectations of the people it serves. This is known as the *explanatory model*. Because of the vast and growing ethnic diversity in the United States, understanding CAM is intimately connected to cultural sensitivity, awareness, and competency. In order to understand the nature and uses of CAM, one must understand the culture

977

and/or explanatory model from which the therapy originated. This makes the study of CAM a daunting task. Although it is not possible or necessary for someone to know all the modalities or systems of healing encompassed in CAM, it is possible for PAs to develop skills to navigate the range of CAM used by their patients.

This chapter does not present detailed information on specific CAM therapies and treatments; rather it discusses broad categories and provides resources. Its main focus is to offer guidelines and suggestions to help PAs learn how to interact and communicate effectively with patients regarding both their beliefs about health, healing, and disease and their use of CAM. It is imperative that PAs gather the tools and learn the skills to support open and honest communication with the goal of providing the best care possible for each patient, which in today's society means asking about a person's belief system and about complementary and alternative medicine.

HISTORY

The existence, use, and popularity of CAM is not a new phenomenon in the United States. It has been part of our history since the early colonial days, and its prevalence has waxed and waned throughout the centuries.

During the colonial days, the early immigrants to this country used mostly lay and folk healers to treat illnesses. *Lay* healers were untrained individuals who took on the role of caregiver and healer in a given community. A *folk* healer usually refers to those individuals who had undergone some training, commonly by apprenticeship, and specialized in a specific form of healing. Clergy were also commonly looked upon to fill the role of healer in a community.[1]

Alternative systems flourished from about 1790 to around 1870, with some lasting well into the early 1900s and beyond. In its earliest appearance in this country, the first recorded use of an alternative system of health care occurred in the late 1700s. The first of these alternative systems was known as Thomsonianism, named after Samuel Thomson. Thomson's approach to treating illness included hot baths and herbs. By today's standards, we would consider him an herbalist.[1]

Another alternative system that gained wide public support was founded by Sylvester Graham; its followers were referred to as Grahamites. Graham held that many forms of illness were initiated or aggravated by the use of calomel, a form of mercury, and the other "poisonous drugs" then commonly used by educated physicians. The Grahamites taught that the maintenance of good health depended on the observance of hygienic measures, the avoidance of alcohol, a diet of "natural" vegetable foods, and the use of whole wheat flour rather than refined flour. The enduring product from this group is still found in supermarkets today— the Graham cracker.[1]

Several other popular systems emerged that are still present today. In the early 1800s, homeopathy flourished. Founded by Samuel Hahnemann, a German physician, the approach to health and healing in this system radically challenged the emerging beliefs and theories then held by conventional medicine. Initially accepted by educated physicians and then rejected, homeopathy has endured. Two of his most prominent theories are "likes cures likes" and "the law of infinitesimals." Hahnemann found through experimentation that large doses of medicine served to aggravate illness and that small doses tended to support the body's own healing ability to overcome the illness. In this way, homeopathy provided a gentler, more natural approach for which patients were seeking.[1] During epidemics of cholera, typhus, and scarlet fever, homeopathy consistently proved its superiority over the punishing conventional treatments of the day. By 1900, 8% to 10% of American-educated physicians used homeopathy.[2,3]

In the late 1800s, the emergence of osteopathy (introduced by an allopathic civil war surgeon Andrew Taylor Still) and chiropractics (introduced by Daniel David Palmer) added to the increasing number of alternatives, which remain available today. These two approaches focus on musculoskeletal manipulation, with the latter focused more specifically on the spine.[2]

Alternative systems continued to crop up despite the increasing number of educated physicians. These other systems of providing treatment for ill patients emerged in reaction to the harsh, brutal, and commonly fatal treatments being used by educated physicians. One need only read the account of George

Washington's death to understand why this was so. In the 1800s, treatments of the day used by educated physicians included bloodletting (induced bleeding), purging (induced vomiting using calomel), blistering (burning the skin to induce blisters to draw out illness), and sweating. During the last 2 days of his life, our first president was bled (more than half of his total volume), purged, and blistered. His death was not a result of his illness (which was a nonfatal viral infection); rather, he died from the treatments.[1]

Because it was common knowledge that it was dangerous, if not fatal, to seek treatment from a physician, the public looked for other ways to address their health and illness needs. In response to the harsh approaches and unsuccessful outcomes offered by educated physicians, more and more Americans chose "alternative" healers because the treatments offered by the alternative systems were gentler and more natural, using herbs, lifestyle changes, nutrition, and an approach that incorporated the whole person.

With the increasing popularity of alternative practices, and as educated physicians began to use some of those practices themselves, conventional medicine found itself in a growing state of disfavor. By 1900, 20% of all practitioners of medicine were "alternative" physicians: 110,000 allopaths (conventional), 10,000 homeopaths, 5000 eclectics, and an additional 5000 practitioners of other alternatives. With more than 20 medical schools teaching homeopathy, conventional medicine was forced to take a hard look at itself. Two events that ushered in significant change were the formation of the American Medicine Association in 1848 and the release of the Flexner Report on Medical Education in 1910. In the early 1900s, the AMA issued a statement to its members stating that it was unethical for physicians and members of the AMA to consult, confer, or interact with "alternative" practitioners. In effect, this created the beginning of the exclusion of any medical approaches or treatments that were not considered within the mainstream of medicine. Alternatives would suffer additional losses with the publication of the Flexner Report. As a result of this report, which publicly documented the disorganized and unregulated state of medical education in the United States, medical schools made huge advances in curriculum development and entrance and graduation requirements. These curricular changes left little room for the inclusion of alternative approaches, such as homeopathy. As scientific medicine began to emerge in both the United States and Europe, the focus of medical education became scientifically based as well. By 1923, the number of U.S. medical schools teaching homeopathy had dropped from 22 to 2.[2]

Other factors also contributed to the near disappearance of these alternatives health approaches, most notably the discovery of the cell theory by Rudolf Virchow and the germ theory by Louis Pasteur in the late 1800s, followed by the discovery of x-rays in the early 1900s, and then penicillin in 1928. Biomedical medicine and scientific research became inseparable and the ensuing discoveries would lead to the technological advances we find today in medicine. The discovery of antibiotics was a pivotal point for the emergence of conventional medicine. With each new discovery that followed, the alternatives lost favor. Patients were now choosing conventional physicians over alternatives, and the use of alternatives almost completely disappeared from 1920 to 1960.

However, beginning around 1970, alternative approaches to health and healing began to resurface. The reemergence of alternative medicine approaches was influenced by several factors:

1. Social and civil rights movements of the 1960s.
2. Growing costs of health care.
3. Emergence of the field of psychology and the role of the mind in relationship to illness and disease.
4. Uncovering of the debilitating and sometimes fatal adverse effects of medications previously thought safe.
5. Emergence of resistant strains of bacteria.
6. HIV/AIDS epidemic.
7. A world that was becoming smaller through technology.

The reasons for choosing alternatives today are not very different than they were more than 200 years ago. Patients are once again looking for a kinder, gentler, more natural approach to health and healing. They are also looking for more choices and greater control in their health decisions, and they are less likely to accept the debilitating adverse effects of biomedical treatments.

Today, as this country begins a new millennium, biomedical medicine finds itself needing to discover ways in which to integrate other (complementary and/or alternative) systems, philosophies, approaches, and treatments into the care offered and provided to the growing diversity of patients.

GOVERNMENT RESPONSE

Owing to the rising use of alternative approaches, a Congressional mandate established the Office of Alternative Medicine (OAM) within the National Institutes of Health (NIH) in 1991. The purpose of this office was to facilitate the evaluation of alternative medical treatment modalities and their effectiveness through research and other initiatives. The initial financial budget for this undertaking was $2 million. However, before it could begin the process of evaluation, the OAM needed a classification system to better identify the alternatives. Initially, there were seven groups, but the classification has since been revised to five major domains, including the following:

1. Alternative health systems.
2. Mind-body interventions.
3. Biologically based therapies.
4. Manipulative and body-based methods.
5. Energy therapies[4] (Table 50-1).

In 1999, the Omnibus appropriations bill resulted in the change of title and status of the OAM from an office to a center—the National Center for Complementary and Alternative Medicine (NCCAM)—within the NIH. This change resulted in a more expansive role that includes establishing a clearinghouse to provide information to providers and patients, conducting and funding research, disseminating health information and other programs with regard to the investigation, and validation of CAM treatments.[4] Its budget for this expanded role was $68 million in 2000; it was increased to $100 million in 2002.

In 2000, President Clinton created the White House Commission on Complementary and Alternative Medicine Policy (WHCCAMP) in response to the national awareness of the growing popularity and use of natural medicines and the paucity of research focusing on CAM treatments. Federal policy was failing to keep up, which was creating a potential consumer safety issue.[5] The commission was charged with formulating recommendations for the President on four issues regarding CAM, including the following:

1. Education and training of health care practitioners in CAM.
2. Coordination of research to increase knowledge among the public about CAM products.
3. Provision of reliable and useful information on CAM to health care professionals.
4. Provision of guidance on appropriate access to and delivery of CAM.

The Commission completed its task in March of 2002 and presented its final report to the President.

Table 50-1 NCCAM's Five Domains of Alternative Medicine

Alternative Health Systems	Mind-Body Interventions	Biologically Based Therapies	Manipulative and Body-Based Methods	Energy Therapies
Traditional	Meditation Imagery	Herbal medicine	Chiropractic	*Qi gong*
Oriental medicine	Hypnosis	Special diets	Osteopathic	Reiki
Ayurvedic (Indian)	Biofeedback	such as Ornish,	Craniosacral therapy	Therapeutic
medicine	Yoga	Pritikin, Weil,	Massage	touch
Tibetan medicine	Tai chi	Atkins, and	Reflexology	Electro-
Native American	*Qi gong*	macrobiotic	Pilates	magnetic
medicine	Prayer	Orthomolecular	Rolfing	therapies
Homeopathy	Spiritual healings	medicine	Trager body work	
Naturopathy	Soul retrieval	Iridology	Alexander technique	
	Intuitive diagnosis			

This report includes recommendations the Commission deemed necessary to make CAM modalities safe and accessible to the American population. Regarding the education of conventional and CAM providers, the Commission believes that because the public uses both conventional and CAM approaches, this should be reflected in the educational training of all health care practitioners. The curricula of conventional health care practitioners should include CAM education, and the curricula of CAM practitioners should include conventional medicine. The result would be conventional providers who can discuss CAM with their patients, provide guidance on CAM use, collaborate with CAM practitioners, and make referrals to them, as well as CAM practitioners who can communicate and collaborate with conventional providers and make referrals to them.[6]

TRENDS

The history of CAM includes several factors that must be taken into consideration here. Although the use of alternatives in our country's history can be traced to as far back as early colonial days, many of the commonly used alternatives today originated thousands of years earlier in ancient cultures.

In the 1800s, medicine in both Europe and the newly formed United States was still an emerging field with no consistency or agreement in theories or treatments. The nature of disease was mostly a mystery and was subject to conjecture and individual philosophies. Therefore, the alternatives that arose during the 19th century resulted because individuals were trying to find more acceptable approaches than the brutal treatments used by conventional medicine. Many of these alternatives were treatments created by individuals who were working from their own combination of personal, cultural, and/or religious beliefs about health and healing.

However, over the past 50 years, many events have led to the erosion of faith and trust that the American people have had regarding our health care system's ability to treat, cure, and/or prevent illness. The increased prevalence of chronic diseases such as osteoarthritis and the general unsatisfactory progress in the multi-million dollar "war on cancer" have caused many to wonder if the range of modern medicine's effectiveness has reached its limits. In addition, there is a heightened awareness of the public to the constantly growing number of studies that demonstrate unnecessary, counterproductive, and dangerous practices in our medical system, including prolonged use of addictive drugs, unnecessary surgeries, and increased numbers of iatrogenic diseases.[7] The event that most recently illuminated the limitations of biomedical medicine despite its vast advances in technology was the beginning of the AIDS epidemic in the 1980s. The current treatments for many of the conditions associated with AIDS are painful and unpleasant and at times do not affect the ultimate outcome; therefore, patients have begun to look for other options and choices, much as they did 200 years ago. Another major factor is that the alternatives that are most popular today reflect the changing tide of immigration to the United States, with increasing use of Asian and Ayurvedic (Indian) approaches and treatments. As our country grows richly diverse and moves away from the *melting pot* philosophy, many immigrants are maintaining and using their country of origin's cultural and/or religious traditions concerning health and healing.

Another factor that has greatly influenced the reemergence and use of alternatives in this country is the explosion of communication technology, combined with the vast political changes that have occurred in other countries. This has enabled the open flow and exchange of cultural and religious customs, and it has provided exposure for all to the health care systems of other countries. Today's patients are better educated and are more aware of the existence of other ways to manage their health or illness beyond that of the biomedical model.

PREVALENCE AND USE OF CAM IN THE UNITED STATES

In the first of two landmark research studies done by David Eisenberg, MD, regarding the use and prevalence of CAM in the United States, 33.8% of Americans were found to have used alternative medicine in 1990. Americans spent more than $13 billion for alternatives, with an estimated $10 billion spent out of pocket, and visits to alternative practitioners (425 million) exceeded visits to primary care physicians (388 million). The most commonly used CAM modalities in 1990 included relaxation techniques, chiropractic care, and massage. An alarming finding was that only 39.8% of patients disclosed their use of these modalities to their primary care providers.[8]

In the follow-up study done in 1997, the usage of CAM had increased to 42.1%, and for adults ages 35 to 49, it was estimated that 1 of every 2 adults used some form of alternatives. Spending also increased to $21 billion, with $12 billion paid out of pocket, and there was a 47.3% increase in total number of visits to alternative practitioners (425 billion to 629 million). Although relaxation techniques, chiropractic care, and massage continued to be popular; the use of herbal medicine, self-help groups, folk remedies, energy healing, and homeopathy had also increased.[8,9] However, the disclosure rate to primary care providers remained relatively unchanged at 38.5%.[9]

In general, patients who use CAM tend to be between the ages of 25 and 65, educated, nonblack, and suffering from chronic types of illnesses. In addition, they may have chosen CAM because conventional medical treatments failed and/or caused unacceptable adverse effects, or there was no conventional treatment available.[10] Those who used CAM tended to want more autonomy in their health care choices and treatments, tended to have a more holistic philosophical orientation, believing in the importance of mind, body, and spirit, and valued environmentalism, spirituality, and personal growth. They also tended to seek health promotion and disease prevention and were more likely to have had a transformation experience that had changed their world view.[11]

Conditions for which CAM treatments or providers were most commonly used included back problems, allergies, fatigue, arthritis, hypertension, insomnia, lung problems, skin problems, digestive problems, depression and anxiety,[8,9] cancer, and human immunodeficiency virus (HIV). Today, commonly used CAM modalities that have moved into mainstay biomedical medicine include massage, acupuncture, relaxation/stress management, and herbs. However, factors such as geographic location, ethnicity, and socioeconomic status all influence the popularity of CAM modalities among patients.

In a more recent study done in 2000, the use of CAM was found to be 44% among those who responded to the survey. The overall disclosure rate of alternative modality use to a conventional practitioner was 43%, and a 25% disclosure rate specifically for the use of herbs and/or vitamins. Speculation regarding the reasons for this lack of disclosure by patients included fear of disapproval, the patient perception that such information was not important, the fact that they don't have the time during the quick office visit, or their belief that the conventional provider won't understand.[12]

In a 2001 study in the *Annals of Internal Medicine,* 79% of patients surveyed who admitted use of both conventional and CAM providers perceived the combination of both treatments to be superior to either treatment alone. However, their reported disclosure rate to the conventional provider regarding their CAM use was only 37%. The main reason offered by patients for the lack of disclosure was that they were concerned about their conventional provider's inability to understand or incorporate CAM therapy into their overall management.[13]

Over the past 12 years, study after study has demonstrated that the use of CAM by people in the United States is here to stay. Unlike some changes within our health care system that have originated from within the system itself, this movement originated and has been sustained by those outside the system—the patients. This use of other health care models, methods, systems, and treatments, in addition to or in lieu of conventional medicine, is not showing any signs of slowing or reversing. However, it is alarming that the disclosure rates of patients have not changed. Patients are still reluctant for a variety of reasons to disclose their use of CAM to conventional providers. This is a trend that physician assistants (PAs) can directly impact.

FUTURE TRENDS

In 1999, the American Academy of Physician Assistants (AAPA) passed a resolution that stated that PAs need to become more knowledgeable about CAM practices. Although most current PA programs do not formally include education about CAM, this is likely to change in the near future based on the recommendation of the White House Commission on Complementary and Alternative Medicine Policy.

In the meantime, it is important for PA students and practicing PAs to begin to educate themselves regarding CAM, especially those approaches or modalities that are being used by their current patients. The continued prevalence and use of CAM in this country indicate that for practitioners to be successful in today's health care arena, knowledge about CAM is vital. A growing quantity of reputable conferences, journals, coursework, and Internet sites offer a wide variety of accurate and up-to-date information about the changing face of medicine and the integration of CAM modalities into everyday practice. It is imperative that physician assistants begin to use these resources.

FASTEST GROWING CAM

Presently, the fastest growing alternative market is herbs, with $1.6 billion spent in 1994 and $4 billion in 1998. Although there was a slight decline in herb sales in 2001 of about 15%, this market continues to be the fastest growing and perhaps the largest of all CAM used today.[14] Between 1990 and 1997, the use of herbal remedies increased by 380%, and the use of high-dose vitamins increased by 130%, so that 1 in 5 Americans were taking prescription medications along with herbs, vitamins, or both.[9] In a more recent study done by Kaufman and associates in 2002, researchers found that 80% of Americans take at least one type of medication, herb, or supplement, and 16% use these substances concomitantly.[15]

The fastest growing herbal use in 2000 included gingko biloba, St. John's wort, saw palmetto, echinacea, ginseng, and garlic. In 2001, the herbs that saw the greatest increase in use included: soy, valerian root, milk thistle, green tea, and black cohash.[14] This rapidly changing market is influenced by several factors, including media information and emerging research information that either supports or refutes the herbs' healing properties. Because trends of CAM modality use vary according to time period, geographic location, and cultural influences, it is important for PAs to be aware of and sensitive to the nature of the population with whom they are routinely working. PAs also need to stay on top of the emerging research being generated by the NIH and the NCCAM regarding specific CAM use and efficacy, as well as those modalities that biomedical medicine is beginning to integrate, such as acupuncture, massage therapy, and stress reduction techniques.

ROLE OF THE PA

Given the knowledge that many patients are using some form of CAM, whether by seeing an acupuncturist, getting regular massage therapy treatments, or taking herbs or vitamins, PAs have the responsibility to open the door to communication. It is no longer acceptable to wait for the patient to disclose. There is the growing concern that without disclosure, the course of patients' treatment may have an unexpected or undesired effect, such as a drug-herb interaction. To effectively navigate the changing face of medicine in today's environment, PAs need to incorporate some adjustments in their approach to *all* patients. The following six recommendations should be considered in every patient encounter:

1. **Ask your patients**   The disclosure rate of the use of CAM by patients to their conventional providers is an alarming statistic that PAs can easily change. The most important thing PAs and PA students can begin to do immediately is to routinely ask *all* their patients about use of CAM. This can easily be integrated into history taking in several areas. First, when asking patients what they have tried to make the symptom better or worse, listen to the patient's response, and then follow up with additional questions such as, *"Other patients have tried alternative approaches such as herbs or massage or another practitioner, have you tried any of those?"* If the patient's response is affirmative, then the PA needs to ask a few more questions such as *"Did the treatments help? Whom did you see? What did the treatments consist of? How long did you use the treatment?"* It is not uncommon for patients to have used or visited a number of alternative providers before making an appointment with a conventional provider.

Another opportunity to explore patients' potential use of CAM, as well as to gain insight into their explanatory model, is in the social history. To better understand patients, it is important that providers know more about their belief systems. These questions should be asked of *all* patients, not just those who are obviously from a different culture or country. Questions could include the following: *"What do you do to stay healthy emotionally, physically, and spiritually? What is most important to you in your life? What to you think might be causing your symptom?"*

The final opportunity to ask about CAM use, which is of critical importance, is when asking about medications. PAs should not be writing a prescription without having asked *every* patient not only about prescription or over-the-counter medication use, but also about the use of herbs, remedies, vitamins, and/or supplements. Don't worry if you may not know the herb or remedy. Patients can offer information, and there are abundant resources now available for PAs to find out more about a product that the patient is using and any potential interactions. Because of the large number of patients using pharmaceuticals and herbs, remedies, vitamins, or supplements, this is a vital question, as research continues to uncover potential synergetic, antagonistic, or negative effects of such combinations.

2. Become knowledgeable

The Code of Conduct for PAs and the AAPA emphasize the importance of staying up-to-date and knowledgeable regarding all health care issues, including CAM. The number of opportunities to learn about CAM is growing (such as by attending conferences and CME activities, talking with or experiencing the work of CAM practitioners, and attempting to locate those practitioners in your area should you decide to refer patients). More and more insurance companies are providing some coverage of CAM; therefore, it is also important to find out which modalities or practitioners may be covered.

3. Be nonjudgmental and open-minded, and make no assumptions

Health care systems in other countries are commonly very different from those in the United States. In fact, 75% of the world's population use folk or lay healers in approaches that include physical and nonphysical components, as well as using aspects of family or ceremony not common to the biomedical model.[16] Although some of these aspects may seem unfamiliar or bizarre, these beliefs and customs have significant and powerful meaning to the patient. Therefore, all inquiries regarding the use of CAM must be asked in an open-minded, open-ended, nonjudgmental way. Patients are very sensitive to and perhaps overly cautious about a conventional provider's negative judgment or disapproval. If a PA dismisses or devalues these methods in front of the patient, irreparable damage can occur in the patient/provider relationship. Therefore, PAs need to be sensitive and compassionate about these differences.

4. Work toward a mutually acceptable treatment plan

Being open, sensitive, and compassionate regarding a patient's beliefs concerning health, healing, and disease allows the conventional provider to work more closely with the patient in creating a treatment plan that incorporates and respects the patient's needs and wishes. Whatever treatment plan is decided upon, follow-up with the patient must occur on a regular basis, especially if the plan includes only alternative modalities or a combination of CAM and conventional approaches. This enhances and maintains the patient/PA relationship so that if the CAM treatments should be unsuccessful and the patient should wish to try a conventional approach or make some adjustment in the treatment plan, the doorway has been left open for him or her to do so. Unfortunately, many times patients feel that if they do not do what the conventional provider recommended, they cannot go back, should they wish later to enlist the help and support of that practitioner.

5. Be willing to communicate directly with CAM providers

It wasn't until 1980 that the American Medical Association (AMA) lifted its statement regarding the interaction between conventional and alternative providers. It has become essential for PAs to interact and communicate with CAM providers whom patients are seeing. This bridge building serves several functions. First, it allows patients to create health care teams that truly reflect and support their needs in the healing process. Second, it provides a resource and possible future relationship from which the PA can learn about a specific CAM modality or provide a referral for other patients. Third, it supports the emerging new health care model of integrated medical approaches and treatments.

6. Last, do not omit or negate your required responsibilities such as making a diagnosis, ordering laboratory or diagnostic studies, utilizing prescriptions or recommending surgery, and using accurate documentation

A patient's statement that he or she is using CAM does not negate or relieve you of your duty to meet and carry out your roles and responsibilities in the manner in which you have been trained. Working with patients who are using or interested in using CAM should not be viewed as an "either/or" situation, that is, either it's the biomedical approach or the alternative approach. Rather, consider the approach of "both-and." It is possible for a patient's treatment to utilize *both* biomedical *and* alternative techniques, and it appears that this is what our patients want.

CASE STUDY 50-1

A 53-year-old man with a history of coronary heart disease is approaching the point of needing surgical intervention despite treatment with medications and dietary changes. During his most recent visit, you review your concerns regarding the progression of his disease, and you discuss the inevitable need for surgical intervention in the near future. He expresses significant concern and fear regarding surgery. He has just learned that his only child is pregnant with their first grandchild, and he wants to make sure he will be around to see this grandchild and any others. He states that his father died on the operating table during surgery and asks if there is anything else he can do, or if he has any other options.

This case describes a very common situation that occurs when patients are uncomfortable with the proposed course of treatment, yet aware that something needs to be done. In this case, as in many situations, the diagnosis of a serious illness provides an opportunity and the motivation for patients to significantly change those aspects or behaviors that may have contributed to the illness in the first place. When a patient asks, *"Is there anything else I can do?"* he or she is communicating a very important

message that PAs need to hear. This may be that the patient is deeply uncomfortable or fearful of the proposed treatment, or that he or she does not agree with it because it creates a conflict with personal beliefs (explanatory model) about health, healing, and illness. PAs need to recognize and explore these possibilities with the patient.

In addition, if the PA is knowledgeable about CAM, he or she can in fact offer more information and options. For example, recent studies have revealed that more and more surgeons and/or hospitals are offering patients CAM modalities before and during surgery that help to reduce both the mental and physiological stresses of surgery. Such modalities presently being used include hypnotherapy, guided imagery, and Reiki. Studies have reported that through a reduction in preoperative stress, postoperative pain and complications are significantly reduced and patients are discharged sooner.[17,18] Another option is the "Dr. Dean Ornish's Opening Your Heart Program," which is specifically designed for patients with coronary artery disease (CAD) who wish to try and manage their disease from a nonsurgical approach. This is the first program of its kind that scientifically documented the reversal of CAD without surgery. The program is located in many cities and is also covered by some insurance plans. The components include techniques of stress management such as yoga and meditation, a low-fat and low-cholesterol diet, cessation of smoking and other addictions, utilizing group therapy and support groups, and exercise.[19]

Finally, in any patient for whom surgery is recommended, it is imperative for the PA to find out if that patient is taking any herbs, supplements, or vitamins. Studies are beginning to document that certain supplements interfere with, potentiate, or negate anesthetic agents or have effects on blood-coagulating properties. For example, the properties of commonly used herbs such as gingko biloba, garlic, and Asian ginseng increase the risk of bleeding; therefore, it is important to know this and to have the patient stop the herb at least 2 weeks before surgery, if possible.[20,21] Conversely, some herbs taken preoperatively, such as vitamins

A and C, zinc, and aloe vera, have been found to be beneficial to the healing and recovery period postoperatively.[17,21]

CASE STUDY 50-2

Evaluation of a slender, active, 52-year-old woman complaining of right knee pain reveals moderate osteoarthritic changes of joint narrowing and minimal spurring on x-ray. She has a history of peptic ulcer disease and has been using acetaminophen for pain relief; however, she reports it is only minimally effective.

The drugs of choice for osteoarthritis are the nonsteroidal anti-inflammatory drugs (NSAIDs), but because of her history of peptic ulcer disease, this class is not recommended. However, if pain relief cannot be obtained with acetaminophen, it is possible to use an NSAID, but it must be combined with a second drug such as misoprostol to protect the stomach. Other possible medications include opioid analgesics; however, the adverse effects may include sedation and drowsiness. Because of the nature of her work, she feels that taking anything that would make her drowsy is not acceptable. She is also concerned about having to take one medication to offset the adverse effects of another, and in fact, doesn't want to take any drugs.

At this point, many conventional providers do not have much else to offer, and the patient may leave the office feeling disappointed. This is one of the motivations for patients when they seek alternatives. However, the PA did ask the appropriate questions and learned that the patient has made significant changes to her eating habits and lifestyle since her diagnosis of peptic ulcer disease, including losing weight and exercising regularly. She meditates regularly and is a vegetarian. She also states that she just started yoga to see if this might help with her knee pain and is interested in working with her body from a more natural approach. She also takes a combination of antioxidant vitamins.

If the PA is unsure of what other options are available for osteoarthritis, a follow-up appointment should be scheduled, which will give the PA time to review the research, consult with colleagues or alternative practitioners or other reliable resources such as NCCAM, and begin to develop a treatment plan. In this way, the patient/provider relationship is maintained even though the patient may not use conventional approaches.

The PA learned that additional options are available that may be more acceptable for this patient and that will provide a mutually acceptable treatment plan. For example, research has shown that the use of glucosamine sulfate significantly reduces the pain of osteoarthritis without the adverse effects of NSAIDs and with minimal adverse effects overall. A trial period during which glucosamine sulfate is used may be more acceptable for this patient because of the lack of adverse effects. However, as with recommending or prescribing any medications, attention is warranted about potential adverse or unwanted interactions or effects. Glucosamine sulfate should be used with caution in patients who are allergic to shellfish and in those on sodium-restricted diets because glucosamine sulfate is made from shellfish and tends to have a high sodium content. The PA also learned that yoga is known to have beneficial effects on flexibility and strength, both of which are important for patients with osteoarthritis, and the patient was encouraged to continue with the yoga.[22]

As with any treatment plan, follow-up should be scheduled to document the progress of the patient. It is important to educate the patient that many CAM approaches may take weeks to months before they take effect, which is another reason to maintain regular follow-up appointments.

CONCLUSION

This chapter serves as an introduction to the complexity of complementary and alternative medicine and the issues currently facing practitioners trained in the biomedical model, including PAs. Today, patients come from diverse belief systems regarding health and healing, and they are better educated and are seeking additional options to be used in lieu of or in combination with conventional medicine. As the health care system of this country attempts to navigate these changes, which involves finding ways to integrate different health care systems, philosophies, and treatments, PAs must also begin to integrate some basic changes into their approach to every patient, including asking about the patient's belief systems and the use of alternatives. In addition, PAs need to take advantage of the emerging research and educational opportunities regarding CAM to better educate themselves and their patients about the use of alternatives. Doing so will serve to enhance and deepen the PA/patient relationship and will play a vital role in the integration of a health care system that honors, recognizes, and respects the validity and viability of different approaches to health and healing.

CLINICAL APPLICATIONS

1. Take a moment to reflect on the following. What were your beliefs about illness when you were a child? Where did those beliefs come from? What did your family of origin believe about the causes of illness and how they should be treated? What are your beliefs now?

2. Have you ever used some form of CAM? Think about the reasons why you did. What CAM modality did you choose? Why that particular one? What was your experience? Did the existence of quantitative research play a role in your decision to use the alternative? Did you or would you share this information with your health care provider? Why or why not?

REFERENCES

1. Bordley J III, McGehee Harvey A. Two Centuries of American Medicine 1776-1976. Philadelphia: WB Saunders, 1976.
2. Jonas W, Levin JS (eds). Essentials of Complementary and Alternative Medicine. Philadelphia: Lippincott, Williams & Wilkins, 1999.
3. Micozzi M (ed). Fundamentals of Complementary and Alternative Medicine. New York: Churchill Livingstone, 1996.
4. National Center for Complementary and Alternative Medicine [database on line]. Major domains of complementary and alternative medicine. Silver Springs, MD: National Institutes of Health, January 2002. Available from http:nccam.nih.gov/fcp/classify.
5. News briefs. Alternative Therapies 2000;6:24.
6. White House Commission on Complementary and Alternative Medicine Policy. Final Report, March 2002. Available at http:whccamp.hhs.gov.
7. Hastings A, Fadiman J, Gordon JS (eds). The Complete Guide to Holistic Medicine: Health for the Whole Person. Colorado: Westview Press, 1980.
8. Eisenberg D, et al. Unconventional medicine in the United States: prevalence, costs and patterns of use. N Engl J Med 1993;238:246.
9. Eisenberg D, et al. Trends in alternative medicine use in the United States. JAMA 1998;280:1569.
10. Eisenberg D. Advising patients who seek alternative medical therapies. Ann Intern Med 1997;127:61.
11. Astin JA. Why patients use alternative medicine. JAMA 1998;279:1548.
12. Oldenkick R, Coker A. Usage of complementary medicine among patients of mainstream physicians. South Med J 2000;93:375.
13. Eisenberg D, Kessler RC, Van Rompay MI, et al. Perceptions about complementary therapies relative to conventional therapies among patients who use both: result from a national survey. Ann Intern Med 2001;135:344.
14. Blumenthal M. Herb sales down 15 percent in mainstream market. Herbalgram 2001;51:69.
15. Kaufman DW, et al. Recent patterns of medication use in the ambulatory adult population of the United States: the Slone survey. JAMA 2002;287:337.
16. Helman CG. Culture, Health and Illness, ed 3. Oxford: Butterworth-Heinemann, 1994.
17. Petry J. Surgery and complementary therapies: a review. Alternative Therapies 2000;6:64.
18. Oz M. Healing from the Heart: A Leading Surgeon Explores the Power of Alternative Medicine. New York: Penguin Putnam, 1998.
19. Ornish D. Program for Reversing Health Disease. New York: Ballantine, 1990.
20. Ang-Lee MK, Moss J, Yuan C-S. Herbal medicine and perioperative care. JAMA 2001;286:208.
21. Pribitkin ED, Boger G. Surgery and herbal therapy: essential guidelines on bleeding, skin reactions, and wound healing. Comp Health Pract Rev 2000;6:29.
22. One Medicine [database on line]. Glucosamine. Newton, MA: Integrative Medicine Communications. Available at http:onemedicine.com. Accessed March 2002.

RESOURCES

Burton Goldberg Group (ed). Alternative Medicine: The Definitive Guide. Washington: Future Medical, 1993. *Good reference source for the definition and basic understanding of many commonly used complementary and alternative modalities.*

Jonas W, Levin JS (ed). Essentials of Complementary and Alternative Medicine. Philadelphia: Lippincott, Williams & Wilkins, 1999. *A well-written and comprehensive text that presents in-depth information regarding the philosophies and* traditional uses of many of the commonly used complementary and alternative approaches.

Micozzi M (ed). Fundamentals of Complementary and Alternative Medicine. New York: Churchill Livingstone, 1996. *A well-rounded text presenting the background, context, and clinical approaches for common complementary and alternative medicine approaches.*

Sierpina VS. Integrative Health Care: Complementary and Alternative Therapies for the Whole Person. Philadelphia: FA Davis, 2001. *An extremely helpful text geared specifically to the provider with valuable information for conventional practitioners in navigating an integrative approach to health care.*

Alternative Therapies in Health and Medicine A Peer Reviewed Journal. California: Innovision Communications. *A bimonthly peer-reviewed journal that is an international scientific forum for the dissemination of peer-reviewed information to health care professionals regarding the use of complementary and alternative therapies in promoting health and healing.*

Herbalgram. Texas: American Botanical Council. Available at www.herbalgram.org. *A quarterly journal published by the American Botanical Council, a nonprofit research and educational organization with the goal of providing solid information and education regarding the medicinal use of herbs.*

Integrative Medicine Select: An Evidence-Based Approach. Alabama: Oakstone Medical Publishing. *Provides monthly continuing medical education (CME) through Johns Hopkins University School of Medicine for health care professionals, with overviews and critical analysis of the most current and clinically useful information available in the literature related to complementary and alternative approaches to heath, well-being, and illness.*

National Center for Complementary and Alternative Medicine at the National Institutes of Health. Available at www.nccam.nih.gov. *Provides information for health care professionals regarding the use of CAM, as well as up-to-date information regarding ongoing research and results.*

The Integrative Medicine Consult. Massachusetts: Integrative Medicine Communications. Available at www.onemedicine.com. *Science-based clinical information for medical professionals on the latest developments in complementary and alternative medicine therapies, with the focus of helping in the integration of complementary and alternative medicine into everyday medical practice. This is a totally independent group that is not sponsored by any manufacturer, and the work is peer reviewed.*

CHAPTER 51

Violence Prevention

Paula Phelps

INTRODUCTION

The focus of this chapter is violence across the life span, in other words, from shaken baby syndrome to elder abuse. In general, the discussion will concern family violence. Family violence is the general heading for violence perpetrated between family members or intimate partners, or at the hands of a caregiver. Family violence is defined as "an all-inclusive expression referring to threatening or overt behaviors presumed to have harmful consequences for those against whom it is directed."[1] It includes verbal and emotional abuse, physical abuse, neglect, and sexual abuse. The victims are babies, children, teenagers, intimate partners, and elders.

Because medical providers are often the first or only professionals to see victims of abuse, they are in a unique position to intervene effectively. Over the past 5 years, the general medical community has recognized this fact and has moved to increase the training of physicians and other health care professionals to recognize and treat victims and potential victims of family violence. In 1997, the president of the Association of American Medical Colleges stated that domestic violence is a problem not only for the judicial system and social services, but also for

"physicians and the health care system." He asserted that "medical schools and teaching hospitals must include in their curricula the knowledge necessary to heighten awareness, to recognize the early and sometimes subtle signs, and to provide appropriate counseling and treatment."[2]

OVERVIEW AND MAGNITUDE OF THE PROBLEM

The exact prevalence of family violence is hard to quantify. Research studies use different definitions and have found a broad range of results. In 1996, 3 million cases of child abuse were reported. Approximately 51,000 to 186,000 cases of elder abuse per year are reported. Depending on the study, there is a lifetime prevalence of 22% to 50% of women who experience violence inflicted by a current or former partner.[1]

Every year, family violence affects a significant segment of the U.S. population. Twenty million women are verbally abused, 5 million women are physically abused, 2 million women are severely abused, and 2000 women are killed.[3]

Each year in the United States, there are 2.8 million victims of child abuse or neglect. Of these children, over half a million (565,000) are seriously injured, 18,000 suffer permanent disability, and an estimated 2000 die.[3]

Elder abuse affects 2 million elderly, with a prevalence that ranges from 1% to 5%.[4] Because only 5% of the elderly are now residing in nursing homes and because our population is rapidly aging, the magnitude of this problem will only worsen over the next decade.

CYCLE OF VIOLENCE

Family violence is cyclical, both on an individual basis and at the generational level. The cycle of violence at the individual level consists of outbursts of violence followed by a honeymoon period, followed by a building up of aggression. Then the cycle begins again with another outburst of violence. During the honeymoon period, the abuser may treat the victim with kindness and gift giving. During the period of building up of aggression, the victim can feel as those she/he is "walking on eggshells" and is waiting for the next explosion of violence.

In the generational cycle of violence, it has been shown that witnessing violence in the home or being a victim of abuse can greatly impact the child, both at the time it occurs and in the future. Fantuzzo and Mohr conclude that, "childhood exposure to domestic violence can be associated with increased display of aggressive behavior, increased emotional problems such as depression and/or anxiety, lower levels of social competence, and poorer academic functioning.[5] This impact on the child is extended into the child's adulthood, and he or she is more likely to have poor parent/child relationships, decreased psychological well-being, and violence within his/her own relationships than are children who did not witness abuse."[6] Likewise, the medical consequences of child sexual abuse are lifelong. These medical conditions may include chronic depression, morbid obesity, marital instability, high utilization of medical care, chronic gastrointestinal distress, and recurrent headaches.[7]

PAs are in the unique role of being able to implement strategies for both primary and secondary prevention of violence. With regard to domestic violence, it has been eloquently stated, "For as long as women have been beaten and injured by their part-ners, doctors have set their bones, sutured lacerations, and sent them home, usually without exploring the underlying problem."[8] A recent study reported that only 29% of domestic violence victims said they had discussed their abuse with their physician or health care provider, and of those 29%, only one in five said the doctor raised the subject.[9]

PREVENTION STRATEGIES

If society as a whole were to address the issue of family violence as a public health concern, a combination of prevention strategies would be used. Primary prevention strategies are those that are aimed at preventing illness before it occurs. Secondary prevention strategies detect an illness before it can cause harm to the individual. Tertiary prevention strives to improve the outcomes of a disease through rehabilitation or treatment.[10] Because of the cyclical nature of family violence, when clinicians can treat existing disease, they are also preventing recurrence in the individual and occurrence in the next generation. In other words, tertiary prevention can also be primary prevention. Therefore, all community prevention programs should use a three-pronged approach: education, screening, and appropriate referral.

Suggested community education to prevent family violence would involve efforts to provide support for parents, spouses, and caregivers, or for future parents, spouses, and caregivers. Education examples include the following:

➤ Teaching about dating violence and parenting issues in high school health education classes.
➤ Prenatal health care providers routinely including education on shaken baby syndrome and domestic violence in their packets of information for obstetrical patients.
➤ Teaching school-aged children to instill violence awareness and to develop conflict resolution skills.
➤ Getting involved in media campaigns that target issues related to the prevention of different kinds of violence (e.g., shaken baby syndrome, child abuse, sexual abuse, domestic violence, and elder abuse).

Screening includes identification of populations at risk for violence and the recognition of signs and symptoms of abuse. Children at high risk for maltreatment include those in the following groups: children living in single-parent homes; from large families; and from families with an annual income of less than $15,000. Children at low risk for abuse include those living with both parents; from single-child families; and from families whose annual income is more than $30,000.[1]

Unlike child abuse, no single profile has been associated with domestic violence. Domestic violence is found in all populations, regardless of demographics for age, sex, sexual orientation, educational background, income, or disability.

Elder abuse risk factors include the following:

➤ Older age.
➤ Lack of access to resources.
➤ Low income.
➤ Social isolation.
➤ Low educational level.
➤ Functional disability.
➤ Substance abuse by caregiver.
➤ Psychological disorder and character pathology.
➤ Previous history of family violence.
➤ Caregiver burnout and frustration.
➤ Cognitive impairment.

Red flags for abuse in any population include inconsistencies between history and physical findings, multiple injuries in various stages of healing, and injuries that suggest a defensive posture (e.g., on face and fore-arms). Some injuries are suggestive of abuse in one population, but not in another. For example, humeral, tibial, or femoral fractures in infants are strongly suggestive or suspicious of abuse but can be accidental in older children. Because homicide is the leading cause of pregnancy-associated death,[11] and because approximately 25% of all obstetrical patients are estimated to be involved in battering relationships,[12] any injury during pregnancy should arouse suspicion of abuse and should be investigated accordingly.

Injuries to the epithelium provide evidence of the weapon used or the abuse endured. Blunt trauma is the most common kind of injury. Other forms of trauma are thermal injury, strangulation, and laceration.

ROLE OF THE PHYSICIAN ASSISTANT

As was discussed previously, physician assistants (PAs) can play a key role in violence prevention, as well as in identification and referral for treatment of victims of violence. Careful and sensitive history taking builds rapport with the patient and provides information that the PA can use for diagnosis and/or prevention.

RADAR is a pneumonic to help caregivers remember to screen for, document, and refer domestic violence situations (see Box). The components of RADAR can be used for other forms of abuse as well.

RADAR: A DOMESTIC VIOLENCE INTERVENTION

R = Routinely screen female patients.
Victims of violence are most likely to disclose abuse to a health care provider, but only if they are asked about it. *Always interview the patient alone.*
A = Ask direct questions.
Ask simple, direct questions in a nonjudgmental way. "Is there anyone who has physically or sexually hurt you or frightened you?" "Have you ever been hit, kicked, or punched by your partner?" "Does your partner try to control your activities or your money?" "I notice you have a number of bruises; did someone do this to you?" "Because violence is so common in many women's lives, we've begun to ask about it routinely."
If patient answers YES, see below for responses and continue with the following steps.
D = Document your findings.
Record a description of the abuse as she has described it to you. Use statements such as "the patient states she was..." If she gives the specific name of the assailant, use it in your record. "She says her boyfriend John Smith struck her..." Record all pertinent physical findings. Use a body map to supplement the written record. Offer to photograph injuries. When serious injury or sexual abuse is detected, preserve all physical evidence. Document an opinion if the injuries were inconsistent with the patient's explanation.

Continued

RADAR: A DOMESTIC VIOLENCE INTERVENTION—cont'd

A = Assess patient safety.

Before she leaves the medical setting, find out if she is afraid to go home. Has there been an increase in frequency or severity of violence? Have there been threats of homicide or suicide? Have there been threats to her children or pets? Is there a gun or other weapon present?

R = Review options and referrals.

If the patient is in imminent danger, find out if there is someone with whom she can stay. Does she need immediate access to a shelter? Offer her access to a private phone to make a call. If she does not need immediate assistance, offer information about hotlines and resources in the community. Remember that it may be dangerous for the woman to have this information in her possession. Do not insist that she take it. *Make a follow-up appointment to see her.*

If the Patient Answers Yes:
- Encourage her to talk about it.
- "Would you like to talk about what has happened to you?" "Would you like help?"
- Listen nonjudgmentally.
- This serves both to begin the healing process for the woman and to give you an idea of what types of referrals she may need.
- Validate her experience.
- "You are not alone." "You do not deserve to be treated this way." "You are not to blame." "What happened to you is a crime." "Help is available to you." "The violence is likely to get worse, and I am worried about you." "If you are not safe, your children are not safe."

If the Patient Answers No, or Will Not Discuss the Topic:
- Be aware of any clinical signs that may indicate abuse:
- Injury to the head, neck, torso, breasts, abdomen, or genitals; bilateral or multiple injuries; delay between onset of injury and time of treatment; explanation by the patient that is inconsistent with the type of injury; injury during pregnancy; previous history of trauma; chronic pain symptoms for which no cause is apparent; psychological distress such as depression, suicidal ideation, anxiety, and/or sleep disorder; a partner who seems overly protective or who will not leave the woman's side; frequent health care visits; substance abuse.
- If any of these clinical signs are present, ask more specific questions. Make sure she is alone.
- "I am worried about you. It looks as though someone may have hurt you. Can you tell me how it happened?" "Sometimes when people feel the way you do, it may be because they are being hurt at home. Is this happening to you?"
- If the patient denies abuse, but you strongly suspect it:
- Document your opinion, and let her know that there are resources available to her should she choose to pursue such options in the future. *Make a follow-up appointment to see her.*

Used with permission. ©1995 RADAR Pocket Card developed by Philadelphia Family Violence Working Group, c/o Physicians for Social Responsibility, 215/765-8703. Adapted from New York Office for Prevention of Domestic Violence. RADAR action steps developed by the Massachusetts Medical Society. ©1992 Massachusetts Medical Society.

What is most important is that PAs remember that the safety of the patient and the family is of utmost concern. PAs must know the laws of the states in which they practice. Child abuse and elder abuse must be reported in all states. Domestic violence is reportable in a few states.

By developing knowledge about the cycle of violence, enhancing history-taking skills with RADAR, and performing physical examinations with the possibility of detecting abuse in mind, PAs can have a profound effect on patients' lives. The following cases illustrate opportunities that PAs may have to recognize and intervene in cases of abuse.

CASE STUDY 51-1

Heidi, a 12-year-old, is brought to an outpatient clinic for menorrhagia and dysmenorrhea over the past year. Menarche was at age 9. Periods are monthly, but last for 2 weeks and are very heavy for 8 days. Before the PA/patient meeting, Heidi's mother wishes to speak to the PA alone. She discloses to the clinician that the girl was sexually abused as an infant, with full vaginal penetration. Although the mother has disclosed this information, the girl is unaware of this and the mother does not want the girl told. The patient is nervous and shy. When asked why she came into the clinic, Heidi says, "because my Mom made me come." How should the PA proceed with the history and physical examination?

Commentary

It is important to find out if the sexual abuse was reported to the legal system and if the child has been seen by a counselor for related issues of abuse. Child abuse is a reportable offense in every state in the country. Even though the abuse occurred before the child was able to remember the event, there may be some long-term manifestations from the trauma, both physically and emotionally. In this case, the girl has been seen by a counselor and treated for attention deficit hyperactivity disorder (ADHD) and bipolar disorder. It is unknown if these psychological conditions are related to the abuse.

As far as the history and physical examination are concerned, it is important that the PA establish a good rapport and gain the trust of the patient. It may even be necessary to postpone the genital examination until a subsequent visit.

CASE STUDY 51-2

Mary is a 45-year-old G4P4, who comes into the clinic for her annual examination. Upon routine domestic violence screening, the patient admits that she is a victim of frequent emotional abuse and occasional physical abuse. Her physical examination is normal, but how does the PA deal with the situation of ongoing abuse in the patient's life?

Commentary

The most important issue here is the safety of the patient and her children. The clinician must respect Mary's autonomy and let her decide if it is safe for her to go home. If Mary feels that it is safe to return home, but she is ready to get out of the abusive relationship, then the PA should refer her to the local domestic violence hotline. If Mary is not ready to leave the relationship, the PA must avoid a judgmental attitude that would discourage future communication. A safety plan should be discussed for future use, no matter what decision Mary makes about the relationship during this visit.

CASE STUDY 51-3

Johnny, a 6-week-old boy, is brought into a family practice clinic by his parents. The baby is crying, and the parents explain that they placed him on the couch to sleep, but he must have awakened and rolled off the couch. They found him on the floor 30 minutes ago crying and brought him right into the office. On x-ray, a spiral fracture of the left femur is found. What aspects of this case should lead the PA to suspect child abuse? What is the PA obligated to do with the information?

Commentary

The first piece of suspicious information is that "Johnny rolled off the couch." A 6-week-old baby is developmentally unable to roll over. Second, a spiral fracture in an infant is suggestive of abuse because of the twisting force that would be needed to cause that injury. Child protective services must be called to investigate the case.

CLINICAL APPLICATIONS

1. Regarding Case Study 51-1, how would you discuss with her mother the importance of informing Heidi of her history of abuse? What issues might Heidi's mother bring to the discussion? How would you present the information to Heidi?

2. Regarding Case Study 51-2, if Mary were your patient, what community resources would be available to her? Research her options, such as domestic violence hotlines, shelters that accept

women with children, legal advice, and financial assistance.

3. In Case Study 51-3, research and discuss the events that would follow a report to child protective services.

4. What do you think you will find challenging and rewarding about taking care of victims of abuse?

REFERENCES

1. Bostock DJ, Auster S. AAFP Home Study. Family Violence. Monograph 274, March 2002.

2. Cohen JJ. Academic medicine: January 1997, President's column. Available at http://www.aamc.org/findinfo/aamcpubs/acadmed/jan1997/janpres.htm.

3. Sedlak. In Many Faces of Family Violence, an unauthored CD-ROM produced by Medulogic, a commercial company that specializes in CME credits for physicians. Preview is available at http://www.mdulogic.com/faces11.html, 1999.

4. Swagerty, Takahashi, Evans. Elder mistreatment. American Family Physician 1999;59:2804.

5. Fantuzzo JW, Mohr WK. Prevalence and effects of child exposure to domestic violence. Future Child 1999;9:21.

6. McNeal C, Amato PR. Parents' marital violence: long-term consequences for children (abstract). Journal of Family Issues 1998;19:123.

7. Flitti VJ. Long-term medical consequences of incest, rape, and molestation (abstract). South Med J 1991;84:328.

8. Community Health Clinics Join the Frontlines in the Fight Against Domestic Violence, May 13, 1999. Available at http://endabuse.org/newsflash/indix.php3?Search+Article&NewsFlashID=65. Accessed 7 August 2002.

9. New Women's Health Survey Finds High Rates of Abuse, May 20, 1999. Available at http://endabuse.org/newsFlash/index.php3?Search+Article&NewsFlashID=65. Accessed 7 August 2002.

10. Campus-Outcalt D. Preventive health examinations. In: Weiss BD (ed). 20 Problems in Primary Care. New York, McGraw-Hill, 1999.

11. Horon IL, Cheng D. Enhanced surveillance for pregnancy-associated mortality—Maryland, 1993-1998. JAMA 2001;285:1455.

12. Salber PR, Taliaferro E. The Physician's Guide to Domestic Violence: How to Ask the Right Questions and Recognize Abuse. Volcano, CA: Volcano Press, 1995.

RESOURCE

2000 National Victim Assistance Academy web page. Available at http://www.ojp.usdoj.gov/ovc/assist/nvaa2000/academy/. *Provides a variety of information useful to people experiencing violence and to clinicians.*

APPENDIX 1

Facts and Timeline in PA History

Appendix Table 1-1	Distribution of Closed Physician Assistant Training Programs by State
State	**Program**
Alabama	University of Alabama, Birmingham
Arizona	Maricopa County Hospital
	Indian HSMC, Phoenix
California	U.S. Navy, San Diego
	Loma Linda University PA Program
Colorado	University of Colorado OB-GYN Associate Program
Florida	Santa Fe Community College PA Program*
Indiana	Indiana University Fort Wayne PA Program
Maryland	Johns Hopkins University Health Associates
Mississippi	University of Mississippi PA Program
Missouri	Stephens College PA Program
North Carolina	Catawba Valley Technical Institute
	University of North Carolina Surgical Assistant Program
North Dakota	University of North Dakota
New Hampshire	Dartmouth Medical School
New Mexico	USPHS Gallup Indian Medic Program
Ohio	Lake Erie College PA Program
	Cincinnati Technical College PA Program
Pennsylvania	Pennsylvania State College PA Program
	Allegheny Community College
South Carolina	Medical University South Carolina
Texas	U.S. Air Force, Sheppard PA Program
Virginia	Naval School Health Sciences
Wisconsin	Marshfield Clinic PA Program

From Oliver DR. Third Annual Report of Physician Assistant Educational Programs in the United States, 1986-1987. Alexandria, VA: Association of Physician Assistant Programs, 1987.
*Transferred to another sponsoring institution (University of Florida, Gainesville).

Appendix Table 1-2   AAPA Presidents

1968-69	William D. Stanhope, PA
1969-70	William D. Stanhope, PA
1970-71	John J. McQueary, PA
1971-72	Thomas R. Godkins, PA
1972-73	John A. Braun, PA
1973-74	Paul F. Moson, PA
1974-75	C. Emil Fasser, PA-C
1975-76	Thomas R. Godkins, PA
1976-77	Roger G. Whittaker, PA*
1977-78	Dan P. Fox, PA
1978-79	James E. Konopa, PA
1979-80	Ron Rosenberg, PA
1980-81	C. Emil Fasser, PA-C
1981-82	Jarrett M. Wise, RPA
1982-83	Ron I. Fisher, PA
1983-84	Charles G. Huntington, RPA
1984-85	Judith B. Willis, MA, PA
1985-86	Glen E. Combs, PA-C
1986-87	R. Scott Chavez, PA-C
1987-88	Ron L. Nelson, PA-C
1988-89	Marshall R. Sinback, Jr., PA-C
1989-90	Paul Lombardo, RPA-C
1990-91	Bruce C. Fichandler, PA
1991-92	Sherri L. Stuart, PA-C
1992-93	William H. Marquardt, PA-C
1993-94	Ann L. Elderkin, PA
1994-95	Debi A. Gerbert, PA-C
1995-96	Lynn Caton, PA-C
1996-97	Sherrie L. McNeeley, PA-C
1997-98	Libby Coyte, PA-C
1998-99	Ron L. Nelson, PA-C
1999-2000	William C. Kohlhepp, MHA, PA-C
2000-2001	Glen E. Combs, MA, PA-C
2001-2002	Edward Friedmann PA-C
2002-2003	Ina S. Cushman, PA-C

From American Academy of Physician Assistants, Alexandria, Virginia, 2002.
*Deceased.

Appendix Table 1-3   AAPA National Conference Locations

1973	Sheppard Air Force Base, Texas
1974	New Orleans, Louisiana
1975	St. Louis, Missouri
1976	Atlanta, Georgia
1977	Houston, Texas
1978	Las Vegas, Nevada
1979	Fort Lauderdale, Florida
1980	New Orleans, Louisiana
1981	San Diego, California
1982	Washington, D.C.
1983	St. Louis, Missouri
1984	Denver, Colorado
1985	San Antonio, Texas
1986	Boston, Massachusetts
1987	Cincinnati, Ohio
1988	Los Angeles, California
1989	Washington, D.C.
1990	New Orleans, Louisiana
1991	San Francisco, California
1992	Nashville, Tennessee
1993	Miami Beach, Florida
1994	San Antonio, Texas
1995	Las Vegas, Nevada
1996	New York, New York
1997	Minneapolis, Minnesota
1998	Salt Lake City, Utah
1999	Atlanta, Georgia
2000	Chicago, Illinois
2001	Anaheim, California
2002	Boston, Massachusetts
2003	New Orleans, Louisiana

From American Academy of Physician Assistants, Alexandria, Virginia, 2002.

Appendix Table 1-4   Student Academy Presidents

1972-73	J. Jeffrey Heinrich
1973-74	John McElliott
1974-75	Robert P. Branc
1975-76	Tom Driber
1976-77	John Mahan
1977-78	Stephen Nunn
1978-79	William C. Hultman
1979-80	Arthur H. Leavitt, II
1980-81	Katherine Carter Stephens
1981-82	William A. Conner
1982-83	Michael J. Huckabee
1983-84	Emily H. Hill
1984-85	Thomas J. Grothe
1985-86	Gordon L. Day
1986-87	Patrick E. Killeen
1987-88	Keevil W. Helmly
1988-89	Toni L. Deer
1989-90	Paul S. Robinson
1990-91	Jeffrey W. Janikowski
1991-92	Kathryn L. Kuhlman
1992-93	Ty W. Klingensmith Flewelling
1993-94	Beth A. Griffin
1994-95	Ernest F. Handau
1995-96	Beth Grivett
1996-97	James P. McGraw, III
1997-98	Stacey L. Wolfe
1998-99	Marilyn E. Olsen
1999-00	Jennifer M. Huey-Voorhees
2000-01	Rodney W. Richardson
2001-02	Abby Jacobson
2002-03	Andrew Booth

From American Academy of Physician Assistants, Alexandria, Virginia, 2002.

Appendix Table 1-5   APAP Presidents

1972-73	Alfred M. Sadler, Jr., MD
1973-74	Thomas E. Piemme, MD
1974-75	Robert Jewett, MD
1975-76	C. Hilmon Castle, MD
1976-77	C. Hilmon Castle, MD
1977-78	Frances L. Horvath, MD
1978-79	Archie S. Golden, MD
1979-80	Thomas R. Godkins, PA
1980-81	David E. Lewis, MEd
1981-82	Regional D. Carter, PhD, PA-C
1982-83	Stephen C. Gladhart, EdD
1983-84	Robert H. Curry, MD
1984-85	Denis R. Oliver, PhD
1985-86	C. Emil Fasser, PA-C
1986-87	Jack Liskin, MA, PA-C
1987-88	Jesse C. Edwards, MS
1988-89	Suzanne B. Greenberg, MS
1989-90	Steven R. Shelton, MBA, PA-C
1990-91	Ruth Ballweg, PA-C
1991-92	Albert F. Simon, Med, PA-C
1992-93	Anthony A. Miller, Med, PA-C
1993-94	Richard R. Rahr, EdD, PA-C
1994-95	Ronald D. Garcia, PhD
1995-96	Janet Hammond, MA, PA-C
1996-97	J. Dennis Blessing, PhD, PA-C
1997-98	Donald L. Pedersen, PhD, PA-C
1998-99	Walter A. Stein, MHCA-PA-C
1999-00	P. Eugene Jones, PhD, PA-C
2000-01	Gloria Stewart, EdD, PA-C
2001-02	David Asprey, PhD, PA-C
2002-03	James F. Cawley, MPH, PA-C

From Association of Physician Assistant Programs, Alexandria, Virginia, 2002.

Appendix Table 1-6   Physician Assistant: A Timeline of the Profession—Physician Assistants in American Medicine

1650	Feldshers, originally German military medical assistants, are introduced into Russian armies by Peter the Great in the 17th century.
1778	Congress provided for a number of hospital mates to assist physicians in the provision of patient care modeled after the "loblolly boys" of the British Royal Navy.
1803	Officers de Santé introduced into France by Renee Fourcroy to help alleviate health care personnel shortages in the military and civilian sectors. Abolished in 1892.
1891	Establishment of the first company for "medic" instruction at Fort Riley, Kansas.
1940	Community Health Aides introduced into Alaska to improve the village health status of Eskimos and other Native Americans.
1959	U.S. Surgeon General identifies shortage of medically trained personnel.
1961	Charles Hudson, in an editorial in the *Journal of the American Medical Association*, calls for a "mid-level" provider from the ranks of former military corpsmen.
	World Health Organization begins introducing and promoting health care workers in developing countries (e.g., Me'decin African, Dresser, Assistant Medical Officer, and Rural Health Technician).
1965	First physician assistant (PA) class enters Duke University, North Carolina.
1966	Barefoot Doctors in China arise in response to Chairman Mao's purge of the elite and intellectual, sending many physicians into the fields to work, leaving peasants without medical personnel.
	Child Health Associate Program begins at University of Colorado.
	Allied Health Professions Personnel Act (PL-751) promotes the development of programs to train new types of primary care providers.
1967	First class of PA graduates.
1968	Alderson-Broaddus (West Virginia) program officially enrolls its first class.
	American Academy of Physician Assistants (AAPA) is established.
	Health Manpower Act (PL-90-490) funds the training of a variety of health care providers.
	Physician Assistants, Volume 1, is published.
1969	MEDEX program launched at University of Washington (Seattle, Washington); first class enters.
1970	Kaiser Permanente becomes first HMO to employ a PA.
1971	American Medical Association recognizes the PA profession, and begins work on national certification and codification of its practice characteristics.
	Comprehensive health Manpower Training Act (PL-92-157) contracts for physician assistant education and deployment.
	First graduates from the University of Washington MEDEX Northwest program.
1972	*The Physician's Assistant: Today and Tomorrow* by Sadler, Sadler, and Bliss is published; first book written on the PA profession.
	The Association of Physician Assistant Programs is established.
	Alderson-Broaddus' first 4-year program graduates its first class.
	"The Essentials" Accreditation standards for PA programs are adopted and the Joint Review Committee on Educational Programs for Physician Assistants (JRC-PA) is formed to evaluate compliance with the standards.
	Federal support for physician assistant education enacted by Health Resources Administration (HRA).
1973	First AAPA Annual Conference held at Sheppard Air Force Base, Texas, with 275 attendees.
	AAPA and Association of Physician Assistant Programs (APAP) establish a national office in Washington, D.C.
	National Commission of Certification of Physician Assistants is established.
	National Board of Medical Examiners administers the first certifying Examinations for Primary Care Physician Assistants.

Appendix Table 1-6 Physician Assistant: A Timeline of the Profession—Physician Assistants in American Medicine—cont'd

1974 AAPA becomes an official organization on the Joint Review Committee on Educational Programs for physician assistants (JRC-PA). The committee reviews physician and surgeon assistant programs and makes accreditation recommendations to the Committee on Allied Health Education and Accreditation.

The American College of Surgeons becomes a sponsoring organization of the JRC-PA.

1975 *The Physician Assistant: A National and Local Analysis,* by Ford, is published.

1976 Federal support of PA education continues under grants from the Health Professions Educational Assistance Act (PL 94-484).

1977 *The New Health Professionals: Nurse Practitioners and Physician's Assistants,* by Bliss and Cohen, is published.

The Physician's Assistant: A Baccalaureate Curriculum, by Myers, is published.

AAPA Education and Research Foundation (later renamed Physician Assistant Foundation) is incorporated to recruit public and private contributions for student financial assistance and to support research on the PA profession.

Rural Health Clinic Services Act (PL 95-210) passed by Congress provides Medicare reimbursement of PA and nurse practitioner services in rural clinics.

Health Practitioner (later renamed *Physician Assistant)* journal begins publication; later distributed to all PAs as the official AAPA publication.

1978 *The Physician's Assistant: Innovation in the Medical Division of Labor,* by Schneller, is published.

AAPA House of Delegates becomes policy-making legislative body of the Academy.

Air Force begins appointing PAs as commissioned officers.

1979 Graduate Medical Education National Advisory Council estimates a surplus of physicians and non-physician providers in the near future.

1980 The AAPA Political Action Committee is established to support candidates for federal office who support the PA profession.

1981 *Staffing Primary Care in 1990: Physician Replacement and Cost Savings,* by Record, documents that PAs in HMO settings provide 79% of the care provided by a primary care physician, at 50% of the cost.

1982 *Physician Assistants: Their Contribution to Health Care*, by Perry and Breitner, is published.

1984 *First Annual Report on Physician Assistant Educational Programs in the United States,* by Oliver and the Association of Physician Assistant programs, is published.

Alternatives in Health Care Delivery, edited by Carter and Perry, is published.

1985 AAPA's first Burroughs Welcome Health Policy Fellowship is created.

Membership of AAPA surpasses 10,000 mark. Membership categories are expanded to include physicians, affiliates, and sustaining members.

AAPA and APAP begin first joint project providing PA graduates with a national job back service: PA JOB FIND.

The Canadian National Forces inaugurates a Canadian Physician Assistant.

University of Colorado PA program awards a master's degree (MPH) to its graduates.

1986 AAPA succeeds in legislative drive for coverage of PA services in hospitals and nursing homes, and for assisting in surgery, under Medicare Part B (Omnibus Budget Reconciliation Act PL 99-210).

Physicians Assistants: New Models of Utilization, edited by Zarbock and Harbert, is published.

Continued

Appendix Table 1-6   Physician Assistant: A Timeline of the Profession—Physician Assistants in American Medicine—cont'd

1987	*The Physician Assistant in a Changing Health Care Environment,* by Schafft and Cawley, is published.
	National PA Day, October 6, is established, coinciding with the anniversary of the first graduating class of PAs from the Duke University PA Program 20 years earlier.
	New AAPA National Headquarters at 950 North Washington Street, Alexandria, VA, is established.
	AAPA contracts to publish *Journal of the American Academy of Physician Assistants (JAAPA).* Editor selected is first PA hired as AAPA professional staff.
	Additional Medicare coverage of PA services (in rural, underserved areas) approved by Congress.
1988	First edition of *JAAPA* published and distributed.
1990	Navy PAs commissioned.
1991	AAPA assumes administrative responsibility of the Accreditation Review Committee on Education for Physician Assistants (formerly the JRC-PA).
1992	Army and Coast Guard PAs commissioned.
1993	*The Role of the Physician Assistant and Nurse Practitioner in Primary Care,* edited by Clawson and Osterwies, is published.
	24,600 PAs are in active practice in 49 states, territories, and the District of Columbia.
1994	*Physician Assistant: A Guide to Clinical Practice,* edited by Ballweg, Stolberg, and Sullivan, is published.
1995	*The Physician Assistant Medical Handbook,* edited by Labus, is published.
	Physician Assistants in the Health Workforce, 1994 (report of the Advisory Group on Physician Assistants and the Workforce [AGPAW]), is published.
1996	American Medical Association (AMA) grants observer status to AAPA in the AMA House of Delegates.
1997	*The Physician Assistant Emergency Medical Handbook,* by Salyer, is published.
	Physician Assistants in American Medicine, by Hooker and Cawley, is published.
1998	The APAP Research Institute is founded by Donald Pedersen, PhD, to fund small, faculty-oriented research activities.
	Perspectives on Physician Assistant Education becomes an indexed journal and is published quarterly.
	Physician Assistant: A Guide to Clinical Practice, second edition, edited by Ballweg, Stolberg, and Sullivan, is published.
2000	The Association of Physician Assistant Programs decides that the master's degree is the appropriate degree for entry level PAs.
	PAs in the Canadian Forces number more than 100.
	The NCCPA makes the PANCE, and PANRE is converted to computer.
2001	A schism develops between the NCCPA and the AAPA over who can credit CME.
	A record 4267 PAs sit for the PANCE for the first time (91.5% pass).
2002	The 35th anniversary of the first graduation of PAs. The event is celebrated in Boston at the AAPA National Conference.
	The AAPA estimates that there are approximately 42,000 clinically active PAs in American medicine.
	Twenty-fifth anniversary of the Association of Physician Assistant Programs. The number of accredited PA programs is 132. The event is celebrated in Fort Lauderdale, FL.
	Physician Assistants in American Medicine, second edition, by Hooker and Cawley, is published.
2003	*Physician Assistant: A Guide to Clinical Practice,* third edition, edited by Ballweg, Stolberg, and Sullivan, is published.

APPENDIX 2

Sample Job Descriptions

The following sample job descriptions for PAs were adapted for this Appendix by Kenneth Harbert from those he developed during his employment at Geisinger Medical Center.

CARDIOLOGY
Primary Function

Perform, under the responsibility and supervision of the physician, diagnostic and therapeutic tasks to allow the physician to extend his or her services through the more effective and efficient use of knowledge in a sphere of decision making required to establish a diagnosis and to plan appropriate therapy. The physician assistant may assist in gathering the data necessary to implement the therapeutic plan of the physician.

Duties and Responsibilities

To assist the physician in the care and evaluation of patients, the physician assistant in cardiology will:
1. Perform and record specific cardiovascular history and physical examinations.
2. Write routine orders for appropriate laboratory tests, x-ray studies, and various consultations.
3. Inform the supervising physician of all changes in the patient's condition.
4. Provide ongoing health education regarding cardiovascular problems for patient and family members.
5. Provide follow-up in monitoring of cardiac catheterization patients when they are admitted to the hospital after having undergone a previous evaluation in the outpatient department.
6. Provide follow-up care and monitoring of electrophysiology study patients when they are admitted to the hospital.
7. Provide evaluation, write routine orders, perform history and physical examination, and provide follow-up care for patients with suspected cardiac disease (e.g., ischemic heart disease, congestive heart failure, arrhythmias, cardiomyopathies).

As indicated by training and experience, the physician assistant performs therapeutic and diagnostic procedures as directed by the physician.

Organizational Relationships

1. Reports clinically to the director of cardiology and/or assigned supervising physician.
2. Reports administratively to the director of physician extender services, or to the designate in his or her absence.

Qualifications

Must have proven ability to work in a team environment. Must have demonstrated a deep concern for the health and well-being of others. Must be able to deal with patients and their families in such a way as to instill confidence and facilitate communication. Must possess the degree of professional training to be qualified both professionally and legally to perform all services indicated under "Duties and Responsibilities." Must have completed an approved CAAHEP program for physician assistants in primary care. Must be eligible or certified by the State Board of Medical Education and Licensure and by the NCCPA. Must be eligible to participate in and/or have completed an approved advanced cardiac life support (ACLS) program within the past 2 years. Must be currently certified in basic life support with an updated cardiopulmonary resuscitation (CPR) card.

Criteria for Performance Evaluation

Performance will be judged by the eagerness to perform and by the effectiveness, efficiency, and accuracy with which responsibilities are initiated and executed; by the extent of cooperation with physicians, nursing personnel, receptionists, and diagnostic testing personnel to ensure a smoothly coordinated effort in the delivery of quality patient care; by the level of productivity within the department that is within the PA's control; by whether the necessary requirements for certification and re-certification have been met; by the degree of support given to the manager of physician extenders, the director of cardiology, and the supervising physician in identifying, communicating, and assisting in the solution of department problems; and most important, by the courtesy shown to all patients within the department of cardiology, both inpatients and outpatients.

CARDIOVASCULAR AND THORACIC SURGERY
Primary Function

Perform, under the responsibility and supervision of the surgeon, diagnostic and therapeutic tasks to allow the physician to extend his or her services through the more effective use of knowledge in the sphere of decision making required to establish a diagnosis and to plan therapy. The physician assistant may assist in gathering the data necessary to implement the therapeutic plan of the surgeon.

Duties and Responsibilities

1. To assist the surgeon in the preoperative care and workup of patients, the PA will:
   a. Conduct and record history and physical examination.
   b. Write routine admission orders and arrange appropriate laboratory and x-ray studies and consultations.
   c. Confirm operating schedule and availability of blood and summarize appropriate data prior to surgery.
   d. Write routine preoperative orders. All orders will be part of a prearranged cardiovascular thoracic surgical service protocol.
2. To assist the surgeon in each surgical procedure, the PA may perform these services as directed by the surgeon: insert monitoring catheters and intravenous lines and close the wound, under the supervision of the surgeon.
3. To participate in postoperative care of patients, being especially knowledgeable in the recognition of postoperative complications, the PA will:
   a. Inform the surgeon of all changes in the patient's condition.
   b. Assess the patient's postoperative course and implement indicated therapy as determined by the CVT surgical service protocol.
   c. Collect data and write pertinent progress notes on charts.
   d. Summarize details of the patient's hospitalization, including operative procedures and follow-up of complications.
   e. Make routine rounds as directed by the surgeon.
4. As indicated by training and experience, to perform therapeutic procedures as directed by the surgeon.
5. To examine preoperative and follow-up patients in the clinic prior to their being seen by the surgeons and to complete admission formalities.
6. To participate in clinical research, review of patient records, and other elected projects.
7. To rotate on a night call schedule as assigned.

Organizational Relationships

1. Reports directly to the clinical director for all patient care–related functions.
2. Reports directly to the director of physician extender services for all nonpatient administrative responsibilities.

Qualifications

1. Must have proven ability to work effectively in a team environment.
2. Must be able to deal directly with patients in such a way as to instill confidence and facilitate communication.
3. Will have satisfactorily completed training as a physician assistant within an approved CAAHEP program.
4. Must be eligible for certification or be certified by the NCCPA.

Criteria for Performance Evaluation

Performance will be judged by the effectiveness and accuracy with which responsibilities are initiated and executed; by the extent of cooperation with physicians, nursing personnel, receptionists, and diagnostic testing personnel to ensure a smoothly coordinated effort in the delivery of quality patient care; by whether the necessary requirements for certification and re-certification are met; by the degree of support given to the clinical director of CVT surgery and to the director of physician extender services in identifying, communicating, and assisting in the solution of department problems; and by the courtesy shown to patients within the department.

NEUROSURGERY
Primary Function

Perform, under the responsibility and supervision of the surgeon, diagnostic and therapeutic tasks to allow the physician to extend his or her services through the more effective use of knowledge in the sphere of decision making required to establish a diagnosis and to plan therapy. The physician assistant may assist in gathering the data necessary to implement the therapeutic plan of the surgeon.

Duties and Responsibilities

1. To assist the surgeon in the preoperative care, operative care, and workup of patients, the PA will:
    a. Conduct and record history and physical examination.
    b. Write routine admission orders, and arrange for appropriate laboratory tests, and x-ray studies, and consultations.
    c. Confirm operating schedule and summarize appropriate data prior to surgery.
    d. Write routine preoperative orders. All orders will be part of a prearranged neurosurgical service protocol.
2. To participate in the postoperative care of patients, being especially knowledgeable in the recognition of postoperative complications, the PA will:
    a. Inform the surgeon of all changes in the patient's condition.
    b. Collect data and write pertinent progress notes on charts.
    c. Summarize details of patient's hospitalization.
    d. Make routine rounds as directed by the surgeon.
    e. Assess the patient's postoperative course and implement indicated therapy as determined by the neurosurgical service protocol.
3. Keep the surgeon and the director of physician extenders informed as to additional needs or problem areas, and make other suggestions for the improvement of the department.
4. Rotate on-call for in-house patient problems, as scheduled.

Organizational Relationships

1. Reports directly to the surgeon for all patient care–related functions.
2. Reports directly to the director of physician extender services for all nonpatient administrative responsibilities.

Qualifications

1. Must have proven ability to work in a team environment.
2. Must have demonstrated a deep concern for the health and well-being of others.
3. Must be able to deal with patients in such a way as to instill confidence and facilitate communication.
4. Must possess sufficient medical training to be qualified legally and professionally to fulfill all demands placed upon him or her.
5. Will have satisfactorily completed training as a physician assistant within an accredited CAAHEP program.

Criteria for Performance Evaluation

Performance will be judged by the effectiveness and accuracy with which responsibilities are initiated and executed; by the extent of cooperation with physicians, nursing personnel, receptionists, and diagnostic testing personnel to ensure a smoothly coordinated effort in the delivery of quality patient care; by the degree of support given to the director of physician extenders and director of neurosurgery in identifying, communicating, and assisting in the solution of department problems; and by the courtesy shown to patients within the department.

OCCUPATIONAL HEALTH/EMPLOYEE HEALTH SERVICE/FAMILY PRACTICE
Primary Function

Perform, under the responsibility and supervision of the physician, diagnostic and therapeutic tasks to allow the physician to extend his or her services through the more effective use of knowledge in the sphere of decision making required to establish a diagnosis and to plan therapy. The physician assistant may assist in gathering the data necessary to implement the therapeutic plan of the physician.

Duties and Responsibilities

1. To assist the physician in the care and evaluation of patients, the PA will:
   a. Conduct pre-employment and focused history and physical examinations on outpatients.
   b. Make complete entries in the medical record, write orders, and record progress notes. Orders will be reviewed/countersigned by supervising physician within 24 hours.
   c. Initiate appropriate laboratory, radiological, and special examinations for tests required for the evaluation of illness or injury.
   d. Communicate with patients by phone and letter regarding their problems, after consultation with the supervising physician.
   e. Provide counseling and instruction to patients regarding their health-related problems.
   f. Prepare and dictate summaries of the clinical care of the patient, as directed by the supervising physician.
   g. Relay telephone orders for the institution or for renewal of medications and treatments in accordance with established protocols.
   h. Monitor infectious disease status, including immunizations, as indicated.
   i. Manage medical emergencies and initiate appropriate therapy until the arrival of a physician.
   j. Provide follow-up and health maintenance care in accordance with protocols or instructions from the supervising physician.
   k. Assist in the training of health care personnel in certain diagnostic, therapeutic, and clinical techniques, as directed by the supervising physician.
   l. Perform clinical procedures under the direction or supervision of the supervising physician.
   m. Keep the director informed as to additional needs or problem areas, and make other suggestions beneficial to the improvement of the department.

2. As indicated by training and experience, perform therapeutic and diagnostic procedures as directed by the supervising physician or designated alternate, including but not limited to the following:
   a. Wound care and dressings and suturing of lacerations.
   b. Venipuncture.
   c. Audiometric, pulmonary function, and visual acuity screenings.
   d. Incision and drainage of small abscesses.
   e. Ear lavage.
   f. Management of acute and chronic injuries or illnesses associated with occupational medicine patients, and provision of comprehensive care.

Organizational Relationships

1. Clinically reports to the departmental clinical director.
2. Administratively reports to the director of physician extender services.

Qualifications

1. Must hold a certificate of completion from an accreditated CAAHEP program for physician assistants.
2. Must be eligible for certification or be certified by the State Board of Medicine and be eligible or certified by the NCCPA.

Criteria for Performance Evaluation

Performance will be judged by the eagerness to perform and by the effectiveness and accuracy with which responsibilities are initiated and executed; by the extent of cooperation with physicians, nursing personnel, receptionists, and diagnostic testing personnel to ensure a smoothly coordinated effort in delivering quality patient care; by ensuring a level of productivity within the department that is within the PA's control; by meeting the necessary requirements for certification and re-certification; by the degree of support given to the clinical director and the director of physician extender services in identifying, communicating, and assisting in the solution of department problems; and by the courtesy shown to patients in the department.

Must have proven ability to work in a team environment. Must be able to deal directly with patients in such a way as to instill confidence and facilitate clear, concise communication.

APPENDIX 3

Matrix for Critical Appraisal

Appendix Table 3-1 Matrix for Critical Appraisal

Please explain your responses to the following questions.

Citations

Step 1. Do I want to evaluate the study? (INR)

Is the study Interesting,

Novel,

Relevant?

Step 2. Study Outline/Method

Research Question

Subjects/Target Population   Temporal and Geographic Characteristics.

                                    Intended Follow-up.

                                    Sampling.

Predictor Variable Defined

Outcome Variable Defined

Findings

Continued

Appendix Table 3-1   Matrix for Critical Appraisal—cont'd

Step 3. Is the Study Finding Believable?

Do the subjects and variables accurately represent the research question?

Subjects:

Predictor Variable:

Outcome variable:

Are findings attributable to other factors? (Chance, Bias, Confounders)

? Chance.

? Bias.

- Bias in Selecting Study Subjects.
- Biases in Following Up on The Study Subjects.
- Biases in Executing or Measuring the Predictor Variable.
- Biases in Measuring the Outcome Variable
- Biases in Analyzing the Data

? Confounders.

Are the findings believable within the context of other knowledge?

? Consistency With Other Literature.

? Biological Plausibility.

? Analogy.

Step 4. What is the Clinically Relevant Finding? (Likelihood Ratios- LR- for diagnostic tests; Disease-specific mortality-DSM-Patient-specific mortality-PSM- and/or Life expectancy-LE- for prognosis; Absolute Risk Reduction-ARR-Number Needed To Treat-NNT-Discounting for Therapy)

Weighing Costs and Benefits

Step 5. Will the Study Help Me in Caring For My Patient?

Are the Subjects Adequately Described and Applicable to My Patient?

Is the Predictor Variable Adequately Described and Applicable to My Patient?

Will the Finding Result in an Overall Net Benefit for My Patient?

Index

Page references followed by "f" indicate figures, "t" indicate tables, and "b" indicate boxes